McGraw-Hill Education
SPECIALTY BOARD REVIEW

Dermatology

A Pictorial Review

NOTICE

McGraw-Hill Education
SPECIALTY BOARD REVIEW

Dermatology

A Pictorial Review

THIRD EDITION

Editor

Asra Ali, MD
Private Practice—Dermatology
Houston, Texas

Mc Graw Hill Education

New York Chicago San Francisco Athens London Madrid Mexico City Milan
New Delhi Singapore Sydney Toronto

McGraw-Hill Education Specialty Board Review
Dermatology: A Pictorial Review, Third Edition

1 2 3 4 5 6 7 8 9 0 CTP/CTP 18 17 16 15 14

ISBN 978-0-07-179323-0
MHID 0-07-179323-2

This book was set in Slimbach by Cenveo® Publisher Services.
The editors were Anne M. Sydor and Robert Pancotti.
The production supervisor was Catherine H. Saggese.
Project management was provided by Hardik Popli, Cenveo Publisher Services.
China Translation & Printing Services, Ltd. was the printer and binder.

Library of Congress Cataloging-in-Publication Data

Dermatology (Ali)
Dermatology : a pictorial review / editor, Asra Ali.—Third edition.
p. ; cm. — (McGraw-Hill specialty board review)
Includes bibliographical references and index.
ISBN 978-0-07-179323-0 (pbk. : alk. paper)
ISBN 0-07-179323-2 (pbk. : alk. paper)
I. Ali, Asra, editor. II. Title. III. Series: McGraw-Hill specialty board review.
[DNLM: 1. Skin Diseases—Atlases. 2. Dermatology—methods—Atlases. WR 17]
RL74.2
616.5—dc23

2014020128

CONTENTS

CONTRIBUTORS

Sumaira Z. Aasi, MD
Professor
Department of Dermatology
Stanford University
Palo Alto, California
Chapter 12

Nnenna G. Agim, MD
Assistant Professor of Dermatology
Children's Medical Center
Dallas and University of Texas Southwestern Medical Center
Pediatric Dermatology
Houston, Texas
Chapters 14, 15

Jennifer Ahdout, MD
Department of Dermatology
UC Irvine
Irvine, California
Director of Dermatology, Lasers, and Skin Care
Spalding Drive Plastic Surgery & Dermatology
Beverly Hills, California
Chapter 1

Carolyn A. Bangert, MD
Associate Professor
Department of Dermatology
University of Texas
Houston, Texas
Chapter 22

Melissa A. Bogle
Director
The Laser & Cosmetic Surgery Center of Houston
Houston, Texas
Clinical Assistant Professor
Department of Dermatology
University of Texas M.D. Anderson Cancer Center
Houston, Texas
Chapters 16, 26

Jerry E. Bouquot, DDS, MSD, FICD, FACD, FRCM (UK)
Adjunct Professor
Department of Diagnostic & Biomedical Sciences
University of Texas School of Dentistry
Houston, Texas
Adjunct Professor
Department of Rural Health & Community Dentistry
West Virginia University School of Dentistry
Morgantown, West Virginia
Director of Research
The Maxillofacial Center for Education & Research, Morgantown, West Virginia
Chapter 4

Kamal Busaidy, BDS, FDSRCS
Associate Professor
Department of Oral and Maxillofacial Surgery
University of Texas-School of Dentistry
Houston, Texas
Chapter 4

John C. Browning, MD, FAAD, FAAP
Assistant Professor of Pediatrics and Dermatology
Baylor College of Medicine
Houston, Texas
Assistant Professor of Pediatrics and Dermatology
University of Texas Health Science Center
San Antonio, California
Chief of Dermatology
Children's Hospital of San Antonio
San Antonio, California
Chapters 13, 15

Christopher T. Burnett, MD
Dermatology Associates of Wisconsin
Milwaukee, Wisconsin
Chapters 24, 28

Stephanie F. Chan
Graduate student in Biostatistics
Harvard University
Cambridge, Massachusetts
Chapter 29

T. Minsue Chen, MD
Mohs Research in Advanced Dermatologic Surgery and Education Fellow
Department of Dermatology
University of Texas M.D. Anderson Cancer Center
Houston, Texas
Chapter 25

Alice Z. Chuang, PhD
Gibson and Martha Gayle Professor
University of Texas Health Science Center
Houston, Texas
Chapter 29

Joseph Constantino, MS
Institute of Human Nutrition-Columbia University
College of Physicians and Surgeons
New York, New York
Chapter 20

Whitney L. DeLozier, MD
Department of Dermatology
University of Texas at Houston
Houston, Texas
Chapter 17

Hafeez Diwan, MD, PhD
Associate Professor and Head of Dermatopathology
Departments of Pathology & Immunology and Dermatology
Baylor College of Medicine
Houston, Texas
Chapter 30

Hung Q. Doan, MD, PhD
Resident
Department of Dermatology
The University of Texas Health Science Center
Houston, Texas
Chapters 10, 20

Libby Edwards, MD
Chief of Dermatology
Carolinas Medical Center
Charlotte, North Carolina
Chapter 5

Dirk M. Elston, MD
Director
Department of Dermatology
Geisinger Medical Center
Danville, Pennsylvania
Chapter 16

Neil Farnsworth, MD, FAAD
Private practice
New Orleans, Louisiana
Chapters 18, 23

Adrienne M. Feasel, MD
Dermatologist
Ladera Park Dermatology
Austin, Texas
Chapters 14, 15

Kristy Fleming, MD
Private Practice
Newport Beach, California
Chapter 35

Pamela Gangar, MD
Clinical Research Fellow
Department of Dermatology
M.D. Anderson Cancer Center
Houston, Texas
Chapter 8

Daniel Gareau, PhD
Instructor in Clinical Investigation
Laboratory of Investigative Dermatology
The Rockefeller University
New York, New York
Chapter 32

Ryan J. Gertz, MD
Surgical Pathology Fellow
Department of Pathology and Laboratory Medicine
University of Wisconsin Hospital and Clinics
Madison, Wisconsin
Chapters 10, 20

Rachel Gordon, MD
Center for Clinical Studies
Texas Medical Center
Houston, Texas
Chapter 17

Sana Hashmi, BA
Medical student
School of Medicine
Stanford University
Stanford, California
Chapter 33

Alyn D. Hatter, DO, MS
Chief Resident Dermatology
University Hospitals Case Medical Center
Case Western Reserve University
Cleveland, Ohio
Chapter 16

Adelaide A. Hebert, MD
Professor & Director of Pediatric Dermatology
Department of Dermatology
The University of Texas Medical School
Houston, Texas
Chapter 14

Whitney A. High, MD, JD, MEng
Associate Professor
Department of Dermatology & Pathology
Director of Dermatopathology (Dermatology)
University of Colorado School of Medicine
Denver, Colorado
Chapters 7, 17, 19

Sharon Jacob, MD
Associate Professor
Department of Dermatology
Loma Linda University
Loma Linda, California
Chapter 6

Richard R. Jahan-Tigh, MD, MS
Assistant Professor
Department of Dermatology
University of Texas Medical School at Houston and MD Anderson Cancer Center
Houston, Texas
Chapter 30

Samer Jalbout, MD
Department of Dermatology
Medical University of Modena and Reggio Emilia
Modena, Italy
Chapter 32

Robert H. Johr, MD
Clinical Professor Dermatology
University of Miami
Miami, Florida
Chapter 31

Farhan Khan, MD, MBA
Medical Director
St. Anthony's Minor Emergency Center
Houston, Texas
Chapters 10, 20

Joy H. Kunishige, MD
Assistant Professor
Department of Plastic Surgery
University of Pittsburgh Medical Center
Zitelli & Brodland Skin Cancer Center
Pittsburgh, Pennsylvania
Chapters 11, 14

Alexander Lazar, MD, PhD
Director
Department of Pathology
The University of Texas M.D. Anderson Cancer Center
Selective (Soft Tissue) Pathology Fellowship Training Program
Houston, Texas
Chapter 11

Michelle Longmire, MD
Department of Dermatology
Stanford University
Stanford, California
Chapter 12

Kurt Q. Lu, MD
Assistant Professor, Department of Dermatology
Case Western Reserve University
Case Medical Center
Cleveland, Ohio
Chapter 27

Laith Mahmood, DDS, MD
Private Practice
Summerwood Oral & Maxillofacial Surgery
Houston, Texas
Chapter 4

Bassel H. Mahmoud, MD, PhD
Resident, Department of Dermatology
Henry Ford Hospital
Detroit, Michigan
Chapter 28

Steven Marcet, MD
Dermatologist
Newnan Dermatology
Newnan, Georgia
Chapter 18

Rana Majd Mays, MD
Department of Dermatology
Baylor College of Medicine
Houston, Texas
Chapter 17

Natalia Mendoza, MD
Department of Dermatology
University of Texas
Medical School at Houston
Houston, Texas
Chapter 17

Denise W. Metry, MD
Associate Professor of Dermatology and Pediatrics
Texas Children's Hospital/Baylor College of Medicine
Houston, Texas
Chapters 13, 15

Jason H. Miller, MD
Resident Physician
Department of Dermatology
University of Texas at Houston Health Science Center
M. D. Anderson Cancer Center
Houston, Texas
Chapters 22, 23

Paradi Mirmirani, MD
Permanente Medical Group
Vallejo, California
University of California
San Francisco, California
Case Western Reserve University
Cleveland, Ohio
Chapter 1

Kiran Motaparthi, MD
Assistant Professor
Department of Dermatology
Baylor College of Medicine
Houston, Texas
Chapter 35

Kaveh A. Nezafati, MD
Department of Dermatology
The University of Texas Southwestern Medical Center
Dallas, Texas
Chapter 9

Tri H. Nguyen, MD, FACMS, FAAD, FACPH
Texas Surgical Dermatology
Houston, Texas
Chapter 25

Roberto A. Novoa, MD
Resident
Department of Dermatology
Case Western Reserve University
Case Medical Center
Cleveland, Ohio
Chapter 27

Amit G. Pandya, MD
Department of Dermatology
The University of Texas Southwestern Medical Center
Dallas, Texas
Chapter 9

Gustavo Pantol, MD
Clinical Assistant Professor
FIU Wertheim College of Medicine
Miami, Florida
Chapter 33

Giovanni Pellacani, MD
Professor
Department of Dermatology
Medical University of Modena and Reggio Emilia
Modena, Italy
Chapter 32

Victor G. Prieto, MD, PhD
Professor
Departments of Pathology and Dermatology
The University of Texas M.D. Anderson Cancer Center
Houston, Texas
Chapter 30

Marigdalia K. Ramirez-Fort, MD
Department of Dermatology
Tufts Medical Center
Boston, Massachusetts
Chapters 10, 20, 32, 33

Ronald P. Rapini, MD
Chernosky Professor and Chair
Department of Dermatology
University of Texas Medical School at Houston and M.D. Anderson Cancer Center
Houston, Texas
Chapter 21

Riva Z. Robinson, MD
Resident Physician
Department of Preventive Medicine
Texas A&M Health Science Center College of Medicine
Round Rock, Texas
Chapters 20, 33

Roger Romero, MD
Department of Dermatology
The University of Texas Southwestern Medical Center
Dallas, Texas
Chapter 9

Mirwat S. Sami, MD
Ophthalmic Plastic and Reconstructive Surgeon, Private Practice
Houston Oculofacial Plastic Surgery
Houston, Texas
Department of Head and Neck Surgery, Division of Surgery
University of Texas M.D. Anderson Cancer Center
Houston, Texas
Department of Surgery, Division of Ophthalmology
Texas Children's Hospital
Houston, Texas
Department of Ophthalmology
Houston Methodist Hospital
Houston, Texas
Chapter 2

Charles S. Soparkar, MD, PhD
Ophthalmic Plastic and Reconstructive Surgery Private Practice
Plastic Eye Surgery Associates
Houston, Texas
Department of Ophthalmology
Baylor College of Medicine
Houston, Texas
Department of Ophthalmology
Weill Cornell Medical College
The Methodist Hospital
Houston, Texas
Chapter 2

Rakhshandra Talpur, MD
Senior Research Scientist, Dermatology Research
Department of Dermatology
University of Texas M.D. Anderson Cancer Center
Houston, Texas
Chapter 8

Marzieh Thurber, MD
Jupiter Medical Center
Jupiter, Florida
Chapter 14

Stephen K. Tyring, MD, PhD
Clinical Professor of Dermatology
University of Texas Health Science Center
Houston, Texas
Chapters 10, 17, 20

Ravi Ubriani, MD
Assistant Professor of Clinical Dermatology
Columbia University
New York, New York
Chapter 3

Kara E. Walton, MD
Assistant Professor
Department of Dermatology
Medical College of Wisconsin
Milwaukee, Wisconsin
Chapter 24

Rungsima Wanitphakdeedecha, MD
Associate Professor
Department of Dermatology
Faculty of Medicine
Siriraj Hospital
Mahidol University
Bangkok, Thailand
Chapter 25

PREFACE

McGraw-Hill Education Specialty Board Review Dermatology: A Pictorial Review is now in its third edition.

The ever-changing field of dermatology demands constant updating of information. To address this need, the third edition presents many new images as well as a new chapter on confocal microscopy. The goal of this edition is similar to that of the previous two editions of the book. Not only is the book an excellent tool for dermatology-related questions on board exams to prepare residents in dermatology, primary care, and other clinical specialties, it will also help practicing dermatologists and other clinicians with their recertification exams.

As an invaluable resource in the clinical setting, the revised and updated new edition of this practical guide provides comprehensive, yet concise, coverage of the diagnosis and management of common dermatologic disorders as well as some less common but important dermatologic conditions. Each chapter is organized in a readable and helpful format. Principles of diagnosis, differential diagnosis, and considerations for therapy are discussed in clinically related chapters.

There are chapters dedicated to cosmetic and surgical procedures with helpful insights. As a result, the book will be useful to more procedure-focused physicians as well. The questions and answers at the end of each chapter were also updated with new questions in order to make the learning process more interactive. It is hoped that the reader will gain from this edition as much as the editor did in preparing it.

CHAPTER 1

HAIR FINDINGS

PARADI MIRMIRANI AND JENNIFER AHDOUT

DEVELOPMENT

- Follicles form during third month of gestation; form first on head
- Lining of follicle = ectodermal origin
- Dermal papilla = mesodermal origin
- Epidermal invaginations occur at an angle to the surface and over sites of mesenchymal cell collections
- Eventually these epidermal cells form a column that surrounds the mesenchymal dermal papilla to form the bulb
- The dermal papilla (along with "stem" cells in the bulge) induces hair follicle formation by the overlying epithelium
- Additionally, 2 or 3 other collections of cells form along the follicle:
  - Upper collection becomes the mantle from which the sebaceous gland will develop
  - Lower swelling becomes the attachment for the arrector pili muscle and where follicle germinal cells reside in telogen phase
  - If a third collection of cells exists, it is found opposite and superior to the sebaceous gland and develops into the apocrine gland

STRUCTURE (FIG. 1-1)

- Longitudinal structure: (superior to inferior)
  - Permanent portion of the hair follicle
    - Infundibulum
    - Area of the sebaceous gland
    - Isthmus: begins at sebaceous gland and ends at the bulge (site of insertion of arrector pili muscle)
    - Area of the bulge: location of follicular stem cells
  - Transient portion of the hair follicle
    - Lower hair follicle
    - Hair bulb: contains the matrix, melanocytes; envelopes the dermal papilla; critical line of Auber is at the widest diameter; below this line is the bulk of mitotic activity

MICROSCOPIC STRUCTURE (FIG. 1-2)

- The hair follicle is arranged in concentric circles (from outer to inner)
  - Basement membrane (glassy membrane): PAS-positive, acellular; thin during anagen and thickens during catagen
  - Outer root sheath (ORS): present the length of the follicle; never keratinizes; stays fixed in place
  - Inner root sheath (IRS): grows toward cell surface and separates from the hair shaft at the level of the sebaceous gland
    - Henle layer: one cell thick and first to cornify
    - Huxley layer: two cells thick; eosinophilic-staining trichohyalin granules
    - Cuticle
- Hair shaft: grows toward cell surface; cornifies without trichohyalin or keratohyalin granules
  - Cuticle: shingle-like hair cells that interlock with cuticle cells of IRS
  - Cortex: arises from cells in center of hair bulb; disulfide bonds in this region give hair its tensile strength; keratinizes to form shaft; contains pigment of hair
  - Medulla: contains melanosomes; found only in terminal hairs
- Hair cycle: human follicles (Fig. 1-1) cycle in an asynchronous pattern (adjacent hairs in different stages)
  - Anagen: growth phase, stages I–VI
    - Eighty-four percent of hair follicles at any one time; last a few months to 7 years
    - Cells in the hair bulb are actively dividing
  - Catagen: transitional or degenerative stage
    - Two percent of hair follicles at any one time
    - Last a few days to weeks
    - Matrix cells have stopped dividing
    - Incomplete keratinization
    - Thickened basement membrane (glassy layer)
    - Transient, lower portion of follicle is broken down
  - Telogen: resting phase
    - Fourteen percent of hair follicles at any one time
    - Lasts about 3 months

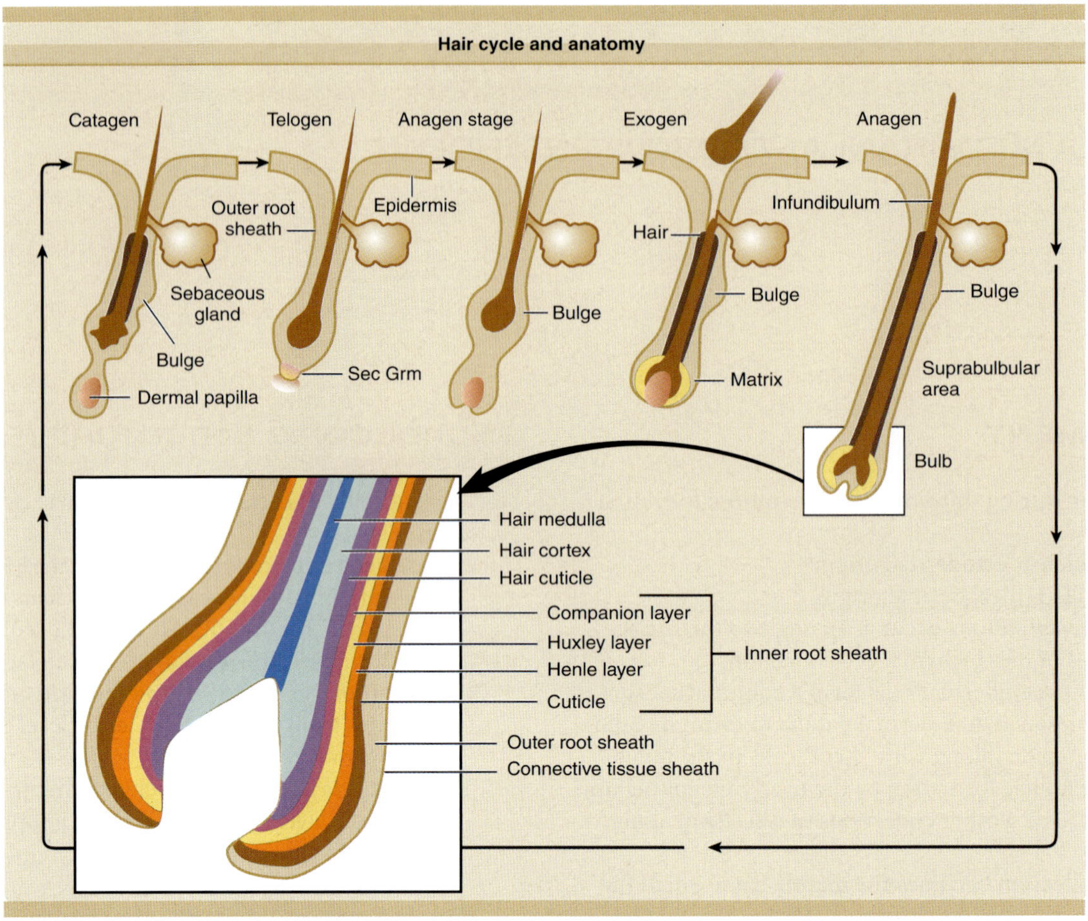

FIGURE 1-1 Hair cycle and anatomy. The hair follicle cycle consists of stages of rest (telogen), hair growth (anagen), follicle regression (catagen), and hair shedding (exogen). The entire lower epithelial structure is formed during anagen and regresses during catagen. The transient portion of the follicle consists of matrix cells in the bulb that generate 7 different cell lineages, 3 in the hair shaft, and 4 in the inner root sheath. (*Reprinted with permission from Goldsmith LA et al*, Fitzpatrick's Dermatology in General Medicine, *8th Ed. New York: McGraw-Hill; 2012*.)

    - "Club hair"; no inner root sheath
    - Dermal papilla retracted to higher position in dermis
- Hair pigmentation
  - Pigment comes from melanocytes located in the matrix, above the dermal papilla
  - Eumelanin: pigment of brown-black hair
  - Pheomelanin: pigment of blonde-red hair
  - Loss of melanocytes and decreased melanosomes cause graying of hair—poliosis (can be seen in regrowth of hair after alopecia areata). In youth, catalase breaks down hydrogen peroxide so that the pigmentation of hair is retained. With aging, the protective function of catalase is lost, and hydrogen peroxide builds up and turns hair gray or white.
- Hair growth
  - Hair grows approximately 0.35 to 0.37 mm/d
  - Longer anagen phase = longer hair

HAIR DISORDERS

Alopecia, Nonscarring

DIFFUSE

1. Telogen effluvium
   - Hair shedding, often with an acute onset
   - Reactive process, response to a physical event (surgery, pregnancy, thyroid disease, iron deficiency, high fever), medications (Table 1-1), or severe mental or emotional stress

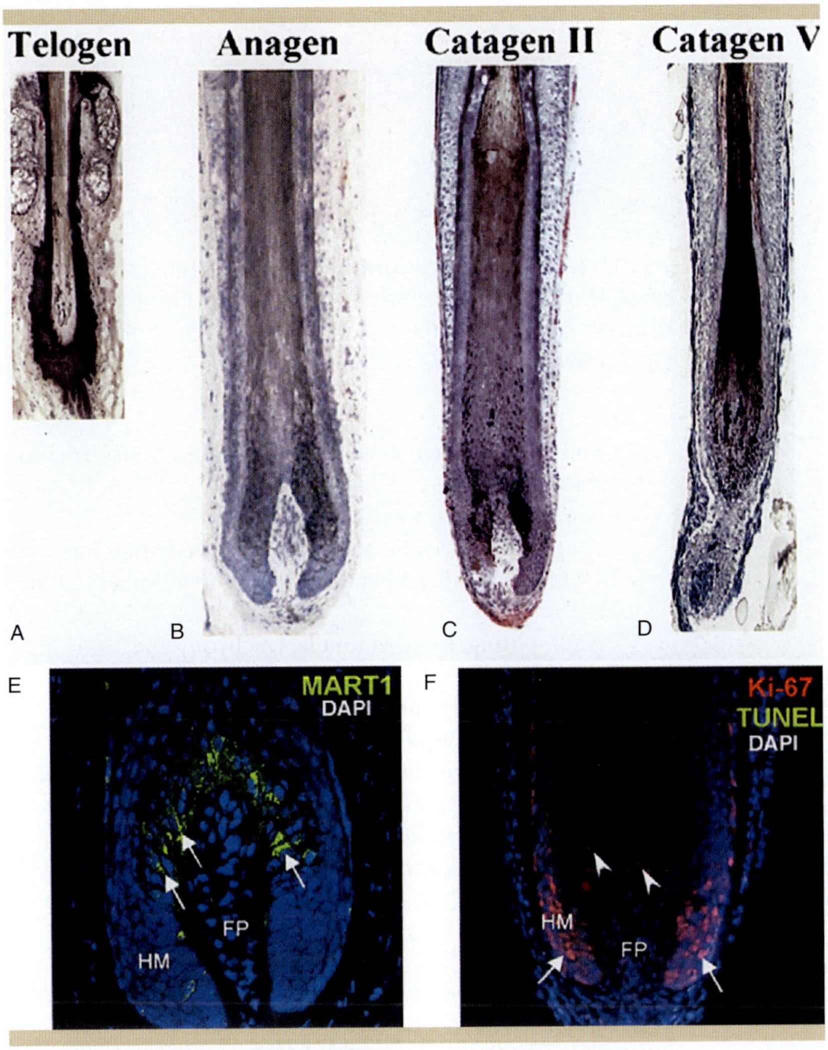

FIGURE 1-2 Morphology and fluorescent microscopy of human hair follicle at distinct hair cycle stages. **A–D**. Morphology of human hair follicle during telogen **(A)**, late anagen **(B)**, and early and late catagen **(C, D)**. **(E)** Immunofluorescent visualization of the melanocytes (arrows) in the hair bulb of late anagen hair follicle with anti–melanoma-associated antigen recognized by T cells antibody. **(F)** Immunofluorescent detection of proliferative marker Ki-67 (arrows) and apoptotic TUNEL+ cells (arrowheads) in early catagen hair follicle. FP = follicular papilla; HM = hair matrix. (*Reprinted with permission from Goldsmith LA et al.* Fitzpatrick's Dermatology in General Medicine, *8th Ed. New York: McGraw-Hill; 2012.*)

- A large number of hairs shift from anagen to telogen at one time
- Telogen hairs move back to anagen in 3 to 4 months following the inciting event; hair density may take 6 to 12 months to return to baseline
- The percentage of hairs in telogen rarely goes beyond 50%
- Positive pull test: more than 6 telogen hairs
- Telogen hairs on hair mount (Fig. 1-3)
- Histology: increased number of telogen hairs
- Prognosis: recovery is spontaneous and occurs within 6 months if inciting cause is reversed. Regrowing hairs with tapered or pointed hairs can be seen in the recovery phase

2. Loose anagen syndrome
   - Fair-haired children with thin, sparse, hair; no need for haircuts; easily dislodgable hair
   - Examination reveals sparse growth of thin, fine hair and diffuse or patchy alopecia
   - Anagen hairs are easily and painlessly pulled from scalp
   - Diagnosis: epilated hairs are predominantly in anagen phase; hair mount shows distorted anagen bulb, ruffled cuticle (Fig. 1-4)
   - Histology: premature and abnormal keratinization of the inner root sheath
   - Improves with age
3. Anagen effluvium (aka anagen arrest)
   - Hair broken off and not shed
   - Radiation therapy and chemotherapy agents; occurs 2 to 4 weeks after treatment
   - Hair shafts are abruptly thinned (Pohl-Pinkus constrictions) and break off at skin surface
   - Other causes: mercury intoxication, boric acid intoxication, thallium poisoning, colchicine, severe protein deficiency
   - Histology: normal follicles

PATCHY

1. Alopecia areata (Fig. 1-5)
   - Abrupt onset

TABLE 1-1 Common Medications Causing Telogen Effluvium

Angiotensin-converting enzyme inhibitors (ACEIs)
Anticancer
Anticoagulation (heparin, coumadin)
Anticonvulsant (sodium valproate, carbamazepine)
Selective serotonin reuptake inhibitors (SSRIs), tricyclic antidepressants (TCAs), and other psychiatric medications (amitriptyline, doxepin, haloperidol, lithium, haloperidol)
Antigout (probenecid, allopurinol)
Antithyroid (methimazole, propylthiouracil)
β-blockers (propanolol, timolol)
Antibiotics (nitrofurantoin, sulfasalazine)
Oral contraceptives: containing progestins with high androgen potential
Other (amiodarone, indomethacin, vitamin A, oral contraceptives)

- Exclamation point hairs which are broken hairs that are tapered at the scalp (Fig. 1-6)
- Pigmented hair affected first, subsequently gray hair may also be targeted (Fig. 1-7)
- Peach- or salmon-colored scalp
- Hair pull test positive for telogen hairs when disease is active

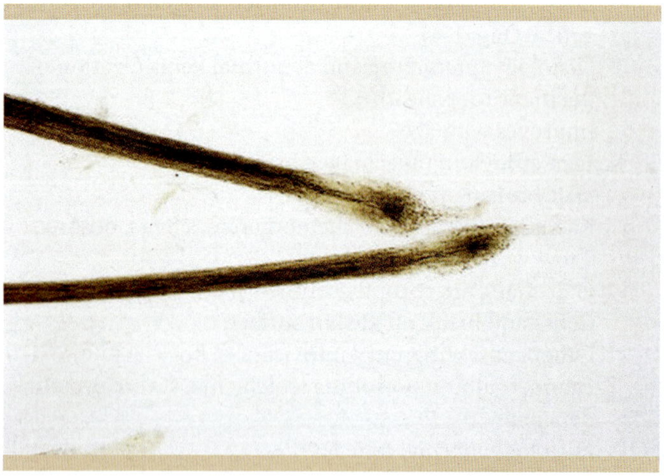

FIGURE 1-3 Hair mount showing a telogen hair. (*Reprinted with permission from Weedon D, ed.* Weedon's Skin Pathology, *3rd Ed. London: Churchill Livingston Elsevier; 2010.*)

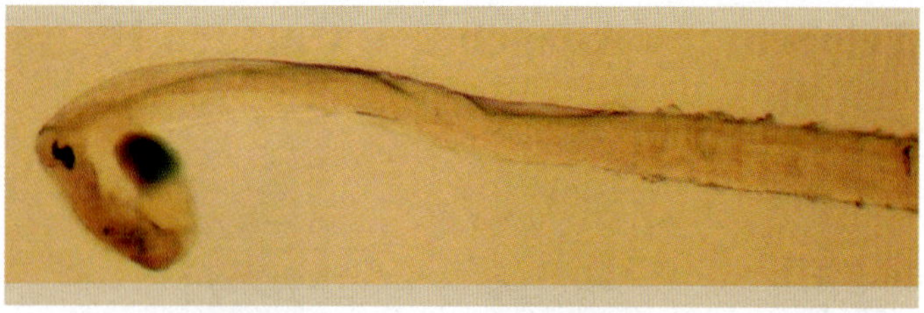

FIGURE 1-4 Hair mount showing a dystrophic anagen hair with a ruffled cuticle in a patient with loose anagen syndrome. (*Used with permission from Dr. Paradi Mirmirani.*)

- Follicular damage in anagen; then rapid transformation into telogen
- Alopecia totalis: total scalp hair loss
- Alopecia universalis: total scalp and body hair loss
- Ophiasis: localized hair loss along the periphery of the scalp
- Nails: pitting, mottled lunula, trachyonychia, or onychomadesis
- Histology: peribulbar infiltrate of T cells and macrophages ("swarm of bees")
- Associations: In the patient: atopic disorders, thyroid disease, vitiligo. In the family: atopic disorders, thyroid disease, vitiligo, diabetes mellitus, pernicious anemia, systemic lupus erythematosus (other autoimmune conditions)

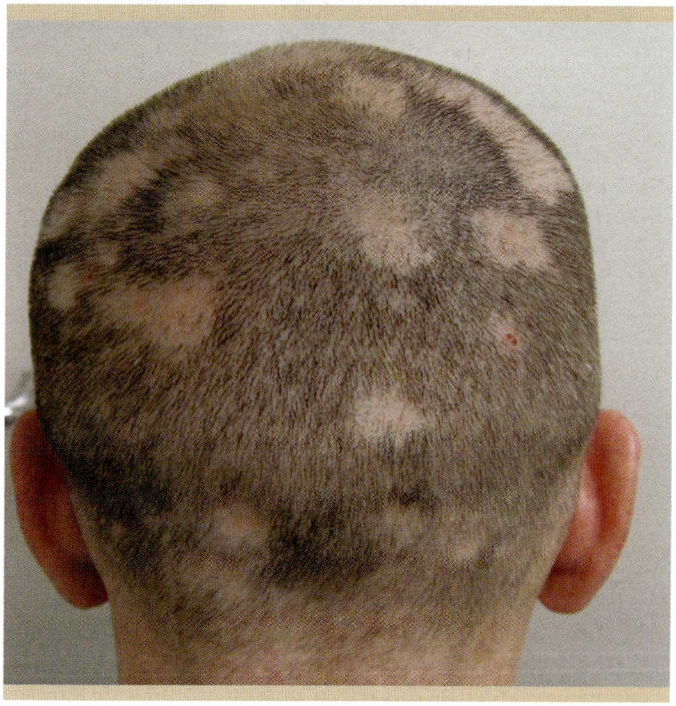

FIGURE 1-5 Patchy alopecia areata. (*Used with permission from Dr. Paradi Mirmirani.*)

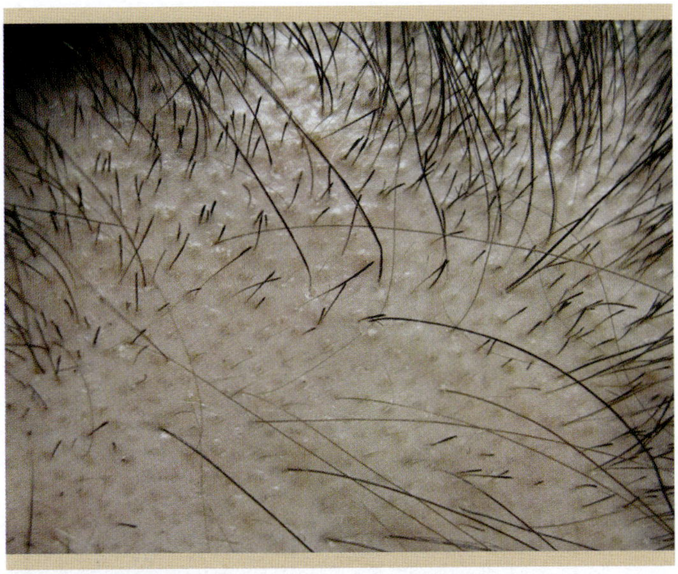

FIGURE 1-6 Exclamation point hairs in alopecia areata. (*Used with permission from Dr. Paradi Mirmirani.*)

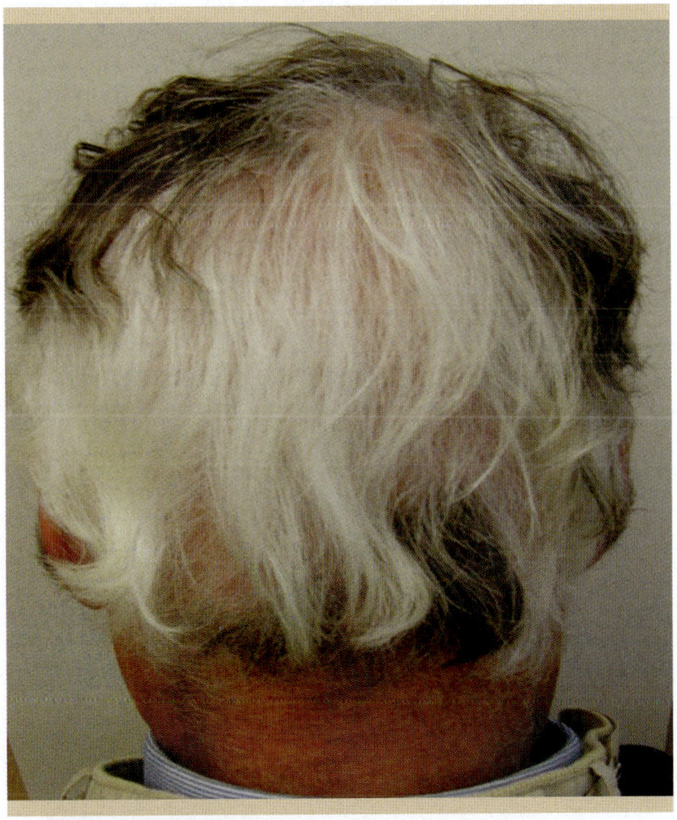

FIGURE 1-7 Alopecia areata primarily affecting pigmented hairs. (*Used with permission from Dr. Paradi Mirmirani.*)

- Treatment: Patchy, or more than 50%: intralesional steroids, minoxidil 5% solution or foam, anthralin, topical steroids. Unresponsive or extensive: topical immunotherapy (squaric acid dibutylester [SADBE] or diphenylcyclopropenone [DPCP]), systemic cortisone (short-term or bridge treatment), psoralen plus ultraviolet A (UV-A), excimer laser.

2. Trichotillomania
   - Impulse-control disorder
   - Repeated plucking or pulling of hairs
   - Confluence of short, sparse hairs within an otherwise normal area of the scalp
   - Varying lengths of regrowth, "friar tuck" distribution of hair loss (Fig. 1-8)
   - Regrowing hair is blunt tipped instead of pointed
   - Eyebrows and upper eyelashes may be affected
   - Often have other habits: nail biting, skin picking
   - Histology: pigment casts, increased catagen hairs, trichomalacia
   - Treatment: psychological intervention and/or psychiatric medication to modify behavior
3. Pityriasis amiantacea (Fig. 1-9)
   - Thick scale, matted hair
   - May mimic severe seborrheic dermatitis or psoriasis; however, hair that is involved is easily dislodged on attempts to physically remove the scale
   - Treatment: keratolytics, corticosteroids, oil, improves with age

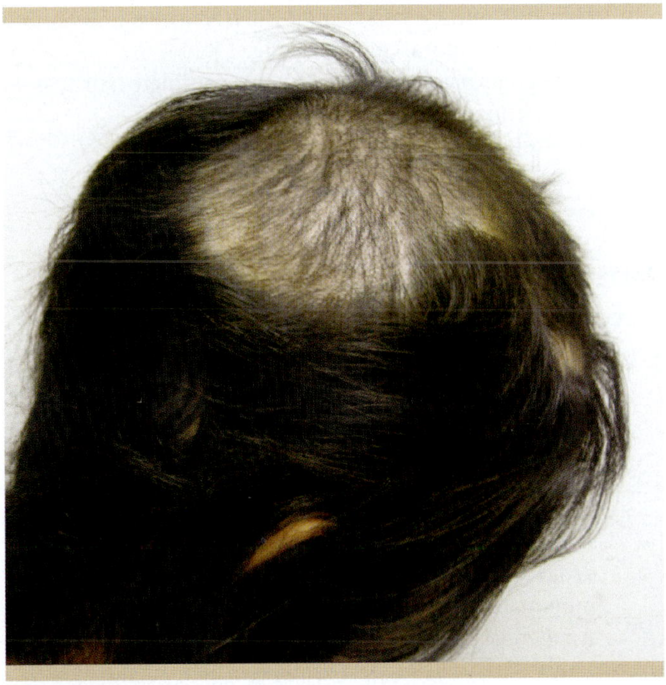

FIGURE 1-8 Trichotillomania. (*Used with permission from Dr. Paradi Mirmirani.*)

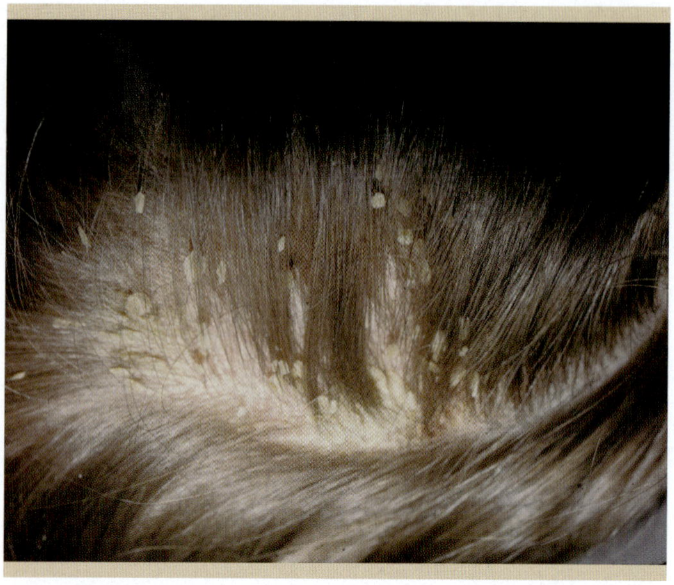

FIGURE 1-9 Pityriasis amiantacea. (*Used with permission from Dr. Adelaide Hebert.*)

4. Traction alopecia
   - Prolonged traction on the scalp by physical pressure: tight braids, foam rollers, tight pony tail, hair extensions
   - The "fringe sign" is characteristic of marginal traction alopecia: the hair along the frontal hairline is retained but is attenuated or finer in caliber. The area of alopecia is behind this "fringe"(Fig. 1-10)
   - Hair loss may be persistent if the traction is unrelenting
5. Triangular (temporal) alopecia (Fig. 1-11)
   - Triangular patch of vellus hairs or complete hair loss—either congenital or appears early in life
   - Frontotemporal region
   - Histology: vellus hairs
   - No treatment, usually persistent

Patterned

1. Androgenetic alopecia, female-patterned hair loss
   - Hereditary thinning in genetically susceptible men and women
   - Circulating testosterone (T) is converted to dihydrotestosterone (DHT) by 5-α-reductase enzyme at the target tissue. DHT is the active androgen causing miniaturization of hairs in androgen-sensitive areas of scalp. In women there may be some additional nonandrogen signals that lead to thinning, especially during menopausal years
   - Anagen is shorter; number of follicles remains the same. Paradoxically DHT enlarges hair in androgen-sensitive areas (beard, chest)
   - Male pattern: potential areas of hair loss are the frontal, temporal, midscalp, and vertex regions

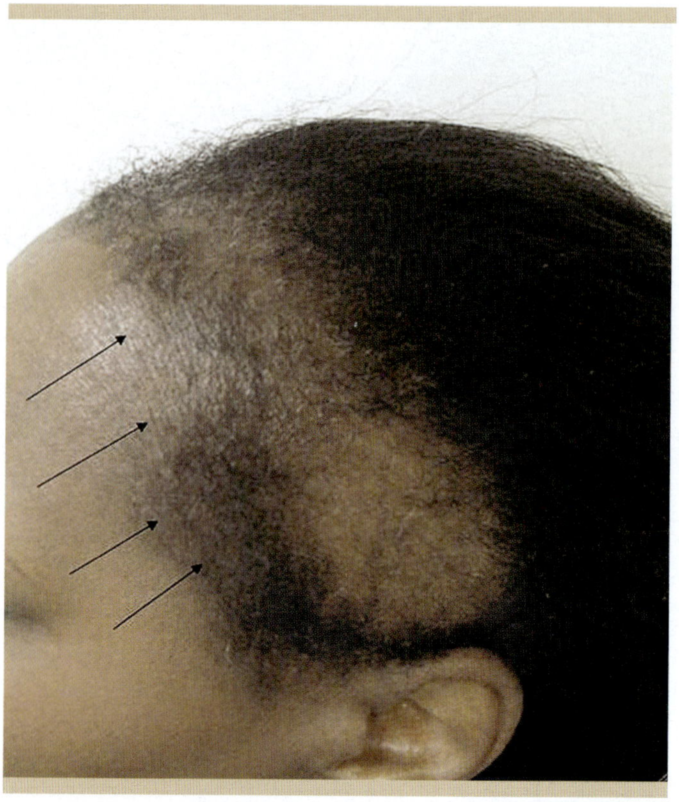

FIGURE 1-10 The "fringe sign" of traction alopecia involving the marginal hairline. (*Used with permission from Dr. Paradi Mirmirani.*)

   - Female pattern: diffuse thinning in the midscalp, vertex, and temporal areas; frontal hairline is retained (Ludwig classification)
   - Histology: miniaturization increased vellus-to-terminal-hair ratio, preserved sebaceous glands

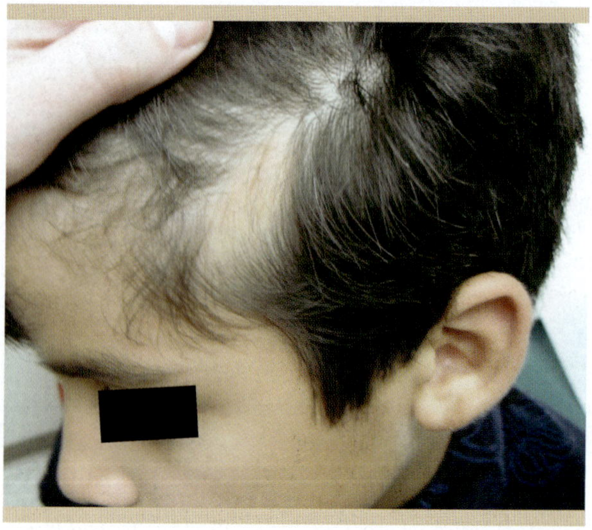

FIGURE 1-11 Triangular alopecia. (*Used with permission from Dr. Adelaide Hebert.*)

- Medical treatment:
  - Finasteride: 5-α-reductase type II inhibited
  - Minoxidil: increases the number of follicles in anagen, enlarges miniaturized hairs
- Surgical treatment: hair transplantation with minigrafts and micrografts

2. Age-related thinning (senescent alopecia)
   - Thinning that starts in the later years may not be androgen dependent
   - May be more diffuse than androgenetic alopecia
   - Treatment: minoxidil, surgical treatment
3. Androgen excess
   - Hair loss in a patterned distribution in those with excess androgens
   - Etiology: pituitary (prolactinoma, Cushing disease), adrenal (adrenal tumor, congenital adrenal hyperplasia), ovarian (polycystic ovary syndrome, ovarian tumor), drug induced
   - Workup: prolactin, total and free testosterone, DHEA-S, 17-OH progesterone
   - Treatment: oral contraceptives, spironolactone, flutamide, cyproterone acetate

Alopecia, Scarring

Classification:

- Primary: hair follicle is the primary target of the immune attack, i.e., lichen planopilaris (LPP), folliculitis decalvans, and acne keloidalis
- Secondary: hair follicle is an innocent bystander which is nonspecifically affected by the inflammatory process, i.e., cutaneous sarcoidosis, burns, and chronic infections.

Further classification of primary cicatricial alopecia is based on histology of predominant infiltrate seen on scalp biopsy.

- End stage: no significant infiltrate
- Predominantly lymphocytic: pseudopelade (of Brocq), lichen planopilaris, central centrifugal cicatricial alopecia (CCCA). Alopecia mucinosa and discoid lupus erythematosus are often included in this category, but these disorders may not be exclusively folliculocentric.
- Predominantly neutrophilic: folliculitis decalvans, dissecting cellulitis
- Mixed infiltrate: acne keloidalis

1. Pseudopelade (of Brocq; Fig. 1-12)
   - Oval- or irregularly shaped atrophic patches which may be mistaken for alopecia areata with patches of hair growth, "footprints in the snow."
   - No scalp redness or perifollicular scale
   - Histology: atrophy, perifollicular inflammation at the level of the infundibulum, fibrosis that extends in to the subcutis
2. Lichen planopilaris (LPP) (Fig. 1-13)
   - Perifollicular erythema and scale at the periphery of the patch of alopecia

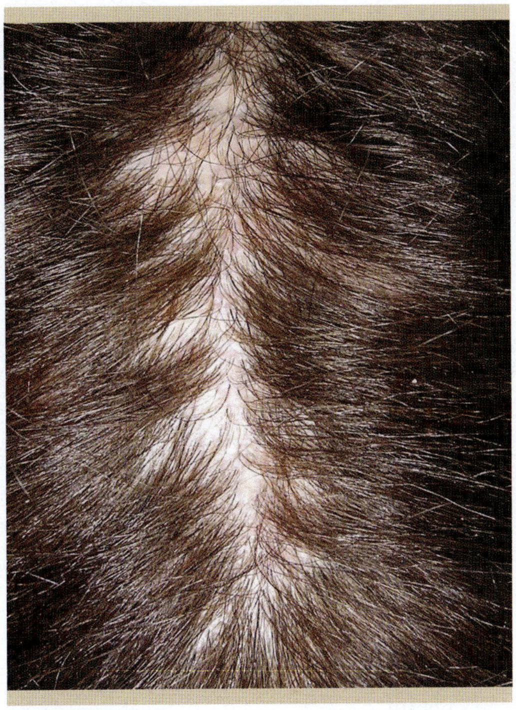

FIGURE 1-12 Pseudopelade (of Brocq). (*Used with permission from Dr. Paradi Mirmirani.*)

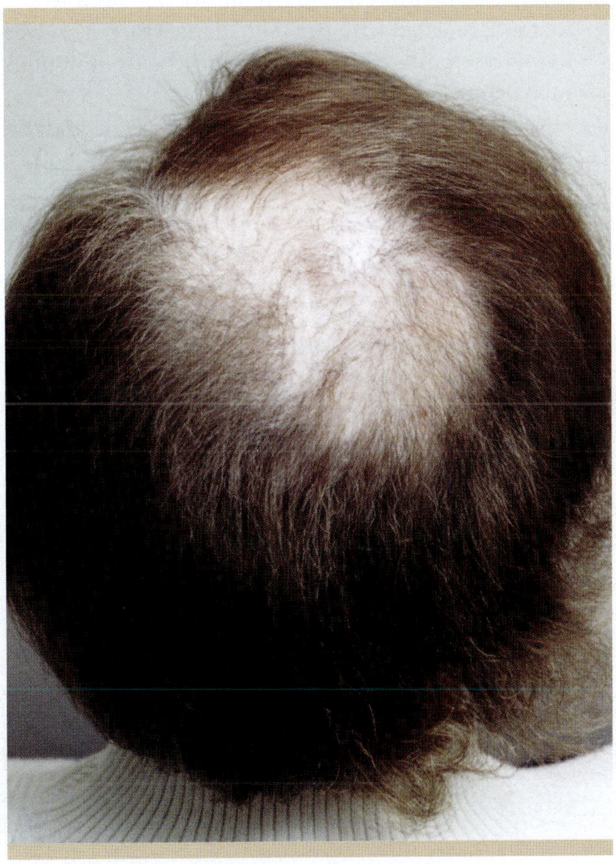

FIGURE 1-13 Lichen planopilaris. (*Used with permission from Dr. Vera Price.*)

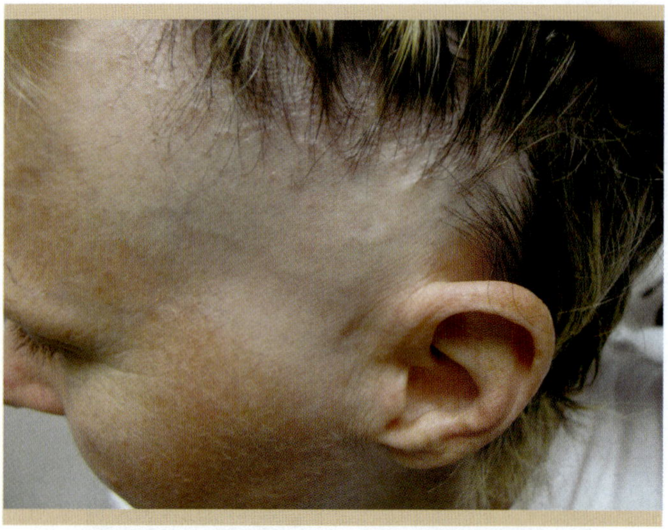

FIGURE 1-14 Frontal fibrosing alopecia. (*Used with permission from Dr. Paradi Mirmirani.*)

- More than 50% associated with cutaneous or oral lichen planus
- Involves scalp alone or scalp and other hair-bearing areas (Graham Little syndrome)
- Frontal fibrosing alopecia: frontotemporal hairline recession and eyebrow loss in postmenopausal women that is associated with perifollicular erythema and scaling, in a bandlike distribution along the frontotemporal hairline (Fig. 1-14)
- Histology: typically same as LPP, may see lichenoid interface dermatitis of the superficial follicular epithelium

3. Lupus erythematosus
    - Chronic cutaneous (discoid) lupus erythematosus (Fig. 1-15): scarring alopecia, erythema, hypo- and hyperpigmentation of the scalp, dilated follicles plus keratin plugs, scaling at the center of the patch of alopecia
    - Systemic lupus erythematosus: diffuse, nonscarring alopecia; broken hairs in frontal region ("lupus hairs")
    - Diagnostic biopsy and direct immunofluorescence
    - Treatment: topical, intralesional, or oral steroids; systemic retinoids; antimalarials

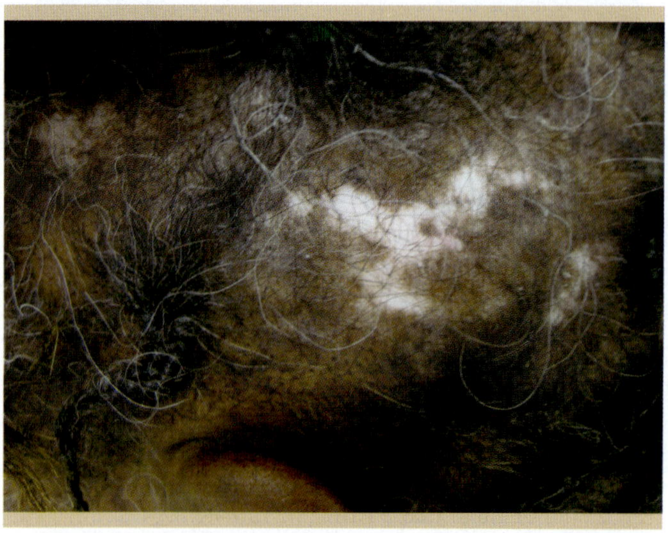

FIGURE 1-15 Discoid lupus. (*Used with permission from Dr. Paradi Mirmirani.*)

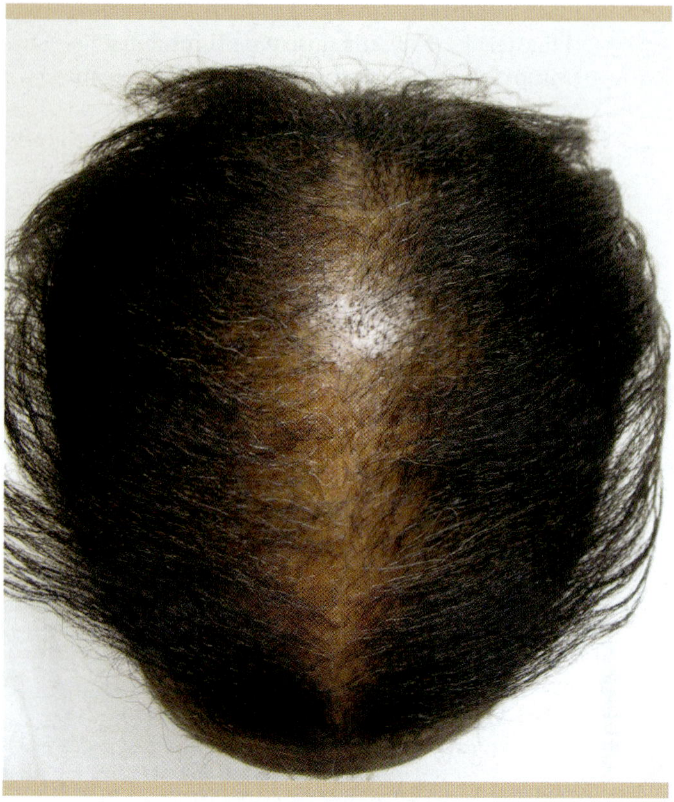

FIGURE 1-16 Central centrifugal cicatricial alopecia. (*Used with permission from Dr. Paradi Mirmirani.*)

4. Central centrifugal cicatricial alopecia (CCCA) (Fig. 1-16)
    - Previously called follicular degeneration syndrome; hot-comb alopecia
    - Follicular loss mainly on the crown of the scalp
    - Possibly secondary to hair care practices
    - Histology: premature desquamation of the inner root sheath, mononuclear infiltrate at the isthmus, loss of the follicular epithelium with fibrosis
5. Alopecia mucinosa (follicular mucinosis)
    - Erythematous plaques or flat patches without hair
    - Children: head and neck, benign, self-resolving
    - Adults: more widespread distribution; may be associated with cutaneous T-cell lymphoma
    - Histology: mucin in the outer root sheath and sebaceous glands, perifollicular lymphohistiocytic infiltrate
6. Dissecting cellulitis: Perifolliculitis capitis abscedens et suffodiens (Fig. 1-17)
    - May be part of the follicular occlusion triad (cystic acne, hidradenitis, dissecting cellulitis)

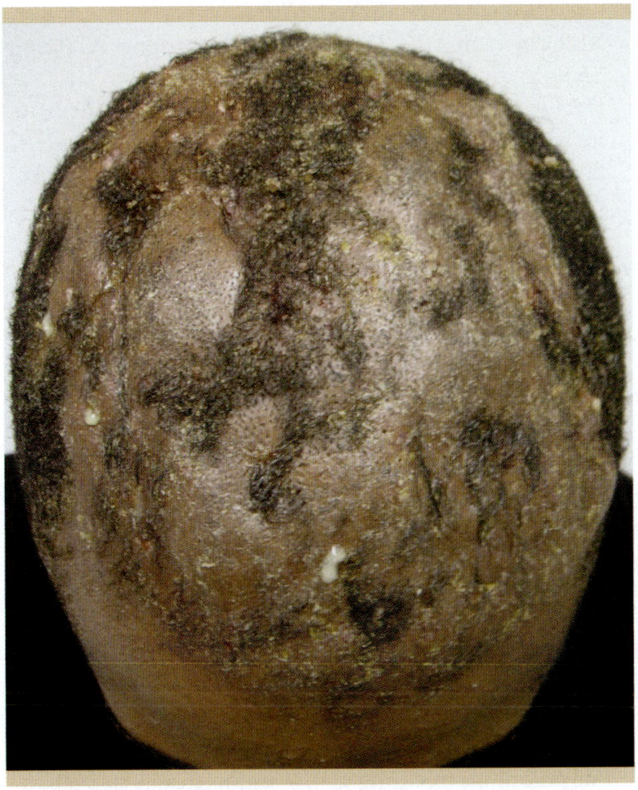

FIGURE 1-17 Dissecting cellulitis. (*Used with permission from Dr. Paradi Mirmirani.*)

- Fluctuant nodules on vertex, occiput, sterile pus
- Histology: sinus tracts, sterile abscesses
- Treatment: systemic steroids, systemic antibiotics, dapsone, retinoids, biologics, surgical excision

7. Folliculitis decalvans (Fig. 1-18)
    - Scarring alopecia with crusting, pustules, and erosions
    - *Staphylococcus aureus* usually cultured

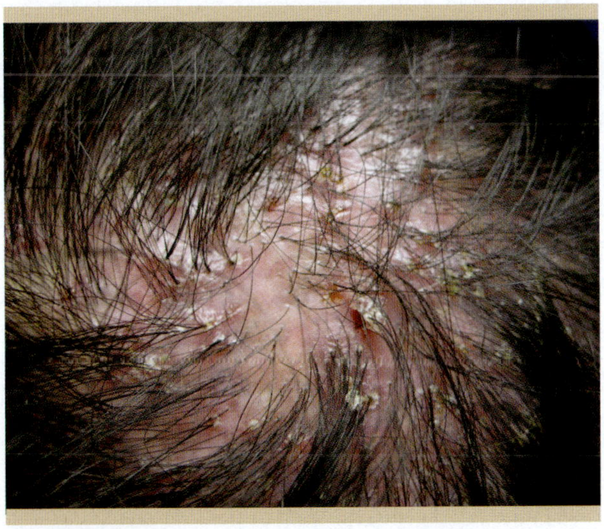

FIGURE 1-18 Folliculitis decalvans. (*Used with permission from Dr. Paradi Mirmirani.*)

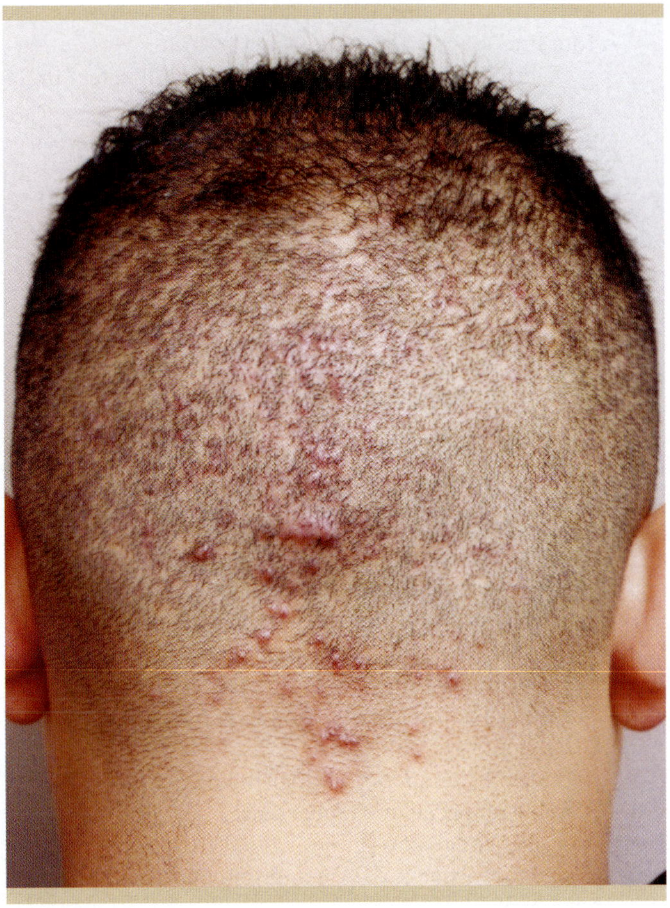

FIGURE 1-19 Acne keloidalis. (*Used with permission from Dr. Adelaide Hebert.*)

    - Histology: acute suppurative folliculits with neutrophils and eosinophils; later mixed with lymphocytes and histiocytes
    - Loss of sebaceous epithelium and perifollicular fibrosis
    - Treatment: staphylococcal eradication: systemic antibiotics with or without rifampin, systemic and/or topical steroids

8. Acne keloidalis (Fig. 1-19)
    - Follicular pustules and papules that progress to firm, keloidal papules
    - Commonly on occiput of patients with coarse and/or curly hair
    - Foreign-body reaction to trapped hair shaft fragments
    - Often bacterial superinfection
    - Histology: follicular dilatation and mixed peri-infundibular infiltrate with follicular rupture and foreign-body granulomas
    - Treatment: systemic antibiotics, topical and/or intralesional steroids

Congenital Disorders Associated With Alopecia

1. Ectodermal dysplasias: abnormal development of the skin, hair, nails, teeth, or sweat glands.

- Anhidrotic ectodermal dysplasia (Christ-Siemens-Touraine syndrome)
  - X-linked recessive form associated with defect in Ectodysplasin, pegged teeth
  - Autosomal recessive forms associated with defect in NEMO gene, immunodeficiency disorders; autosomal dominant form is rare
  - Thin, sparse hair
  - Absent pilosebaceous units in Blaschko lines
  - Hypohidrosis, atopic dermatitis, nail dystrophy
  - Abnormal facies: saddle nose, frontal bossing, thick lips, and peg teeth
  - Hair has longitudinal groove on electron microscopy
- Hidrotic ectodermal dysplasia (Clouston syndrome)
  - Autosomal dominant defect in gap junction protein (connexin 30)
  - Thin, sparse hair after puberty
  - Palmoplantar keratoderma, nail dystrophy, bulbous fingertips, tufted terminal phalanges
  - Normal sweating, facies, and dentition

2. KID syndrome
   - Autosomal dominant mutation in gap junction protein GJP2 (connexin 26)
   - Keratitis (± blindness), ichthyosis, and deafness
   - Scarring alopecia, dystrophic nails
3. Aplasia cutis congenita
   - Congenital absence of skin and subcutaneous tissue; may involve cranium
   - Coin-sized defect or larger
   - Often midline scalp vertex
   - Hair collar sign: ring of dark hair encircling aplasia lesion; suggests neural tube defect

Hair Shaft Disorders (Table 1-2)

1. Argininosuccinic aciduria
   - Autosomal recessive
   - Decrease in argininosuccinase
   - Most common urea cycle defect
   - Hyperammonemia, failure to thrive, hepatomegaly, seizures, ataxia, mental retardation
   - Trichorrhexis nodosa: brush-like ends in opposition (Fig. 1-20)
   - Low-protein diet and arginine supplementation may reverse hair anomalies
2. Björnstad syndrome (Fig. 1-21)
   - Missense mutations in the *BCS1L* gene on chromosome 2q34–36: abnormal mitochondrial function, leads to the production of reactive oxygen species
   - Pili torti (spares eyelashes): closely grouped twists seen on hair mount (Fig. 1-22)
   - Bilateral sensorineural deafness correlates with the severity of hair defects
   - Crandall syndrome: pili torti, deafness, hypogonadism
3. Menkes kinky hair syndrome
   - XLR defect in *MKHD* gene (copper transport ATPase 7A)
   - Decreased serum copper and ceruloplasmin with increased copper in all organs *except* the liver
   - Sparse, light-colored, "steel wool" hair; pili torti (most common), trichorrhexis nodosa
   - Skin is pale with laxity and a "doughy" consistency
   - Progressive cerebral degeneration
   - Radiologic findings: wormian bones in cranial sutures, metaphyseal widening, spurs in long bones
   - Tortuous arteries, genitourinary anomalies
4. Monilethrix (Fig. 1-23)
   - Autosomal dominant defect in keratins 1 and 6
5. Netherton syndrome
   - Autosomal recessive defect in *SPINK5* gene
   - Ichthyosis linearis circumflexa, atopic dermatitis
   - Trichorrhexis invaginata (bamboo hair) is the most common hair abnormality, but trichorrhexis invaginata is the most characteristic
6. Trichothiodystrophy
   - Autosomal recessive defect in *XPB/ERCC3* DNA repair transcription gene (analogous to xeroderma pigmentosum group D)
   - Ataxia but no freckling or UV-induced skin cancers
   - Trichoschisis, banding with polarized microscopy ("tiger tail")
   - Hairs have 50% reduction in sulfur (cysteine) content
   - IBIDS: intellectual impairment, brittle hair, ichthyosis, decreased fertility, and short stature
7. Uncombable hair syndrome
   - Autosomal dominant or sporadic
   - Defect: an abnormal configuration of inner root sheath that keratinizes before the hair shaft
   - Blond, shiny, "spun glass" hair
   - Microscopy: pili trianguli et canaliculi, longitudinal groove (Fig. 1-24A), triangular and kidney bean shape on cross section (Fig. 1-24B)
   - Lashes and brows are not affected
   - Biotin may help symptoms
8. Wooly hair (Fig. 1-25)
   - Autosomal dominant
   - Negroid hair on the scalp of person of non-Negroid background
   - Involves only scalp hair
   - Microscopy: hair shaft tightly coiled
   - Improves with age
   - Associations: Naxos syndrome, Carvajal syndrome
9. Bubble hair (Fig. 1-26)
   - Brittle, fragile hair from excessive heat
   - Hairdryers, straightening irons
10. Acquired progressive kinking
    - Tight coiling and kinking of the hair shaft
    - May occur in the setting of AIDS, drugs (retinoids)

TABLE 1-2 Hair Shaft Disorders

Hair Finding	Microscopic Description	Associations
Trichorrhexis nodosa (Fig. 1-20)	Brooms stuck end to end	Most common hair shaft dystrophy Congenital or acquired: Argininosuccinic aciduria, Menkes kinky hair syndrome, citrullinemia, trichothiodystrophy Acquired disease: Proximal: common in black female hair after chemical or hot comb straightening Distal: excessive brushing
Pili torti (Fig. 1-22)	Hair flattened and twisted from 90 to 360 degrees at *irregular* intervals	Björnstad syndrome, citrullinemia, Menkes kinky hair syndrome, Crandall syndrome, Bazex syndrome, Salamon syndrome, Beare syndrome, trichothiodystrophy, isotretinoin therapy
Monilethrix (Fig. 1-23)	Elliptical nodes with a *regular* periodicity of 0.7–1 mm between nodes, hair shaft is constricted (fractures common)	AD, short, brittle hairs emerging from keratotic follicular papules
Trichorrhexis invaginata	"Bamboo hair" with intussusception of the hair shaft (ball and socket)	Netherton syndrome
Trichoschisis	Clean transverse break along hair shaft where a local absence of cuticle is present	Trichothiodystrophy
Tiger tail	Zigzag alternating light and dark transverse bands on polarized microscopy	Trichothiodystrophy
Pili trianguli et canaliculi (Fig. 1-24)	Hair has triangular cross section with longitudinal groove on electron microscopy	Uncombable hair syndrome
Pili annulati	"Zebra-striped hair" with alternating segments of light and dark color due to air cavities	Pili annulati
Flag sign	Intermittent reddish discoloration of hair	Kwashiorkor, anorexia nervosa

Infectious Disorders

1. Tinea capitis (Table 1-3)
   - Clinical spectrum: asymptomatic carrier state, seborrheic type with scaling of the scalp, "black dot" type with areas of broken hair, and inflammatory kerion (Fig. 1-27). It can mimic scarring alopecia (Fig. 1-28)
     - Risk factors: African-American children, atopy, or autoimmune disorders
     - Treatment: Griseofulvin, terbinafine, or itraconazole; may add oral prednisone in case of kerion
2. Piedra
   - Gritty nodules on the hair in temperate climates
   - White piedra is caused by *Trichosporon beigelii*
   - Black piedra is caused by *Piedraia hortai*
3. Syphilis (Fig. 1-29)
   - "Moth-eaten" alopecia

Hypertrichosis

- Excessive hair growth in nonandrogen–dependent areas

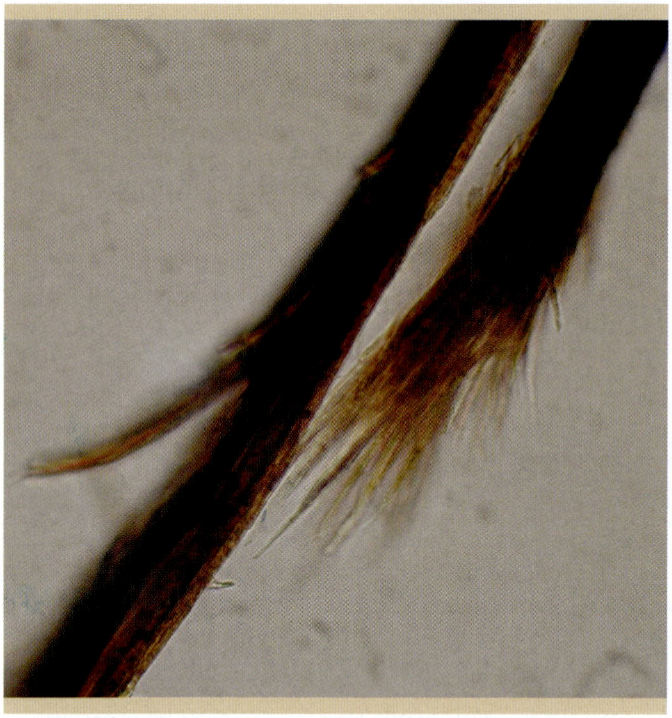

FIGURE 1-20 Hair mount showing trichorrhexis nodosa. (*Used with permission from Dr. Paradi Mirmirani.*)

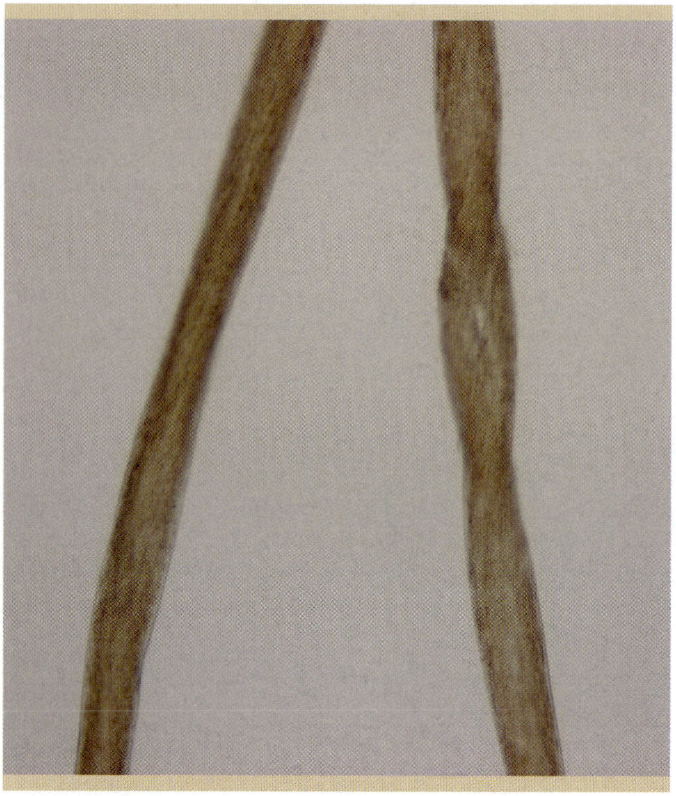

FIGURE 1-22 Hair mount showing pili torti. (*Used with permission from Dr. Paradi Mirmirani.*)

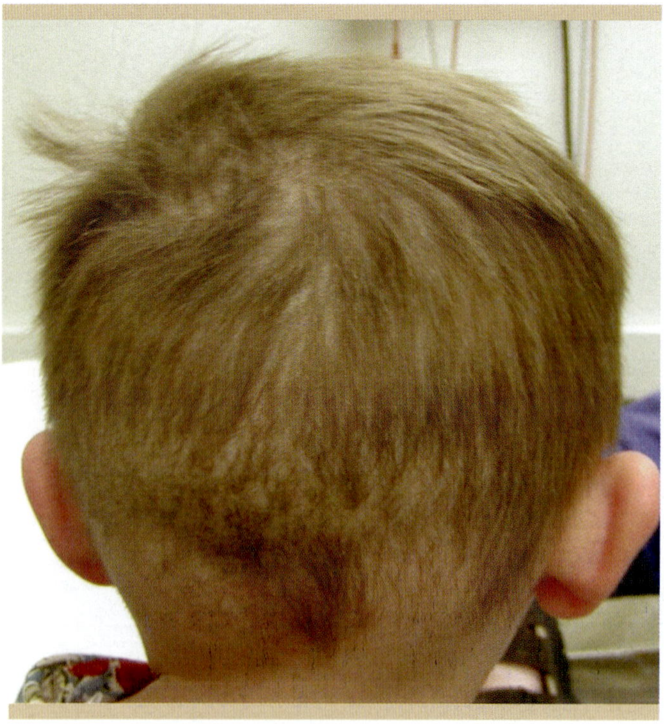

FIGURE 1-21 Björnstad syndrome. (*Used with permission from Dr. Paradi Mirmirani.*)

- Local congenital or acquired hypertrichosis: melanocytic nevi, Becker nevus (smooth muscle hamartoma), meningioma, porphyria, spinal dysraphism
- Generalized congenital hypertrichosis: X-linked dominant congenital hypertrichosis lanuginosa, fetal hydantoin syndrome, fetal alcohol syndrome
- Generalized acquired hypertrichosis: acquired hypertrichosis lanuginosa, internal malignancy, Rubenstein-Taybi,

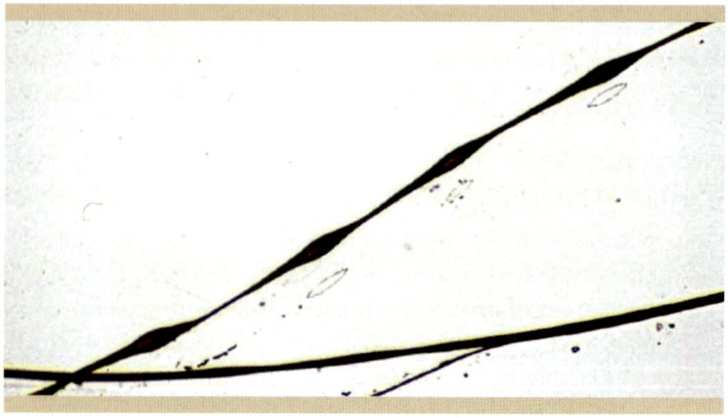

FIGURE 1-23 Hair mount showing Monilethrix. (*Used with permission from Dr. Vera Price.*)

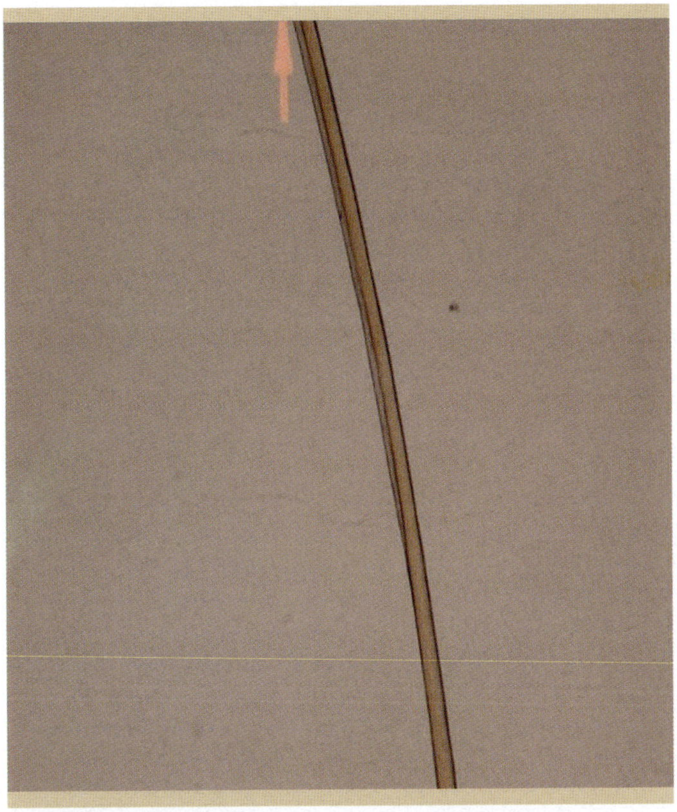

FIGURE 1-24A Hair mount showing longitudinal groove along hair shaft in uncombable hair syndrome. (*Used with permission from Dr. Sarah Chamlin.*)

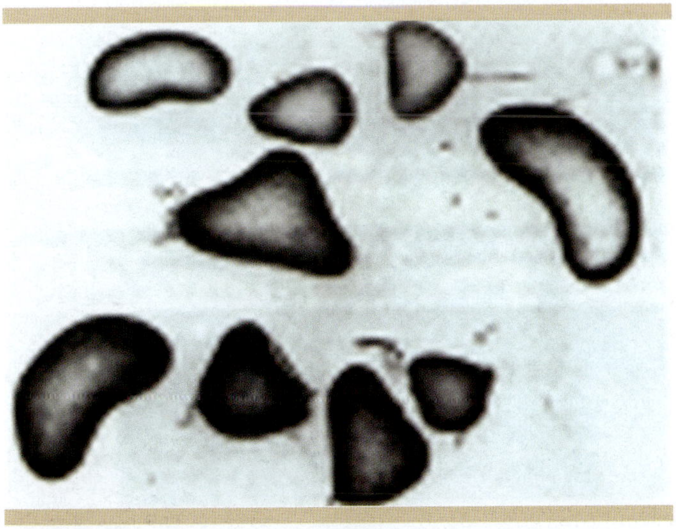

FIGURE 1-24B Cross-section of hair shaft showing triangular formation. (*Used with permission from Dr. Vera Price.*)

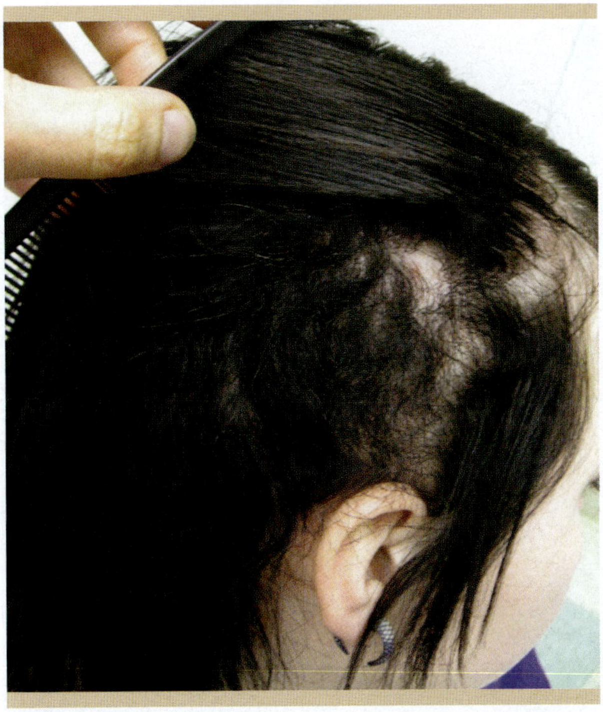

FIGURE 1-25 Wooly hair. (*Used with permission from Dr. Paradi Mirmirani.*)

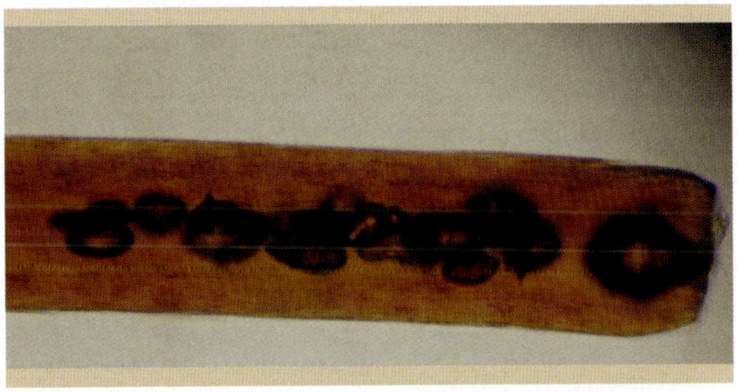

FIGURE 1-26 Hair mount showing bubble hair. (*Used with permission from Dr. Paradi Mirmirani.*)

TABLE 1-3 Presentations of Tinea Capitis

Tinea	Fungus
"Black dot" tinea: alopecia with pinpoint black dots (infected hairs that have broken off)	*Trichophyton tonsurans, endothrix*
Kerion: boggy lesions with crust, severe inflammatory reaction (Fig. 1-27)	*Trichophyton mentagrophytes* *Trichophyton verrucosum*
Favus: large crust of matted hyphae (scutula)	*Trichophyton schoenleinii*

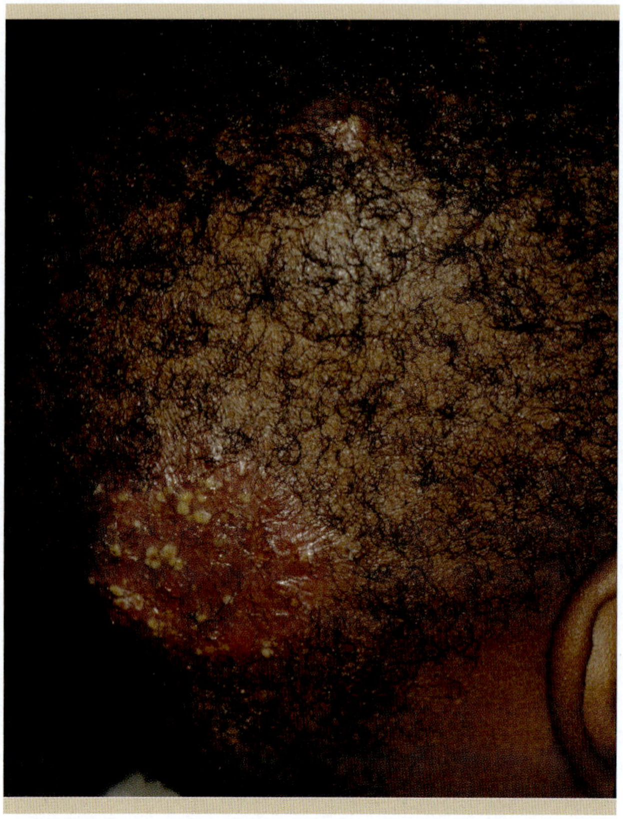

FIGURE 1-27 Kerion on scalp. (*Used with permission from Dr. Adelaide Hebert.*)

Cornelia de Lange, minoxidil, cyclosporine, phenytoin, anorexia nervosa
- Eyelash trichomegaly-HIV

Hirsuitism

- Excessive terminal hair growth in androgen-dependent areas
- Usually related to hyperandrogenism, but may be idiopathic
- Polycystic ovarian syndrome: hirsuitism, acne, abnormal periods, obesity
- Ovarian, adrenal, pituitary tumors
- Medications: androgens, high-progesterone oral contraceptives, minoxidil
- Treatment: waxing, plucking, shaving, bleaching, cream hair removal, electrolysis, laser, spironolactone, eflornithine cream

Miscellaneous

1. Pseudofolliculitis (Fig. 1-30)
    - Occurs at any site where hair is shaved, most common on beard
    - Ingrown hairs, foreign-body reaction
2. Green hair
    - Reaction to copper in pools
    - Treat with chelating agents

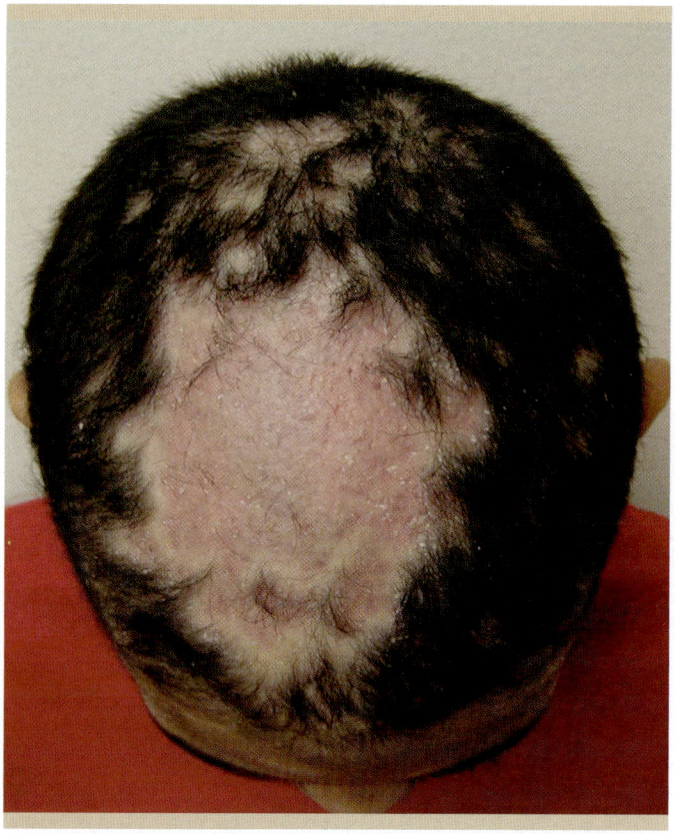

FIGURE 1-28 Tinea capitis mimicking cicatricial alopecia. There was full regrowth after treatment with a course of oral antifungals. (*Used with permission from Dr. Paradi Mirmirani.*)

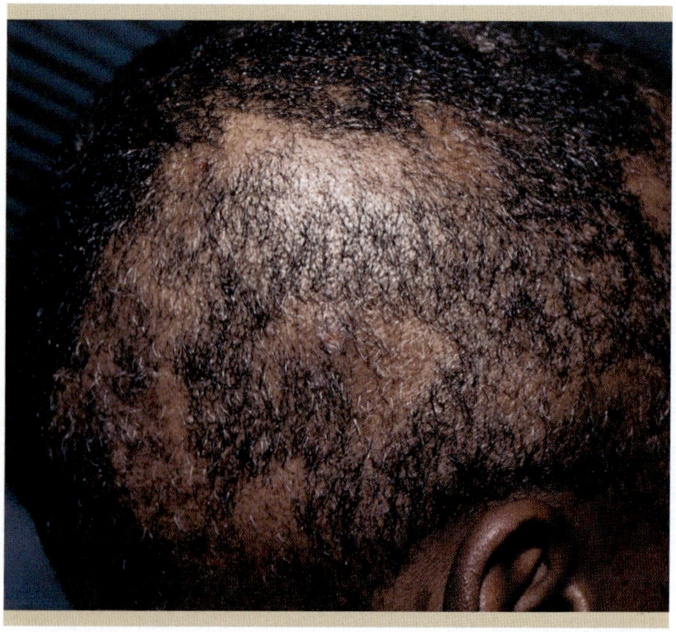

FIGURE 1-29 Syphilis. (*Used with permission from Dr. Robert Jordon.*)

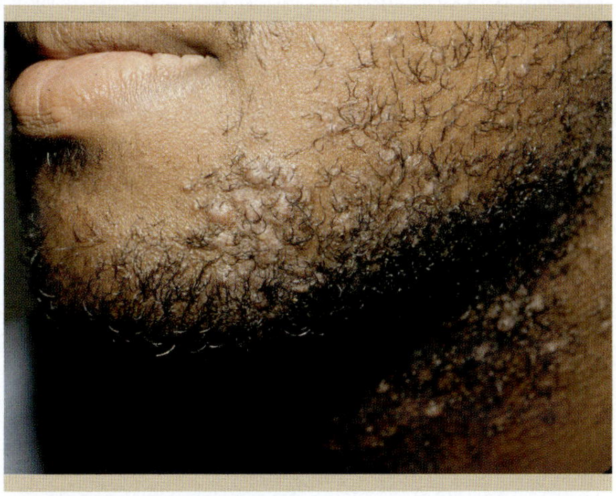

FIGURE 1-30 Pseudofolliculitis. (*Used with permission from Dr. Robert Jordon.*)

3. Piebaldism
   - Autosomal dominant defect in *C-KIT* gene
   - White forelock, depigmented patches on ventral midline
4. Halo scalp ring
   - Temporary nonscarring alopecia attributed to caput succedaneum
   - Occurs perinatally, mothers are primigravidae

QUIZ

Questions

1. A 42-year-old woman presents with concern regarding excessive hair growth on her face. She reports a history of regular menstrual periods and reports that at her most recent annual gynecologic examination, she was told that her ovaries were normal in size. What is the most logical next step?

   A. Check serum androstenedione and testosterone
   B. Check 21-hydroxylase level
   C. Skin biopsy
   D. Referral to endocrinology
   E. CT abdomen

2. A 24-year-old woman is seen with gradual hair thinning over the past few years. On examination her frontal hairline is retained but the central part is widened, and there are many hairs of varied length and caliber. The follicular markings are intact and there is no scaling or erythema of the scalp. A pull test is negative. A scalp biopsy will likely show:

   A. Peribulbar lymphocytic inflammation
   B. An increased catagen/telogen ratio
   C. Premature desquamation of the inner root sheath
   D. Miniaturized hair follicles with preserved sebaceous glands

3. A 6-year-old girl is sent home from school for having "lice" and presents to you for evaluation and treatment. On examination, there are freely mobile structures noted along the hair shaft. What is the most likely diagnosis?

   A. Pediculosis
   B. Hair casts
   C. Trichoptilosis
   D. Monilethrix
   E. Pili annulati

4. A 6-year-old girl is brought in by her mother who is concerned that she has never needed a haircut. There is no family history of similar hair problems. Her daughter does not complain of any scalp itching. The blond girl has fine textured hair that covers her scalp well but is barely past her ears in length. She has no patchy or diffuse hair loss. A hair pull is done and many hairs are easily extracted. A hair mount is done. The most likely finding is:

   A. Exclamation point hairs
   B. A telogen club hair
   C. Dystrophic anagen hair with a ruffled cuticle
   D. Trichorrhexis nodosa

5. Match the syndrome on the right with most common hair findings on the left:

A. Pili torti	i. Trichothiodystrophy
B. Trichorrhexis invaginata	ii. Menkes kinky hair syndrome
C. Pili trianguli et canaliculi	iii. Netherton syndrome
D. Trichoschisis	iv. Uncombable hair syndrome
E. Trichorrhexis nodosa	v. Argininosuccinic aciduria

6. A significantly increased number of "club hairs" on a pull test is indicative of:

   A. Anagen effluvium
   B. Telogen effluvium
   C. Normal hair anatomy
   D. Alopecia areata
   E. Androgenetic alopecia

7. A 60-year-old woman with previously "salt-and-pepper" hair comes in to the office complaining that her hair "turned white overnight." Examination shows diffuse hair loss but the follicular markings are intact. There is no scaling or erythema of the scalp. A pull test is positive. A hair mount shows telogen club hairs. Your diagnosis is:
   A. Alopecia areata
   B. Telogen effluvium
   C. Anagen effluvium
   D. Androgenetic alopecia

8. A 54-year-old postmenopausal woman is seen with a complaint of a "receding hairline." Her scalp is itchy. On examination there is a band of alopecia at the frontal hairline and extending to the temporal hairline. Where the hairline used to be, the skin is atrophic and white with loss of follicular markings. Along the current hairline there is perifollicular scaling and erythema. A scalp biopsy is done showing a dense lymphocytic infiltrate at the level of the isthmus. Your diagnosis:
   A. Hair loss due to excess androgens
   B. Folliculitis decalvans
   C. Alopecia areata in an ophiasis pattern
   D. Frontal fibrosing alopecia

9. Regarding androgens in women, which of the following statements is NOT correct?
   A. There are no differences in eyelashes, eyebrows, and vellus hair-bearing areas in men and women
   B. Eyebrows, eyelashes, and vellus hairs are androgen dependent
   C. The conversion of testosterone to DHT at the follicle leads to androgen action
   D. Testosterone binds the androgen receptor

10. The following hair shaft disorders are associated with increased hair fragility and breakage:
    i. Trichorrhexis nodosa
    ii. Trichorrhexis invaginata
    iii. Pili annulati
    iv. Pili trianguli et canaliculi
    v. Monilethrix

    A. i and ii
    B. All of the above
    C. iii and iv
    D. i, ii, and v

Answers

1. A. In the case of idiopathic hirsutism, women will present with the clinical signs of androgen excess, however, with normal menses, normal-sized ovaries, normal adrenal function, and no evidence of adrenal or ovarian tumors. They may often have a slightly elevated level of plasma androstenedione and testosterone, making this the next logical step in workup.
2. D. The description of hair loss fits best with a clinical diagnosis of androgenetic alopecia. The histologic findings seen in androgenetic alopecia are miniaturized follicles with retained sebaceous glands.
3. B. Hair casts present most commonly in young girls between 2 and 8 years old. These casts are nonadherent and thus slide freely along the hair shaft in contrast to the nits from pediculosis capitis which are adherent to the hair and do not slide. Trichoptilosis is the result of chemical or physical damage to the hair and are commonly referred to as "split ends."
4. C. The clinical scenario is that of a patient with loose anagen syndrome. There is no alopecia, but the hair is somewhat sparse and fails to grow long. Hairs that are easily extracted show a hook-shaped appearance (dystrophic anagen) with a ruffled cuticle.
5. A-ii; B-iii, C-iv, D-i, E-v.
6. D. "Club-shaped" hairs are characteristic of telogen hairs. An increased number of telogen hairs on hair pull would be suggestive of telogen effluvium. In contrast to telogen hairs, anagen hairs have a curled appearance at the root. While it may be normal to find a small number of telogen hairs, a significantly increased number would represent telogen effluvium.
7. A. The clinical scenario describes a patient with alopecia areata. Alopecia areata not uncommonly will affect pigmented hair first, thus giving the appearance of "going white overnight." In active alopecia areata telogen hairs or broken hairs may be seen on hair mount.
8. D. Frontal fibrosing alopecia is a primary cicatricial alopecia, lymphocytic type, thought to be a variant of lichen planopilaris. The typical patient is a postmenopausal woman with a bandlike area of hair loss along the frontotemporal rim; loss of eyebrows is variably seen. At the active border of hair loss, there is perifollicular erythema and scaling.
9. B. The hair follicle requires conversion of testosterone to DHT for expression of androgen action. Only testosterone and DHT bind the androgen receptor. The growth and development of eyebrows, eyelashes, and vellus hairs are NOT androgen dependent. Therefore, there are no differences between these areas in men and women.
10. D. Hair shaft disorders are typically divided into those that cause increased fragility/breakage and those that do not. Patients with trichorrhexis nodosa, trichorrhexis invaginata, and monilethrix typically present with short, broken hair.

REFERENCES

Alkhalifah A, Alsantali A, Wang E, McElwee KJ, Shapiro J: Alopecia areata update: part I. Clinical picture, histopathology, and pathogenesis. *J Am Acad Dermatol* Feb 2010;62(2):177–188, quiz 189–190. PMID: 20115945.

Blume-Peytavi U et al; Skin Academy: European Consensus on the evaluation of women presenting with excessive hair growth. *Eur J Dermatol* Nov-Dec 2009;19(6):597–602. Epub 2009 Sep 2.

Cotsarelis G, Millar SE: Towards a molecular understanding of hair loss and its treatment. *Trends Mol Med* Jul 2001;7(7):293–301.

Goldsmith LA, Katz SI, Gilchrest BA, Paller AS, Leffell AS, Wolff K: *Fitzpatrick's Dermatology in General Medicine*, 8th Ed. New York: McGraw-Hill; 2012: 960–1009.

Han A, Mirmirani P: Clinical approach to the patient with alopecia. *Semin Cutan Med Surg* Mar 2006;25(1):11–23.

Mirmirani P, Huang KP, Price VH: A practical, algorithmic approach to diagnosing hair shaft disorders. *Int J Dermatol* Jan 2011;50(1):1–12.

Price VH: Treatment of hair loss. *N Engl J Med* Sep 23 1999;341(13): 964–973.

Price VH, Mirmirani P: *Cicatricial Alopecia: An Approach to Diagnosis and Management*. New York: Springer; 2011.

Sperling LC, Cowper SE, Knopp EA: *An Atlas of Hair Pathology with Clinical Correlations*. 2nd Ed. *Informa Healthcare*; 2012.

Weedon D, ed. *Weedon's Skin Pathology*, 3rd Ed. London: Churchill Livingston Elsevier; 2010.

CHAPTER 2

EYE FINDINGS

MIRWAT S. SAMI
CHARLES S. SOPARKAR

EYELID ANATOMY (FIG. 2-1)

Eyelids

- Unique and distinct in their anatomy
- Five layers superficial to deep: skin, orbital septum, eyelid retractors, tarsal plates, conjunctiva
- Skin
  - Unique because it is the thinnest in the body, few vellus hair follicles, no subcutaneous fat layer with loose attachments to underlying tissue
- Orbicularis oculi
  - Main protractor, or closing muscle of the eyelid; motor innervation by cranial nerve VII (facial nerve)
  - Three anatomic parts: pretarsal and preseptal (together comprising the palpebral portion of orbicularis) and orbital parts. The pretarsal and preseptal parts involved with involuntary blink; orbital portion involved with voluntary for forced eye closure
  - Concentric muscle fibers shaped like a horse-shoe, covering entire eyelid; insert at medial and lateral canthal tendons and orbital portion interdigitates with frontalis, corrugator, and procerus muscles in the forehead
- Orbital septum
  - Dense fibrous sheath of mesodermal origin forming middle lamella of eyelid
  - Extension of periosteum of orbital bones; extends from arcus marginalis at bony rim toward the tarsus; attaches to levator aponeurosis and capsulopalpebral fascia in upper and lower eyelids, respectively
  - Keeps orbital fat in posterior compartment and acts as a barrier between orbit and eyelid, preventing postseptal spread of infection
- Eyelid retractors
  - Attach to tarsal plates and serve to retract or open eyelids
  - Upper eyelid: levator palpebrae superioris, Müller muscle
  - Lower eyelid: capsulopalpebral fascia, inferior tarsal muscle
- Tarsal plates
  - Dense connective tissue plates in each eyelid, responsible for structural integrity and contour of eyelids; contain meibomian glands
  - Rigid attachments to orbital rim periosteum by lateral and medial canthal tendons
- Conjunctiva
  - Divided into palpebral and bulbar conjunctiva
  - Mucosal membrane with numerous mucin-producing goblet cells, blood vessels, nerve endings, and loose underlying stromal tissue (substania propria)
  - Palpebral conjunctiva is the posterior-most lining of the eyelids and is firmly adherent to tarsal plates
  - Palpebral conjunctiva continues to the cul-de-sac or fornices of the eyelids where it is reflected to form the bulbar conjunctiva that covers the globe
  - Bulbar conjunctiva is delicate and freely movable except where it fuses with the globe at the limbus
- Preaponeurotic fat pads
  - Lie immediately posterior to orbital septum
  - Upper lid: 2 fat pads anterior to levator aponeurosis; nasal smaller and paler than central pad
  - Lower lid: 3 fat pads anterior to capsulopalpebral fascia; lateral pad is small; nasal and middle pads separated by inferior oblique muscle
- Sensory innervation of the eyelids
  - Cranial nerve V (trigeminal nerve) via terminal branches of ophthalmic (V_1) and maxillary (V_2) divisions
- Canthal tendons
  - Medial and lateral tendons attaching to orbital rim periosteum
  - Complex arrangement of fibrous tendon with muscular component from orbicularis muscle, attaching tarsal plates of each eyelid to orbital rim
  - Attachments are important for proper orientation and apposition of eyelids to globe
  - Lateral canthus is 2 to 3 mm superior to medial canthus
  - Elongation, weakening, or transection of tendons will produce eyelid instability
- Eyelid Margin
  - Eyelashes
    - Each lid margin has 2 to 3 rows of eye lashes located anterior to the tarsus
    - About 100 in the upper lid and 50 in the lower lid; 10-week growth period with 5-month resting phase

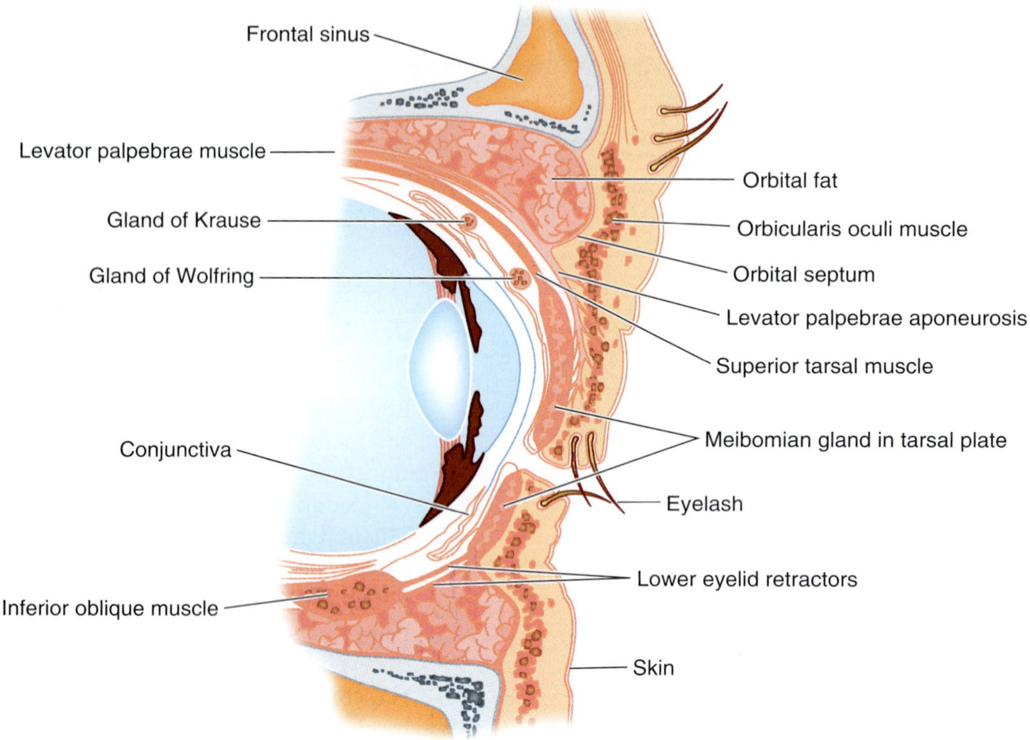

FIGURE 2-1 Eyelid anatomy. (*Redrawn with permission from Riordan-Eva P, Richter JP:* Vaughan & Ashbury's General Ophthalmology, *17th Ed. New York: McGraw-Hill; 2008.*)

- Glands of the eyelids (posterior to anterior)
  - Meibomian glands: sebaceous glands located within the tarsus; secrete lipid layer of tear film
  - Glands of Moll: modified sweat glands; apocrine glands that lubricate cilia
  - Glands of Zeis: modified sebaceous glands associated with the cilia; secrete lipid and lubricate cilia
- Interpalpebral fissure:
  - Fusiform space between the eyelid margins; measure of actual distance between upper and lower eyelids; typically 10 to 11 mm vertically and 20 mm horizontally in adults

Upper Eyelid

- Upper eyelid retractors: levator palpebrae superioris, Müller muscle
- Levator palpebrae superioris
  - Main retractor of upper eyelid; divided into muscular and aponeurotic portions
  - Aponeurosis attaches to anterior surface of tarsus and also sends attachments to orbicularis and skin, forming upper eyelid crease
  - Innervated by cranial nerve III (oculomotor nerve)
  - Thinning or disinsertion of levator leads to ptosis of the upper eyelid and higher eyelid crease, as seen in involutional ptosis
- Müller muscle
  - Minor retractor; smooth muscle with cervical sympathetic innervation
  - Lies posterior to levator aponeurosis at superior tarsal border
- Upper eyelid tarsal plate: 29 mm long, 1 mm thick; 10 mm in vertical height; 30 to 40 meibomian glands in plate with orifices at eyelid margin
- Upper eyelid crease: formed by attachments of levator aponeurosis to skin through septum and orbicularis

Lower Eyelid

- Lower eyelid retractors: capsulopalpebral fascia and inferior tarsal muscle
- Capsulopalpebral fascia
  - Analogous to derived from the capsulopalpebral head of the inferior rectus muscle
  - Fuses with septum and inserts into inferior tarsal
- Inferior tarsal muscle
  - Analogous to Müller muscle; weak retractor
  - Sympathetic innervation

- Lower eyelid tarsal plate: 29 mm long, 1 mm thick; 4 to 5 mm in vertical height; 20 to 30 meibomian glands in plate with orifices at eyelid margin
- Lower eyelid crease: less prominent than upper eyelid crease due to lack of attachments of skin to underlying structures; indicates the inferior edge of the tarsus

DISORDERS OF EYELID MALPOSITION

Dermatochalasis (Fig. 2-2)

- Redundancy of eyelid skin with orbital fat prolapse due to involutional changes
- May cause visual field compromise if excessive enough to obstruct pupillary aperture
- Treatment is surgical excision of redundant skin by blepharoplasty procedure

Blepharoptosis (Fig. 2-3)

- Lower position of eyelid; may cause functional vision loss
- Causes:
  - Involutional: age-related dehiscence of the levator muscle
  - Myogenic: causes include myasthenia gravis, myotonic dystrophy, chronic progressive external ophthalmoplegia
  - Neurogenic: causes include cranial nerve III palsy, Horner syndrome, multiple sclerosis
  - Traumatic: due to trauma to levator muscle
  - Mechanical: mass effect of orbital or eyelid tumors, dermatochalasis, blepharochalasis, cicatrix
- Treat underlying cause if possible; most cases require surgical correction of ptosis by levator advancement or repair, or use of frontalis sling

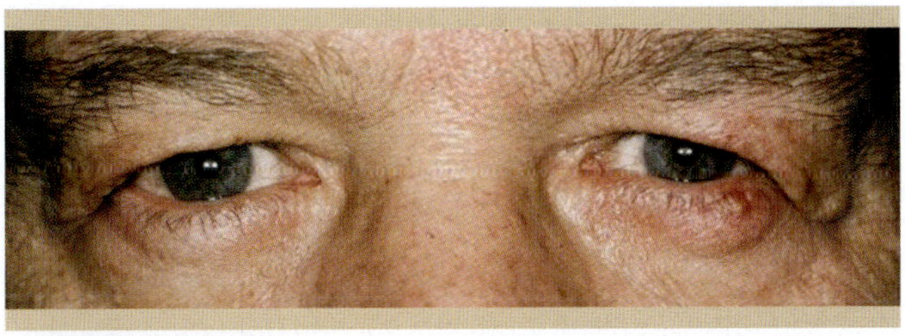

FIGURE 2-2 Dermatochalasis of upper lids and herniation of orbital fat of lower lids. (*Used with permission from Dr. Mirwat S. Sami.*)

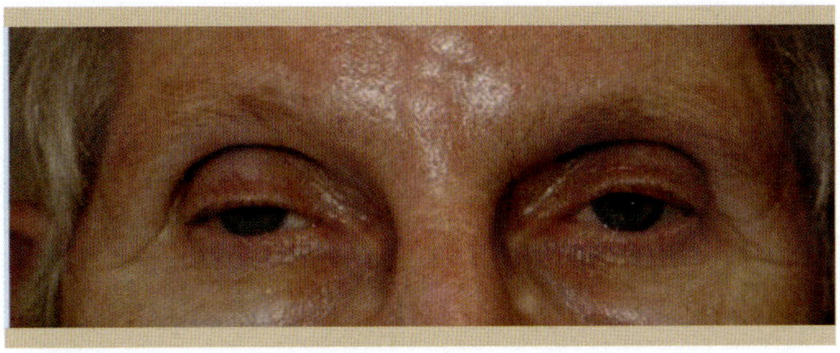

FIGURE 2-3 Bilateral involutional ptosis of upper eyelids with visual field decline. High eyelid crease indicative of levator dehiscence and attenuation. (*Used with permission from Dr. Mirwat S. Sami.*)

Entropion (Fig. 2-4)

- Inversion of eyelid margin causing ocular irritation
- Causes: involutional (most often canthal tendon laxity), cicatricial, spastic, congenital
- Treatment is directed toward symptomatic relief with ocular lubrication, treating underlying cause and/or surgically stabilizing eyelid and reapproximating it to globe

Ectropion (Fig. 2-5)

- Eversion of eyelid margin causing keratinization and hypertrophy of conjunctiva due to prolonged eye exposure and dryness
- Causes: involutional (most often canthal tendon laxity), paralytic (CN VII palsy), cicatricial, mechanical
- Treatment is directed toward symptomatic relief with ocular lubrication, treating underlying cause, and/or surgically stabilizing eyelid and reapproximating it to globe

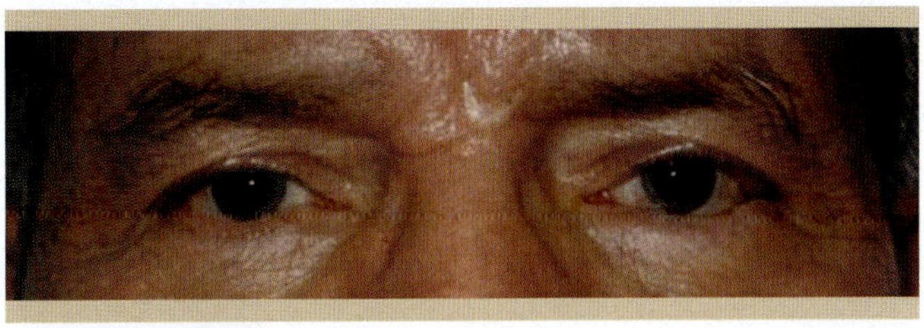

FIGURE 2-4 Involutional entropion of left lower eyelid resulting in keratopathy from eyelashes rubbing against cornea. (*Used with permission from Dr. Mirwat S. Sami.*)

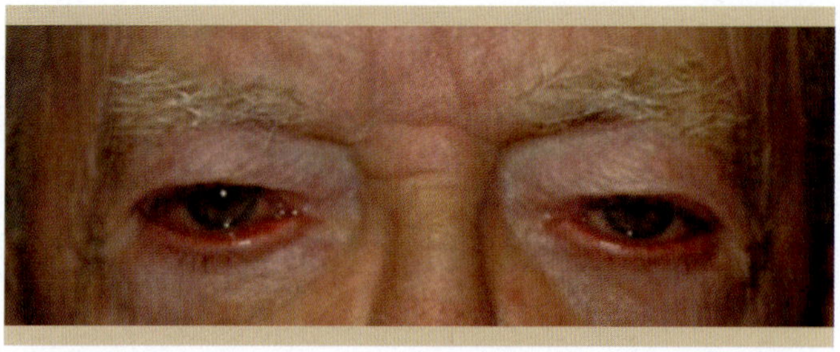

FIGURE 2-5 Bilateral lower eyelid involutional ectropion resulting in exposure keratopathy, tearing, and dry eyes. (*Used with permission from Dr. Mirwat S. Sami.*)

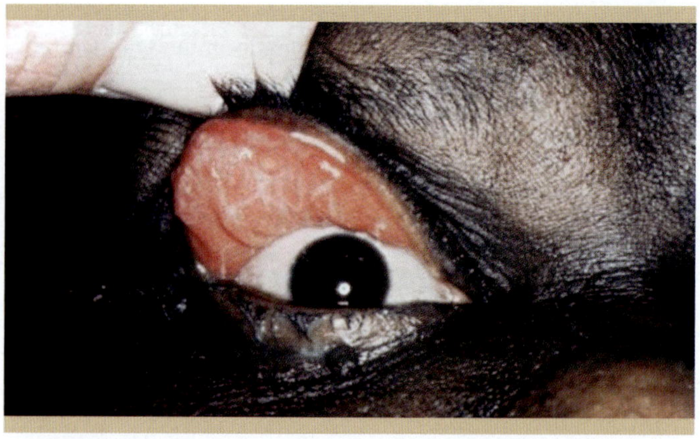

FIGURE 2-6 Floppy eyelid syndrome with easy eversion and distraction of eyelid from globe. Fibrosis of palpebral conjunctiva develops secondary to chronic papillary conjunctivitis and irritation. (*Used with permission from Dr. Charles S. Soparkar.*)

Blepharochalasis

- Idiopathic inflammatory edema of eyelids
- Characterized by recurrent attacks of transient, painless edema, typically bilateral, resulting in atrophy, wrinkling and redundancy of eyelid skin with prolapse of orbital fat pads and lacrimal glands
- Familial variant of angioneurotic edema, seen most often in young women; in rare cases, associated with Ascher syndrome (progressive enlargement of upper lip and thyromegaly), renal agenesis, vertebral abnormalities, or congenital heart anomalies
- Histopathology reveals dermal lymphocytic perivascular infiltrates with IgA deposition and elastolytic changes
- Treatment is aimed at surgically correcting the resulting dermatochalasis and ptosis but should be avoided until the disease is quiescent

Floppy Eyelid Syndrome (Fig. 2-6)

- Characterized by easily everted, flaccid eyelids
- Chronic papillary conjunctivitis due to lid autoeversion during sleep with mechanical irritation from bedsheets, resulting in nonspecific irritative symptoms
- Associated with sleep apnea, obesity, hyperglycemia, keratoconus, allergic conjunctivitis with excessive eye rubbing
- Marked decrease in number of elastin fibers in the tarsus
- Treatment is lubrication and patching of lids during sleep or surgical horizontal eyelid tightening and stabilization

DISORDERS OF EYELID MARGIN

Blepharitis

- Inflammation of eyelid margin, typically a chronic condition that can be controlled but not completely cured
- Due to staphylococcal or seborrheic inflammation
- Associated with rosacea, dry eyes, and chalazia
- Symptoms of ocular irritation, redness, burning, and tearing
- Erythematous, thickened and sometimes irregular eyelid margins, dilated vessels
- Meibomian gland inflammation results in inspissation, thickened secretions, and dry eyes
- Eyelashes affected with madarosis, trichiasis, or poliosis; base of lashes frequently surrounded by hard scale and debris, called collarettes, that are hallmark of staphylococcal blepharitis
- Treatment includes warm compresses, cleansing of eyelid margin, ocular lubrication, topical antibiotic ointment (for infectious etiology); consider systemic tetracycline/doxycycline for blepharitis associated with rosacea

Trichiasis

- Misdirection of eyelashes with contact with ocular surface
- Can be congenital or acquired
- Acquired causes include chronic blepharitis, herpes zoster, OCP, Stevens-Johnson syndrome, chemical eye injuries, entropion, and trauma
- Treat underlying cause; epilation or destruction of misdirected eyelashes may also be required

Distichiasis

- Aberrant growth of eyelashes through meibomian gland orifices
- Can be congenital or acquired
- Acquired cases result from chronic inflammation of eyelids such as rosacea, OCP, Stevens-Johnson syndrome
- Treat underlying cause; epilation or destruction of eyelashes may also be required

Madarosis

- Loss of eyelashes due to local or systemic disorders
- Localized or diffuse
- May be associated with abnormalities in hair growth on other parts of the body
- May be associated with inflammation, scarring, tumors, infections, medications, or endocrine disorders (hypothyroidism, hypopituitarism)

Poliosis

- Premature whitening of eyelashes/eyebrows
- Can be associated with vitiligo (common acquired idiopathic depigmentation of skin)
- Associated with Vogt-Koyanagi-Harada syndrome, sympathetic ophthalmia, Waardenburg syndrome, tuberous sclerosis, radiation, and dermatitis

Chalazion (Fig. 2-7)

- Localized, chronic lipogranulomatous lesion of the eyelid; considered sterile but may become secondarily infected
- Obstruction of meibomian gland with accumulation of secretions causes inflammatory response with lipogranuloma formation
- Pathology demonstrates epithelioid and giant cells surrounding empty lipid vacuoles and zonal granulomatous inflammation
- Treatment includes warm compresses and eyelid hygiene in the acute stage; secondary infections can be treated with topical antibiotics
- Treatment of chronic chalazia frequently requires surgical excision of cyst-like lesion and granulomatous tissue; steroid injections to excisional bed can be useful in treating recurrent chalazia

Hordeolum (Fig. 2-8)

- Acute, suppurative infection of inspissated sebaceous glands of eyelid; *Staphylococcus aureus* and *Staphylococcus epidermidis* are most common pathogens

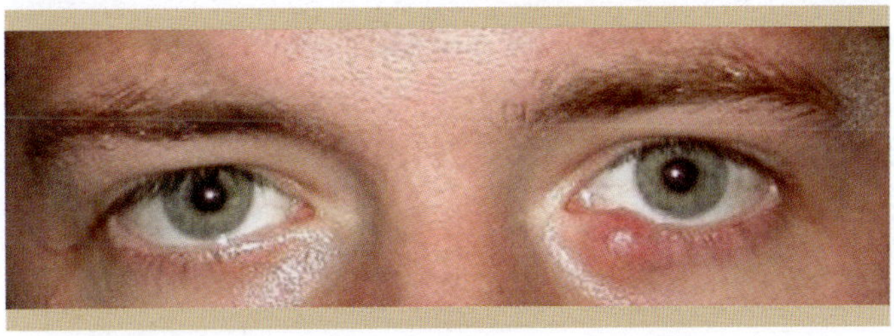

FIGURE 2-7 Chalazion of left lower eyelid. (*Used with permission from Dr. Mirwat S. Sami.*)

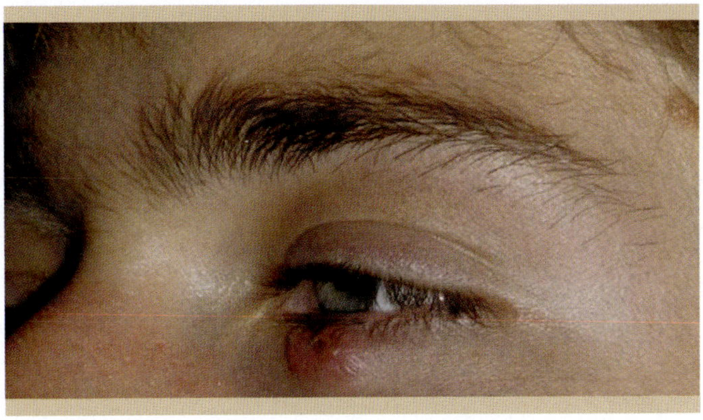

FIGURE 2-8 External hordeolum of left lower eyelid with suppurative inflammation. (*Used with permission from Dr. Charles S. Soparkar.*)

- External hordeolum (stye) when glands of Zeis or Moll are affected
- Internal hordeolum when meibomian glands are affected
- Associated with seborrhea, rosacea, and blepharitis
- Treatment includes warm compresses, eyelid hygiene, topical antibiotics; if medical management fails, surgical incision and drainage can be performed

Phthiriasis Palpebrum/Pediculosis

- Infestation of eyelashes with *Phthirus pubis*, which is also responsible for pubic lice
- Spread by direct contact, usually sexually transmitted
- Infestation causes blepharoconjunctivitis with redness, burning, and itching
- Slit-lamp examination reveals tiny pearl-colored eggs (nits) or adult lice attached to eyelash base; eyelid margins may be covered with reddish-brown granules consisting of louse feces and dried blood; follicular conjunctivitis and preauricular lymphadenopathy is also frequently noted
- Treatment includes mechanical removal of nits and lice; topical ointment (physostigmine) to smother adult lice; delousing creams and shampoos

Molluscum Cantagiosum

- Dome-shaped, waxy nodules with central umbilication along eyelid margin; multiple lesions are typical
- Usually asymptomatic; can cause follicular conjunctivitis and punctate keratitis with resulting ocular irritation, burning, and dry eyes
- Double-stranded DNA poxvirus responsible for infection following direct contact with skin
- Pathology reveals lobular acanthosis with large intracytoplasmic inclusion bodies in infected epidermal cells,

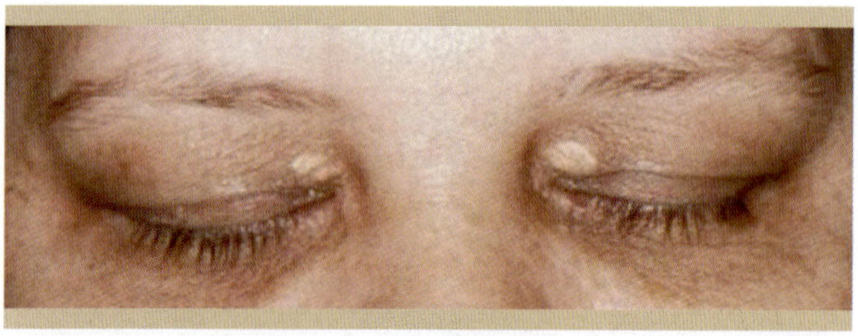

FIGURE 2-9 Bilateral medial upper eyelid xanthalesmas. (*Used with permission from Dr. Charles S. Soparkar.*)

surrounded by lymphocytic infiltration; inclusion bodies are filled with viral nucleic acids
- Usually self-limited with spontaneous resolution in 3 to 12 months
- Treatment includes surgical excision, curettage, and cryotherapy

Xanthelasma Palpebrarum (Fig. 2-9)

- Yellow, slightly elevated soft plaques located in upper or lower eyelids; usually bilateral and medial in location
- Unknown pathogenesis; two-thirds of patients have normal serum lipids
- May occur in hyperlipidemic states such as familial hypercholesterolemia, juvenile xanthogranuloma, or histiocytosis X
- Pathology reveals benign, lipid-laden macrophages (foam cells) located around dermal blood vessels
- Erdheim Chester disease (lipoid granulomatosis)
    - Multisystemic disease with lipogranuloma formation in liver, heart, kidneys, lungs, and bone
    - Ocular findings include proptosis and xanthalesma-like lesions
- Treatment is cosmetically driven, requiring full-thickness excision; recurrence is common

PERIOCULAR ADNEXAL TUMORS (SEE CHAPTER 11)

Hidrocystoma (Fig. 2-10)

- Small, round cystic lesions, sometimes found in clusters around lower eyelids and canthal regions; usually translucent, filled with serous fluid
- Most are eccrine, arising from ductal dilation of sweat glands
- Can be apocrine, arising from glands of Moll, in which case they are true adenomas

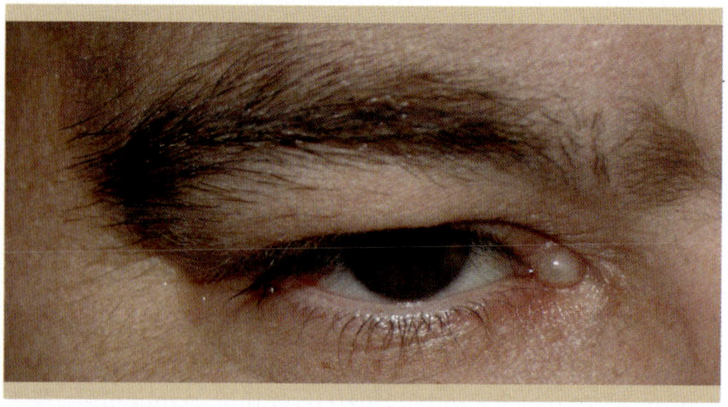

FIGURE 2-10 Apocrine hidrocystoma in right medial canthal region. (*Used with permission from Dr. Mirwat S. Sami.*)

- Often enlarge in conditions of increased heat and humidity that stimulate perspiration
- Schopf-Schulz-Passarge syndrome
    - Rare, autosomal recessive disorder with multiple eyelid hidrocystomas
    - Systemic findings of hypotrichosis, hypodontia, nail abnormalities, palmarplantar eccrine syringofibroadenomas
- Treatment consists of surgical excision of entire cyst, including cyst wall

Syringoma (Fig. 2-11)

- Multiple, small, waxy nodules on lower eyelids and cheeks
- Most often in young women
- Benign proliferation of eccrine ductal structures
- Treatment includes surgical excision of entire cyst or carbon dioxide laser

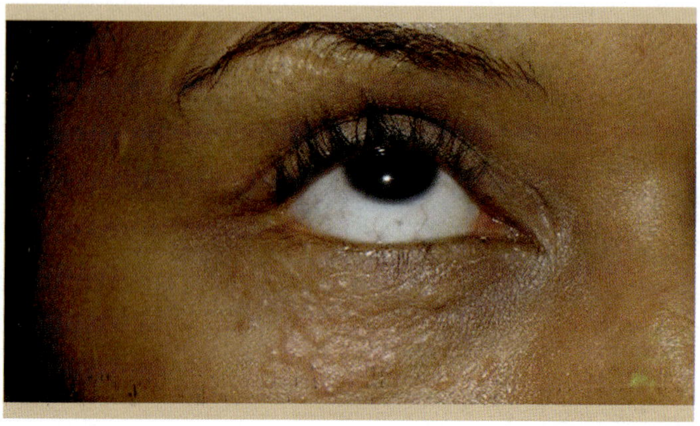

FIGURE 2-11 Lower eyelid syringomas. (*Used with permission from Dr. Mirwat S. Sami.*)

CONGENITAL ABNORMALITIES

Albinism (See Chapter 9)

- Oculocutaneous albinism: lack of pigment of skin, hair, and eyes
- Ocular albinism: lack of pigment limited to eyes
- Ocular findings: decreased vision, iris transillumination defects, foveal hypoplasia, hypopigmented fundus, nystagmus, photophobia, high myopia, strabismus

Nevus of Ota (Ocular Melanocytosis or Melanosis Oculi) (See Chapter 9)

- Unilateral congenital pigmentary lesion of sclera (bluish or slate gray) with periocular skin hyperpigmentation
- May involve eyelid or adjacent skin with dermal hyperplasia (commonly seen in Asians)
- Higher incidence of glaucoma and possibly malignant melanoma (mostly Caucasians)

Incontinentia Pigmenti (Bloch-Sulzberger Syndrome) (See Chapter 9)

- X-linked dominant disorder, occurring exclusively in females (lethal in males)
- Ocular findings: proliferative retinal vasculopathy, retinal detachment, retrolental membrane formation, cataracts, glaucoma, microphthalmos, nystagmus, strabismus
- Also skin lesions, alopecia, dental, and CNS abnormalities

Juvenile Xanthogranuloma (JXG)

- Benign skin condition affecting young children, usually younger than 2 years
- Histiocytic proliferation in skin with Touton giant cells resulting in yellow-orange nodules, ranging from 1 to 20 mm in diameter; regressed lesions become flat and hypopigmented
- In 75%, skin lesions will be only manifestation of disease
- Noncutaneous sites include muscles, salivary glands, pericardium, lungs, viscera, bones, testes, ovaries, kidneys, and CNS
- Ocular involvement is the most common noncutaneous site
- Ocular findings include eyelid skin lesions, iris lesions resulting in heterochromia, spontaneous hyphema (blood in anterior chamber of eye), glaucoma, uveitis, orbital masses
- Treatment: skin lesions usually regress; treatment of intraocular lesions is geared toward management of hyphema, glaucoma, and uveitis; iris lesions can be irradiated or surgically excised if discrete

Down Syndrome (See Chapter 14)

- Trisomy 21
- Ocular findings: Brushfield spots (tan iris hamartomas), epicanthal folds, high refractive errors, glaucoma, cataracts, amblyopia

Cockayne Syndrome (See Chapter 14)

- Autosomal recessive disorder mapped to chromosome 10
- Ocular findings: cataracts, retinitis pigmentosa, optic atrophy

Goldenhar Syndrome (Oculo-Auriculo-Vertebral Dysplasia)

- Ocular findings: limbal dermoids, dermolipomas, lower lid coloboma; microphthalmos (presence indicates increased risk of mental retardation)
- Hypoplasia of malar, maxillary, and mandibular regions, pretragal auricular appendages (Fig. 2-12), vertebral abnormalities, and fistula between mouth and ear

Treacher Collins Syndrome (Mandibulofacial Dysostosis) (Fig. 2-13)

- Autosomal dominant disorder due to defect in first and second branchial arch structures
- Ocular findings: lateral lid defects (lower lid colobomas), absent lateral canthal tendon, poorly developed puncta, and lid structures like meibomian glands and eyelashes, antimongoloid slant
- Hypoplastic midface: bilateral and symmetric mandibular and zygomatic hypoplasia, micrognathia; dental and ear abnormalities

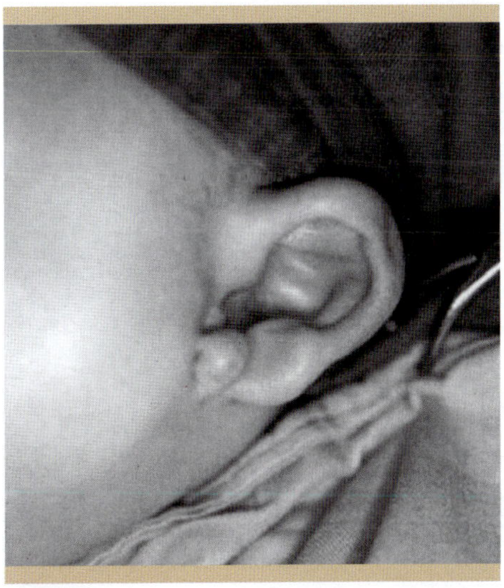

FIGURE 2–12 Pretragal auricular appendages in Goldenhar syndrome. (*Used with permission from Dr. Charles S. Soparkar.*)

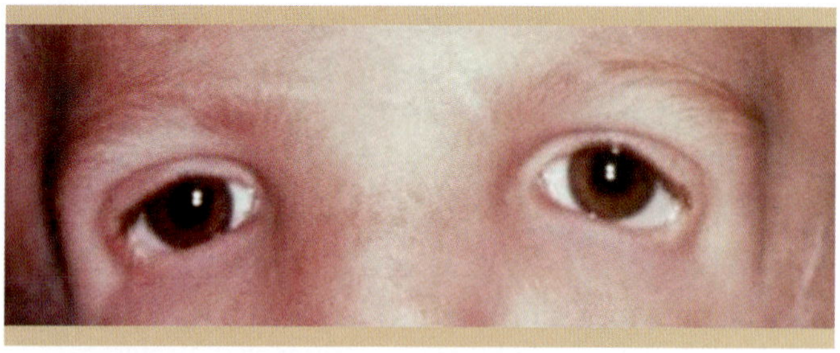

FIGURE 2-13 Treacher Collins syndrome with bilateral lateral lid defects, absent lateral canthal tendons, absent lashes, antimongoloid slant, and ectropion. (*Used with permission from Dr. Charles S. Soparkar.*)

Crouzon Syndrome (Craniofacial Dysostosis) (Fig. 2-14)

- Autosomal dominant or sporadic disorder resulting in absence of forward development of the cranium and midface
- Ocular findings: proptosis, hypertelorism, exotropia, nystagmus, optic atrophy
- Other findings include mental retardation, parrot's beak nose, high arched palate, ear deformities

Apert Syndrome (Fig. 2-15)

- Crouzon syndrome with syndactyly and enlarged anterior segment of eye (anterior megalophthalmos)
- Associated with increased paternal age

Ankyloblepharon

- Autosomal dominant disorder (autosomal recessive and sporadic forms also found) resulting in complete or partial fusion of eyelid margins, usually temporally and bilateral

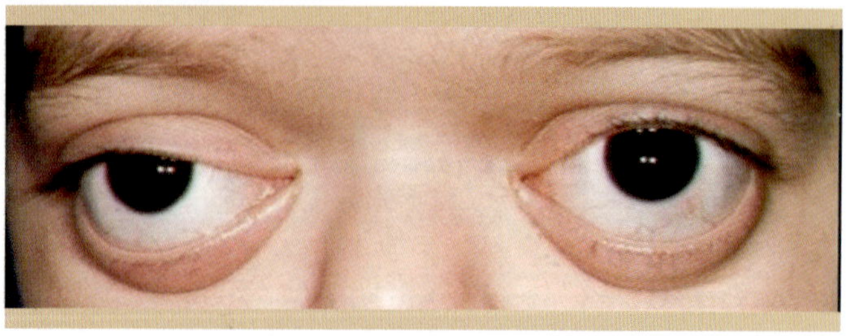

FIGURE 2-14 Crouzon syndrome. (*Used with permission from Dr. Charles S. Soparkar.*)

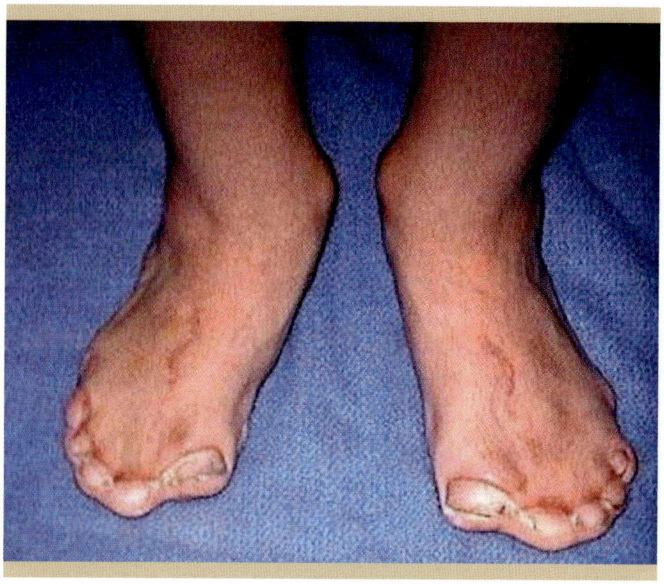

FIGURE 2-15 Apert syndrome with syndactyly. (*Used with permission from Dr. Charles S. Soparkar.*)

- Associated with heterogenous group of congenital, nonprogressive disorders known as ectodermal dysplasia characterized by abnormalities of ectodermally derived tissues like hair, teeth, nails, sweat glands
- CHANDS syndrome (autosomal recessive): Curly hair, ankyloblepharon, nail dysplasia (hypoplastic nails)
- Hay-Wells syndrome (autosomal dominant): Ankyloblepharon-ectodermal dysplasia-clefting (AEC) syndrome with ankyloblepharon, cleft lip and palate, sparse eyelashes

Waardenburg Syndrome (See Chapter 9)

- Autosomal dominant disorder resulting in defect of neural crest cell migration and differentiation
- Ocular findings: lateral displacement of inner canthi (dystopia canthorum—most common), confluent eyebrows, heterochromia iridis, fundus hypopigmentation
- Also sensorineural deafness, white forelock

CONNECTIVE TISSUE DISORDERS

Ehlers-Danlos Syndrome (See Chapter 14)

- Abnormalities in the synthesis and metabolism of collagen
- Most ocular abnormalities occur in the kyphoscoliosis type (previously known as type VI)
- Retinal detachments, microcornea, myopia, blue sclera, angioid streaks, keratoconus, myopia, lens subluxation, and ocular fragility can lead to a ruptured globe/blindness

Marfan Syndrome (See Chapter 14)

- Autosomal dominant disorder mapped to chromosome 15q21, resulting in defect in fibrillin

- Ocular findings: lens subluxation (50–80%), glaucoma, cataracts, flat cornea, increased axial length of the globe resulting in myopia (nearsightedness), and retinal detachment
- Other findings include tall stature, cardiac disease, dissecting aortic aneurysm

Osteogenesis Imperfecta (Van der Hoeve syndrome) (See Chapter 14)

- Autosomal dominant with variable expression
- Blue sclera is common in all subtypes; due to thinning of sclera allowing visualization of underlying uvea
- Also may present with keratoconus, megalocornea, anterior embryotoxon, congenital glaucoma, zonular cataract, dislocated lens, choroidal sclerosis, retinal hemorrhage

Pseudoxanthoma Elasticum (PXE) (See Chapter 14)

- Autosomal recessive disorder resulting in defect in *ABCC6* gene
- Skin and subcutaneous tissue abnormalities, calcification of arteries, gastrointestinal bleeding all due to increased calcification of elastic tissue
- Typical findings: angioid streaks, breaks in calcified, and thickened Bruch membrane; these radiate from the optic nerve; also, macular degeneration, retinal hemorrhage, choroidal ruptures
- Classic skin findings resembling skin of plucked chicken

Thyroid-Associated Ophthalmopathy (TAO) (Figs. 2-16, 2-17, and 2-18) (See Chapter 23)

- Also known as thyroid eye disease (TED) and Graves ophthalmopathy
- Autoimmune-mediated inflammation of the extraocular muscle and periorbital connective tissue resulting in glycosaminoglycan and collagen deposition
- Most common cause of unilateral or bilateral proptosis in adults; most common cause of acquired strabismus and diplopia in adults
- Women affected 8 to 10 times more often than men

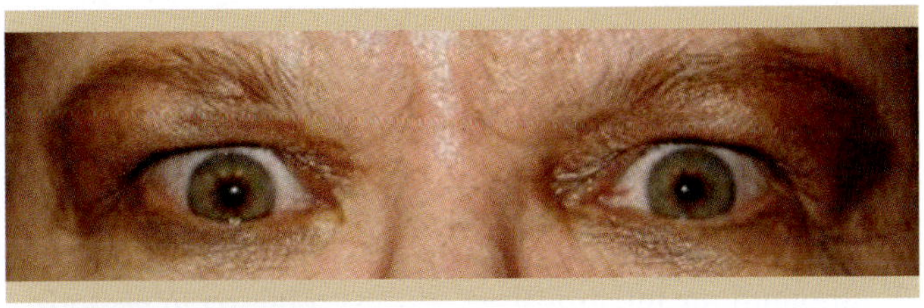

FIGURE 2-16 Bilateral upper eyelid retraction and proptosis in a middle-aged woman with TED. (*Used with permission from Dr. Mirwat S. Sami.*)

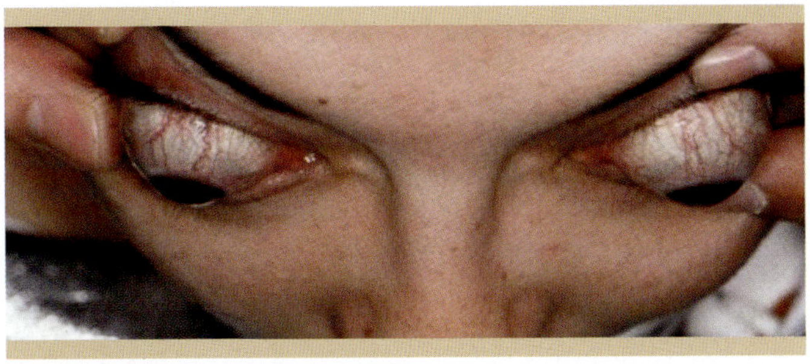

FIGURE 2-17 Thyroid eye disease with severe exophthalmos bilaterally. (*Used with permission from Dr. Mirwat S. Sami.*)

- Among patients with TAO, 90% have Graves hyperthyroidism, 6% are euthyroid, 3% have Hashimoto thyroiditis, and 1% have primary hypothyroidism
- Clinical findings: eyelid retraction (most common feature) (Fig. 2-16), lateral flare, scleral show, exophthalmos (Fig. 2-17 and Fig. 2-18), chemosis, periorbital edema, exposure keratopathy, dry eyes, ocular dysmotility (restrictive myopathy, inferior rectus most often affected, followed by medial rectus, superior rectus, lateral rectus, and obliques), lid lag on downgaze (von Graefe sign), lagophthalmos (incomplete closure of eye)

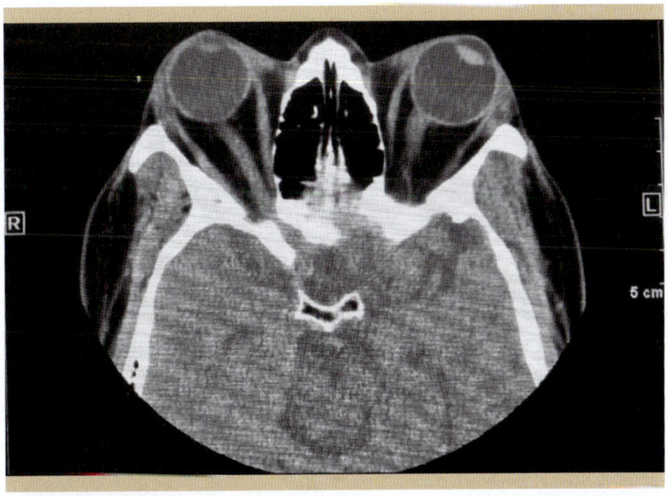

FIGURE 2-18 CT scan of a patient who has TED with severe exophthalmos bilaterally and suffers from compressive optic neuropathy. Note the increase in intraconal fat with fat stranding and modest extraocular muscle enlargement. (*Used with permission from Dr. Mirwat S. Sami.*)

- Optic neuropathy results from crowding of engorged periorbital and muscles at orbital apex resulting in compression; in severe cases, proptosis can cause stretch neuropathy
- Pretibial myxedema and acropachy can also be present
- Pathology reveals patchy infiltrates of lymphocytes, monocytes, and fibroblasts in extraocular muscles and periorbital; increased mucopolysaccharides resulting in increased fluid retention and orbital congestion
- CT findings: enlargement of extraocular muscle bellies with sparing of tendon; increase in retroorbital and intraconal fat potentiating exophthalmos; intraconal fat stranding in acute inflammatory phase; sometimes associated with dilation of superior ophthalmic vein; crowding at orbital apex by muscles and fat resulting in optic nerve compression
- Risk factors include history of thyroid disorder, family history, race (African American), advancing age, gender, smoking, environmental risk factors
- Treatment: aggressive ocular lubrication; cessation of smoking; corticosteroids, radiotherapy, or orbital decompression surgery for compressive optic neuropathy
- Once the disease is inactive or quiescent, rehabilitative measures can be carried out electively to correct exophthalmos and exposure with decompression surgery, strabismus surgery for restrictive dysmotility, and eyelid surgery to correct retraction or other eyelid malposition

Melkersson-Rosenthal Syndrome (Fig. 2-19)

- Rare neurologic disorder of unknown etiology, characterized by classic triad of recurrent orofacial and/or periorbital swelling, lingua plicata (fissured tongue), and unilateral or bilateral facial paralysis
- Females more commonly affected than men; seen in adults but may occur in children

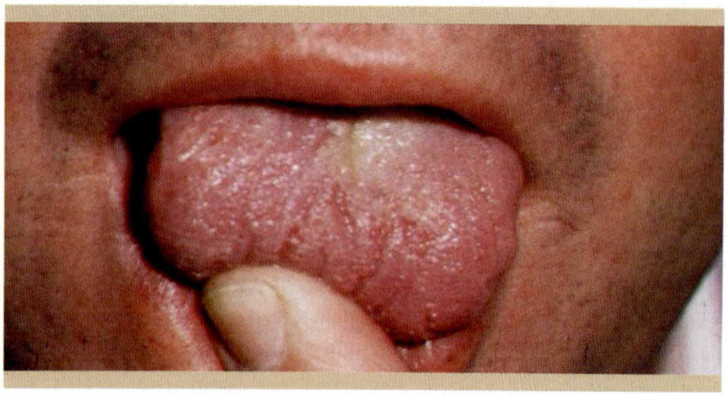

FIGURE 2-19 Melkersson-Rosenthal syndrome with lingua plicata (fissured tongue). (*Used with permission from Dr. Charles S. Soparkar.*)

- Nonpitting facial edema and lingua plicata tend to occur several years before facial palsy that is indistinguishable from Bell palsy
- Histopathology: edema, noncaseating granuloma, perivascular mononuclear infiltration and fibrosis; intralymphatic and perilymphatic granulomatous infiltrates are very characteristic
- Recurs intermittently and may become a chronic disorder
- Poorly understood etiology and treatment is largely symptomatic including NSAIDs, corticosteroids, antibiotics, and immunosuppressants

COLLAGEN-VASCULAR DISEASES (SEE CHAPTER 22)

Sjögren Syndrome (See Chapter 22)

- Autoimmune condition (SSA [Ro] and SSB [La] antigens) of lacrimal and salivary glands
- Associated with HLA-B8, DR3, DQw2, and DRw52 antigens
- Ocular findings: xerophthalmia, keratoconjunctivitis sicca, punctate keratopathy, uveitis, optic neuritis, scleritis
- One of the few conditions to produce bilateral enlargement of lacrimal (and salivary) glands

Relapsing Polychondritis (See Chapter 22)

- Episodic inflammatory condition involving cartilaginous structures, associated with HLA-DR4
- Inflammation of almost every part of the eye: conjunctivitis, episcleritis, scleritis, uveitis, retinopathy, diplopia, and eyelid swelling, all occur in a relapsing fashion

Polyarteritis Nodosa (PAN) (See Chapter 22)

- Autoimmune condition resulting in necrotizing inflammation of medium- or small-sized arteries
- Ocular findings: interstitial keratitis, scleritis, marginal corneal ulceration, CN palsies, occlusive retinal arteritis, ischemic retinopathy resulting in visual loss

Dermatomyositis (DM) (See Chapter 22)

- Autoimmune disorder resulting in inflammatory myopathy with cutaneous lesions
- Ocular findings: heliotrope rash, most prominent on upper eyelids; rarely, myositis of extraocular muscles resulting in ophthalmoplegia; retinopathy may occur in juvenile dermatomyositis

Wegener Granulomatosis (Fig. 2-20) (See Chapter 22)

- Autoimmune inflammatory process resulting in necrotizing granulomas with localized destruction
- Antineutrophil cytoplasmic antibodies (c-ANCA) directed at neutrophil proteinase 3 (PR-3)

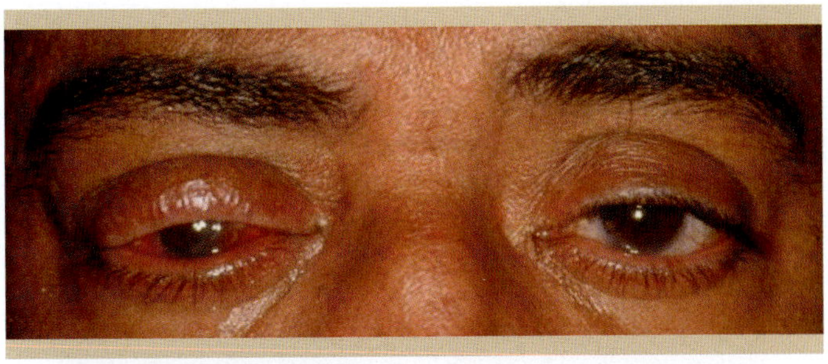

FIGURE 2-20 Wegener granulomatosis with chemosis, scleritis, eyelid inflammation, and bony erosion resulting in "lethal midline granuloma" and saddle-nose deformity (*Used with permission from Dr. Charles S. Soparkar.*)

- Ocular involvement in 29 to 58%; can be localized to the orbit
- Ocular findings: uveitis, nodular scleritis, peripheral keratitis, retinal vasculitis; nasolacrimal duct stenosis; orbital pseudotumor causing refractile proptosis, pain, and loss of vision

BULLOUS DERMATOSES (SEE CHAPTER 10)

Ocular Cicatricial Pemphigoid (OCP) (Fig. 2-21)

- Chronic autoimmune disorder affecting mucous membranes and skin with scarring
- Average age of onset is 65 years; female to male ratio is 2:3

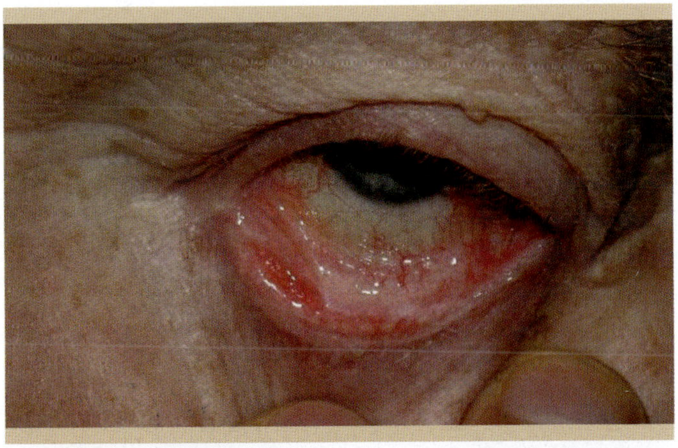

FIGURE 2-21 Ocular cicatricial pemphigoid with chronic cicatricial changes resulting in symblepharon formation and shortening of the fornix. (*Used with permission from Dr. Charles S. Soparkar.*)

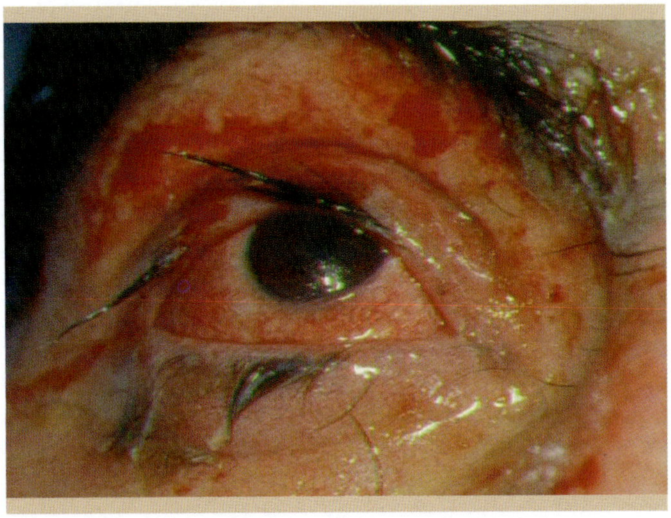

FIGURE 2-22 Stevens-Johnson syndrome in young male with conjunctival and extensive systemic involvement resulting in large areas of denuded skin. (*Used with permission from Dr. Charles S. Soparkar.*)

- Oral cavity is most commonly affected site; ocular involvement is more common in patients with oral involvement (75%) versus skin without oral involvement (25%)
- Autoantibodies directed against epithelial basement membrane; linear pattern of fluorescein staining on immunhistochemical analysis indicates deposition of IgG at this level
- Ocular findings: chronic recurrent conjunctivitis leading to conjunctival shrinkage, symblepharon, and trichiasis

Stevens-Johnson Syndrome (Erythema Multiforme) (Fig. 2-22)

- Complex immunologic syndrome resulting in vasculitis triggered by microbial, neoplastic, or pharmacologic agents
- Other causes: infection, vaccination, systemic diseases, physical agents
- Incidence in HIV patients is 3 times higher than that of the general population
- Ocular findings: conjunctivitis, chemosis, vesicles, bullae, conjunctival membranes, corneal ulceration, subepithelial fibrosis, vascularization, opacification, and rarely, perforation, trichiasis, distichiasis, lagophthalmos
- Characteristic target skin lesions, wheals, bullae, mucosal erosions; tracheal, renal, and CNS involvement with very poor prognosis

Xeroderma Pigmentosum (See Chapter 14) (Fig. 2-23)

- Rare, autosomal recessive disorder due to enzymatic defect in DNA repair (UV light endonuclease)

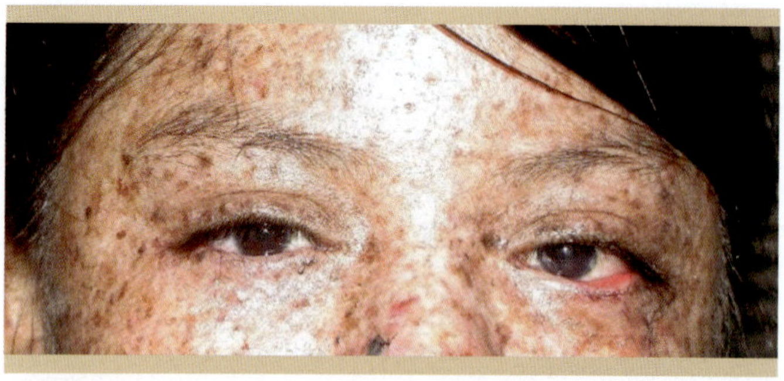

FIGURE 2-23 Xeroderma pigmentosum with corneal opacities and extensive cicatricial skin changes and actinic keratosis in sun-exposed areas. (*Used with permission from Dr. Charles S. Soparkar.*)

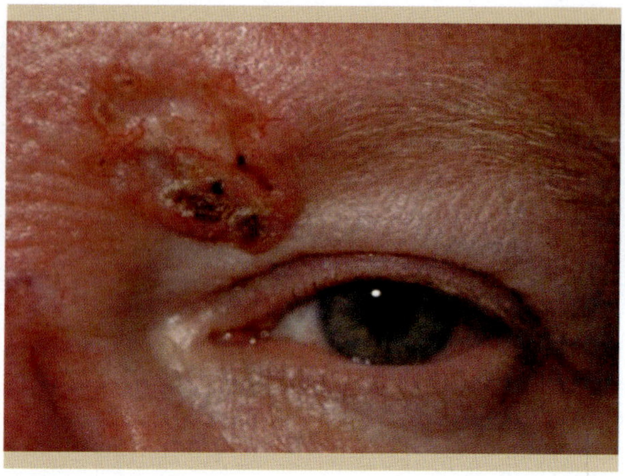

FIGURE 2-24 Basal cell carcinoma of left brow and upper eyelid region. (*Used with permission from Dr. Mirwat S. Sami.*)

- Cellular hypersensitivity to ultraviolet radiation leading to multiple cutaneous malignancies; basal cell carcinoma is most common; also squamous cell carcinoma, mucoepidermoid carcinoma and malignant melanoma
- Ocular findings include thin eyelid skin with photophobia, tearing, dry eyes, cicatricial eyelid changes with resulting ectropion, entropion, and trichiasis
- Also increased incidence of ocular surface tumors like conjunctival and corneal squamous cell carcinoma
- Blistering of skin with sun-exposure, progressing to areas of hypo- or hyperpigmentation, xerosis, and scaling; skin infections can lead to sepsis and death
- Ocular therapy includes sun protection, aggressive lubrication, treatment of infections, and suspicious lesions

EYELID TUMORS

Basal Cell Carcinoma (BCC) (Fig. 2-24) (See Chapter 12)

- Most common epithelial tumor of the eyelid
- Most common location is the lower eyelid (48.9–72.1%)
- Highest recurrence in lesions arising from the medial canthus (60%)
- Nodular BCC most common type

Squamous Cell Carcinoma (SCC) (See Chapter 12)

- Approximately 5% of malignant eyelid tumors
- Incidence of metastasis is 0.23 to 2.4% of cases
- Location of lesion most common on lower eyelid, than lid margin

Sebaceous Cell Carcinoma (Fig. 2-25) (See Chapter 11)

- May arise from meibomian glands (most common), Zeis glands, or glands associated with the caruncle; predilection for the upper lid due to greater number of sebaceous glands
- Can masquerade and be misdiagnosed as recurrent chalazia or chronic blepharitis
- Locally invasive with distant lymphatic and hematogenous spread
- Yellowish, firm, painless, indurated papule, or ulceration with skip areas

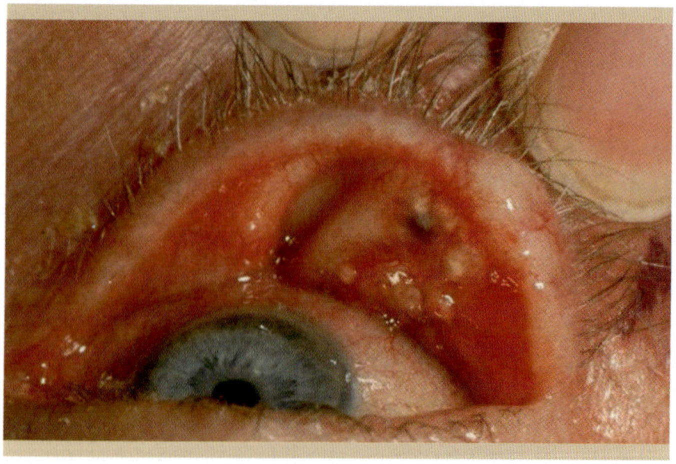

FIGURE 2-25 Sebaceous cell carcinoma of left upper eyelid. (*Used with permission from Dr. Mirwat S. Sami.*)

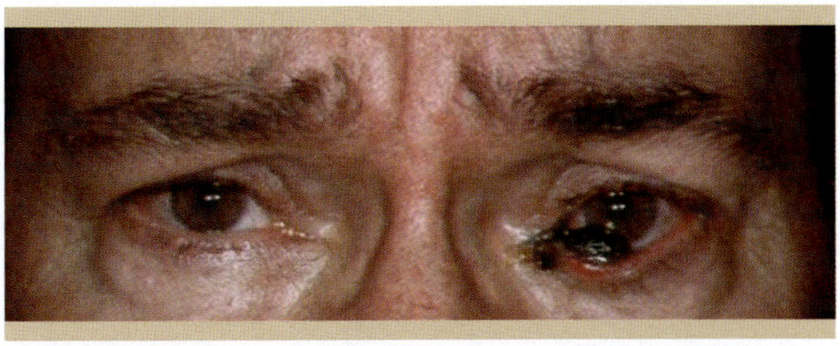

FIGURE 2-26 Malignant melanoma of left lower eyelid with conjunctival extension. (*Used with permission from Dr. Charles S. Soparkar.*)

- Large anaplastic cells with open vesicular nuclei and prominent nuclei set in foamy or frothy cytoplasm, pagetoid spread

Melanoma (Fig. 2-26) (See Chapter 12)

- Rare pigmented eyelid tumor; less than 1% of all eyelid tumors
- Most common melanoma in eyelid is nodular; more aggressive with early vertical invasion
- Change in the appearance of a pigmented lesion warrants excisional biopsy of the lesion

Merkel Cell Carcinoma (Fig. 2-27) (See Chapter 12)

- Rare vascular, violaceous, well-demarcated nodule with little epidermal change

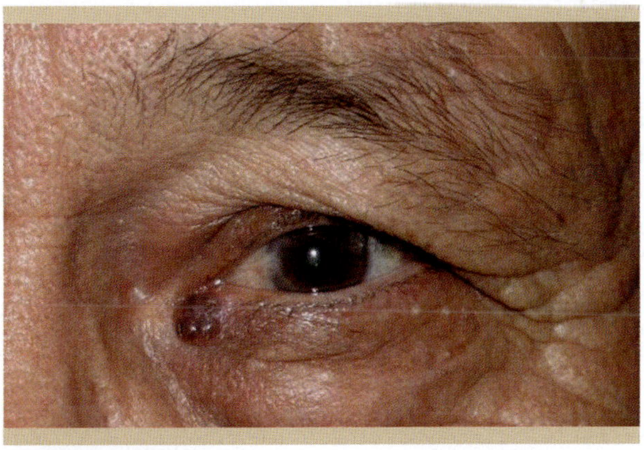

FIGURE 2-27 Merkel cell carcinoma of left lower eyelid and caruncle. (*Used with permission from Dr. Charles S. Soparkar.*)

- Usually occurs in upper eyelid; occurs in elderly
- Rapidly growing tumor with metastasis and death in 30% of patients

METABOLIC DISORDERS (SEE TABLE 2-1) (SEE CHAPTER 23)

Hepatolenticular Degeneration (See Chapter 27)

- Wilson disease; autosomal recessive disorder of copper metabolism
- Ocular findings: Keyser-Fleischer ring, greenish-brown deposits of copper in Descemet membrane of cornea

Homocystinuria (See Chapter 27)

- Autosomal dominant disorder resulting in deficiency of cystathionine-β-synthetase
- Ocular findings: dislocation of crystalline lens (ectopia lentis), myopia, scleral rupture, retinal detachment

Primary Amyloidosis (Myeloma Associated) (See Chapter 27)

- Amyloid protein (AL) derived from immunoglobulin light chains
- Periorbital purpuric plaques ("pinch purpura")
- Amyloid deposition in the corneal stroma, conjunctiva, and eyelid nodules

VIRAL DISEASES (SEE CHAPTER 17)

Varicella and Herpes Zoster Ophthlmicus (See Chapter 17)

- Varicella-zoster virus (VZV): Human herpes virus 3 (HHV3) that causes both varicella (chicken pox) and herpes zoster (shingles). Herpes zoster ophthalmicus occurs later in life; more common in immunosuppressed individuals
- Ophthalmic branch of the trigeminal nerve is commonly involved (Fig. 2-28); nasociliary branch involvement results in conjunctivitis, keratitis, episcleritis, and uveitis
- Hutchinson sign: involvement of nasal tip or nasal sidewall, innervated by branch of nasociliary nerve; signifies ocular involvement
- Prodrome of pain over the affected dermatome. eruption may resent as maculopapular, vesiculopapular, ulcerative, and may form a crust with possible scarring
- Ocular complications such as keratitis and uveitis occur in 50% of patients with cutaneus eruption and appear within 3 weeks of developing rash
- Acute retinal necrosis has been reported following chicken pox and herpes zoster infection in healthy patients
- Anterior uveitis is treated with topical steroids and cycloplegics

TABLE 2-1 Metabolic Disorders

Disease	Inheritance	Gene Defect	Characteristic Ocular Finding
Alkaptonuria	Autosomal recessive	Homogentisic acid oxidase	Blue-black sclerae (Osler sign)
Fabry disease	X-linked recessive	α-galactosidase	Whorled corneal opacities
Wilson disease	Autosomal recessive	Copper transporter ATP7β	Keyser-Fleisher rings
Homocystinuria	Autosomal recessive	Cystathionine-β-synthetase	Downward ectopia lentis
Richner-Hanhart syndrome (Tyrosinemia II)	Autosomal recessive	Hepatic tyrosine aminotransferase	Corneal clouding, pseudoherpetic corneal ulcers
Mucopolysaccharidoses	AR (Hunter XLR)	Varies	Corneal clouding, pigmented retinopathy in some

Herpes Simplex Keratitis (See Chapter 17)

- Primary ocular herpes occurs as a follicular conjunctivitis, regional lymphadenitis, and ulcerative blepharitis
- Recurrent episodes of keratitis are common
- Dendritic corneal ulcers are pathognomonic
- Recurrent stromal keratitis causes structural damage to cornea resulting in corneal opacities often requiring corneal transplant
- Most common cause of corneal blindness in the United States

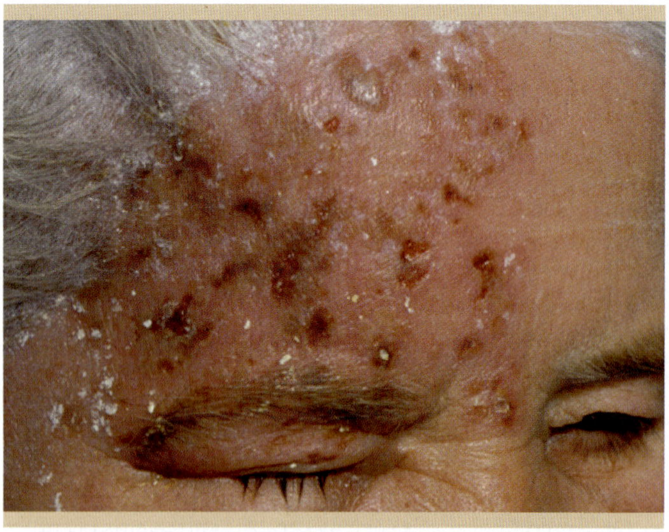

FIGURE 2-28 Herpes zoster ophthalmicus with vesicular eruption in dermatome of ophthalmic branch of trigeminal nerve (cranial nerve V). (*From Wolff K, Johnson RA:* Fitzpatrick's Color Atlas and Synopsis of Clinical Dermatology, *6th Ed. New York*: *McGraw-Hill; 2009, p. 845.*)

Rubella (See Chapter 17)

- When congenital, cataracts, or glaucoma may develop (bilateral in 75% of patients)
- Other ocular findings include salt-and-pepper fundus retinopathy

Measles (Rubeola) (See Chapter 17)

- Conjunctivitis (part of the 3 Cs: cough, coryza, conjunctivitis)
- Koplik spots may be seen on the conjunctiva

Mumps

- Dacryoadenitis (inflammation of lacrimal glands)

BACTERIAL DISEASES (SEE CHAPTER 18)

Cat-Scratch Disease (Oculoglandular Syndrome of Parinaud)

- Due to *Bartonella henselae*; also causes bacillary angiomatosis
- Characterized by malaise, fever, painful regional lymphadenopathy
- Ocular findings: conjunctival hyperemia, anterior uveitis, retinal granulomas, optic nerve edema followed by pallor (neuroretinitis)
- Generally good visual prognosis unless significant neuroretinitis
- Unilateral granulomatous conjunctivitis

Syphilis (See Chapter 18)

- Caused by the spirochete *Treponema pallidum*
- Congenital syphilis: interstitial keratitis
- Secondary syphilis: anterior uveitis

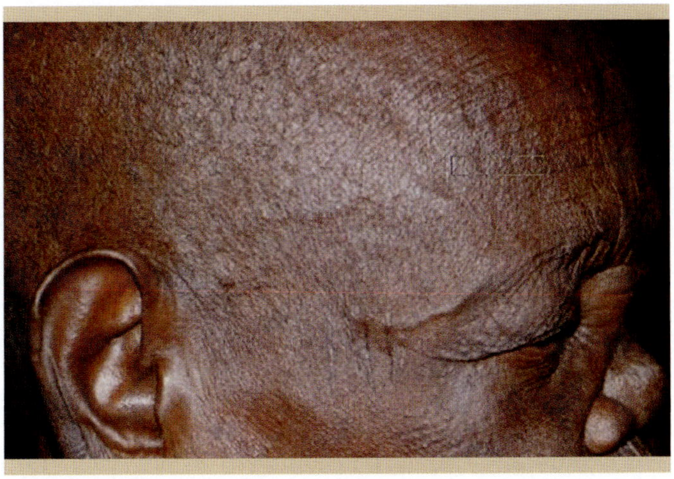

FIGURE 2-29 Lepromatous leprosy with diffuse dermal infiltration, madarosis, leonine facies, and saddle-nose deformity. (*Used with permission from Dr. Charles S. Soparkar.*)

- Neurosyphilis: Argyll Robertson pupil: small, irregular pupil that reacts normally to accommodation but not to light

Miliary Tuberculosis (See Chapter 18)

- Caused by *Mycobacterium tuberculosis*
- Can cause choroidal tubercles in the retina (discrete yellow nodules)

Leprosy (Fig. 2-29) (See Chapter 18)

- Caused by *Mycobacterium leprae*
- Twenty to fifty percent of leprosy patients with ocular involvement (mostly patients with lepromatous leprosy); if left untreated, leads to blindness
- Ocular findings: loss of eyebrows (71%), diminished sensitivity of cornea (63%), lagophthalmos (inability to close the eye, more common in tuberculoid leprosy) (44%), and madarosis (41%)

Lyme Disease (See Chapter 18)

- Systemic infection caused by spirochete *Borrelia burgdorferi,* transmitted by the bite of an infected *Ixodes* tick
- Stage 1: conjunctivitis and photophobia
- Stage 2: CN VII palsy (Bell palsy), blurred vision due to papilledema, optic atrophy, optic or retrobulbar neuritis, or pseudotumor cerebri
- Stage 2 or stage 3: episcleritis, symblepharon, keratitis, iritis, pars planitis, vitreitis, chorioretinitis, exudative retinal detachment, retinal pigment epithelial detachment, cystoid macular edema, and branch artery occlusion

Actinomyces (See Chapter 18)

- *Actinomyces israelii* is a gram-positive anaerobic bacillus; found in soil, brackish water
- In the United States, keratitis associated with contact lens use, especially when tap water is used to cleanse lenses; can also cause conjunctivitis and blepharitis
- Can cause canaliculitis (infectious inflammation of proximal tear drainage system); pathognomonic findings include stone formation and sulfur granules

FUNGAL DISEASES (SEE CHAPTER 19)

Candidiasis

- Occurs in debilitated, immunocompromised patients on hyperalimentation and in IV drug abusers
- Systemic candidiasis carries a 30% risk of ocular involvement
- Ocular findings: anterior uveitis, chorioretinitis with fluffy white lesions in the vitreous ("string of pearls") signifying necrotizing granulomatous vitreoretinitis, retinal infiltrates, and hemorrhages
- Treatment is systemic antifungal treatment, typically amphotericin B; surgical interventions, including intravitreal antifungal placement and vitrectomy to debulk infection and membranes, are considered in patients not responding to maximal medical management

Mucormycosis

- Most common and virulent fungal orbital disease
- Occurs in immunocompromised patients, especially poorly controlled diabetics
- Mucorales order of phycomycetes includes *Rhizopus, Mucor, Absidia* species; *Rhizopus* is most commonly identified in these infections, not *Mucor* species
- Direct tissue inoculation or spread from oral, nasal, or sinus infections in immunocompromised patients
- Usually fulminant disease with 50% mortality within 2 weeks, despite treatment
- Display affinity for blood vessels, causing thrombosis, infarction, and necrosis, resulting in typical black eschar visible in nose or mouth
- Ocular findings: rapidly growing orbital mass or proptosis, orbital ischemia with multiple cranial neuropathies, severe pain, decreased vision, corneal anesthesia, retinal vascular occlusions, ophthalmic artery occlusion with blindness
- Treatment includes surgical debridement, antifungals, and control of underlying disease

PHAKOMATOSES (SEE CHAPTER 14)

Ataxia-Telangiectasia (Louis-Bar Syndrome) (See Chapter 14)

- Autosomal recessive, defect in *ATM* gene on 11q22-23
- Telangiectasias of the bulbar conjunctiva (first appear between 2 and 5 years of age and become more pronounced with time)

- Other ocular findings include ocular dysmotility, including inability to initiate voluntary saccades (oculomotor apraxia), impaired convergence and nystagmus
- Visual acuity, pupillary reflex responses, and fundi are normal
- Thymic hypoplasia results in IgA and other immunoglobulin deficiencies leading to recurrent infections and malignancy
- Systemic telangiectasias, dysarthria, skin lesions, growth, and mental retardation

Sturge-Weber Syndrome (Encephalofacial Angiomatosis) (See Chapter 13)

- Nonhereditary condition characterized by facial angiomatous malformations known as "nevus flammeus" or port-wine stain found in the first 2 divisions of trigeminal nerve
- Usually unilateral and present at birth, darkens with age and becomes nodular
- Ocular findings: conjunctival and episcleral hemangiomas, ipsilateral iris hyperchromia with prominent iris processes, choroidal hemangiomas resulting in exudative retinal detachment
- Ipsilateral glaucoma develops in 30% of patients, usually before 2 years of age, due to iris neovascularization, immature angle structures, or increased episcleral venous pressure
- Klippel-Trenaunay-Weber: variant of Sturge-Weber with nevus flammeus, intracranial hemangiomas, cerebral calcification, hemiparesis, seizures, mental deficiency, and soft tissue and skeletal hemihypertrophy

Tuberous Sclerosis (Bourneville Disease) (See Chapter 14)

- Autosomal dominant or sporadic (66%), mapped to chromosome 9q34 (hamartin) and 16p13 (tuberin)
- Typical triad of adenoma sebaceum, mental retardation, and epilepsy, usually during the first 3 years of life; associated with early mortality
- Ocular findings: astrocytic hamartomas of the retina and optic nerve; mulberry shaped with calcifications
- Cutaneous findings of facial angiofibroma, ash-leaf spots, shagreen patches, periungual fibromas, may have café au lait spots
- CNS findings of subependymal hamartomas, cerebral calcifications, intracranial hamartomas, seizures, and mental retardation
- Other findings include cardiac rhabdomyomas, renal angiomyolipoma, cystic bone lesions, and parenchymal pulmonary cysts that spontaneously rupture causing pneumothorax

Neurofibromatosis (See Chapter 14)

- Autosomal dominant disorder with variable expressivity
- Disorder of Schwann cells and melanocytes with hamartomas of eye, skin, and CNS

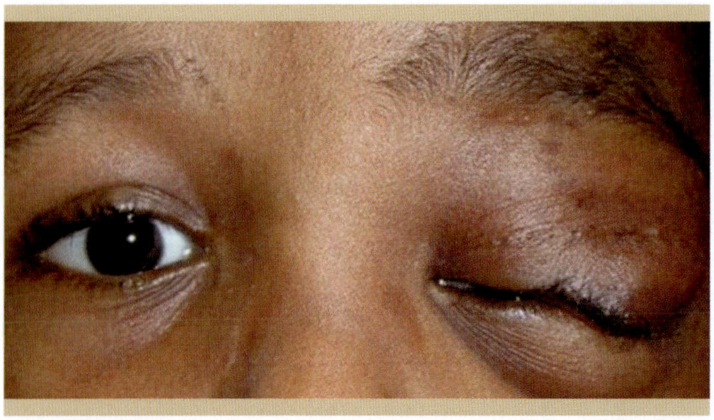

FIGURE 2-30 Neurofibromatosis I with plexiform neurofibromas of left upper and lower eyelid resulting in blepharoptosis. (*Used with permission from Dr. Mirwat S. Sami.*)

- Two types:
  - NF-1 (von Recklinghausen syndrome) (Fig. 2-30)
    - mapped to chromosome 17q11; 50% are sporadic
    - more common form
    - café au lait spots, neurofibromas, plexiform neurofibromas, intertriginous freckling, optic nerve glioma, iris Lisch nodules, osseous lesions (sphenoid bone dysplasia, thinning of long bone cortex)
    - Plexiform neurofibromas found in the upper eyelids result in typical S-shaped ptosis; feel like "bag of worms"; also ipsilateral glaucoma
    - Also retinal astrocytic hamartoma, choroidal nevus, ectropion uveae
    - Absence or dyplastic sphenoid wing results in pulsating exophthalmos
  - **NF-2**
    - Mapped to chromosome 22q; less common
    - Bilateral cerebellar-pontine angle tumors such as acoustic neuromas resulting in hearing loss, ataxia, headaches in second to third decade
    - Also posterior subcapsular cataract, ocular dysmotility, meningioma, schwannoma, neurofibroma, pheochromocytoma
    - No Lisch nodules

Angiomatosis Retinae (von-Hippel–Lindau Syndrome) (See Chapter 14)

- Autosomal dominant with incomplete penetrance; mapped to VHL gene on chromosome 3
- Congenital hamartomas of eye, brain (cerebellum), and kidney/adrenal gland
- Von Hippel disease: only ocular involvement
- Ocular findings: retinal hemangioblastomas characterized by typical appearance of orange-red mass fed by dilated

tortuous retinal artery and drained by engorged vein; leak heavily resulting in serous retinal detachments and edema
- Retinal angiomas have a poor prognosis unless treated with laser photocoagulation, cryotherapy, irradiation, or vitreous surgery
- Also associated with cerebellar hemangioblastomas and tumors of kidney, pancreas, liver, adrenal glands, including renal cell carcinoma and pheochromocytoma

DERMATOUVEITIDES

Sarcoidosis (See Chapter 8)

- Chronic, idiopathic, multisystem, noncaseating granulomatous inflammation primarily affecting lungs, skin, and eyes
- More common among young African-Americans
- All parts of the eye can be affected, from external to intraocular structures
- Eyelid skin granulomas are typically firm, reddish-brown, waxy nodules; chronic dacryoadenitis (lacrimal gland inflammation) is also common
- Elevated, yellowish conjunctival lesions, mostly in palpebral conjunctiva
- Anterior uveitis is the most common eye finding with mutton-fat keratic precipitates, iris nodules, cataract formation, and glaucoma; usually bilateral
- Posterior segment inflammation results in pars planitis, vitritis, choroidal lesions, retinal periphlebitis described as "candlewax drippings," retinal neovascularization, optic nerve granulomas
- Neurosarcoidosis can also affect cranial nerves III, IV, and VI (oculomotor, trochlear, and abducens nerves) resulting in paresis of extraocular muscles, ocular dysmotility, and thus diplopia and ptosis
- Systemic involvement results in fever, erythema nodosum, hilar lymphadenopathy, arthralgias, hepatosplenomegaly, hypercalcemia, parotid gland infiltration, and facial nerve palsy
- Löfgren syndrome
  - Fever, erythema nodosum, bilateral hilar adenopathy, and arthralgias
  - Associated with anterior uveitis in 6% of patients
- Heerfordt syndrome (uveoparotid fever)
  - Fever, uveitis, which may precede the parotid enlargement, and facial nerve palsy
- Mikulicz syndrome
  - Lacrimal, parotid, submandibular, and sublingual glands affected resulting in sicca syndrome

Behçet Disease

- Chronic recurrent autoimmune condition characterized by multisystemic involvement, resulting in relapsing inflammation and occlusive vasculitis
- Associated with HLA-B51
- Typically seen in young adults, males more than females; more common in Japan and Mediterranean countries
- Characterized by triad of oral ulcers, genital ulcers, and inflammatory eye disease with poor visual outcomes despite treatment
- Ocular findings: nongranulomatous panuveitis (inflammation of all parts of eye), conjunctivitis, episcleritis, keratitis, recurrent vascular occlusion with retinal hemorrhages, exudates, ischemic optic neuropathy; traction RD, glaucoma, cataract
- Systemic features: oral aphthous ulcers, skin lesions, genital ulcers, arthritis, intestinal symptoms, aortitis, CNS symptoms
- Pathology: lymphocytic infiltration and occlusive vasculitis with thrombus formation resulting in tissue destruction
- Diagnosis based on major and/or minor criteria
- Major criteria: recurrent oral aphthous ulcers (at least 3 in a 12-month period), skin lesions (erythema nodosum), genital ulcers, ocular inflammation
- Minor criteria: arthritis, GI findings (intestinal ulcers), migratory thrombophlebitis, CNS involvement (brain stem, spinal cord, peripheral nerves), intersitital lung disease, vascular occlusive, obliterative or aneurysmal disease
- Treatment involves immunosuppressants for eye involvement such as azathioprine or cyclosporine A

Vogt-Koyanagi-Harada Syndrome (See Chapter 9)

- Rare autoimmune disorder characterized by granulomatous inflammatory process targeting melanocytes
- Distribution in all races but more common in Asians, American Indians, and Hispanics, between 30 and 50 years of age; may have female preponderance
- HLA-DR1 and 4
- Characterized by uveitis, encephalitis, skin pigmentary changes, and auditory disturbance
- Harada disease: ocular involvement only
- Prodrome: typically begins with a viral-like prodrome of fever and nausea accompanied by neurologic changes such as meningismus and seizures; soon after, followed by acute granulomatous uveitis with serous retinal detachments
- Chronic stage: sunset fundus (depigmented fundus), Dalen-Fuchs nodules (yellow retinal spots), perilimbal vitiligo (Sugiura sign)
- Recurrent stage: recurrence of anterior uveitis
- Treatment: corticosteroids, immunosuppressive agents

Uveitis Associated With HLA-B27 (See Chapter 22)

- Nongranulomatous acute uveitis is seen with the following HLA-B27–associated conditions:
  - Ankylosing spondylitis
  - Reiter syndrome
  - Psoriatic arthritis
  - Inflammatory bowel disease (IBD)—associated (ulcerative colitis, Crohn disease)

- Conjunctivitis is most common eye finding; uveitis may progress to visual impairment
- Systemic features of the respective disease can be found; interestingly, uveitis does not occur in psoriasis without arthritis

Toxoplasmosis

- Congenital or acquired, due to infection with *Toxoplasma gondii*
- Results in a primary retinal infection with coagulative necrosis and granulomatous uveitis and vitritis
- Most common cause of posterior uveitis; most common cause of pediatric uveitis
- Congenital infection is due to transplacental spread; other findings include stillbirth, mental retardation, seizures, intracranial calcification, hepatosplenomegaly
- Acquired infection presents with flu-like symptoms, rash, and meningoencephalitis
- Diagnosis: ELISA or IFA for *Toxoplasma* IgG or IgM

NUTRITION-RELATED DISORDERS (SEE CHAPTER 20)

Vitamin A Deficiency

- Major role of this vitamin in vision, growth, and immunity
- Ocular findings: night blindness (nyctalopia), dry eyes (xerophthalmia), Bitot spots, corneal thinning, and ulceration (keratomalacia)
- Bitot spots: foamy areas on conjunctiva from accumulation of keratin or bacteria

Vitamin B Deficiency

- Vitamin B_1 (thiamine) deficiency: (also known as Beriberi)
  - Seventy percent have ocular abnormalities: dry eyes, vision loss from optic nerve atrophy
- Vitamin B_2 (riboflavin) deficiency:
  - Ocular findings: seborrheic blepharitis, corneal vascularization, and interstitial keratitis

Vitamin C (Ascorbic Acid) Deficiency

- Ocular features include dry eyes, subconjunctival hemorrhage, and hemorrhage within the optic nerve sheath

QUIZ

Questions

1. Staged treatment for a patient with severe TED is best done in which order?

   A. Decompression, strabismus, lid repair
   B. Strabismus, decompression, lid repair
   C. Lid repair, decompression, strabismus
   D. Decompression, lid repair, strabismus

2. Which of the following is the most common epithelial eyelid tumor?

   A. Basal cell carcinoma
   B. Squamous cell carcinoma
   C. Sebaceous cell carcinoma
   D. Melanoma

3. Which of the following signs is most likely to be present in a patient with TED?

   A. Exophthalmos
   B. Extraocular dysmotility
   C. Eyelid retraction
   D. Optic neuropathy

4. All the following tumors have a significant risk of metastasis except:

   A. Squamous cell carcinoma
   B. Basal cell carcinoma
   C. Sebaceous cell carcinoma
   D. Merkel cell carcinoma

5. Neurofibromatosis I is associated with all the following except:

   A. Café au lait spots
   B. Plexiform neurofibromas
   C. Optic nerve glioma
   D. Adenoma sebaceum

6. Cicatricial ectropion is generally associated with:

   A. Trichiasis
   B. Anterior lamellar shortening
   C. Blepharospasm
   D. Symblepharon

7. Which of the following syndromes is associated with glaucoma

   A. Tuberous sclerosis
   B. CHANDS syndrome
   C. Sturge-Weber syndrome
   D. Albinism

8. All the following can be found in Vogt-Koyanagi Harada syndrome except:

   A. Auditory disturbance
   B. Meningismus
   C. Sunset fundus
   D. Arthritis

9. What is the causative organism of Oculoglandular disease of Parinaud?

   A. *Phthirus pubis*
   B. *Bartonella henselae*
   C. *Mycobacterium avium intracellulare*
   D. *Demodex*

10. What is the most common causative organism of canaliculitis?

    A. *Staphylococcus aureus*
    B. *Neisseria gonorrhea*
    C. *Actinomyces israelii*
    D. *Hemophilus influenza*

Answers

1. A. Decompression, strabismus, lid repair.
2. A. Basal cell carcinoma.
3. C. Eyelid retraction.
4. B. Basal cell carcinoma.
5. D. Adenoma sebaceum is associated with tuberous sclerosis and not with neurofibromatosis I.
6. B. Anterior lamellar shortening. All the other options will cause entropion.
7. C. Sturge-Weber syndrome.
8. D. Arthritis.
9. B. *Bartonella henselae.*
10. C. *Actinomyces israelii.*

REFERENCES

American Academy of Ophthalmology: *Orbit, Eyelids and Lacrimal System*, vol 7. San Francisco: AAO; 2004.

Colombo F, Holbach LM, Junemann AGM, Schlotzer-Schrehardt U, Naumann GOH: Merkel cell carcinoma: clinicopathologic correlation, management, and follow-up in five patients. *Ophthal Plast Reconstr Surg* 2000;16(6):453–458.

Dutton JS: *Atlas of Clinical and Surgical Orbital Anatomy*. Philadelphia: WB Saunders; 1994.

Foster CS, Vitale AT: *Diagnosis and Treatment of Uveitis*. Philadelphia: WB Saunders; 2002.

Gold DH, Lewis RA: *Clinical Eye Atlas*. AMA Press; 2002

Goldsmith LA, Katz SI, Gilchrest BA, Paller AS, Leffell DJ, Wolff K: *Fitzpatrick's Dermatology in General Medicine*, 8th Ed. New York: McGraw-Hill; 2012.

Kanski JJ: *Clinical Ophthalmology: A Systematic Approach*, 6th Ed. Burlington, Massachusetts: Butterworth-Heinemann; 2007.

Liesegang TJ: Herpes simplex virus epidemiology and ocular importance. *Cornea* 2001;20(1):1–13.

Liesegang TJ: Herpes zoster virus infection. *Curr Opin Ophthalmol* 2004;15(6):531–536.

Mannis M, Macsai M, Huntley A: *Eye and Skin Disease*, 1st Ed. Philadelphia: Lippincott-Raven; 1996.

Mithal S, Pratap VK, Gupta AR: Clinico-histopathological study of the eye in leprosy. *Indian J Ophthalmol* 1988;36(3):135–139.

Riordan-Eva P, Whitcher JP: *Vaughan and Asbury's General Ophthalmology*, 16th Ed. New York: McGraw-Hill; 1999.

Shields JA, Shields CL: *Intraocular Tumors: A Text and Atlas*. Philadelphia: WB Saunders; 1992

Spitz JL: *Genodermatoses: A Clinical Guide to Genetic Skin Disorders*, 2nd Ed. Philadelphia: Lippincott Williams & Wilkins; 2005.

Yanoff M, Fine BS: *Ocular Pathology*, 5th Ed. Philadelphia: Mosby; 2002.

Zvulunov A, Barak Y, Metzker A: Juvenile xanthogranuloma, neurofibromatosis, and juvenile chronic myelogenous leukemia. World statistical analysis. *Arch Dermatol* 1995;131(8):904–908.

CHAPTER 3

NAIL FINDINGS

RAVI UBRIANI

NAIL ANATOMY (FIG. 3-1)

- Nail plate
  - Forms from keratinization of the nail matrix epithelium and is firmly attached to the nail bed
  - Dorsal nail plate is produced by the nail matrix
  - Ventral portion is produced by the nail bed
  - Nail thickness depends on the length of the nail matrix and nail bed
  - Pink color owing to underlying nail bed blood vessels
  - Onychocorneal band: most distal portion of firm attachment of the nail plate to the nail bed
  - Onychodermal band: pink band that lies between the onychocorneal band and the nail plate white free edge
- Proximal nail fold
  - Dorsal portion: thinner than skin of the digit, devoid of pilosebaceous units
  - Ventral portion: in continuity with the matrix, adheres to the nail plate surface, and keratinizes with a granular layer
  - Horny layer forms the cuticle and prevents the separation of the plate from the nail fold
  - Dermis contains numerous capillaries that run parallel to the surface of the skin; morphology can be altered in connective tissue diseases
- Nail matrix
  - Lies above the midportion of the distal phalanx
  - Keratinization of the proximal nail matrix cells produces the dorsal nail plate
  - Keratinization of the distal nail matrix cells produces the ventral nail plate
  - Lunula: where the distal matrix is not completely covered by the proximal nail fold but is visible through the normal nail plate as a white half-moon-shaped area
  - Cells are able to synthesize both "soft," or skin-type, and "hard," or hair-type, keratins—the matrix expresses keratins Ha1, K1, K10
  - Alteration in the color of lunula can be an indication of either a cutaneous or systemic disorder or a systemic drug side effect
- Nail bed
  - Extends from the distal margin of the lunula to the onychodermal band
  - Completely visible through the nail plate
  - Epithelium is adherent to the nail plate, 2 to 5 cell layers
  - Nail bed keratinization produces a thin horny layer that attaches to the ventral nail plate
  - The bed expresses keratins K6, K16, K17
  - No granular layer is present
- Hyponychium
  - Anatomic area between the nail bed and the distal groove, where the nail plate detaches from the dorsal digit
- Dermis
  - No subcutaneous tissue, no pilosebaceous units
  - Condensed connective tissue that forms a tendon-like structure connecting the matrix to the periosteum of the phalangeal bone
- Blood and nerve supply
  - Blood supply provided by the lateral digital arteries, arches supply the matrix and nail bed
  - Sensory nerves: originate from the dorsal branches of the paired digital nerves, run parallel to the digital vessels
- Nail growth
  - Fingernails: 3 mm/mo, 0.1 mm/d, take 5 to 6 months to regrow
  - Toenails: 1 mm/mo, 0.03 mm/d, take 12 to 18 months to regrow
  - After nail plate is avulsed, it takes 40 days before new fingernail will first emerge

NAIL DISORDERS

Chromonychia

- Abnormality in color of the substance and/or the surface of the nail plate and/or subungual tissue
- Systemic cause: all digits are usually involved
- Endogenous cause: edge of color corresponds to shape of lunula (concave)
- External contact: edge of color follows the shape of the proximal nail fold (convex)

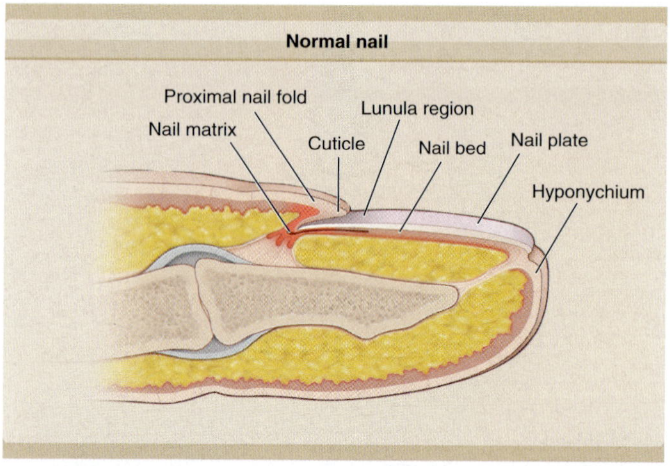

FIGURE 3-1 Drawing of a normal nail. (*Redrawn from De Berker D et al:* Keratin expression in the normal nail unit: Markers of regional differentiation. *Br J Dermatol. 2000;142:89.*)

1. Blue lunula
   - Causes of this condition include the following:
     - Wilson disease
     - Argyria, silver nitrate
     - Drugs: azidothymidine (AZT), quinacrine, busulfan, phenolphthalein
2. Red lunula (Fig. 3-2)
   - Causes of this condition include the following:
     - Cardiac failure

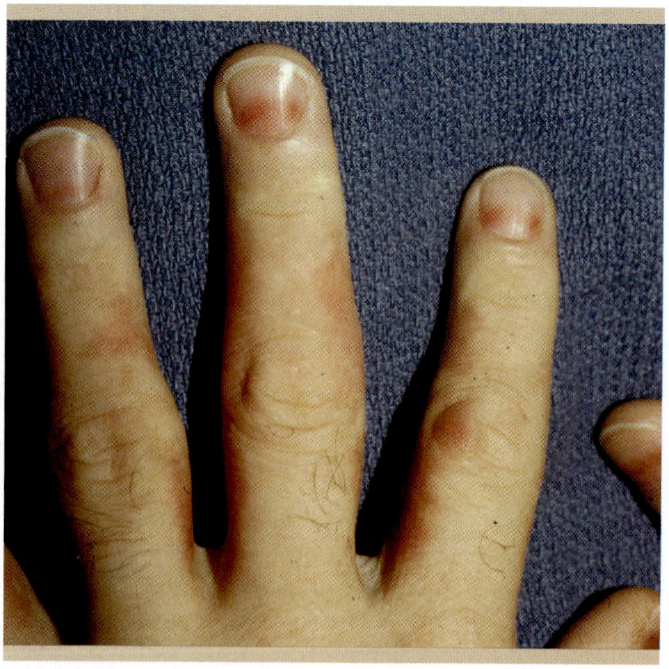

FIGURE 3-2 Red lunulae. (*Used with permission from Dr. Adelaide Hebert.*)

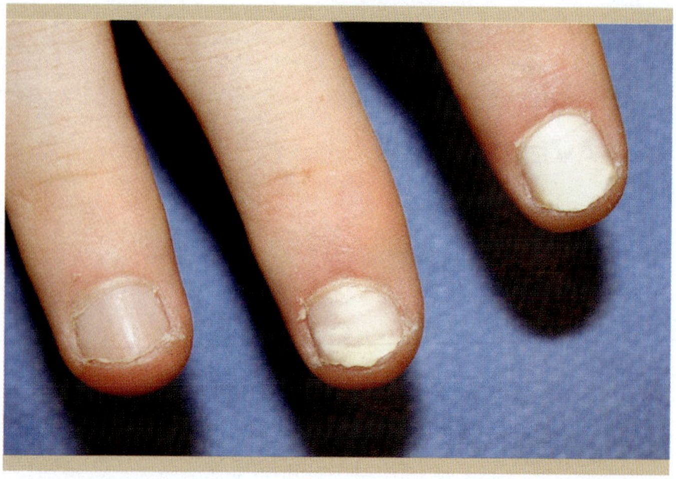

FIGURE 3-3 Leukonychia. (*Used with permission from Dr. Ravi Ubriani.*)

     - Rheumatoid arthritis
     - Alopecia areata
     - Lupus
     - Polycythemia vera
     - Carbon monoxide poisoning
3. Leukonychia (Fig. 3-3)
   - Can be caused by defective keratinization of the distal matrix with persistent parakeratosis in the ventral nail plate
   - White color of nail in 5 patterns: total leukonychia (inherited usually), distal portion still appears pink, transverse leukonychia (systemic disorder), punctate (from minor trauma), longitudinal (associated with Darier disease)
   - One hereditary form is autosomal dominant and may be associated with epithelial cysts and renal calculi. There are also reported families with leukonychia and acquired sensorineural deafness
4. Longitudinal melanonychia (Fig. 3-4)
   - Presence of a pigmented stripe, usually brown or black
   - Deposition of melanin in the nail plate from a variety of causes
     - Melanotic macule is the most common cause
     - Bands of nevocellular nevi
     - Nevi, pigmented fungal infections, or melanoma
     - Drugs
   - Azidothymidine (AZT): develops between 8 weeks to 1 year
   - Antimalarials
   - Laugier-Hunziker syndrome (findings include longitudinal melanonychia, and macular pigmentation of the lips, mouth, and anogenital area)
   - Trauma
   - Pregnancy
   - Radiation induced

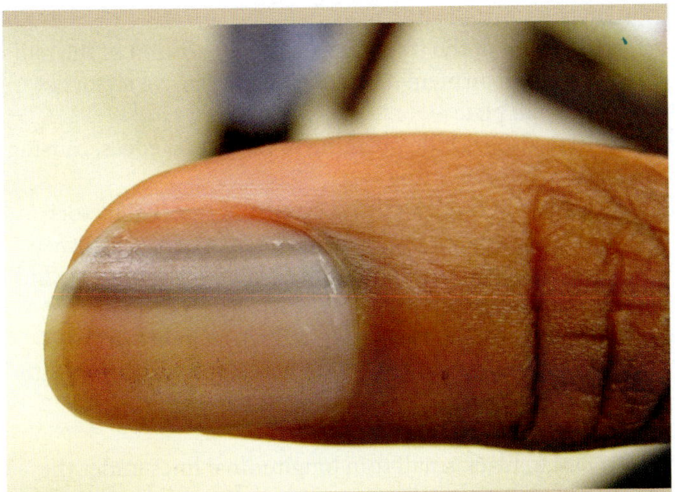

FIGURE 3-4 Longitudinal melanonychia. (*Used with permission from Dr. Ravi Ubriani.*)

- Inflammatory nail disorders (lichen planus, onychomycosis, chronic radiation dermatitis, pustular psoriasis, or Hallopeau disease)
- Systemic diseases: acquired immune deficiency syndrome (pigmentation unrelated to AZT treatment), Addison disease, Cushing syndrome, hyperthyroidism, hemosiderosis, hyperbilirubinemia, alkaptonuria, systemic lupus erythematosus, scleroderma, and porphyria
- Nutritional disorders
  - Vitamin B_{12} or folate deficiency
  - Bluish-black pigmentation
  - Pigmentation is completely reversible after correction of the vitamin deficiency

5. Subungual melanoma
   - Broad band, dark brown to black in color with indistinct lateral borders
   - 0.7 to 3.5% of cutaneous melanomas. Most common type of melanoma in Asian and African-American populations—the rate is the same as in Caucasian populations, but is overrepresented because the frequency of other types of melanoma is low
   - Longitudinal black or brown bands with different hues
   - Commonly affects thumbs and great toes
   - Hutchinson sign: spread of pigmentation onto the nail folds
   - Pigmentation in a single digit, especially the index finger, thumb, or great toe
   - Usually occurs at age 50 or older
6. Subungual hemorrhage (Fig. 3-5)
   - Reddish to reddish-black pigment depending on the age of the bleed
   - Progressively grows out distally as the nail plate grows
   - Can be due to trauma

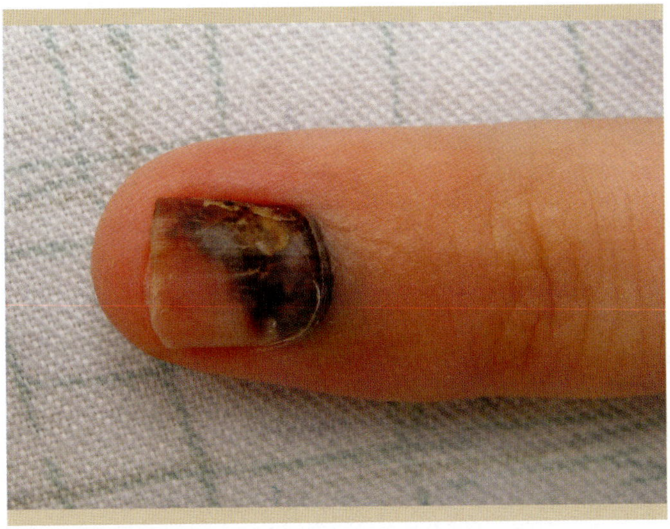

FIGURE 3-5 Subungual hemorrhage. (*Used with permission from Dr. Ravi Ubriani.*)

   - Nail tumors can be preceded by or first recognized after trauma and may bleed
   - May need to be biopsied to rule out subungual melanoma if hemorrhage does not grow out with the nail or if it recurs at the same place

External Factors Causing Nail Disorders

1. Habit-tic deformity (Fig. 3-6)
   - Multiple transverse grooves (Christmas-tree pattern) with a central depression
   - Usually affects thumbnails
   - Chronic mechanical injury to the cuticle and underlying matrix
2. Onychogryphosis (Fig. 3-7)
   - Curved, thickened nail plate without attachment to the nail bed

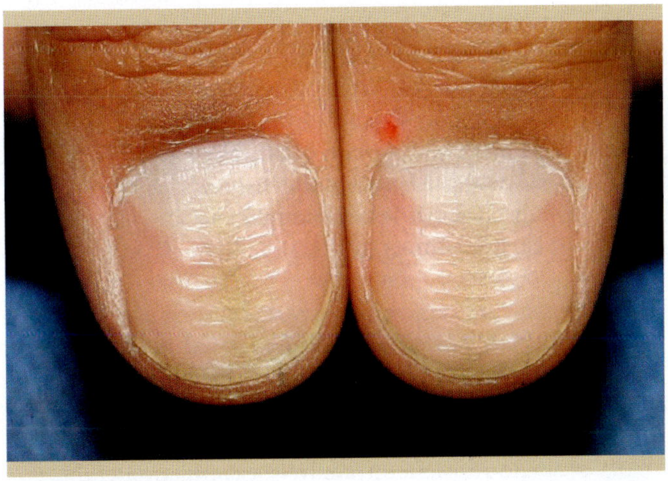

FIGURE 3-6 Habit tic. (*Used with permission from Dr. Ravi Ubriani.*)

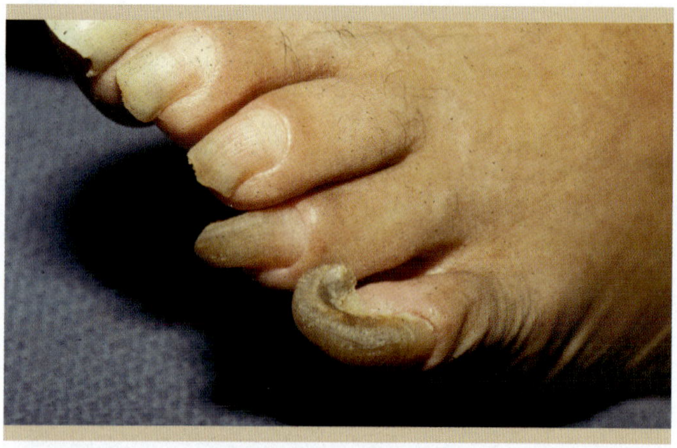

FIGURE 3-7 Onychogryphosis. (*Used with permission from Dr. Richard Krathen.*)

- Opaque, yellow-brown with an oyster shell appearance
- Nail keratin is produced by the nail matrix at uneven rates, with the faster-growing side determining the direction of the deformity
- Ill-fitting footwear, self-neglect, trauma, age, occasionally inherited as an autosomal dominant trait
- Hemionychogryphosis with lateral deviation of the nail plate results from congenital malalignment of the big toenail

3. Onycholysis
   - Separation of the nail plate from the bed
   - Yeast and bacteria usually colonize underlying space
   - Primary causes
     - Trauma
     - Idiopathic
   - Secondary causes
     - Dermatologic and systemic conditions: onychomycosis, diabetes mellitus, thyroid disorders, pregnancy, porphyria, pellagra, scurvy, psoriasis, scleroderma, lupus, hidrotic ectodermal dysplasia, chronic contact dermatitis, pompholyx, herpes simplex, sarcoidosis, amyloidosis
     - Photo-induced onycholysis: tetracyclines (demecycline highest, doxycycline next, minocycline least), psoralens, 8-MOP, fluoroquinolones, chloramphenicol
     - Nail bed tumors
     - Congenital
   - Treatment: Remove underlying cause. If traumatic, emphasize nontraumatic nail practices and reduce wetwork. Concurrent use of topical anti-yeast medications can reduce colonization and hasten reattachment. There is no role for oral antifungals. In cases of single-resistant onycholysis, examination of the underlying nail bed with biopsy may be necessary to rule out underlying malignancy
4. Onychoschizia/brittle nails
   - Splitting of the free edge and distal portion of the nail plate impairment of intercellular adhesive factors of the nail plate
   - May also include breaking of the lateral edges, causing transverse splitting
   - Causes of onychoschizia consist of external factors that dissolve or break the coherence between corneocytes: immersion/desiccation, chemicals, trauma, and fungi
   - Treatment: in some cases, reduction in use of nail cosmetics may be helpful. Oral supplementation with biotin or silicone may be helpful as well
5. Splinter hemorrhages
   - Red to black small thin longitudinal lines under the nail plate
   - Most commonly located in the distal nail plate
   - Disruption of longitudinal blood vessels in the nail bed
   - Caused by injury to the nail (most common cause) or by certain drugs, and/or inflammatory nail disorders
   - Resolves spontaneously
   - Treatment: if no underlying cause, reassurance as to benign nature of condition. Otherwise, treat underlying condition
6. Ingrown nails
   - Great toenails are particularly vulnerable
   - Improper nail trimming, tight shoes, or poor posture can cause a corner of the nail to curve downward into the skin
   - Can lead to inflammation, granulation tissue formation, and infection
   - Treatment: nonsurgical treatments try to separate the lateral nail fold from the nail plate with barriers or by taping the lateral nail fold away from the plate. Surgical treatment includes phenol destruction of the lateral part of the nail plate leading to a narrowed nail. In acute cases, antibiotics and/or drainage of purulent collection may be necessary
7. Transverse overcurvature (pincer or trumpet nail)
   - Nail displays an increase in curvature along the nail bed
   - May be associated with subungual exostosis
   - Overcurvature may extend to the point of encompassing a cone of nail bed soft tissue
   - Treatment: nonsurgical bracing treatments can slowly flatten the nail plate. Surgical treatment includes phenol destruction of the lateral part of the nail plate leading to a narrowed nail. In acute cases, antibiotics and/or drainage of purulent collection may be necessary
8. Chronic paronychia (Fig. 3-8)
   - Inflammation of the proximal nail fold with painful periungual erythema

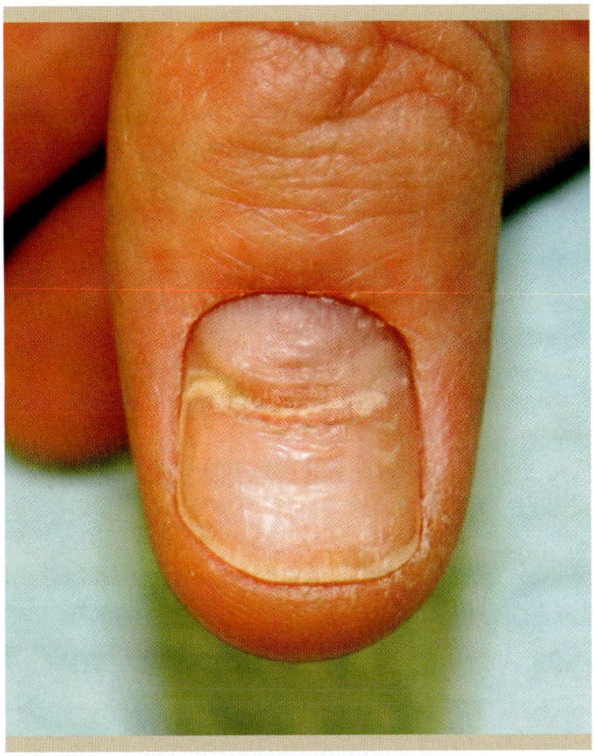

FIGURE 3-8 Chronic paronychia. (*Used with permission from Dr. Ravi Ubriani.*)

- Nail detaches from the distal portion of the proximal nail fold, which has lost its cuticle
- May result in *Candida* invasion with discolored nail plate and cross-ridged lateral edges
- Can be acute or chronic
- Acute: usually caused by infection (see "Infections of the Nails" section below)
- Chronic: Occurs in patients whose hands are subjected to moist local environments or in patients who damage the cuticle through traumatic nail practices. Thought to be an irritant or allergic contact dermatitis of the proximal nail fold due to entry of irritants or allergens under the proximal nail fold after loss of the cuticle
- Can be a side effect of epidermal growth factor receptor inhibitors (Fig. 3-9)
- Treatment: acute cases: (see "Infections of the Nails" below); chronic cases: reduction of wetwork and contact with irritants and discontinuation of traumatic nail practices is necessary. Short-term use of high-potency topical steroids. Topical anti-yeast medications have become less favored, but can be used in addition. Oral antifungal medications should not be used as single therapy, but have not been disproven as adjuncts to above therapy

9. Onychomadesis (nail shedding)
    - Spontaneous separation of the nail plate from the nail bed beginning from the proximal nail end

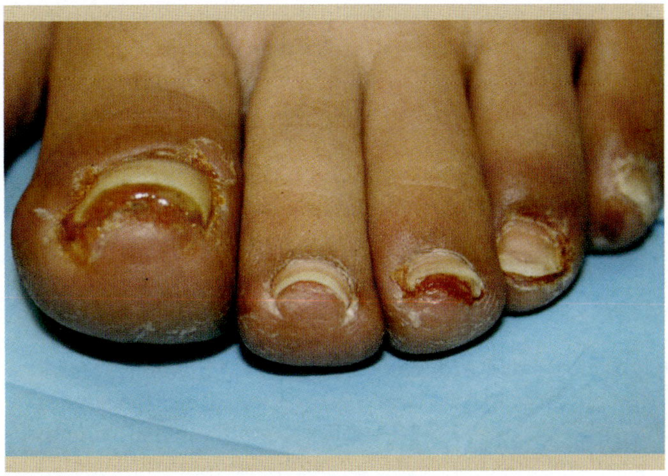

FIGURE 3-9 Epidermal growth factor inhibitor dermatitis. (*Used with permission from Dr. Ravi Ubriani.*)

    - Associated with: systemic lupus erythematosus, pemphigus vulgaris, mycosis fungoides, alopecia areata universalis, epidermolysis bullosa, keratosis punctata palmaris et plantaris, thrombocytopenia, neurologic disease, peritoneal dialysis, penicillin anaphylaxis, chemotherapy, retinoids (dose-related nail matrix damage), lead intoxication, and carbamazepine
    - When associated with systemic illness, generalized skin disease, or drug therapy, the condition may be considered a severe form of Beau lines. (Temporary slowing or cessation of nail plate production)
    - Nail plate shows a transverse split but continues growing for some time
    - Eventually the nail is cast off after losing the connection to the underlying nail bed
    - Treatment: reassurance as to eventual resolution if related to a one-time event. Treat underlying cause if still active or related to an underlying disease

10. Allergic contact dermatitis (Fig. 3-10)
    - Fingertip, nail bed, and nail fold dermatitis, paronychia, onycholysis, and nail dystrophy
    - Usually caused by acrylates used in false nails and nail glues
    - Treatment: confirm diagnosis by patch testing if in doubt. High-potency topical steroids for control of dermatitis. Complete avoidance of acrylic nails and nail glues should alleviate the problem, but underlying issues that prompted use of artificial nails will remain.

Genetic Syndromes

1. Keratosis follicularis (Darier disease) (Fig. 3-11)
    - Autosomal dominant
    - Defect in ATPase 2A2, which encodes sarco (endo)plasmic reticulum Ca^{2+}-ATPase (SERCA2), a calcium pump

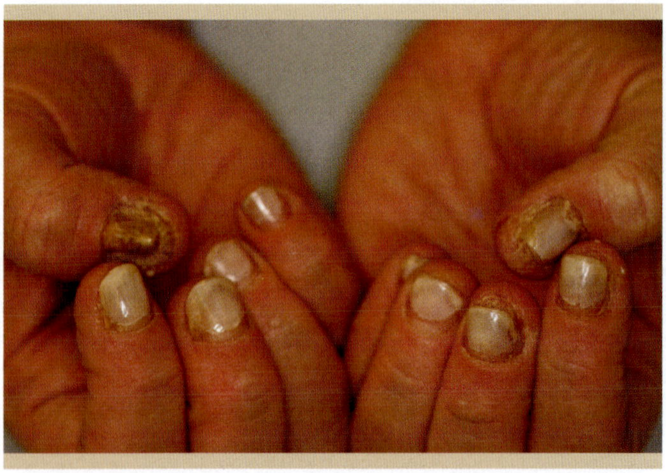

FIGURE 3-10 Allergic contact dermatitis to acrylic nails. (*Used with permission from Dr. Ravi Ubriani.*)

- Nails: red and white longitudinal streaks, wedge-shaped nicking of the distal nail plate, subungual hyperkeratosis
- May be related to acrokeratosis verruciformis of Hopf (acral Darier disease): multiple warty lesions resembling plane warts typically observed on the dorsum of the hands and feet

2. Nail-patella syndrome
   - Also known as HOOD or Fong syndrome
   - Autosomal dominant
   - Defect in *LMX1B* gene
   - Nails: triangular lunula, hypoplasia of nails, may involve all fingernails (thumbs are the most severely affected)
   - Hypoplastic or absent patella, bilateral posterior iliac horns, radial head subluxation, scoliosis, palmoplantar hyperhidrosis
   - Glomerulonephritis ± renal failure
   - Eyes: heterochromic irides, Lester iris, cataract
3. Dyskeratosis congenita
   - X-linked form associated with *DKC1* gene, located at Xq28, encodes for *dyskerin* protein (essential in ribosome biogenesis and telomerase assembly)
   - Autosomal dominant form associated with *hTERC* gene
   - Classical tetrad of progressive bone marrow failure, reticulated skin hyperpigmentation, nail dystrophy, and oral leukoplakia
   - Nails: ridging, longitudinal fissuring, thin and dystrophic—first component of syndrome to appear
4. Congenital malalignment
   - Lateral deviation of the long axis of nail growth relative to the distal phalanx
   - Subsequent ingrowing and possible hemionychogryphosis if untreated
   - Acquired traumatic malposition may follow acute trauma
5. Hereditary ectodermal dysplasia
   - Primary epidermal disorders in which one of the following signs occur: hypotrichosis, hypodontia, onychodysplasia, and anhidrosis
   - Nails are most commonly short, thickened, and hypoplastic
6. Epidermolysis bullosa (EB)
   - Junctional and dystrophic forms may produce anonychia
   - Abnormalities of the nail matrix and nail bed associated with the pathologic genetic alterations of the dermal-epidermal junction
7. Pachyonychia congenita (PC) (Fig. 3-12)
   - Autosomal dominant
   - Nail changes: severe nail thickening, yellow-gray color, transversely overcurved with subungual hyperkeratosis mainly at the distal portion of the nails

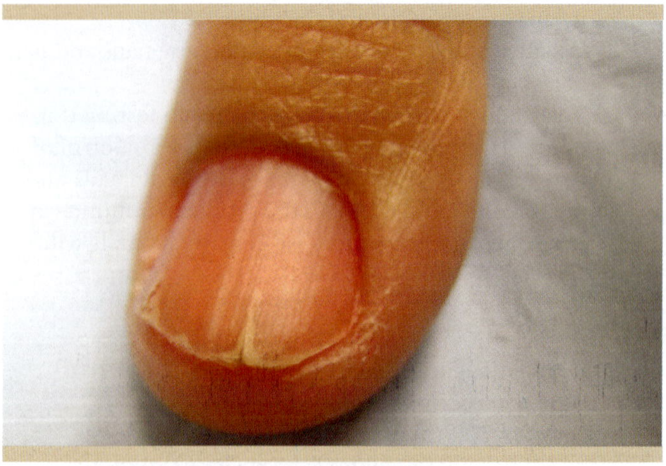

FIGURE 3-11 Darier nail. (*Used with permission from Dr. Adelaide Hebert.*)

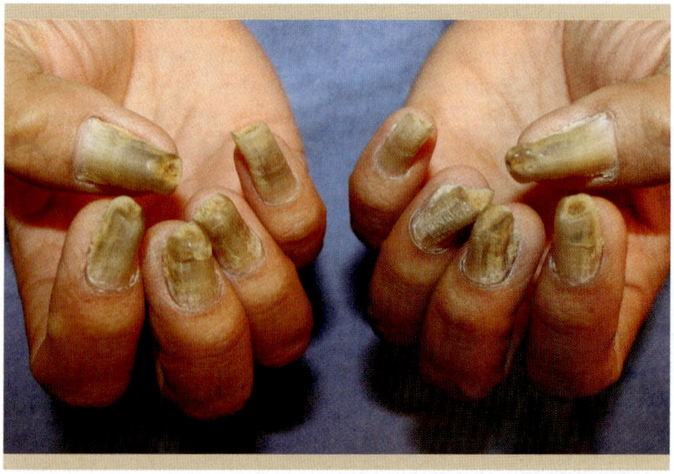

FIGURE 3-12 Pachyonychia congenita. (*Used with permission from Dr. Ravi Ubriani.*)

- Two main clinical subtypes, PC-1 and PC-2, and other rare variants:
  - Type I PC: Jadassohn-Lewandowsky (more common)
    - ▲ Keratins 6A and 16 defects
    - ▲ Palmoplantar and follicular hyperkeratosis, benign oral leukoplakia
  - Type II PC: Jackson-Lawler
    - ▲ Keratins 6B and K17 defects
    - ▲ Type I PC symptoms plus bullae on palms and soles, early dentition/natal teeth, steatocystoma multiplex
  - Type III: Schafer-Branauer
    - ▲ Type I symptoms plus corneal dystrophy, cataracts
  - Type IV: pachyonychia congenita tarda
    - ▲ Late onset, hyperpigmentation around the neck, waist, and flexures

8. Coffin-Siris syndrome
   - Rare, clinically heterogenous disorder associated with developmental delay, hirsutism, and coarse facial features
   - Nail changes: hypoplastic fifth fingernails or toenails

Infections of the Nails

1. Onychomycosis (Fig. 3-13)
   - Clinical features depend on type of infection present
     - Distal subungual onychomycosis: *Trichophyton rubrum*, *Trichophyton interdigitale*
       - ▲ Distal onycholysis with subungual hyperkeratosis and yellow discoloration
     - Proximal subungual onychomycosis: *T. rubrum*, *Fusarium* sp., *Aspergillus* sp., *Scopulariiopsis* sp.
       - ▲ Proximal leukonychia with normal nail plate surface
       - ▲ Associated with AIDS
     - Superficial white onychomycosis: *T. interdigitale*, *Fusarium* sp., *Aspergillus* sp.
       - ▲ Superficial areas of friable opaque leukonychia
       - ▲ More common in children and HIV-positive individuals

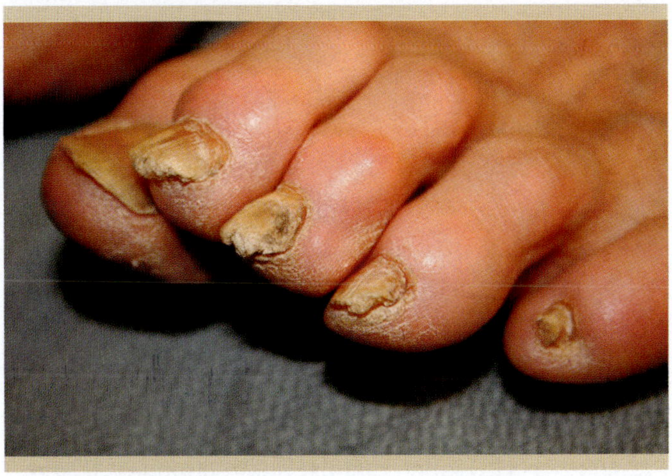

FIGURE 3-13 Onychomycosis. (*Used with permission from Dr. Ravi Ubriani.*)

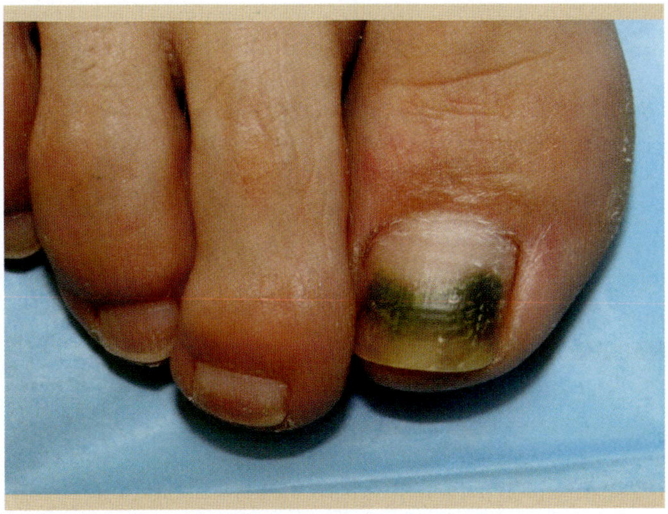

FIGURE 3-14 *Pseudomonas* nail. (*Used with permission from Dr. Ravi Ubriani.*)

   - Treatment: oral antifungals or topical antifungal nail lacquer should be used if no contraindications with appropriate laboratory monitoring

2. Green nails (*Pseudomonas* nail infection) (Fig. 3-14)
   - *Pseudomonas aeruginosa* (gram-negative bacteria) can infect the dorsal or ventral nail plate of the nail
   - Presents with green (pyocyanin) or yellow (fluorescein) nail pigmentation
   - Can happen more frequently to patients with underlying onycholysis or onychomycosis
   - Treatment: topical vinegar soaks, floxacin, or gentamicin can be used to treat the infection. Treat underlying condition if onycholysis or onychomycosis is present
3. Acute paronychia (Fig. 3-15)
   - Associated with direct or indirect trauma to the cuticle or nail fold

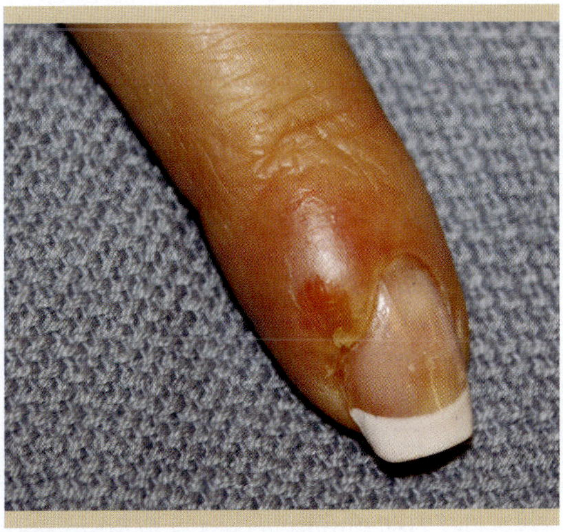

FIGURE 3-15 Acute paronychia. (*Used with permission from Dr. Ravi Ubriani.*)

- May start in the paronychium (lateral nail fold) at the side of the nail with local redness, swelling, and pain
- Most common causative pathogen is *Staphylococcus aureus*, less commonly *Streptococcus pyogenes*, *Pseudomonas pyocyanea*, *Proteus vulgaris*, or herpes simplex virus
- Treatment: incision and drainage with culture and appropriate antibiotics for staph and strep infection. Consideration should be given to diagnostic procedures for HSV as acute paronychia can be caused by HSV

Nail Signs of Systemic Disease

1. Nail pitting
   - Depressions in the nail plate that vary in morphology and distribution
   - Characteristic of psoriasis, alopecia areata, and eczema
   - Easily detachable parakeratotic cells in the superficial layers of the nail plate, as the nail plate grows outward, these parakeratotic foci are exposed to the surrounding environment and there is a gradual sloughing of these cells, leaving a distinct depression within the nail plate
   - Indicates a disturbance in the maturation and keratinization of the proximal nail matrix
   - Alopecia areata (Fig. 3-16)
     - Nail findings are seen in 20% of adults and 50% of children
     - Geometric nail pitting (most common); pits are small and regularly distributed along longitudinal and transverse lines
     - Twenty-nail dystrophy or trachyonychia (generalized nail roughness) seen mainly in patients with alopecia totalis or alopecia universalis
   - Psoriasis
     - Deep and irregularly distributed pits
   - Atopic dermatitis
     - Deep and irregularly distributed pits
   - Treatment: topical psoriasis medications applied to the proximal nail fold or injection of steroid into the proximal matrix may be helpful, but side effects may limit use to only the most motivated patients
2. Koilonychia
   - Nail plate is concave with raised edges (spoon nails)
   - Iron-deficiency anemia associated with Plummer-Vinson syndrome
   - Normal finding in childhood
   - Can be seen in patients with Mal de Meleda (keratoderma palmoplantaris transgrediens): painful glove-and-stocking keratoderma, psoriasiform hyperkeratotic plaques, koilonychia, onychogryphosis, and fissured tongue/lingua plicata
3. Lichen planus
   - Affects one or more nails in 10% of cases
   - Acute nail changes: ridging, distal splitting, thinning, subungual hyperkeratosis (Fig. 3-17)
   - Late nail changes: pterygium formation (adhesion of the proximal nail fold to the proximal nail bed) and loss of nail. These changes are permanent once they occur. (Fig. 3-18)
   - Treatment: injections of steroid or systemic prednisone may be necessary to prevent development of pterygium, but side effects must be balanced on an individual basis
   - Histology mirrors that of lichen planus in the skin, demonstrating a lichenoid infiltrate with apoptosis of keratinocytes. Spongiosis, focal parakeratosis, and scarring are more common in lichen planus of the nails

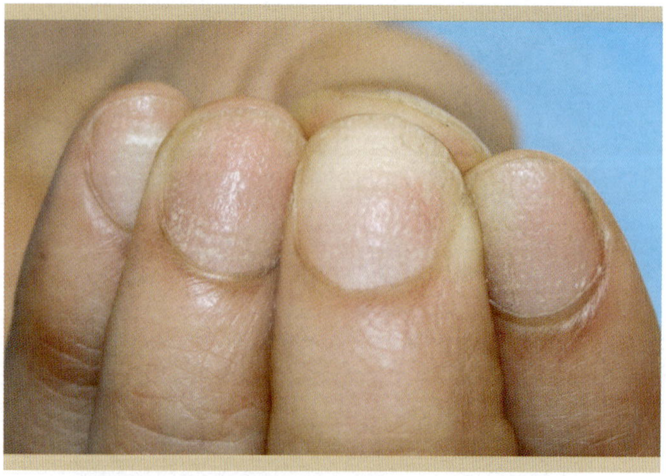

FIGURE 3-16 Nail pitting. (*Used with permission from Dr. Ravi Ubriani.*)

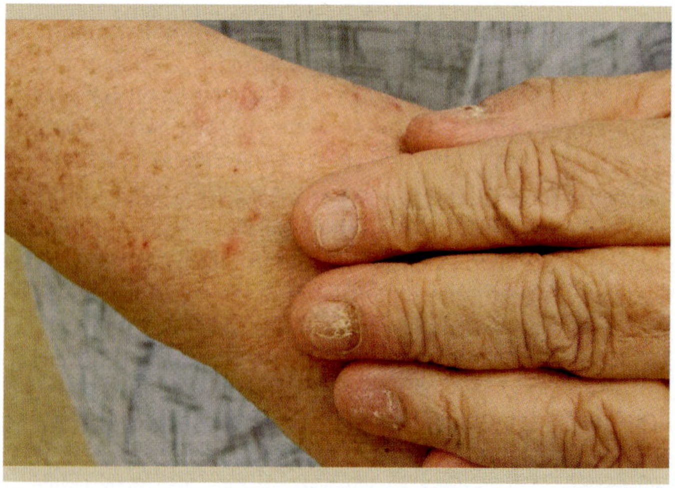

FIGURE 3-17 Lichen planus, acute changes. (*Used with permission from Dr. Ravi Ubriani.*)

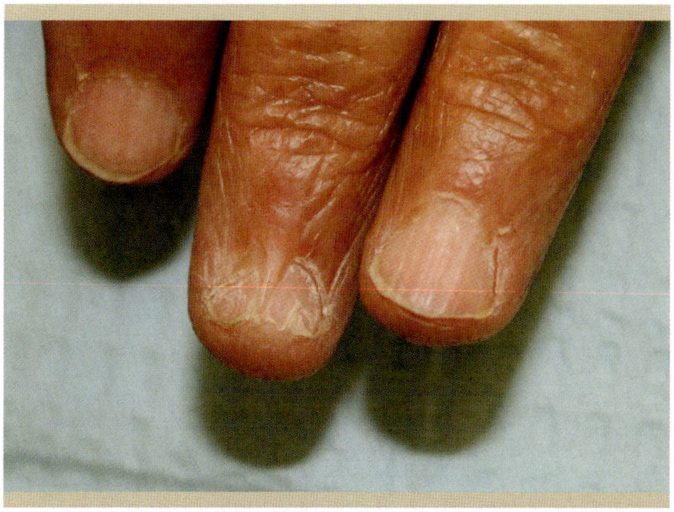

FIGURE 3-18 Pterygium. (*Used with permission from Dr. Ravi Ubriani.*)

4. Lindsay's nail (half and half nail)
    - Distal nail bed: brown to pink; proximal nail bed (40–80%) white
    - Associated with the following conditions: Azotemia, chronic renal failure with uremia
5. Mees lines
    - Transverse white bands
    - Grow out with nail
    - Appear after an episode of poisoning with arsenic, thallium, or other heavy metals
6. Muehrcke lines
    - Nonspecific finding that may be associated with periods of metabolic stress, which transiently impairs the ability of the body (and particularly of the liver) to synthesize proteins
    - Paired white bands parallel to the lunula, and do *not* grow out with nail
    - Associated with: hypoalbuminuria, nephritic syndrome, chemotherapy, malnutrition, cirrhosis
7. Nail fold telangiectasias (nail fold capillary loops)
    - Can be visualized by nail fold capillaromicroscopy or dermatoscopy
    - Dermatomyositis: enlargement of capillary loops, loss of capillaries, disorganization of the normal distribution of capillaries, "budding" ("bushy") capillaries, twisted enlarged capillaries, and capillary hemorrhages
    - Scleroderma (SSc): architectural disorganization, giant capillaries, hemorrhages, loss of capillaries, angiogenesis, and avascular areas found in more than 95% of patients
    - Systemic lupus erythematosus: morphological alterations of capillary loops, venular visibility, and sludging of blood with variability of capillary loop length
    - Antiphospholipid syndrome: symmetrical microhemorrhages
    - Sjögren syndrome: abnormalities range from nonspecific findings (crossed capillaries) to more specific findings (confluent hemorrhages and pericapillary hemorrhages) or SSc-type findings
8. Terry's nail
    - 1- to 2-mm distal pink band, proximal nail is opaque (white, ground-glass-like opacity)
    - Lunula is obliterated
    - Associated with hepatic failure, hyperthyroidism, malnutrition, liver cirrhosis, hypoalbuminemia congestive heart failure, diabetes mellitus
9. Twenty-nail dystrophy (trachyonychia)
    - Term used to describe nail plate roughness, pitting, and ridging that may affect 1 to 20 nails
    - Autosomal dominant inherited form: present at birth and gets worse with age
    - Alopecia areata, psoriasis, lichen planus, atopic dermatitis, ichthyosis vulgaris, immunoglobulin A deficiency, or idiopathic
    - Histology demonstrates spongiosis most often
10. Yellow nail syndrome (YNS) (Fig. 3-19)
    - Pathogenesis unknown, lymphatic vessel alterations may play a role in some cases
    - Spontaneous partial or total remission in 7 to 30% of cases, however, relapse often occurs
    - Nail improvement is often concomitant with improvement of the respiratory pathology
    - Characterized by the triad of characteristic nail changes, chronic respiratory disorders (bronchiectasis, pleural effusion, bronchial hyperresponsiveness, bronchiectasis, chronic bronchitis), and primary lymphedema
    - Total or distal yellow discoloration, with slow growth and loss of the cuticle and lunula. Other characteristics

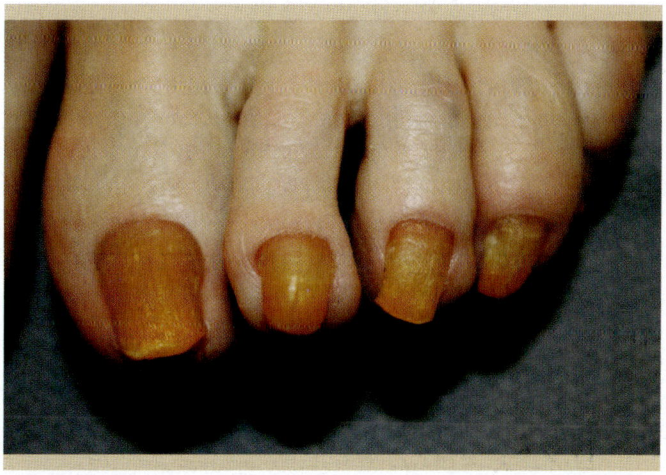

FIGURE 3-19 Yellow nails. (*Used with permission from Dr. Ravi Ubriani.*)

include thickening, hardening, longitudinal overcurvature, transverse ridging associated with variations in the ungual growth rate, and onycholysis that may lead to shedding
- Erythema and edema of the proximal nail fold or chronic paronychia may occur
- Most cases reported are idiopathic; however, the syndrome has been described in association with malignancy
- Familial occurrence of YNS has been reported
- Treatment: case reports have suggested itraconazole or high-dose vitamin E as treatments, but these must be balanced against side effects on an individual basis

11. Psoriasis
    - Affects 10 to 55% of adults
    - Nail matrix disease: pitting (most common nail finding), leukonychia, red spots in lunula, nail plate crumbling, Beau lines (occurs in lesions of the matrix of short duration, often caused by intermittent inflammation), onychorrhexis (occurs in lesions of the matrix of long duration)
    - Nail bed disease: oil drop (salmon patch) discoloration (due to psoriatic lesions contained entirely within the nail bed that can be seen through the overlying nail plate), onycholysis, nail bed hyperkeratosis (from the deposition and collection of cells under the nail plate that have not undergone desquamation), and splinter hemorrhage
    - Acrodermatitis continua of Hallopeau (ACH): rare pustular eruption on the distal portions of the fingers and less often, on the toes. Classified as a form of acropustular psoriasis that tends to be resistant to treatment
    - Histology mirrors that of psoriasis in the skin, except that hypergranulosis is more often a feature
12. Beau lines (Fig. 3-20)
    - Interruption of growth in the nail matrix will produce transverse linear depressions in the nail plate separated by areas of normal nail
    - Can be seen in the following conditions: chronic paronychia, chemotherapy, use of systemic retinoids, fever, illness, Raynaud disease, pemphigus, trauma
13. Median canaliform dystrophy of Heller (Fig. 3-21)
    - Midline split with backward-angled ridges ("fir tree")
    - Beginning at or distal to the proximal nail fold
    - Etiology unknown, occasionally associated with prior local trauma or the initiation of treatment with isotretinoin
    - May be related to habit-tic deformity
    - Enlarged lunula resulting from pressure on the base of the nail
14. Pterygium ("angel-wing" deformity)
    - Has been described on both dorsal and ventral aspects of the nail plate

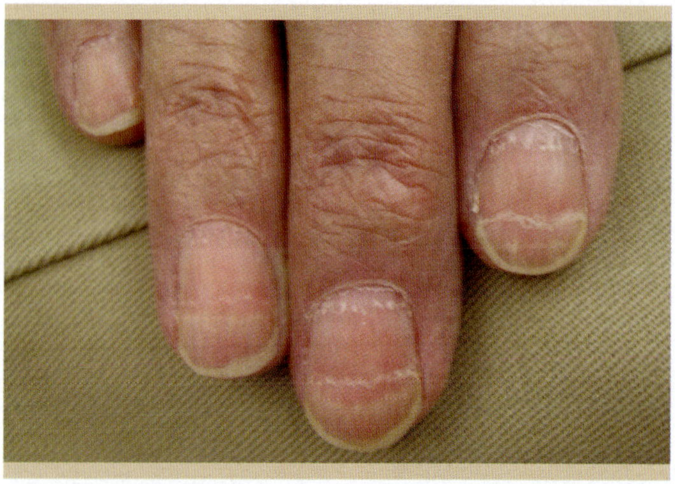

FIGURE 3-20 Beau lines. (*Used with permission from Dr. Sharon Hymes.*)

    - Dorsal nail plate: gradual progressive thinning of the nail plate and secondary fissuring caused by the fusion of the proximal nail fold to the matrix and then to the nail bed
        - Portions of the divided nail plate progressively decrease in size as the pterygium widens
        - Total loss of the nail with permanent atrophy
        - Associated with: lichen planus, bullous disorders, radiotherapy, digital ischemia, trauma, and congenital disorders
    - Ventral nail plate: distal extension of the hyponychial tissue that is anchored to the undersurface of the nail,

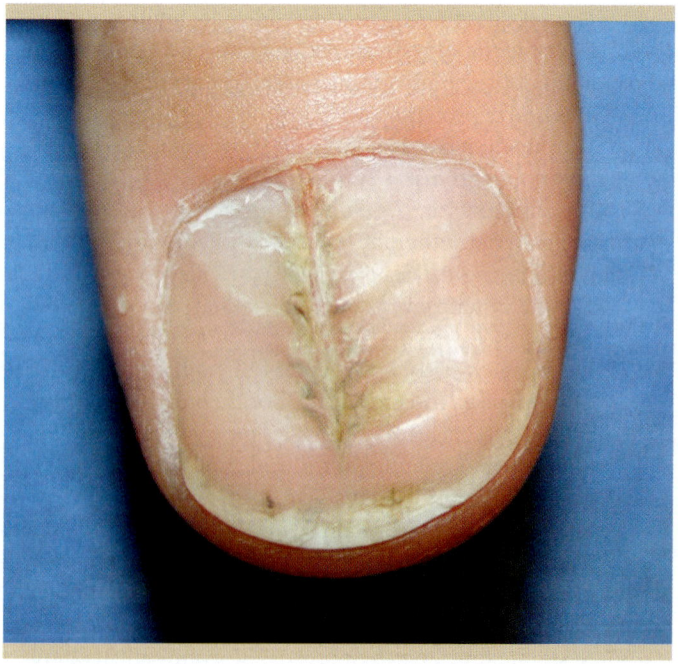

FIGURE 3-21 Median canaliform dystrophy. (*Used with permission from Dr. Ravi Ubriani.*)

thereby obliterating the distal groove. Also known as pterygium inversum unguis
  - Associated with: scleroderma, Raynaud's disease, median nerve causalgia (sympathetic maintained pain), formaldehyde/nail polish, trauma, and congenital disorders

15. Brachyonychia/racquet nail
    - Short nails, the width of nail plate and nail bed is greater than length, occurs with a congenitally short distal phalanx
    - Thumb involvement is common, may be bilateral
    - Autosomal dominant trait secondary to obliteration of the epiphyseal line
    - Associated with: acroosteolysis, Down syndrome, Rubenstein-Taybi syndrome, nail biting, bone resorption in hyperparathyroidism, or psoriatic arthropathy
16. Onychorrhexis
    - Longitudinal nail ridging (aged nails)
    - Abnormalities in epidermal growth and keratinization of the proximal nail matrix
    - Associated with the following disorders: lichen planus, alopecia areata, rheumatoid arthritis, graft-versus-host disease, drugs: isotretinoin, thallium poisoning
17. Clubbing (Fig. 3-22)
    - Increased transverse and longitudinal nail curvature
    - Hypertrophy of the soft tissue components of the digit pulp
    - Hyperplasia of the fibrovascular tissue at the base of the nail
    - Early clubbing obliterates the normal diamond-shaped window formed at the base of the nail beds when there is opposition of the dorsum of 2 fingers from opposite hands. The angle that the proximal nail fold makes with the proximal nail plate is called Lovibond angle. Normally this is about 160 degrees. In clubbing, it exceeds 180 degrees

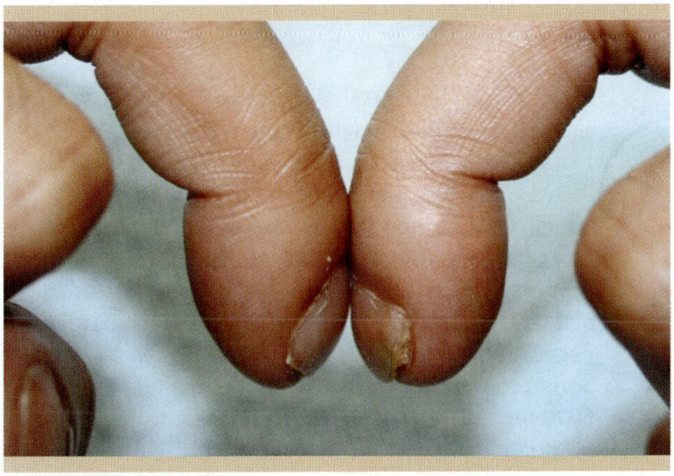

FIGURE 3-22 Clubbing. (*Used with permission from Dr. Ravi Ubriani.*)

    - Associated with: inflammatory bowel disease, pulmonary malignancy, asbestosis, chronic bronchitis, chronic obstructive pulmonary disease (COPD), cirrhosis, congenital heart disease, endocarditis, atrioventricular malformations, fistulas
18. Anonychia
    - Absence of all or part of one or several nails
    - May be congenital (with underlying bone abnormalities) or acquired (usually associated with lichen planus)
    - Occurs sporadically or may have a dominant or recessive inheritance pattern
19. Acrokeratosis paraneoplastica (Bazex syndrome)
    - Multiple, well-defined, psoriasiform, scaly, erythematous patches and plaques, distributed symmetrically over dorsa of hands and feet, helices of ears with similar lesions
    - Palms and soles with keratoderma-like lesions
    - Nail changes: ridging, thickening, yellow discoloration, onycholysis, paronychia
    - Clinical course: acrokeratosis on the hands, feet, ears, and nose that spreads progressively to the arms, legs, and trunk as the tumor grows
    - More than half of acrokeratosis paraneoplastica—associated malignancies are found in the upper aerodigestive tract (upper parts of the respiratory and gastrointestinal tracts)
    - Regional lymphadenopathy is often present
    - In nearly two-thirds of cases, cutaneous lesions precede the symptoms or diagnosis of malignancy
    - Cutaneous manifestations disappear during the treatment of the tumor

Tumors of the Nail Area

1. Periungual and subungual warts (Fig. 3-23)
    - Hyperkeratotic papules with a rough surface: caused by human papilloma virus, most frequently types 1, 2, and 4
    - Most common nail tumor that affect fingernails more often than toenails
    - Direct trauma usually causes innoculation of the virus and initiates the localized viral infection; penetration of papilloma viruses into the skin is favored by skin abrasion or maceration
    - Clinical development of warts occurs a few weeks to more than 1 year after inoculation
    - Subungual warts may appear as a nodule under the nail plate and may result in onycholysis; it may present as a linear growth under the nail plate causing a longitudinal band of onycholysis with splinter hemorrhages
    - Warts may produce slight matrix damage due to compression, resulting in nail plate ridging and grooving
    - Periungual warts are asymptomatic; however, there may be pain associated with subungual warts

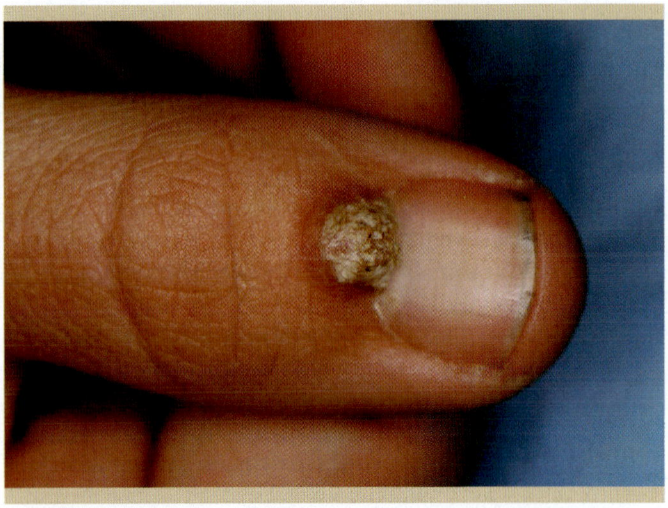

FIGURE 3-23 Periungual wart. (*Used with permission from Dr. Ravi Ubriani.*)

- Located around the nail fold, usually extend under the nail plate and may lie adjacent to the nail matrix
- Histology: hyperkeratosis with columns of parakeratosis overlying elongated papillae, hypergranulosis, and koilocytic changes
- Bowen disease and squamous cell carcinoma have been reported to occur in long-standing periungual warts

2. Epidermal inclusion cyst
   - Occurs secondary to traumatic impregnation of the dermis with epidermal cells
   - Cyst is lined with epidermis and filled with keratin
   - Occasionally observed under the nail following trauma (such as a complication of nail surgery)
   - Can erode adjacent structures, including bone
   - Often asymptomatic, however, rupture of the cyst wall can elicit a foreign-body giant-cell reaction
   - May appear as a subungual tumor raising the nail plate or causing a bulbous enlargement of the terminal phalanx
   - X-ray will show a sharply demarcated, round defect
   - Treatment by surgical removal of the cyst contents and the wall of the cyst
3. Onychomatricoma
   - Uncommon benign tumor of the nail matrix
   - Longitudinal band of yellow thickening of the nail plate with longitudinal ridging and multiple holes at the distal nail
   - Increased transverse curvature of the nail, splinter hemorrhages of the proximal nail plate
   - Villous tumor projections in the nail plate, MRI shows tumoral core in the matrix area and invagination of the lesion into the funnel-shaped nail plate
   - Filiform tumor that consists of nail matrix epithelium over a connective tissue core
   - Epithelium may show clear cell change
   - Treatment
     - Simple retraction of the proximal nail fold allows superficial removal of the tumor from the matrix
4. Subungual and periungual keratoacanthoma
   - May occur as solitary or multiple tumors
   - Rare, benign, rapidly growing, and locally aggressive
   - Usually situated below the edge of the nail plate or in the most distal portion of the nail bed
   - Lesion may start as a small and painful keratotic nodule visible beneath the free edge of the nail plate; occasionally it occurs under the proximal nail fold
   - Rapid growth to a 1- to 2-cm lesion within 4 to 8 weeks
   - The tumor can erode the bone, radiographically; it appears as a well-defined, crescent-shaped lytic defect (MRI is superior to radiographic studies in detecting an erosion of the distal phalanx)
   - Treatment: removal of the entire tumor with histologic control of the resection margins. The patient should be followed to rule out a recurrence
5. Acquired periungual fibrokeratoma
   - Asymptomatic nodule with a hyperkeratotic tip, narrow base
   - Possibly caused by trauma
   - Variant of acquired digital fibrokeratoma
   - Emerges from beneath the proximal nail fold, grows on the nail, and causes sharp longitudinal depressions
   - Some of these lesions originate from within the matrix and thus grow in the nail plate, eventually to emerge in the middle of the nail. (also called "dissecting ungual fibrokeratoma")
   - Histology demonstrates a hyperkeratotic and acanthotic epithelium with prominence of the granular layer overlying a dense and hypocellular collagenous tissue core
   - Immunohistochemistry shows that the fibroblasts are vimentin positive, and many of them stain with HHF35 (monoclonal antibody, specific for muscle actin)
   - Treatment: excision
6. Koenen tumor
   - Periungual fibroma
   - Develops in about 50% of the cases of tuberous sclerosis (epiloia or Bourneville-Pringle disease)
   - Usually appear between the ages of 12 and 14 years and increase progressively in size and number with age
   - Small, round, smooth, flesh colored, asymptomatic, more frequent on toes than on fingers
   - Tumors grow out of the nail fold, overgrow the nail bed, and destroy the nail plate. May cause longitudinal depressions in the nail plate
   - Sometimes tumors also grow in the nail plate
   - Histology: similar to that of fibrokeratoma as described above with atypical stellate myofibroblasts in the tissue core
   - Treatment: Excessively large tumors often are painful and should be excised at their base

7. Infantile digital fibromatosis
   - 1- to 2-cm round, smooth, dome-shaped, shiny, firm red dermal nodules
   - Dorsal and axial surfaces of the fingers and toes
   - Not painful but can lead to functional deformity of a joint or cause limited mobility
   - It may be present at the time of birth or develop within the first year of life
   - Slow growth in the first month, followed by a rapid phase of growth (10–14 months), then be spontaneous involution
   - Conservative approach unless IDF causes a problem with mobility
   - Histology: scattered cells with eosinophilic cytoplasmic inclusions on routine hematoxylin and eosin staining. Inclusions are typically juxtanuclear and may even indent the adjacent nucleus
8. Bowen disease (in situ epidermoid carcinoma)
   - Carcinoma in situ of the nail that differs from other variants of squamous cell carcinoma
   - Etiology linked to human papillomavirus (HPV)-16, -34, and -35; arsenic also may play a role (also think about association with genital warts), exposure to x-ray
   - Presents as a circumscribed plaque with a warty surface extending from the nail groove both under and around the nail, periungual swelling due to deep tumor proliferation
   - Commonly presents with subungual involvement with extensive hyperkeratosis of the nail bed, associated with partial or total nail loss
   - Less common presentations: longitudinal melanonychia, lifting of the nail plate by subungual pseudofibrokeratoma
   - Nail dystrophy develops when the matrix is affected
   - Carcinoma cuniculatum: rare variant of squamous cell carcinoma with low biologic malignancy
   - Treatment: imiquimod, photodynamic therapy, methotrexate, radiation therapy, Mohs micrographic surgery, excisional surgery, bone involvement requires amputation of the distal phalanx
9. Myxoid cyst (digital mucoid cyst) (Fig. 3-24)
   - Asymptomatic, smooth nodule that enlarges slowly
   - Typically located at the distal interphalangeal (DIP) joints or in the proximal nail fold
   - A split or groove in the nail develops distally
   - Incision of the cyst results in extrusion of clear jelly-like material
10. Subungual exostosis and osteochondroma
   - Subungual exostoses are not true tumors but rather are outgrowths of normal bone or calcified cartilaginous remains
   - Location: commonly in the dorsomedial aspect of the tip of the great toe, although subungual exostoses may also occur in lesser toes or, less commonly, thumb, or index fingers

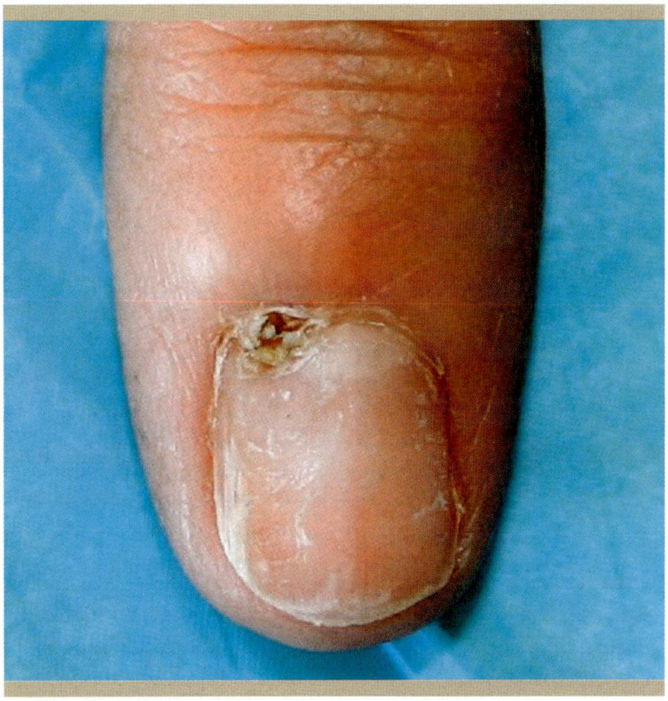

FIGURE 3-24 Myxoid cyst. (*Used with permission from Dr. Ravi Ubriani.*)

   - Triad of pain (the leading symptom), nail deformation, and radiographic features is usually diagnostic
   - Trauma is the main cause
   - Begin as small elevations on the dorsal aspect of the distal phalanx and may eventually emerge from under the nail edge or destroy the nail plate
11. Osteochondroma
   - Bone-hard tumor, confirmed by x-ray
   - History of trauma, growth rate is slow
   - Radiographic studies show a well-defined, circumscribed, pedunculated or sessile bone growth projecting from the dorsum of the distal phalanx near the epiphyseal line
   - Therapy of subungual exostosis and osteochondroma consists of local curettage or excision
12. Giant cell tumor of the tendon sheath
   - Solitary, often lobulated, slow-growing, skin-colored, and smooth-surfaced nodule that tends to feel firm and rubbery
   - Usually occurs on the dorsum of the distal interphalangeal joint; rarely, it can present in the region of the lateral nail fold and may interfere with nail growth
   - Periodic inflammation and drainage may occur
   - Histopathology shows a cellular tumor composed of histiocytic and fibroblastic cells with a variable number of giant cells and some foam cells in a hyalin stroma with siderophages
   - Treatment is surgical excision

Vascular Tumors

1. Pyogenic granuloma
   - Eruptive hemangioma usually seen following trauma
   - Small, benign, eruptive bluish/red nodule develops rapidly on the periungual skin, may develop distally in the hyponychium region or in the nail bed, especially associated with onycholysis of the toe
   - Tenderness and a tendency to bleed are characteristic features
   - Lesion becomes necrotic and forms a collarette of macerated white epithelium
   - Granulation tissue can be secondary to systemic retinoids, antiretroviral medications, cyclosporine, or epidermal growth factor receptor inhibitors. These medications can all cause similar side effects in the nails: paronychia, xerosis, desquamation, and periungual granulation tissue
   - Remove by excision at its base followed by electrodesiccation or application of Monsel or aluminum chloride solution. CO_2 or pulsed dye lasers can also be used
2. Glomus tumor (Fig. 3-25)
   - Triad: pain, tenderness, temperature sensitivity
   - Around 75% of glomus tumors occur in the hand, especially in the fingertips and in particular in the subungual area. One percent to two percent of all hand tumors are glomus tumors
   - Intense, often pulsating pain that may be spontaneous or provoked by the slightest trauma or changes in temperature
   - Tumor is seen through the nail plate as a small bluish to reddish-blue spot several millimeters in diameter: longitudinal erythronychia with a distal fissured nail plate, usually in a single digit in middle-aged women
   - One-half of the tumors cause minor nail deformities, ridging, and fissuring. About 50% cause a depression on the dorsal aspect of the distal phalangeal bone or possibly a cyst, visible on radiographic study
   - Transillumination may help localize the tumor; MRI has the highest sensitivity to localize the tumor
   - Histology: tumor with afferent arteriole and vascular channels lined with endothelium and surrounded by irregularly arranged cuboidal cells with round dark nuclei and pale cytoplasm; positive for vimentin, a 42-kD muscle actin (with HHF 35), a smooth muscle actin (CGA 7), and myosin
   - Treatment: surgical removal, recurrences occur in 10 to 20% of cases

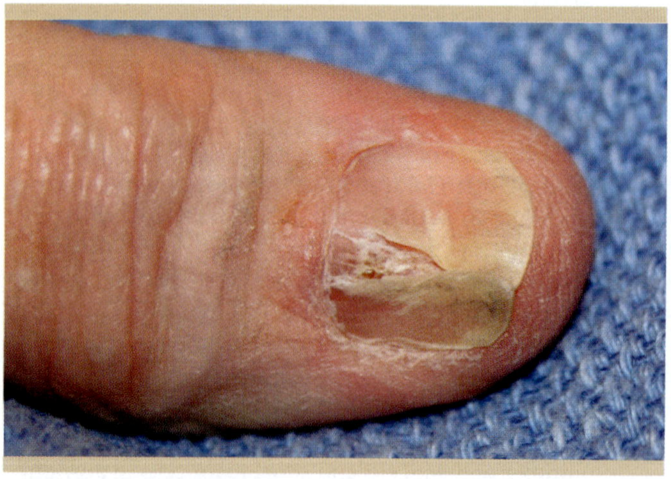

FIGURE 3-25 Glomus tumor. (*Used with permission from Dr. Ravi Ubriani.*)

Vitamins and Nail Disease

- There is circumstantial evidence that vitamin and mineral supplementation can be beneficial in nail disease. A review from August 2007 suggests that there is no role for vitamin or mineral supplementation in healthy nails. Clinical cases such as nail changes in hemodialysis, anorexia, bulemia, and genodermatoses provide the circumstantial evidence of the role of vitamins and minerals in nail health
- Biotin: shown in multiple well-designed studies to be an effective treatment for brittle nail syndrome, but takes 2 to 3 months to have an effect
- Vitamin E: case reports have shown success in yellow nail syndrome, but the supplementation was in conjunction with other treatments
- Retinoids and Vitamin A: deficiency can be associated with eggshell nails. Overdosage or systemic retinoid therapy can result in numerous nail problems, including acute paronychia, pyogenic granulomas, plate fragility and thinning, onychorrhexis, onychoschizia, onychomadesis, median canaliform dystrophy, transverse leukonychia, and a desquamative erythroderma with complete destruction of the nails. Topical retinoids are beneficial in nail psoriasis and can have a role in pachyonychia congenita
- Vitamin D: topical use is beneficial in nail psoriasis
- Vitamin B_{12}: deficiency can result in hyperpigmentation of the nail
- Calcium: severe deficiency can lead to a transverse leukonychia
- Iron: deficiency can result in koilonychia, as in Plummer-Vinson syndrome. Supplementation can reduce brittleness of the nails, even when laboratory evaluation reveals no iron deficiency
- Zinc: supplementation improves nail changes in acrodermatitis enteropathica. Acute onset deficiency can lead to a transverse leukonychia or Beau lines
- Selenium: super-therapeutic selenium administration can lead to multiple nail problems, including brittle nails, transverse yellowish-white or red streaks, or longitudinal streaks
- Silicon: supplementation has been shown to decrease nail brittleness in well-designed studies

- Claims have been made regarding benefits from gelatin, L-methionine, keratin , collagen, panthothenic acid, salt, chromium, rhodanates, pyridoxine, vitamin C, or primrose oil, but the review did not find enough evidence to support a role for any of these supplements

Drug Reactions Affecting the Nails

- Many drug reactions can cause problems with the nails. Drug reactions in the nails can differ from other cutaneous drug reactions because the kinetics of nail formation can result in delayed or prolonged abnormalities
- Teratogenesis: nail hypoplasia and anonychia may result from drugs taken during pregnancy. Anticonvulsants and anticoagulants are the most common causes
- Beau lines and onychomadesis: result from acute severe toxicity to the nail matrix keratinization. They are clinically noted weeks after administration of the drug because of the slow growth of the nail. The most common causes are chemotherapy and radiation but these have been described with many different medications
- Nail fragility: chemotherapy, retinoids, and antiretroviral agents
- Slowed nail growth: cyclosporine, heparin, lithium, methotrexate, and zidovudine
- Increased nail growth: fluconazole, itraconazole, levodopa, and oral contraceptives
- Transverse leukonychia: results from retention of nuclei in the nail plate due to transient impairment of keratinization in the matrix. When they present as bands along the entire width of the nail plate, they are known as Mees lines. This finding has been reported with many medications including chemotherapy, cyclosporine, and retinoids, and can be seen in arsenic or thallium poisoning. Apparent leukonychia that does not migrate with nail growth and fades with compression is called Muehrcke lines. It is associated with low albumin and can be seen in patients treated with chemotherapy even with normal albumin levels
- Onycholysis and photo-onycholysis: Result from acute toxicity to the nail bed epithelium. Onycholysis with subungual abscess has been reported most frequently with taxane chemotherapy, but has also been reported with methotrexate, retinoids, and infliximab. Photo-onycholysis is seen with PUVA, tetracyclines, fluoroquinolones, oral contraceptive pills, thiazide diuretics, and captopril
- Acute paronychia: can be seen with methotrexate, antiretrovirals (indinavir and lamivudine), retinoids (especially isotretinoin), and epidermal growth factor receptor inhibitors (gefitinib, erlotinib, and cetuximab)
- Pyogenic granulomas: causes are similar to acute paronychia. Can be caused by cyclosporine, indinavir, and epidermal growth factor receptor inhibitors
- Ischemic changes: Beta-blockers (especially propanolol) and bleomycin can produce ischemic and Raynaud phenomenon. Bleomycin effects can be seen several months after treatment
- Subungual hemorrhages: antithrombotics, anticoagulants, taxanes, tetracyclines, and ganciclovir
- Nail atrophy: prolonged application of high-potency topical steroids
- Melanonychia: zidovudine, chemotherapy, hydroxyurea, psoralens all can cause activation of melanocytes and appearance of melanonychia. Radiation therapy can cause melanonychia even when used remote from the affected area
- Pigmentation: deposition of agents in the nails and subungual tissue can produce pigmentary changes. Tetracycline (yellow), gold salts (yellow), and clofazimine (dark-brown) deposit in the nails—these deposits will grow out with the nails and will be parallel to the lunula. Minocycline (blue-gray) and antimalarials (blue-brown) can deposit in the subungual tissues—these deposits will not grow out with nail growth. Tar and anthralin can stain the superficial layers of the nail plate and have a proximal border parallel to the cuticle as they are not dependent on endogenous deposition

QUIZ

Questions

1. A 56-year-old woman presents with a nonpainful abnormal appearing second great toenail. She reports that this has been present for many years and denies a history of trauma. Examination reveals a thickened and yellow nail with multiple holes at the distal margin. Surgical exploration reveals a soft filiform papule in the matrix and cavities in the nail plate. Pathological examination of the tumor is most likely to reveal which diagnosis:

   A. Blue nevus
   B. Glomus tumor
   C. Myxoid cyst
   D. Onychomatricoma
   E. Squamous cell carcinoma

2. Paronychia, periungual pyogenic granulomas, and xerosis are associated with which of the following medications?

   A. Epidermal growth factor receptor inhibitors
   B. Hedgehog signaling pathway inhibitors
   C. Histone deacetylase inhibitors
   D. Serine/threonine-specific protein kinase inhibitors
   E. Tumor necrosis factor inhibitors

3. Dorsal pterygium is associated with which of the following diseases?

   A. Alopecia areata
   B. Lichen planus
   C. Lupus
   D. Psoriasis
   E. Scleroderma

4. A 60-year-old man develops diffuse yellow thickening of all his nails. The most appropriate consultation would be to:

   A. Cardiologist
   B. Dentist
   C. Gastroenterologist
   D. Nephrologist
   E. Pulmonologist

5. What is the approximate growth rate of normal toenails?

   A. 0.01 mm/d
   B. 0.02 mm/d
   C. 0.03 mm/d
   D. 0.04 mm/d
   E. 0.05 mm/d

6. What medicine has the highest rate of photo-induced onycholysis?

   A. Demeclocycline
   B. Doxycycline
   C. Minocycline
   D. Oxsoralen
   E. Tetracycline

7. A 30-year-old man has long-standing abnormalities of his fingernails. On examination, there is severe nail thickening, yellow-gray color, and massive subungual hyperkeratosis. Follicular hyperkeratosis is seen on the elbows and knees. You correctly diagnose pachyonychia congenita. What is the most likely oral finding?

   A. Benign oral leukoplakia
   B. Black hairy tongue
   C. Oral hairy leukoplakia
   D. Oral melanoacanthoma
   E. Oral squamous cell carcinoma

8. An 18-year-old girl has numerous progressively enlarging smooth flesh-colored papules at the periungual folds of the nails on the hands and feet. This finding is associated with which of the following diseases?

   A. Bazex syndrome
   B. Nail-patella syndrome
   C. Plummer-Vinson syndrome
   D. Rubenstein-Taybi syndrome
   E. Tuberous sclerosis complex

9. Match the following nail findings with the most likely causative clinical scenario.

i. Red lunula	A. Wilson disease
ii. Blue lunula	B. Trauma
iii. Green nails	C. Antimalarial treatment
iv. Blue-brown nails	D. Pseudomonas infection
v. White spots on the nail	E. Carbon monoxide poisoning

10. Match the following nail findings with the most likely causative genetic disorder.

i. Severe nail thickening, yellow-gray color, subungual hyperkeratosis	A. Coffin-Siris syndrome
ii. Short, thickened, and hypoplastic nails	B. Keratosis follicularis
iii. Triangular lunula, hypoplasia of nails	C. Pachyonychia congenita
iv. Hypoplastic fifth fingernails	D. Fong syndrome
v. Red and white longitudinal streaks, wedge-shaped nicking of the distal nail plate, subungual hyperkeratosis	E. Hereditary ectodermal dysplasia

Answers

1. D (onychomatricoma). Onychomatricoma is an uncommon benign tumor of the nail matrix that produces characteristic changes in the nail plate. Glomus tumors are usually painful. Myxoid cysts can be stable but will not produce a filiform tumor and usually present with a groove in the nail plate. Squamous cell carcinoma is usually progressive.
2. E (tumor necrosis factor inhibitors). Paronychia, periungual pyogenic granulomas, and xerosis are associated with epidermal growth factor receptor inhibitors.
3. B (lichen planus). Dorsal pterygium is associated with lichen planus. Pterygium inversum unguis is associated with scleroderma and lupus.
4. E (pulmonologist). Yellow nail syndrome has an unknown pathogenesis, but is associated with chronic respiratory disorders. It can also be associated with lymphedema.
5. C (0.03 mm/d). Fingernails grow at 3 mm/mo (0.1 mm/d) and take 5 to 6 months to regrow. Toenails grow at 1 mm/mo (0.03 mm/d) and take 12 to 18 months to regrow.
6. A (Demeclocycline). The rate of photo-onycholysis for tetracyclines is as follows: Demeclocycline > doxycycline > tetracycline > minocycline.
7. A (benign oral leukoplakia). The most common type of pachyonychia congenita (Jadassohn-Lewandowsky, Type I) has benign oral leukoplakia as a finding. One of the less common types (Type II PC: Jackson-Lawler, Type II) can have early dentition/natal teeth as a finding.
8. E (tuberous sclerosis complex). These nail changes are periungual fibromas, also known as Koenen tumors. They develop in 50% of patients with tuberous sclerosis, and usually begin to appear around ages 12 to 14.
9. i-E; ii-A, iii-D, iv-C, v-B.
   i. Red lunulae are associated with carbon monoxide poisoning, cardiac failure, rheumatoid arthritis, alopecia areata, polycythemia vera, and lupus

ii. Blue lunulae are associated with Wilson disease, argyria, silver nitrate, and drugs including azidothymidine, quinacrine, busulfan, and phenolphthalein
iii. Green nails are associated with *Pseudomonas* infection
iv. Blue-brown nails are associated with antimalarial medications. Minocycline can cause blue-gray discoloration. AZT and HIV (independently) can cause longitudinal melanonychia.
v. Punctate leukonychia is associated with minor trauma, and is distinguishable from total leukonychia, transverse leukonychia, and longitudinal melanonychia, which are associated with underlying conditions.

10. i-C; ii-E; iii-D; iv-A; v-B.
i. Severe nail thickening, yellow-gray color, and massive subungual hyperkeratosis are all findings of pachyonychia congenita.
ii. Short, thickened, and hypoplastic nails are a feature of many of the hereditary ectodermal dysplasias.
iii. Nail-patella syndrome, also known as HOOD or Fong syndrome, is an autosomal dominant disorder with a defect in the *LMX1B* gene. Findings include triangular lunula and hypoplastic nails. Non-nail findings include absent patella, glomerulonephritis, and Lester iris.
iv. Hypoplastic fifth fingernails and toenails are a feature of Coffin-Siris syndrome, along with developmental delay, hirsutism, and coarse facial features.
v. Keratosis follicularis or Darier disease is an autosomal dominant disorder with a defect in the ATPase 2A2. Nail findings are red and white longitudinal streaks, wedge-shaped nicking of the distal nail plate, and subungual hyperkeratosis.

REFERENCES

André J, Lateur N: Pigmented nail disorders. *Dermatol Clin* 2006;24(3):329–339.

Baran R, Richert B: Common nail tumors. *Dermatol Clin* 2006;24(3):297–311.

Braun RP et al. Diagnosis and management of nail pigmentations. *J Am Acad Dermatol* 2007;56(5):835–847. Epub 2007 Feb 22.

Cutolo M, Sulli A, Secchi ME, Paolino S, Pizzorni C: Nailfold capillaroscopy is useful for the diagnosis and follow-up of autoimmune rheumatic diseases. A future tool for the analysis of microvascular heart involvement? *Rheumatology (Oxford)* 2006; 45(Suppl 4):iv43–iv46.

Daniel CR: Nail pigmentation abnormalities. *Dermatol Clin* 1985;3: 431–443.

Faergemann J, Baran R: Epidemiology, clinical presentation and diagnosis of onychomycosis. *Br J Dermatol* 2003;149:1–4.

Fistarol SK, Itin PH: Nail changes in genodermatoses. *Eur J Dermatol* 2002;12:119–128.

Goldsmith LA, et al. *Fitzpatrick's Dermatology in General Medicine*, 8th Ed. New York: McGraw-Hill; 2012.

Hasan T, Khan AU: Phototoxicity of the tetracyclines: photosensitized emission of singlet delta dioxygen. *Proc Natl Acad Sci USA* 1986;83(13):4604-4606.

Herzberg AJ: Nail manifestations of systemic diseases. *Clin Podiatr Med Surg* 1995;12:309–318.

James WD, Berger TG, Elston DM: *Andrews' Diseases of the Skin: Clinical Dermatology*, 10th Ed. Philadelphia: Elsevier-Saunders; 2006.

Jiaravuthisan MM, Sasseville D, Vender RB, Murphy F, Muhn CY: Psoriasis of the nail: anatomy, pathology, clinical presentation, and a review of the literature on therapy. *J Am Acad Dermatol* 2007;57(1):1–27.

McKee PH: *Pathology of the Skin: With Clinical Correlations*, 3rd Ed. London: Mosby-Wolfe; 2005.

McLean WH: Genetic disorders of palm skin and nail. *J Anat* 2003;202:133–141.

Mehra A, Murphy RJ, Wilson BB: Idiopathic familial onychomadesis. *J Am Acad Dermatol* 2000;43(2):349–350.

Pappert AS, Scher RK, Cohen JL: Nail disorders in children. *Pediatr Clin North Am* 1991;38:921–940.

Perrin C, Goettmann S, Baran R: Onychomatricoma: clinical and histopathologic findings in 12 cases. *J Am Acad Dermatol* 1998;39(4 Pt 1):560–564.

Piraccini BM, Iorizzo M, Starace M, Tosti A: Drug-induced nail diseases. *Dermatol Clin* 2006;24(3):387–391.

Razi E: Familial yellow nail syndrome. *Dermatol Online J* 2006;12(2):15.

Rich P: Nail disorders. Diagnosis and treatment of infectious, inflammatory, and neoplastic nail conditions. *Med Clin North Am* 1998;82:1171–1183.

Scheinfeld N, Dahdah MJ, Scher R: Vitamins and minerals: their role in nail health and disease. *J Drugs Dermatol* 2007;6(8):782–787.

Scher RK, Daniel CR: *Nails*, 3rd Ed. Philadelphia: Elsevier-Saunders; 2005.

Sharma V, Sharma NL, Ranjan N, Tegta GR, Sarin S: Acrokeratosis paraneoplastica (Bazex syndrome): case report and review of literature. *Dermatol Online J* 2006;12(1):11.

Telfer NR: Congenital and hereditary nail disorders. *Semin Dermatol* 1991;10:2–6.

Tosti A, Piraccini BM: Warts of the nail unit: surgical and nonsurgical approaches. *Dermatol Surg* 2001;27(3):235–239.

van de Kerkhof PC et al. Brittle nail syndrome: a pathogenesis-based approach with a proposed grading system. *J Am Acad Dermatol* 2005;53(4):644–651.

CHAPTER 4

ORAL PATHOLOGY

KAMAL BUSAIDY
JERRY BOUQUOT
LAITH MAHMOOD

UNIQUE TONGUE CHANGES

Hairy Tongue (Black Hairy Tongue) (Fig. 4-1)

- Etiology: elongation of keratin on filiform tongue papillae from inadequate oral hygiene, dry mouth, or microbial overgrowth. Also associated with smoking, antibiotic therapy, extended hospital stays, and poor general health status
- Clinical findings: white, black, or brown hair-like projections on dorsal tongue, more concentrated toward posterior and often associated with halitosis. There may be a burning sensation from secondary candidiasis
- Treatment: scrape off daily with floss or a tongue scraper; eliminate smoking; improve oral hygiene; treat burning symptoms with antifungals

Hairy Leukoplakia (Fig. 4-2)

- Etiology: HIV in AIDS
- Clinical findings: vertical or randomly oriented, asymptomatic white keratotic thickening of the lateral border of the tongue, usually unilateral. No other evidence of biting trauma and no ulceration
- Treatment: treat the HIV infection; this lesion will disappear with systemic treatment of the AIDS

Fissured Tongue (Scrotal Tongue; Lingua Plicata; Hamburger Tongue) (Fig. 4-3)

- Etiology: developmental anomalies; becomes more pronounced over decades
- Associated frequently with: Melkersson-Rosenthal syndrome; Down syndrome; benign migratory glossitis (geographic tongue)
- Clinical findings: irregular, often deep fissures of the tongue dorsum, often with a fissure down the midline; may be symptomatic (burning sensation, pain with spicy foods) if associated with secondary candidiasis
- Treatment: maintain good oral hygiene; antifungals if symptomatic

Bifid Tongue (in Oral-Facial-Digital Syndrome Type I)

- Etiology: x-linked dominant inherited trait with multiple malformations of the face, oral cavity, and digits
- Clinical appearance (oral): multiple deep clefts along border of tongue give the illusion of border lobules, sometimes with a deep central fissure; hamartomas or lipomas of the ventral tongue; cleft of the hard or soft palate; accessory gingival frenula, hypodontia
- Treatment: surgical correction of clefts, as needed

Ankyloglossia (Tongue Tie) (Fig. 4-4)

- Etiology: developmental defect fusing ventral tongue to oral floor
- Clinical findings: attachment of the ventral tongue to the floor of the mouth, even to the gingivae of the lower incisors; limits tongue movement but seldom interferes with speech
- Treatment: usually none is needed, but attachment can be surgically corrected if there is a speech defect or anterior mandibular gingiva becomes inflamed or deteriorated

Lingual Varicosities (Fig. 4-5)

- Etiology: chronically increased hydrostatic pressure in the superficial veins of the ventral tongue; etiology unknown but not related to varicose veins of the extremities
- Clinical findings: asymptomatic, undulating, slightly elevated blue superficial veins of the ventral tongue (sometimes lip mucosa or vestibule); sometimes present as 2 to 3 mm blue/purple papules ("caviar spots"). Lesion blanches

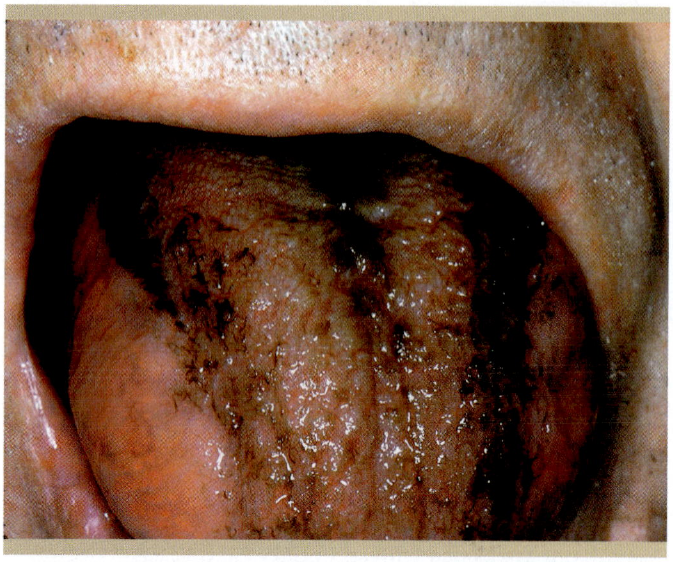

FIGURE 4-1 Black hairy tongue. (*Used with permission from Dr Nadarajah Vigneswaran.*)

with pressure on the posterior portion of the vessel; usually bilateral

- Treatment: none needed unless it becomes tender or painful, which indicates that a thrombus has occurred in the affected vein; if so, surgical excision of a portion of the vessel can be done

Papillary Tip Melanosis (Black Lingual Bumps) (Fig. 4-6)

- Etiology: developmental or drug-induced pigmentation of the tips of the fungiform (sometimes filiform) papillae

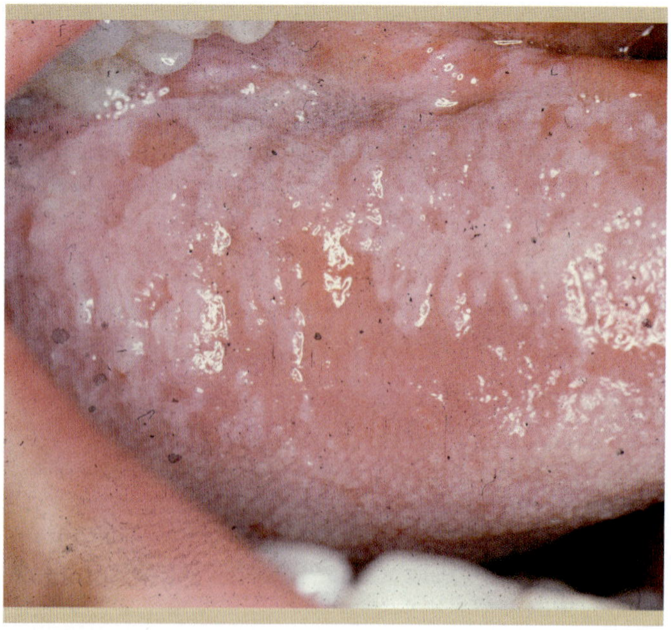

FIGURE 4-2 Hairy leukoplakia. (*Used with permission from Dr. Bela Toth.*)

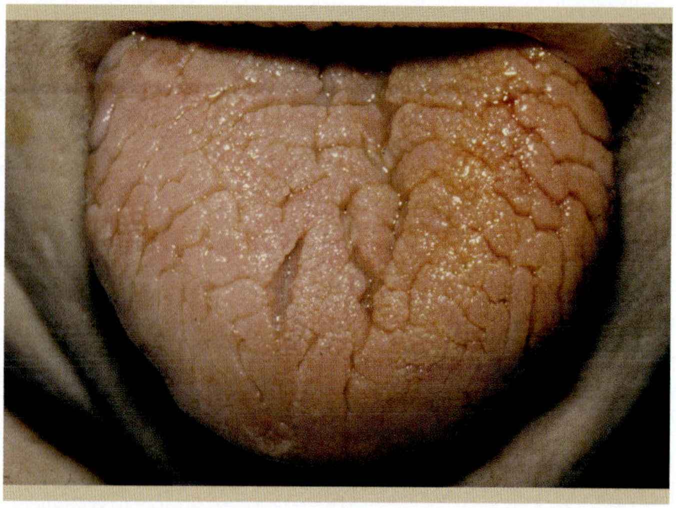

FIGURE 4-3 Fissured tongue.

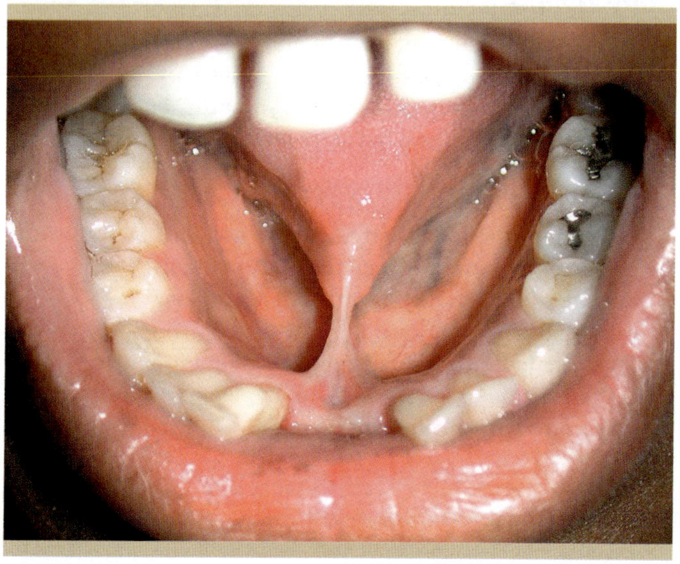

FIGURE 4-4 Ankyloglossia.

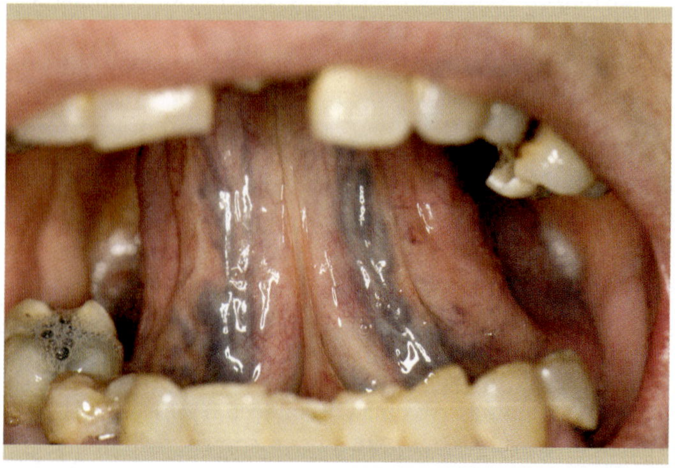

FIGURE 4-5 Lingual varicosities.

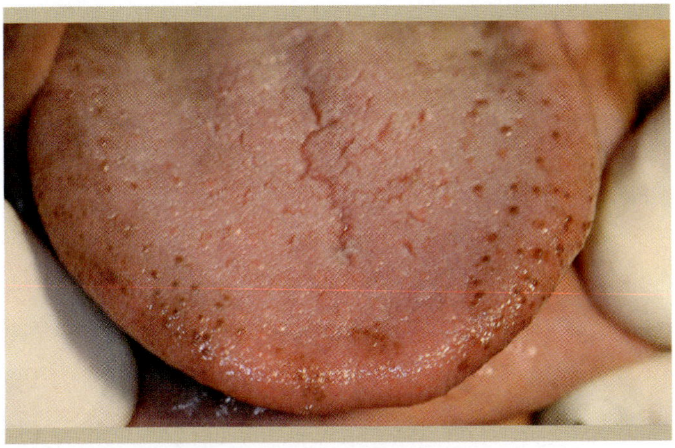

FIGURE 4-6 Papillary tip melanosis.

- Clinical findings: asymptomatic light or dark brown pigmentation of the tops of the fungiform papillae, usually clustered in 1 region of the lingual dorsum
- Treatment: no treatment is needed; may disappear with cessation of drug use, otherwise no change over time

Geographic Tongue (Benign Migratory Glossitis) (Fig. 4-7)

- Etiology: unknown, but appears to be a variant of psoriasis, although it occurs in only 10% of persons with skin psoriasis
- Clinical appearance: single or multiple focal loss of filiform papillae surrounded by a small grove, usually with a serpiginous white line along the outer border; affected areas heal and develop on other tongue surfaces; sometimes circular or serpiginous red or white thin lines are seen on buccal or lip mucosae; if associated with a burning sensation, consider secondary candidiasis

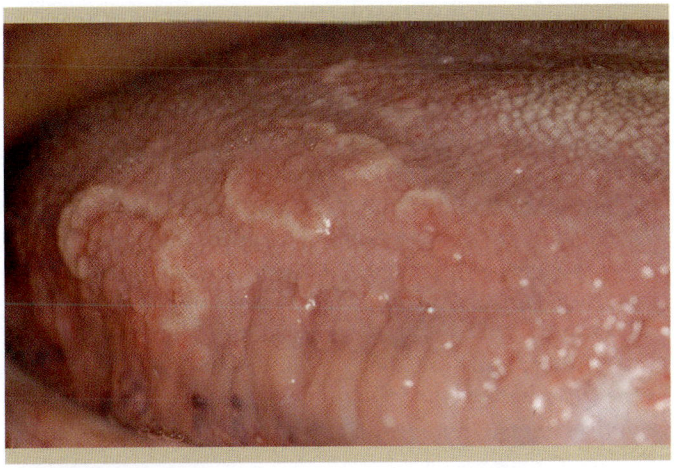

FIGURE 4-7 Benign migratory glossitis (geographic tongue).

- Histology: Psoriasiform mucositis; elongation of the rete ridges is noted with associated hyperparakeratosis and acanthosis; absence of filiform papillae in center; clustering of neutrophils within the epithelium (Munro microabscesses)
- Treatment: none, unless secondary atrophic candidiasis occurs, then topical or systemic antifungals; antibiotics and corticosteroids may also be helpful, if antifungals are ineffective

Chronic Lingual Papulosis (Fig. 4-8)

- Etiology: mouth breathing, tongue thrust habit (rubbing tongue against the teeth), associated with geographic tongue (benign migratory glossitis)
- Clinical appearance: numerous 2 to 4 mm fibroma-like, asymptomatic, moderately firm masses (enlarged filiform papillae) scattered diffusely or in clusters on the anterior dorsum of the tongue, often associated with geographic tongue
- Treatment: none required, unless secondary candidiasis developed in the grooves around the masses, in which case antifungals should be used

Atrophic Glossitis (Dry Mouth Syndrome; Burning Tongue Syndrome) (Fig. 4-9)

- Etiology: systemic medications (anticholinergic effects: diuretics, sedatives, hypnotics, antihistamines, antihypertensives, antipsychotics, antidepressants, anticholinergics, appetite suppressants); radiotherapy to head and neck (H&N); salivary gland surgery; autoimmune disorders (HIV infection, systemic lupus erythematosus, rheumatoid arthritis, Sjögren syndrome); idiopathic xerostomia; anemias (vitamin B, especially B_{12}, iron deficiency); endocrine disorders (diabetes, hyperthyroidism)

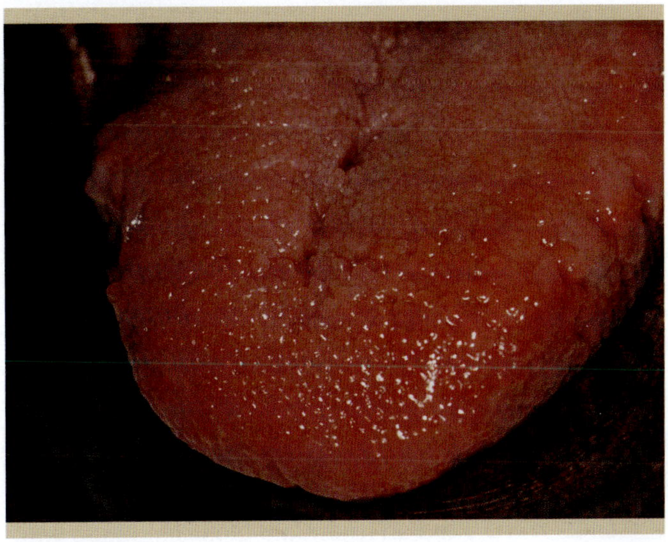

FIGURE 4-8 Chronic lingual papulosis.

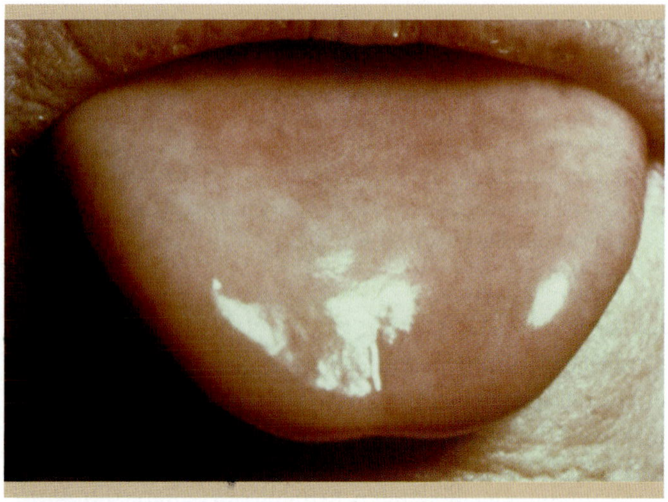

FIGURE 4-9 Atrophic glossitis.

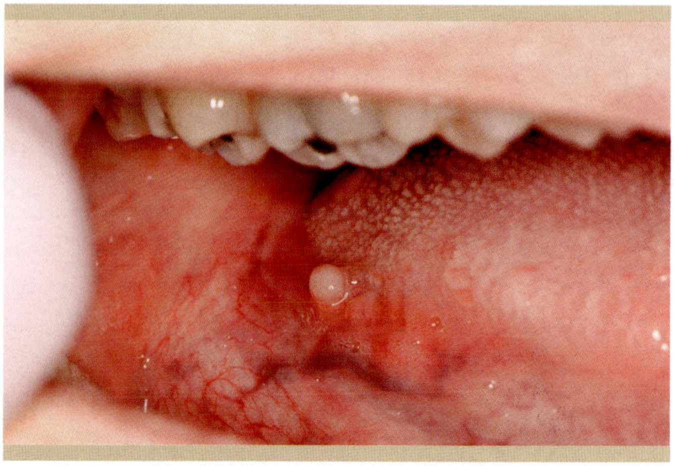

FIGURE 4-11 Lymphoepithelial cyst.

- Clinical findings: dry, possibly glossy atrophic mucosa, often with burning tongue and loss of papillae of the tongue
- Treatment: discontinue offending medication; commercial saliva substitute; fluoride supplementation for caries prevention; treat underlying anemias or other systemic disorders

Median Rhomboid Glossitis (Fig. 4-10)

- Etiology: developmental defect of tuberculum impar which increases susceptibility of posterior lingual dorsal mucosa to candidiasis
- Clinical appearance: smooth pink or red oval or rhomboid-shaped region of the lingual dorsum, in the posterior midline (anterior to the foramen cecum); may be painful with spicy food or have burning sensation if affected by secondary candidiasis
- Treatment: none required, unless symptomatic from candidiasis, then use systemic antifungal drugs

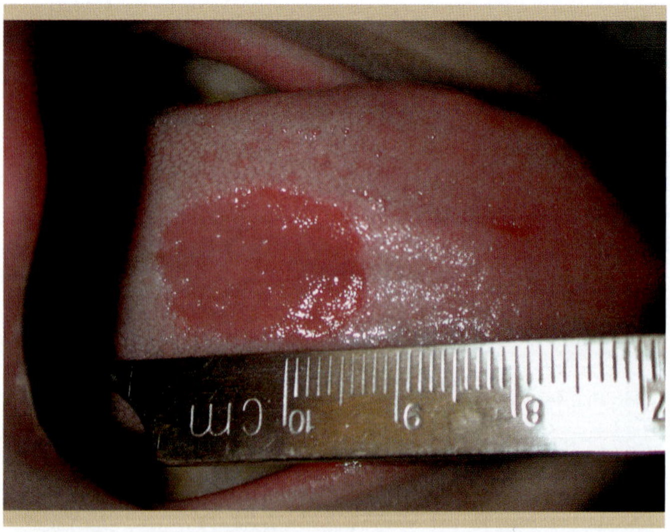

FIGURE 4-10 Median rhomboid glossitis. (*Used with permission from Dr. Kamal Busaidy.*)

Lymphoepithelial Cyst (Fig. 4-11)

- Etiology: entrapment of sloughed keratin in a crypt of a chronically hyperplastic lingual tonsil, with eventual separation of the crypt epithelium from the surface and subsequent cyst formation
- Clinical findings: smooth, asymptomatic whitish-yellow papule almost always less than 5 mm in diameter, typically with adjacent or surrounding lobulated and enlarged lingual tonsil
- Treatment: conservative surgical excision, but the cyst typically remains small and innocuous

Hyperplastic Lingual Tonsil (Fig. 4-12)

- Etiology: Chronic enlargement of normal lymphoid tissues of the lingual tonsils from repeated pharyngitis or "flue."
- Clinical findings: Asymptomatic lobulated soft, sessile or pedunculated masses of the posterior lateral tongue near its attachment; masses may be bilateral and are often semitranslucent or red, but may be pink. **Caution:** if unilateral and firm or ulcerated, may represent *squamous cell carcinoma*; the posterior lateral tongue is the most common site of this cancer. Also, occasionally the lingual tonsils are involved with *lymphoma*.
- Treatment: No treatment is needed unless interferes with chewing or speaking, then conservative surgical removal is the treatment of choice, with biopsy interpretation to rule our *carcinoma* or *lymphoma*

Hyperplastic Circumvallate Papillae (Fig. 4-13)

- Etiology: nonsyndromic developmental anomaly

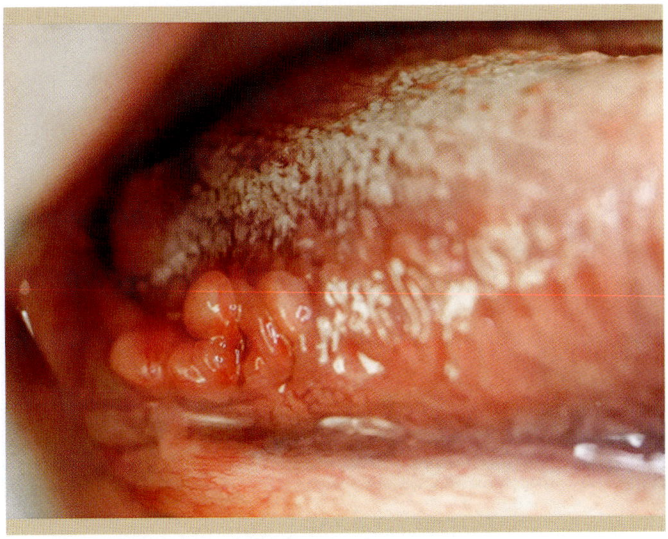

FIGURE 4-12 Hyperplastic lingual tonsil.

- Clinical findings: v-shaped line of 3 to 5 mm diameter pink, asymptomatic papules across the posterior dorsum of the tongue
- Treatment: no treatment required

MUCOSAL DISCOLORATIONS

Leukoplakia (Leukokeratosis, Erythroleukoplakia) (Fig. 4-14)

- Etiology: unknown, but associated with tobacco smoking and ultraviolet radiation (lip vermilion lesions only). This is a premalignant lesion with an approximate 4% lifetime risk of transforming into carcinoma; lesions of oral floor or with irregular/granular surface or admixture of red and white patches have a higher risk

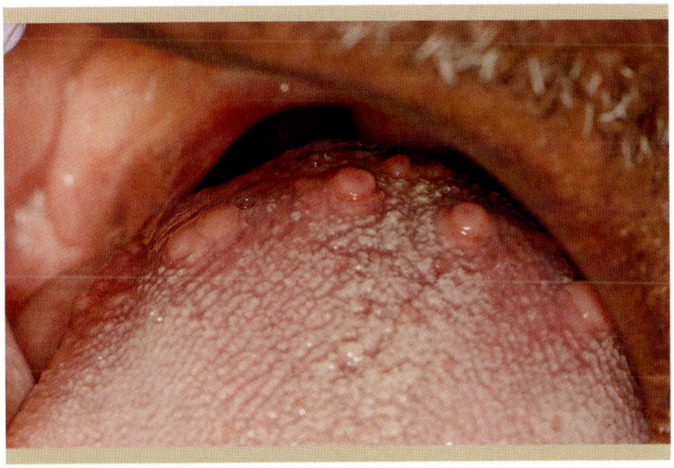

FIGURE 4-13 Hyperplastic circumvallate papillae.

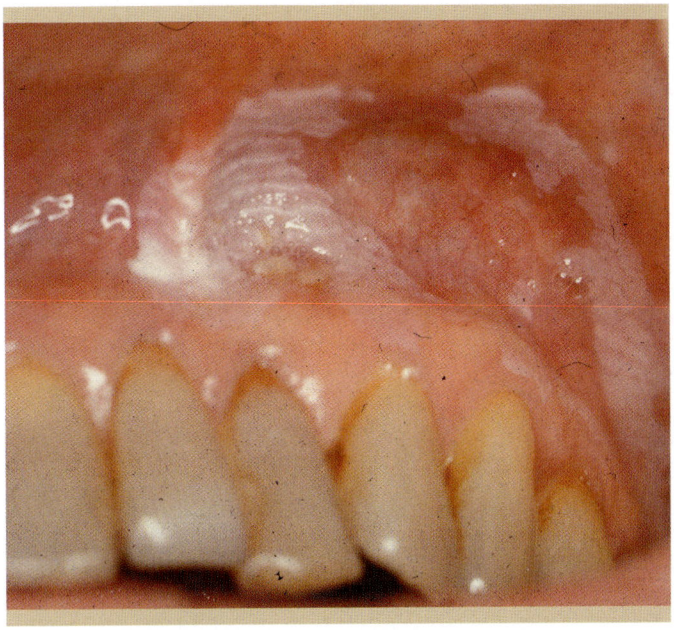

FIGURE 4-14 Leukoplakia. (*Used with permission from Dr. Bela Toth.*)

- Clinical findings: white or red patch varies from flat, smooth, and slightly translucent macular areas to thick, firm, rough-surfaced, and fissured raised plaques.
- Histology: thickened surface parakeratin with or without dysplasia of the more basal cells
- Treatment: conservative excision, when possible, with lose surveillance thereafter. The use of toluidine blue stains or autofluorescence devices may be helpful to identify areas of dysplasia

Frictional Keratosis (Chronic Cheek Bite) (Fig. 4-15)

- Etiology: surface keratin thickening in response to chronic, mild trauma (adjacent sharp teeth, cheek biting habit, tongue thrust habit, etc.)
- Clinical findings: asymptomatic, thickened white, corrugated or velvety, diffuse plaques, usually on buccal mucosa or lateral tongue
- Histology: hyperkeratosis and acanthosis, with intracellular "edema" of superficial epithelial cells (a form of spongiosis)
- Treatment: no treatment is necessary except removal of local irritant. There is no cancer potential if left untreated

Nicotine Palatinus (Piper Smoker Palate) (Fig. 4-16)

- Etiology: hyperkeratosis and sialadenitis of the hard palate from the thermal effects of pipe or cigar smoking; may also occur with heavy cigarette smoking (>2 ppd)
- Clinical findings: diffuse white keratotic thickening of the entire hard palate mucosa, with small papules with central red dots representing inflamed minor salivary glands,

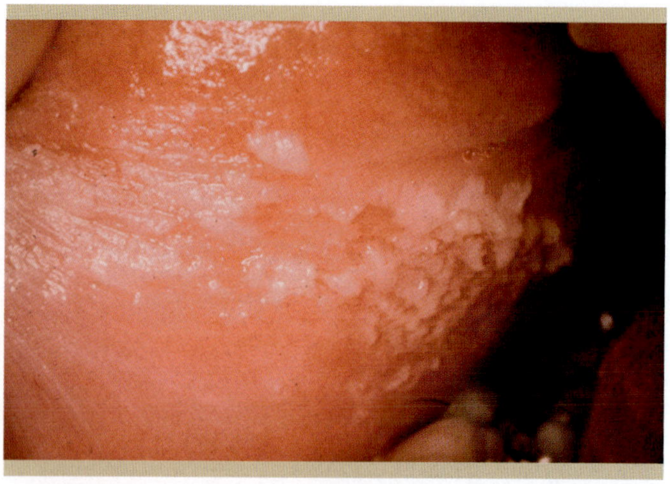

FIGURE 4-15 Chronic cheek bite (frictional keratosis). (*Used with permission from Dr. Robert Gorlin.*)

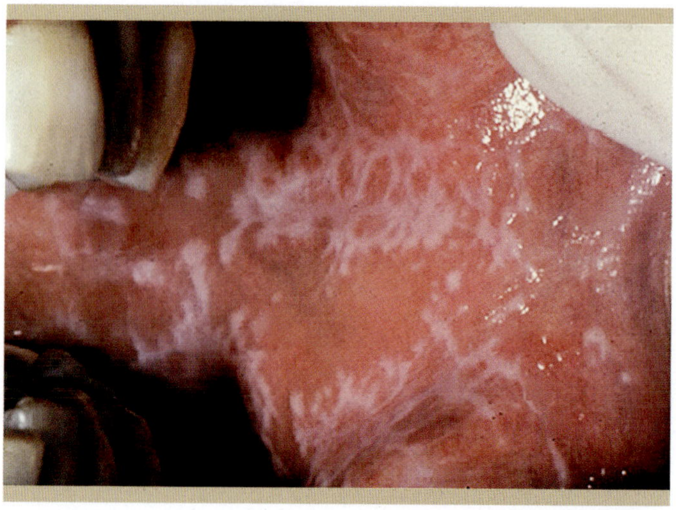

FIGURE 4-17 Lichen planus—reticular type.

which are located only in the posterior 2/3 of the hard palate)

- Treatment: none required but will gradually fade to normal after smoking cessation. **Caution:** this is not considered to be a precancer but any white keratotic patches remaining 4 months after habit cessation should be rediagnosed as *leukoplakia* (see above) and treated accordingly

Lichen Planus (Fig. 4-17)

- Etiology: autoimmune attack, primarily from T-lymphocytes against the oral mucosal epithelium at the level of the basement membrane. Fifteen percent of patients with oral lesions have coincident skin lesions, (purple pruritic polygonal papules). There is an unexplained association with hepatic diseases such as *hepatitis C virus (HCV) infection, autoimmune chronic active hepatitis,* and *primary biliary cirrhosis*

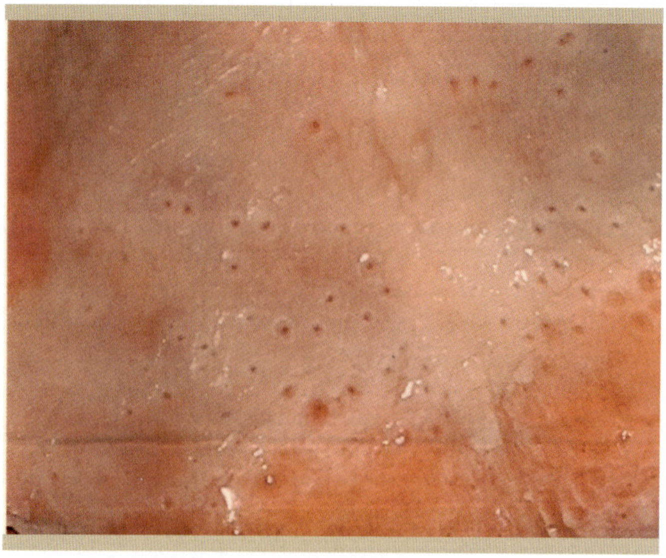

FIGURE 4-16 Nicotine palatinus.

- Clinical findings: reticular white keratotic streaks with fine "sunburst" streaking perpendicular to the larger lines; lines are mistakenly referred to as *Wickham striae.* Usually affects buccal, vestibular, lingual mucosa. Multiple clinical presentations include the *reticular form*; erosive or atrophic form, with an asymptomatic or moderately tender erythematous background behind the white reticular streaks; *ulcerated* and/or *bullous form*, with breakdown ulcers and/or large blister formation. When only gingival tissue are involved, the disease may generically be called *desquamative gingivitis,* a term also applied to gingival pemphigoid cases
- Treatment: there is no cure for lichen planus, but symptomatic cases can be helped by use of topical and systemic corticosteroids or by use of nonsteroidal anti-inflammatory drugs (NSAIDs), especially sulfonylureas, antimalarials, β-blockers, and some angiotensin-converting enzyme (ACE) inhibitors. Erosive forms should be biopsied to evaluate *epithelial dysplasia.* Caution: Lichenoid hypersensitivity reactions (see below) must be ruled out prior to applying a lichen planus designation, Caution: *erosive* and *ulcerative forms* have a 1:200 risk of developing into *squamous cell carcinoma*; the *reticular form* is not considered to be premalignant

Lichenoid Reaction (Cinnamon Reaction) (Fig. 4-18)

- Etiology: topical hypersensitivity response to dental materials, oral hygiene products, food, gum, or candies (especially those with cinnamon or peppermint, or "hot" feeling)
- Clinical findings: same appearance as erosive lichen planus (see above), perhaps with ulceration and pain

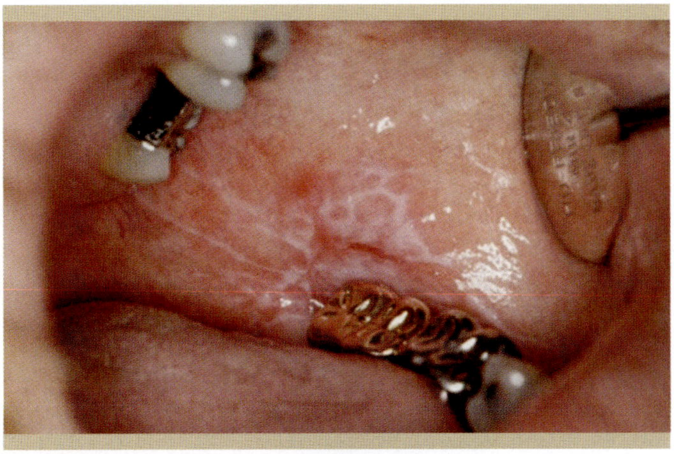

FIGURE 4-18 Lichenoid reaction.

or tenderness, located in area(s) of contact with foreign materials; the localized pattern is what separates this from *lichen planus*—the histopathology is essentially identical for both

- Treatment: none necessary if symptoms are mild; may disappear over time. Usually, however, identification of the allergen (gold, amalgam, cinnamon, or peppermint flavorings) is required, with subsequent removal from the mouth. Chronic cases may become self-perpetuating

Actinic Cheilosis/Cheilitis (Fig. 4-19)

- Etiology: damage from long-term exposure to ultraviolet (UV) light (actinic radiation); often considered to be a premalignant condition with a low risk of transformation into squamous cell carcinoma
- Clinical findings: diffuse puffiness and irregular patchwork of red and pale areas, almost exclusively on the lower lip vermilion. Vertical lines are often identified in the vermilion, along with surface leukoplakia, crusting of the mucosa and ulcers that may be shallow and non-tender

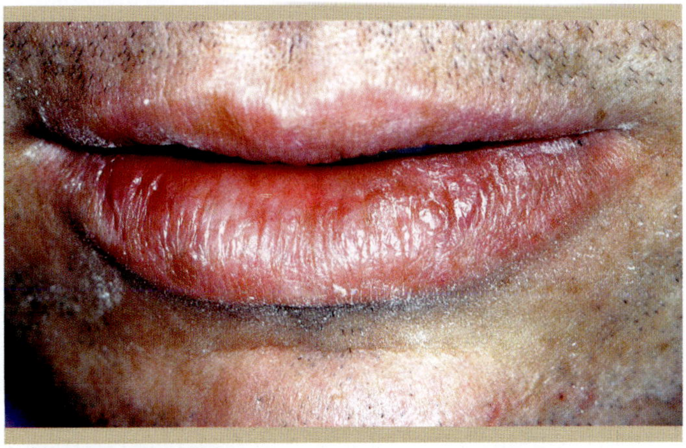

FIGURE 4-19 Actinic cheilosis. (*Used with permission from Dr. Nadarajah Vigneswaran.*)

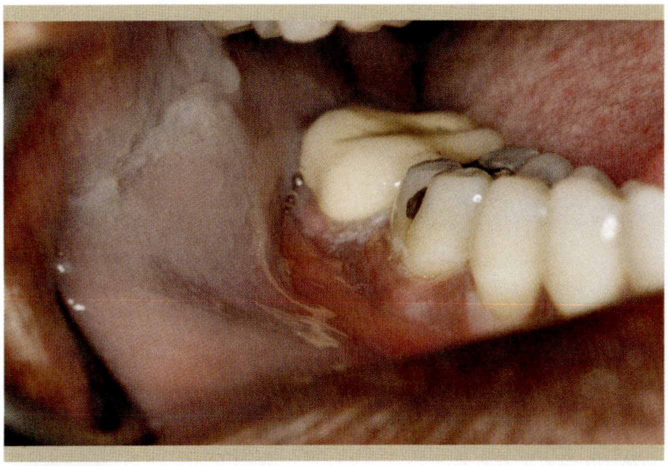

FIGURE 4-20 Leukoedema.

- Histology: hyperkeratosis usually is accompanied by dysplasia and superficial invasion
- Treatment: lip stripping procedure; liquid nitrogen, imiquimod cream 5%, 5-fluorouracil, surgical excision. Long-term follow-up for carcinoma development

Leukoedema (Fig. 4-20)

- Etiology: familial developmental anomaly
- Clinical findings: asymptomatic, symmetric, corrugated or velvety, diffuse white plaques, usually on buccal mucosa. Lesions disappear when the cheek is stretched. May also be seen across the soft palate
- Histology: hyperkeratosis and acanthosis, with intracellular "edema" of superficial epithelial cells (a form of spongiosis)
- Treatment: no treatment is necessary

White Sponge Nevus (Fig. 4-21)

- Etiology: autosomal dominant defect of keratins 4 and 13, causing prolonged retention of surface keratinocytes
- Clinical findings: symmetric, thickened, white, corrugated or velvety, diffuse plaques, usually on buccal mucosa, but maybe on ventral tongue, labial mucosa, soft palate, alveolar mucosa, or floor of the mouth
- Histology: hyperkeratosis and acanthosis, with intracellular "edema" of superficial epithelial cells (a form of spongiosis)
- Treatment: no treatment is necessary

Smokeless Tobacco Keratosis (Tobacco Pouch, Snuff Pouch) (Fig. 4-22)

- Etiology: combined mild chemical burn and mechanical abrasion of the mucosa secondary to chronic and direct contact with chewing tobacco or snuff or betel quid
- Clinical findings: diffuse asymptomatic, poorly demarcated soft white keratosis, often wrinkled, of the

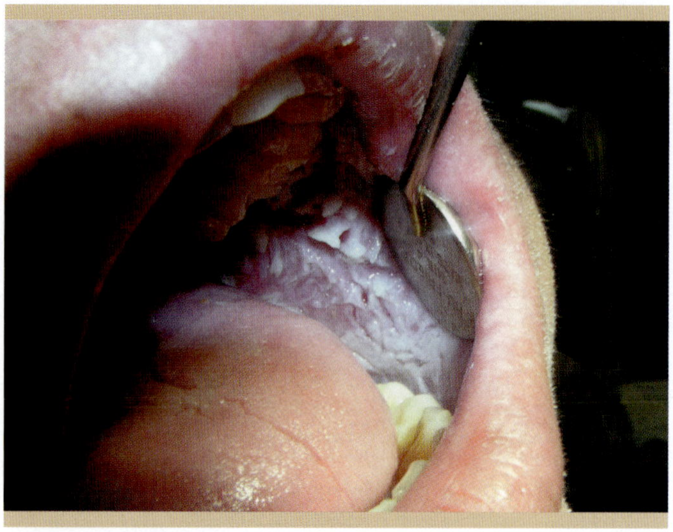

FIGURE 4-21 White sponge nevus. (*Used with permission from Dr. Kelly Peters.*)

vestibule in the area of chronic tobacco placement; no ulceration or induration are seen. Caution: this carries a low-grade risk of development of oral *squamous cell carcinoma* (see below) or *verrucous carcinoma* (see below)
- Treatment: no treatment is needed unless induration, ulceration, or mass formation occurs. Self-palpation can be performed by the patient monthly, with a follow-up professional examination every 6 to 12 months while the tobacco habit remains, with biopsy of any abnormalities. The lesion will slowly fade to normal with cessation of the tobacco habit. Caution: any white patches remaining in the area 4 months after cessation should be rediagnosed as *leukoplakia* and treated accordingly

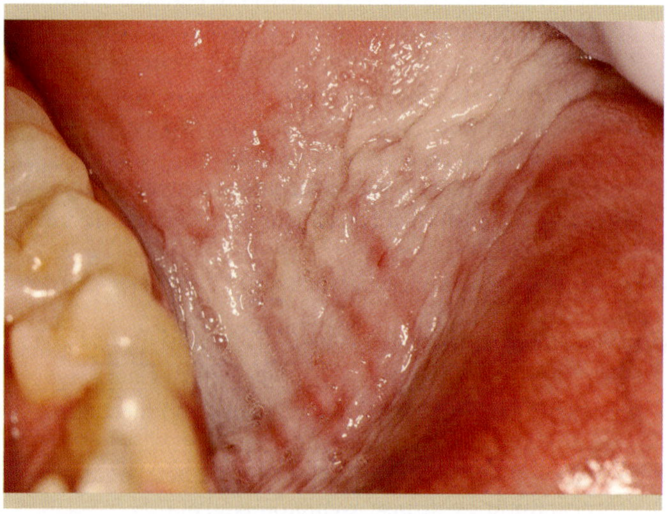

FIGURE 4-22 Smokeless tobacco keratosis.

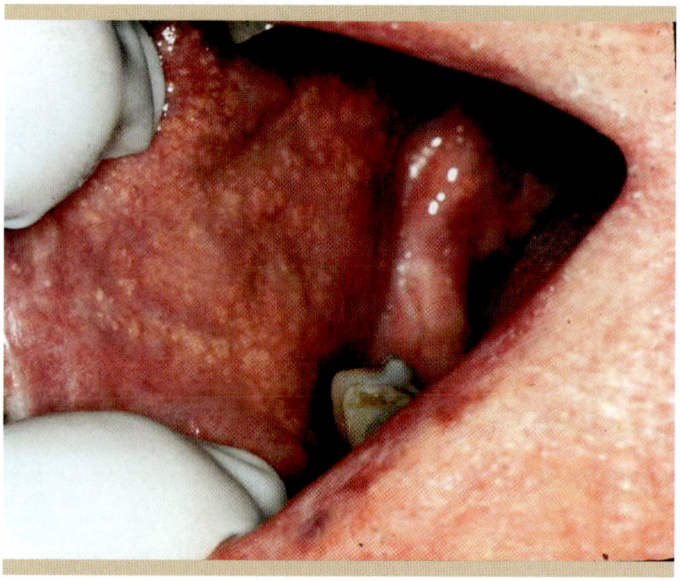

FIGURE 4-23 Fordyce spots. (*Used with permission from Dr. Nadarajah Vigneswaran.*)

Fordyce Granules (Fordyce Spots) (Fig. 4-23)

- Etiology: ectopic sebaceous glands (single or scores of glands)
- Clinical findings: yellow papules, usually on the buccal mucosa (often bilateral) or the interface of the vermilion border and the skin of the upper lip (sometimes referred to as Fox-Fordyce disease). There is no associated taste dysfunction
- Histology: submucosal sebaceous glands, usually without a visible duct
- Treatment: none needed, lesion remain small indefinitely; lip lesions may be surgically removed for aesthetic reasons

Oral Candidiasis (Thrush) (Fig. 4-24)

- Etiology: caused by *Candida albicans*; predisposing factors: dry mouth, immunodeficiency, certain medications (antibiotics, corticosteroids, antidepressants, antipsychotics), diabetes mellitus, vitamin deficiency (especially vitamins B and iron), chemotherapy, radiotherapy, or Sjögren syndrome
- Clinical findings: velvety white plaques in the mouth and on the tongue. Lesions may be rubbed off to leave behind an inflamed base that may be painful and may bleed. Usually a mild and self-limited illness
- Treatment: Oral antifungal agents; use topicals first, then systemic agents for recalcitrant lesions

Subcorneal Acantholytic Keratosis (Fig. 4-25)

- Etiology: may be idiopathic, but often is the result of a mild chemical burn of the oral mucosa secondary to one of the products in toothpaste (especially whitening toothpastes), mouthwash or topical fluoride use; occasionally

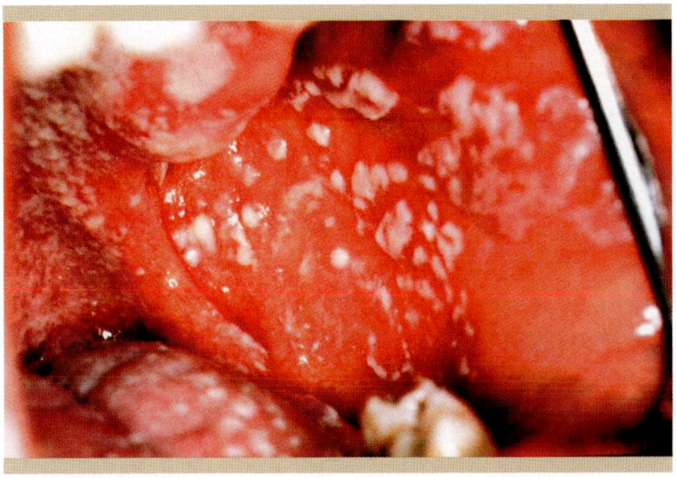

FIGURE 4-24 Pseudomembranous candidiasis (thrush). (*Used with permission from Dr. Nadarajah Vigneswaran.*)

results from chronic placement of cocaine in the lower vestibule
- Clinical findings: mild, asymptomatic diffuse grayish-white alteration of the mucosa, usually in the mandibular vestibule or the oral floor; may be partially scraped off daily to reveal a normal appearing mucosa
- Treatment: no treatment is necessary but will quickly fade to normal with cessation of use of the dental product; idiopathic cases often go on for years without change or increase in severity

Erythroplakia (Carcinoma In Situ) (Fig. 4-26)

- Etiology: premalignancy, often associated with tobacco smoking. High risk of transformation into invasive squamous cell carcinoma
- Clinical findings: red, smooth, soft macule, perhaps with a pebbled surface change, and perhaps with white keratotic patches (erythroleukoplakia)

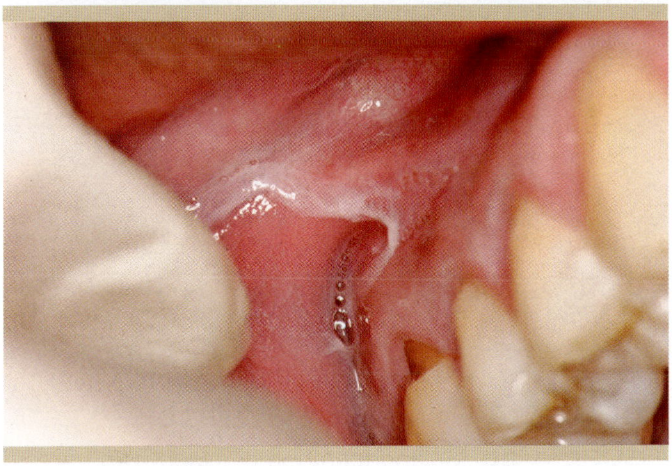

FIGURE 4-25 Subcorneal acantholytic keratosis.

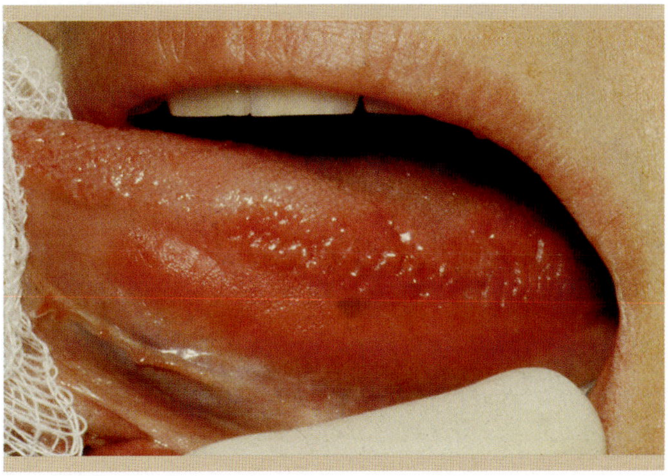

FIGURE 4-26 Erythroplakia (Carcinoma in situ).

- Histology: anaplasia with or without hyperkeratosis; no invasion beyond basement membrane
- Treatment: surgical excision. Close surveillance required due to potential for malignant transformation

Oral Melanosis (Fig. 4-27)

- Causes: physiologic pigmentation (normal racial brown, systemic medications (AZT, chloroquine, tranquilizers, etc.); tobacco smoking (smoker's melanosis)
- Clinical findings: single or multiple asymptomatic brown macules, usually with irregular outline, possibly with poorly demarcated borders, possibly with areas in increased darkness; physiologic pigmentation has childhood onset and no change after 20 years of age

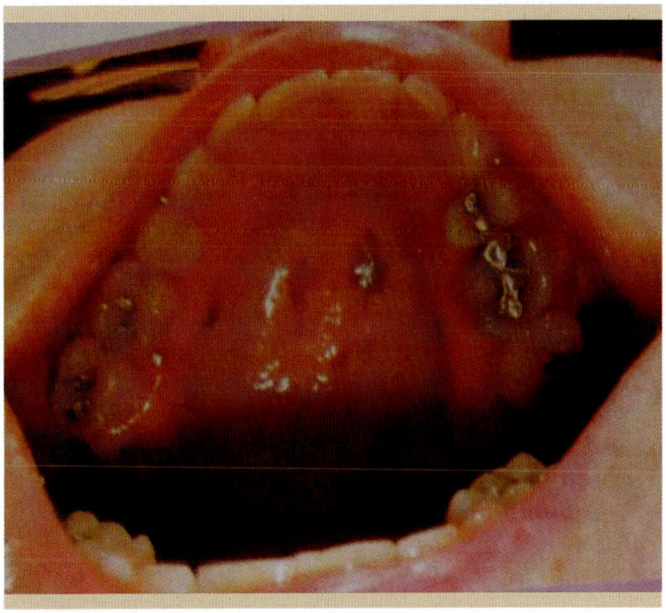

FIGURE 4-27 Focal melanosis. (*Used with permission from Dr. Mark Wong.*)

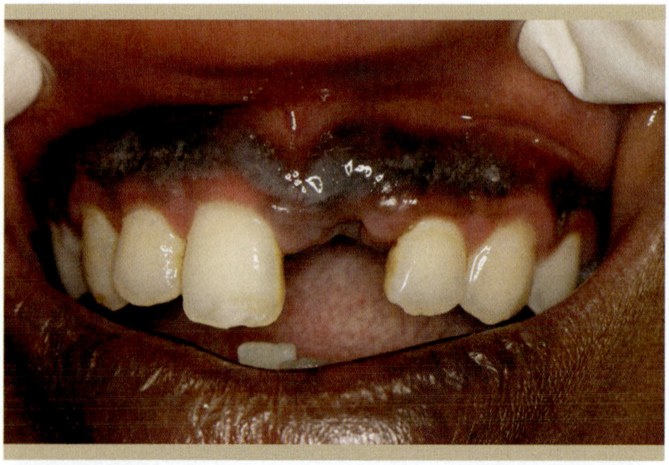

FIGURE 4-28 Physiologic (Racial) melanosis, with whitish-gray keratin covering from cocaine placement.

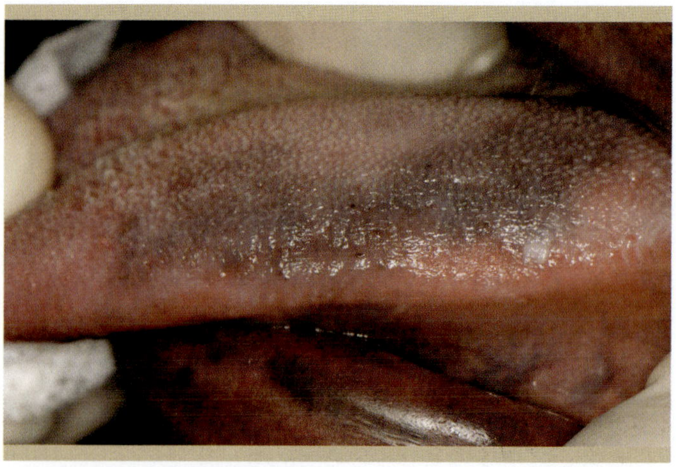

FIGURE 4-29 Drug-induced pigmentation (grayish-brown discoloration from AZT for HIV; patient also has leukoedema (see Fig. 4-20).

- Histology: increased melanin in basal layer, otherwise normal appearance
- Treatment: none required; drug-induced melanosis usually disappears with cessation of drug use

Physiologic Melanosis (Racial Pigmentation) (Fig. 4-28)

- Etiology: normal increased melanin deposition in the basal layer of the oral epithelium, especially in persons with normally dark skin pigmentation
- Clinical findings: light to dark brown, well demarcated, evenly colored macules of the gingival or any other oral surface except the vermilion borders of the lips; childhood onset, becomes more pronounced up to and sometimes beyond puberty
- Treatment: no treatment is needed once there is confirmation of the long-term presence since childhood. Caution: any oral melanosis of less than a year's duration in an adult should be biopsied to make absolutely sure it is not an early *melanoma*, since the survival from that disease is dismal unless caught at the earliest possible stage

Drug-Induced Pigmentation (Fig. 4-29)

- Etiology: melanin deposits within the epithelium or precipitation of unknown compounds immediately beneath the epithelium as a secondary response to systemic drugs; not a sign of overdose or adverse side effects
- Clinical findings: irregular, asymptomatic, nonhemorrhagic, brown or gray discoloration of any mucosal surface, but usually the palate or gingivae
- Treatment: no treatment needed but will slowly fade away with discontinuation of the systemic medication

Melanoacanthoma, Melanoacanthosis (Fig. 4-30)

- Etiology: unknown, but considered a reactive process; not related to melanoacanthosis of the skin
- Clinical findings: brown/black pigmentation of gingiva, tongue, palate. Macules can be several centimeters in diameter
- Histology: acanthosis with dendritic melanocytes scattered between keratinocytes throughout all epithelial layers
- Treatment: none required; will gradually return to normal over 3 to 6 weeks

Amalgam Tattoo (Fig. 4-31)

- Etiology: traumatic impaction of amalgam particles into submucosal regions
- Clinical findings: gray or bluish gray macule with moderately well-demarcated borders

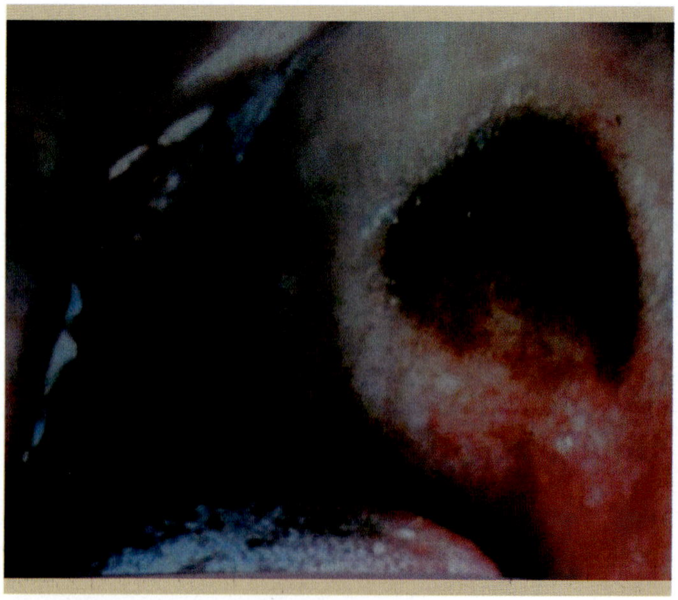

FIGURE 4-30 Melanoacanthoma. (*Used with permission from Dr. Nadarajah Vigneswaran.*)

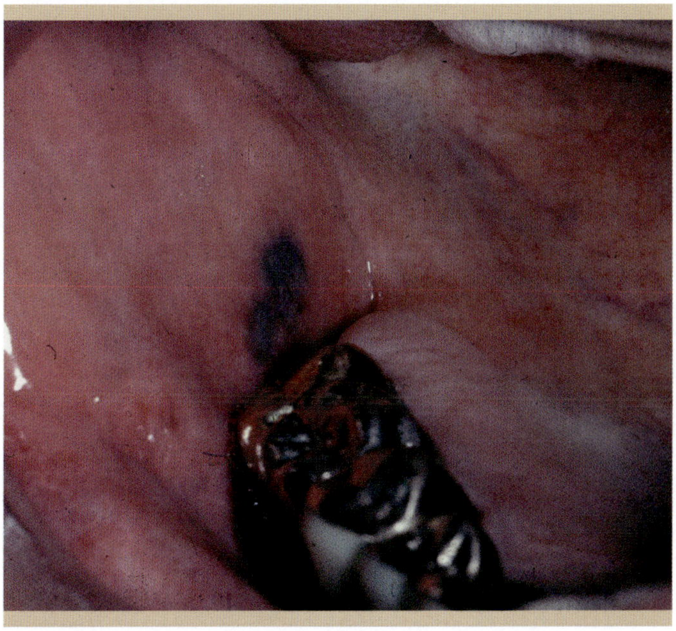

FIGURE 4-31 Amalgam tattoo. (*Used with permission from Dr. Bela Toth.*)

- Histology: black fragments of metal within submucosa, usually without an inflammatory response
- Treatment: no treatment necessary

MUCOSAL ULCERS

Aphthous Stomatitis (Canker Sore) (Fig. 4-32)

- Etiology: autoimmune disease, hypersensitivity response, nutritional deficiency, sometimes part of a systemic disorder (ulcerative colitis, Crohn disease; Behçet syndrome); often a strong familial component. Typically enhanced by stress; may be triggered by minor trauma

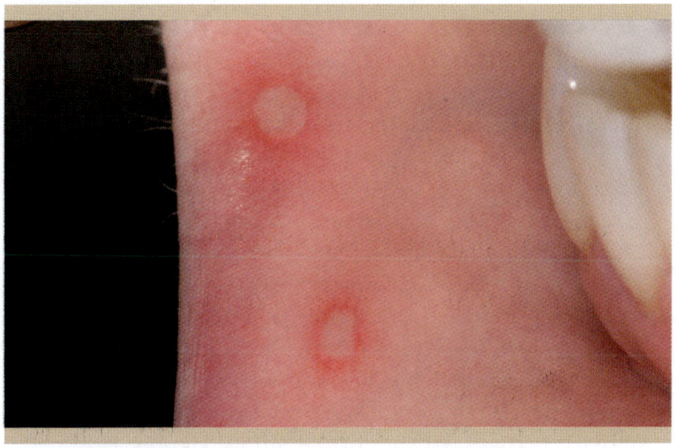

FIGURE 4-32 Aphthous stomatitis (canker sores).

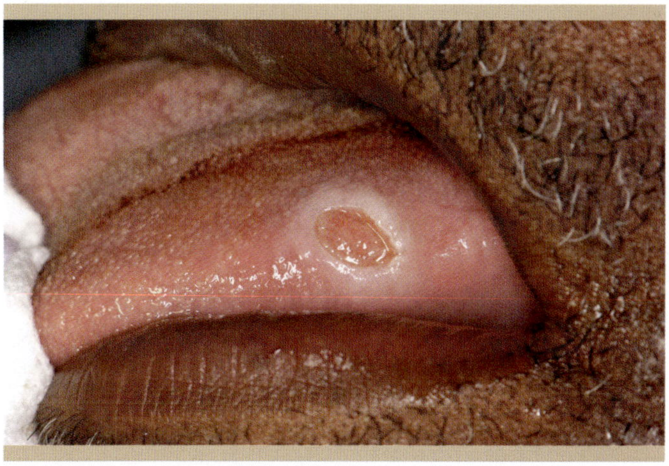

FIGURE 4-33 Traumatic ulcer.

- Clinical findings: very painful ulcers of any mucosal site except mucosa overlying jawbone. Often a 1 to 2 day prodromal tenderness or erythema. Ulcers are 2 to 30 mm, have red inflammatory halos for first 4 to 5 days and have saucerized ulcer beds. There are 3 forms: recurrent aphthous ulcers (RAU) minor (80% of all cases); RAU major (numerous ulcers, large ulcers, may produce scars); herpetiform RAU (occurs in clusters that mimic may consist of tens or hundreds of minute ulcers)
- Treatment: topical corticosteroids are the mainstay of treatment, with systemic steroids for refractory cases. Colchicine (0.6 mg tid) if associated with arthralgias; Cimetidine (200 mg bid/qid); Azathioprine (50 mg qd) if ocular lesions; Thalidomide (requires special FDA approval for use)

Traumatic Ulcer (Fig. 4-33)

- Etiology: acute trauma to mucosa
- Clinical findings: abrupt onset ulcer has clean ulcer bed initially but the bed quickly becomes white from surface necrosis and develops inflammatory red halo. May be very deep
- Treatment: topical anesthesia as needed; heals spontaneously in 3 to 7 days

Traumatic Ulcerative Granuloma With Stromal Eosinophilia (TUGSE; Traumatic Eosinophilic Ulcer) (Fig. 4-34)

- Etiology: unknown but usually initiated by trauma or irritation. Eosinophils may be from muscle damage in this deep ulcer
- Clinical findings: 2 to 3 cm, deep, mildly tender ulcer with minimal inflammatory red halo and very long duration (months). Occasional lesions are ulcerated masses, similar to pyogenic granuloma (see below)
- Treatment: remove local causes of recurring trauma, then conservative surgical excision. Recurrences are common and required somewhat more aggressive surgical removal

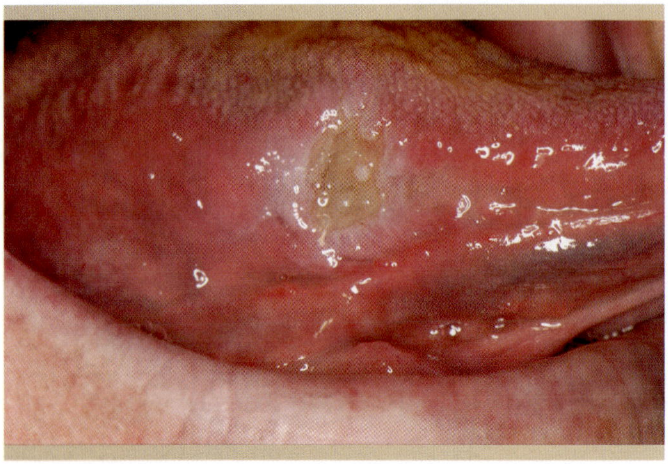

FIGURE 4-34 Traumatic ulcerative granuloma with stromal eosinophilia (TUGSE).

Bisphosphonate-Related Osteonecrosis of the Jaws (BRONJ) (Fig. 4-35)

- Etiology: unknown, but presumed to be from surface trauma to mucosa overlying ischemic alveolar bone "damaged" by long-term use of bisphosphonates, especially those given intravenously
- Clinical findings: chronic (>6 weeks) exposure of bone in the mouth in a patient taking bisphosphonate drugs for metastasis, multiple myeloma, or osteoporosis. It may be free of pain or excruciatingly painful. Mucosa at the edge of the ulcer often shows a remarkable lack of erythema and edema but may mimic a "rolled border." Often a history of recent dental extraction or trauma in the area
- Treatment: conservative debridement of loose bone fragments and good oral hygiene related to soft tissues on ulcer edge. antibiotics if superinfected

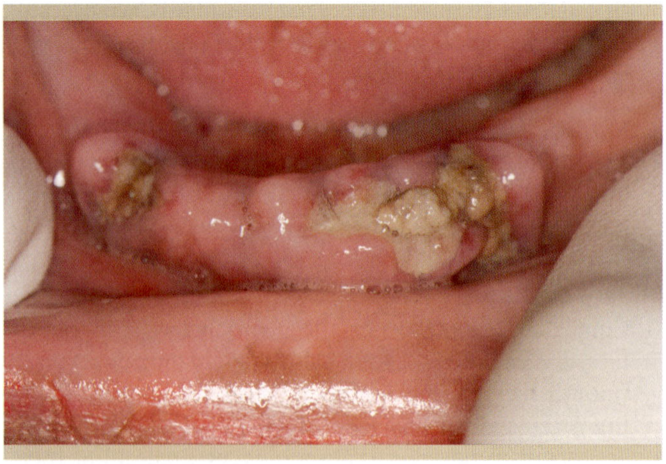

FIGURE 4-35 Bisphosphonate-related osteonecrosis of the jaws (BRONJ).

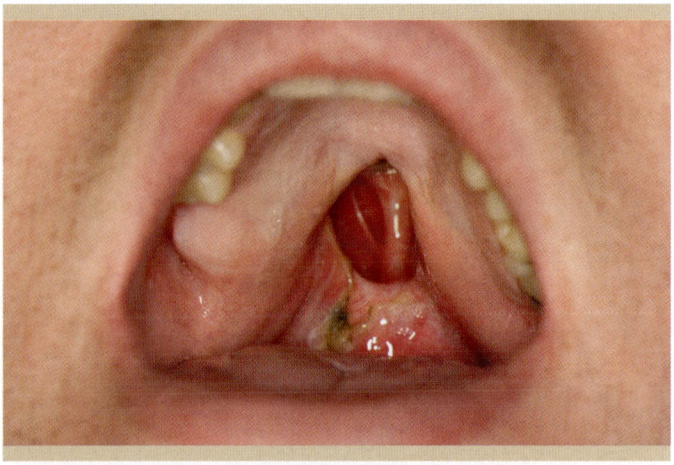

FIGURE 4-36 Perforated palate from phycomycosis.

Mucormycosis (Phycomycosis) (Fig. 4-36)

- Etiology: infection by phycomycosis or any other deep fungus, almost always in persons who are immune compromised, especially in AIDS and the terminal stage of malignancy. A variety of other disorders may cause painless palatal perforation, especially tertiary syphilis, tuberculosis, Wegener granulomatosis, midline lethal granuloma (angiocentric T-cell lymphoma), and chronic sniffing of cocaine
- Clinical findings: painless deep ulceration of the hard palate mucosa with little or no red inflammatory halo around it and typically with fatty tissue in the ulcer bed. There is eventual destruction of the palatal bone and possible extension onto the soft palate
- Treatment: systemic antifungals with probably surgical removal of residual diseased tissues and with reconstructive surgery once the infection is controlled

Squamous Cell Carcinoma (Fig. 4-37)

- Etiology: malignant neoplasm of stratified squamous epithelium with multistep, multifactorial features, associated primarily with tobacco use, alcohol abuse, and possibly, human papillomavirus
- **Clinical findings**: early lesions look like small, indurated ulcers without a surrounding inflammatory halo, or may look like leukoplakia, erythroplakia, or ulcerated indurated mass, like a pyogenic granuloma. Late lesions are larger, painless ulcers, ulcerated or fungating mass, or verrucous or papillary mass. Usually has been present more than a year prior to diagnosis
- **Histology**: dysplastic, invading squamous epithelium of varying levels of dysplasia, with pleomorphic, enlarged and hyperchromatic nuclei, large and pleomorphic cells, keratin pearls (abnormal keratinization), increased mitotic activity, perhaps with abnormal mitotic figures
- **Treatment**: surgical excision, radiation therapy

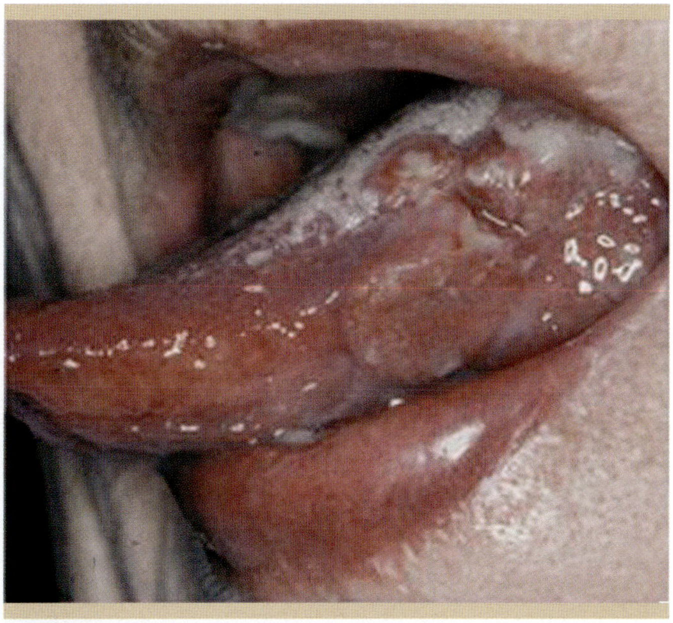

FIGURE 4-37 Squamous cell carcinoma. (*Used with permission from Dr. Bela Toth*).

Primary Herpetic Gingivostomatitis (Fig. 4-38)

- Etiology: initial infection by type I herpes simplex; by adulthood, more than 90% of U.S. citizens have antibodies against the virus. Complete or partial immunity is imparted for a lifetime, with recurrences being much less severe
- Clinical findings: multiple scattered, painful, small, flat-based ulcers (vesicles if seen prior to rupture), 2 to 3 mm in diameter, with a white ulcer bed and surrounding erythematous inflammatory halo.Vesicles can affect any surface but erythematous and edematous gingivitis is always seen with this condition. Low-grade fever often occurs; pain usually disappears in 4 to 6 days; ulcers heal completely without scar formation
- Treatment: none is effective, so palliation and assurance of its short duration are provided; parents should watch for lethargy, psychosis, or other signs of herpetic encephalitis (very, very small risk). Antibiotics can be used for secondary bacterial infections producing high fever or enlarged, tender cervical nodes

Recurrent Herpes Labialis (Fever Blisters) (Fig. 4-39)

- Etiology: recurrence of type 1 herpes simplex; probably induced by stress or decreased immune surveillance of the virus, which remains indefinitely in the trigeminal nerve after the primary infection
- Clinical findings: clustered small flat-based, painful ulcers (vesicles, if seen prior to rupture) of the para-vermilion skin and vermilion borders of the lips; may be bilateral at the commissures. For 1 to 2 days before vesicles appear, the area may show prodromal tenderness or erythema. Vesicles are all present within a day, and then take 4 to 5 days to become nonpainful; vesicles heal without scar formation. There is a rare intraoral version called *recurrent intraoral herpes simplex*, which presents as a cluster of vesicles on bone bound tissue, usually the gingivae
- Treatment: keep the affected skin dry and apply a cold compress (ice cube held in a tee shirt works well). If identified at the earliest manifestation or prodromal, topical and/or systemic antivirals may be used

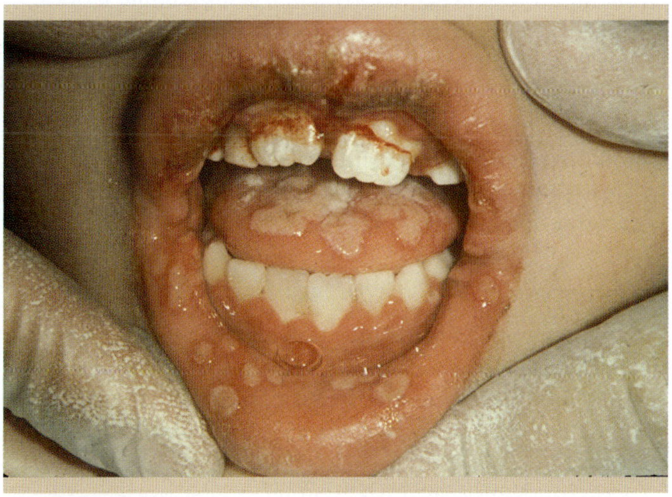

FIGURE 4-38 Primary herpetic gingivostomatitis, with vesicles and acute gingivitis (red, enlarged gingiva).

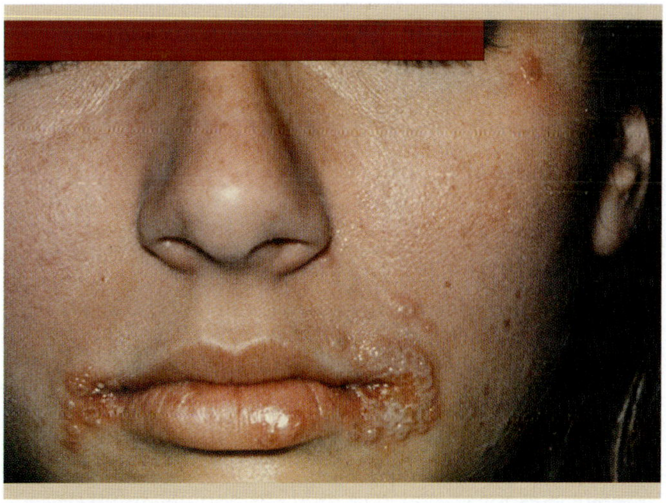

FIGURE 4-39 Recurrent herpes labialis (small vesicles of the tip of tongue are not part of the recurrence—this was the first sign of leukemia in the young patient).

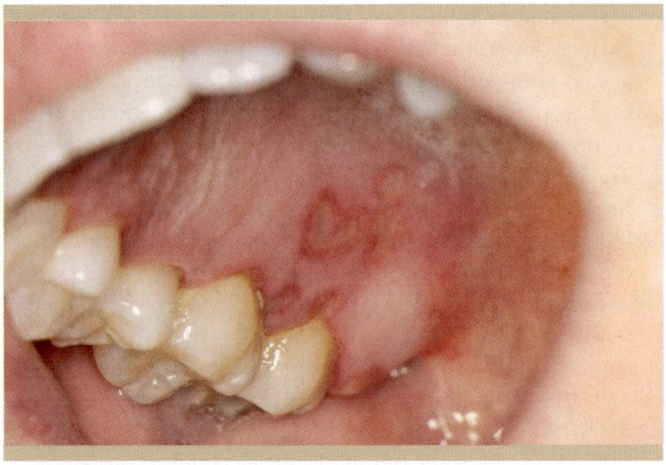

FIGURE 4-40 Herpes zoster (shingles) of the right hard palate, triggered by very hot soup.

Herpes Zoster (Shingles) (Fig. 4-40)

- Etiology: recurrent infection by the varicella-zoster virus. The primary attack is varicella (chickenpox), which is quite generalized but recurrences typically follow a dermatome pattern—in the H&N region it follows a branch of the trigeminal nerve. Cause of recurrence is unknown but may be related to stress, immunosuppression, or trauma (including dental restorative procedures)
- Clinical findings: widely scattered, small (<3 mm), painful ulcers (vesicles if seen prior to rupture) of a region of the oral mucosa; almost always unilateral. Differs from other oral viral diseases in that new vesicles occur for days, often while older vesicles are well into their healing phase. Duration is 1 to 4 weeks with healing occurring without scar formation. Caution: possible *post-herpetic neuralgia* may develop several months to a few years later in a small proportion of patients
- Treatment: Palliation is usually ineffective. The same antivirals used for skin involvement are used for oral infections

Cicatricial Pemphigoid (Mucous Membrane Pemphigoid) (Fig. 4-41)

- Etiology: self-limiting autoimmune disorder, similar to the skin variant, but only a small proportion of patients develop skin lesions, but eye and genital membranes may be involved as well
- Clinical findings: moderate to large bullae, almost always broken, with a flat white ulcer bed and minimal red inflammatory halo or edema of mucosa at the margins
- Histology: subepidermal separation with minimal inflammatory response; may be a mild eosinophilic infiltrate. Direct immunofluorescence of intact mucosa shows IgG globular deposits along the basement membrane
- Treatment: corticosteroid therapy: oral and/or topical; immunosuppressive therapy

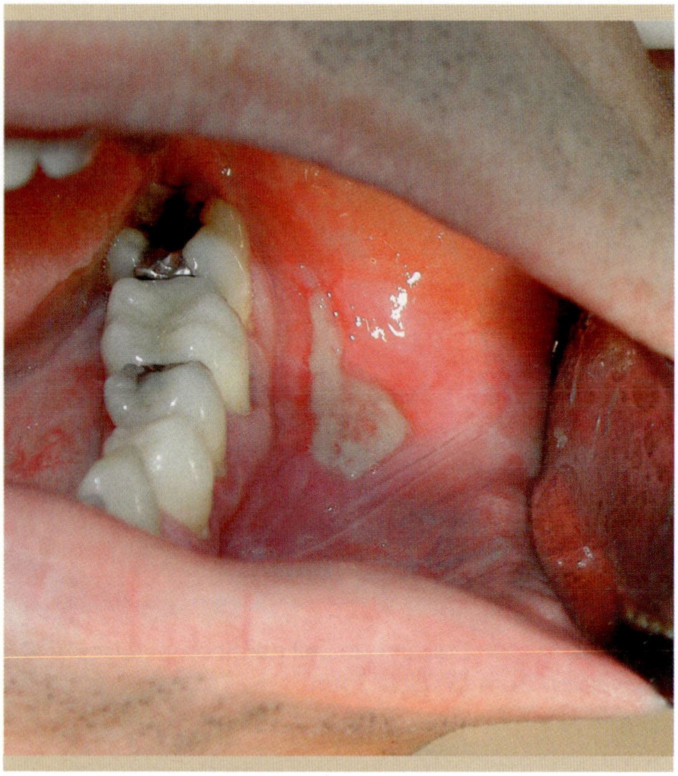

FIGURE 4-41 Mucous membrane (cicatricial) pemphigoid with bulla base in mandibular vestibule. (*Used with permission from Dr. Kamal Busaidy.*)

Erythema Multiforme (Fig. 4-42)

- Etiology: appears to be a hypersensitivity response, especially to herpetic viral infection and certain drugs (NSAIDs, sulphonamides, penicillamine)
- Clinical findings: shallow oral ulcerations, crusted bleeding lips, often erythematous skin lesions ("target lesions"). Steven-Johnson syndrome is a more severe form of EM and is associated with conjunctivitis and genital ulceration
- Histology: subepithelial or intraepithelial lysis with edema and mixed inflammatory infiltrate of stroma
- Treatment: systemic corticosteroids; hydration; analgesia; self-limiting usually

Actinomycosis (Fig. 4-43)

- Etiology: opportunistic infection by facultatively or strictly anaerobic gram-positive bacilli, actinomyces, a bacteria with fungi-like structures that is part of the normal flora of the upper respiratory, gastrointestinal, and female genital tracts. Usually associated with dental or periodontal disease or oral trauma
- Clinical findings: single or multiple chronically draining abscesses and interconnecting sinus tracts, often with sulfur granules (colonies appearing as small yellowish

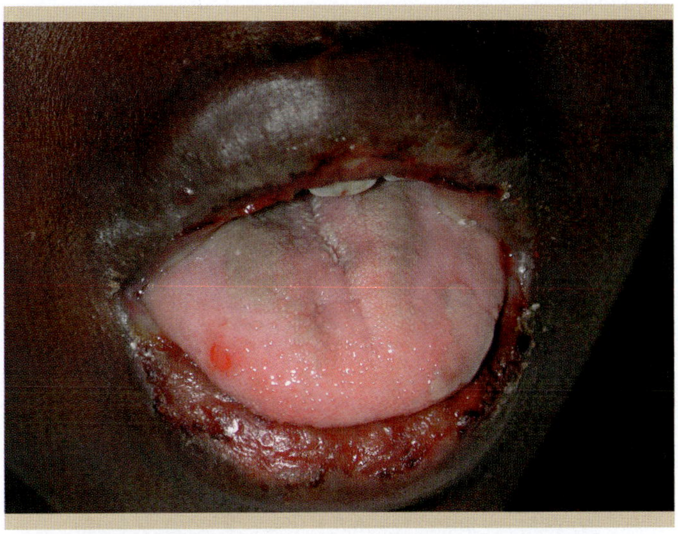

FIGURE 4-42 Erythema multiforme, with erythema and mucosal ulceration of the tongue, with crusting of the vermilion borders.

"rice granules"). Cervicofacial actinomycosis is the most common form
- Treatment: surgical debridement and long-term antibiotic therapy (susceptible to penicillin). May consider prophylactic antibiotics prior to future surgical procedures

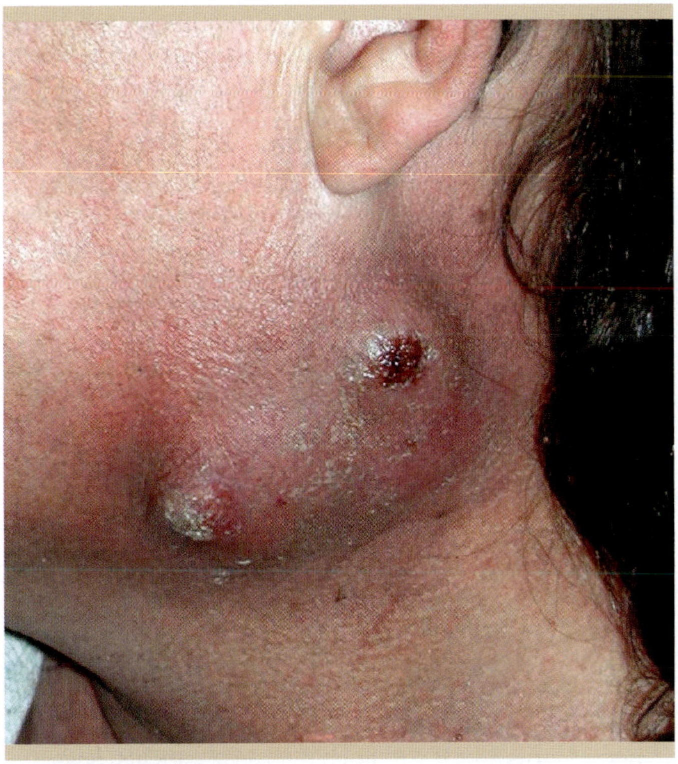

FIGURE 4-43 Actinomycosis.

Radiotherapy and Chemotherapy-Induced Oral Mucositis

- Etiology: damage via cytokine release and reduced cell division from therapeutic irradiation to the oral region or from chemotherapy drugs, especially those affecting hematopoietic tissue, antimetabolites such as fluorouracil, methotrexate, and purine antagonists
- Clinical findings: multifocal, very painful mucosal erythema and breakdown ulceration or erosions, sometimes with a fibrinous pseudomembrane covering. May become colonized by mixed flora, especially *Candida*
- Treatment: analgesics and nutritional support, antimicrobial treatment for secondary infection, tocopherol (vitamin E; accelerates mucosal healing), ice chips, induce local vasoconstriction; reduce amount of fluorouracil delivered to oral mucosal cells, palifermin-synthetic keratinocyte growth factor

MASSES WITH IRREGULAR SURFACES

Pyogenic Granuloma (Fig. 4-44)

- Etiology: proliferative inflammatory response to chronic trauma or irritation
- Clinical findings: smooth or lobulated red to purple mass that may be either pedunculated or sessile; commonly on the gingiva but can occur anywhere in the mouth
- Histology: proliferating granulation tissue with vascular channels, edema, and a mixed inflammatory infiltrate
- Treatment: surgical excision, laser excision. Removal of underlying irritant

Epulis Fissuratum (Denture Injury Tumor) (Fig. 4-45)

- Etiology: proliferative fibrous tissue from chronic, constant, low-grade trauma of a denture edge on the mucosa of the vestibule

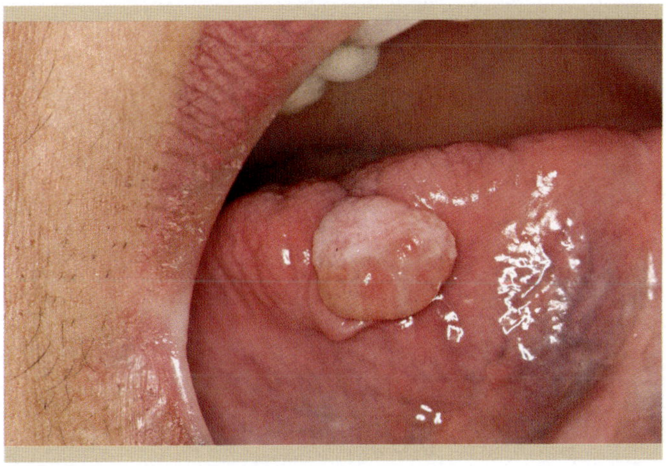

FIGURE 4-44 Pyogenic granuloma.

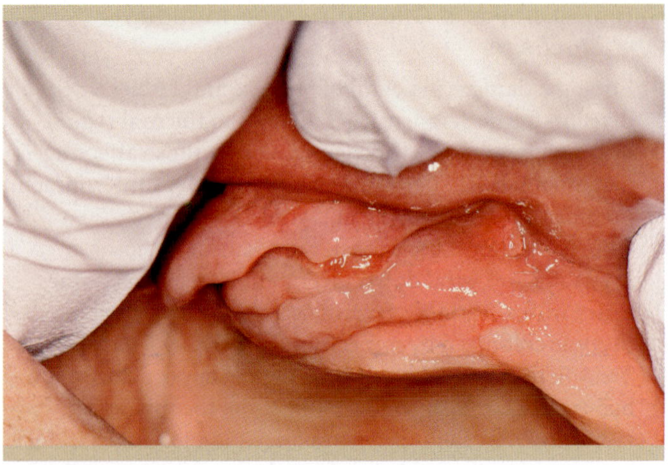

FIGURE 4-45 Epulis fissuratum (denture injury tumor).

- Clinical findings: asymptomatic, linear, lobulated, pink and focally red mass parallel to the alveolus; may have multiple "waves" of linear masses ("redundant tissue"). Usually found in the anterior mandibular or maxillary vestibule; associated with an old, loose denture. May be ulcerated
- Treatment: surgical excision, laser excision, with repair or remake of the offending denture; no cancer potential

Peripheral Ossifying Fibroma (Fig. 4-46)

- Etiology: inflammatory proliferation of periodontal ligament cells from chronic local inflammation; may occur in recent extraction socket (clinical term for inflammatory mass in socket is epulis granulomatosum)
- Clinical Findings: firm, often ulcerated mass occurring exclusively on the gingivae or alveolar mucosa, especially near the anterior teeth. May look more vascular, similar to a pyogenic granuloma, which is less firm. May show internal calcification on radiograph and may spread teeth apart.
- Histology: fibrous, cellular proliferation with variable amounts of bone formation, often with osteoblastic rimming
- Treatment: excision down to and including periosteum; scrape root surface; if in socket, curette thoroughly, including removal of residual periodontal ligament

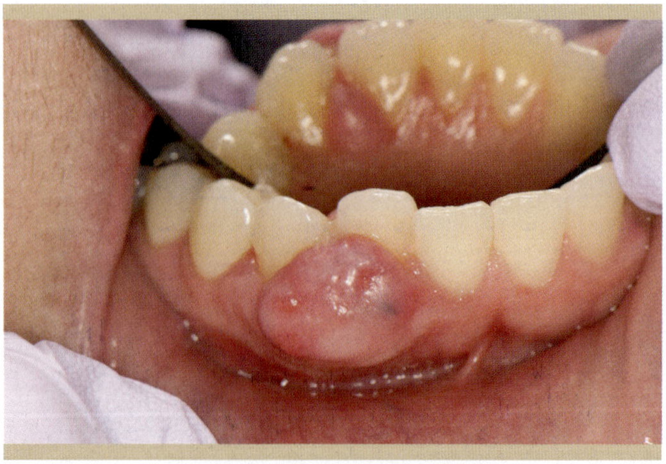

FIGURE 4-46 Peripheral ossifying fibroma.

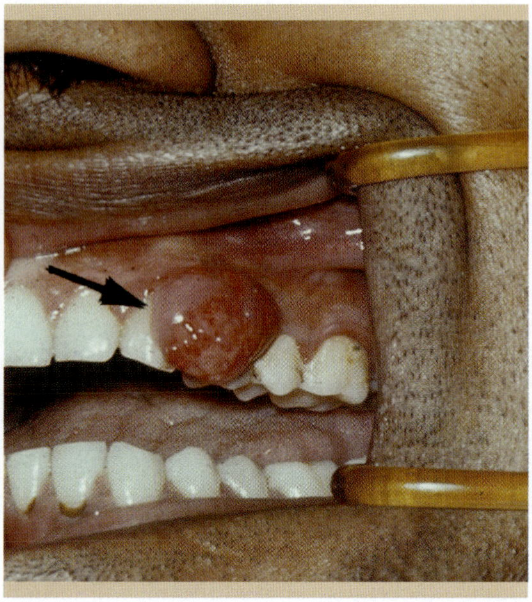

FIGURE 4-47 Peripheral giant cell granuloma.

Peripheral Giant Cell Granuloma (Fig. 4-47)

- Etiology: inflammatory proliferation of periodontal ligament cells from chronic local inflammation; may occur in recent extraction socket (clinical term for inflammatory mass in socket is epulis granulomatosum)
- Clinical findings: lobulated, asymptomatic, red or brown, usually ulcerated, firm mass, often similar to appearance of pyogenic granuloma. Always located on the gingivae or alveolar mucosa. May push adjacent teeth aside
- Histology: similar to central giant cell granuloma with multinucleated giant cells and extravasated erythrocytes in a background of uniform but immature spindle-shaped mesenchymal cells; may have abundant new bone formation near periphery
- Treatment: excision and removal of underlying irritant, including scraping the root surface

Kaposi Sarcoma (Fig. 4-48)

- Etiology: vascular proliferation induced by human herpes virus 8 (HHV 8) in HIV positive patients; not a true sarcoma

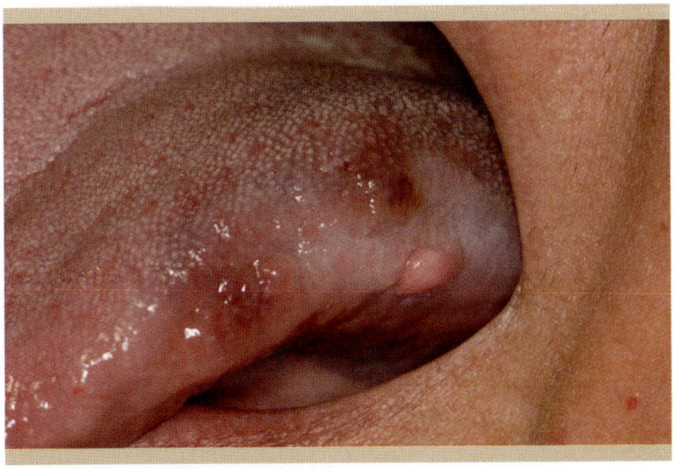

FIGURE 4-48 Kaposi sarcoma in AIDS (with unrelated irritation fibroma of lateral tongue).

- Clinical findings: brown, red, or purple macules, usually on the hard palate or gingiva but can be found on the tongue, uvula, tonsils, pharynx, and trachea. The macule may become a lobulated discolored, perhaps ulcerated mass. Some lesions start de novo as masses
- Treatment: excision of the local lesion; highly active antiretroviral therapy (HAART) or intralesional chemotherapy

Hemangioma (Fig. 4-49)

- Etiology: developmental hamartoma or benign neoplasm (if postnatal onset) of blood vessels. Sometimes results from abnormal healing after trauma

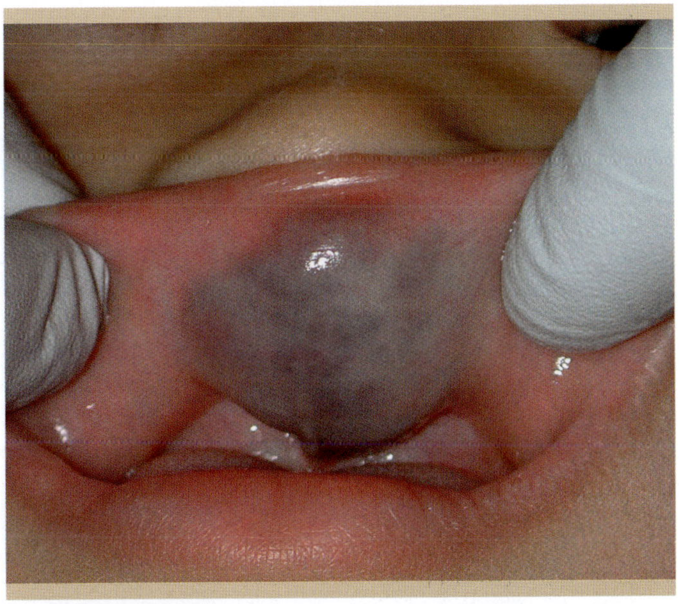

FIGURE 4-49 Hemangioma. (*Used with permission from Dr. Kamal Busaidy.*)

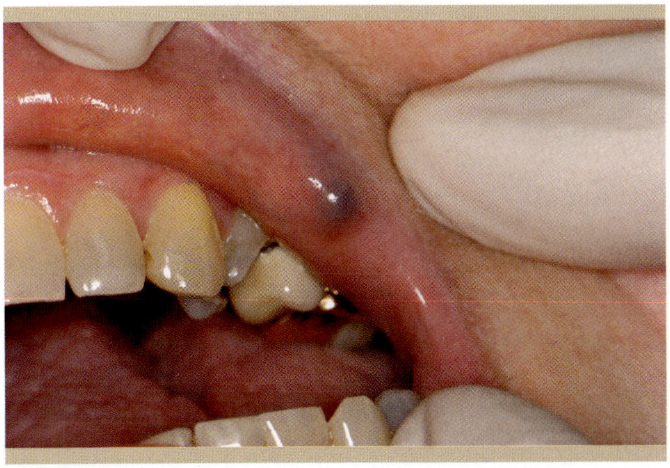

FIGURE 4-50 Traumatic angiomatous lesion (venous pool).

- Clinical findings: occurs usually in childhood, presenting as a lobulated red, purple, or bluish, soft mucosal mass strawberry hemangioma. Capillary types are firmer, with small, more uniform lobules, while cavernous type are soft and often fluctuant, with more of a tendency to be blue
- Treatment: capillary types commonly involute in time. Cavernous types do not involute, and require excision if causing functional or cosmetic disturbance

Traumatic Angiomatous Lesion (Venous Lake) (Fig. 4-50)

- Etiology: ballooned weak spot in a superficial vein secondary to acute trauma
- Clinical findings: small, asymptomatic, sessile, blanching mass of the lower lip vermilion or mucosa (rarely on upper lip); develops quickly and remains unchanged indefinitely
- Treatment: surgical excision for esthetic reasons, otherwise no treatment needed because the lesion remains very small

Lymphangioma (Fig. 4-51)

- Etiology: developmental hamartoma of lymphatic vessels; occasionally, induced by improper healing after injury
- Clinical findings: clusters vesicle-like, nonblanching, soft mass, usually less than 4 cc. Tongue and buccal are the most common sites of involvement
- Treatment: surgical excision or produce scarring with chemicals or lasers; ganciclovir, topical retinoids.

Papilloma (Squamous Papilloma) (Fig. 4-52)

- Etiology: a benign epithelial proliferation induced by human papillomavirus, especially types 6 and 11. Occasionally, an HIV positive person develops numerous oral papillomas

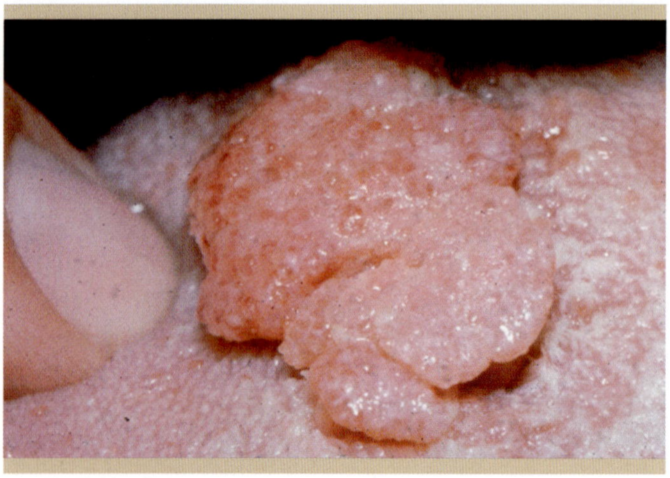

FIGURE 4-51 Lymphangioma of lingual dorsum.

- Clinical findings: single, usually less than 5 mm, soft, asymptomatic pedunculated, and verruciform or papillary mass of any mucosal surface; usually reaches full size within a few months and remains indefinitely thereafter. Minimally contagious, seldom shows as multiple lesions
- Treatment: conservative surgical excision or laser ablation; almost no risk of recurrence. This is not an aggressive or precancerous lesion

Verrucous Carcinoma (Fig. 4-53)

- Etiology: low-grade, slow growing malignancy of squamous epithelium, usually in response to topical placement of smokeless tobacco; may be idiopathic
- Clinical findings: white, firm, asymptomatic oral mass with papillary or verruciform surface projections, usually in a region of chronic placement of snuff or chewing tobacco. Seldom ulcerated but often destroys underlying jawbone

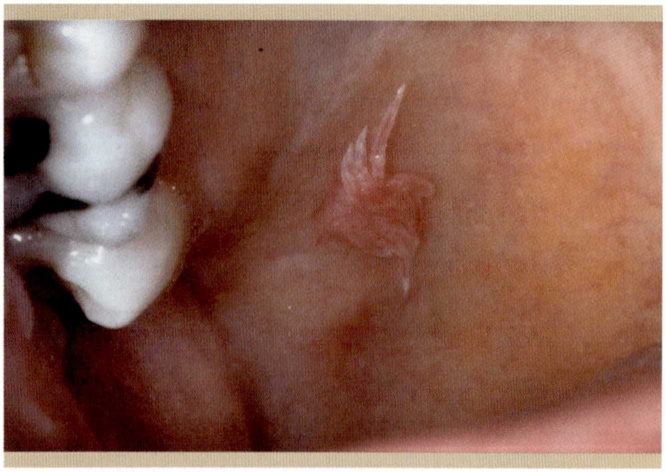

FIGURE 4-52 Papilloma (squamous papilloma) of soft palate.

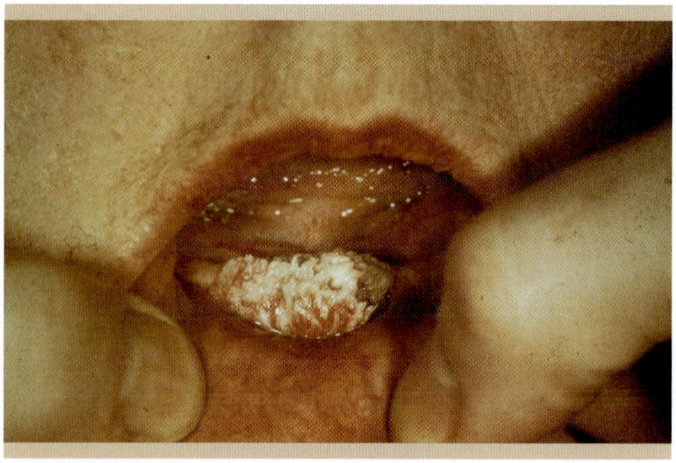

FIGURE 4-53 Verrucous carcinoma. (*Used with permission from Dr Robert Gorlin.*)

- Treatment: Aggressive surgical removal, including at least 1 cm of normal surrounding soft and hard tissues; this cancer seldom metastasizes until late in development (years), but recurrence is common

MASSES WITH SMOOTH SURFACES

Mucocele (Mucus Retention Phenomenon) (Fig. 4-54)

- Etiology: traumatic rupture of a minor salivary gland duct, with spillage of mucus into the submucosal stroma producing a large pool surrounded by granulation tissue. A very large similar lesion of the oral floor, ranula, arises from rupture of the submandibular duct

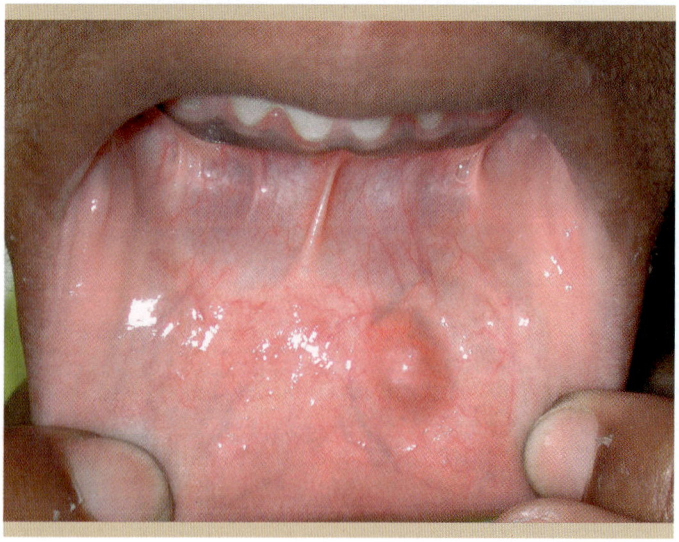

FIGURE 4-54 Mucocele of lower lip. (*Used with permission from Dr. Kamal Busaidy.*)

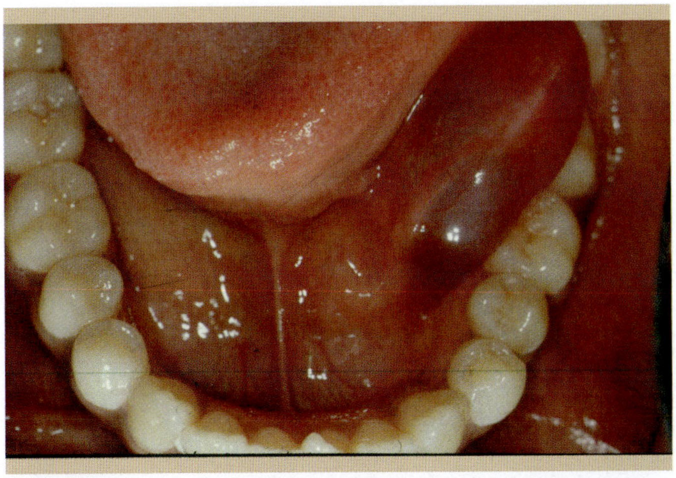

FIGURE 4-55 Ranula (mucocele of submandibular gland).

- Clinical findings: dome-shaped, soft, painless, translucent bluish mass, most commonly on lower lip but occasionally on buccal mucosa, palate or ventral tongue. Usually less than 1 cm in diameter but when arising from the glands of the ventral tongue, which are deep in the muscle, the lesion can get to be 3 to 4 cm; in this location it is often referred to as a *cyst of Blandin-Nuhn*
- Treatment: surgical excision, including the underlying ruptured gland. Recurrence may occur because of inadvertent scalpel damage to adjacent normal glands. Usually the gland is just above the muscle, but with a cyst of Blandin-Nuhn a much deeper excision is required or else recurrence is common

Ranula (Fig. 4-55)

- Etiology: traumatic rupture of the submandibular gland duct, with spillage of mucus above the muscles of the oral floor producing a large pool of mucus with no epithelial lining. This is, essentially, a very large mucocele
- Clinical findings: Large, often tender, often fluctuant, soft sessile mass of the oral floor, off the midline. Color can vary from pink to blue to purple and the mass may appear semitransparent; may be so large as to push the tongue and interfere with eating or speaking
- Treatment: may try to find the broken duct and suture it to the overlying mucosa or may marsupialize the mucus pool, but definitive treatment typically requires removal of the offending submandibular gland located below the muscles of the oral floor

Traumatic Fibroma (Fig. 4-56)

- Etiology: proliferative, avascular fibrous overgrowth in response to acute or chronic trauma of the submucosa; not a true neoplasm but, rather, an inflammatory fibrous hyperplasia

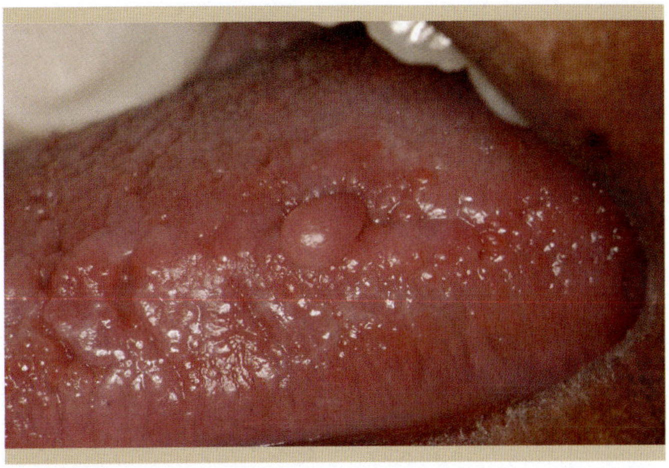

FIGURE 4-56 Irritation (traumatic) fibroma, in area of chronic lingual papulosis.

- Clinical findings: asymptomatic, usually pedunculated, firm or soft, pink mass; found most commonly on the buccal and labial mucosae; usually less than 1 cm in diameter
- Treatment: conservative surgical excision; slight chance of recurrence, especially if the causative trauma continues

Giant Cell Fibroma (Fig. 4-57)

- Etiology: proliferative, avascular fibrous overgrowth in response to acute or chronic trauma of the submucosa; not a true neoplasm but, rather, an inflammatory fibrous hyperplasia; differs from the traumatic fibroma in that it has histopathologically unique fibroblasts and typically has a lobulated or mildly papillary surface change
- Clinical findings: asymptomatic sessile or pedunculated, firm or soft, pale or white mass, often with lobulation or multiple small surface papules (may look like a *papilloma*).

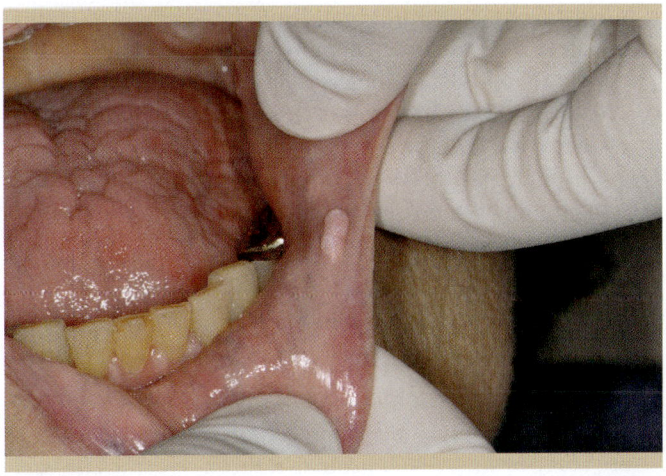

FIGURE 4-57 Giant cell fibroma of lip commissure.

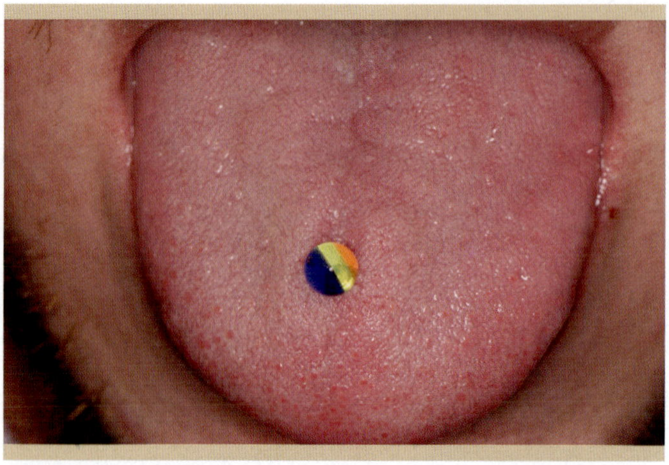

FIGURE 4-58 Lingual barbell (tongue jewelry).

Found on any mucosal surface but most commonly on the buccal and labial mucosae; usually less than 1 cm in diameter

- Microscopic findings: avascular collagen with scattered atypical fibroblasts beneath the epithelium. Lesional fibroblasts are large and angular or stellate, with a slightly hematoxylin cytoplasm and often with multiple nuclei; mitotic figures are not found
- Treatment: conservative surgical excision; slight chance of recurrence

Lingual Barbell (Tongue Jewelry) (Fig. 4-58)

- Etiology: surgical puncture of the anterior tongue midline, with placement of a barbell-shaped metal or plastic foreign object or "jewel." Usually this can be done with little or no anesthesia because the lingual midline comprises dense fibrous tissue without sensory nerve fibers
- Clinical findings: colorful ball on the dorsum midline of the tongue, with similar ball of the ventral midline, connected by a thin rod. There are no symptoms unless the fistula in which the connecting rod is placed becomes infected, which seldom happens; may see red granulation tissue around the fistulous opening
- Treatment: no treatment is necessary unless infected, in which removal of the jewelry typically is enough for cure; the fistula typically closes without surgical repair, but may remain indefinitely. **Caution**: the ventral portion of the device may chronically impact the backs of the lower incisors, either chipping the teeth or damaging the periodontal tissues

Granular Cell Tumor (GCT) (Fig. 4-59)

- Etiology: benign proliferation of macrophage-like granular cells, probably of Schwann cell origin; lesional cells are reactive with S-100 protein, neuron-specific enolase, and NK1-C3, myelin-associated P0 and P2 proteins,

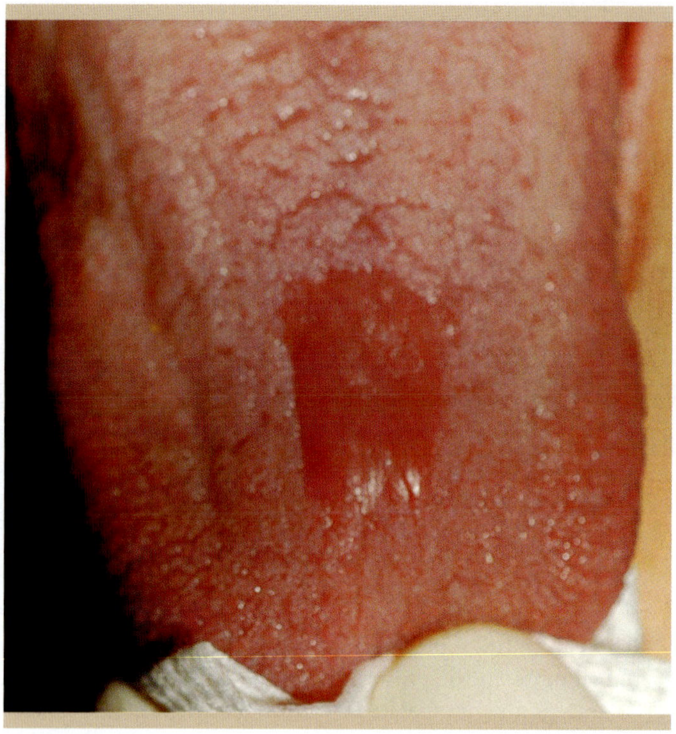

FIGURE 4-59 Granular cell tumor.

myelin basic protein and Leu-7. There is a malignant counterpart
- Clinical findings: sessile, pale, moderately firm mass with minimal elevation, usually on the dorsum of the tongue (25% of all cases occur on the tongue); adult onset, limited size, seldom larger than 1 cm.
- Treatment: conservative surgical excision; 2 to 8% risk of recurrence; Ki-67 immunoreactivity, seen in 10% of lesions, suggested increased risk

Neurofibromatosis (Fig. 4-60)

- Etiology: benign neurofibromas and schwannomas occur as part of von Recklinghausen syndrome (neurofibromatosis; MEN I)
- Clinical findings: sessile or pedunculated, soft, asymptomatic masses of any oral mucosa, but typically on the tongue; begin developing in childhood, with slow enlargement over years and with new masses developing over time. Usually there are few such masses in the mouth, as opposed to the numerous ones on the skin
- Treatment: surgical excision if a mass interferes with eating or speaking, or if begins to enlarge after a period of inactivity (malignant transformation may occur, but is uncommon)

Inflammatory Papillary Hyperplasia (Fig. 4-61)

- Etiology: chronic, mild trauma and/or low-grade mucosal inflammatory secondary to a loose denture which is

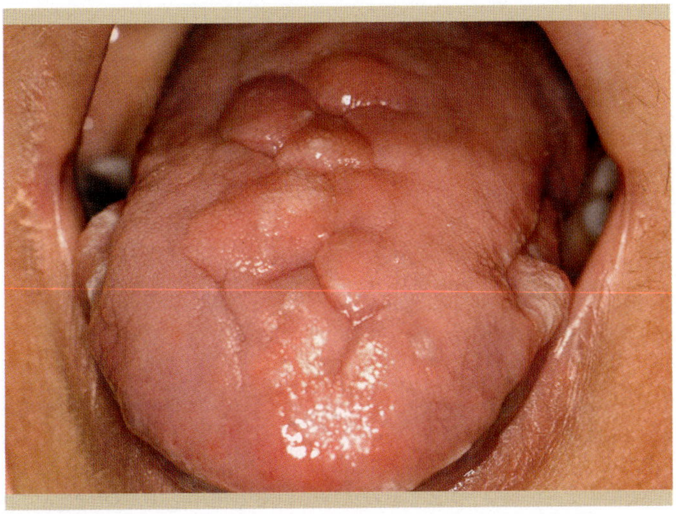

FIGURE 4-60 Neurofibromatosis with multiple neurofibromas of the tongue.

typically not removed overnight, as is typically suggested for dentures

- Clinical findings: multiple asymptomatic sessile or pedunculated papules and nodules of the vault of the hard palate, often with a diffuse mucosal erythema surrounding them. Early lesions are edematous and appear semitranslucent, while older lesions are pale pink and firm to palpation. If burning sensation is felt, suspect a secondary candidiasis
- Treatment: replace or reline denture and keep it out overnight. Small nodules do not have to be removed but larger ones must be surgically removed or laser ablated prior to remake of the denture; with new or well-fitted denture, recurrence is very unlikely

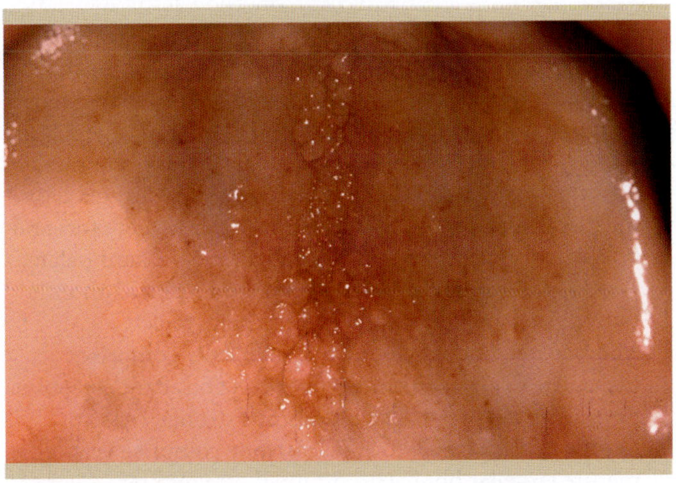

FIGURE 4-61 Inflammatory papillary hyperplasia.

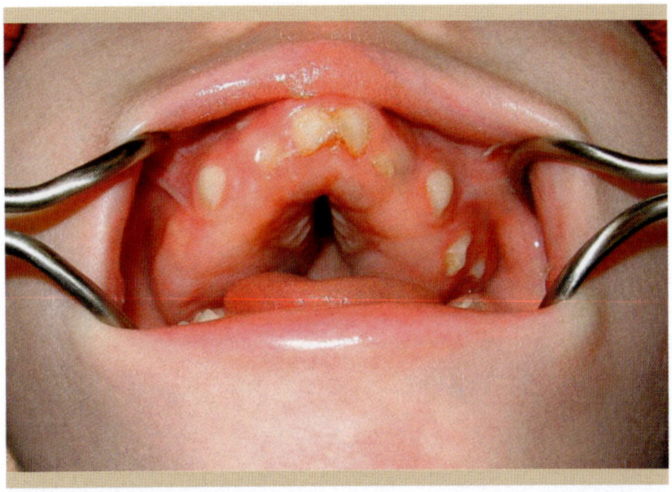

FIGURE 4-62 Drug-induced gingival hyperplasia. *(Used with permission from Dr Mark Wong.)*

Drug-Induced Gingival Hyperplasia (Fig. 4-62)

- Etiology: fibrous proliferation induced by long-term use of phenytoin (Dilantin), cyclosporine or nifedipine, among others; risk increases with poor oral hygiene and gingivitis
- Clinical findings: slow, painless enlargement of gingivae in 1 or all 4 quadrants, perhaps with erythema and edema of the edges touching the teeth; may be so severe as to cover the teeth
- Treatment: improved oral hygiene with regular dental cleanings; discontinuation of precipitating drugs when possible; surgical or laser resection of gingival tissue for severe cases; recurrence is diminished if oral hygiene is improved

BONY HARD MASSES

Torus Mandibularis (Mandibular Torus) (Fig. 4-63)

- Etiology: focal proliferations of cortical bone probably results from piezo-type stimulation of bone at regions of torque, from clenching, grinding teeth; etiology may be unknown in some cases
- Clinical findings: adult onset sessile or pedunculated, asymptomatic, very slowly enlarging, bony hard mass on the lingual cortex of the mandible, near the premolars and first molars; often bilateral. May have painful surface ulceration from trauma during eating hard foods (hard crust on bread, potato chips, fish bones, etc.)
- Treatment: no treatment required unless interferes with denture wearing or oral hygiene, or develops infection from surface mucosal traumatic ulceration; may then be surgically removed. Slowly enlarges, typically, for decades and is susceptible to bisphosphonate-related osteonecrosis of the jaws (BRONJ)

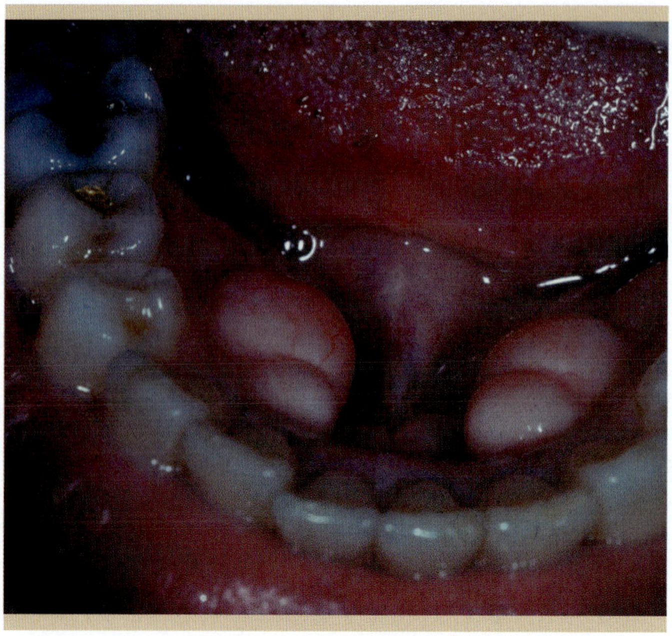

FIGURE 4-63 Bilateral torus mandibularis. (*Used with permission from Dr. Bela Toth.*)

Torus Palatinus (Palatal Torus) (Fig. 4-64)

- Etiology: unknown cause for this focal proliferation of cortical bone in the palatal midline
- Clinical findings: adult onset sessile or pedunculated, asymptomatic, very slowly enlarging, bony hard mass of the midline of hard palate; may completely fill the palatal vault. May become ulcerated from surface injury during eating

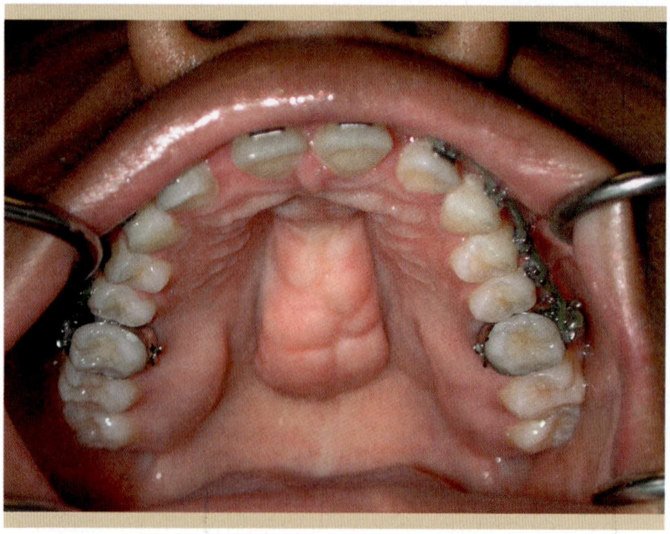

FIGURE 4-64 Torus palatinus. (*Used with permission from Dr. Kamal Busaidy.*)

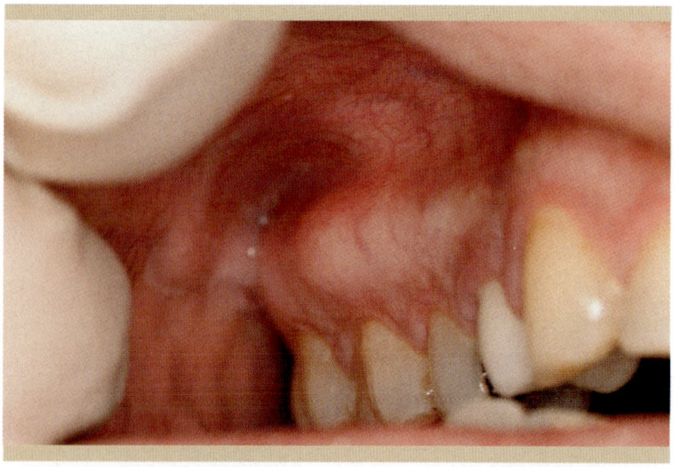

FIGURE 4-65 Buccal exostoses (multiple bone masses over the teeth).

- Treatment: no treatment required unless interferes with denture wearing or oral hygiene, or develops infection from surface mucosal traumatic ulceration; may be surgically removed. Slowly enlarges for decades and is susceptible to bisphosphonate-related osteonecrosis of the jaws (BRONJ)

Buccal Exostoses (Fig. 4-65)

- Etiology: unknown cause for these focal proliferations of cortical bone, but presumed to be from pressures produced by clenching or grinding the teeth over many years.
- Clinical findings: Sessile, asymptomatic, very slowly enlarging, bony hard masses on the facial cortex immediately centered over one or more teeth
- Treatment: No treatment required unless interferes with denture wearing or oral hygiene, or develops infection from surface mucosal traumatic ulceration; may be surgically removed. May slowly enlarge for decades but usually reaches maximum size within a few years

Reactive Exostosis (Fig. 4-66)

- Etiology: Relatively rapid (over weeks, months) focal proliferation of cortical bone, presumably from abnormal healing after surface trauma
- Clinical findings: Sessile or pedunculated, asymptomatic or mildly tender, gradually enlarging, bony hard mass on a cortical surface other than those surfaces where tori and buccal exostoses are found; usually found on hard palate, develops to full size (up to 4 cm) within a 3- to 5-month period; surface mucosa may be erythematous
- Microscopic findings: bony mass typically comprises immature or newly formed bone with abundant osteoblastic activity and a background fibrous stroma; older lesions may resemble tori, that is, they comprise very mature lamellar bone with minimal osteoblastic activity and marrow filling the spaces within the bone.

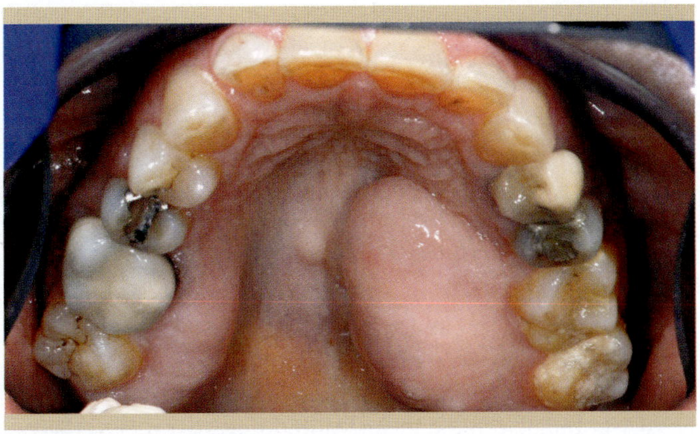

FIGURE 4-66 Reactive exostosis of left hard palate.

Caution: may mimic parosteal osteosarcoma clinically and microscopically

- Treatment: conservative surgical removal with biopsy to rule out low-grade or parosteal osteosarcoma

Osteoma (Fig. 4-67)

- Etiology: Benign neoplasm of cortical bone
- Clinical findings: Sessile or pedunculated, asymptomatic, bony mass of any jawbone surface, or within the sinuses; childhood onset; usually dense radiopaque but sometimes filled with marrow so appears normally dense on radiographs
- **Caution:** multiple jaw osteomas may be associated with Gardner syndrome, an autosomal dominant disorder with gastrointestinal polyps, multiple osteomas, supernumerary teeth, and epidermoid cysts or fibromas. Facial osteoma is often the first diagnosed presentation

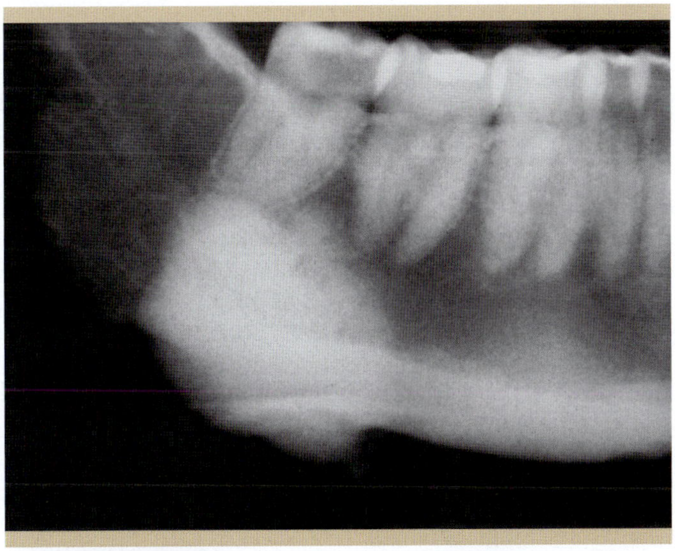

FIGURE 4-67 Osteoma. (*Used with permission from Dr. Mark Wong.*)

- Treatment: none. May require excision if severely deforming or interfere with function; work up for Gardner syndrome if in a child

QUIZ

Questions

Unique Tongue changes

1. A 24-year-old man, on routine examination is found to have nonpainful, sessile masses in the posterior lateral tongue bilaterally. Further inspection shows them to be soft and pink. He is recovering from a recent upper respiratory infection. What is the most likely histological finding when biopsying this tissue?

   A. Invasive islands and cords of malignant squamous-epithelial cells
   B. Thick layer of parakeratin with underlying koilocytes
   C. Normal lymphoid tissue
   D. Dense irregular connective tissue

2. An otherwise healthy 42-year-old man presents with a 5-year history of intermittent tongue pain. The pain is worse when eating and he describes the latest exacerbation after eating at an Indian restaurant. Examination shows a single, irregular deep fissure running down the mid dorsum of the tongue that is moderately tender to palpation. What therapy might be of help with his symptoms?

   A. Nystatin lozenges
   B. Partial glossectomy
   C. Antibiotics
   D. Chlorhexidine mouth wash

3. A concerned mother brings her 6-year-old daughter to your clinic for evaluation of a lingual frenum. Her daughter has met all her milestones and does very well in school. She is wondering if her daughter will require surgical correction of this developmental defect. Oral examination shows a ventral tongue fused to the floor of the mouth with very minimal extension of the frenum to the lingual gingival. What is the best advice to give her?

   A. Treatment is recommended as this condition usually progresses to causes speech problems later in life.
   B. Treatment is necessary as swallowing and chewing will be affected once she begins her growth spurt
   C. Usually no treatment is needed
   D. She may elect for treatment, which will consist of topical steroid therapy

Mucosal Discolorations

1. A 45-year-old former smoker presents with a 1-year history of a white lesion along the buccal mucosal area adjacent to his first left mandibular molar. Histological examination after incisional biopsy shows thickened surface parakeratin without basal cell dysplasia. What is the cancer risk of this lesion?

   A. Greater than 75% lifetime risk of malignancy
   B. Unknown risk
   C. No risk of malignancy
   D. Approximately 4% risk of malignant development

2. Which of the following is considered a therapy that may be used to help with symptoms of lichen planus?

   A. Antibiotics
   B. Antivirals
   C. Antifungals alone
   D. Antifungals combined with steroids

3. Which of the following is not a known cause of oral candidiasis?

   A. Poor oral hygiene
   B. AIDS
   C. Drug-induced xerostomia
   D. Diabetes mellitus

Mucosal Ulcerations

1. A patient presents to you with painful mouth sores. Examination shows moderately sized mucosal ulcerations along the buccal mucosa bilaterally. The lesions have a white base with a mild red halo at the margins. What is the likely histological finding after biopsy?

   A. Subepidermal separation
   B. Dysplasia invading squamous epithelium, keratin pearls
   C. Prickle cell necrosis
   D. Hyperkeratosis with keratin plugging

2. A patient presents 1 week after elective oral surgery with painful sores around her lips and lesions on the palmar surface of her hands. Further inspection of the palms shows the lesions having a background pink center with intense erythema at the periphery. What is the recommended treatment?

   A. Antibiotic ointment
   B. Antifungal ointment
   C. Systemic corticosteroids
   D. NSAIDs

3. Which of the following would not be considered as an underlying condition in a patient with recurrent major aphthous ulcers?

   A. Behçet syndrome
   B. Crohn disease
   C. Ulcerative colitis
   D. Sjögren syndrome

Masses With Irregular Surfaces

1. Which of the following is characteristic of a clinical presentation of peripheral ossifying fibroma?

   A. Lobulated red and purple fluctuant mass on the anterior maxillary mucogingival margin
   B. Hard mass overlying the gingival margin near the anterior mandibular teeth
   C. Lobulated, liner, flesh-colored mass parallel to the maxillary alveolus
   D. Smooth purple mass in between teeth 9 and 10 on the gingival margin

2. A 58-year-old truck driver presents with a painless mass in his anterior mandibular vestibule. It has grown in size in the past 6 months. Examination shows a 3 × 4 cm white-gray lesion with an irregular surface. Social history is positive for a 35-year chewing tobacco habit. What is the likely treatment for this lesion?

   A. Observation
   B. Antifungal lozenges
   C. Aggressive surgical resection
   D. Systemic steroids

Masses With Smooth Surfaces

1. Which of the following describes a cyst of Blandin-Nuhn?

   A. An asymptomatic, sessile, soft white mass with lobulations found on the buccal mucosa
   B. Sessile, pale moderately firm mass on the dorsum of the tongue, measuring 6 mm
   C. Sessile, soft, asymptomatic mass on the dorsum of the tongue found in childhood with multiple masses developing over time
   D. Dome-shaped, soft, asymptomatic, translucent 4-cm mass on the ventral tongue

2. A 74-year-old edentulous female nursing home patient presents with an incidental finding of multiple small nodules on her hard palate. The palate is also erythematous. Her daughter is concerned about the cause of the condition. What is the recommended treatment?

   A. Palatal resection to prevent spread
   B. Chemo radiation
   C. New dentures and avoiding denture retention overnight
   D. Antifungal lozenges

Bony Hard Masses

1. A concerned mother brings her 6-year-old son to be evaluated for multiple hard lesions on his maxilla. Examination shows 2 small, hard, painless growths in the maxillary vestibule bilaterally as well as a hard lesion beneath the left inferior orbital rim. His father has similar symptoms. What other likely findings are to be found on physical examination?
   A. Sessile, soft masses on the tongue and skin with light brown patches
   B. Congenitally missing teeth
   C. Vesicular, painful clusters on the lower vermilion border
   D. Numerous polyps in the large intestine

2. A 42-year-old woman presents with a 4-month history of a hard lesion in the hard palate. She recalls having a burn on her palate from eating pizza that took quite some time before it healed, after which she began noticing this current lesion developing. What is the likely histological finding upon biopsy?
   A. Avascular collagen with scattered atypical fibroblasts beneath the epithelium
   B. Immature bone in a background of fibrous stroma
   C. Multinucleated giant cells in background of uniform and immature spindle-shaped mesenchymal cells
   D. Proliferating granulation tissue with vascular channels and a mixed inflammatory infiltrate

Answers

1. C. A nonpainful, soft, semitranslucent bilateral lesion on the posterior lateral tongue in an otherwise healthy young man with history of pharyngitis should lead one to suspect hyperplastic lingual tonsil. It is due to chronic enlargement of normal lymphoid tissues of the lingual tonsils from repeated pharyngitis or "flue." The histology is that of normal lymphoid tissue. Choice A corresponds to squamous cell carcinoma. Choice B corresponds to lymphoma. Choice D corresponds to irritation fibroma.
2. A. This patient has fissured tongue. The condition can develop pain in later years. Pain can be attributed to spicy foods and secondary candidal infection. Antifungal medication may be of some help to this patient. Also, you can advise avoiding spicy foods.
3. C. Ankyloglossia usually requires no treatment unless there is evidence of speech impediment or if the gingival attachment is causing periodontal pathology. This girl seems to have no speech problems because she is doing well in school and the gingival attachment is minimal. Thus surgical correction can be deferred at this time.

Mucosal Discolorations

1. D. This is an example of leukoplakia. Commonly seen with a patient having a history of tobacco use; It is considered a premalignant lesion with approximate 4% risk of transforming into a carcinoma. Oral floor lesions or those with mixed colorations of red/white are at higher risk of transformation. Treatment is with conservative excision and close surveillance.
2. D. Topical steroid application can be used to treat mild forms of lichen planus. More severe cases require systemic steroid usage. Other drugs that can be used include nonsteroidal anti-inflammatory drugs (NSAIDs), especially sulfonylureas, antimalarials, β-blockers, and some angiotensin-converting enzyme (ACE) inhibitors.
3. A. The following are known causes of oral candidiasis: xerostomia (dry mouth), immunodeficiency, antibiotics, corticosteroids, antidepressants, antipsychotics, diabetes mellitus, vitamin deficiency, chemotherapy, radiation therapy, and Sjögren syndrome.

Mucosal Ulcerations

1. A. The clinical presentation is most characteristic of cicatricial pemphigoid. Clinical findings are moderate to large bullae that are often broken, thus showing a flat ulcerative lesion. There is an inflammatory halo of mucosa at the margins. Histology shows subepithelial separation with minimal inflammatory response. Choice B corresponds to squamous cell carcinoma. Choice C corresponds to erythema multiforme. Choice D corresponds to systemic lupus.
2. C. The clinical presentation is characteristic of erythema multiforme. This hypersensitivity reaction may have been the result of postoperative pain medications prescribed to her after her surgery (NSAIDs are known causes). One should discontinue any possible offending agents and begin systemic corticosteroids along with hydration and analgesia. This condition is usually self-limiting.
3. D. Sjögren syndrome is an autoimmune disease with resultant destruction of the salivary and lacrimal glands. It may be associated with other autoimmune diseases such as rheumatoid arthritis, systemic lupus erythematosus, and polymyositis. It does not produce the oral lesions associated with aphthous ulcers. The other conditions listed should be ruled out in a patient presenting with recurrent major aphthous ulcers.

Masses With Irregular Surfaces

1. B. Peripheral ossifying fibroma is an inflammatory mediated proliferation of periodontal ligament cells. Histology shows a fibrous, cellular proliferation usually with osteoblastic rimming. Choice C is representative of epulis fissuratum. Choice A is characteristic of a hemangioma. Choice D is characteristic of a pyogenic granuloma.
2. C. This description is characteristic of verrucous carcinoma. It is a low-grade slow growing malignancy of squamous epithelium closely associated with chewing

tobacco use. Treatment is surgical resection with margins of at least 1 cm.

Masses With Smooth Surfaces

1. D. A cyst of Blandin-Nuhn is a mucocele that has formed deep within the tongue musculature. Choice A describes a giant cell fibroma. Choice B is characteristic of a granular cell tumor. Choice C describes a neurofibroma.
2. C. This condition is typical of inflammatory papillary hyperplasia due to old dentures that are chronically worn overnight and often ill fitting. Large lesions can require intervention; however, smaller lesions are not usually treated. The dentures should be removed while sleeping. Relining the existing denture or fabrication of a new, better-fitting set, is also helpful.

Bony Hard Masses

1. D. The childhood presentation of facial and intraoral osteomas with an autosomal dominant inheritance raises the suspicion for Gardner syndrome. One must do a thorough work up to look for the other manifestations of the condition, including gastrointestinal polyps, multiple osteomas, supernumerary teeth, and epidermoid cysts or fibromas.
2. B. This lesion is typical of reactive exostosis. It is a rapid proliferation of focal bone after abnormal healing from surface trauma. Histological findings can vary according to the age of the lesion. Choice B represents findings in early presentation while older lesions resemble tori. Choice A represents a giant cell fibroma. Choice C is characteristic of peripheral giant cell granuloma. Choice D represents a pyogenic granuloma.

REFERENCES

Adibi S, Suarez P, Bouquot J: Papillary tip melanosis (pigmented fungiform lingual papillae). *Texas Dent J* 2011;128:572–573, 576–578.

Akpan A, Morgan R: Oral candidiasis. *Postgrad Med J* 2002;78: 455–459.

Andrews BT, Trask DK: Oral melanoacanthoma: a case report, a review of the literature, and a new treatment option. *Ann Otol Rhinol Laryngol* 2005;114:677–680.

Arduino PG, Porter SR: Oral and perioral herpes simplex virus type I (HSV-I) infection: review of its management. *Oral Dis* 2006;12:254–270.

Baccaglini L, Atkinson JC, Patton LL, et al. Management of oral lesions in HIV-positive patients. *Oral Surg Oral Med Oral Pathol Oral Radiol* 2007;103 (Suppl 1):S50.e1–S50.e23.

Bhaskar SN, Jacoway JR: Pyogenic granuloma—clinical features, incidence, histology, and result of treatment: report of 242 cases. *J Oral Surg* 1966;24:391–398.

Bouquot JE, Adibi SA, Sanchez M: Chronic lingual papulosis—new "independent" entity or chronic version of transient lingual papillitis? *Oral Surg Oral Pathol Oral Med Oral Radiol* 2012;113:111–117.

Bouquot JE, Ephros H: Erythroplakia: the dangerous red mucosa. *Pract Perio Aesth Dent* 1995;7:59–68.

Bouquot JE, Farthing PM, Speight PM: The pathology of oral cancer and precancer revisited. *Curr Diag Path* 2006;12:11–21.

Bouquot JE, Horn N, Wan S-F: Herpes zoster. *Texas Dent J* 2007;124:132, 136–138.

Bouquot JE, Muller S, Nikai H: Lesions of the oral cavity. In: Gnepp DG, ed. Diagnostic surgical pathology of the head and neck, 2nd Ed. Philadelphia; W.B. Saunders: 2009, pp 191–309.

Bouquot JE, Suarez P, Vigneswaran N: Oral precancer and early cancer detection in the dental office—review of new technologies. *J Implant Advanced Clin Dent* 2010;2:47–63.

Buchner A, Merrell PW, Carpenter WM: Relative frequency of solitary melanocytic lesions of the oral mucosa. *J Oral Pathol Med* 2004;33:550–557.

Cherry-Peppers G, Daniels CO, Meeks V, et al. Oral manifestations in the era of HARRT. *J Nat Med Assoc* 2003;95:21S–32S.

Deshpande RB, Bharucha MA: Median rhomboid glossitis: secondary to colonization of the tongue by Actinomyces (a case report). *J Postgrad Med* 1991;37:238–240.

Fanburg-Smith JC, Meis-Kindblom JM, Fante R, Kindblom LG: Malignant granular cell tumor of soft tissue: diagnostic criteria and clinicopathologic correlation. *Am J Surg Pathol* 1998;22(7):779–794.

Fettig A, Pogrel MA, Silverman S Jr, et al. Proliferative verrucous leukoplakia of the gingiva. *Oral Surg Oral Med Oral Pathol Oral Radiol Endod* 2000;90:723–730.

Goldsmith LA et al. *Fitzpatrick's Dermatology in General Medicine*, 8th Ed. New York: McGraw-Hill; 2012.

Gu GM, Epstein JB, Morton TH Jr: Intraoral melanoma: long-term follow-up and implication for dental clinicians. A case report and literature review. *Oral Surg Oral Med Oral Pathol Oral Radiol Endod* 2003;96:404–413.

Hatch CL: Pigmented lesions of the oral cavity. *Dent Clin North Am* 2005;49:185–201.

Johnson N, Schmid S, Franceschi S, et al. Squamous cell carcinoma of the oral cavity and oropharynx. In: Barnes L, Eveson JW, Reichart P, Sidransky D, eds. *WHO Classification of tumours: pathology & genetics of head and neck tumors*. Lyon, France: IARC; 2005, p. 169–175.

Kerr R, et al, eds. *Clinician's Guide to Oral Cancer and Potentially Malignant Oral Lesions*. Decker Publ, 2010.

McKee PH: *Pathology of the Skin: With Clinical Correlations*. London: Mosby-Wolfe; 1996.

Medina JE, Dichtel W, Luna MA: Verrucous-squamous carcinomas of the oral cavity: a clinicopathologic study of 104 cases. *Arch Otolaryngol* 1984;110:437–440.

Menta Simonsen Nico M, Rivitti EA, Lourenco SV: Actinic cheilitis: histologic study of the entire vermilion and comparison with previous biopsy. *J Cutan Pathol* 2007;34:309–314.

Neville D, Allen B: Oral and Maxillofacial Pathology, 3rd Ed. Philadelphia: W.B Saunders; 2008.

Samaranayake LP, Cheung LK, Samaranayake YH: Candidiasis and other fungal diseases of the mouth. *Dermatol Ther* 2002;15:251–269.

Seo IS, Azzarelli B, Warner TF, et al. Multiple visceral and cutaneous granular cell tumors: ultrastructural and immunocytochemical evidence of Schwann cell origin. *Cancer* 1984;53(10):2104–2110.

Shapiro SD, Abramovitch K, Van Dis ML, et al. Neurofibromatosis: oral and radiographic manifestations. *Oral Surg Oral Med Oral Pathol* 1984;58:493–498.

Spellberg B, Edwards J, Ibrahim A: Novel perspectives on mucormycosis: pathophysiology, presentation and management. *Clin Microbiol Rev* 2005;18:556–569.

Williams HK, Williams DM: Oral granular cell tumours: a histological and immunocytochemical study. *J Oral Pathol Med* 1997;26:164–169.

Zain RB, Fei YJ: Fibrous lesions of the gingiva: a histopathologic analysis of 204 cases. *Oral Surg Oral Med Oral Pathol* 1990;70:466–470.

CHAPTER 5

GENITAL DERMATOLOGY

LIBBY EDWARDS

RED LESIONS

Eczema/Atopic Dermatitis/Neurodermatitis/Lichen Simplex Chronicus

- Common genital dermatosis
- Symptom of excruciating pruritus with pleasure upon rubbing and scratching
- Frequent history of atopy and extragenital eczema
- Posterior scrotal, any vulvar, and perianal locations, sometimes proximal, medial thighs
- Variable morphology; lichenification and erosions which are often subtle (Fig. 5-1)
- Diagnosis is by morphology, pruritus, and response to therapy
- Therapy by ultrapotent corticosteroid ointments, nighttime sedation, avoidance of irritants

Contact Dermatitis (CD)

- Common, especially irritant CD in older incontinent patients
- For irritant CD, symptoms of irritation, rawness, and burning
- For allergic CD, symptom of itching, sometimes irritation/pain from scratching
- Morphology is usually nonspecific erythema for chronic CD, blisters or erosions for severe or acute CD
- Uncommon but unique morphology is small, monomorphous, discrete erosions; when chronic, these can become red, eroded papules (Jacquet diaper dermatitis, granuloma gluteale infantum or adultorum) (Fig. 5-2)
- Common etiologies for chronic irritant CD are incontinence, over washing, medication creams and gels; most common for acute irritant CD are medications for topical agents for anogenital warts
- Common allergens for the specific sensitization of allergic CD are medication (benzocaine, diphenhydramine, neomycin), panty liners (formaldehyde- and formalin-releasing agents), fragrances, preservatives, and stabilizers in hygiene products
- Diagnosis is by morphology, history and setting, and response to therapy
- Therapy by removal of irritants, bland emollients, and for allergic CD, also ultrapotent corticosteroid ointment or systemic corticosteroids; for irritant CD, midpotency corticosteroids may be useful; nighttime sedation if pruritic

Seborrhea/Seborrheic Dermatitis

- Uncommon genital eruption in adults; most often in homeless, neurologically compromised, HIV infected
- Symptoms can be absent, or consist of itching or irritation depending upon severity and individual patient
- Morphology is nonspecific genital redness, with accentuation in skin folds/crural creases; accompanied by extragenital seborrhea with yellowish scale in axilla, scalp, face, etc.
- Etiology is unknown; inability to bathe frequently and *Pityrosporum ovale* are possible
- Diagnosis is by setting, presence of typical extragenital disease, and response to therapy
- Therapy is frequent bathing, vigorous removal of scalp scale, and topical corticosteroids for the genital skin. Ketoconazole cream sometimes stings on anogenital skin

Psoriasis

- Common skin disease that often affects anogenital skin because of local irritation
- Symptoms include pruritus in some, and cosmetic annoyance and irritation in many
- Morphology is that of red, usually well-demarcated plaques (Fig. 5-3), with subtle scale; most often but not always accompanied by extragenital disease with dense white scale, nail abnormalities
- Etiology is autoimmune in origin
- Increased risk of accompanying metabolic syndrome, obesity, and arthritis
- Diagnosis is by morphology, the presence of typical extragenital disease, and, when needed, skin biopsy

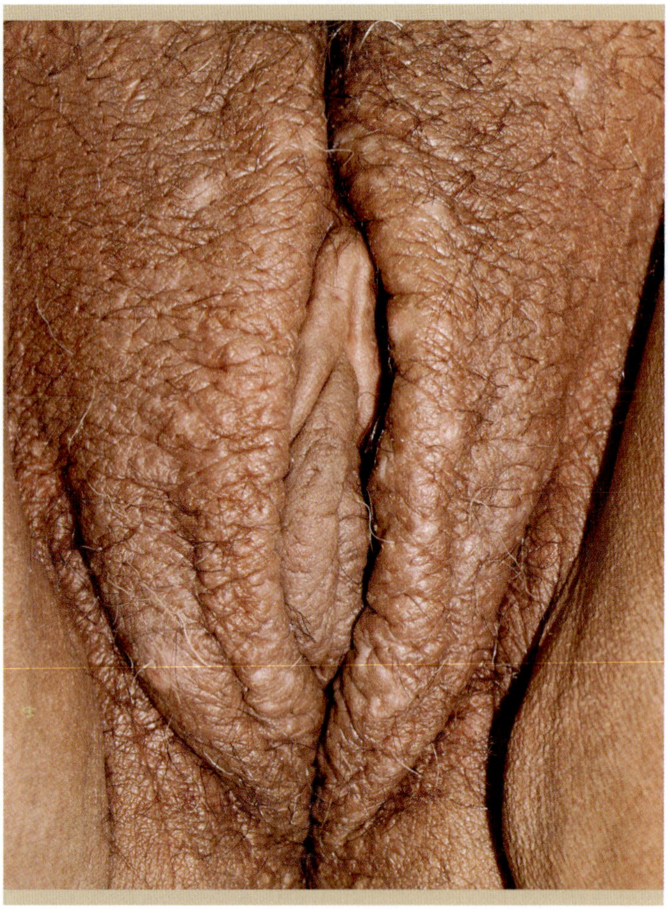

FIGURE 5-1 Thickened skin with lichenification and prurigo nodules, but no obvious erythema in this dark complexioned woman. (*Used with permission from Dr. Libby Edwards*.)

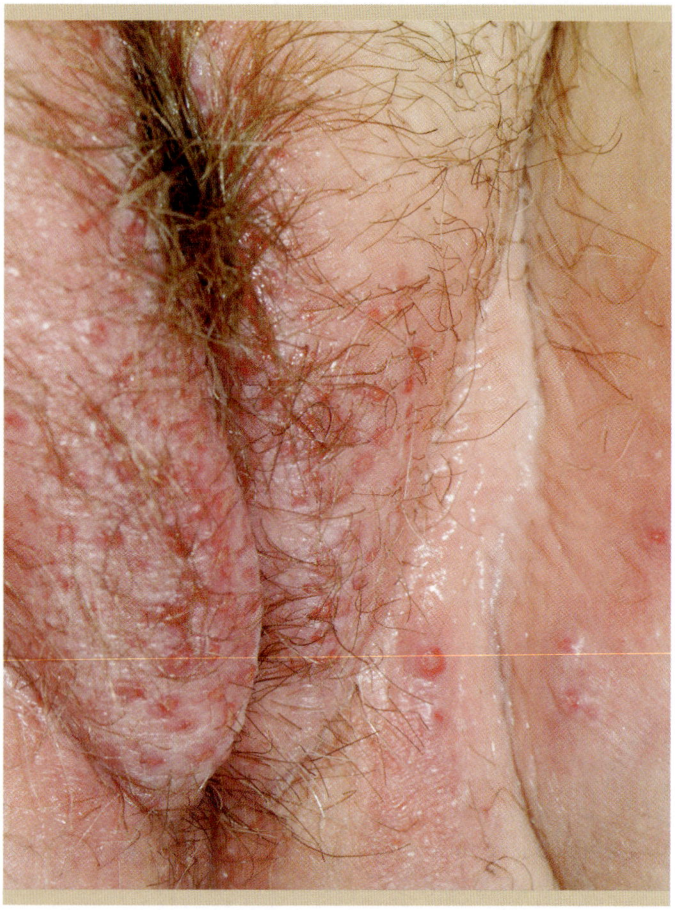

FIGURE 5-2 A unique morphology of contact dermatitis of the vulva consists of small, monomorphous erosions; there are nodules of granuloma gluteale in this photo as well. (*Used with permission from Dr. Libby Edwards*.)

- Therapy includes topical corticosteroid ointments with careful follow-up to evaluate for atrophy
- Topical tacrolimus and pimecrolimus are useful in some but often produce unacceptable stinging with application
- Tars, anthralin, salicylic acid too irritating for anogenital psoriasis
- Systemic therapy in severe disease, especially methotrexate and biologic agents
- Attention to diagnosis and management of secondary infection, especially Candidiasis

Tinea Cruris

- Eruption that is fairly common in men, rare in women
- Symptoms include pruritus in many, but some patients are asymptomatic
- Morphology is well-demarcated plaques of erythema and scale, with accentuation of scale at the border; located on the proximal, medial thighs extending to the crural crease. Unless immunosuppressed, spares the scrotum and penis
- Some exhibit follicular papules, pustules, or crusts of fungal folliculitis

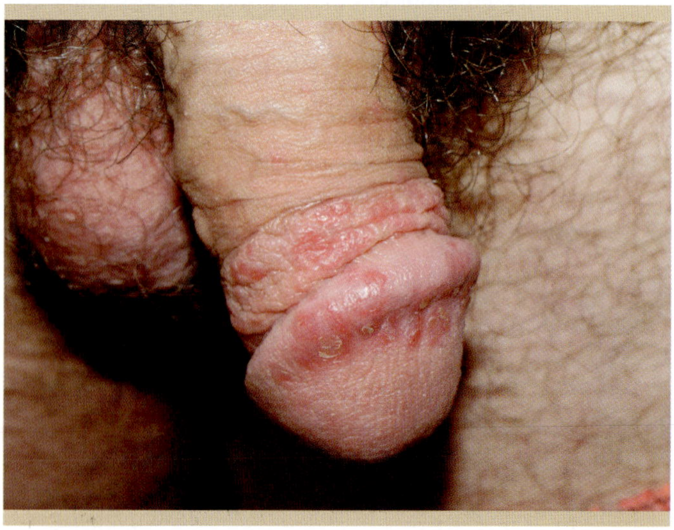

FIGURE 5-3 Psoriasis of the genitalia does not exhibit the classic silvery scale of psoriasis on dry keratinized surfaces. (*Used with permission from Dr. Libby Edwards*.)

- Usually with accompanying typical onychomycosis
- Etiology is infection by any of several dermatophytes; most common are *Epidermophyton floccosum* and *Trichophyton rubrum*, with *Trichophyton mentagrophytes* and *Trichophyton verrucosum* at times
- Diagnosis is by the classic morphology, with identification of fungi on a skin scraping in unclear cases
- Therapy is a topical antifungal agent to include any azole, terbinafine, Naftin (not nystatin). Oral therapy with fluconazole, itraconazole, terbinafine, or griseofulvin when fungal folliculitis is present

Erythrasma

- Infrequent eruption; more common in men than women
- Morphology mimics that of tinea cruris; pink or tan, well-demarcated plaques on the proximal, medial thighs to the crural crease; subtle scale without peripheral accentuation
- Etiology is infection by the bacterium *Corynebacterium minutissimum*
- Diagnosis is by morphology and confirmed by coral fluorescence under Wood lamp
- Therapy consists of topical erythromycin, clindamycin, or fusidic acid

Candidiasis

- Common vaginal infection in women; prominent vulvar disease and infection in men less often unless diabetic, incontinent, immunosuppressed, or obese
- Symptoms include pruritus, with rawness and irritation in more severe disease
- Redness of the introitus; more extensive infection exhibits red plaques in the crural crease, on the vulva, scrotum, and penis. Plaques are sometimes superficially eroded with satellite erosions, papules, or collarettes
- The etiology is an infection with *Candida albicans* or *Candida tropicalis*; non-albicans *Candida* infections are generally mucosal only
- The diagnosis is by morphology and confirmed by a fungal preparation or culture and response to therapy, since this can mimic psoriasis and seborrhea
- Therapy consists of the topical antifungal therapies of any azole or nystatin, and oral therapy with fluconazole is effective as well; griseofulvin is not beneficial

Plasma Cell Vulvitis/Balanitis (Zoon's Vulvitis/Balanitis, Vulvitis and Balanitis Plasmacellularis Circumscripta)

- Under-recognized dermatosis on mucous membranes
- Symptoms include pruritus, rawness, and burning
- Morphology is that of one or more deeply red, purpuric, or rusty red/brown, smooth, shiny, and usually well-demarcated patches of the glans penis, or the vulva, primarily the introitus or periurethral mucosa (Fig. 5-4); sometimes appears erosive

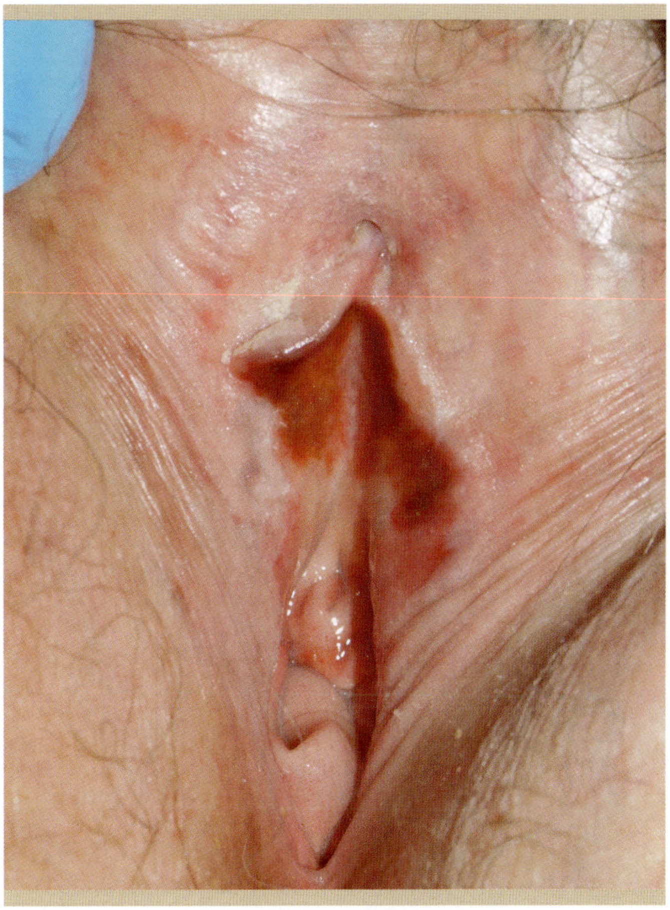

FIGURE 5-4 Deep, rusty red glistening plaque of plasma cell vulvitis. (*Used with permission from Dr. Libby Edwards.*)

- Plasma cell vulvitis/balanitis is unassociated with extragenital disease
- The etiology is unknown, but inflammatory and noninfectious in nature; perhaps related to lichen planus
- The diagnosis is by morphology, confirmed by a biopsy showing an upper dermal plasma cell infiltrate and a flattened, thinned epithelium with lozenge-shaped epithelial cells
- There is no association with malignancy and no scarring
- Therapy consists of potent/ultrapotent topical corticosteroids and intralesional corticosteroids. There is anecdotal evidence for benefit with calcineurin inhibitors, imiquimod, and circumcision

High Grade Squamous Intraepithelial Lesion (HSIL, old terminologies are vulvar intraepithelial neoplasia/VIN III, penile intraepithelial lesion/PIN III, anal intraepithelial lesion/AIN III, bowenoid papulosis, squamous cell carcinoma in situ/SCCIS)

- Common tumor that often mimics anogenital warts
- Often asymptomatic; sometimes with pruritus or irritation/burning

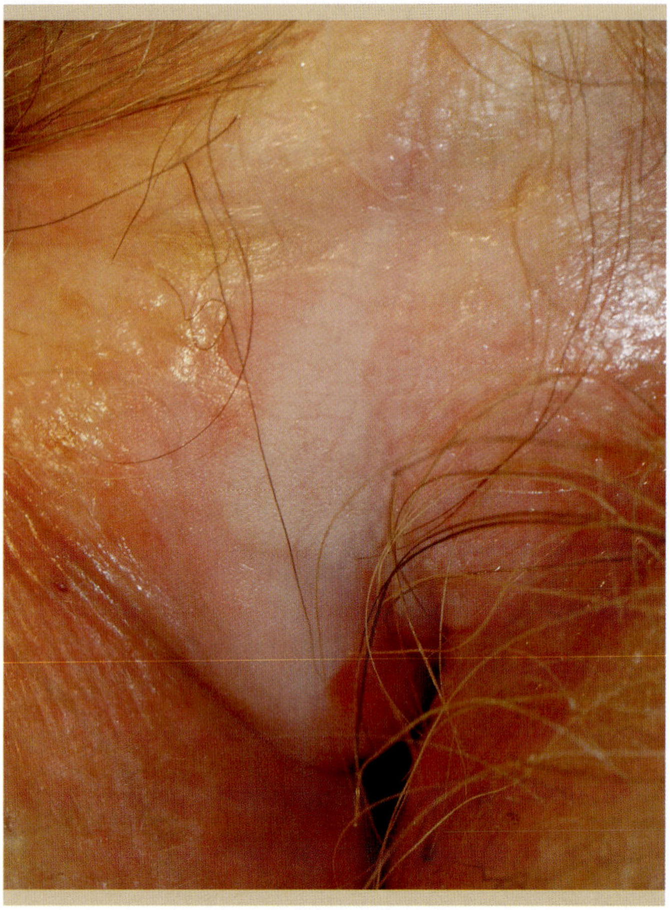

FIGURE 5-5 This differentiated vulvar intraepithelial neoplasia (squamous cell carcinoma in situ) is manifested by both a white, thickened plaque and a central red, atrophic plaque (arrow). (*Used with permission from Dr. Libby Edwards*.)

- Morphology most often flat, brown papules
- Etiology is high risk human papillomavirus (HPV) infection
- The diagnosis is by biopsy
- Therapy is destruction or excision in an immunocompetent person, as well as cervical surveillance in women
- Unrelated are differentiated VIN, PIN, AIN that represent SCCIS associated with underlying lichen sclerosus or lichen planus, and is far more aggressive. Manifested by red, white, or brown plaques (Fig. 5-5) in patients with longstanding lichen planus or lichen sclerosus, and treated with excision.

Extramammary Paget Disease

- Uncommon malignant disease that is often mistaken for eczema or psoriasis
- Morphology is that of a red plaque, often moist and exudative, classically with white islands of hyperkeratosis and located generally anywhere on the vulva, or sometimes the keratinized anogenital, scrotal, or penile skin (Fig. 5-6)

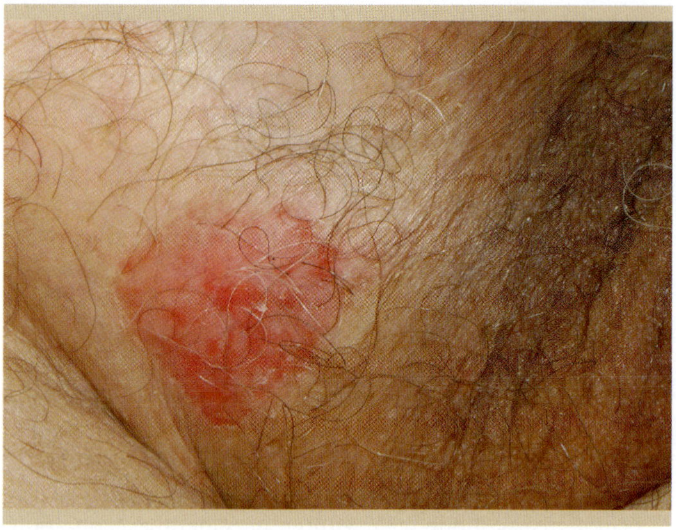

FIGURE 5-6 This scrotal plaque of primary Paget disease shows a typical red, scaling plaque with erosions. (*Used with permission from Dr. Libby Edwards*.)

- Primary form is unassociated with internal malignancy; 10 to 20% of Paget disease is secondary, associated with underlying genitourinary or gastrointestinal adenocarcinoma
- The etiology is controversial; primary is most likely a malignancy of Toker cells or sweat gland origin; secondary is from migration of underlying adenocarcinoma
- Therapy consists of excisional surgery as well as surveillance for underlying urogenital or gastrointestinal malignancy, which occurs in about 15% of patients. Recent evidence suggests benefit with imiquimod and photodynamic therapy

Perianal Streptococcal Disease (Perianal Streptococcal Cellulitis)

- Seen most often in boys at about age 3 to 5 years, this condition is often confused with candidiasis and dermatophytosis
- The primary symptoms are irritation, burning, painful defecation, often with associated constipation from avoidance of defecation
- The usual morphology is that of a discrete pink lightly scaling perianal plaque, but more severe disease shows deep redness and crusting (Fig. 5-7). Sometimes, fissuring is present. Occasionally, there is associated bacterial vaginitis, and involvement of the vulva or scrotum
- The cause is most often group A β-hemolytic *Streptococcus*, but *Staphylococcus aureus* has become much more common

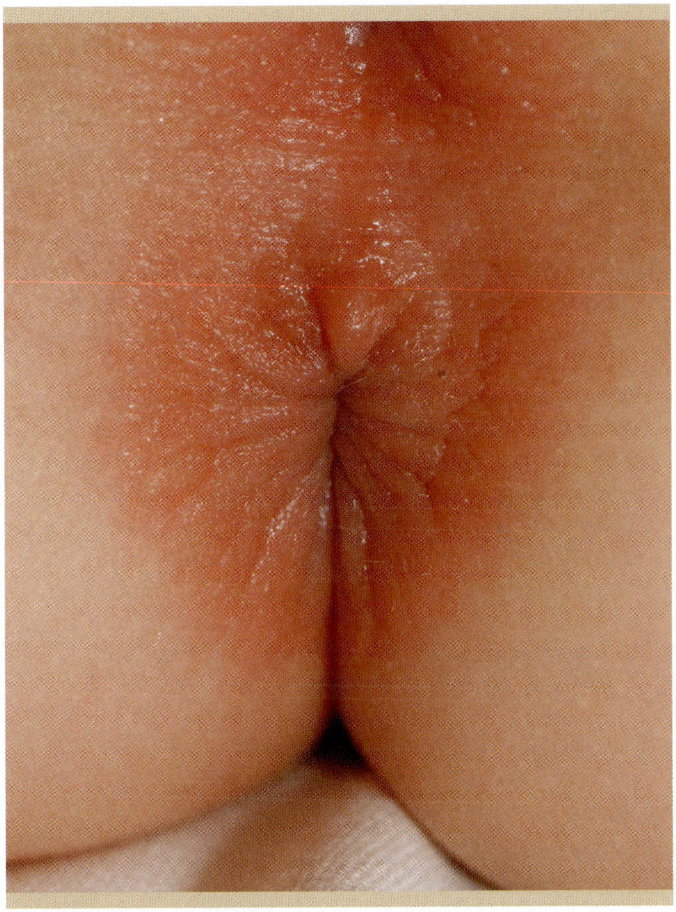

FIGURE 5-7 This perianal streptococcal disease exhibits a red, edematous plaque. (*Used with permission from Dr. Libby Edwards*.)

- The diagnosis is made by the clinical presentation and confirmed on culture
- Cefuroxime is superior to oral penicillin and amoxicillin for the treatment of this condition, but those patients with *S. aureus* should be treated according to culture results. Hydrocortisone 1% ointment can hasten improvement in symptoms, and the stool softener docusate improves constipation and painful defecation

EROSIVE AND BLISTERING LESIONS (SEE ALSO CONTACT DERMATITIS, CANDIDIASIS, PAGET DISEASE, ZOON'S VULVITIS)

Lichen Planus

- Erosive vulvovaginal lichen planus is a fairly common dermatosis in postmenopausal women, and much less often seen in men, especially those who are circumcised
- Symptoms include itching, burning, and dyspareunia

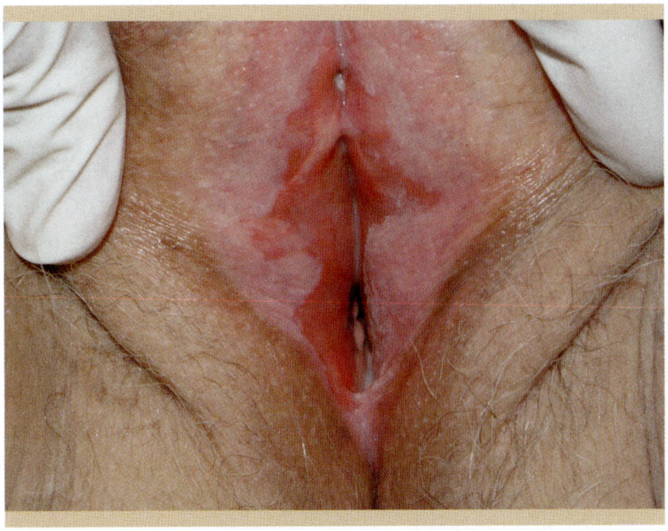

FIGURE 5-8 Erosive genital lichen planus is most often on the modified mucous membranes of the vulva, often with surrounding white epithelium. (*Used with permission from Dr. Libby Edwards*.)

- Morphology is usually that of superficial nonspecific erosions (Fig. 5-8); classic but less often is white lacy or fern-like papules. Lichen planus of the glans often appears as red papules that mimic yeast and HSIL (Fig. 5-9). Mucous membrane and modified mucous membranes of the external genitalia and vagina as well as the mouth are generally affected, and loss of vulvar architecture, vaginal synechiae, and phimosis are common. Esophageal lichen planus and secondary squamous cell carcinoma are increasingly recognized

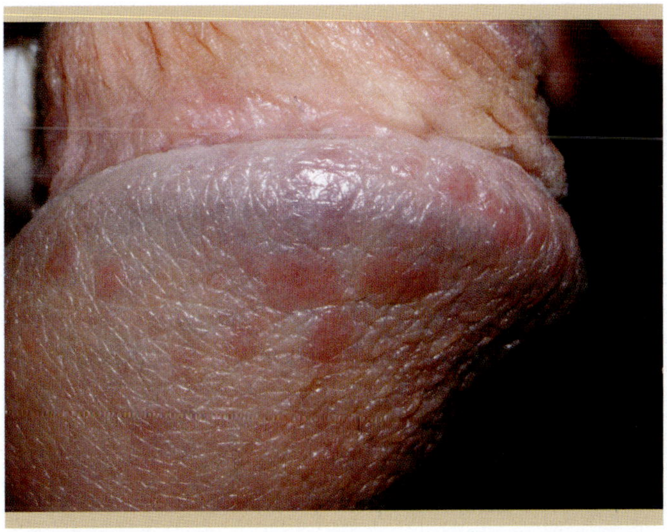

FIGURE 5-9 Pink, flat-topped papules are typical of lichen planus on the glans of a circumcised male. (*Used with permission from Dr. Libby Edwards*.)

- The etiology is one of cell-mediated autoimmunity
- The diagnosis is made by the morphology and distribution, and confirmed by a biopsy showing either lichen planus or lichenoid dermatitis and differentiating from immunobullous diseases and lichen sclerosus
- Treatment is primarily with ultrapotent topical corticosteroid ointments, and tacrolimus and pimecrolimus can be useful when tolerated. Systemic immunosuppressives are used with variable success, and surveillance for cutaneous squamous cell carcinoma is important

Fixed Drug Reaction

- Uncommon recurrent, same site skin reaction that can occur on keratinized skin as well as on the mucous membrane of the mouth, glans penis, or vulva
- On keratinized skin, a blister or round, edematous plaque is typical
- On the vulva and penis, this blister erodes immediately (Fig. 5-10)
- Etiologies include tetracyclines, sulfonamides, analgesics, sedatives, oral contraceptives, metronidazole, as well as phenolphthalein found in some over-the-counter laxatives
- Therapy consists of discontinuation of the offending medication, with bland emollients, soaks, and pain medication

Pemphigus Vulgaris and Cicatricial Pemphigoid (Benign Mucous Membrane Pemphigoid)

- Autoimmune blistering diseases that promptly erode and regularly affect mucous membranes
- Can be indistinguishable from erosive lichen planus when unaccompanied by extra-mucosal blisters
- Regularly accompanied by genital scarring
- Diagnosed by routine biopsy of the edge of a blister or erosion, with characteristic direct immunofluorescence of perilesional skin
- Management with systemic corticosteroids and steroid-sparing immunosuppressive agents, with local therapy to control infection and other accompanying conditions

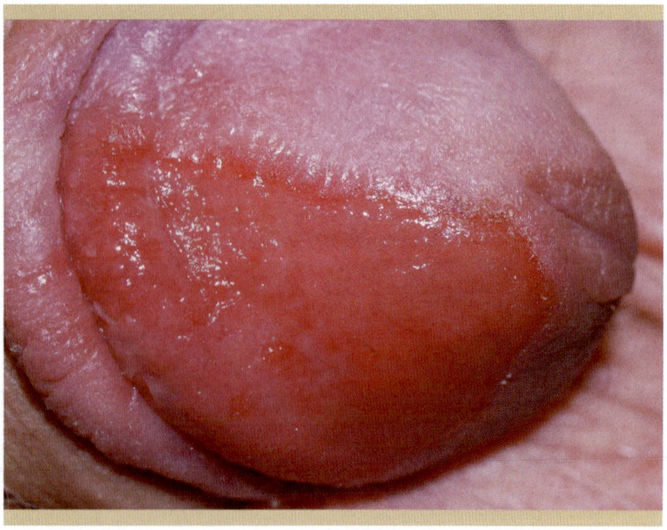

FIGURE 5-10 A fixed drug eruption occurs as an acute or recurrent same site well-demarcated erosion. (*Used with permission from Dr. Libby Edwards.*)

Herpes Simplex Virus Infection

- Very common infection that is most often latent but often exhibits recurrent eruptions
- Symptoms include a tingling prodrome followed by burning, painful vesicles, and erosions
- Morphology consists of scattered vesicles that quickly erode into round erosions with a primary occurrence, followed by grouped and coalescing vesicles and round erosions on any area of anogenital skin, as well as on the lower back or buttocks
- The etiology is the virus *Herpesvirus hominis*
- The management consists of oral acyclovir, famciclovir, or valacyclovir in various regimens to shorten outbreaks, suppress recurrences, and decrease viral shedding

NONINFECTIOUS ULCERS

Aphthae

- Under-recognized cause of genital ulcers
- Most common in young girls between about 11 and 18 years
- Characterized by pain; in young girls, often with a prodrome of fever, malaise, sore throat
- Morphologic appearance is one or more ulcers, from 2 to 3 mm to about 2 cm, occurring primarily at the introitus and modified mucous membranes (Fig. 5-11). Sometimes affects nearby keratinized skin, and occurs primarily on the scrotum in men
- Can produce marked scarring
- Adults often have recurrent disease; young girls most often experience a solitary episode
- Aphthae in eastern and mideastern countries frequently occur as 1 sign of Behçet disease; true Behçet disease with inflammatory eye findings, neurologic disease, inflammatory arthritis, pathergy, end-organ damage, etc. is rare in western countries.
- Etiology is unknown, perhaps cell-mediated response to a brisk response to a viral or bacterial infection
- The diagnosis can be made by the presentation and morphology
- Therapy consists of immediate institution oral corticosteroids until pain subsides. If frequently recurrent, suppressive therapy with dapsone is useful; colchicine, thalidomide, or tumor necrosis factor α-blockers can be useful

Crohn Disease

- Rare but characteristic cause of vulvar ulcers

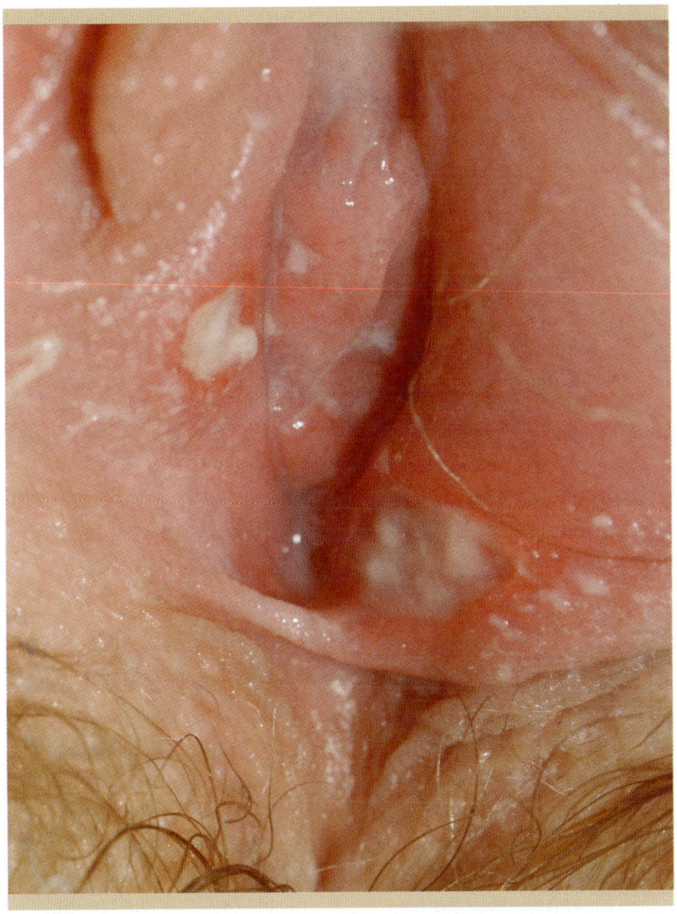

FIGURE 5-11 Aphthae of the vulva exhibit well-demarcated painful ulcers with a white fibrin base. (*Used with permission from Dr. Libby Edwards*.)

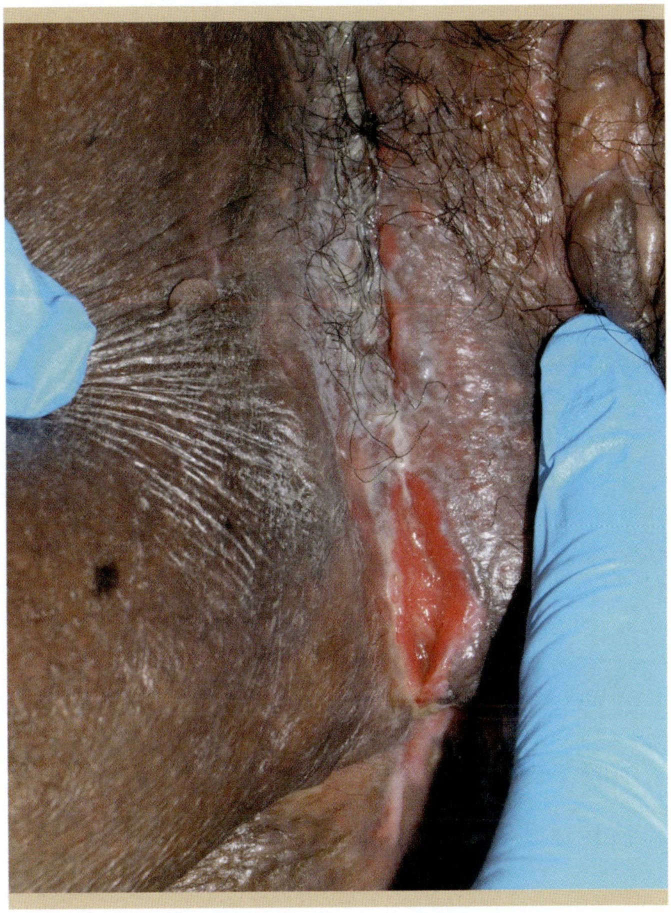

FIGURE 5-12 This linear skin-fold ulceration is classic for vulvar Crohn disease. (*Used with permission from Dr. Libby Edwards*.)

- Most common morphology is draining perianal fistulae; less common is firm, nonpitting, nonspecific edema. Although uncommon, the linear "knife-cut" skin-fold ulcerations are pathognomonic (Fig. 5-12).
- The diagnosis is made by the appearance of the ulcers, which usually are found in a setting of known Crohn disease. Perianal fistulae and edema raise the suspicion of Crohn disease, and a biopsy shows granulomatous inflammation. The diagnosis is confirmed with a gastrointestinal evaluation yielding a diagnosis of intestinal Crohn disease
- Systemic therapy is managed by a gastroenterologist

MISCELLANEOUS

Lichen Sclerosus (Et Atrophicus)

- Anogenital skin disease that is most common in postmenopausal women; it occurs in men only if uncircumcised
- Symptoms are primarily itching, with rubbing and scratching producing pain and rawness; dyspareunia is common
- Classic morphology is that of well-demarcated hypopigmented plaques with crinkled texture change (Fig. 5-13); some plaques exhibit a waxy surface, smooth, shiny skin, or irregular white hyperkeratosis
- Location is the modified mucous membranes and keratinized skin of the vulva, and the glans penis and distal shaft of men; perianal and perineal skin is regularly involved in women but rarely occurs in men
- Long-standing or severe disease produces loss of vulvar architecture and phimosis in men
- Nearly always spares the vagina and mouth
- Diagnosis is by classic morphology, biopsy is indicated if the diagnosis is not clear
- Management consists of circumcision for men. For women, therapy is ultrapotent topical corticosteroids applied once or twice daily until skin findings, then either midpotency topical corticosteroids daily, or thrice weekly ultrapotent medications to maintain control
- Recalcitrant disease can be improved with tacrolimus or pimecrolimus
- Surveillance for intercurrent squamous cell carcinoma is important

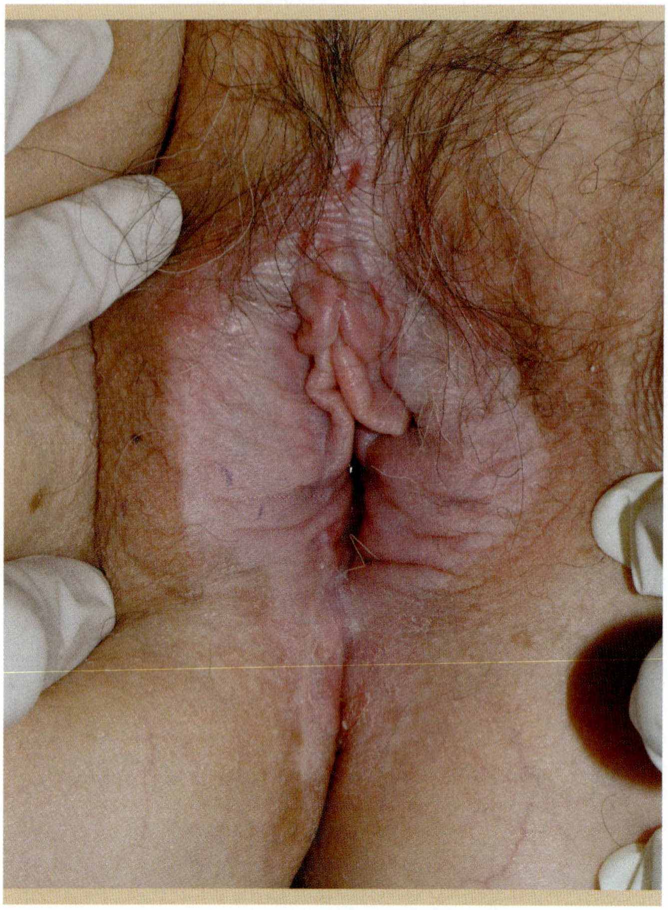

FIGURE 5-13 Lichen sclerosus typically exhibits a white, crinkled plaque that includes perianal skin. (*Used with permission from Dr. Libby Edwards.*)

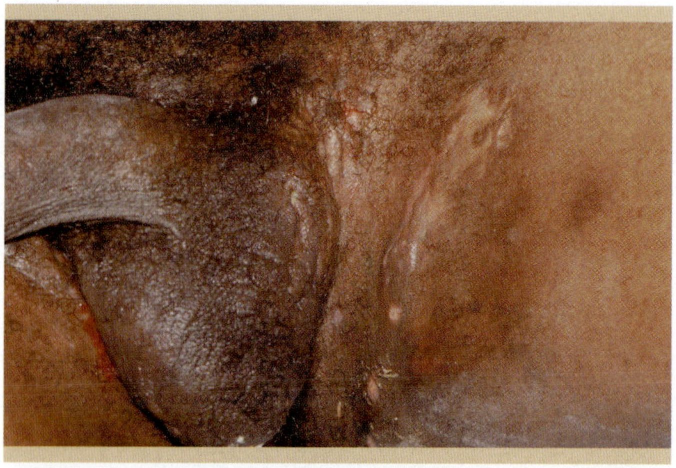

FIGURE 5-14 Hidradenitis suppurativa is characterized by chronic red nodules and draining sinus tracts. (*Used with permission from Dr. Libby Edwards.*)

Hidradenitis Suppurativa

- Common disease of variable severity, sometimes called "inverse acne"
- More common in individuals of African descent
- More common in women, often more severe in men
- Symptoms include pain and itching
- Morphology consists of epidermal cysts that become inflamed, erode, and drain, forming chronic sinus tracts. Comedones are often present (Fig. 5-14)
- Location of lesions include the proximal medial thighs, scrotum, vulva, lower abdomen, and axillae
- Scarring is usual and can be severe; squamous cell carcinoma occurs rarely
- Sometimes associated with cystic acne or dissecting cellulitis; the "follicular retention triad"
- Etiology multifactorial, including hereditary factors, hormonal factors, obesity, and smoking
- The diagnosis is made by the morphology of red nodules and comedones, the chronic nature, location, scarring, cultures that show no pure growth of a pathogen, and poor short-term response to antibiotics
- Management consists of chronic anti-inflammatory antibiotics including tetracyclines, sulfas, macrolides, and clindamycin. Discontinuation of smoking and weight loss are beneficial. More recently, metformin and tumor necrosis factor α-antagonists have been reported to be useful. Surgery, both to remove or unroof small recalcitrant areas, or to remove an entire area of involvement, is a mainstay of therapy

Genital Melanosis/Lentiginosis

- This uncommon condition can appear indistinguishable from cutaneous melanoma, but it is unassociated with the development of malignancy of any kind
- Genital melanosis is asymptomatic
- The morphology consists of patches of well-demarcated brown and black patches. The color and borders are often irregular, and can show wild discoloration at times (Fig. 5-15)
- Most often located on the modified mucous membranes and introitus of the vulva, and the glans penis of men, although the shaft can be affected
- The cause is unknown, but this is often associated with vulvar lichen sclerosus
- The diagnosis is made by biopsy of any area of the hyperpigmentation
- Management is reassurance

Genital Warts

- Usually sexually transmitted, this condition occurs in about 1% of adults
- Usually asymptomatic, although pruritus or irritation are occasionally present
- These are located on any area of anogenital mucous membranes or keratinized skin

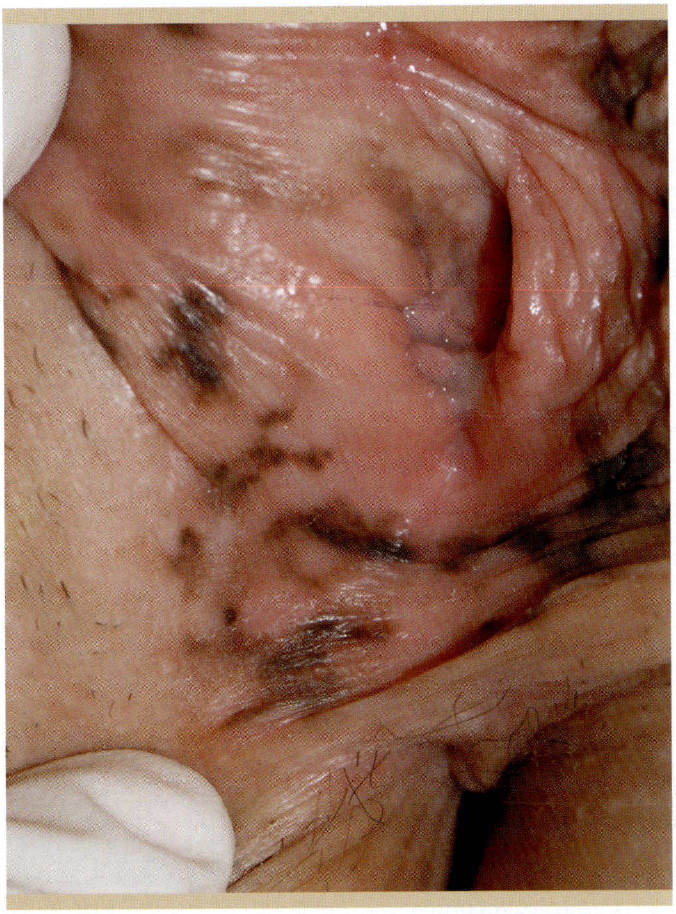

FIGURE 5-15 Genital lentiginosis mimics melanoma with brown patches that are irregular in color, borders, and size. (*Used with permission from Dr. Libby Edwards.*)

- Genital warts occur in several morphologies; although skin colored in white patients, those who are naturally darkly complexioned often exhibit brown warts. Genital warts are often filiform (spiky) papules, but they may also be dome shaped papules or multilobular, resembling a raspberry. Some warts are nearly flat. An occasional patient exhibits large, globular warts
- Anogenital warts are produced by many different HPV types. HPV types 6 and 11 account for most warts in this location, and for all low-risk types. HPV types 16 and 18 account for most warts that are associated with HSIL (squamous cell carcinoma in situ) and cervical and anal squamous cell carcinoma
- The management of anogenital warts is primarily patient education. The home-applied therapies imiquimod, sinecatechins, and podophyllotoxin are commonly used. Office-applied therapies include bi- and trichloroacetic acid, podophyllum resin. Cryotherapy, excision, and laser are used as well
- Recurrence is usual, although most patients are clear of the virus in the first year

Vulvodynia/Penodynia/Scrotodynia/Anodynia

- Idiopathic vulvar pain is well recognized to be a common phenomenon, with a prevalence of about 8%; penile and scrotal pain are under-reported but probably common. Information on male genital pain is inferred from research and experience with vulvar pain
- These are defined as chronic sensations of burning, rawness, irritation, or soreness (not itching) in the absence of relevant clinical or laboratory findings; most experience dyspareunia
- Additional symptoms include the frequent occurrence of additional pain syndromes such as headaches, fibromyalgia, irritable bowel syndrome, interstitial cystitis, and temporomandibular joint disease. Anxiety, depression, and sexual dysfunction are usual
- An examination of the area shows normal skin except for mild erythema in some
- Cultures are normal
- The etiology is unknown. Pelvic floor dysfunction is one factor, as is neuropathic pain. Anxiety and depression are operative in most
- Therapy includes patient education, pelvic floor physical therapy, and medications for neuropathic pain, such as tricyclic medications (up to 150 mg), gabapentin (up to 1200 mg 3 times a day), venlafaxine extended release 150 mg daily, duloxetine 60 mg daily, and pregabalin (up to 300 mg twice daily). Counseling and support are important

QUIZ

Questions

1. A 73-year-old uncircumcised man presents with a burning, solitary, well-demarcated, red-brown, shiny plaque on the glans. A fungal culture is negative, and there are no other abnormalities of mucous membranes. The most likely diagnosis is:

   A. Lichen planus
   B. Irritant contact dermatitis
   C. Zoon's vulvitis
   D. HSIL (PIN)

2. An 81-year-old woman has lichen sclerosus which is improving with clobetasol ointment. However, her anterior vulva remains irritated and raw. Management of her symptoms will improve with:

   A. Application of topical benzocaine (Vagisil) for pain control
   B. Washing the vulva after each urination and drying with a hair dryer
   C. Management of incontinence
   D. Changing laundry detergent and double rinsing clothes

3. Diseases associated with vulvar lichen sclerosus include:
   A. Hypertension
   B. Hypothyroidism
   C. Vitiligo
   D. Squamous cell carcinoma

4. Appropriate choices to treat inverse genital psoriasis include:
   A. Topical tar
   B. Salicylic acid shampoos for scalp psoriasis
   C. Topical corticosteroid ointment
   D. Ultraviolet light

5. A 64-year-old woman presents with a 1-year history of large painful burning and erosions of the vulva and the mouth. She is otherwise healthy, and on no medications except for thyroid replacement, calcium, and vitamin D. Appropriate diagnostic investigation is:
   A. A fungal culture of the base of erosion
   B. A biopsy of the edge of erosion for routine histology and a biopsy of adjacent uninvolved skin for direct immunofluorescence
   C. A biopsy of the base of erosion for routine histology and a biopsy of the edge for direct immunofluorescence
   D. Thyroid functions

6. A 43-year-old man reports excruciatingly itchy fungus of the scrotum unrelieved by over-the-counter topical antifungal therapy. He experiences pleasure with scratching, and his examination shows redness lichenification of the posterior scrotum. His medial thighs and toenails are normal. The best strategy is:
   A. A superpotent corticosteroid twice daily
   B. A biopsy to rule out squamous cell carcinoma
   C. Oral antifungal therapy since topical medication was ineffective
   D. A fungal culture

7. A healthy 11-year-old girl presents with a 2-day history of vulvar pain preceded by fever, malaise, and sore throat. She has 3-round, 1-cm, well-demarcated ulcers on the medial labia minora. She is best managed by:
   A. A herpes culture and oral acyclovir
   B. A dark-field microscopic examination of a scraping of the base of the ulcer, and a VDRL; then penicillin while awaiting laboratory results
   C. Prednisone 40 mg each morning until pain resolves
   D. Topical hydrocortisone cream twice a day to the ulcer

8. A 31-year-old woman presents with a 3-year history of recalcitrant and unremitting vulvar burning and dyspareunia, unresponsive to antifungal and antibiotic therapy. Her examination is normal except for mild redness of the introitus. Her most likely diagnosis is:
   A. Allergic contact dermatitis
   B. Resistant yeast infection
   C. Subclinical HPV infection
   D. Vulvodynia

9. A 26-year-old healthy but overweight male smoker seeks a diagnosis and treatment for recurrent boils in the groin and perianal skin, present for the past 5 years. These are painful and improve with amoxicillin, but then recur. Strategies that will probably improve his bois include all except:
   A. Smoking cessation
   B. Cephalexin 500 mg bid for 1 week, with mupirocin in the nares tid 1 week each month
   C. Weight loss
   D. Ongoing doxycycline

10. A 69-year-old woman reports to the office with vulvar pain; on examination she exhibits erosions and narrowing of the vestibule, loss of the labia minora, and erosions of the gingivae and the posterior buccal mucosae with surrounding white striae. Most likely, she also has involvement of:
   A. The scalp
   B. The nails
   C. The vagina
   D. The conjunctivae

Answers

1. C. This patient exhibits the characteristic appearance of plasma cell mucositis or Zoon's balanitis. A well-demarcated plaque of irritant contact dermatitis is unlikely in an uncircumcised man, and lichen planus may have this morphology but generally is not a solitary plaque without oral disease. A biopsy is indicated to rule out PIN, but it is only solitary in a setting of lichen planus or lichen sclerosus, which are not described here.
2. C. Urinary incontinence is an extremely common cause of irritant contact dermatitis in the elderly. Contact dermatitis is a common secondary phenomenon in the management of vulvar symptoms. A common cause is the application of medications, and benzocaine is a prominent cause of allergic contact dermatitis and should be avoided. Laundry detergent is not a usual cause of contact dermatitis, and would produce dermatitis of other areas that touch clothing. Over washing and incontinence are typical irritants in older women.
3. Lichen sclerosus has no association with hypertension. Because lichen sclerosus is partly autoimmune in origin; however, there is an association with hypothyroidism and vitiligo, other autoimmune conditions. About 3%

of women with uncontrolled lichen sclerosus develop squamous cell carcinoma.

4. C. Genital psoriasis usually responds well to topical corticosteroids and is first-line therapy. The ointment vehicle is preferred as creams often burn with application. Frequent reevaluation and prompt decrease in the potency of the topical corticosteroid are important in preventing steroid atrophy. Topical tar and salicylic acid are too irritating for genital skin. Ultraviolet light is useful for psoriasis in general, but is impractical in the genital area, and ultraviolet light is known to increase the risk of cutaneous squamous cell carcinoma, so is best avoided.
5. B. Erosions are nonspecific, so that laboratory evaluation is needed to make a diagnosis. Chronic large, well-demarcated erosions of the mouth and vulva are not consistent yeast infections. A biopsy is required to make this diagnosis, but if the base of erosion is sampled, the lack of epidermis will prevent the pathologist from making a diagnosis. Direct immunofluorescent biopsies are best taken from adjacent normal skin.
6. A. The lichenification responds best to a potent steroid, but he should be advised to use it sparingly, to wear briefs rather than boxers to prevent spread to the medial thighs, and to return in 3 to 4 weeks for reevaluation to assess for improvement and occurrence of steroid side effects. A biopsy is not needed if the only physical finding is lichenification, and fungal infection is a very unlikely cause of his eruption. Unless immunosuppressed, tinea generally affects the medial thighs rather than the scrotum, and he did not respond to good first-line topical therapy.
7. C. The setting and morphology of the ulcer, as well as the rarity and painless nature of a chancre allow for the clinical diagnosis of aphthous ulcer in this child. Prednisone is the treatment of choice. Hydrocortisone provides insufficient anti-inflammatory effects, and the cream base burns open skin.
8. D. Vulvodynia is a common pain syndrome characterized by chronic sensations of vulvar burning and dyspareunia, most often introital and called the vestibulodynia pattern (formerly called vulvar vestibulitis). Patchy redness of the vestibule (introitus) is usual. Allergic contact dermatitis is pruritic rather than painful (except for pain from scratching), and this should produce abnormalities of redness and scaling or erosion on examination. Yeast infection is usually recurrent and pruritic rather than chronic burning and rawness sensation, and the lack of response to antifungals indicate an alternate diagnosis. Subclinical HPV has been disproved as a cause of chronic burning by molecular studies for HPV.
9. D. This patient has hidradenitis suppurativa, or inverse cystic acne. A 1-week course of an antibiotic will not affect his disease, since this is not an infectious disease. However, smoking and obesity are known to worsen hidradenitis, so that eliminating these factors will probably improve his disease. Doxycycline has anti-inflammatory properties and is a standard therapy for hidradenitis. Otherwise, surgery and tumor necrosis factor α-blockers can be used.
10. C. She has lichen planus, which regularly affects the mouth, vulva, and vagina (called the vulvo-vaginal-gingival syndrome). However, erosive vulvar lichen planus can, but usually does not, exhibit lichen planopilaris or lichen planus of keratinized extragenital skin, or nails. Eye involvement is uncommon, but esophageal involvement is increasingly recognized.

REFERENCES

Clément E, Sparsa A, Doffoel-Hantz V, et al. Photodynamic therapy for the treatment of extramammary Paget's disease. *Ann Dermatol Venereol* 2012;139:103.

Fox LP, Lightdale CJ, Grossman ME: Lichen planus of the esophagus: what dermatologists need to know. *J Am Acad Dermatol* 2011;65:175.

Hanami Y, Motoki Y, Yamamoto T: Successful treatment of plasma cell cheilitis with topical tacrolimus: report of two cases. *Dermatol Online J* 2011;17:6.

Heath C, Desai N, Silverberg NB: Recent microbiological shifts in perianal bacterial dermatitis: Staphylococcus aureus predominance. *Pediatr Dermatol* 2009;26:696–700.

Herranz P, Sendagorta E, Feito M, Gómez-Fernandez C: Sustained remission of extramammary Paget disease following treatment with imiquimod 5% cream. *Actas Dermosifiliogr* 2012 [Epub ahead of print].

Letsinger JA, McCarty M, Jorizzo JL: Complex aphthosis: a large case series with evaluation algorithm and therapeutic ladder from topicals to thalidomide. *J Am Acad Dermatol* 2005;52:500.

Meury SN, Erb T, Schaad UB, Heininger U: Randomized, comparative efficacy trial of oral penicillin versus cefuroxime for perianal streptococcal dermatitis in children. *J Pediatr* 2008;153:799.

Reed BD, Harlow SD, Sen A, et al. Prevalence and demographic characteristics of vulvodynia in a population-based sample. *Am J Obstet Gynecol* 2012;206:170.

Shear NH: Pharmacologic interventions for hidradenitis suppurativa: what does the evidence say? *Am J Clin Dermatol* 2012;13:283.

Sideri M, Jones RW, Heller DS, et al. Comment on the Article: Srodon M, Stoler MH, Baber GB, et al. The distribution of low and high-risk HPV types in vulvar and vaginal intraepithelial neoplasia (VIN and VaIN). *Am J Surg Pathol* 2006;30:1513–1518. *Am J Surg Pathol* 2007;31:1452.

van Kessel MA, van Lingen RG, Bovenschen HJ: Vulvitis plasmacellularis circumscripta in pre-existing lichen sclerosus: treatment with imiquimod 5% cream. *J Am Acad Dermatol* 2010;63:c11.

Verdolini R, Clayton N, Smith A, Alwash N, Mannello B: Metformin for the treatment of hidradenitis suppurativa: a little help along the way. *J Eur Acad Dermatol Venereol* 2012 [Epub ahead of print].

CHAPTER 6

CONTACT DERMATITIS

MELISSA A. BOGLE
GIUSEPPE MILITELLO
SHARON E JACOB

CONTACT DERMATITIS

- Inflammatory response of the skin to an antigen (allergen) or irritant
- Allergic contact dermatitis (ACD)
  - Delayed type hypersensitivity reaction (type IV)
  - Dermal Dendritic cells play a central role in processing and presenting antigen complexes in the sensitization phase
  - Individuals previously sensitized to the allergen can develop a cutaneous response with subsequent exposure to the allergen. These responses can be incrementally more severe with each exposure.
  - Common allergens include plants from the *Toxicodendron* genus (e.g., poison ivy), nickel sulfate, fragrances, preservatives, and rubber additives
  - Acute ACD: lesions appear within 24 to 96 hours of exposure to the allergen in sensitized individuals
- Irritant contact dermatitis (ICD)
  - Irritants are cytotoxic to the keratinocyte, disrupt the lipid architecture, and promote the release of inflammatory mediators
  - ICD will only occur in areas of the skin that has been in direct contact with the offending chemical agent
  - Subsequent inflammatory response in the dermis
  - Two types:
    - Mild irritants: require prolonged or repeated exposure before inflammation is noted (e.g., soap)
    - Strong irritants: strong acids, alkalis, can produce immediate reactions similar to thermal burns
- Clinical Presentation
  - Acute contact dermatitis: clear fluid–filled vesicles or bullae that appear on bright red edematous skin, pruritic. ICD generally occurs within the area of contact with the chemical, whereas ACD can extend beyond the borders of the contact area
  - Subacute contact dermatitis: less edema and formation of papules, pruritic
  - Chronic contact dermatitis: minimal edema, scaling, skin fissuring, and lichenification
  - Histology
  - Dermis with perivascular lymphocytes and other mononuclear cells and epidermal spongiosis are seen in ACD. Cytotoxicity more commonly seen in ICD
  - Chronic ACD: acanthosis with hyperkeratosis and parakeratosis. Difficult to distinguish, clinically and histologically, allergic contact from irritant contact dermatitis in the chronic phase

CONTACT URTICARIA

- An immunoglobulin E (IgE)—mediated immediate hypersensitivity reaction (type I)
- Immediate release of inflammatory mediators, resulting in a wheal-and-flare reaction
- Rubber latex currently is the most important source of allergic contact urticaria

PHOTOSENSITIVITY INDUCED BY EXOGENOUS AGENTS

- Photodermatitis
  - Diagnosed by the presence of lesions limited to sun-exposed body areas (sparing of the submental chin, posterior auricular area, and inner arms can be clues). Certain substances transform into allergens (photoallergic) or irritants (phototoxic) by ultraviolet light
- Photoallergic reaction
  - Delayed-type hypersensitivity reaction (type IV); a form of allergic contact dermatitis whose distribution is limited to sun-exposed areas of the body
  - Onset delayed as long as 24 to 96 hours after exposure to the drug and light

- Amount of inciting substance (chemical allergen, drug, etc.) required to elicit photoallergic reactions is considerably smaller than that required for phototoxic reaction
- Irradiation of certain substances by ultraviolet light results in the transformation of the substance into allergens
- Examples of agents that can cause a photoallergic reaction (Tables 6-1 and 6-2)

- Phototoxic reaction
  - Chemically induced nonimmunologic acute skin irritation with damage to to cell membranes from the effects of light-activated compounds
  - Active chemical may enter the skin via topical administration or via ingestion, inhalation, or parenteral administration. Often occurs within minutes or hours of light exposure
  - Most compounds are activated by wavelengths within the ultraviolet A (UV-A) (320–400 nm) range
  - Does not require prior sensitization
  - Clinical appearance: an exaggerated sunburn reaction
  - Examples of agents that can cause phototoxic reactions (Tables 6-3 and 6-4)
- Photopatch test
  - Used to find causative agent of photoallergic reaction
  - Photopatch testing protocol
  - Day 1: Determine minimal erythema doses (MEDs), and apply 2 sets of patches
  - Day 2: Read MEDs
  - Day 2: Remove patches, read, and irradiate 1 set (10 J/cm^2 UV-A)
  - Day 4: First reading
  - Days 5–9: Second reading

FRAGRANCE-RELATED ALLERGENS

1. Balsam of Peru (also referred to as *Myroxylon pereirae*)
   - Wood extract derived from *Myroxylon balsamum* tree
     - Contains:
     - Cinnamein (cinnamic acid, cinnamyl cinnamate, cinnamic aldehyde, benzyl benzoate, benzoic acid, and vanillin)
     - Polymers of coniferyl alcohol with benzoic acid and cinnamic acid
   - Found in the following products: fragrances, flavorings/spices, pharmaceuticals (antifungal and antibacterial products), diaper powders and ointments, cough medicines, aperitifs
   - Cross-reacts with colophony, turpentine, benzoin, wood tar
2. Fragrance Mix I
   - Used as a screening tool for detecting fragrance allergy
   - Contains 8 allergens constituent: α-amylcinnamic alcohol, cinnamic alcohol, cinnamic aldehyde, eugenol, geraniol, hydroxycitronellal, isoeugenol, oak moss absolute
   - Along with balsam of Peru, Fragrance Mix I detects the majority of patients with a fragrance allergy
3. Fragrance Mix II
   - Second fragrance mixture for patch testing
   - Constituents: hydroxyisohexyl 3-cyclohexene carboxyaldehyde (Lyral), Citral, farnesol, citronellol, hexyl cinnamal, coumarin
   - Lyral is the most common sensitizer in the mix
4. Cinnamic aldehyde
   - Fragrance and flavor agent; constituent of cinnamon oil
   - When found in toothpaste, mouthwash, gum, patients may experience perioral dermatitis, tongue swelling, mouth ulceration
   - Flavoring in beverages (cola)
   - Spices: causes hand dermatitis in bakers
   - Components of essential oils: balsam of Peru, hyacinth, myrrh, patchouli, ceylon, and cassia oil
5. Lily of the valley
   - Allergen: hydroxycitronellal (synthetic)
   - Found in perfumes, soaps, cosmetics, eye cream, aftershaves
   - Also used in insecticides and antiseptics
6. Musk ambrette
   - Fixative in perfumes
   - Photoallergen
7. Oak moss absolute
   - *Evernia prunastri:* lichen oak moss
   - Main allergen: atranorin
   - Essential oil from lichens can contain the following other allergens: evernic acid and fumarprotocetaric acid
   - "Masculine" odor in aftershaves
8. Geraniol
   - *Sweet floral* odor of rose
   - Constitutes a large portion of rose and palmarose oil, geranium oil, lavender oil, jasmine oil, and citronella oil
   - Most widely used fragrance in perfumes, colognes, facial makeup, and skin-care products
9. Eugenol
   - Powerful spicy odor of clove with a pungent taste
   - Found in oils of clove and cinnamon leaf
   - Also found in roses, carnations, hyacinths, and violets
   - Fragrance in perfume, cosmetics; flavoring in toothpaste, mouthwash; and food flavorings, dental cement, insecticidal and fungicidal properties—used to preserve meats and other foods

HAIR-RELATED ALLERGENS

1. Paraphenylenediamine (PPD)
   - Dark permanent hair dye: hand dermatitis in hairdressers, scalp/hairline dermatitis in clients

TABLE 6-1 Topical Photoallergens

Group	INCI Name/Chemical Name/Trade Name*
Sunscreens	*UVB absorbers:*
	para-Aminobenzoic acids (*PABA*):
	Amyl dimethyl PABA (*Padimate A; Escalol 506*)[†]
	PABA (*Pabanol*)[†]
	Ethylhexyl dimethyl PABA (octyl dimethyl PABA; *Padimate O; Escalol 507*)[†]
	Cinnamates:
	Cinoxate (2-ethoxyethyl-*p*-methoxycinnamate; *Phiasol*)
	Ethylhexyl methoxycinnamate (octyl methoxycinnamate; *Parsol MCX; Escalol 557*)
	Salicylate:
	Homosalate (metahomomenthyl salicylate; *Eusolex HMS*)
	UVA absorbers:
	Anthranllate:
	Menthyl anthranilate (cyclohexanol; *Trivent MA*)
	Benzophenones (partial UVB absorption):
	Benzophenone-3 (oxybenzone; *Escalol 567*)[†]
	Benzophenone-4 (sulisobenzone; *Escalol 577*)[†]
	Dibenzoylmethane:
	Butyl methoxydibenzoylmethane (avobenzone; *Parsol 1789*)[†]
Fragrances	6-Methylcoumarin[†]
	Musk ambrette[†]
	Sandalwood oil
Antibacterials	Dibromosalicylanilide (dibromsalan; DBS)[†]
	Tetrochlorosalicylanilide (TCSA; *Impregon; Irgasan BS200*)[†]
	Tribromosalicylanilide (tribromsalan; TBS)*
	Chlorhexidine (*Hibiclens*)
	Dimethylol-dimethyl hydantoin
	Hexachlorophene (*pHisoHex*)
	Bithionol (thiobisdichlorophenol; bisphenol; *Actamar*)[†]
	Dichlorophene (G4)
	Triclosan (*Irgasan DP300*)

(*Continued*)

TABLE 6-1 Topical Photoallergens (Continued)

Group	INCI Name/Chemical Name/Trade Name*
Antifungals	Fentichlor (thiobischlorophenol)*
	Jadit (butylchlorosalicylamide; buclosamide)
	Multifungin (bromochlorosalicylanilide; BCSA)
Others	Chlorpromazine (*Thorazine*)*
	Clioquinol
	Ketoprofen (*Orudis*)
	Olaquindox
	Promethazine (*Phenergan*)*
	Quinidine (*Cardioquin; Quinidex*)
	Thiourea (thiocarbamide)

*INCI: International Nomenclature of Cosmetic Ingredients.
†Commonly reported photoallergens.
Reprinted with permission from Freedberg IM et al. *Fitzpatrick's Dermatology in General Medicine,* 6th Ed. New York: McGraw-Hill; 2003, p. 1305.

- Dyed furs, photographic developers, photocopy, printing ink, dark cosmetics, black rubber (rubber antioxidant), leather processing
- Cross-reacts with PABA, ester anesthetics, sulfa medications, azo dyes (textile dermatitis)
- *Black henna*: formulations are available that contain PPD and sometimes lead to an allergic reaction (Type IV hypersensitivity)
- Natural henna is derived from the *Lawsonia alba* plant and does not usually lead to ACD
- Patch test with PPD

2. Glycerol thioglycolate (GTG)
    - Acidic (salon) permanent wave solutions and hair straighteners
    - Chemical remains in hair shaft for months: chronic dermatitis in hairdressers and clients
    - Note: Alkaline (home) permanent solutions contain ammonium thioglycolate (ATG) and are also irritating

TABLE 6-2 Systemic Photoallergens

Property	Generic Name (US Trade Name)
Antifungal	Griseofulvin (*Fulvicin-U/F*)
Antimalarial	Quinine
Antimicrobials	Quinolone: Enoxacin (*Penetrex*), sulfonamides
Cardiac medication	Quinidine (*Quinaglute, Quinidex*)
Nonsteroidal	Ketoprofen (*Orudis, Oruvall*)
	Piroxicam (*Feldene*)
Vitamin	Pyridoxine hydrochloride (vitamin B_6)

Reprinted with permission from Freedberg IM et al. *Fitzpatrick's Dermatology in General Medicine,* 6th Ed. New York: McGraw-Hill; 2003, p. 1305.

TABLE 6-3 Topical Phototoxic Agents

Agent	Exposure
Rose bengal	Ophthalmologic examination
Antimicrobials	Occur naturally in plants, fruits, and vegetables (lime, lemon, celery, fig, parsley, and parsnip); used in perfumes and cosmetics; used for topical photochemotherapy
Tar	Topical therapeutic agent; roofing materials

Reprinted with permission from Freedberg IM et al. *Fitzpatrick's Dermatology in General Medicine,* 6th Ed. New York: McGraw-Hill; 2003, p. 1301.

TABLE 6-4 Systemic Phototoxic Agents

Property	Generic Name (US Trade Name)
Antianxiety drugs	Alprazolam (*Xanax*)
	Chlordiazepoxide (*Librax; Librium; Limbitrol*)
Anticancer drugs	Dacarbazine (*DTIC-Dome*)
	Fluorouracil (*Adrucil*)
	Methotrexate (*Rheumatrex*)
	Vinblastine (*Velban*)
Antidepressants	Tricyclics:
	Amitriptyline *(Elavil; Limbitrol; Triavil)*
	Desipramine *(Norpramin)*
	Imipramine *(Tofranil)*
Antifungal	Griseofulvin (*Fulvicin; Grifulvin V; Gris-PEG*)
Antimalarials	Chloroquine *(Aralen)* Quinine
Antimicrobials	Quinolones:
	Ciprofloxacin *(Cipro)*
	Enoxacin *(Penetrex)*
	Gemifloxacin
	Lomefloxacin *(Maxaquin)**
	Moxifloxacin *(Avelox)*
	Nalidixic acid *(NegGram)**
	Norfloxacin *(Chibroxin; Noroxin)*
	Ofloxacin *(Floxin; Ocuflox)*
	Sparfloxacin *(Zagam)**
	Suifonamides
	Tetracyclines
	Demeclocycline (*Declomycin)**
	Doxycycline *(Monodox; Periostat; Vibramycin)**
	Minocycline *(Dynacin; Minocin)*
	Tetracycline *(Helidac; Sumycin)*
	Trimethoprim *(Bactrim; Polytrim; Septra)*
Antipsychotic drugs	Phenothiazines:
	Chlorpromazine *(Thorazine)**
	Perphenazine *(Triavil; Trilafon)*

(Continued)

TABLE 6-4 Systemic Phototoxic Agents (Continued)

Property	Generic Name (US Trade Name)
	Prochlorperazine *(Compazine)**
	Thioridazine *(Mellaril)*
	Trifluoperazine *(Stelazine)*
Cardiac medications	Amiodarone *(Cordarone; Pacerone)**
	Quinidine *(Quinaglute; Quinidex)*
Diuretics	Furosemide *(Lasix)**
	Thiazides:
	Bendroflumethiazide *(Corzide)*
	Chlorothiazide (*Aldoclor; Diuril*)*
	Hydrochlorothiazide *(Accuretic; Aldactazide; Aldoril; Atacana Avalide; Capozide; Dlovan; Dyazide; HydroDIURIL)**
Dye	Fluorescein (*AK-Fluor; Fluor; Fluor-I-Strip Fluorescite)*
	Methylene blue *(Urised)*
Furocoumarins	Psoralens:
	5-Methoxypsoralen*
	8-Methoxypsoralen (Oxsoralen-Ultra
	4,5′,8-Trimethylpsoralen*
Hypoglycemics	Sulfonylureas:
	Acetohexamide
	Chlorpropamide (*Diabinase*)
	Glipizide (*Glucotrol)*
	Glyburide (*DiaBeta; Glucovance Glynase Pres Tab; Micronase)*
	Tolazamide (*Tolinase)*
	Tolbutamide (*Orinase)**
NSAIDs	Acetic acid derivative:
	Diclofenac (*Arthrotec; Cataplan Voltaren)*
	Anthranilic acid derivative:
	Mefenamic acid (*Ponstel)*
	Enolic acid derivative:
	Piroxicam (*Feldene)**
	Propionic acid derivatives:
	Ibuprofen *(Advil; Motrin; Nuprin Vicoprofen)*

(Continued)

TABLE 6-4 Systemic Phototoxic Agents (Continued)

Property	Generic Name (US Trade Name)
	Ketoprofen *(Orudis; Oruvail)*
	Naproxen *(Aleve; Naprelan; Naprosyn)**
	Oxaprozin *(Daypro)*
	Tiaprofenic acid
	Salicylic acid derivative:
	Diflunisal *(Dolobid)*
	Others:
	Celecoxib *(Celebrex)*
	Nabumetone *(Relafen)**
Photodynamic therapy agents	Porfimer *(Photofrin)**
	Verteporfin *(Visudyne)**
Retinoids	Acitretin *(Soriatane)*
	Isotretinoin *(Accutane)*
	Etretinate
Other	Flutamide *(Eulexin)*
	Hypericin
	Pyridoxine (vitamin B6)
	Ranitidine *(Zantac)*

*Commonly reported.
Reprinted with permission from Freedberg IM et al. *Fitzpatrick's Dermatology in General Medicine*, 6th Ed. New York: McGraw-Hill; 2003, p. 1302.

3. Ammonia persulfate
    - Peroxide hair bleaches
    - Bleached baking flour
    - Contact urticaria and anaphylactoid reactions
4. Cocamidopropyl betaine
    - Allergen may be dimethylaminopropylamine or amidoamine (residues from synthesis)
    - Surfactant
    - Shampoo (dermatitis in hair dressers), liquid soaps

MEDICINE-RELATED ALLERGENS

1. Tixocortol pivalate
    - Used to test for allergy to group A steroids (e.g., prednisone, hydrocortisone)
    - Short-chain esters
2. Budesonide
    - Screening agent for allergy to groups B (e.g., triamcinolone) and D2 (e.g., HC-17 butyrate) steroids
    - Cross reactions may be seen between Groups A and D2, and between budesonide and group D2
    - Long-chain steroids
3. Ethylenediamine dichloride
    - Stabilizer in topical creams, medicines, dyes, rubber, resin, waxes, insecticides, asphalt, fungicides
    - Previously found in nystatin cream
    - Cross-reacts with aminophylline, antihistamines (hydroxyzine, cetirizine), meclizine (antivert)
4. Glutaraldehyde
    - Cold sterilizing solution (medical/dental equipment)
    - Embalming fluid, electron microscopy, cosmetics, waterless hand cleansers, wallpaper, liquid fabric softener, leather tanning

5. Wool alcohols
    - Lanolin and lanolin alchol
    - From the sebum of sheep
    - Lanolin consists of 95% wool esters: alcohols (52%) and acids (48%)
    - Wool alcohols are used to test for lanolin allergy
    - Topical creams (e.g., Eucerin), cosmetics, adhesives, topical steroids
6. Propylene glycol
    - A dimer alcohol used to make drugs more soluble, also used in packaged foods
    - Vehicle base in pharmaceuticals (Valium, ECG, and lubricant jelly), cosmetics, food, and topical medications (corticosteroid creams, ointments, foams, gels, and solutions)
    - Brake fluid, tobacco formulations, antifreeze
7. Thimerosal
    - Mercury-containing organic compound (an organomercurial)
    - Made from the combination of ethyl mercuric chloride, thiosalicylic acid, sodium hydroxide, and ethanol
    - Preservative used in vaccines: thimerosal has been removed from all vaccines routinely recommended for children 6 years of age or younger, with the exception of inactivated influenza vaccine
    - Also found in antitoxins, immunoglobulins
    - False-positive intradermal testing (e.g., to tuberculosis) can occur if material is preserved with thimerosal
    - Eye/ear drops, nasal sprays, contact lens solutions: conjunctivitis, eyelid dermatitis
    - Cosmetics, liquid soap, oral hygiene products, pesticides
    - Cross-reacts with piroxicam, mercury
    - Most reactions seen with patch testing are not currently clinically relevant and are indicative of prior exposure (e.g., vaccines)
8. Neomycin sulfate
    - Antibiotic in the aminoglycoside group
    - Used topically in ointments, creams, ear drops, and eye drops
    - Cross-reacts with gentamycin, tobramycin, streptomycin, or any systemic aminoglycoside
    - Often co-reactivity to bacitracin (Fig. 6-1)
9. Triclosan
    - Antibacterial agent
    - Soap, shampoo, mouthwash
10. Benzocaine
    - Topical anesthetic (remedies for hemorrhoids, sunburn, toothaches, sore throats, athlete's foot)
    - Cross-reacts with ester anesthetics, PABA, paraphenylenediamine, sulfa medications
    - Patch test with caine mix: benzocaine, dibucaine hydrochloride, and tetracaine hydrochloride

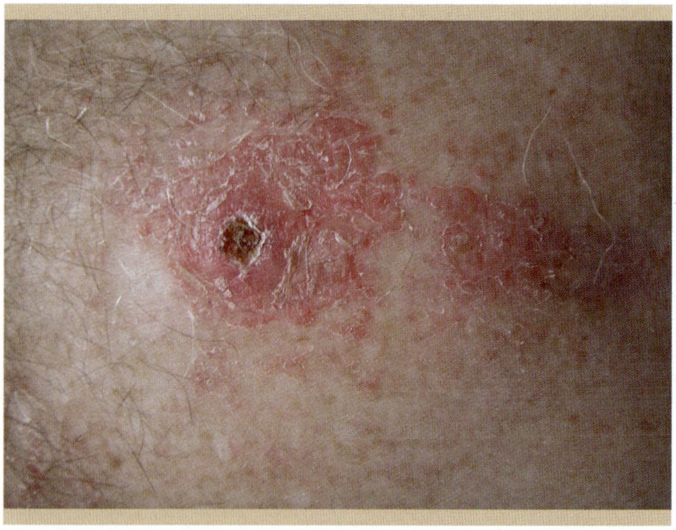

FIGURE 6-1 ACD to bacitracin following a biopsy. *(Used with permission from Dr. Sharon E. Jacob.)*

NAIL-RELATED ALLERGENS

- Contact dermatitis to nail allergens may present as chronic paronychia, onychodystrophy, fingertip dermatitis, or face and neck dermatitis (ectopic dermatitis)

1. Ethyl cyanoacrylate
    - Instant glue ("Super Glue"), artificial nail glue
    - Liquid bandages, sealant for ileostomy appliances
    - Electronic circuit boards, aircrafts, automobiles
2. Methyl methacrylate
    - Clear, rigid plastic (artificial nails, hard contact lenses, hearing aids, dentures, dental fillings/sealants)
    - Glue for surgical prostheses/artificial joints: dermatitis in orthopedic surgeons
    - Cross-reacts with ethyl methacrylate
3. Toluene-sulfonamide (tosylamide) formaldehyde resin
    - Used in nail polishes
    - Nail polish: eyelid, face, neck, finger dermatitis

PLANT-RELATED ALLERGENS

1. *Pinaceae*
    - Pine trees (i.e., *Pinus* species) and spruce trees
    - Source of colophony (or wood rosin)
        - Main allergens of colophony are oxidation products of abietic acid and its isomer primaric acid
        - Found in medical adhesives, cosmetics, athletic grip aids, dental cement, violin bow rosin, newsprint/magazine paper, soldering materials, nail coating (construction workers)
        - Cross-reacts with balsam of Peru
    - Source of turpentine, oleoresin also contains irritants, such as α-pinene, and allergens, such as Δ-3-carene

2. *Alliaceae*
   - Genus *Allium*
   - Includes onions, garlic, and chives
   - Allergens: diallyldisulfide, allylpropyl disulfide, and allicin
   - Fresh garlic is both an allergen and a potent irritant
   - Causes second- and third-degree burns when applied to injured skin
   - Most common cause of fingertip dermatitis in housewives and caterers
3. Lichens
   - Allergens: usnic acid, atranorin, evernic acid, fumarprotocetraric acid
   - Forest workers, gardeners, woodcutters
   - Lichen extracts (oak moss, tree moss): dermatitis from aftershave products
4. *Primulaceae*
   - *Primula obconica*: primrose
   - Allergen is primin
   - Highly allergenic petals and sepals
   - May cross-react with other quinones: orchids or tropical woods, such as teak, rosewood
5. Family *Asteraceae* (previously *Compositae* family) (Fig. 6-2)
   - Ragweed, chrysanthemum, feverfew and carrot weed, daisy, sunflower, dandelion, artichoke, lettuce, and endives
   - Gardeners, florists, farmers, cooks: airborne or summer-exacerbated dermatitis
   - Allergen: *Sesquiterpene lactones (SQLs) and bisabolol*
     - Found in the leaves, stems, flowers, and some pollen
     - Cross-reactivity occurs randomly
     - SQL mix (i.e., alantolactone, dehydrocostus lactone, costunolide) is a biologically variable and may have low sensitivity
     - Compositae mix (arnica, yarrow, tansy, German chamomile and feverfew) may be a more sensitive screening agent
   - Ragweeds (*Ambrosia* species)
     - Oleoresin is thought to cause airborne contact dermatitis
     - Typically occurs in atopic patients
   - Feverfew and carrot weed (*Parthenium hysterophores*)
   - Chrysanthemum (*Dendranthema grandiflorum* cv.): most common *Asteraceae* plants that cause occupational contact dermatitis
   - Sunflower (*Helianthus annuus*)
     - 1-0-methyl 1-4,5-dihydroniveusin A
     - Trichomes, or small hairs, on the surfaces of the leaf secrete the allergen
     - Windblown trichomes from dry plants can cause airborne contact dermatitis
   - Dandelion (*Taraxacum officinale*)
     - Airborne allergic contact dermatitis
     - Allergen is taraxinic acid (1-0-*b*-glucopyranoside)

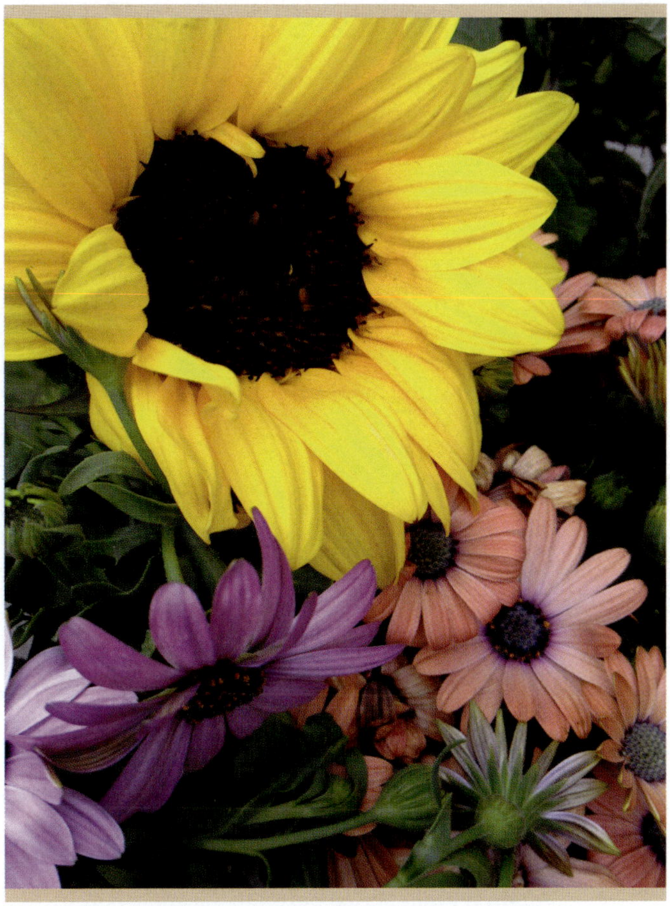

FIGURE 6-2 Family *Asteraceae*. (*Used with permission from Dr. Sharon E. Jacob.*)

6. Toxicodendron species (*Rhus*); family (*Anacardiaceae*)
   - Poison ivy, poison oak, poison sumac, Brazilian pepper tree, Indian marking nut, mango, ginkgo, cashew, Japanese lacquer tree, and pistachio.
   - Allergens are pentadecylcatechols, found in the plant sap
     - Urushiol (milky secretion)
     - Oleoresin (dry resin)
     - Cathecols are soluble in rubber
     - Particles suspended in smoke can carry urushiol
     - Blister fluid does not contain urushiol
     - Nonleaf portions of the plant can induce dermatitis
   - Most common cause of contact dermatitis in children
   - Poison ivy
     - *Toxicodendron radicans:* climbing vine, eastern United States (Fig. 6-3)
     - *Toxicodendron rydbergii*: nonclimbing dwarf shrub, the northwestern United States
   - Poison oak
     - *Toxicodendron diversilobum*: western United States
     - *Toxicodendron toxicarium*: eastern United States

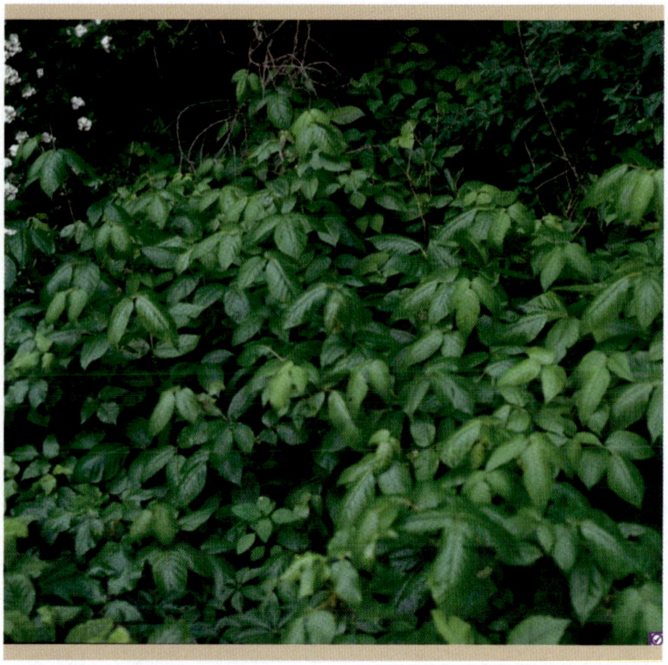

FIGURE 6-3 Poison ivy. (*Used with permission from Dr. Sharon E Jacob.*)

- Poison sumac: *Toxicodendron vernix*
- Identification
  - *Poison ivy and poison oak*: 3 to 5 leaflets per compound leaf
  - *Poison sumac*: 7 to 13 leaflets per leaf; have smooth edges
- Cross-reacting substances
  - Cashew and pistachio nut tree: entire tree except for the nut
  - Indian marking tree: black juice (used as a laundry marker, causes Dhobi itch)
  - Japanese lacquer tree: viscous sap that is used for varnishing wood; polymerized urushiol persists in the lacquer
  - Brazilian pepper tree: sap and crushed berries
  - Mango tree: skin of the fruit and the leaves, bark, and stems of the plant contain sensitizing resorcinols; pulp of the fruit is nonallergenic
  - Ginkgo tree: anacardic acid, which is present in the seed pulp

7. *Liliaceae*
   - Tulips, hyacinths, and asparagus
   - Allergen: tuliposide A is converted to tulipalin A, the allergen, by means of acidic hydrolysis
   - Tulip fingers; combined allergic and irritant contact dermatitis
8. *Alstroemeriaceae* family (Peruvian lily)
   - Tuliposide A and B are found in virtually all portions of the plant
   - Flowers contain more allergen than the stems; the leaves have the smallest amount of allergen
   - Most common cause of allergic hand dermatitis in florists

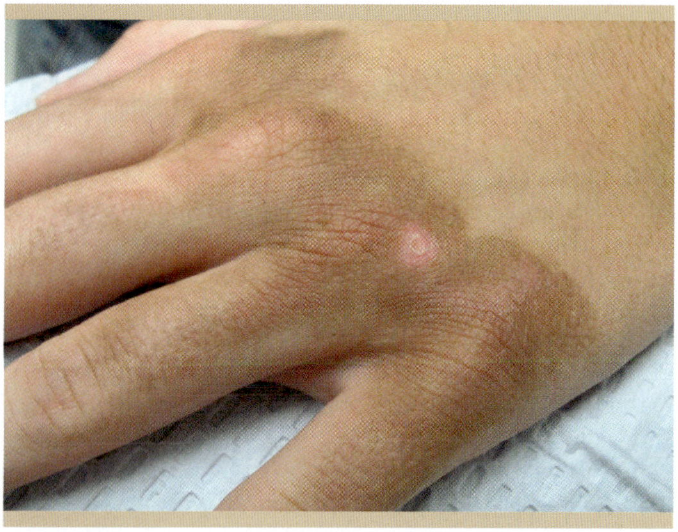

FIGURE 6-4 Phytophotodermatitis. (*Used with permission from Dr. Asra Ali.*)

9. Phytophotodermatitis
   - Phytophotodermatitis results in hyperpigmentation (Fig. 6-4)
   - *Berloque dermatitis* is due to bergamot oil; UV light reacts with bergapten (a furocoumarin) and induces melanogenesis
   - Most common plant families to cause phytophotodermatitis are *Umbiliferae* (most common), *Rutaceae,* and *Moraceae*
     - *Umbiliferae*: cow parsley, parsley, celery, carrot, fennel, cow parsnip, hogweed, parsnip
     - *Rutacea*: lime, lemon, grapefruit, mokihana (Hawaiian leis), rue
     - *Moracea*: fig
   - Allergens can be found in perfumes and fragrances, cosmetics, toiletries, soap, household cleaners, detergents, air fresheners
10. Contact urticaria from plants
    - Roasted chili peppers contain capsaicin
    - *Urticaceae* family: stinging nettle (*Urtica dioica*)
    - Irritant chemicals, which include acetylcholine, histamine, and 5-hydroxytryptamine
11. Chemical irritant dermatitis
    - Most common dermatitis in florists
    - *Dieffenbachia picta* (*Araceae*), also known as dumb cane: calcium oxalate
    - Daffodil itch: calcium oxalate in the sap

Rubber Allergens

1. Latex
   - Milky fluid derived from rubber tree *Hevae brasiliensis*

- Composed primarily of *cis*-1,4-polyisoprene
- Reaction can involve irritant dermatitis, immediate (type I) hypersensitivity; rarely may cause delayed (type IV) hypersensitivity
- Multiple episodes of contact urticaria with scratching can lead to clinical appearance of chronic dermatitis
- Gloves, condoms, balloons, rubber adhesives
- Corn starch powder—with which gloves are dusted—is a potent carrier of latex proteins
- Health care workers, rubber industry workers, children with spina bifida or urogenital abnormalities
- In vitro tests: radioimmunoassay tests (RAST) for IgE
- Cross-reaction
  - Food: bananas, avocados, chestnuts, kiwis
  - Shared IgE epitopes: ragweed, grasses, and *Ficus* trees

2. Rubber additives
   - *Rubber accelerators*
   - Rubber accelerators are chemicals used to speed up the manufacturing process of rubber (vulcanization); sulfur cross-links the polymer chains in the latex
   - Carbamates (carba mix)
     - Diphenylguanidine, zinc-dibutyldithiocarbamate, and zinc-diethyldithiocarbamate in equal parts
     - Rubber dermatitis in bleached fabrics (waistbands, bra straps)
     - Consumer rubber products (condoms, swimwear, makeup sponges, eyelash curlers, gloves, shoes)
     - Crosss-reacts with thiurams
   - Mercaptobenzothiazole (MBT)
     - Most common cause of allergic shoe dermatitis
     - Rubber products: gloves, makeup sponges, rubber in undergarments/clothing, swimwear
     - Also in tires, condoms, antifreeze, fungicides, flea and tick powders, photographic film emulsions, adhesives, bactericides, and is an anticorrosive agent in cutting oils and greases
   - Mercapto mix
     - Composed of 3 chemical accelerators: benzothiazole sulfenamide derivatives
     - *N*-Cyclohexylbenzothiazyl-sulfenamide, dibenzothiazyl disulfide, and morpholinylmercaptobenzothiazole
   - Thiuram mix
     - Composed of 4 substances in equal parts: Tetramethylthiuram monosulfide, tetramethylthiuram disulfide, disulfiram, dipentamethylenethiuram disulfide
     - Most common rubber additives to cause a type IV reaction
     - Found in almost all rubber products, shoes, gloves, condoms, elastic bands, and ingredients of pesticides, insect repellents, antiscabies medication, fungicides, wood preservatives, paint additives, lubricating oils, and the drug disulfiram (Antabuse)
   - Thiourea
     - Commonly tested with a dialkyl thiourea mix
     - Common source is neoprene rubber

Antioxidants

- Added to decrease the rate of rubber degradation
- Substituted phenols are used for latex gloves
- Black rubber mix
  - Allergens: *N-Phenyl-N'-cyclohexyl-p-phenylenediamine* (CPPD), *N-Isopropyl-N'-phenyl-p-phenylenediamine* (IPPD) and *N,N'-Diphenyl-p-phenylenediamine* (DPPD)

PRESERVATIVES

1. Formaldehyde (Fig. 6-5)
   - Released from the proallergen *N*-hydroxymethyl succinimide
   - Cleaved into succinimide and formaldehyde when it comes in contact with the transepidermal water on the surface of the skin
2. Formaldehyde is the active allergenic compound
   - Textile resins
     - Permanent press or wrinkle-resistant textiles (urea-formaldehyde, melamine formaldehyde)
   - Cosmetics, household products, ink, latex paint, pathology fixatives, fertilizer, embalming solution, insulation
   - Formaldehyde resins
     - *p-tert*-butylphenol formaldehyde resin (common shoe glue allergen)

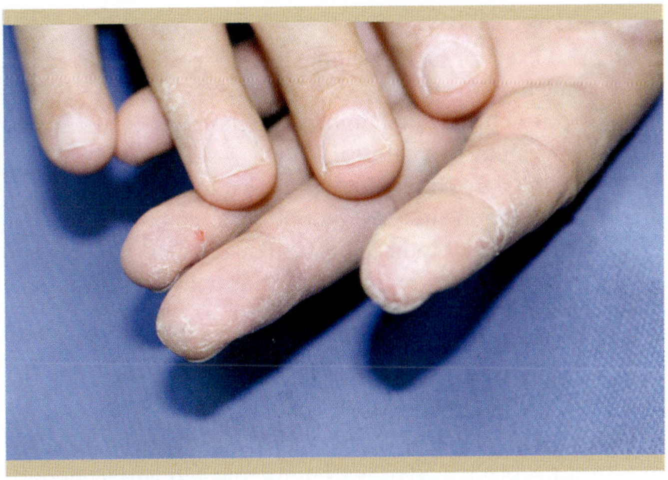

FIGURE 6-5 Chronic fingertip dermatitis due to formaldehyde allergy in pathologist. (*Used with permission from Dr. Sharon E Jacob.*)

- Leather and foam adhesive
- Other uses: waterproof glues and finishes
- Formaldehyde-releasing preservatives
  - Quaternium-15 (most common): cosmetics, lotions, creams, shampoos and soaps, polishes, cleaners, cutting fluids, and paints
  - Imidazolidinyl urea (Germall 115, Euxyl K200)
  - Diazolidinyl urea (Germall II)
  - DMDM hydantoin
  - 2-Bromo-2-nitropane-1, 3-diol (Bronopol)
  - Sodium hydroxymethyl glycinate

3. Non–formaldehyde-releasing preservatives
   - Methyldibromo glutaronitrile (MDBGN)
   - Parabens
     - Most used topical preservatives worldwide
     - Paraben paradox: some sensitized patients only react to parabens when applied to dermatitic skin (e.g., leg ulcer patients)
     - Medical creams, lotions, pastes, and several cosmetics and skin-care products; food preservatives; industrially in oils, fats, and glues
   - Isothiazolinones
     - Kathon CG: combination of methylchloroisothiazolinone and methylisothiazolinone
     - Cosmetics and commercial household products such as shampoos, creams, lotions, cleaners, and washing materials; it is also a widely used industrial preservative for cutting fluids

METAL ALLERGENS

1. Nickel
   - Most common cause of patch test reactions
   - Jewelry, clothing (snaps, zippers, and buttons), coins, keys, other metals; gold less than 18 carats can contain nickel
   - Also used for nickel plating, to color ceramics, to make some batteries
   - Foods naturally high in nickel include chocolate, soybeans, nuts, and oatmeal
   - Dimethylglyoxime spot test is used to detect nickel
     - Rub on the item; if solution turns color (pink to reddish), it indicates a positive reaction
     - Indicates the presence of nickel in a concentration of at least 1:10,000
2. Potassium dichromate
   - Chromates (chrome)
   - Usually found as chrome salts
   - Cement, leather tannin, ceramics, paint, match heads, suture, bleach/detergents, numerous industrial chemicals, green felt of card tables, glues
   - Green tattoo and cosmetic pigments
   - Green textile dyes (military green, green pool table felt)
3. Gold
   - A gold salt, gold sodium thiosulfate, is used for patch testing
   - A common allergen in eyelid dermatitis
   - Positive reactions may not be clinically relevant (patients with positive patch reactions, usually tolerate their gold jewelry)
4. Cobalt
   - used in dental amalgams, to make drills, cutting tools and mechanical parts, in glass, pottery and porcelain, and a component of the synthesis of vitamin B_{12}
   - Commonly see co-sensitization with nickel
   - A disodium-1-nitroso-2-naphthol-3,6-disulfonate spot test is used to detect cobalt
   - Foods high in cobalt: apricot, beans, beer, beets, cloves, cocoa, coffee, liver, and nuts

COLORS AND DYE ALLERGENS

Tattoos

- Ink particles are found within large phagosomes in the cytoplasm of both keratinocytes and phagocytic cells
- Allergic reactions to red tattoo pigments are most common and are associated with cinnabar (mercuric sulfide); however, nickel contamination has been reported in a variety of pigment colors (Table 6–5)
- Photoaggravated reactions: most commonly yellow dye
- Cutaneous reactions: eczematoid dermatitis within the tattoo, foreign-body reaction, and tattoo-induced pseudolymphoma

TABLE 6-5 Tattoo Components

Tattoo Color	Component
Blue	Cobalt aluminate
Brown	Ferric oxide
Green	Chromic oxide, lead chromate, phthalocyanine dyes
Red	Cinnabar (mercuric sulfide), sienna (ferric hydrate), sandalwood, Brazilwood, organic pigments (aromatic azo compounds)
Yellow	Cadmium sulfide
Black	Carbon (India ink), iron oxide, logwood
Purple	Manganese, aluminum
White	Titanium oxide, zinc oxide

Dyes

Aniline textile dyes (disperse dyes). Blue 106 and 124 are the most common dye allergens in textile dermatitis

ADHESIVES

Epoxy Resin

- Two-component adhesives
- Most common allergens: bisphenol A and epichlorohydrin
- Glue, laminates, eyeglass frames, vinyl gloves, handbags, plastic necklaces, dental bonding agents, microscopy immersion oil, floor coverings

PATCH TESTING

- T.R.U.E. test (allergen patch test) (Table 6-6, Fig. 6-6)
  - Commercially available, ready-to-use contact allergen test containing 35 allergens and allergen mixes and 1 negative control
  - Allergen mixes incorporated into hydrophilic gels attached to a waterproof polyester patch backing
  - Perspiration and transepidermal water loss rehydrate the dried gel layer, thereby releasing the allergens onto the skin
  - T.R.U.E. test is removed after 48 hours and reactions are again interpreted at 72 to 96 hours after test application
- Comprehensive Patch Systems
  - Allows for customized patch testing and flexibility
  - Employs a multi-well aluminum or plastic patch containers applied to Scanpor tape in 2 rows of 5 (Fig. 6-7)

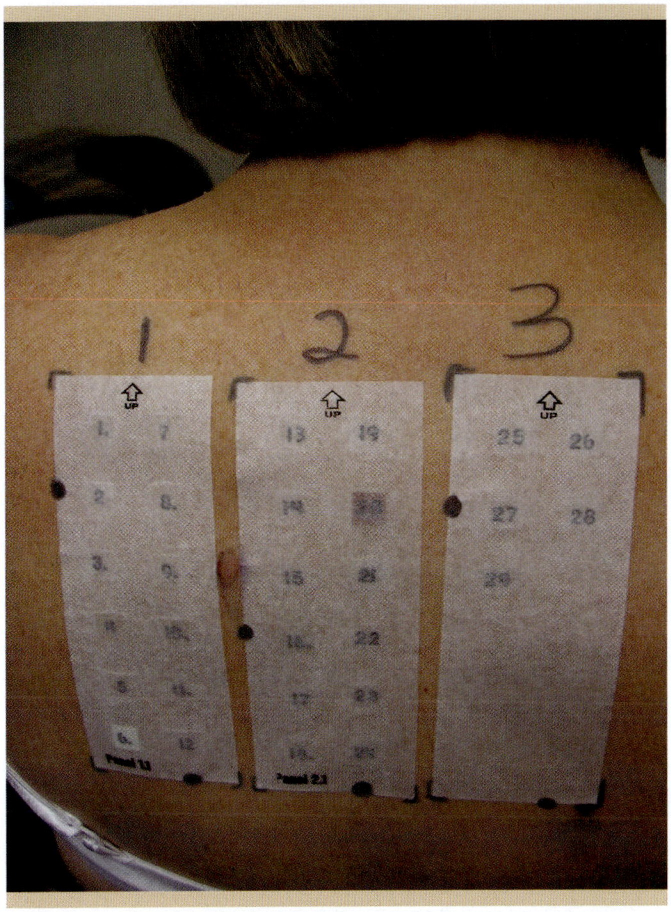

FIGURE 6-6 T.R.U.E. patch testing system for patch testing. (*Used with permission from Dr.* Sharon E. Jacob.)

TABLE 6-6 T.R.U.E. Test Panels

Panel 1.2	Panel 2.2	Panel 3.2
Nickel sulfate	p-tert-Butylphenol formaldehyde resin	Diazolidinyl urea
Wool alcohols	Epoxy resin	Quinoline mix
Neomycin sulfate	Carba mix	Tixocortol-21-pivalate
Potassium dichromate	Black rubber mix	Gold sodium thiosulfate
Caine mix	Cl^+ Me^- isothiazolinone (MCI/MI)	Imidazolidinyl urea
Fragrance mix	Quaternium-15	Budesonide
Colophony	Methyldibromo glutaronitrile	Hydrocortizone-17-butyrate
Paraben mix	p-Phenylenediamine	Mercaptobenzothiazole
Negative control	Formaldehyde	Bacitracin
Balsam of Peru	Mercapto mix	Parthenolide
Ethylenediamine dihydrochloride	Thimerosal	Disperse blue 106
Cobalt Dichloride	Thiuram mix	2-Bromo-2-nitropropane-1,3-diol (Bronopol)

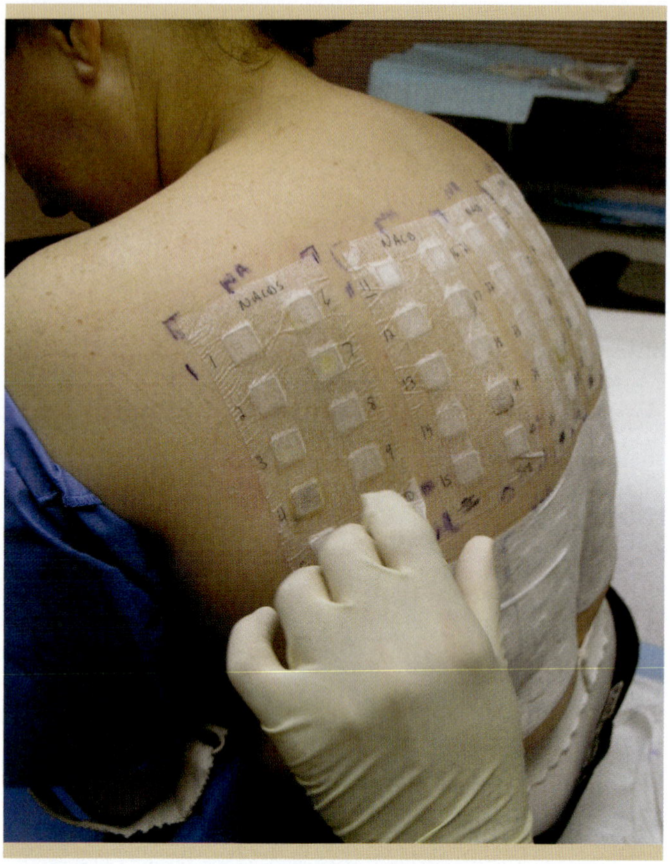

FIGURE 6-7 Comprehensive patch testing system for patch testing. (*Used with permission from Dr. Sharon E. Jacob.*)

- Each well is filled with an aliquot amount of the standard allergen being tested, and the patch is taped to normal skin on the patient's upper back
- After 48 hours, the patch is removed, and an initial reading is taken, with a delayed second reading made at 72 to 96 hours.
- Patch Test Evaluation (Reading)
    - Macular erythema, 1+ (induration), 2+ (induration with discrete papules), 3+ (coalescing papules +/– bullae on an indurated base)
- Repeat open application test (ROAT)
    - For individuals who develop weak or 1+ positive reactions to a chemical on a patch test
    - Useful in determining whether the reaction is significant or in personal product testing (only leave-on products should be tested)
    - Consists of rubbing in the product twice daily for 5 to 7 days to the skin of the antecubital fossa
    - Grading is analogous to epicutaneous patch testing
    - Samples of the individual ingredients used by the cosmetic manufacturer may be requested and tested on the individual

QUIZ

Questions

1. Which of the following is in the *Rutaceae* family of plants?

    A. Cow parsley
    B. Fennel
    C. Parsnip
    D. Mokihana
    E. Celery

2. The following plant is a member of the *Compositae* family?

    A. Poison ivy
    B. Mango
    C. Artichoke
    D. Indian marking nut
    E. Brazilian pepper tree

3. Which of the following is the most sensitizing fragrance in Fragrance Mix II?

    A. lyral
    B. Cinnamic alcohol
    C. Eugenol
    D. Geraniol
    E. Hydroxycitronellal

4. Which of the following is a screening agent for hydrocortisone allergy?

    A. Tixocortol pivalate
    B. Budesonide
    C. Clobetasol proprionate
    D. Hydrocortisone butyrate
    E. Desoximetasone

5. Sesquiterpene lactone is the allergen found in which plant?

    A. Garlic
    B. Lichen
    C. Ragweed
    D. Mango
    E. Peruvian lily

6. Which of the following is used to screen for hair dye allergy?

    A. Ethyl acrylate
    B. Glutaraldehyde
    C. Dimethylaminopropylamine
    D. Para-phenylenediamine
    E. Fragrance Mix

7. Which of the following spot test is used to detect cobalt in metal objects?
   A. Dimethyl glyoxime
   B. Hydroxycitronellal
   C. Diglycidyl ether of bisphenol A
   D. Disodium-1-nitroso-2-naphthol-3,6-disulfonate
   E. Diazolidinyl urea

8. Which of the following metals is found in green-colored tattoos?
   A. Chromic oxide
   B. Cobalt aluminate
   C. Cinnabar (mercuric sulfide)
   D. Ferric oxide
   E. Cadmium sulfide

9. Which of the following professions is at a higher risk for allergic contact dermatitis to glyceryl thioglycolate?
   A. Florist
   B. Chef
   C. Car mechanic
   D. Dental assistant
   E. Hairdresser

10. Which of the following is the most sensitizing formaldehyde-releasing preservative?
    A. Methylisothiazolinones
    B. DMDM hydantoin
    C. Methyldibromoglutaronitrile
    D. Quaternium 15
    E. Melamine formaldehyde

Answers

1. D. The most common plant families to cause phytophotodermatitis are *Umbelliferae* (most common), *Rutaceae*, and *Moraceae*. The *Umbelliferae* family includes cow parsley, parsley, celery, carrot, fennel, cow parsnip, hogweed, and parsnip. The *Rutaceae* family includes lime, lemon, grapefruit, mokihana (Hawaiian leis), and rue. The *Moraceae* family includes fig.
2. B. The *Asteraceae* family of plants is significant plant sources of allergic contact dermatitis. The members of this family include Ragweed, chrysanthemum, feverfew and carrot weed, daisy, sunflower, dandelion, artichoke, lettuce, and endives. The other choices are all members of the *Toxicodendron* (urushiol) family.
3. A. Fragrance Mix I is a screening mix for fragrance allergy. It contains 8 allergen constituents: α-amylcinnamic alcohol, cinnamic alcohol, cinnamic aldehyde, eugenol, geraniol, hydroxycitronellal, isoeugenol, and oak moss absolute. Fragrance Mix II is also a screening mix for fragrance allergy. It contains hydroxyisohexyl 3-cyclohexene carboxaldehyde (Lyral), Citral, farnesol, citronellol, hexyl cinnamal, and coumarin. Lyral is the most common sensitizer in the mix.
4. A. Corticosteroids are organized into 5 groups according to chemical structure. Group A consists of hydrocortisone, hydrocortisone acetate, prednisone, and methylprednisolone. Tixocortol pivalate and hydrocortisone are the screening agent for group A allergy. Group B includes triamcinolone, fluocinolone acetonide, desonide, and budesonide. The screening agents for this group are budesonide and triamcinolone. Group C steroids include desoximethasone and clocortolone pivalate; this is the least allergenic class. Group D is subcategorized into D1 and D2 classes. Clobetasol is in group D1, while hydrocortisone butyrate and valerate are found in group D2. Group D2 may cross-react with group A and budesonide.
5. C. Sesquiterpene lactone is the allergen found in the *Asteracea* family of plants such as ragweed, feverfew, and daisies. Garlic contains the allergen diallydisulfide and is a common cause of fingertip dermatitis in chefs and food handlers. Mango is a *Toxicodendron* species (*Rhus*) of the family (*Anacardiaceae*), as are poison ivy, poison oak, poison sumac, Brazilian pepper tree, Indian marking nut, ginkgo, cashew, and Japanese lacquer tree. Peruvian lily belongs to the *Alstroemeriaceae* family. The allergens are tuliposide A and B and are found in virtually all portions of the plant. Notably, the flowers contain more allergen than the stems. Peruvian lilies are the most common cause of allergic hand dermatitis in florists.
6. D. The most common causative agent in hair dye allergy is para-phenylenediamine (PPD). It is used as the primary screening agent. Ethyl acrylate is a screening agent for acrylic plastics or polymers. Contact dermatitis is frequently encountered in nail cosmetics. Glutaraldehyde is cold sterilizing solution and is used as a disinfectant. Allergic reactions are commonly seen in workers involved in cleaning medical equipment such as dental assistants. Dimethylaminopropylamine is a by-product in the manufacture of cocamidopropylbetaine, a surfactant in shampoos. The fragrance mixes are used to screen for fragrance allergy.
7. D. The disodium-1-nitroso-2-naphthol-3,6-disulfonate spot test is used to detect cobalt in metal objects. While the dimethyl glyoxime spot test is used to detect nickel. To use, a drop of solution is placed on a cotton swab and rubbed on the object in question. A pink-red color indicates the presence of the respective metal.
8. A. Chromic oxide is used as a tattooing pigment to achieve a green color. Notably, a significant number of tattoo-allergic reactions are to the red pigment, cinnabar (mercuric sulfide). Other metals are used as tattooing pigments: cobalt aluminate (blue), ferric oxide (brown), carbon (black), titanium (white), manganese (purple), and cadmium sulfide (yellow).

9. E. Glyceryl thioglycolate (GTG) is an acidic permanent wave solutions used in professional hair salons. The chemical is known to remain in hair shaft for months and can cause chronic dermatitis in hairdressers and clients.
10. D. Formaldehyde-releasing preservatives are common in cosmetic products and topical medicaments. These include diazolidinyl urea, imidazolidinyl urea, quaternium 15, DMDM hydantoin, and sodium hydroxymethyl glycinate. Quaternium 15 is the most sensitizing. Methylisothiazolinone and methyldibromoglutaronitrile are preservatives which don't release formaldehyde. Melamine formaldehyde is one of several formaldehyde releasers used as a finishing resin in permanent press or "wrinkle-free" clothing. Patients may react to the resin or the formaldehyde itself.

REFERENCES

Baran R: Nail cosmetics: allergies and irritations. *Am J Clin Dermatol* 2002;3:547–555.

Chan EF, Mowad C: Contact dermatitis to foods and spices. *Am J Contact Dermat* 1998;9(2):71–79.

Fisher A, Rietschel R, Fowler J: *Fisher's Contact Dermatitis*, 6th Ed. Baltimore: Williams & Wilkins; 1995.

Frosch PJ, Menne T, Lepoittevin JP: *Contact Dermatitis*, 4th Ed. Berlin: Springer; 2006.

Marks J Jr, Elsner P, DeLeo V: *Contact and Occupational Dermatology*, 3rd Ed. St. Louis: Mosby; 2002.

McCleskey PE, Swerlick RA: Clinical review: thioureas and allergic contact dermatitis. *Cutis* 2001;68:387–396.

Thiboutot DM, Hamory BH, Marks JG Jr: Dermatoses among floral shop workers. *J Am Acad Dermatol* 1990;22:54–58.

Van der Walle HB, Brunsveld VM: Dermatitis in hairdressers. *Contact Dermatitis* 1994;30:217–221.

CHAPTER 7

AUTOIMMUNE BULLOUS DISEASES

WHITNEY A. HIGH

TERMINOLOGY AND CONCEPTS

Indirect Immunofluorescence

- Goal: to detect circulating autoantibodies in serum by purposefully incubating it with a test substrate
- Method: *serum* from a patient is collected and directed against a substrate (such as monkey esophagus, rat bladder, or salt-split skin), followed "indirectly" by the addition of fluorescein-conjugated antibodies directed against specific complement fractions and immunoglobulins to label any resultant complexes

Direct Immunofluorescence

- Goal: to detect antibody and immunoreactants already deposited in tissue of the patient
- Method: *tissue* from a patient is incubated "directly" with fluorescein-conjugated antibodies directed against specific complement fractions and immunoglobulins (IgG, IgM, and IgA) to label any resultant complexes

Use of Salt-Split Skin

- Goal: to differentiate among autoimmune bullous conditions via the level of any deposition of immunoreactants within salt-split skin (i.e., deposition either "above" or "below" the lamina lucida, where the split occurs)
- Methods:
  - Direct: incubate the patient's skin in 1 molar saline to induce a split through the lamina lucida; add fluorescein-conjugated antibodies to label any resultant complexes; identify the level of deposition ("roof" or "floor")
  - Indirect: incubate the patient's serum with normal skin already presplit with 1 molar saline; add fluorescein-conjugated human anti-immunoglobulin to label any resultant complexes; identify the level of deposition ("roof" or "floor")
- Immunoreactants deposit in the "roof" ("above" the split) in:
  - bullous pemphigoid
- Immunoreactants deposit in the "floor" ("below" the split) in:
  - Bullous systemic lupus erythematosus (SLE)
  - Antiepiligrin cicatricial pemphigoid (autoantibodies to laminin-5)
  - Anti-p105 pemphigoid (autoantibodies to 105-kDa lower lamina lucida protein)
  - Anti-p200 pemphigoid (autoantibodies to a 200-kDA protein of the C-terminus of laminin γ1 although the pathogenicity of the antibody is disputed)
  - Ghohestani disease (autoantibodies to α-5 chain of type IV collagen)
  - Epidermolysis bullosa acquisita (EBA)

Nikolsky Sign ("direct" Nikolsky sign)

- Positive: pressure applied laterally at the edge of lesion results in blister extension
- Indicative of epidermal fragility
- Diseases with a "positive" direct Nikolsky sign include the following:
  - Pemphigus foliaceus
  - Pemphigus vulgaris
  - Staphylococcal scalded skin syndrome (Ritter disease)
- Recent evidence shows that a "direct" Nikolsky sign is moderately sensitive but highly specific for pemphigus
- The "marginal" variant of the Nikolsky sign involves lateral extension of the blister via either pulling of the lateral remnants or rubbing at the edge of a lesion

Pseudo-Nikolsky Sign

- Positive: separation of the epidermis from the dermis by lateral pressure (rubbing) on erythematous skin (but not a blister itself—see "marginal" Nikolsky sign)
- Diseases with a "positive" pseudo-Nikolsky sign include the following:
  - Stevens-Johnson syndrome (SJS)
  - Toxic epidermal necrolysis (TEN)

Asboe-Hansen Sign ("indirect" Nikolsky sign)

- Positive: pressure applied to the top of a lesion results in lateral extension of the blister
- Diseases with a "positive" Asboe-Hansen sign include:
  - bullous pemphigoid

AUTOIMMUNE BULLOUS DISEASES

Bullous Pemphigoid (Fig. 7-1)

- Autoimmune, subepidermal, blistering skin disease
- Bullous pemphigoid (BP) is the most common autoimmune bullous condition in dermatology
- Antigens
  - Bullous pemphigoid antigen 230 (BP230, formerly BPAg1)
    - 230 kDa
    - Intracellular portion of hemidesmosome plaque, part of the plakin superfamily
  - Bullous pemphigoid antigen 180 (BP180, formerly BPAg2)
    - 180 kDa (type XVII collagen)
    - Transmembranous protein with a collagenous extracellular domain
- Clinical
  - Most often occurs in older patients (average age is 65 years) with comorbidities
  - Mucosal disease is uncommon (10–25% of cases)
  - Yields tense blisters and bullae
  - Blisters are often more prominent in flexural/intertriginous areas
  - May present or begin as an urticarial eruption that is intensely pruritic
  - In infants/children the disease may often involve the palms/soles/face
  - "Positive" Asboe-Hansen sign, "negative" direct Nikolsky sign

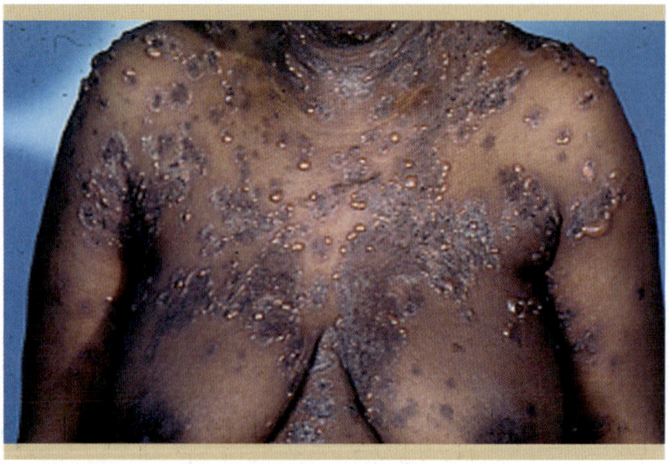

FIGURE 7-1 Bullous pemphigoid. (*Used with permission from Dr. Robert Jordon.*)

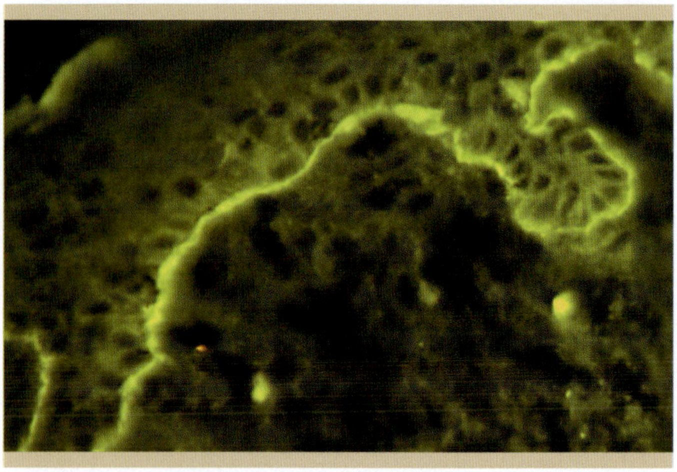

FIGURE 7-2 Bullous pemphigoid immunofluorescence. (*Used with permission from Dr. Robert Jordon.*)

- Diagnosis
  - Light microscopy
  - Subepidermal vesiculation
  - Often with prominent but superficial dermal eosinophils
  - Eosinophils may also be present in the blister cavity
  - There may be an associated eosinophilic spongiosis
  - Immunofluorescence (**Fig. 7-2**)
  - Optimal location for biopsy for DIF is from perilesional skin
  - False-negative results may be observed if testing is performed on lesional skin
  - Linear deposition of C3 (90–100% of patients) and IgG (70–90% of patients) at basement membrane zone (BMZ)
  - Salt-split skin (DIF or IIF) reveals IgG deposition on the blister "roof"
  - IIF performed on monkey esophagus also shows linear deposition at the DEJ
  - ELISA testing
    - Circulating antibodies are detected in about 70% of patients
    - Correlation exists between clinical disease activity and antibody levels to BP180
- Associations
  - BP may be associated with certain drugs, including captopril, furosemide, ibuprofen, nonsteroidal anti-inflammatory agents, penicillamine, some antibiotics
- Treatment
  - Topical steroids (potent)
  - Oral prednisone
  - Tetracycline derivatives +/− nicotinamide
  - Other medications/interventions sometimes employed include azathioprine, cyclophosphamide, dapsone, IVIG, methotrexate, mycophenolate mofetil, plasmapheresis, and rituximab

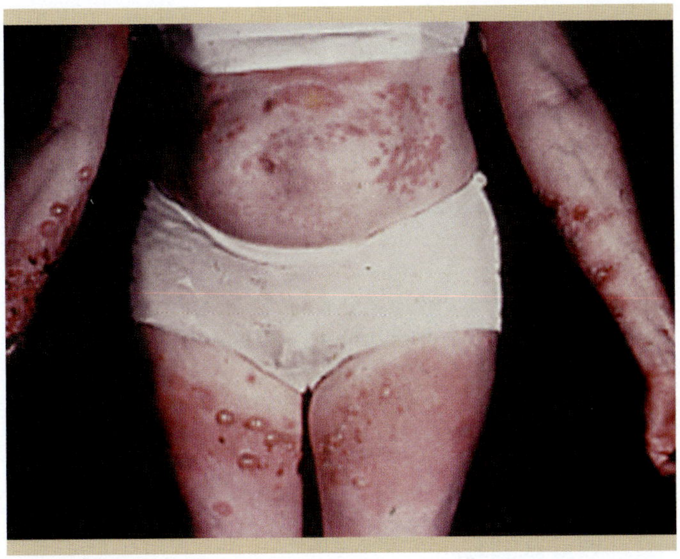

FIGURE 7-3 Pemphigoid gestationis. (*Used with permission from Dr. Robert Jordon.*)

- Course/prognosis
  - Generally a self-limited disease, often with remission in 1.5 to 6 years
  - High levels of BP180 by ELISA is considered a risk factor for relapse

Pemphigoid Gestationis (Herpes Gestationis) (Fig. 7-3)

- Autoimmune, subepidermal, blistering skin disease of pregnancy
- Rare disorder affecting about 1 in 50,000 pregnancies in the United States
- No relationship to herpes infection (essentially bullous pemphigoid in pregnancy)
- Antigens
  - Antigens are similar to those of bullous pemphigoid (BP180 and BP230)
  - Sera may contain antibodies for up to 5 epitopes within BP180
- Clinical
  - Condition occurs during the second and third trimesters
  - Pruritic lesions typically begin as "hive-like" plaques located periumbilically
  - Rash spreads peripherally, often sparing the face, palms/soles, and mucosa
  - The condition eventuates as tense bullae
  - In some cases lesions may appear after parturition only
  - There is often relative quiescence of disease in late pregnancy, followed by a flare at parturition or in the immediate postpartum period (75% of cases)
  - Infants born to affected mothers may develop lesions as well (10% of cases)
- Diagnosis
  - Light microscopy
    - Subepidermal vesiculation
    - Often with prominent but superficial dermal eosinophils
    - Eosinophils may also be present in the blister cavity
    - There may be an associated eosinophilic spongiosis
  - Immunofluorescence
    - Optimal location for biopsy for DIF is from perilesional skin
    - Linear deposition of C3 and IgG (about 25–50% of patients) at basement membrane zone (BMZ)
    - IIF reveals linear deposition of C3 in 90% of cases and IgG in 25% of cases
    - Salt-split skin (DIF or IIF) reveals IgG deposition on the blister "roof"
  - Complement fixation assay
    - Serum demonstrates affirmative "HG factor" in up to 90% of cases
    - HG-factor is a heat-stable form of IgG that binds normal human complement
  - ELISA testing
    - Circulating antibodies can often be detected (similar to BP)
    - Correlation exists between clinical disease activity and antibody levels for BP180 when measured by ELISA
    - In one study ELISA showed higher sensitivity and specificity than IIF
- Treatment
  - Oral corticosteroids (the mainstay of treatment in HG)
    - Dosage is often increased at delivery to control an anticipated flare
    - Prednisone is considered relatively safe during gestation
    - Betamethasone and dexamethasone are often avoided (cross placenta)
  - Topical steroids may be helpful in early urticarial lesions or premenstrual flares
  - Minocycline or doxycycline with nicotinamide may be used in nonbreastfeeding mothers with refractory disease but only after delivery
  - Other medications/interventions sometimes employed include azathioprine, cyclosporine, cyclophosphamide, dapsone, IVIG, methotrexate, plasmapheresis, and rituximab
- Associations
  - Some HLA haplotypes are associated with the disease (DR3 61–85%, DR4 52%)
  - Mothers demonstrate an increased risk of Graves disease (not concurrently)
- Course/prognosis
  - Maternal mortality is unaffected
  - Fetal consequences may include premature delivery or smaller infants

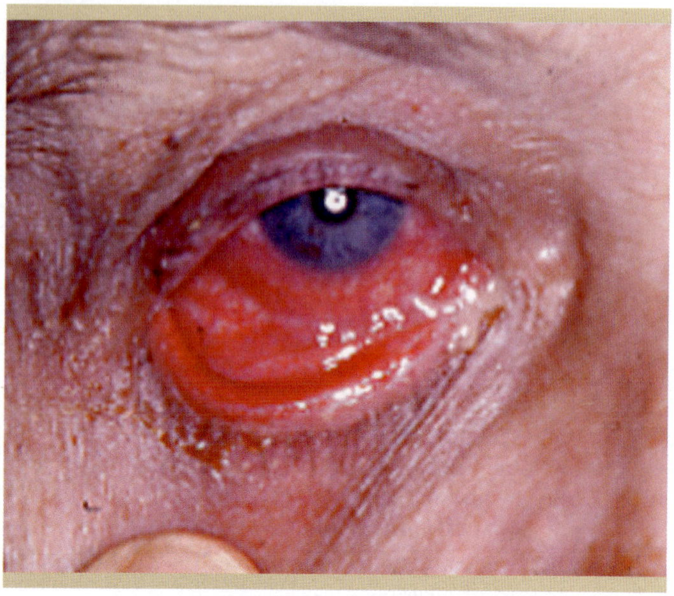

FIGURE 7-4 Cicatricial pemphigoid. (*Used with permission from Dr. Robert Jordon.*)

- Early onset of disease and blister formation may be associated with an increased risk of adverse pregnancy outcomes
- May recur in subsequent pregnancies, usually appearing earlier, being more severe, and lasting longer postpartum
- "Skip pregnancies" may be attributed to changes in paternity
- Postpartum flares may be precipitated by resumption of menses or use of oral contraceptives

Cicatricial Pemphigoid (Fig. 7-4)

- Rare autoimmune, subepidermal, blistering skin disease
- Antigens
  - Bullous pemphigoid antigen 180 (BP180)
  - Epiligrin (laminin-5)
  - Bullous pemphigoid antigen 230 (BP230)
  - B4 integrin (exclusively ocular forms)
  - EBA antigen (type VII collagen)
- Clinical
  - Often involves mucous membranes (mucous membrane pemphigoid)
  - May include the nasopharynx, larynx, esophagus, genitalia, and rectal mucosa
    - In the oropharynx the gingivae are most often involved
    - Lesions of the upper airway/larynx may result in hoarseness or dysphagia
    - Lesions of the esophagus may lead to stenosis or require dilatation
  - Lesions of the conjunctival mucosa may yield
    - Symblepharon (fibrous tracts tethering bulbar and conjunctival epithelium)
    - Synechiae (adhesion of the iris to the cornea or lens)
    - Corneal opacification (leading to blindness)
  - Skin involvement in one-third of patients (often involving the scalp, face, and upper trunk)
  - Bullae are tense and located upon an erythematous base
  - Bullae often occur repeatedly in the same place (even after temporary resolution), with resultant scarring
- Diagnosis
  - Light microscopy
    - Relatively pauci-inflammatory subepidermal vesiculation
    - Neutrophils may be seen near to the dermoepidermal junction
    - Eosinophils are few in comparison to most forms of bullous pemphigoid
    - There may be underlying dermal fibrosis indicative of scarring
    - Similar histologic features may be present in forms of cell-poor bullous pemphigoid (BP) or epidermolysis bullosa acquisita (EBA)
  - Immunofluorescence
    - Optimal location for biopsy for DIF is from perilesional skin
    - DIF shows linear deposition of C3 along the basement membrane
    - Deposition of IgG (25%) or IgA (20%) or IgM may be detected in some cases
    - Similar deposition is seen in BP and EBA (DIF alone cannot differentiate)
    - IIF detects circulating IgG in about 20% of patients (typically in low titer)
    - Salt-split skin reveals linear deposition in the "floor" of the blister cavity
- Variant
  - Brunsting-Perry form (**Fig.** 7-5)
    - Lacks mucosal involvement
    - Occurs on the head, neck, and scalp of older men
    - Consists of erosions that heal with scarring (often confused with skin cancer)
  - Associations
    - Some forms may occur as a paraneoplastic phenomenon
    - Some cutaneous cases associated with penicillamine use
    - Some ocular cases associated with use of systemic practolol, or topical epinephrine, echothiophate iodide, or pilocarpine
- Treatment
  - Topical steroids (including ophthalmic preparations)
  - Oral prednisone
  - Dapsone (particularly for ocular disease)
  - Other medications sometimes employed include azathioprine, cyclosporine, cyclophosphamide, dapsone, IVIG, methotrexate, and mycophenolate mofetil

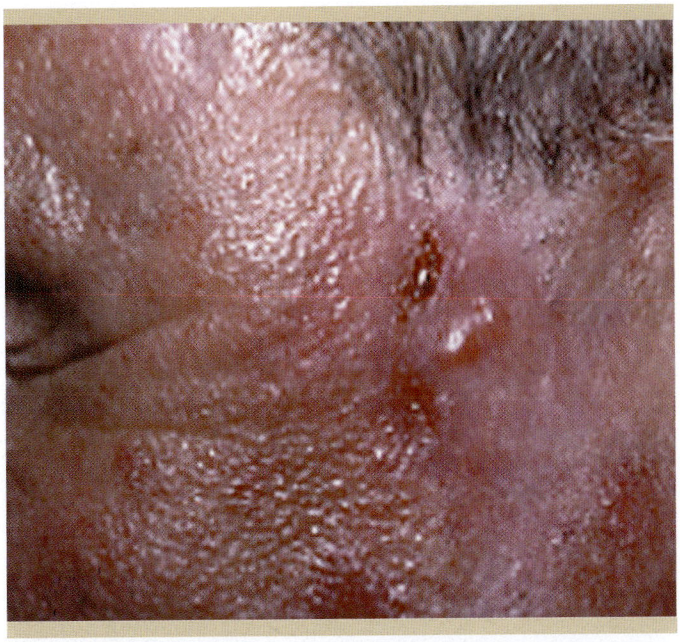

FIGURE 7-5 Cicatricial pemphigoid Brunsting-Perry. *(Used with permission from Dr. Robert Jordon.)*

- Course/prognosis:
  - Disease activity may be waxing and waning
  - Many cases may be chronic and progressive
  - Proper management may require assistance from ophthalmology/oral medicine

Bullous Lupus Erythematosus

- Autoimmune subepidermal blistering disorder occurring in the setting of systemic lupus erythematosus (SLE)
- Bullous SLE (BSLE) is more common in women and blacks
- Antigens
  - In most cases it is the noncollagenous (NC) domain of type VII collagen
  - Subdivided for classification into:
    - Type 1: with identifiable circulating and/or tissue-bound antibodies to type VII collagen by IIF, immunoblotting, immunoprecipitation, or ELISA
    - Type 2: without identifiable circulating and/or tissue-bound antibodies to type VII collagen by IIF, immunoblotting, immunoprecipitation, or ELISA
- Clinical
  - Development of BSLE may coincide with a flare of preexisting SLE, or it may first present commensurate with a new diagnosis of SLE
  - Patients must otherwise meet ACR criteria for SLE
  - Typically presents as an extensive bullous eruption developing relatively suddenly
  - Lesions range in size from small vesicles to large hemorrhagic bullae
  - Bullae favor the upper trunk, proximal upper extremities, face, and neck
  - Cutaneous lesions may be pruritic, and oral lesions may be painful
- Diagnosis
  - Light microscopy
    - Subepidermal vesiculation
    - Inflammation is not marked, but there is typically a neutrophilic infiltrate with nuclear dust located in the upper dermis near the DEJ
    - Vacuolization of basilar keratinocytes, a thickened basement zone, or other features of cutaneous lupus erythematosus are not usually observed
  - Immunofluorescence
    - Optimal location for biopsy for DIF is from perilesional skin
    - DIF with linear but course deposition of IgG along BMZ
    - Often with similar deposition of IgM, IgA, and C1q (a positive "lupus band")
    - Salt-split skin with deposition of immunoreactants on "floor" of the blister cavity
- Treatment
  - Dapsone
  - Oral prednisone (particularly if the patient is intolerant of dapsone)
  - Other medications sometimes employed include azathioprine, methotrexate, mycophenolate mofetil, and rituximab
- Course/prognosis
  - Bullous aspects of the disease often respond rapidly to dapsone
  - An internist/rheumatologist should be involved with management of any systemic manifestations of systemic lupus erythematosus

Linear IgA Bullous Dermatosis (LABD) (Fig. 7-6)

- Autoimmune, subepidermal, blistering skin disease
- Most often a disease of adults (> 30 years), but the condition may occur also in infants or children (formerly "chronic bullous disease/dermatosis of childhood")
- Antigens
  - 97-kDa extracellular portion of BP180 (formerly called "LAD-1")
  - 120-kDa antigen also described
  - 97- and 120-kDa antigens may represent cleaved fragments of BP180
  - A 250-kd dermal antigen (corresponding to collagen VII of anchoring fibrils) has also been described in a small subset of patients
- Clinical
  - Annular or grouped papules, vesicles, and/or bullae distributed symmetrically upon extensor surfaces ("cluster of jewels")

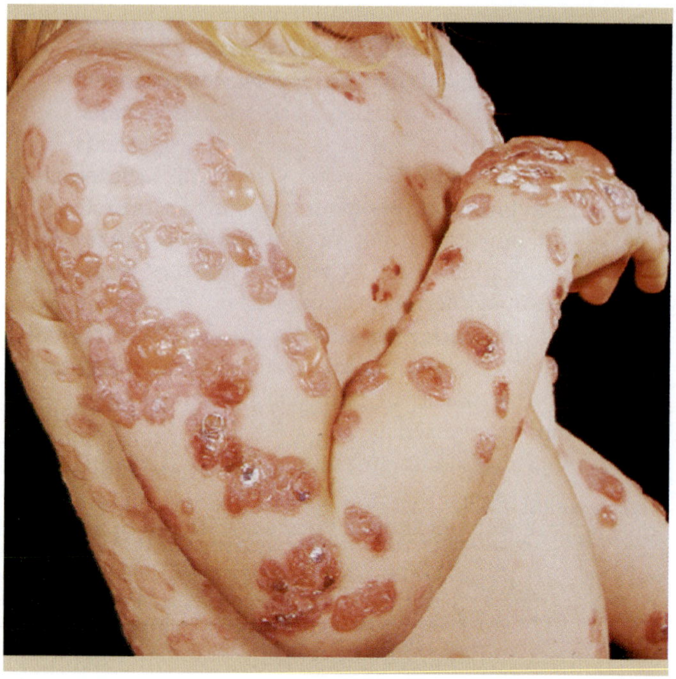

FIGURE 7-6 Linear IgA bullous dermatosis. (*Reprinted with permission from Goldsmith LA et al.* Fitzpatrick's Dermatology in General Medicine, *8th Ed. New York: McGraw-Hill; 2012, p. 627.*)

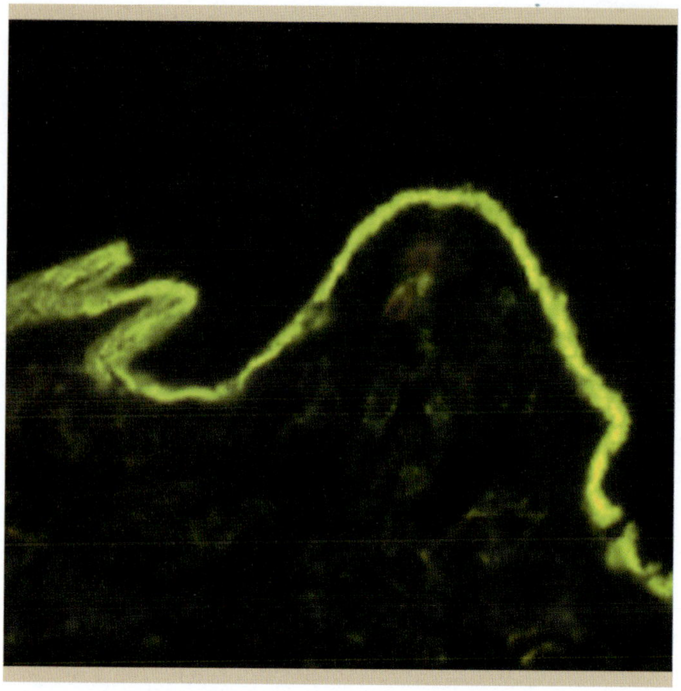

FIGURE 7-7 Linear IgA bullous dermatosis immunofluorescence. (*Used with permission from Dr. Robert Jordon.*)

- Typically abrupt in onset, with tense bullae on an erythematous base
- Some patients may experience a prodrome of pruritus or burning before vesicles
- In adults vesicles may involve perioral areas (50–80%) or the perineum
- Clinically lesions may be indistinguishable from dermatitis herpetiformis

- Diagnosis
  - Light microscopy
    - Subepidermal vesiculation
    - Collections of neutrophils along the basement membrane
    - Often there are relatively fewer eosinophils than most cases of bullous pemphigoid
    - However, cases with lymphocytes, eosinophils, and papillary microabscesses of neutrophils (similar to dermatitis herpetiformis) may occur
  - Immunofluorescence
    - DIF with linear deposition of IgA along the basement membrane (possibly with some codeposition of IgG and C3) (**Fig 7-7**)
    - Optimal location for biopsy for DIF is from perilesional skin
    - IIF is less likely to be positive in adults than in children (about 30% vs. 75%), and hence, it is not very often employed
    - IIF on salt-split skin reveals IgA antibody bound to "roof" of the blister cavity, similar to bullous pemphigoid
- Associations:
  - Vancomycin (most common single drug association)
  - Some cases are also associated with use of amiodarone, amoxicillin/clavulanate, ampicillin, captopril, cyclosporine, diclofenac, interferon, IL-2, iodinated contrast media, lithium, moxifloxacin, penicillin, phenytoin, somatostatin, sulfamethoxazole/trimethoprim, other sulfonamides, and vigabatrin
- Treatment
  - Dapsone
  - Prednisone
  - Sulfapyridine (sometimes effective when dapsone is not)
  - Colchicine
  - Other immunosuppressive medications (mycophenolate mofetil, etc.)
  - Tetracycline antibiotics (doxycycline or minocycline) and nicotinamide
- Course/prognosis
  - Variable and unpredictable
  - Disease spontaneously remits in some instances (64% children, < 48% adults)
  - Most drug-induced cases respond to discontinuance (within about 2 weeks)

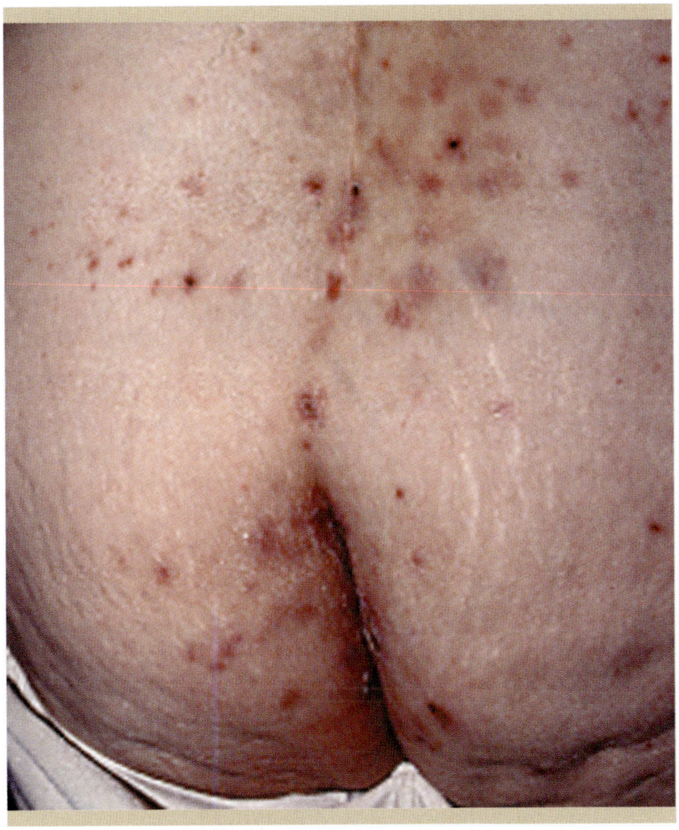

FIGURE 7-8 Dermatitis herpetiformis. (*Used with permission from Dr. Robert Jordon.*)

- There is no association with celiac disease (unlike dermatitis herpetiformis)

Dermatitis Herpetiformis (DH) (Fig. 7-8)

- Autoimmune, subepidermal, blistering skin disease
- Antigen
  - Gluten-tissue transglutaminase (t-TG) in the gut leads to development of IgA-based antibodies that cross-react with epidermal transglutaminase (e-TG/TG-3)
- Clinical
  - Onset typically between 20 and 40 years of age, but the condition may occur late life or childhood as well
  - Eruption may be preceded by burning or intense pruritus
  - Eruption yields pruritic, grouped vesicles (with a "herpetiform" appearance)
  - Pruritus may often be so severe that no "intact" vesicles exist
  - Symmetric distribution often includes the extensor surfaces, elbow/knees, buttocks, posterior hairline, and nuchal areas
  - Mucosal involvement is extremely rare
- Diagnosis
  - Histology
    - Subepidermal vesiculation
    - Neutrophilic microabscesses forming in in the tips of dermal papilla
    - Sometimes with fibrin deposition and rarely with eosinophils
  - Immunofluorescence
    - Both lesion and nonlesional skin may be utilized for testing
    - Granular IgA deposits in dermal papillae of lesional and nonlesional skin
    - The pattern of deposition is often likened to a "picket fence" (**Fig. 7-9**)
    - Deposition of immunoreactants diminishes with a gluten-free diet, but does not diminish with dapsone treatment alone
  - ELISA testing
    - Testing for tTG antibodies is highly specific (100%) and highly sensitive (96.6%) for the detection of DH
    - Testing for tTG antibodies may be falsely negative in those less than 3 years old
    - Testing for eTG (TG-3) antibodies is highly specific (100%), but poorly sensitive (44.8%) for the detection of DH

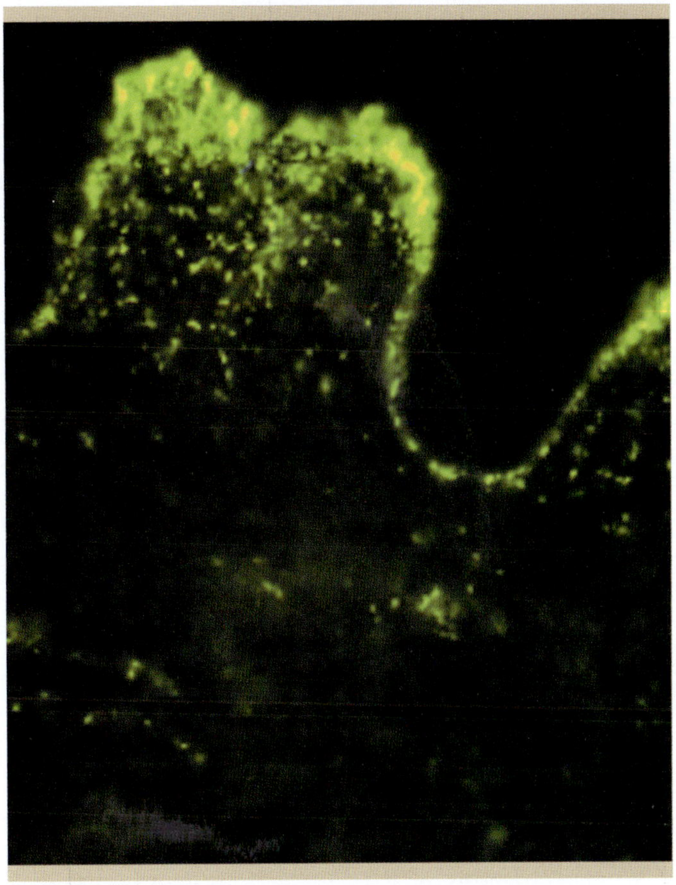

FIGURE 7-9 Dermatitis herpetiformis immunofluorescence. (*Used with permission from Dr. Robert Jordon.*)

- Tests are normally performed for IgA, but screening for IgG antibodies must be performed if the patient is IgA deficient (occurs in 2–3% of those with DH)
- Other testing
  - Anti-endomysial reactivity is a different lab assay, using serum and primate esophageal tissue, which detected the same tTG antibodies
- Associations
  - There is an association between DH and HLA-DQ2 and HLA-DQ8 haplotypes
  - Patients with DH have a higher incidence of other autoimmune disorders, including thyroid disease, diabetes mellitus (type I), Sjögren syndrome, systemic lupus erythematosus, and vitiligo
  - Iodides and some NSAIDS may exacerbate DH (ibuprofen is safe in most cases)
- Treatment
  - A strict gluten-free diet, while difficult to maintain, results in disease remission
  - Dapsone is the premier pharmaceutical intervention
  - Sulfapyridine may be used in those unable to tolerate dapsone
  - Other agents sometimes employed include azathioprine, colchicine, cyclosporine, and prednisone
  - Cyclosporine is generally avoided as it may potentiate an increased risk of intestinal lymphomas already observed in those with gluten-sensitive enteropathy
- Course/prognosis
  - Untreated and without dietary modifications the disease may persists indefinitely
  - Often it waxes and wanes without treatment as well
  - Several studies have shown an increased incidence of GI lymphoma in DH that may be mitigated by a gluten-free diet, but not by medical management

Epidermolysis Bullosa Acquisita (EBA)

- A rare autoimmune, subepidermal, blistering skin disease
- Differs from congenital forms of epidermolysis bullosa, which are due to mutations in constituents of the basement membrane zone
- EBA is acquired and immunologically mediated, and is not inherited
- Antigens
  - The NC1 domain of type VII collagen (a major component of anchoring fibrils)
- Clinical
  - The disease presents nearly exclusively in adults
  - Primarily involves the skin, but may also affect mucous membranes
  - Trauma-prone areas of the skin tend to be involved (the extensor surfaces of elbows, knees, ankles, and buttocks)
  - Bullous lesions heal with scarring and milia formation
  - The disease may lead to permanent nail destruction and hair loss
  - Involvement of mucous membranes may yield ulceration and periodontal disease
- Diagnosis
  - Light microscopy
    - Subepidermal vesiculation, usually it is pauci-inflammatory in nature
    - There may be neutrophils in close proximity to the DEJ
    - Some cases may be more inflammatory and may even resemble bullous pemphigoid
    - Dermal fibrosis may be present in older lesions (correlates with scarring)
  - Immunofluorescence
    - Optimal location for biopsy for DIF is from perilesional skin
    - DIF shows band IgG and lesser extent C3 deposited in linear fashion at the BMZ
    - IIF reveals circulating IgG autoantibodies to type VII collagen
    - IIF with salt-split skin shows deposition of immunoreactants upon the "floor" of the blister (a key distinction from bullous pemphigoid and LABD)
- Associations
  - EBA often occurs concurrently with other systemic diseases, including:
  - Inflammatory bowel disease (strongest association)
  - Systemic lupus erythematosus
  - Amyloidosis, thyroiditis
  - Multiple endocrinopathy syndrome
  - Rheumatoid arthritis
  - Pulmonary fibrosis
  - Chronic lymphocytic leukemia
  - Thymoma
  - Diabetes
- Treatment
  - Patients must also be instructed in skin protection and basic wound care
  - Common medications/interventions often employed to treat EBA include the following:
    - Prednisone (and other systemic corticosteroids)
    - Azathioprine
    - Cyclosporine
    - Cyclophosphamide
    - Dapsone
    - Colchicine (often avoided with concurrent IBD)
    - Methotrexate
    - IVIG
    - Rituximab
    - Plasmapheresis
- Course/prognosis:
  - EBA is notoriously difficult to treat and it is often refractory to pharmacologic interventions
  - Often the disease follows a protracted and chronic course with multiple exacerbations and remissions

Inherited Epidermolysis Bullosa

- Inherited/congenital disorders caused by mutation that impairs the production and/or function of constituents of the dermoepidermal junction and basement membrane zone
- See Tables 7-1 to 7-3 for details

Pemphigus Vulgaris (PV) (Fig. 7-10)

- Autoimmune, intraepidermal, blistering skin disease

TABLE 7-1 Revised Classification of Inherited Epidermolysis Bullosa, Based on Clinical Phenotype and Genotype, for the Most Commonly Observed and Well-Characterized Variants or Subtypes of This Disease

Major EB Type	Major EB Subtype	Protein/Gene Systems Involved
EBS ("epidermolytic EB")	EBS-WC	K5, K14
	EBS-K	K5, K14
	EBS-DM	K5, K14
	EBS-MD	Plectin
JEB	JEB-H	Laminin-5*
	JEB-nH	Laminin-5; type XVII collagen
	JEB-PA†	α6β4 Integrin‡
DEB ("dermolytic EB")	DDEB Type VII	Collagen
	RDEB-HS	Type VII collagen
	RDEB-nHS	Type VII collagen

DDEB, dominant dystrophic EB; *EBS-DM*, EBS, Dowling-Meara; *EBS-K*, EBS, Köbner; *EBS-MD*, EBS with muscular dystrophy; *EBS-WC*, EBS, Weber-Cockayne; *JEB-H*, JEB, Herlitz; *JEB-nH*, JEB, non-Herlitz; *JEB-PA*, JEB with pyloric atresia; *RDEB-HS*, recessive dystrophic EB, Hallopeau-Siemens; *RDEB-nHS*, RDEB, non–Hallopeau-Siemens.

*Laminin-5 is a macromolecule composed of 3 distinct (α_3, β_3, γ_2) laminin chains; mutations in any of the encoding genes result in a JEB phenotype.

†Some cases of EB associated with pyloric atresia may have intraepidermal cleavage or both intralamina lucida and intraepidermal clefts.

‡$\alpha_6\beta_4$ Integrin is a heterodimeric protein; mutations in either gene have been associated with the JEB-PA syndrome.

TABLE 7-2 Genetic Modes of Transmission in Inherited Epidermolysis Bullosa*

Major EB Type	Usual Mode(s) of Transmission	Rare Modes of Transmission
EBS†	Autosomal dominant	Autosomal recessive
JEB	Autosomal recessive	—
DEB	Autosomal dominant	Autosomal dominant/ autosomal recessive heterozygosity
	Autosomal recessive	

*Excluding de novo mutations, which have been reported to occur in most forms of inherited EB.

†An x-linked recessive disorder, referred to as Mendes da Costa disease, which was once included among the many variants of EBS, is no longer considered to be a subtype of any form of inherited EB.

- Antigens
  - Desmoglein 3 (a desmosomal core protein)
    - 130-kDa glycoprotein (member of cadherin supergene family)
  - Less commonly
    - Desmoglein 1: seen in patients with cutaneous and mucosal disease
    - Plakoglobin: 85-kDa plaque protein found in desmosomes
- Clinical
  - A bullous condition involving the skin and mucous membranes
  - Not uncommonly PV begins in the mouth, even months before skin disease
  - Prior to the advent of oral corticosteroids the condition had a high mortality
  - The condition results in flaccid blisters that progress rapidly to erosions/ulcerations
  - Intact bullae are rare due to the fragility of the intraepidermal process
  - Lesions of pemphigus vulgaris may develop excess granulation tissue or crusting
  - Nikolsky sign ("direct" or "marginal" Nikolsky sign) is positive
- Diagnosis
  - Light microscopy
    - Biopsy for traditional light microscopy should be performed at bulla margin overlapping slightly onto normal-appearing skin

TABLE 7-3 Ultrastructural Findings Among Major Types and Selected Subtypes of Inherited Epidermolysis Bullosa

EB Type or Subtype	Ultrastructural Site of Skin Cleavage	Other Ultrastructural Findings
EBS		
EBS-WC	Intrastratum basale	Split may spread to the suprabasilar layer
EBS-DM	Intrastratum basale, just superficial to the HD	Dense, circumscribed clumps of keratin filaments (most commonly observed within lesional biopsy sites)
EBS-MD	Predominantly in the stratum basale, above the level of the HD attachment plaque	Lack of integration of keratin filaments with HD
EBS-AR	Intrastratum basale	Absent keratin filaments within basal keratinocytes
EBSS	Intrastratum granulosum	—
JEB		
JEB-H	Intralamina lucida	Markedly reduced or absent HD; absent SBDP
JEB-nH	Intralamina lucida	Variable numbers or rudimentary appearance of HDs
JEB-PA	Both intralamina lucida and lower stratum basale, above the level of the HD plaque	Small HD plaques often with attenuated SBDP, and reduced integration of keratin filaments with HD
DDEB		
DDEB	Sublamina densa	Normal or decreased numbers of AF
DDEB-TBDN	Sublamina densa	Electron-dense stellate bodies within stratum basale; reduced AF
RDEB		
RDEB-HS	Sublamina densa	Absent AF
RDEB-nHS	Sublamina densa	Reduced or rudimentary-appearing AF

AF, anchoring fibril; *HD*, hemidesmosome; *SBDP*, subbasal dense plate; for explanation of other abbreviations, see footnote to Table 7-1.
Modified from Fine J-D, Smith LT: Non-molecular diagnostic testing of inherited epidermolysis bullosa: current techniques, major findings, and relative sensitivity and specificity, In: Fine J-D, Bauer EA, McGuire J, Moshell A, eds. *Epidermolysis Bullosa: Clinical, Epidemiologic, and Laboratory Advances, and the Findings of the National Epidermolysis Bullosa Registry*. Baltimore: Johns Hopkins University Press; 1999, p. 52.

  - Histologic features include suprabasilar acantholysis leading to a "tombstone" appearance of residual keratinocytes along DEJ
  - Eosinophils are often present
  - There may be tracking of acantholysis down adnexal structures
- Immunofluorescence
  - Biopsy for DIF should be performed from perilesional skin
  - DIF shows net-like intracellular deposition IgG and C3 with the epidermis (Fig. 7-11)
  - IIF can be performed using monkey esophagus and it shows a similar pattern
- ELISA testing
  - Antibody levels for DG3 may be measured and correlate with disease activity
- Variations
  - Pemphigus vegetans (**Fig. 7-12**)
    - A vegetating form of PV most common in the intertriginous regions (particularly the axilla and inguinal folds)
    - Histologically, it comprise the features of pemphigus vegetans but with prominent epidermal acanthosis and with marked eosinophilic abscesses
- Associations

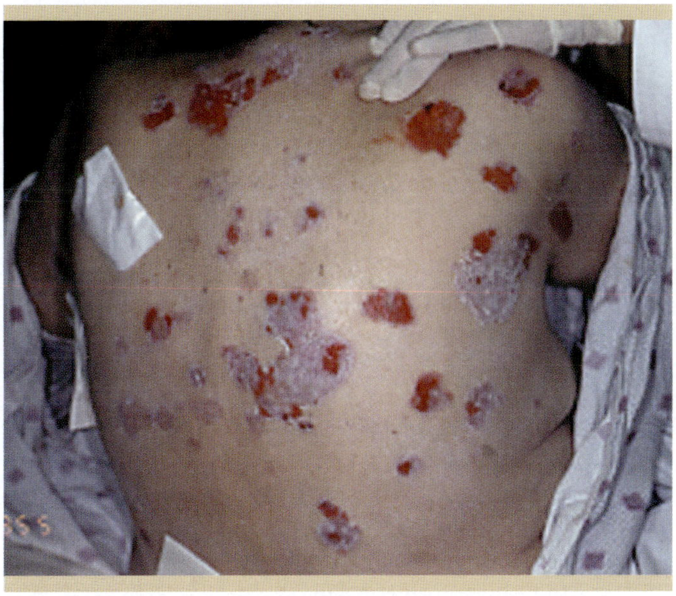

FIGURE 7-10 Pemphigus vulgaris. (*Used with permission from Dr. Robert Jordon.*)

- Drug-induced pemphigus vulgaris is associated with penicillamine, captopril, cephalosporin, nonsteroidal anti-inflammatory drugs (NSAIDs), pyrazolones, and other thiol-containing compounds or cysteine-like chemical structure
- Treatment
  - Systemic corticosteroids are the mainstay of treatment
    - Prednisone (≥1 mg/kg per day to begin therapy)
  - Once a response is achieved it is standard to transition to a steroid-sparing agent
  - Immunosuppressive medications/interventions that may be employed include azathioprine, cyclophosphamide, cyclosporine, dapsone, IVIG, methotrexate, mycophenolate mofetil, plasmapheresis, rituximab

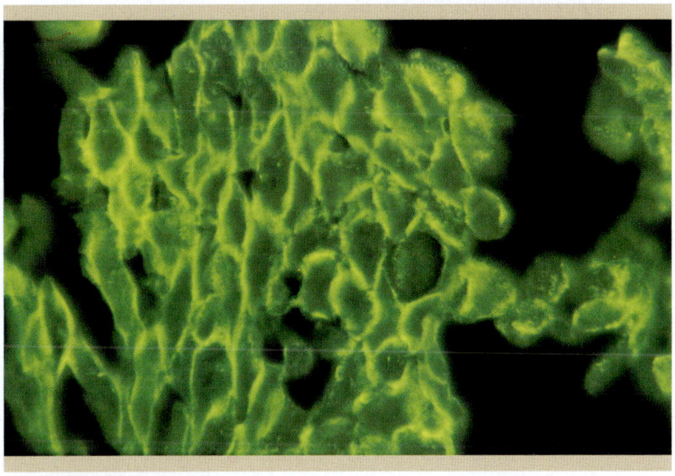

FIGURE 7-11 Pemphigus vulgaris immunofluorescence. (*Used with permission from Dr. Robert Jordon.*)

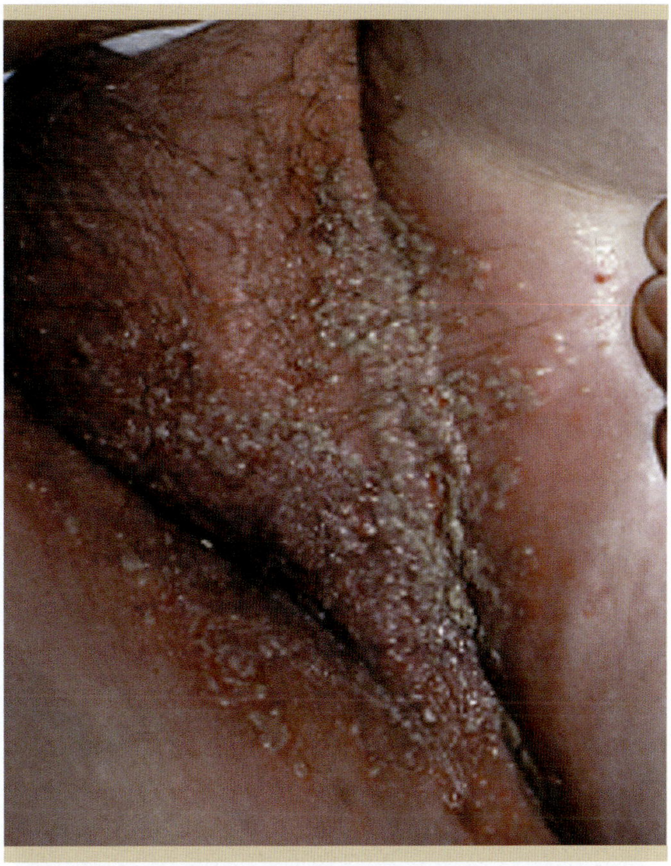

FIGURE 7-12 Pemphigus vegetans. (*Used with permission from Dr. Robert Jordon.*)

- Course/prognosis
  - Prior to development of corticosteroids patients with PV had high mortality
  - Even with modern treatment modalities, the mortality in PV is about 3-fold higher than that of the general population
  - Complications secondary to the use of systemic corticosteroids often contribute to morbidity and mortality
  - The prognosis is worse in those patients with extensive disease or in older patients
  - Chronic immunosuppression may also elevate the risk of a lymphoma/leukemia

Pemphigus Foliaceus (PF) (Fig. 7-13)

- Autoimmune, intraepidermal, blistering skin disease
- Antigens
  - Desmoglein 1 (a desmosomal core protein)
    - 160-kDa glycoprotein (member of cadherin supergene family)
  - Less commonly
  - Plakoglobin: 85-kDa plaque protein found in desmosomes

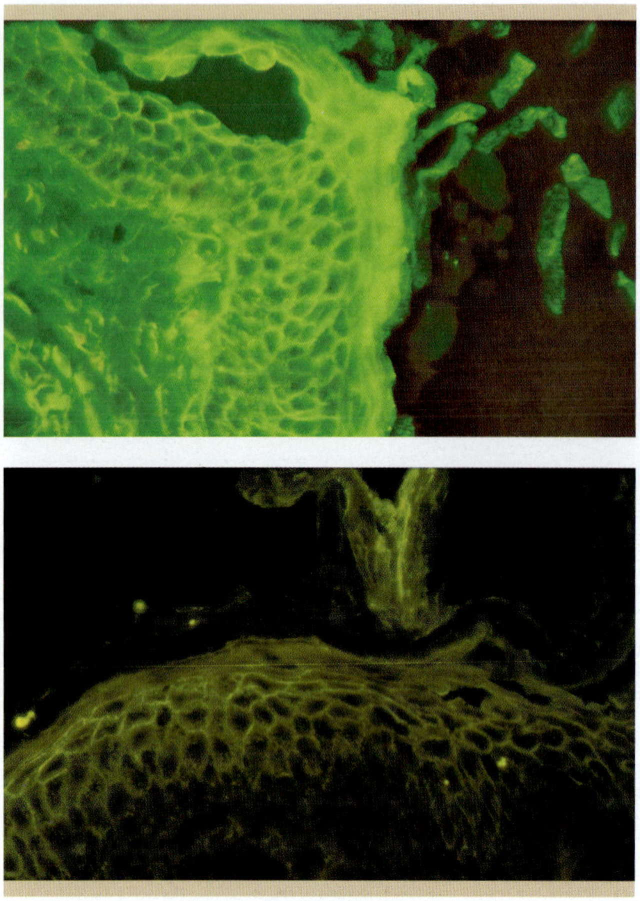

FIGURE 7-13 Pemphigus foliaceus. (*Used with permission from Dr. Robert Jordon*.)

- Clinical
  - A bullous condition involving the skin (but not often the mucous membranes)
  - The condition may be localized or generalized
  - The condition results in flaccid blisters that progress rapidly to erosions/ulcerations
  - Intact bullae are rare due to the fragility of the intraepidermal process
  - Sometimes all that is present is a collarette (the residuum) of a ruptured blister and the condition may even be confused with papulosquamous disease
  - Sun and/or heat may exacerbate disease
  - Nikolsky sign ("direct" or "marginal" Nikolsky sign) may be positive, if it can be performed at all
- Diagnosis
  - Light microscopy
    - Biopsy for traditional light microscopy should be performed at bulla margin overlapping slightly onto normal-appearing skin
    - Histologic features include a chiefly subcorneal acantholysis, although in some cases there may be more widespread acantholysis, with similarities to PV
    - Eosinophils may be present
  - Immunofluorescence
    - Biopsy for DIF should be performed from perilesional skin
    - DIF shows net-like intracellular deposition IgG and C3 in the upper epidermis
    - IIF can be performed using guinea pig esophagus, and it shows a similar pattern
    - Sometimes the distribution of immunoreactants, particularly in DIF, is not particularly zonal in the epidermis, and it may not be possible to discriminate between PV and PF using this technique alone (clinical correlation is helpful)
  - ELISA testing
    - Antibody levels for DG1 may be measured and may correlate with disease activity
- Variants
  - Fogo selvagem (Portuguese for "wild fire")
    - Endemic form of PF that occurs in persons living in the Amazon river basin
    - There is an observed relationship to the bite of black fly *Simulium nigrimanum*
    - Often several persons in a village may be affected at the same time
  - Pemphigus erythematosus (Senear and Usher)
    - Variant of PF with erythematous patches and vesiculation
    - Most often located upon the cheeks, forehead, sternum/upper chest, and upper back (photoexposed distribution)
    - May have positive antinuclear antibody (ANA), but rarely have other stigmata of systemic lupus erythematosus
- Associations
  - Drug-induced pemphigus foliaceus may be associated with penicillamine, angiotensin convertase inhibitors, nifedipine, nonsteroid anti-inflammatory agents, and penicillamine/bucillamine
  - Some cases of PF have been associated with thymoma
- Therapy
  - Topical glucocorticosteroids
  - Systemic corticosteroids
  - Other medications or interventions employed include azathioprine, cyclophosphamide, cyclosporine, dapsone, IVIG, mycophenolate mofetil, plasmapheresis rituximab, and tetracyclines (doxycycline or minocycline) with nicotinamide
  - Photoprotection is appropriate for patients with a photoexposed trigger
- Course/prognosis
  - Because mucosal disease is general absent, and the disease of often more limited, PF is not associated with the same adverse prognosis as PV
  - Given the lesser morbidity and mortality, therapy for PF is often less aggressive than that of PV

Paraneoplastic Pemphigus

- A paraneoplastic blistering skin disorder that also has elements of a lichenoid and vacuolar dermatitis
- Tumor antigens are hypothesized to evoke an immune response that leads to the development of oral erosions or ulcerations
  - Antigens
    - Desmoplakin I (250 kDa)
    - BP230 (230 kDa)
    - Desmoplakin II (210 kDa)
    - Envoplakin (210 kDa)
    - Periplakin (190 kDa)
    - HD1/plectin (500 kDa)
    - Unidentified 170-kDa protein
    - DGI (160 kDa)
    - DGIII (130kDa)
- Clinical
  - Cutaneous lesions are highly variable
  - There is often diffuse erythema, vesiculobullous lesions, papules, scaly plaques, exfoliative erythroderma, erosions, or ulcerations
  - Severe mucosal disease (most often severe lingual ulceration and other stomatitis) is a requirement of all classification schemes
- Diagnosis
  - Light microscopy
    - Suprabasilar acantholysis similar to that of PV
    - But with an underlying lichenoid infiltrate, vacuolization of basilar keratinocytes, lymphocytic exocytosis, and dyskeratotic keratinocytes with satellitosis
  - Immunofluorescence (**Fig. 7-14**)
    - DIF with IgG and C3 deposits both within the intercellular spaces (as in PV) but also along the BMZ as well
    - IIF testing with rat bladder (transitional epithelium) is often employed as a screening test for paraneoplastic pemphigoid
  - ELISA testing
    - Interesting as it will show positivity for both BP230, but also DG1 and DG3
- Associations
  - Most cases are related to a leukemia or non-Hodgkin lymphoma (NHL)
  - Fewer cases are associated with Waldenström macroglobulinemia, sarcomas, thymomas, and Castleman disease
  - Castleman disease is the most common cause of paraneoplastic pemphigus in children
- Treatment
  - High-dose systemic corticosteroids (prednisone)
  - Other medications/interventions often employed include azathioprine, cyclophosphamide, cyclosporine, IVIG, plasmapheresis, rituximab (anti-CD20 antibody)

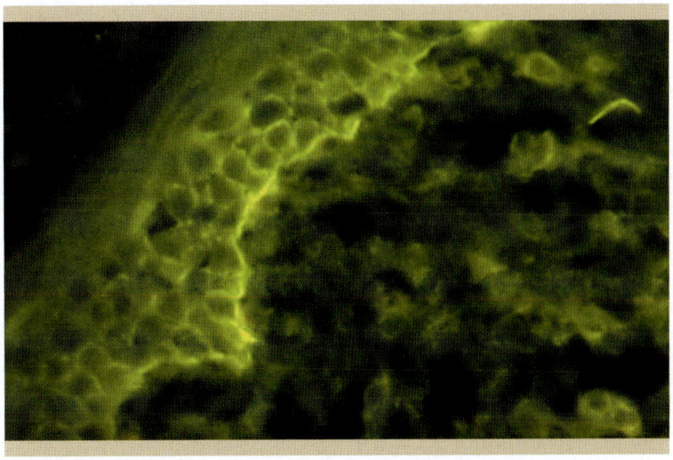

FIGURE 7-14 Paraneoplastic pemphigus immunofluorescence. *(Used with permission from Dr. Robert Jordon.)*

- Course/prognosis
  - The prognosis of the disease, partly because of its severity and partly because of the general lack of reserve in cancer patients, is typically quite grave
  - Published mortality has been in the range of 75 to 80%
  - Even when the disease responds to management, it will often recur with recurrences of the cancerous condition
  - Ultimately, very often, involvement of respiratory tract epithelium may lead to respiratory insufficiency due to bronchiolitis obliterans and this may lead to death

QUIZ

Questions

1. Which of the following statements regarding bullous pemphigoid is true?

   A. The condition is most common in patients older than 60 years
   B. The condition often begins in the mouth
   C. Prior to the advent of corticosteroids the disease was often fatal
   D. Ocular involvement may often lead to symblepharon or blindness
   E. Skin lesions often heal with scarring or milia

2. In linear IgA bullous dermatosis, DIF examination of perilesional skin most often demonstrates:

   A. IgA deposition in a linear band along the dermoepidermal junction
   B. IgA deposition in a granular pattern intermittently within the papillary dermis
   C. IgG accumulation in a net-like pattern in the epidermis

D. IgG accumulation in a linear band along the dermoepidermal junction
E. C3 accumulation in a granular pattern along the dermoepidermal junction

3. The Brunsting-Perry variant of cicatricial pemphigoid most often involves what type of patient?
A. A young man
B. A young woman
C. An elderly man
D. An elderly woman
E. An elderly person of either sex

4. IIF examination of salt-split skin demonstrates deposition of immunoreactants along the *roof* of the blister cavity in:
A. Anti-epiligrin cicatricial pemphigoid
B. Bullous pemphigoid
C. Bullous lupus erythematosus
D. Epidermolysis bullosa acquisita
E. Epidermolysis bullosa simplex

5. In dermatitis herpetiformis, DIF examination of affected skin most often demonstrates:
A. Linear deposition of IgG and C3 along the dermoepidermal junction
B. Linear deposition of IgA along the dermoepidermal junction
C. Granular IgA deposition intermittently in the papillary dermis
D. Net-like deposition of IgG and C3 in the upper epidermis
E. Net-like deposition of IgG and C3 in the lower epidermis

6. Which of the following grains contains no gluten, and can be consumed on a gluten-free diet designed to manage dermatitis herpetiformis?
A. Barley
B. Rice
C. Rye
D. Kamut
E. Wheat

7. Which material is often used in indirect immunofluorescence as a screening material for paraneoplastic pemphigus?
A. Guinea pig esophagus
B. Guinea pig bladder
C. Monkey esophagus
D. Monkey bladder
E. Rat bladder

8. The pathologic effects of pemphigus vulgaris are attributed to antibodies to which antigen?
A. Desmocollin 1
B. Desmocollin 3
C. Desmoglein 1
D. Desmoglein 3
E. Desmoplakin

9. By definition, paraneoplastic pemphigus requires involvement of what anatomic site?
A. Conjunctiva
B. Genital mucosa
C. Oral mucosa
D. Scalp
E. Skin

10. While epidermolysis bullosa acquisita may be associated with all of the following conditions, for which condition is the association strongest and most prevalent?
A. Amyloidosis
B. Chronic lymphocytic leukemia
C. Inflammatory bowel disease
D. Rheumatoid arthritis
E. Thyroiditis

Answers

1. A. Patients with bullous pemphigoid are typically older (> 60 years old) with comorbidities. Unlike pemphigus, most cases of bullous pemphigoid do not begin in the mucosa. Prior to the advent of systemic corticosteroids, it was pemphigus vulgaris that was often fatal. Ocular involvement leading to symblepharon is more common in cicatricial pemphigoid. Epidermolysis bullosa acquisita heals with scarring and milia.
2. A. In linear IgA bullous dermatosis, DIF most often reveals linear deposition of IgA along the dermoepidermal junction. Similarly linear deposition of linear IgG and C3 deposition is more common in bullous pemphigoid. Intermittent and course deposition of IgA in the papillary dermis is more common in dermatitis herpetiformis. Net-like intraepidermal deposition of immunoreactants is seen in pemphigus.
3. C. The Brunsting-Perry variant of cicatricial pemphigoid most often affects the scalp of elderly men. For this reason, it may often be confused with non-melanoma skin cancer.
4. B. Because cleavage occurs through the lamina lucida, DIF, or IIF examination of salt-split skin from bullous pemphigoid demonstrates deposition of immunoreactants on the roof of the blister cavity.
5. C. In DIF studies, dermatitis herpetiformis demonstrates intermittent and granular accumulation of IgA in the papillary dermis. Linear deposition of IgA would be

definitional for linear IgA bullous dermatosis, and linear deposition of IgG and C3 is common to bullous pemphigoid. Net-like deposition of immunoreactants in the epidermis is common to pemphigus.

6. B. Rice contains no gluten. All the other grains are thought to contain some gluten. The presence of gluten in oats is variable and controversial, and it may depend upon processing techniques, but it is not the "best" answer. Rice is a principal grain in any gluten-free diet.
7. E. Rat bladder if the tissue used in IIF screening tests for paraneoplastic pemphigus.
8. D. The clinical condition in pemphigus vulgaris is dictated chiefly by antibodies to DG3 (130 kDa), and in fact, measurement of this antibody by ELISA titrate to disease activity.
9. C. Paraneoplastic pemphigus always involves the oral mucosa, usually with severe ulcerations of the tongue. In fact, severe painful stomatitis is one of the principal criteria for diagnosis of the disease in all diagnostic schema.
10. C. While all the listed conditions can be seen in association with epidermolysis bullosa acquisita, in the literature, the disorder is most tightly associated with inflammatory bowel disease.

REFERENCES

Amagai M: Pemphigus, In: Bolognia JL, et al, eds. *Dermatology*. New York: Mosby; 2012, pp. 449–462.

Bickle K, Roark TR, Hsu S: Autoimmune bullous dermatoses: a review. *Am Fam Physician* 2002;65(9):1861–1870.

Borradori L, Bernard P: Pemphigoid group, in Bolognia JL, Jorizzo JL, Rapini RP, eds. *Dermatology*. New York: Mosby; 2003, pp. 463–477.

Goldsmith LA et al. *Fitzpatrick's Dermatology in General Medicine*, 8th Ed. New York: McGraw-Hill; 2012.

Herron MD, Zone JJ: Dermatitis herpetiformis and linear IgA bullous dermatosis, in Bolognia JL, Jorizzo JL, Rapini RP, eds. *Dermatology*. New York: Mosby; 2003, pp. 479–489.

McKee PH: *Pathology of the Skin: With Clinical Correlations*. London: Mosby-Wolfe; 1996.

CHAPTER 8

DISORDERS OF CORNIFICATION, INFILTRATION, AND INFLAMMATION

PAMELA GANGAR
RAKHSHANDRA TALPUR

CUTANEOUS DISORDERS OF CORNIFICATION

Ichthyoses

- Group of disorders characterized by generalized scaling of the skin
- Pathogenesis: increased cohesiveness of cells of the stratum corneum, abnormal keratinization, and abnormal proliferation

Ichthyosis Vulgaris (Fig. 8-1)

- Epidemiology: most common disorder of cornification; AD
- Pathogenesis
  - Loss of function mutation in filaggrin (FLG) gene
  - Increased adherence of the stratum corneum and scale formation is thought to result from a lack of water-retaining amino acids that derive from filaggrin metabolism
- Clinical features
  - Not present at birth; onset during infancy/childhood
  - Fine white, flaky scales develop on the extremities, especially the extensor surfaces with sparing of the groin and flexural areas due to increased humidity
  - Improves with advancing age
  - Associated with keratosis pilaris and atopic triad of asthma, hay fever, and eczema
- Pathology
  - Thirty to fifty percent of affected individuals lack a granular layer on light microscopy and profilaggrin-containing keratohyalin granules by EM
- Treatment
  - Emollients and humectants
  - Keratolytics—be careful with salicylic acid to avoid salicylism
  - Topical retinoids—can be irritating

Lamellar Ichthyosis (Fig. 8-2)

- Epidemiology: AR
- Pathogenesis
  - In the majority of patients, it is caused by transglutaminase-1 deficiency due to deleterious mutations in the *TGM1* gene
  - Has also been mapped to the ATP-binding cassette transporter gene (ABCA12) and the cytochrome P450 family 4, subfamily F, polypeptide 22 gene (CYP4F22)
- Clinical features
  - Apparent at birth and persists throughout life
  - Collodion baby
  - Characterized by large, dark-brown, and plate-like scales that form a mosaic pattern with minimal to no erythroderma
  - Ectropion, eclabium, and significant hypoplasia of nasal and auricular cartilage due to tautness of facial skin
  - Variable palmoplantar keratoderma (PPK), may have alopecia and nail dystrophy
- Treatment
  - Oral retinoids may be necessary from early childhood if severe
  - Keratolytics limited secondary to irritation and systemic absorption

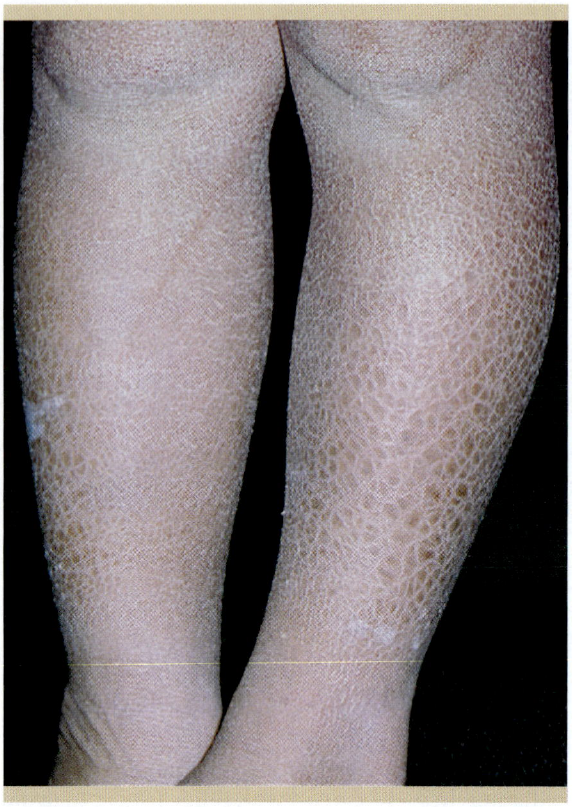

FIGURE 8-1 Ichthyosis vulgaris. (*Reprinted with permission from Freedberg IM et al:* Fitzpatrick's Dermatology in General Medicine, *6th Ed. New York: McGraw-Hill; 2003, p. 487.*)

- Topical vitamin D_3 derivatives, tazarotene, and formulations containing lactic acid and propylene glycol in a lipophilic cream base
- Palliation for heat intolerance
- Ophthalmologic evaluation

Non-Bullous Congenital Ichthyosiform Erythroderma:

- Epidemiology: AR
- Pathogenesis
  - Mapped to 6 different genes: transglutaminase 1, ALOXE3, ALOX12B, ABCA12, CYP4F22, and NIPAL4.
  - 12-LOX and eLOX sequentially function to generate epoxy alcohol metabolites, which are necessary for formation of the epidermal lipid barrier
- Clinical features
  - Presents at birth with a collodion membrane
  - Persists throughout life
  - Characterized by intense erythroderma, white small powdery scale, ectropion, and scarring alopecia
  - Palms and soles have diffuse, fissuring keratoderma
  - Obstruction of sweat ducts and pores results in hypohidrosis and heat intolerance
- Pathology
  - Increased lamellar bodies, accumulation of lipid droplets in the stratum corneum, and disorganized intercellular lipid lamellae
- Treatment
  - See "Lamellar Ichthyosis"
  - Erythrodermic patients need supplemented fluid, calories, iron, and protein to balance increased loss through the skin

X-Linked Ichthyosis

- Epidemiology: XLR; affects males almost exclusively
- Pathogenesis
  - Decreased or absent steroid sulfatase activity
  - Results in impaired hydrolysis of cholesterol sulfate and DHEA-S with subsequent accumulation of cholesterol 3-sulfate in the epidermis, which may inhibit TGM-1
- Clinical features
  - In women pregnant with an affected fetus, steroid sulfatase deficiency in the fetal placenta causes low or absent levels of estrogen, which causes failure of progression of labor
  - Presents within first weeks after birth with mild erythroderma and generalized peeling of large, translucent scale
  - The typical large, polygonal, dark-brown scale with tight adherence develops during infancy and is distributed symmetrically on the extremities, trunk, and neck
  - Palms, soles, and face spared—except preauricular areas
  - Asymptomatic corneal opacities in 10–50%
  - Twenty-fold increase of cryptorchidism and are thought to be at higher risk for testicular cancer and hypogonadism
- Treatment
  - Emollients
  - Topical keratolytics
  - Topical retinoids

Ichthyosis Bullosa of Siemens

- Epidemiology: AD
- Pathogenesis: heterozygous mutations in gene for keratin 2 (expressed only in the uppermost spinous and granular cell layers of the epidermis)
- Clinical features
  - At birth—may appear normal or show mild blistering
  - Trauma induced blistering in infancy
  - Hyperkeratosis develops in early childhood
  - Predilection for skin overlying joints, flexures, and dorsa of hands/feet—spares palms and soles
  - Characteristic feature is superficially denuded areas with collarette-like borders
- Pathology: clumping of tonofilaments on EM
- Treatment: see "Bullous Congenital Ichthyosiform Erythroderma"

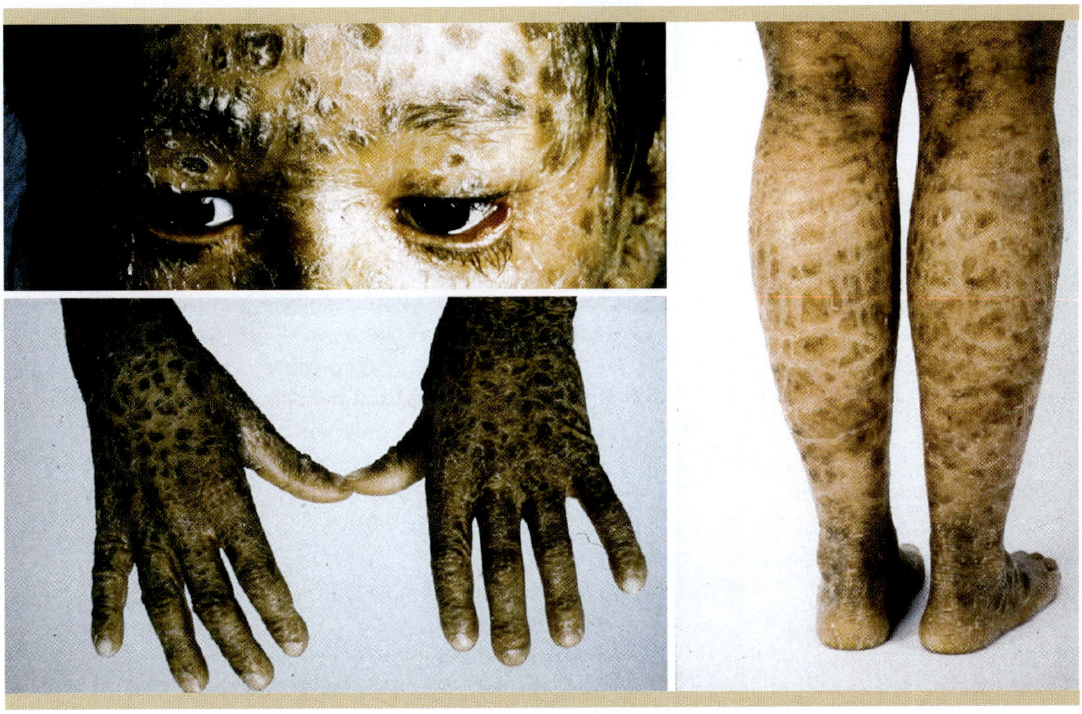

FIGURE 8-2 Lamellar ichthyosis. (*Reprinted from Russell LJ et al. Linkage of autosomal recessive lamellar ichthyosis to chromosome 14q.* Am J Hum Genet *1994;55:1146.*)

Bullous Congenital Ichthyosiform Erythroderma

- Epidemiology: AD; ~50% occur sporadically (new mutations)
- **Pathogenesis**
  - Heterozygous mutations in keratins 1 and 10, which are expressed in the suprabasal and granular layers of the epidermis
  - KRT1 is associated with severe PPK
  - KRT10 spares the palms/soles—not expressed there
  - Epidermal acantholysis and hyperkeratosis result from hyperproliferation, decreased desquamation, and other factors
- Clinical features
  - Presents at birth with erythroderma, erosions, peeling, and widespread areas of denuded skin
  - Over time, blistering and erythroderma resolve, and hyperkeratosis prevails
  - Increased transepidermal water loss and bacterial colonization of the stratum corneum due to disturbed barrier function
  - Sepsis and fluid and electrolyte imbalances account for perinatal morbidity and mortality
  - Pungent body odor
- Pathology: epidermolytic hyperkeratosis—massive, dense orthokeratotic hyperkeratosis, acanthosis with hypergranulosis and cytolysis of the suprabasal and granular layers
- Treatment
  - NICU during neonatal period
  - Keratolytics—limited due to irritation and salicylism
  - Topical emollients, tretinoin, and vitamin D
  - Antibiotics as needed for bacterial infection; antiseptics or antibacterial soaps
  - Systemic retinoids

Ichthyosis Hystrix Curth-Macklin

- Epidemiology: AD
- Pathogenesis: mutations in the keratin 1 gene
- Clinical features
  - No skin fragility
  - Ranges from severe, mutilating PPK to generalized hystrix-like hyperkeratosis
  - Pseudoainhum, starfish-like hyperkeratoses, knuckle pads, flexural digital contractures, and secondary bacterial infections have been described
- Treatment: systemic retinoids and topical keratolytic agents
- Ichthyosis hystrix—descriptive name for a clinically and genetically heterogenous group of skin disorders with massive hyperkeratosis that has a verrucous surface or protruding, porcupine-like spines

Harlequin Fetus

- Epidemiology: AR
- Pathogenesis
  - Massive cell retention in the stratum corneum, abnormal or absent lamellar bodies, and lack of intercellular lipid lamellae
  - Loss of function mutations in the ABC transporter gene ABCA12-codes for lamellar bodies involved in energy-dependent lipid transport

- Clinical features
  - Born prematurely and die within a few days or weeks after birth due to respiratory insufficiency or sepsis
  - Encased in a hard armor-like thickened stratum corneum that immobilizes the baby
  - A few days later, cracks form large, yellow, adherent plates separated by broad, deep, and intensely red fissures
  - Ectropion, eclabium, and rudimentary development of ear and nasal cartilage due to tautness of skin
  - Hands/feet are edematous and swollen
  - Increased transcutaneous water loss and heat results in dehydration, electrolyte imbalance (e.g., hypernatremia), and temperature instability
  - Intelligence is usually normal
- Pathology: hair follicles show marked, concentric accumulation of keratotic material around hair shafts, which is considered a diagnostic feature
- Treatment
  - ICU care
  - Ophthalmology for severe ectropion
  - Systemic retinoids

Sjögren-Larsson Syndrome

- Epidemiology: AR
- Pathogenesis: deficiency of microsomal enzyme fatty aldehyde dehydrogenase (FALDH), which catalyzes the NAD-dependent oxidation of long-chain aliphatic aldehydes
- Clinical features
  - Presents at birth with varying degrees of erythema and ichthyosis
  - Rare collodion membrane
  - After infancy, erythema fades, while hyperkeratosis and scaling become more prominent
  - Predilection sites are the lower abdomen, side and nape of neck, and flexures
  - Seventy percent develop PPK
  - Associated with persistent pruritus
  - Presence of perifoveal glistening white dots in the ocular fundus
  - Involvement of the CNS manifests in the first year of life with delayed motor development, abnormal gait, pyramidal signs, and spasticity
  - Progressive neurologic decline results in di- or tetraplegia and severe MR
- Treatment
  - Topical keratolytics and topical Vitamin D
  - Skin hydration
  - Systemic retinoids
  - 5-lipoxygenase inhibitors—for pruritus
  - Symptomatic treatment for CNS effects

Refsum Disease

- Epidemiology: AR
- Pathogenesis
  - Excessive accumulation of phytanic acid caused by a deficiency of peroxisomal enzyme phytanoyl-CoA hydroxylase
  - Two genes are implicated: PHYH and PEX7
- Clinical features
  - Cutaneous symptoms are variable and tend to develop during childhood or adolescence
  - Starts with insidious neurologic symptoms
  - Waxes and wanes with resulting gradual neurologic deterioration
  - Cardinal features are atypical retinal pigmentosa leading to concentric visual field constriction, hypo- or anosmia peripheral polyneuropathy, cerebellar dysfunction, and elevated protein in CSF
- Pathology: diagnosis established by detecting increased phytanic acid levels in serum
- Treatment
  - Reducing dietary phytanic acid intake (in dairy products and animal fats)
  - Retinal changes are irreversible
  - Therapeutic plasma exchange may be useful for acute toxicity

Neutral Lipid Storage Disease With Ichthyosis

- Epidemiology: AR
- Pathogenesis
  - Inborn error of lipid metabolism with multiorgan accumulation of triglycerides
  - Germline mutations in CGI-58 gene
- Clinical features
  - Congenital generalized ichthyosis, myopathy, cataracts, and sensorineural deafness
  - Widespread tissue deposition of neutral lipids results in a broad array of systemic manifestations in childhood
  - Prognosis depends on the course of liver disease and extent of hepatic fibrosis
- Pathology: diagnostic feature is the presence of numerous lipid-containing vacuoles in circulating granulocytes (Jordan anomaly)
- Treatment
  - Topical emollients and keratolytics
  - Systemic retinoids
  - Fat-restricted diets

Conradi-Hünermann Syndrome

- Epidemiology: XLD
- Pathogenesis
  - Caused by a primary defect in cholesterol biosynthesis
  - Distinct mutations in EBP gene encoding emopamil-binding protein
- Clinical features
  - Generalized erythema with thick adherent scale and linear or whorled hyperkeratosis at birth

- Erythroderma resolves substantially or completely within first weeks/months of life
- In older children, hyperkeratosis is replaced by linear or patchy follicular atrophoderma
- Skeletal abnormalities are usually asymmetric
- Widespread calcifications manifest as stippled epiphyses (chondrodysplasia punctata)—typically involves the trachea and vertebra; can be detected on radiographs in childhood, but not apparent when bone maturation progresses
- Unilateral cataracts
- Normal life expectancy and intelligence
- Treatment
  - Emollients, urea, or lactic acid-containing products
  - Orthopedic and ophthalmology consults **Howel-Evans Syndrome**

CHILD (Congenital Hemidysplasia With Ichthyosiform Erythroderma [or Nevus] and Limb Defects)

- Epidemiology: XLD
- Pathogenesis: inactivating mutation in NSDHL—encodes 3β-hydroxysteroid-dehydrogenase
- Clinical features
  - Presents at birth or neonatal period with striking unilateral erythema and skin thickening with a waxy surface or yellowish adherent scale
  - Often involves right side of body and sharply demarcated at midline
  - Spares the face
  - Ipsilateral skeletal abnormalities range from hypoplasia of digits or ribs to complete amelia
  - Stippled epiphyses can be seen on radiographs in early infancy but resolve during childhood
  - Asymmetric organ hypoplasia affects brain, kidney, heart, and lungs
- Treatment
  - Multidisciplinary depending on organ involvement
  - Topical tretinoin, systemic retinoids, or surgical excision

Netherton Syndrome (Ichthyosis Linearis Circumflexa)

- Epidemiology: AR
- Pathogenesis: caused by mutation in the SPINK5 gene—encodes multi-domain serine protease inhibitor LEKT1, predominantly expressed in lamellar granule system of epithelia and lymphoid tissue
- Clinical features
  - Presents at or soon after birth with generalized erythroderma and scaling
  - Collodion membrane usually not present
  - Usually, ichthyosis evolves into serpiginous or circinate scaling and erythematous plaques which are bordered by a double-edged scale
  - Hair shaft abnormalities develop during infancy and improve with age—include trichorrhexis invaginata and trichorrhexis nodosa
  - Increased levels of IgE, eosinophilia, and increased allergic reactions
  - Increased susceptibility to skin, respiratory tract, or systemic infections
- Treatment
  - Symptomatic
  - May require NICU
  - Topical emollients, keratolytics, tretinoin, calcipotriene, and corticosteroids
  - Avoid topical tacrolimus due to percutaneous absorption
  - Treatment of bacterial/fungal infections as needed

Erythrokeratodermia Variabilis (Mendes da Costa Disease)

- Epidemiology: AD
- Pathogenesis: mutations in the connexin genes GJB3 and GJB4—encode gap junction proteins connexin 31 and connexin 30.3
- Clinical features
  - Hallmark is the coexistence of transient erythematous patches and more stable hyperkeratosis
  - Erythematous component more prevalent during childhood
  - Individuals lesions persist for minutes to hours
  - Over time, hyperkeratosis develops
  - Stabilizes after puberty
  - May be triggered by other factors, including stress, temperature changes, friction, and sun exposure
- Treatment
  - Keratolytic agents for mild disease
  - Systemic retinoids for extensive disease

Keratosis-Ichthyosis-Deafness (KID) Syndrome

- Epidemiology: AD, majority (> 90%) of reported cases have been sporadic
- Pathogenesis: mutations in GJB2 encoding connexin 26
- Clinical features
  - First manifest with transient erythroderma at birth or infancy
  - Symmetrically distributed, well-demarcated hyperkeratotic plaques with an erythematous base and rough, ridged or verrucous surface develop later
  - Stippled PPK
  - Nonprogressive congenital sensorineural hearing impairment—generally severe and bilateral
  - Eye symptoms manifest at birth, infancy, or early childhood and worsen with age
  - Increased susceptibility to mucocutaneous bacterial, viral, and fungal infections (especially *Candida albicans*)
  - SCC of the skin and oral mucosa is a serious complication that may shorten life expectancy

- Treatment
  - Emollients, keratolytics, and topical retinoids
  - Mixed success with systemic retinoids—may aggravate keratitis and neovascularization
  - Hearing aids and cochlear implants have been used successfully
  - Corneal transplants aren't very successful due to revascularization

Palmoplantar Keratodermas (PPKs)

Unna-Thost Syndrome (Non-epidermolytic hyperkeratosis)

- Epidemiology: AD
- Pathogenesis: keratin 1 mutation
- Clinical features
  - Initially erythema of palmoplantar skin with eventual thick yellow hyperkeratosis that expands to involve the lateral aspects of the hands and feet
  - Usually well developed by age 3 to 4
  - Nontransgredient
  - Hyperhydrosis, secondary dermatophyte infections and pitted keratolysis are common
- Treatment
  - Keratolytics
  - Mechanical debridement
  - Variable improvement with systemic retinoids

Vörner Syndrome (Epidermolytic Hyperkeratosis)

- Epidemiology: AD
- Pathogenesis: keratin 9 mutation
- Clinical features: see NEPPK; blisters occasionally reported
- Pathology: epidermolytic hyperkeratosis, clumped tonofilaments
- Treatment: see NEPPK

Howel-Evans Syndrome

- Epidemiology: AD
  - Type A: late onset PPK and increased risk of esophageal carcinoma
  - Type B: early onset PPK and benign course
- Clinical features
  - PPK often limited to pressure areas
  - Associated with keratosis pilaris, dry rough skin, and oral leukokeratosis
  - Esophageal carcinoma arises in the fifth decade

Vohwinkel Syndrome (Mutilating Palmoplantar Keratoderma)

- Epidemiology: AD
- Pathogenesis
  - Mutation in gene encoding loricrin, a major cornified envelope protein
  - Mutation in connexin 26
- **Clinical features**
  - Honeycombed, diffuse hyperkeratosis of the palms of soles that appears in infancy and becomes transgredient
  - Early childhood development of constricting bands of the digits, which may lead to autoamputation (pseudoainhum)
  - Starfish-shaped keratoses over the knuckles of the fingers and toes
  - Moderate hearing loss

Mal de Meleda

- Epidemiology: AR; inhabitants off the Dalmatian coast
- Pathogenesis: SLURP-1 mutation
- Clinical features
  - Onset of diffuse palmar and plantar thickening with an erythematous border, shortly after birth
  - Progressive and transgredient with knee and elbow involvement
  - Severe hyperhidrosis and malodor
  - Complicated by fissuring and secondary fungal or bacterial infections

Papillon-Lefevre Syndrome

- Epidemiology: AR
- Pathogenesis: Mutations in cathepsin C
- Clinical features
  - Diffuse transgredient PPK
  - Destructive periodontitis beginning in childhood
  - Frequent cutaneous and systemic pyogenic infections

Richner-Hanhart Syndrome

- Epidemiology: AR
- Pathogenesis: mutations in gene encoding hepatic tyrosine aminotransferase
- Clinical features
  - Photophobia, dendritic keratitis with corneal ulcerations in the first year of life
  - Elevated serum and urine tyrosine levels
  - Painful, focal hyperkeratotic plaques on the palms and soles
  - Progressive mental retardation
- Treatment: diet restricted in tyrosine and phenylalamine will clear the keratitis and skin lesions and may delay or prevent cognitive impairment

Bart-Pumphrey Syndrome

- Epidemiology: AR
- Pathogenesis: mutation in GJB2 gene that encodes connexin 26
- Clinical features
  - Profound hearing impairment from birth
  - Early childhood development of diffuse PPK (pitted or stippled) and knuckle pads
  - Variable leukonychia that improves with age

Hidrotic Ectodermal Dysplasia (Clouston Syndrome)

- Epidemiology: AD
- Pathogenesis: mutations of GJB6 gene that encodes connexin 30
- Clinical features
  - Diffuse PPK in conjunction with hypotrichosis and nail dystrophy
  - Thickened skin may develop over the knuckles, knees, and elbows
  - Loss of hair shaft cuticle

Olmsted Syndrome

- Epidemiology: AD and XLR
- Clinical features
  - Well-defined erythematous hyperkeratotic plaques in the perioral, inguinal, genital, and intergluteal areas during the first year of life
  - PPK that begins in infancy that becomes diffuse and severe
  - Autoamputation may result from constricting PPK and SCC or melanoma may occur

Naxos Disease

- Epidemiology: AR
- Pathogenesis: deletion of the plakoglobin gene
- Clinical features: arrhythmogenic right ventricular cardiomyopathy, mild nontransgradient nonepidermolytic PPK, and wooly hair

Carvajal Syndrome

- Epidemiology: AR
- Pathogenesis: mutation in gene that encodes desmoplakin
- Clinical features: striate epidermolytic PPK, left ventricular dilated cardiomyopathy, and wooly hair
- Treatment: need cardiac evaluation—as do patients with Naxos disease

Darier Disease

- Epidemiology: AD; men and women equally affected
- Pathogenesis
  - Mutations in the endoplasmic reticulum Ca^{2+} ATPase ATP2A2-protein product SERCA2
  - Defects in Ca^{2+} sequestration into the endoplasmic reticulum produce acantholysis by impairing the normal processing of junctional proteins (desmoplakins)
  - Keratinocyte ER Ca^{2+} depletion is also associated with apoptosis
- **Clinical features**
  - Peak onset during puberty
  - Primary lesions are keratotic, red to brown papules in a seborrheic distribution, involving the trunk, scalp, face, and lateral neck
  - Malodor is frequent
  - Nail changes include longitudinal red and/or white lines, longitudinal ridging, subungual hyperkeratosis, and V-shaped notches
  - Worsens in summer and with lithium
  - Chronic course without spontaneous remission
  - Prone to secondary infection, including bacteria, yeast, dermatophytes, or Kaposi varicelliform eruption (HSV)
  - Oral salivary gland obstruction
  - Subtypes
    - Acral hemorrhagic type—Develop red to blue-black, irregularly shaped, sharply demarcated macules on the palms and soles as well as the dorsal aspects of the hands (hemorrhage into acantholytic vesicles)
    - Segmental types—distribution of lesions along Blaschko lines
- Pathology
  - Acantholysis and dyskeratosis
  - Corps ronds—acantholytic enlarged keratinocytes in malpighian layer with darkly staining and partially fragmented nuclei surrounded by a clear cytoplasm and encircled by a bright ring of collapsed keratin bundles
  - Grains—small, oval cells in the stratum corneum characterized by a strongly eosinophilic cytoplasm composed of collapsed keratin bundles containing shrunken parakeratotic nuclear remnants
- Treatment
  - Lightweight clothing and sunscreen
  - Topical retinoids and emollients
  - Antimicrobial washes and intermittent use of antibiotics/antifungals
  - Systemic retinoids
  - Excision followed by STSG, dermabrasion, or laser removal

POROKERATOSES (FIG. 8-3)

- Epidemiology: AD
- Pathogenesis: clonal hyperproliferation of atypical keratinocytes; causes cornoid lamella, which expands peripherally and forms the raised boundary between abnormal and normal keratinocytes
- Clinical features: five clinical variants
  - Classic porokeratosis Mibelli
    - Infancy or childhood, asymptomatic
    - Small, brown to skin-colored papule that gradually enlarges over years to form a plaque
    - May occur anywhere, including the mucous membranes
  - Disseminated superficial porokeratosis (DSP) and disseminated superficial actinic porokeratosis (DSAP)
    - Most common type
    - Multiple thin papules in a widespread pattern

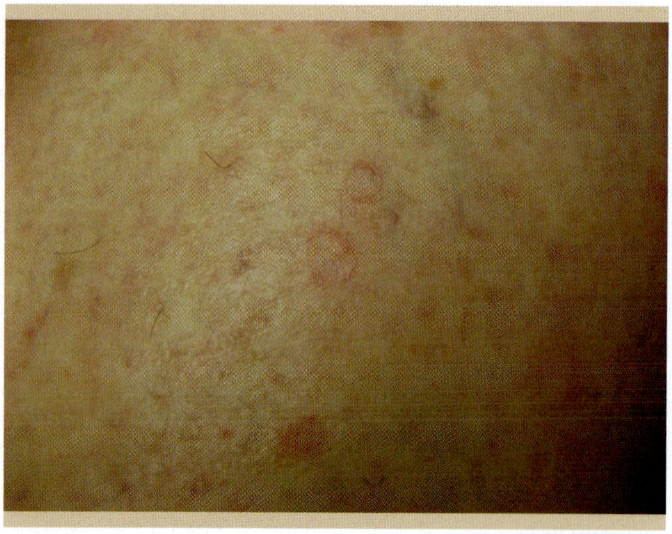

FIGURE 8-3 Porokeratosis. (*Used with permission from Dr. Asra Ali.*)

    - DSP—occurs on the extremities bilaterally and symmetrically, sparing the palms, soles, and mucous membranes
    - DSAP—exclusively involves the sun-exposed areas, most commonly on the lower legs; lesions more prominent and erythematous in the summer
    - Appear during the third to fourth decades of life
  - Linear porokeratosis
    - Infancy or early childhood
    - Plaques follow the lines of Blaschko, most commonly on the extremities
  - Punctate porokeratosis
    - Appears during or after adolescence as 1 to 2 mm papules on the palms and soles
  - Porokeratosis palmaris et plantaris disseminata (PPPD)
    - Uncommon
    - Variation of punctate porokeratosis, buy any surface, including mucous membranes, may be involved
- Pathology
  - Cornoid lamella: thin column of tightly packed parakeratotic cells within a keratin-filled epidermal invagination; extends at an angle away from the center of the lesion
  - Epidermis, beneath the parakeratotic column, has keratinocytes that are irregularly arranged with atypical nuclei
  - Papillary dermis with a moderately dense lymphocytic infiltrate and dilated capillaries
- Treatment
  - Cryotherapy, topical 5-fluorouracil, topical retinoids in combination with 5-FU, topical imiquimod, photodynamic therapy, CO_2 and other lasers, shave excision, curettage, linear excision, and dermabrasion
  - If widespread or refractory, oral acitretin

Pityriasis Rubra Pilaris (PRP)

- Epidemiology: AD
- Pathogenesis: vitamin A deficiency and abnormal vitamin A metabolism
- Clinical features
  - Both sexes equally affected
  - Disease self limited, resolving within 3 to 5 years (classic forms)
  - Follicular hyperkeratosis on an erythematous base
  - Orange-red or salmon-colored plaques with islands of uninvolved skin; can progress to erythroderma
  - Distinctive orange-red waxy keratoderma of the palms and soles
  - Nails: distal yellow-brown discoloration and subungual debris
  - Mucous membrane: diffuse whitish appearance of the buccal mucosa, lacy whitish plaques, and erosions
  - Griffith's classification
    - Type I: classic adult, most common and good prognosis
    - Type II: atypical adult, palmoplantar keratoderma
    - Type III: classic juvenile, good prognosis
    - Type IV: circumscribed juvenile, most common juvenile form
    - Type V: atypical juvenile
    - Type VI: HIV-associated
- Pathology
  - Hyperkeratosis with alternating orthokeratosis and parakeratosis forming a checkerboard pattern in the stratum corneum
  - Focal or confluent hypergranulosis; follicular plugging with perifollicular parakeratosis forming a shoulder effect
  - Thick suprapapillary plates; broad rete ridges; narrow dermal papillae; and sparse superficial dermal lymphocytic perivascular infiltration, acantholysis
- Treatment: Isotretinoin, acitretin, methotrexate

Lichen Simplex Chronica (Fig. 8-4)

- Epidemiology
  - Older adults
- Pathogenesis
  - Secondary to habitual scratching/rubbing of skin
  - Predisposing factors: xerosis, atopy, stasis dermatitis, anxiety, obsessive-compulsive disorder, and pruritus related to systemic disease
- Clinical features
  - Hyperpigmented, lichenified, well-circumscribed leathery plaques
  - Predilection for the posterior neck, occipital scalp, anogenital region, shins, ankles, and dorsal aspects of the hands, feet, and forearms

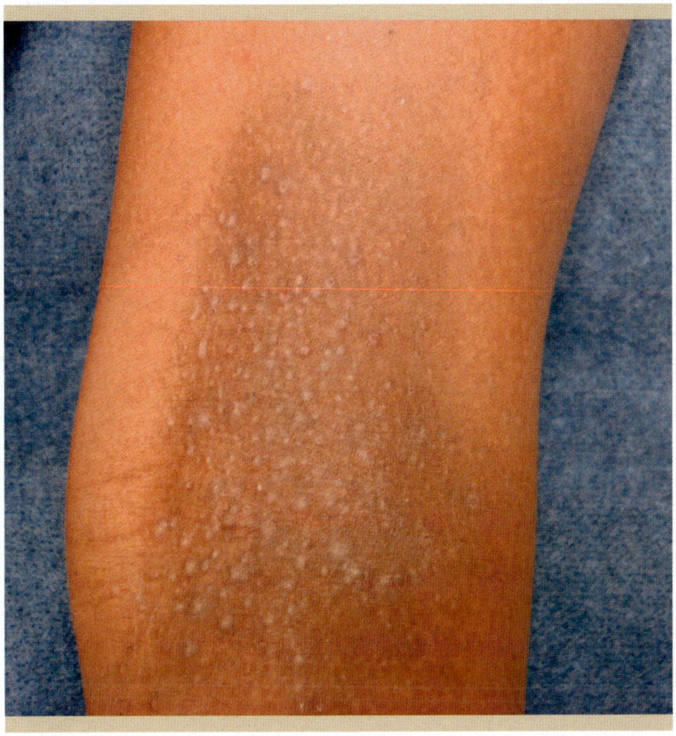

FIGURE 8-4 Lichen simplex. (*Used with permission from Dr. Asra Ali.*)

- Pathology
  - Hyperkeratosis, acanthosis with irregular elongation of the rete ridges, and hypergranulosis
- Treatment
  - Identify and treat underlying pruritic disorders
  - Topical corticosteroids, with or without occlusion
  - Intralesional corticosteroids
  - Topical calcineurin inhibitors
  - Manage pruritus with antihistamines and topical antipruritics
  - SSRIs or informal insight-oriented psychotherapy in patients with OCD

Tyloma (Callus)

- Pathogenesis
  - Caused by chronic external pressure
- Pathology
  - Prominent hyperkeratosis, usually without parakeratosis

Clavus (Corn)

- Pathogenesis
  - Caused by chronic pressure at the site of bony prominences
- Clinical findings
  - Hyperkeratotic lesion
- Pathology
  - Hyperkeratosis with parakeratosis
  - Epidermis is centrally atrophic and peripherally acanthotic
  - Perivascular infiltration of upper dermis

Pityriasis Lichenoides (Fig. 8-5)

- Epidemiology
  - More common in children and males

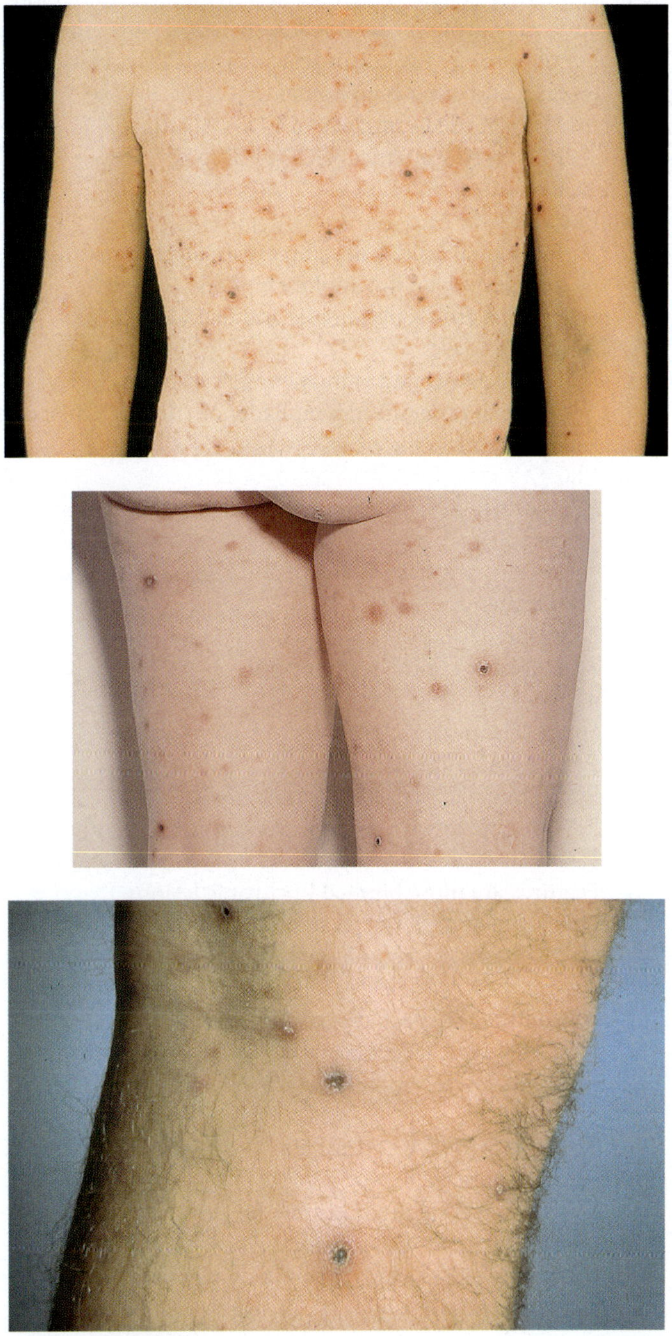

FIGURE 8-5 Pityriasis lichenoides. (*Reprinted with permission from Freedberg IM et al.* Fitzpatrick's Dermatology in General Medicine, *6th Ed. New York: McGraw-Hill; 2003, p. 459.*)

- Pathogenesis
  - Postulated to be a response to foreign antigens (infection, drugs)
  - Two forms
    - Acute: pityriasis lichenoides et varioliformis acuta (PLEVA; Mucha-Habermann disease)
    - Chronic: pityriasis lichenoides chronica (PLC; Guttate Parapsoriasis)
  - Contain lesional T-cell infiltrates that may exhibit clonality; may explain occasional association with other lymphoproliferative disorders such as CTCL, Hodgkin disease, and other lymphomas.
    - PLEVA: predominance of CD8+ T cells
    - PLC: predominance of CD4+ T cells
- Clinical features
  - PLEVA
    - Individual lesions develop crusts/ulcers/pustules/vesicles → heal to varioliform scars
    - Lesions are asymptomatic and usually resolve within weeks
    - Rarely associated with systemic symptoms: fever, malaise, generalized lymphadenopathy, arthritis, or bacteremia
  - PLC
    - Red/brown scaly papules → heal to hypopigmented macules
    - Lesions are more indolent and regress over weeks to months
  - Duration of disease
    - Diffuse < central < peripheral
- Pathology
  - Superficial perivascular interface dermatitis
  - Focal parakeratosis
  - Epidermal damage: edema to necrosis
  - Erythrocyte extravasation with occasional lymphocytic vasculitis
  - Features are more blunted in chronic lesions
  - Lymphoid atypia is not a standard feature of PL; if present, consider lymphomatoid papulosis
- Treatment
  - Discontinue suspected responsible agent
  - First line: topical corticosteroids, topical coal tar preparations, tetracycline, erythromycin (for children), phototherapy
  - Antibiotics are for anti-inflammatory rather than antibiotic effects
  - Low dose weekly methotrexate for fulminant cases
  - Cases with systemic symptoms—give systemic corticosteroids, IVIg, or cyclosporine, once infection has been excluded

Pityriasis Rosea (Pityriasis rosea Gilbert) (Fig. 8-6)

- Epidemiology
  - Healthy adolescents and young adults

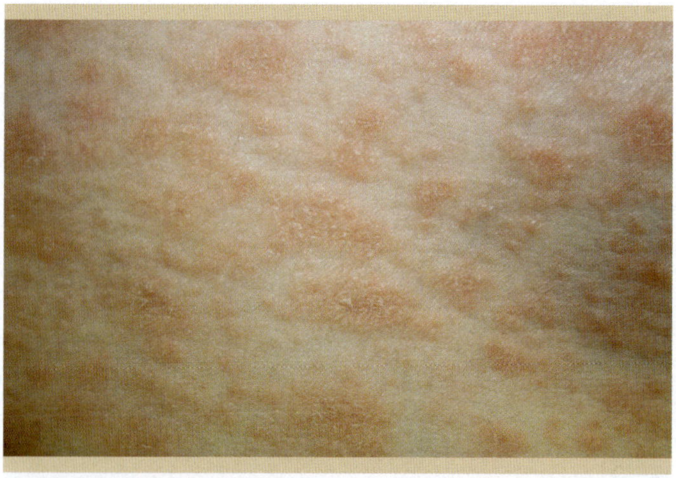

FIGURE 8-6 Pityriasis rosea. (*Used with permission from Dr. Toni Smith.*)

  - Female > male
  - May peak in spring/fall
- Pathogenesis: May have viral etiology as suggested by occasional prodromal symptoms, clustering of cases, and complete absence of recurrent episodes (immunologic defense?); historically HHV-6 and HHV-7 were considered but not proven.
- Clinical features
  - Herald patch: solitary lesion on trunk that predates the remainder of the eruption by hours/days; pink/salmon patch/plaque with central fine scale and marginal trailing collarette of scale with free edge pointing inward
  - Few have mild prodromal symptoms
  - Blossoming of lesions on trunk/proximal extremities: numerous, smaller, thinner than herald patch; usual round/oval; long axis follows the Langer lines of cleavage → posterior trunk = "fir tree" or "Christmas tree" pattern
  - Face/palms/soles = usually spared
  - Persists 6 to 8 weeks with spontaneous resolution; if lesions last more than 5 months → may possibly be PLC instead
  - Variants: inverse PR (occurs in axillae/inguinal areas, more common in younger children and darker skin), urticarial, vesicular, purpuric, pustular
- Pathology
  - Nonspecific: small mounds of parakeratosis, spongiosis, and mild lymphohistiocytic perivascular and interstitial papillary dermal infiltrate; mild erythrocyte extravasation
  - Most patients do not have biopsies as clinical picture may be classic and histology is nonspecific
- Treatment
  - Education/reassurance
  - Counterirritant antipruritic lotions/low- to medium-strength topical corticosteroids
  - If severe, UVB light and oral antihistamines

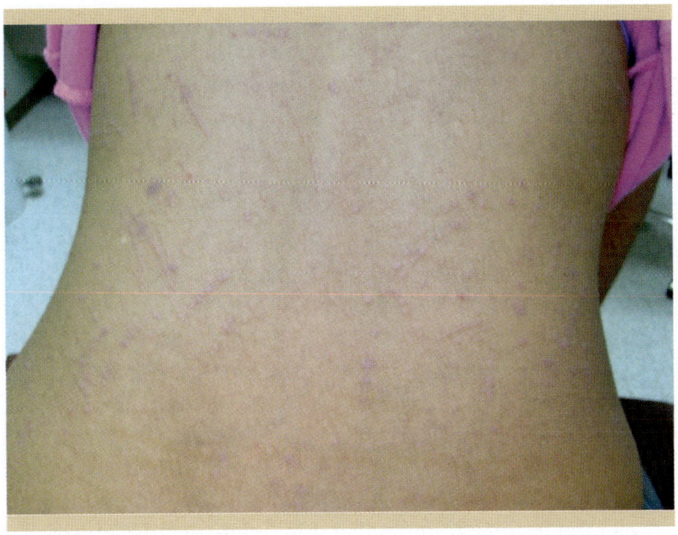

FIGURE 8-7 Lichen planus. (*Used with permission from Dr. Asra Ali.*)

Lichen Planus (Fig. 8-7)

- Epidemiology
  - No racial/gender predisposition
- Pathogenesis
  - T-cell-mediated autoimmune damage to basal keratinocytes that express altered self-antigen on their surface secondary to exposure to exogenous agents
  - Exogenous agents
    - Hepatitis C virus (associated with HLA-DR6)
    - Transfusion-transmitted virus (TTV)
    - HHV-6
    - HBV vaccine
    - Oral contact allergens (metallic dental restorations/reconstructions [amalgam/mercury, copper, gold])
    - Drugs: captopril, enalapril, labetalol, methyldopa, propranolol, chloroquine, hydroxychloroquine, quinacrine, chlorothiazide, HCTZ, gold salts, penicillamine, quinidine
    - Paraneoplastic process
- Clinical features
  - Peak onset in fifth to sixth decade
  - Pruritic violaceous papules—small, polygonal, flat-topped, occasionally umbilicated; shiny/transparent surface
  - Fine white lines = Wickham striae
  - Distribution: flexor surface of wrists/forearms, dorsal surface of hands, anterior lower legs, neck, and presacral areas
  - Mucosal involvement in ~75% of patients with cutaneous LP
  - Variants:
    - Actinic LP/LP tropicus/lichenoid melanodermatitis: occurs in spring/summer on sun-exposed skin with red/brown plaques; majority of reported patients have been from Middle Eastern countries
    - Acute LP/exanthematous LP/eruptive LP: widely distributed with rapid dissemination
    - Annular LP: papules spread peripherally and central area resolves; annular edge is raised and purple to white in color. Usually on axilla or penis
    - Atrophic LP: papules coalesce to form larger plaques that become centrally depressed/atrophic with residual hyperpigmentation; secondary to thinning epidermis and not due to degeneration of elastic fibers
    - Bullous LP: bullous or vesiculobullous lesions develop within preexisting LP
    - LP pemphigoides: bullous or vesiculobullous lesions develop on previously uninvolved skin; have circulating IgG autoantibodies
    - Hypertrophic LP/LP verrucosus: extremely pruritic, thick hyperkeratotic plaques on shins/dorsal foot; may have fine adherent scale; usually symmetric and chronic; may lead to squamous cell carcinoma
    - Inverse LP: violaceous papules/plaques in intertriginous zones
    - LP pigmentosus: occurs in patients with skin types III to IV as brown/gray macules in sun-exposed areas of face/neck; reticulated pigmentation; can have linear distribution following Blaschko lines
    - Lichen planopilaris/follicular LP/LP acuminatus: multiple hyperkeratotic plugs with narrow violaceous rim primarily on scalp resulting in scarring and alopecia. Women > Men
    - Linear LP: spontaneously occur within the lines of Blaschko
    - LP-lupus erythematosus overlap syndrome: prefers acral sites
    - Nail LP: lateral thinning, longitudinal ridging, and fissuring; can lead to dorsal pterygium formation
    - Oral LP: reticular pattern is the most common = whitish linear lines in a lace-like pattern or rings with short radiating spines; buccal mucosa > gingival; check for esophageal and genital involvement
    - Ulcerative LP: ulcerations within palmoplantar LP lesions, particularly those on the soles; chronic ulcers at risk of developing SCC
    - Vulvovaginal LP: erosions; can evolve into malignancy
    - Drug-induced LP: latent period of several months from drug introduction to onset of cutaneous eruption
- Pathology
  - Hyperkeratosis without parakeratosis
  - Focal increases in granular cell layer
  - Irregular acanthosis with a "saw-tooth" appearance
  - Liquefactive degeneration of the basal cell layer

- Band-like lymphocytic infiltrate at dermal-epidermal junction
- Small separations between dermis and epidermis (Max-Joseph spaces)
- Oral LP: parakeratosis rather than hyperkeratosis

- Treatment
  - Consider drug-induced LP before starting therapy
  - Spontaneous remission of cutaneus LP in two-thirds of patients after 1 year; whereas oral LP lasts ~5 years (erosive form rarely resolves)
  - Mild cases—topical corticosteroids and oral antihistamines
  - Children—topical corticosteroids
  - Hypertrophic LP—intralesional corticosteroids or topical steroids under occlusion
  - Vulvovaginal LP—topical superpotent (class I) corticosteroids and calcineurin inhibitors, but if they fail, oral immunosuppressives drugs and/or low-dose oral prednisone may be required
  - Oral LP—inhaled corticosteroids, tacrolimus 0.1% ointment, topical sirolimus
  - Severe, acute cases—systemic corticosteroids, acitretin
  - Severe recalcitrant LP—newer TNF-α inhibitors
  - Misc: griseofulvin, metronidazole, hydroxychloroquine oral sulfasalazine, methotrexate, cyclosporine, mycophenolate mofetil, thalidomide
  - Phototherapy

Lichenoid Keratosis (Lichen Planus-Like Keratosis)

- Epidemiology
  - Individuals aged 35 to 65 years old; women > men
  - Mostly Caucasians
- Pathogenesis
  - Thought to represent inflammation of a benign lentigo (benign lichenoid keratosis, BLK), actinic keratosis (lichenoid actinic keratosis), or SK (irritated SK)
  - Suggested that lichenoid infiltrate of lymphocytes is secondary to a stimulus from Langerhans cells after their processing of an unidentified epidermal antigen (similar to mechanism for lichen planus)
- Clinical features
  - Solitary pink to red/brown, often scaly, papules ranging 0.3 to 1.5 cm in diameter; most closely resembles a BCC or Bowen disease (most frequent reason for biopsy)
  - Usually asymptomatic but can have slight pruritus/stinging
  - Distribution: forearm and upper chest > shins (women), chronically sun-exposed areas
- Pathology
  - lichenoid infiltrate of lymphocytes with scattered histiocytes
  - Interface dermatitis: basal vacuolar alteration, melanin incontinence, colloid bodies
  - May see parakeratosis (unlike lichen planus)
  - Sometimes frank separation of epidermis from dermal infiltrate → subepidermal blister/cleft
- Treatment: none necessary; can destroy any remaining lesions by any method

Lichen Nitidus

- Epidemiology: rare disease—poor data
- Pathogenesis: limited study; no causative agents discovered
- Clinical features
  - Tiny discrete skin-colored uniform pinhead-sized papules with occasional central depression; usually flat with shiny surface
  - Distribution: flexor surface of upper extremities, genitalia, chest, abdomen, dorsal hands
  - Oral lesions: minute, flat, gray/white papules on soft mucosa or white plaques on tongue/hard palate
  - Nails (10%): pitting, rippling, longitudinal ridging, terminal splitting, increased longitudinal linear striations, occasional periungual papules
  - Exhibits Koebner phenomenon
- Pathology
  - Well-circumscribed infiltrate of lymphocytes, epithelioid cells, and occasional Langhans giant cells are "clutched" by surrounding hyperplastic rete ridges in a "ball and claw" configuration
  - Epidermis is atrophic +/− parakeratotic "cap" centrally
  - Absence/thinning of granular layer
  - Liquefactive degeneration of basal layer
- Treatment
  - Most patients have spontaneous clearing within one to several years
  - Primarily symptomatic (topical steroids, oral antihistamines)
  - Topical calcineurin inhibitors (children)
  - Narrowband UVB or PUVA

Lichen Striatus (Linear Lichenoid Dermatoses/ Blaschko Linear Acquired Inflammatory Skin Eruptions [BLAISE]) (Fig. 8-8)

- Epidemiology: female > male; primarily children (4 months–15 years)
- Pathogenesis: theory: during fetal development, aberrant clones of epidermal cells produced by somatic mutation migrate out along lines of Blaschko → exposure to infectious agent triggers intolerance by inducing novel membrane antigen
- Clinical features
  - Typically asymptomatic
  - Continuous/interrupted band of discrete/clustered pink/skin-colored/tan papules that are flat topped/smooth/scaly, 2 to 4 mm in size
  - Typically a single unilateral streak on an extremity

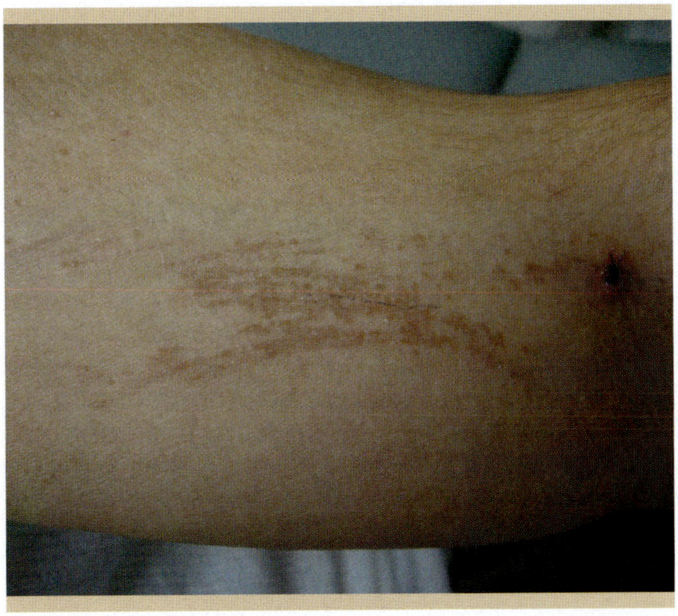

FIGURE 8-8 Lichen striatus. (*Used with permission from Dr. Jason Miller.*)

- Appears suddenly → develops over days/weeks → spontaneous resolution after year or more with postinflammatory hypopigmentation
- Pathology
  - Depends on age of lesion
  - Lichenoid tissue reaction with parakeratosis, dyskeratosis, and focal/diffuse lysis of basal layer
  - Langerhans cells are decreased (early) or increased (late)
- Treatment: not needed except for significant pruritus
  - Topical corticosteroids under occlusion to hasten resolution

Erythema Dyschromicum Perstans (Ashy Dermatoses/Dermatitis)

- Epidemiology
  - Darkly pigmented Latin Americans > Asians, whites
  - Favors skin types III + IV
  - Onset: first to third decade
- Pathogenesis: sporadic case reports of temporal associations with ingestion of ammonium nitrate, whipworm infestation, and HIV seroconversions
- Clinical features
  - Gray/brown/blue macules/patches
  - Uncommon erythematous peripheral margin measuring 1 to 2 mm in width
  - Lesion is usual oval in shape with long axes following skin cleavage lines (similar pattern to pityriasis rosea)
  - Distribution: neck, trunk, proximal arms; usually symmetric; sparing of palms, soles, scalp, nails, and mucous membranes
  - Spontaneous clearing can occur in children but usually persists for years in adults
- Pathology
  - Border of active lesions: vacuolization of basal layer, occasional colloid bodies, lichenoid infiltrate of varying degrees
    - Immunofluorescence: IgM, IgG, fibrinogen, C3 staining colloid bodies (like in LP)
  - Inactive ashy-colored lesions: pigment incontinence, variable epidermal change, including atrophy and effacement of epidermal ridges
- Treatment
  - Usually not effective
  - Sun protection
  - Topical corticosteroids/retinoids
  - Vitamin C, chemical peels, oral antibiotics, vitamin A, dapsone, antimalarials, griseofulvin, oral corticosteroids

Transient Acantholytic Dermatosis (Grover Disease)

- Epidemiology
  - White men, more than 40 years old
  - Peak in winter months
- Pathogenesis
  - Exact etiology unknown; may be secondary to acute/chronic radiation (UV or ionizing), excessive sweating (on the back of a febrile bedridden patient), heat, and xerosis
  - Predisposition with asteatotic, atopic, and allergic contact dermatitis
- Clinical features
  - Discrete round papules/papulovesicles: skin-colored or erythematous, crusted, extremely pruritic
  - Distribution: upper/mid trunk > lower trunk/proximal extremities
  - Can be acute, chronic, or relapsing
  - Exacerbations with heat, friction, sweating, and sunlight exposure, xerosis, ionizing radiation
- Pathology
  - Focal acantholysis and dyskeratosis in association with intraepidermal clefting and vesicle formation
  - Four histological variants (> 1 pattern can be seen in the same biopsy specimen)
    - Darier disease-like
      - ▲ Suprabasal cleft formation
      - ▲ Most pronounced dyskeratotic changes (corps ronds and grains)
    - Hailey-Hailey disease-like
      - ▲ Clefting in stratum spinosum
    - Pemphigus vulgaris or foliaceous-like
      - ▲ PV-like: subrabasal cleft formation
      - ▲ PF-like: clefting in superficial epidermis
    - Spongiotic with acantholysis
  - Direct immunofluorescence is negative

- Treatment
  - Avoid exacerbators—sunlight, exercise, occlusive fabrics, heat
  - Topical agents (e.g., corticosteroids, pramoxine, calcineurin inhibitors, vitamin D analogues) and oral antihistamines
  - Occasionally, oral retinoids, PUVA, and UVA1

FIGURATE ERYTHEMAS

Erythema Annulare Centrifugum (Erythema Figuratum)

- Epidemiology: peak incidence during the fifth decade of life
- Pathogenesis
  - "Hypersensitivity" to one of many antigens
  - Incidentally, there is a relationship between EAC and infectious agents, parasites, ectoparasites, drugs, pregnancy, particular foods, autoimmune endocrinopathies, hypereosinophilic syndrome, and neoplasms
  - TNF-α and IL-2 may have a role (interferon resolves lesions)
- Clinical features
  - Begin as firm pink papules that expand centrifugally and then develop central clearing
  - Trailing scale is present on the inner aspect of the advancing edge
  - Localized or generalized; favors the thighs and hips, spares palms, soles, scalp, and mucous membranes
  - Persist for weeks to months
- Pathology: intense, superficial, and deep lymphocytic or lymphohistiocytic perivascular infiltrate in a coat-sleeve fashion in the middle and lower dermis
- Treatment: self-limited; treat underlying disorder; topical or systemic corticosteroids

Erythema Gyratum Repens (EGR)

- Epidemiology: in more than 80% of patients, associated with underlying neoplasm, most commonly of the lung, breast, esophagus, or stomach
- Pathogenesis
  - Immune reaction in which there is a cross-reaction between tumor and cutaneous antigens
- Clinical features
  - Findings: wood-grain appearance; concentric mildly scaling bands of patches or plaques of erythema; rapid migration (up to 1 cm/day); intense pruritus
  - Course of rash closely mirrors the course of the underlying illness
- Pathology
  - Hyperkeratosis, focal parakeratosis, moderate patchy spongiosis, and a mild superficial perivascular lymphohistiocytic infiltrate, with eosinophils and macrophages
- Treatment: resolves when the associated neoplasm is successfully treated

Urticaria

- Epidemiology
  - Any age
  - More common in women: chronic urticaria, dermographism, cold urticaria
  - More common in men: pressure urticaria
- Pathogenesis
  - High affinity IgE receptors are cross-linked, which initiates a chain of calcium/energy-dependent steps leading to fusion of storage granules with the cell membranes and externalization of contents (degranulation)
  - Degranulation can also be stimulated by anti-IgE and anti-IgE receptor antibodies, opiates, C5a anaphylatoxin, stem cell factor, neuropeptides (substance P)
  - Mast cell granules contain histamine, cytokines (TNF-α, interleukins [3, 4, 5, 6, 8, 13]), GM-CSF, proinflammatory eicosanoids (prostaglandin [PG] D2, leukotrienes [LTC4, D4, E4])
- Clinical features
  - Multiple pruritic wheals of different sizes erupt anywhere on the body and then fade within 2 to 24 hours without bruising; often appears in evening or upon waking; most intense at night
  - In severe cases: can be associated with fatigue, lassitude, sweats, chills, indigestion, arthralgias
    - Acute urticaria
      - ▲ Duration less than 6 weeks
      - ▲ Triggers: 50% idiopathic, 40% viral URI, 9% drugs, and 1% food
      - ▲ Common in children with atopic dermatitis
    - Chronic urticaria
      - ▲ Duration more than 6 weeks and continuous (occurs at least 2 times per week when off of treatment)
      - ▲ Associations with HLA-DR4 and HLA-DQ8, *Helicobacter pylori* gastritis, and intestinal strongyloidiasis
      - ▲ Triggers: 60% ordinary (autoimmune, pseudoallergic, infection-related, idiopathic), 35% physical, and 5% vasculitic
    - Episodic urticaria
      - ▲ Duration more than 6 weeks but less frequent
    - Physical urticaria: induced by exogenous physical stimulus; lesions occur within minutes of provocation and generally resolve < 2 hours and are localized to the stimulated area
      - ▲ Triggered by mechanical stimuli
        - △ Dermographism (factitious urticaria)
        - △ Delayed pressure urticaria (DPU)
        - △ Vibratory angioedema (see "Angioedema (AE)")

      - ▲ Triggered by temperature changes
        - △ Heat/stress = cholinergic urticaria
        - △ Adrenergic urticaria
        - △ Localized heat contact urticaria
        - △ Primary/secondary cold contact urticaria
        - △ Reflex cold urticaria
        - △ Familial cold urticarial
      - ▲ Triggered by sweating or stress
        - △ Heat contact urticaria
        - △ Cold contact urticarial
          - Primary
          - Secondary (cryoglobulins, cryofibrinogen)
      - ▲ Triggered by other exposures
        - △ Primary/secondary solar urticaria
        - △ Aquagenic urticaria
    - Contact Urticaria
      - ▲ Immunologic (allergic reaction with specific IgE): sensitized to environmental allergens (grass, animals, foods)
      - ▲ Nonimmunologic (IgE-independent): secondary to direct effects of urticants on blood vessels (cinnamic aldehyde in cosmetics, nettle stings)
- Pathology: perivascular infiltrate of lymphocytes and eosinophils with some neutrophils with extension of eosinophils into the dermmis, arrayed between collagen bundles
- Treatment
  - Antipruritic lotions and avoidance of triggers
  - First line: antihistamines (first H_1 antihistamine, then add H_2 antagonist if necessary)
  - Second line: systemic corticosteroids (for emergencies; avoid in chronic urticaria), epinephrine (for severe throat angioedema/anaphylaxis only), doxepin combos, montelukast, thyroxine, colchicine, and sulfasalazine
  - Third line: immunotherapy (for severe refractory autoimmune urticaria only): plasmapheresis, IVIG, cyclosporine

Angioedema (AE)

- Epidemiology: hereditary form is AD
- Pathogenesis
  - Hereditary AE: AD mutation in structural gene for C1 inhibitor leading to
    - Reduced quantity (type 1) secondary to trans inhibition of the normal allele or increased catabolism of C1 INH
    - Reduced function (type 2)
    - Heterozygous gain of function mutation in gene that encodes FX11 (type 3)
  - Acquired AE: secondary to formation of inhibitory autoantibodies against C1 INH or persistent low-level activation of C1q by anti-idiotypic antibodies
- Clinical features:
  - Can merge with wheals, especially at eyelids
  - Can be a feature of anaphylaxis if the throat is involved
  - AE without wheals is a separate clinical entity as this occurs in C1 INH deficiency, ACEi or NSAID reactions, and are managed differently
  - Hereditary AE: low C4
  - Acquired AD: low C4 and low serum C1q
  - Vibratory AE: hereditary (AD) or acquired; vibratory stimulus (jogging, motorcycles) lead to localized swelling and erythema in minutes
  - Food/Exercise-induced anaphylaxis: occurs within minute of exercise after prior ingestion of specific food or within 4 hours of a heavy meal
- Treatment
  - See urticaria treatment section above
  - For C1 esterase inhibitor deficiency:
    - Emergency: give C1 inhibitor concentrate or FFP (life-saving) (acquired deficiency patients need more than hereditary)
    - Antihistamines, corticosteroids, and epinephrine do NOT work.
    - Treatment of choice: anabolic steroids (stanozolol or danazol)

Urticarial Vasculitis

- Epidemiology: middle-aged women
- Clinical features
  - Actually considered an urticarial dermatosis and not urticaria
  - Lesions last more than 24 hours (unlike urticaria) although clinically appears like urticaria
  - Lesions be pruritic and/or painful (burning sensation)
  - Often occurs at pressure points and may resolve with residual purpura
  - Forty percent develop angioedema; 50% develop arthralgia (transient/migratory)
  - Course is unpredictable and usually more severe in hypocomplementemic patients
  - Acute hemorrhagic edema of childhood: urticarial vasculitis with prominent cutaneous hemorrhage in young children
- Pathology
  - Evidence of leukocytoclastic vasculitis, fibrinoid deposits in/around blood vessels, extravasation of red cells, endothelial cell swelling, perivenular cellular infiltrate rich in neutrophils
  - Need to biopsy a lesion that is less than 24-hour old for accuracy
- Treatment
  - No universally effective therapy (no randomized trials)
  - Antihistamines are usually insufficient except in mild cases
  - Fifty percent improve with NSAIDs
  - Isolated positive reports with colchicine, dapsone, hydroxychloroquine, methotrexate, plasmapheresis

Other Figurate Erythemas (Covered in Separate Chapters)

- Bullous pemphigoid
- Erythema annulare centrifugum
- Erythema multiforme
- Glucagonoma syndrome
- Granuloma annulare
- Lupus erythematosus, subacute cutaneous
- Lyme disease
- Pityriasis rubra pilaris
- Psoriasis, plaque
- Tinea corporis

Id Reaction (Autoeczematization, Disseminated Eczema)

- Epidemiology: exact prevalence unknown
- Pathogenesis
    - Exact cause of the id reaction is unknown
    - Abnormal immune recognition of autologous skin antigens
    - Increased stimulation of normal T-cells by altered skin constituents
    - Lowering of the irritation threshold
    - Dissemination of infectious antigen with a secondary response
    - Hematogenous dissemination of cytokines from a primary site
- Clinical features
    - Symmetric, pruritic, erythematous, maculopapular, or papulovesicular eruption at a site distant from the primary infection or dermatitis
    - Begins 1 to 2 weeks after primary infection or dermatitis
- Pathology
    - Superficial perivascular lymphohistiocytic infiltrate with a spongiotic epidermis and vesiculation
    - Infectious agents not found in the specimens
- Treatment
    - Systemic or topical corticosteroids
    - Wet compresses
    - Systemic or topical antihistamines

Acrokeratosis Verruciformis of Hopf

- Epidemiology: AD
- Clinical features: flat wart-like papules on the dorsal aspects of the extremities; debatable if truly a separate disease versus part of Darier disease

Hailey-Hailey Disease

- Epidemiology: AD
- Pathogenesis
    - Mutations in the gene ATP2C1 that encodes the Golgi-associated Ca^{2+} ATPase
    - Golgi Ca^{2+} depletion may impair complete processing of junctional proteins, resulting in a loss of cellular adhesion in the statum spinosum (acantholysis)
- Clinical features
    - Initial symptoms and lesions usually develop during the second or third decade
    - Sites of predilection include intertriginous areas, lateral neck
    - Initial lesion is a flaccid vesicle on erythematous or normal skin, which easily ruptures
    - Blisters give rise to macerated or crusted erosions, which spread peripherally
    - Healing occurs with scarring and dyspigmentation
    - Pruritus and malodor are common
    - Friction, heat, and sweating worsen disease
    - Bacterial colonization and secondary bacterial, fungal, and viral infections can complicate—be aware for Kaposi's varicelliform eruption
    - Rarely malignant transformation
- Pathology: "Dilapidated brick wall" appearance of epidermis due to acantholysis
- Treatment
    - Lightweight clothing to avoid friction
    - Topical and systemic antimicrobials as needed
    - Topical corticosteroids
    - Wide excision with grafting
    - Dermabrasion
    - PDT or laser resurfacing

Granuloma Faciale (Fig. 8-9)

- Epidemiology: idiopathic; predominantly in middle-aged white men
- Pathogenesis: unknown
- Clinical features

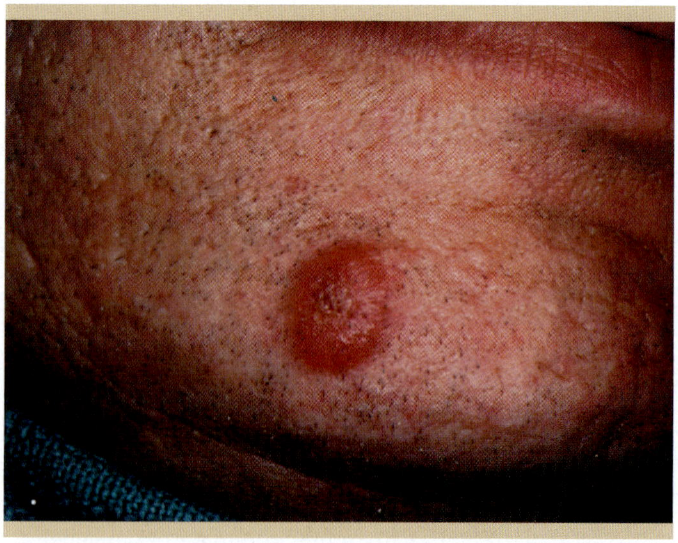

FIGURE 8-9 Granuloma faciale. (*Reprinted with permission from Freedberg IM et al.* Fitzpatrick's Dermatology in General Medicine, *6th Ed. New York: McGraw-Hill; 2003, p. 967.*)

- Solitary, asymptomatic smooth red-brown to violaceous plaque on the face
- Predominantly on the face
- Chronic and only occasionally spontaneously resolve
- Not associated with systemic disease
- Pathology: normal epidermis, Grenz zone and a dense, nodular and diffuse infiltrate of lymphocytes, neutrophils, plasma cells, and eosinophils in the dermis
- Treatment
  - Often resistant to therapy
  - IL corticosteroids
  - Oral dapsone or clofazimine
  - PUVA

Sweet syndrome (Acute Febrile Neutrophilic Dermatosis) (Fig. 8-10)

- Epidemiology
  - Worldwide distribution
  - Female predominance 4:1
  - Average age of onset 30 to 60 years
  - Up to 20% have internal malignancies (no female predominance)
  - Drug induced occurs more often in women
- Pathogenesis: unknown
- Clinical features
  - Initial cutaneous lesions are tender, nonpruritic, erythematous plaques, or papules, which may coalesce
  - Vesiculobullous variant most frequently associated with myelogenous leukemia and can break down to ulceration
  - Favors the head, neck, and upper extremities, but tends to be more widespread when associated with malignancy
  - An upper respiratory tract infection or flu-like illness frequently precedes the development of the syndrome
  - Fever is common
  - Extracutaneous involvement common, including ocular involvement, arthralgias, myalgias, arthritis, neutrophilic pulmonary alveolitis, multifocal sterile osteomyelitis
  - Associated diseases include the following:
    - Streptococcal infection
    - GI yersiniosis
    - Hematologic malignancy (especially AML)
    - Solid tumors—carcinoma of the GU tract, breast, and colon
    - Inflammatory bowel disease
    - Drugs (GM-CSF, furosemide, hydralazine, minocycline, Bactrim, and all-trans-retinioic acid)
    - Autoimmune disease: systemic lupus erythematosus (SLE), Behçet autoimmune thyroid disease, dermatomyositis, sarcoid
- Diagnostic criteria: Requires 2 major and 2 minor
  - Major criteria
    - Abrupt onset of typical cutaneous lesions
    - Histopathology consistent with Sweet's syndrome
  - Minor criteria
    - Preceded by one of the associated infections or vaccinations; accompanied by one of the associated malignancies or inflammatory disorders; associated with drug exposure or pregnancy
    - Presence of fever and constitutional signs and symptoms
    - Leukocytosis
    - Excellent response to corticosteroids
- Pathology
  - Papillary dermal edema
  - Dense diffuse dermal nodular and perivascular neutrophilic infiltrate without vasculitis
- Treatment
  - Cutaneous lesions may involute spontaneously
  - Recurrences occur in 30% (with or without treatment)
  - Treatment of underlying condition
  - Oral prednisone (0.5–1 mg/kg/d) for 4 to 6 weeks

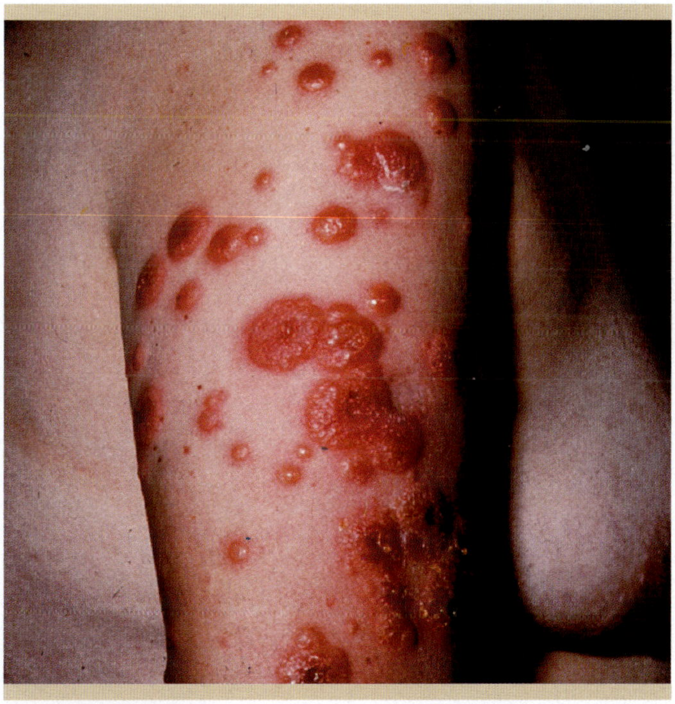

FIGURE 8-10 Acute febrile dermatosis (Sweet syndrome). (*Reprinted from Honigsmann et al. Akute febrile neutrophile Dermatose.* Wien Klin Wochenschr *1979;91:842.*)

Pyoderma Gangrenosum (Fig. 8-11)

- Epidemiology
  - Most commonly in women between 20 to 50 years
  - Fifty percent have underlying systemic disease (IBD, arthritis, and myeloproliferative disorders)

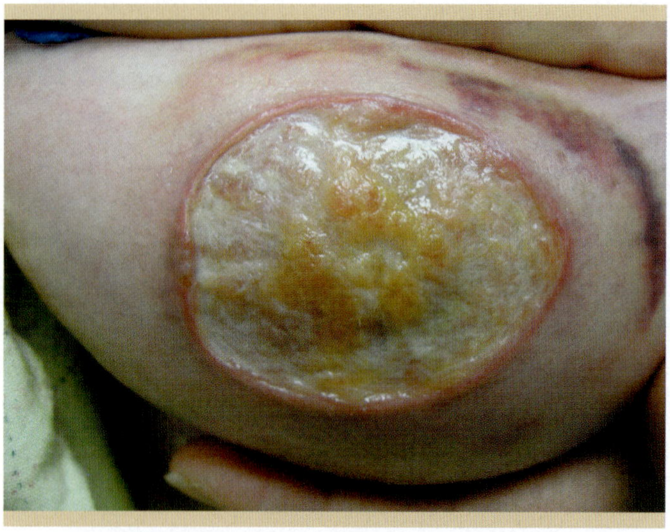

FIGURE 8-11 Pyoderma gangrenosum. (*Used with permission from Dr. Jason Miller.*)

- Pathogenesis
  - Idiopathic in 25 to 50%
  - Immunologic abnormality (autoimmune)
  - Fifteen percent have monoclonal gammopathy (usually IgA)
  - PAPA syndrome (pyogenic sterile arthritis, PG, and acne): mutations in CD2-binding protein 1, which is thought to lead to an abnormal inflammatory response
- **Clinical features**
  - Painful cutaneous lesions that occur on lower extremities (pretibial) but can occur anywhere
  - Start as a tender papulopustule/bulla/nodule with surrounding erythematous/violaceous base
  - All lesions undergo necrosis leading to a central shallow/deep ulcer with a purulent base and irregular, undermined/overhanging gunmetal-colored border that extends centrifugally
  - Re-epithelialization occurs from the margins and heal with atrophic cribriform pigmented scars
  - Lesion number varies from one to over a dozen and can coalesce
  - Classically described as rapidly expanding but can be more indolent
  - Variants
    - Vesiculobullous form (atypical or bullous PG)
      - ▲ Associated with AML, myelodysplasia, and myeloproliferative disorders (CML)
      - ▲ Favors face and upper extremities (dorsal hands)
    - Pustular PG
      - ▲ Associated with IBD
      - ▲ Multiple small sterile pustules that regress without scarring
    - Superficial granulomatous PG
      - ▲ Associated with trauma, that is, surgery
      - ▲ Localized superficial vegetative/ulcerative lesion; favors the trunk
  - Pyostomatitis vegetans: associated with IBD; chronic vegetative sterile pyoderma of labial/buccal mucosa
  - Children: favors head, genital, and perianal areas
- Pathology
  - Nonspecific, especially if partially treated or minimally inflamed
  - Early lesions: neutrophilic vascular reaction that may be folliculocentric
  - Active lesions: neutrophilic infiltrates with leukocytoclasia
  - Fully developed ulcers: necrosis with surrounding mononuclear cell infiltrates and fibrosing inflammation at the edge of the ulcer
- Treatment
  - First line: local +/- systemic corticosteroids +/- adjunctive systemic therapies
  - Second line: cyclosporine, tacrolimus, thalidomide
  - For concomitant Crohn disease: infliximab
  - Total colectomy for ulcerative colitis is not a guaranteed cure for associated PG

GRANULOMATOUS PROCESSES

Granuloma Annulare (pseudorheumatoid nodule) (Fig. 8-12)

- Epidemiology
  - Two-thirds are less than 30 years of age
  - Female:male = 2:1

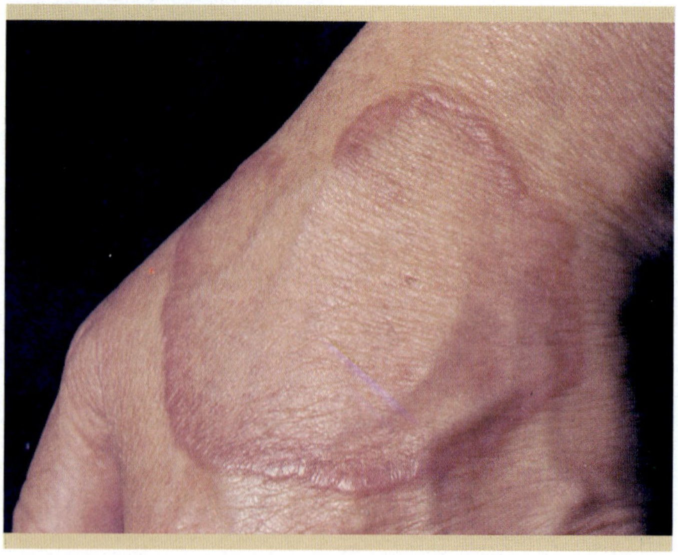

FIGURE 8-12 Granuloma annulare. (*Reprinted with permission from Goldsmith LA et al.* Fitzpatrick's Dermatology in General Medicine, *8th Ed. New York: McGraw-Hill; 2012, p.469.*)

- Pathogenesis
  - Etiology unknown but postulated to be a delayed-type hypersensitivity reaction to an unknown antigen (possibly a Th1-mediated inflammatory reaction)
  - Thought to be primarily a disorder of elastic tissue injury
  - Rare familial cases reported: associated with HLA-Bw35
- Clinical features
  - Self-limited benign disease
  - Arciform/annular plaques that favor the extremities: hands/arms > legs/feet > upper/lower extremities > trunk
  - Plaques can be skin-colored, violaceous, or pink and are composed of individual small papules that can be umbilicated
  - Seen primarily in children and young adults
  - Variants
    - Generalized (disseminated) GA: symmetric distribution on trunk and extremities; later age of onset; poorer response to therapy; increased prevalence of HLA-Bw35 allele; 45% have lipid abnormalities
    - Perforating GA: small papules with central umbilications/crusts/ulcerations on dorsal hands/fingers; exhibits transepidermal elimination of degenerating collagen histologically
    - Deep dermal/subcutaneous GA: large, painless, skin-colored nodules = "pseudorheumatoid nodules"; more common in children 5 to 6 years
    - Patch GA: patches of erythema on extremities/trunk or symmetrical lesions on dorsal feet; can lack annular configuration
    - Paraneoplastic GA: associated with solid tumors, Hodgkin disease, non-Hodgkin lymphoma, and granulomatous mycosis fungoides
  - Classic GA and perforating GA can occur in herpes zoster scars
- Pathology
  - Focal degeneration of collagen and elastic fibers, mucin deposition, and a perivascular/interstitial lymphocytic infiltrate in the upper/mid dermis
  - Histiocytes patterns
    - Infiltrative/interstitial: scattered histiocytes between collagen fibers with mucin deposition between collagen bundles (highlighted with Alcian blue and colloidal iron stains)
    - Palisading granulomas: with central connective tissue degeneration surrounded by histiocytes and lymphocytes; mucin is abundant in the center of the granuloma. More common in deep GA
    - Epithelioid histiocytic nodules (like sarcoidosis)
  - Vascular changes: variable; can have fibrin, C3, and IgM deposition in vessel walls with occlusion; can be predictive of associated systemic disease
- Treatment
  - Localized/asymptomatic disease: reassurance/observation
  - First line: high-potency topical corticosteroids +/− occlusion, intralesional corticosteroid injections
  - Cryosurgery, PUVA/UVA1, CO_2 laser.
  - Spontaneous resolution in 50% but recurrence in 40% (occurs at original sites but clear more rapidly)
  - Systemic agents reserved for severe cases include oral niacinamide, isotretinoin, antimalarials, dapsone, and pentoxifylline

Actinic Granuloma (Annular Elastolytic Giant Cell Granulomas)

- Clinical presentation
  - Annular/serpiginous areas with raised erythematous borders
  - Located on heat/sun-damaged skin
  - Present with 1 to 10 plaques
  - Predominantly in middle-aged women
- Pathology: may lack the classic palisaded arrangement observed in GA; elastosis is abundant in the mid-dermis outside the granuloma; elastic tissue is absent from the center

Chondrodermatitis Nodularis Helices (Ear Corn)

- Epidemiology: occurs in adults more than 40 years of age
- Pathogenesis
  - Predisposing factors: actinic damage, cold exposure, trauma, local ischemia, radiotherapy
  - Helical lesions: may begin with perichondritis/folliculitis
  - Antihelical lesions: may begin with pressure-induced ischemia, involving the cartilage secondarily
- Clinical features
  - Skin-colored to erythematous dome-shaped nodules with central crusts or keratin-filled craters
  - Most occur on upper helical rim or the mid-lower antihelical rim; sites often correspond to outermost portions of pinna
  - Often exquisitely tender to palpation
  - Women: commonly on antihelix
  - Men: commonly on helix
  - Lesion confused with CNH are squamous cell carcinoma, basal cell carcinoma, actinic keratosis, cutaneous horns, and weathering nodules
- Pathology
  - Well-circumscribed area of acanthosis, parakeratosis, and hypergranulosis
  - Central crater with epidermal disruption +/- keratotic plug/dermal debris
  - Lymphohistiocytic infiltrate extends into thickened perichondrium

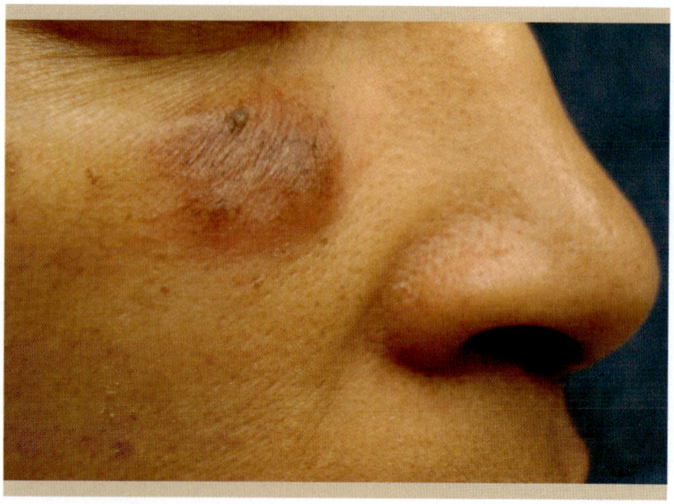

FIGURE 8-13 Sarcoidosis. (*Used with permission from Dr. Asra Ali.*)

- Treatment
  - Relieve/eliminate pressure (special pillows)
  - Topical corticosteroids/antibiotics
  - Surgery: cryosurgery, electrodessication, and curettage, full-thickness excision, CO_2 laser ablation

Sarcoidosis (Fig. 8-13)

- Epidemiology
  - Bimodal age distribution: peaks at 25 to 35 years and 45 to 65 years
  - In United States, higher incidence in African-Americans, who have more acute and severe disease (commonly 40 years AA female)
  - New onset most common in winter/spring
- Pathogenesis
  - Up-regulation of CD4+ T-helper cells of Th1 subtype after antigen presentation → epithelioid granulomas
  - Etiology unknown: may be autoimmune or infectious
  - Genetic susceptibility: HLA-1, HLA-B8, HLA-DR3 alleles; ACE gene polymorphisms
- Clinical features
  - Papules/plaques—red/brown, yellow/brown, erythematous, or violaceous (lupus pernio)
  - Favor the face, lips, neck, and upper trunk/extremities
  - Usually fairly symmetric without scale
  - Commonly develop within preexisting scars or sites of prior trauma
  - Upon diascopy, pressure induces blanching and lesions appear to have "apple jelly" color
  - Can have prominent telangiectasias = angiolupoid sarcoidosis
  - Variants
    - Darier-Roussy sarcoidosis: painless, firm, mobile nodules without epidermal involvement
    - Lupus pernio: papulonodules/plaques in areas affected by cold (nose, ears, cheeks); often with beaded appearance on nasal rim; 75% have lung involvement; 50% have upper respiratory tract involvement
  - Löfgren syndrome: erythema nodosum with hilar adenopathy, fever, migrating polyarthritis, and acute iritis
  - Nail changes: clubbing, subungual hyperkeratosis, onycholysis
  - Heerfordt syndrome: parotid gland enlargement, uveitis, fever, and cranial nerve palsies (usually of the facial nerve)
  - Kveim test: intradermal injection of tissue from spleen or lymph node of a patient with sarcoidosis; biopsy sample is obtained from the area 4 to 6 weeks after injection
- Pathology
  - Superficial and deep dermal epithelioid cell granulomas without any lymphocytes or plasma cells (naked tubercles)
  - No central caseation
  - Multinucleated giant cells are usually Langhans type, with nuclei arranged in a peripheral arc
    - Asteroid bodies: eosinophilic stellate inclusions, likely engulfed collagen
    - Schaumann bodies: rounded laminated basophilic inclusions, likely degenerating lysosomes
- Treatment
  - Corticosteroids (topical, intralesional, or systemic)
  - Hydroxychloroquine, chloroquine
  - Methotrexate, thalidomide, isotretinoin, minocycline, allopurinol

Foreign-Body Granulomas

- Epidemiology: occurs in both children and adults and the general health of the patient is unaffected
- Pathogenesis: foreign body granulomas occur because material remains undigested
- Clinical features
  - Located in areas of trauma and surgery
  - Small, firm nodules, often surrounded by inflammation
  - Red, red-brown, or color of normal skin
  - Ulcerations and fistula
- Pathology
  - Foreign bodies (suture material, keratin, hair, traumatic foreign material)
  - Chronic inflammation with giant multinuclear histiocytes and granulocytes; some foreign bodies (silica, wood, suture material, glass) are birefringent (identify with polarized light)
- Treatment: surgical removal of the foreign body

CUTANEOUS DISORDERS OF INFILTRATION

Scleromyxedema (Generalized and Sclerodermoid Lichen Myxedematosus)

Chronic idiopathic disorder characterized by numerous firm papules and areas of induration that are due to dermal mucin deposition in association with an increase of dermal collagen

- Epidemiology: affects middle-aged adults of both sexes equally
- Pathogenesis: unknown; significance of monoclonal gammopathy is uncertain
- Clinical features
  - Numerous 2 to 3 mm firm, waxy closely spaced papules develop in a widespread symmetrical distribution pattern
  - Most common sites are hands, forearms, and neck
  - Doughnut sign due to skin thickening over the proximal interphalangeal joints
  - Almost always associated with paraproteinemia, monoclonal gammopathy—IgG with γ light chains
  - Less than 10% progress to multiple myeloma
  - Can have internal manifestations: muscular, neurologic, rheumatologic, pulmonary, renal, and cardiovascular
- Pathology
  - Diffuse deposit of mucin in the upper and mid reticular dermis
  - Increase in collagen
  - Marked proliferation of irregularly arranged fibroblasts
- Treatment
  - Monthly courses of melphalan
  - IL and topical corticosteroids
  - PUVA, systemic retinoids, ECP, thalidomide, electron beam radiation
  - Autologous stem cell transplant

Localized Variants of Lichen Myxedematosus

- Clinical features
  - Small, firm, waxy papules limited to a few sites (upper and lower limbs and trunk)
  - Skin is the only site of involvement
  - Not associated with sclerosis, paraproteinemia, systemic involvement, or thyroid disease
  - Four subtypes
    1. Discrete popular form
    2. Acral persistent popular mucinosis
    3. Cutaneous mucinosis of infancy
    4. Pure nodular form
- Associated with HIV, exposure to toxic oil, or L-tryptophan, HCV

Colloid Milium (Colloid Degeneration of Skin, Elastosis Colloidalis Conglomerate)

- Clinical features
  - Grouped whitish papules on sun-exposed skin—dorsal hands, face, neck, ears
  - Three forms: nodular, adult onset, and juvenile (AD)
- Pathology
  - Nodular fissured masses of amorphous eosinophilic material in the superficial dermis
  - Congo red and crystal violet often stain positive

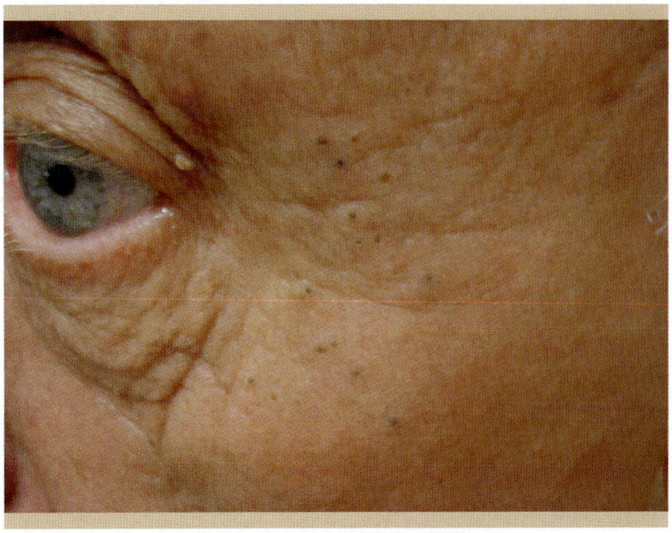

FIGURE 8-14 Favre-Racouchot syndrome. *(Used with permission from Dr. Asra Ali.)*

- Treatment: laser therapy, dermabrasion, cryotherapy, diathermy

Favre-Racouchot Syndrome (Fig. 8-14)

- Clinical features
  - Multiple large open comedones develop on the lateral in inferior aspects of the periorbital area
  - Associated with marked solar elastosis
- Pathology: dilated pilosebaceous openings and cyst-like spaces filled with horny material

Erythema Elevatum Diutinum

- Epidemiology
  - Any age but more common in middle-aged and older adults
  - Male to female ratio is equal
  - No racial predilection
- Pathogenesis
  - Associated infections: β-hemolytic streptococcus, HIV, HBV
  - Associated autoimmune or inflammatory conditions: Wegener granulomatosis, inflammatory bowel disease, relapsing polychondritis, SLE, RA
  - Associated hematologic disorders: plasma cell dyscrasias, myelodysplasia, myeloproliferative disorders, hairy cell leukemia
  - Immune complex deposition as a result of chronic antigenic exposure or high circulating antibody levels are thought to be the underlying pathologic mechanism
- Clinical features
  - Red-violet to red-brown papules, plaques, and nodules that favor extensor surfaces
  - Arthralgias can develop in underlying joints
  - Chronic course, but majority resolve spontaneously more than 5 to 10 years

- Pathology
  - LCB with neutrophilic infiltrate in the upper and mid dermis with eosinophils
  - Classic finding in late stage lesions with extracellular cholesterol deposits and fibrosis
- Treatment
  - Dapsone with relapse upon discontinuation
  - NSAIDs, niacinamide, tetracyclines, chloroquine, colchicines, plasmapheresis
  - IL corticosteroids

Scleredema

Symmetrical diffuse induration of the upper part of the body caused by a thickened dermis and depositions of mucin

- Epidemiology
  - Affects all races
  - Form associated with diabetes is more common in men
  - Other forms more common in women
- Pathogenesis
  - Diabetes mellitus
  - Irreversible glycosylation of collagen and resistance to degradation by collagenase may lead to an accumulation of collagen
  - Excess stimulation by insulin, microvascular damage, and hypoxia may increase the synthesis of collagen and mucin
  - Streptococcal hypersensitivity, injury to lymphatics, and paraproteinemia may play a role
- Clinical features
  - First type—affects primarily middle-aged women and children and is preceded by fever, malaise, and upper or lower respiratory tract infection (usually Streptococcal); Cervicofacial region skin hardens and extends to trunk and proximal upper limbs; can get tongue and pharyngeal involvement; resolves in a few months
  - Second type—same as first but with more subtle onset, without a preceding illness and persists for years; associated with monoclonal gammopathy
  - Third type—affects obese, middle-aged men with insulin-dependent DM; subtle onset with persistent involvement; primarily involves posterior neck and back, has even proved fatal when there was internal involvement
  - Systemic manifestations include serositis, dysarthria, dysphagia, myositis, parotitis, ocular, and cardiac abnormalities
  - Associated with hyperparathyroidism, RA, Sjögren syndrome, malignant insulinoma, MM, gall bladder carcinoma, HIV
- Pathology
  - Thickening of the reticular dermis with large collagen bundles separated by clear spaces filled with mucin
  - No increase in the number of fibroblasts
  - Mucin accumulates in the skeletal muscle and heart
- Treatment
  - Control of hyperglycemia does not influence cutaneous involvement
  - No specific treatment available

Cutaneous Myxoma

- Clinical features
  - Papular lesion
  - May be seen in Carney complex (33% patients)
  - Perifollicular in orientation
  - Includes subungual myxomas
  - Propensity for local recurrence if incompletely excised
- Pathology
  - Myxoid and variably cellular
  - Localized accumulation of mucin within the reticular dermis

CALCIUM DEPOSITS

Subepidermal Calcifying Nodule (Solitary Congenital Nodular Calcification, Winer Nodular Calcinosis)

- Epidemiology: idiopathic (dystrophic calcification); most common in children
- Pathogenesis: trauma in utero, calcification of preexisting milia, eccrine duct hamartoma, or nevi
- Clinical features
  - Solitary firm nodule
  - Most often found on head and neck, most common on ears
  - Lateral aspects of the digits
- Pathology: focal amorphous masses of calcium with inflammatory infiltrate
- Treatment: surgical removal if lesions are symptomatic

Calciphylaxis (Fig. 8-15)

- Epidemiology: predominant in females and diabetics; patients with poor obesity and poor nutritional status at higher risk
- Pathogenesis
  - Necrosis of skin secondary to calcification and occlusion of small cutaneous arterioles
  - Associated with chronic renal failure, hypercalcemia, hyperphosphatemia, an elevated calcium-phosphate product, and secondary hyperparathyroidism; common in patients with endstage renal disease (ESRD)
- Clinical features
  - Early lesions are violaceous reticulated patches
  - Bullae may develop with tissue necrosis and ulcer formation
  - Lesions are extremely painful
  - Lower extremities (below the knees) most common location (90%); proximal greater than distal, where body fat is most abundant
  - Mortality rate of calciphylaxis is reported to be as high as 60 to 80%; the leading cause of death is sepsis from infected, necrotic skin lesions

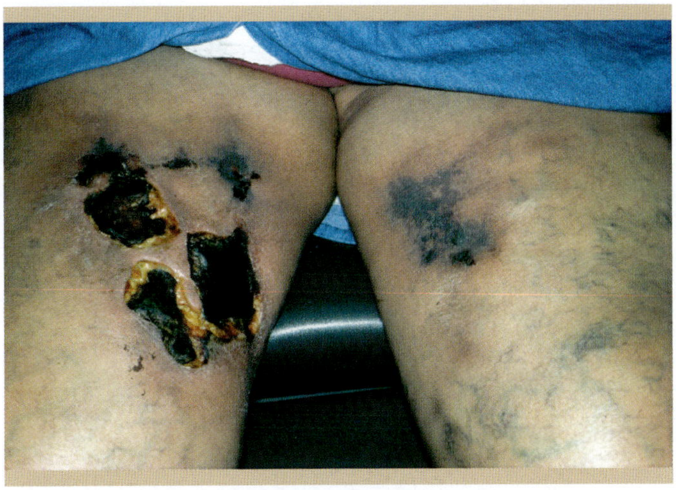

FIGURE 8-15 Calciphylaxis. (*Reprinted with permission from Freedberg IM et al.* Fitzpatrick's Dermatology in General Medicine, *6th Ed. New York: McGraw-Hill; 2003, p. 1493.*)

- Calcium-phosphate product frequently exceeds 60 to 70 mg^2/dL^2
- Laboratory tests for blood urea nitrogen and creatinine levels; calcium, phosphate, alkaline phosphatase, and albumin levels; parathyroid hormone level and coagulation factors: prothrombin time (PT), activated partial thromboplastin time (aPTT), protein C, protein S, anticardiolipin, lupus anticoagulant, factor V Leiden, and homocysteine

- Pathology: calcium deposits within the walls of blood vessels, mixed inflammatory infiltrate; subcutaneous calcium deposits with lobular panniculitis and fat necrosis vascular microthrombi, epidermal necrosis
- Treatment
  - Supportive with appropriate wound care and surgical debridement
  - Serum calcium and phosphate concentrations must be brought to low-normal levels; aggressive wound care, parathyroidectomy, hyperbaric oxygen, low calcium dialysis and systemic corticosteroids with cimetidine

Osteoma Cutis (Cutaneous Ossification)

- Epidemiology
  - Equal incidence in men and women
  - Four genetic disorders that features cutaneous or subcutaneous ossification
  - Fibrodysplasia ossificans progressive (FOP)
  - Progressive osseous heteroplasia (POH)
  - Plate-like osteoma cutis (POC)
  - Albright hereditary osteodystrophy (AOH)
- Pathogenesis
  - Intramembranous ossification begins in the dermis
  - Familial occurrence of Albright hereditary osteodystrophy (pseudohypoparathyroidism and pseudopseudohypoparathyroidism) may be present
- Clinical features
  - Face, extremities, scalp, digits, and subungual regions
  - POH is rare, more progressive, and has associated morbidity due to extensive ossification, lesions are symptomatic papules and nodules
  - POC has one or few areas of involvement, nonprogressive
  - AHO associated with pseudohypoparathyroidism and brachydactly
- Pathology: mature bone is found in the dermis or extends into the subcutaneous tissue
- Treatment
  - Underlying abnormalities of calcium/phosphorus should be addressed
  - Excision of the neoformed bone
  - Recurrence is common in genetic disorders that result in ossification of skin

Calcinosis Cutis (Cutaneous Calcification)

- Pathogenesis
  - Calcium and phosphorus deposits form in the skin
  - Insoluble compounds of calcium (hydroxyapatite crystals or amorphous calcium phosphate) are deposited within the skin
- Clinical features: 4 major types
  - Dystrophic: due to trauma, inflammatory processes, tumors, infections
  - Metastatic: abnormal calcium or phosphate metabolism
  - Iatrogenic: secondary to a treatment or procedure
  - Idiopathic: no causative factor identifiable
    - Ectopic calcification can occur in the setting of hypercalcemia and/or hyperphosphatemia (if calcium-phosphate product exceeds 70 mg^2/dL^2)
    - Multiple, firm, whitish dermal papules, plaques, nodules, or subcutaneous nodules
    - Laboratory studies: serum calcium, inorganic phosphate, alkaline phosphatase, and albumin
- Pathology: granules and deposits of calcium are seen in the dermis, with or without a surrounding foreign-body giant cell reaction
- Treatment: correct the underlying problem

Gout

- Epidemiology
  - More common in men
  - Patients with obesity, excessive alcohol intake, hypertension, diabetes, hyperlipidemia, chronic kidney disease, or the metabolic syndrome are at increased risk for developing gout
- Pathogenesis
  - Over 99% of cases associated with decreased renal excretion of uric acid

  - Rarely, overproduction of uric acid (*Lesch–Nyhan syndrome* with self-mutilation)
  - Secondary elevation in leukemia, polycythemia, hemolytic anemia, tumor chemotherapy; diuretics, chronic renal disease, and ketoacidosis (DM, fasting)
- Clinical features
  - Acute arthritis with exquisite pain, swelling; most often involves great toe (*podagra*) (60%), less often other digits (10%), feet (10%), or other joints. Renal stones a risk
  - Cutaneous findings include uric acid deposits (*tophi*) most often on ears or periarticular; in later case, differential diagnostic considerations include rheumatoid nodule
  - Four clinical stages include (1) asymptomatic hyperuricemia, (2) acute gouty arthritis, (3) intercritical gout (intervals between attacks, which progressively become shorter in duration), and (4) chronic tophaceous gout
- Pathology
  - Epidermis normal or ulcerated; large deposits of amorphous, basophilic material with parallel, needle-shaped clefts within the dermis and subcutis; lymphohistiocytic infiltrate, often with granulomatous foreign-body reaction
  - Fixation in 100% ethanol, crystals are birefringent; crystals dissolve if tissue fixed with formaldehyde; the fixation fluid can be tested for presence of urates
- Treatment: acute flares treated with NSAID or colchicine; prophylaxis with diet, probenecid, or allopurinol

Hemosiderin

- Pathogenesis
  - Intradermal deposits of iron (hemosiderin), chemical degradation
  - Associated with hemorrhage (purpura, hemochromatosis, stasis dermatitis)
- Clinical features
  - Clinical: brown, reddish-brown macules, patches
  - Skin pigmentation in hemochromatosis is caused by epidermal melanin, but hemosiderin is present as well
- Pathology: siderosis around foreign bodies (Perl's iron stain)
- Treatment: focuses on limiting the effects of the underlying disease leading to continued deposition. In hemochromatosis, this entails frequent phlebotomy*

PERFORATING DISORDERS

Kyrle Disease

- Epidemiology
  - Adult onset
  - Occurs in up to 10% of dialysis patients
  - Usually in association with diabetes mellitus and/or pruritus of renal failure
  - Rarely occurs with the pruritus of liver disease or internal malignancy
  - May represent end stage of perforating folliculitis
- Pathogenesis
  - Increased fibronectin levels are found in diabetics and patients with uremia
  - Fibronectin binds to type IV collagen and keratinocytes and may incite epithelial proliferation and perforation
- Clinical features: occurs most commonly on the legs
- Pathology
  - Plug of crusting or hyperkeratosis with variable parakeratosis
  - Transepidermal elimination of elastic fibers and collagen
- Treatment
  - Phototherapy
  - Intralesional steroids
  - Oral/topical retinoids

Perforating Folliculitis

- Epidemiology: more common in women
- Clinical features
  - Onset in young adulthood
  - Primarily affects the trunk and extremities
  - May be ordinary folliculitis with follicular rupture
- Pathology: necrotic material extruded
- Treatment
  - Intralesional corticosteroids
  - Oral/topical retinoids

Elastosis Perforans Serpiginosa (EPS)

- Epidemiology
  - Begins during childhood or early adulthood
  - Forty percent of cases occur in association with genetic disorders, including:
    - Down syndrome
    - Ehlers-Danlos syndrome
    - Osteogenesis imperfecta
    - Marfan syndrome
    - Pseudoxanthoma elasticum
    - Rothmund-Thompson syndrome
    - Cutis laxa
    - Acrogeria
  - Can be induced by penicillamine
- Clinical features
  - Keratotic 2 to 5 mm papules, arranged in a serpiginous pattern
  - Most commonly on the lateral neck, face, arms, and flexural areas
  - Minimal pruritus

__Phlebotomy__ may refer to: phlebotomy, the practice of collecting blood samples, usually by venipuncture.

- Pathology
  - Plug of hyperkeratosis +/− parakeratosis
  - Elastic fibers are seen within the plug or epidermis
  - If penicillamine induced, characteristic lumpy-bumpy elastic fibers with lateral buds seen in lesional and non-lesional skin
- Treatment
  - Inherited forms are often mild and don't require treatment
  - Local cryotherapy
  - Tangential excision
  - Electrosurgical destruction
  - Cellophane tape stripping

Reactive Perforating Collagenosis

- Epidemiology: very rare, more common in black women.
- Clinical features
  - Begins during childhood
  - After superficial trauma, patients develop keratotic papules over the following 3 to 4 weeks
  - Koebnerization can occur
  - Arms and hands most commonly involved
  - Tend to spontaneously resolve over 6 to 8 weeks
  - Rare familial variant: verrucous perforating collagenoma in which severe trauma triggers the formation of verrucous papules with transepidermal elimination of collagen
- Pathology
  - Plug of hyperkeratosis with or without parakeratosis
  - Collagen fibers seen in the epidermis and in the plug
  - Dermal connective tissue adjacent to the plug is normal
- Treatment: inherited form remains mild and rarely needs treatment

OTHER DISORDERS

Flegel Disease (Hyperkeratosis lenticularis perstans)

- Epidemiology: AD or sporadic
- Pathogenesis: lamellar granules (Odland bodies) are absent or altered on EM, which results in hyperkeratosis
- Clinical features
  - Numerous symmetric keratotic papules on the dorsal aspects of the feet and distal arms and legs, including the palms and soles
  - Attached scale, more prominent at periphery—removal may result in bleeding
  - Associated with endocrine disorders such as DM and hyperthyroidism
- Pathology: focal parakeratosis and hypogranulosis, lichenoid infiltrate in the papillary dermis
- Treatment
  - Topical 5-fluorouracil cream
  - PUVA with topical calcipotriol

Malignant Atrophic Papulosis (Degos Disease)

- Epidemiology: equal incidence in men and women; typically occurs between the second and fourth decades
- Clinical features
  - Vaso-occlusive disorder that affects the skin, gastrointestinal tract, and CNS
  - Skin lesions begin as crops of small 2 to 5 mm erythematous papules on the trunk or extremities that over 2 to 4 weeks evolve to have a central depression and porcelain white scar with a rim of telangiectasias
  - Skin findings usually precede systemic findings
- Pathology: wedge-shaped area of altered dermis with a sparse perivascular lymphocytic infiltrate and atrophic epidermis
- Treatment: no proven treatment—consider aspirin with or without pentoxifylline

Anetoderma (Fig. 8-16)

- Epidemiology: more frequently in women aged 15 to 25 years

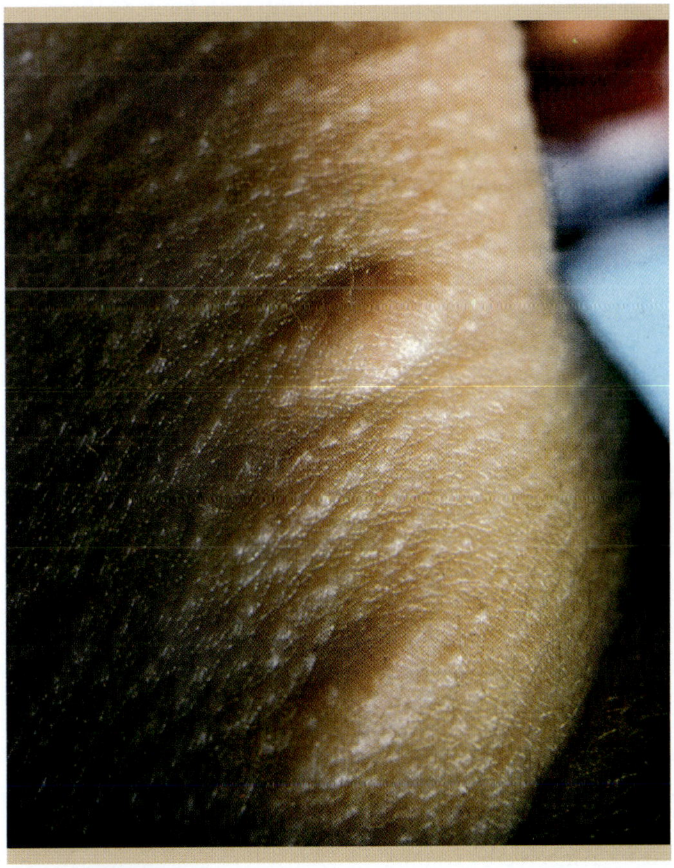

FIGURE 8-16 Anetoderma. (*Reprinted with permission from Freedberg IM et al.* Fitzpatrick's Dermatology in General Medicine, *6th Ed. New York: McGraw-Hill; 2003, p. 1028.*)

- Clinical features
  - Primary anetoderma occurs when there is no underlying disorder—there are 2 types:
    - Jadassohn-Pellizzari type—with preceding inflammatory lesions
    - Schweninger-Buzzi type—without preceding inflammatory lesions
  - Secondary anetoderma occurs in the same site as a pervious skin lesion or in associated with underlying disease (including HIV or antiphospholipid antibody syndrome)
  - Characteristic lesions are flaccid-circumscribed areas of slack skin that are a reflection of markedly reduced or absent dermal elastic fibers—can appear as depressions, wrinkling, or sac-like protrusions
  - "Buttonhole sign" present
  - Chest, back, neck, and upper extremities are sites of predilection
  - Described in premature infants and possibly related to the use of cutaneous monitoring leads or adhesives
- Pathology: focal, complete loss of elastic tissue in the papillary, and/or midreticular dermis
- Treatment: intralesional steroids, aspirin, dapsone, phenytoin, and surgical excision in patients with limited lesions

Idiopathic Atrophoderma of Pasini and Pierini (Scleroderma Atrophique d'emblée)

- Epidemiology
  - Women:men = 6:1
  - Starts insidiously during the second or third decade of life
- Pathogenesis: possible role for Borrelia burgdorferi (+ serology in 40–60%)
- Clinical features
  - Lesions appear on the trunk, especially the back and lumbosacral regions
  - Often symmetric and bilateral, but can appear along Blaschko lines
  - The borders or edges are sharply defined with "cliff-drop" borders
  - Perilesional skin is normal
  - The course is progressive
- Treatment
  - No treatment has been proven effective
  - PCN has been used with inconclusive results
  - Q-switched alexandrite laser for hyperpigmentation

Ainhum (Dactylolysis Spontanea, Bankokerend and Sukhapakla): Autoamputation of Digit

- Epidemiology
  - Triggered by trauma
  - Black men in Africa
  - Pathogenesis: fibrotic band develops from a flexural groove and progressively encircles the toe until spontaneous autoamputation occurs
  - Clinical features: most commonly the fifth toe
  - Pathology: fissuring and epidermal hyperkeratosis and parakeratosis, followed by a fibrotic reaction under the deepening fissure; as scar tissue contracts, it constricts and narrows neurovascular bundles
  - Treatment: no current treatment appears to halt the progression of ainhum
  - Surgical correction by Z-plasty has produced good results
  - Intralesional injection of corticosteroids

Pseudoainhum (Amniotic band syndrome)

- Epidemiology: may be acquired or congenital
- Pathogenesis
  - Due to a collagen band around the affected area
  - Occurs as a secondary event resulting from certain hereditary and nonhereditary diseases leading to annular constriction of digits
  - Can occur after premature rupture of the amniotic membrane
- Clinical features
  - Ring-like constriction bands, presenting as circumferential grooves of variable depth on the digits, extremities, neck, or trunk
  - Early in gestation can result in the body wall complex, characterized by body wall defects with evisceration of thoracic and/or abdominal organs, irregular anencephaly/encephaloceles, and bizarre facial clefting
  - Treatment: plastic surgery to release bands or intralesional injection of corticosteroids

Pseudoxanthoma Elasticum (PXE) (Gronbald-Strandberg syndrome) (Fig. 8-17)

- Epidemiology: AR; occurs in all races without geographic predilection and appears to have a slight female predilection
- Pathogenesis: inactivating mutations in the ABCC6 gene
- Clinical features
  - Affects the elastic fiber network of the skin, eyes, and cardiovascular system
  - Discrete, flat, yellowish papules in the flexural areas appear in the first or second decade of life
  - Lateral neck usually affected first—"plucked skin appearance"
  - Mucosal involvement most prominent on the inner aspect of the inner lip
  - Angioid streaks result from breaks in the calcified elastic lamina of Bruch membrane, which results in neovascularization, hemorrhage, and scarring and ultimately in progressive loss of visual acuity and rarely, legal blindness
  - Affects medium-sized arteries, predominantly of the extremities

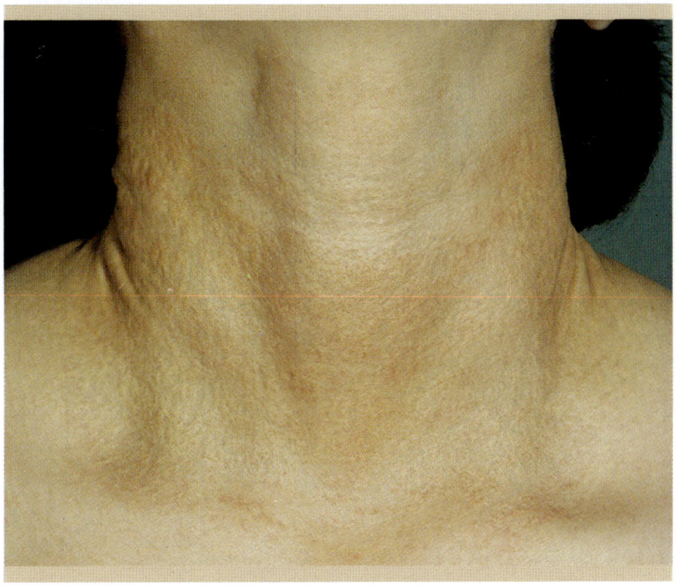

FIGURE 8-17 Pseudoxanthoma elasticum. (*Reprinted with permission from Goldsmith LA et al.* Fitzpatrick's Dermatology in General Medicine, *8th Ed. New York: McGraw-Hill; 2012, p. 1635.*)

  - Frequent sequelae include intermittent claudication, loss of peripheral pulses, renovascular hypertension, angina pectoris, and MI
  - Calcified blood vessels of the gastric and intestinal mucosa may increase the propensity for rupture and hemorrhage leading to GI bleeding
- Pathology: calcified elastic fibers in the mid and reticular dermis
- Treatment
  - Reconstructive surgery for skin sagging
  - Ophthalmology referral
  - Regular exercise, weight control, avoidance of smoking and excessive alcohol, and treatment of dyslipidemia and hypertension

Hypertrophic Osteoarthropathy (HOA)

Divided into primary (pachydermoperiostosis) and secondary (hypertrophic pulmonary osteoarthropathies) forms

- Epidemiology
  - Pachydermoperiostosis (PDP): autosomal dominant; accounts for 5% of all cases
  - Hypertrophic osteoarthropathy (pulmonary hypertrophic osteoarthropathy): associated with underlying cardiopulmonary diseases and malignancies
  - Digital clubbing and subperiosteal new bone formation
  - Associated with polyarthritis, cutis verticis gyrata, seborrhea, and hyperhidrosis
- Treatment: NSAIDs or corticosteroids may alleviate the polyarthritis associated with PDP

Dermatofibrosis Lenticularis Disseminata (Buschke-Ollendorf Syndrome)

- Epidemiology: AD
- Pathogenesis: due to loss of function mutation in LEMD3 gene
- Clinical features
  - Multiple skin-colored or slightly yellowish papules
  - Osteopoikilosis (stippled appearance to the bones) represents islands of increased bone density
  - Nasolacrimal duct obstruction, amblyopia, strabismus, benign lymphoid hyperplasia, hypopigmentation, and short stature
- Pathology: poorly demarcated area of increased dermal collagen bundles in a haphazard array

Pseudocyst of the Auricle

- Epidemiology: middle-aged men
- Clinical features
  - Usually arises in the scaphoid fossa
  - Usually unilateral
  - Present as a painless swelling and tend to arise over a course of a few weeks
- Pathology
  - Cavity within the auricular cartilage that contains clear fluid
  - Cartilage lining may show degenerative changes
- Treatment
  - Aspiration, with or without intralesional corticosteroids
  - I&D with destruction of the cavity

ULCERATION

Pressure Sores (Ulcers)

- Epidemiology: common in patients more than 70 years who are confined to hospital (fractured neck of femur)
- Pathogenesis
  - Prolonged immobility and recumbency (e.g., caused by paraplegia, arthritis, or senility)
  - Vascular disease (e.g., atherosclerosis)
  - Neurological disease causing diminished sensation (e.g., in paraplegia)
  - Malnutrition, severe systemic disease, and general debility
- Clinical features
  - Occur in immobilized patients
  - Due to chronic pressure in tissues overlying bony prominences
  - Lumbosacral region, greater trochanters, and heels are the most common areas
  - Tissue ischemia and neural damage lead to necrosis
  - Varying degrees
    - I: erythema
    - II: induration, blisters

    - III: shallow ulcers
    - IV: deep necrosis of fat and muscle
    - V: bone destruction
  - Underlying a small skin defect, there can be vast necrosis of deep tissues and proliferation of granulation tissue
- Pathology: epidermal necrosis, subepidermal bulla, vascular proliferations, often secondary inflammation
- Prevention: by turning recumbent patients regularly
- Treatment
  - Treatment of malnutrition and the general condition
  - Debridement
  - Regular cleansing with normal saline or 0.5% aqueous silver nitrate
  - Antibacterial, absorbent dressings and semipermeable dressings such as Opsite, if there is no infection
  - Appropriate systemic antibiotic if an infection is spreading
  - Plastic surgical reconstruction may be indicated in the young when the ulcer is clean

QUIZ

Questions

1. Granuloma faciale is associated with all the following *EXCEPT*:

   A. Middle-aged white men
   B. Idiopathic cutaneous disorder
   C. Systemic disease
   D. Eosinophilic granuloma
   E. A prominent grenz zone narrow band of papillary dermal sparing separates epidermis from the dermal infiltrate

2. Common manifestation of Sweet syndrome includes all *EXCEPT*:

   A. Fever
   B. Leukocytosis
   C. Arthralgia
   D. Arthritis
   E. Myalagias
   F. Pancreatitis

3. Which of the following major criteria for classic ulcerative pyoderma gangrenosum

   A. Rapid progression of a painful, necrolytic cutaneous ulcer with irregular violaceous and undermined border.
   B. History suggestive of pathergy.
   C. Histopathological findings of sterile dermal neutrophilia, mixed inflammation.
   D. Rapid response to systemic corticosteroids.

4. Granuloma Annulare synonyms include:

   A. Pseudorheumatoid nodule
   B. Subcutaneous granuloma annulare variant
   C. Generalized granuloma annulare
   D. Disseminated granuloma annulare
   E. All of the above

5. Calciphylaxis is common in following patients:

   A. End stage renal disease
   B. Chronic obstructive pulmonary disease
   C. Hypophosphatemia
   D. None of the above

6. Pseudoxanthoma elasticum is characterized by which of the following:

   A. Autosomal recessive disorder
   B. Mucosal involvement, inner aspect of the lip
   C. Affects medium-sized arteries
   D. All of the above
   E. None of above

7. Which of the following are inherited in an autosomal dominant manner?

   A. Sjögren-Larsson syndrome
   B. Erythrokeratodermia variabilis
   C. Ichthyosis vulgaris
   D. B and C only
   E. All of the above

8. In which of the following diseases can stippled epiphyses be identified on radiologic examination?

   A. CHILD syndrome
   B. Conradi-Hünermann syndrome
   C. Sjögren-Larsson syndrome
   D. A and B only
   E. All of the above

9. Diet modifications can improve the outcome of which of the following diseases?

   A. Refsum disease
   B. Netherton syndrome
   C. Neutral lipid storage disease with ichthyosis
   D. A and C only
   E. All of the above

10. Malignancy is associated with which of the following diseases:

    A. Erythema gyratum repens
    B. Howel-Evans syndrome
    C. Grover disease
    D. A only
    E. A and B only

Answers

1. C. Granuloma Faciale is not associated with systemic disease.
2. F. Sweet syndrome manifestation does not include pancreatitis. Other extracutaneous involvement include ocular, arthralgias, myalgias, arthritis, neutrophilic pulmonary alveolitis, and multifocal sterile osteomyelitis.
3. A. The 2 major criteria for pyoderma gangrenosum are rapid progression of a painful, necrolytic cutaneous ulcer with irregular violaceous and undermined border. Other causes of cutaneous ulceration have been excluded.
4. E. Granuloma annulare synonyms include pseudorheumatoid nodule, subcutaneous granuloma annulare variant, generalized granuloma annulare, and disseminated granuloma annulare.
5. Calciphylaxis occurs in chronic renal failure with type 2 diabetes and obesity.
6. Pseudoxanthoma elasticum has all the features mentioned.
7. D. Erythrokeratodermia variabilis and ichthyosis vulgaris are inherited in an autosomal dominant manner. Sjögren-Larsson syndrome is inherited in an autosomal recessive manner.
8. D. CHILD—ipsilateral skeletal abnormalities range from hypoplasia of digits or ribs to complete amelia; congenital or secondary scoliosis may also occur. Stippled epiphyses can be identified on radiologic examination in early infancy but tend to resolve during childhood. Conradi-Hünermann syndrome—skeletal anomalies are usually asymmetric. They include frontal bossing, malar hypoplasia, a flat nasal bridge, a short neck, rhizomelic shortening of the limbs, and scoliosis. Widespread premature calcifications manifesting as stippled epiphyses (chondrodysplasia punctata) typically involve the trachea and vertebrae and can be detected on radiographs during infancy. These are not apparent once bone maturation progresses.
9. E. Refsum disease—drastic reduction of dietary phytanic acid intake (< 5 mg daily; found mainly in dairy products and animal fats) can both prevent acute attacks and arrest neurologic progression, although retinal changes are usually irreversible. Netherton syndrome—Eosinophilia and allergic reactions to various foods and other antigens are common, with clinical manifestations ranging from an exacerbation of eczematous skin lesions to urticarial and angioedema to anaphylactic shock. Neutral lipid storage disease with ichthyosis—a fat-restricted diet (e.g., low in long-chain but enriched in medium-chain fatty acids) has been reported to be beneficial in a few patients.
10. E. Howel-Evans syndrome (type A) is associated with a higher risk of esophageal carcinoma. In at least 80% of patients, erythema gyratum repens is associated with an underlying neoplasm, most commonly of the lung, breast, esophagus, or stomach.

REFERENCES

Almond SL, Curley RK, Feldberg L: Pseudoainhum in chronic psoriasis. *Br J Dermatol* 2003;149(5)1064–1066.

Arpey CJ, Patel DS, Stone MS, Qiang-Shao J, Moore KC: Treatment of atrophoderma of Pasini and Pierini-associated hyperpigmentation with the Q-switched alexandrite laser: a clinical, histologic, and ultrastructural appraisal. *Lasers Surg Med* 2000;27(3)206–212.

Ganemo A, Virtanen M, Vahlquist A: Improved topical treatment of lamellar ichthyosis: a double-blind study of four different cream formulations. *Br J Dermatol* 1999;141:1027–1032.

Ghadially R, Williams ML, Hou SY, Elias PM: Membrane structural abnormalities in the stratum corneum of the autosomal recessive ichthyoses. *J Invest Dermatol* 1992;99:755–763.

Giro MG, Duvic M, Smith LT: Buschke-Ollendorff syndrome associated with elevated elastin production by affected skin fibroblasts in culture. *J Invest Dermatol* 1992;99(2)129–137.

Goldsmith LA et al. *Fitzpatrick's Dermatology in General Medicine*, 8th Ed. New York: McGraw-Hill; 2012.

Guldbakke KK, Khachemoune A: Calciphylaxis. *Int J Dermatol* 2007;46:231.

Hofmann B, Stege H, Ruzicka T, Lehmann P: Effect of topical tazarotene in the treatment of congenital ichthyoses. *Br J Dermatol* 1999;141:642–666.

Hoque SR, Ameen M, Holden CA: Acquired reactive perforating collagenosis: four patients with a giant variant treated with allopurinol. *Br J Dermatol* 2006;154(4)759–762.

Kim YJ, Chung BS, Choi KC: Calciphylaxis in a patient with end-stage renal disease. *J Dermatol* 2001;28(5)272–275.

Lebwohl M, Phelps RG, Yannuzzi L: Diagnosis of pseudoxanthoma elasticum by scar biopsy in patients without characteristic skin lesions. *N Engl J Med* 1987;317:347–350.

Marcoval J, Moreno A, Peyr J: Granuloma faciale: a clinicopathological study of 11 cases. *J Am Acad Dermatol* 2004;51(2)269–273.

McKee PH: *Pathology of the Skin: With Clinical Correlations*. London: Mosby-Wolfe; 1996.

Richard G: Molecular genetics of the ichthyoses. *Am J Med Genet* 2004;131C(1):32–44.

Richie RC: Sarcoidosis: a review. *J Insur Med* 2005;37(4)283–294. Review.

Sangueza OP, Pilcher B, Martin Sangueza J: Erythema elevatum diutinum: a clinicopathological study of eight cases. *Am J Dermatopathol* 1997;19(3):214–222.

CHAPTER 9

PIGMENTARY DISORDERS

KAVEH A. NEZAFATI
ROGER ROMERO
AMIT G. PANDYA

MELANOCYTES

- Epidermal melanocytes are dendritic cells derived from neural crest cells
- Their migration and differentiation is influenced by a number of signaling molecules: steel factor (stem cell factor, c-Kit ligand), Wnt, bone morphogenic proteins (BMPs), and hepatocytes growth factor
- Provide melanin for 36 neighboring basal and spinous layer keratinocytes = one epidermal melanin unit
- Number and distribution are the same in all skin types and ethnicities
- Concentration and distribution/retention of melanosomes in keratinocytes cause different skin colors
- Types of melanin:
  - *Pheomelanin*: red-yellow
  - *Eumelanin*: brown-black
- Melanosomes
  - Membrane-bound organelles, site of melanin synthesis and storage
  - Found in melanocytes; they move from melanocytes to keratinocytes
- Types of melanosomes:
  - *Eumelanosomes*: large, elliptical in shape and contain organized fibrillar glycoprotein matrix needed for eumelanin synthesis
  - *Pheomelanosomes*: smaller, spherical in shape, loose fibrillar glycoprotein matrix
  - Four stages of melanosome maturation:
    - *Stage I melanosomes (premelanosomes)*
      - ▲ Found in the cytoplasm of melanocytes
      - ▲ Amorphous matrix; contain unprocessed glycoprotein known as Pmel17 (gp100)
    - *Stage II melanosomes*
      - ▲ Found in the cytoplasm of melanocytes
      - ▲ Fully formed melanosome matrix, fibrils elongate and assemble into parallel sheets
      - ▲ Contain tyrosinase
      - ▲ No active melanin synthesis in eumelanosomes; melanin synthesis (not melanogenesis) in pheomelanosomes
    - *Stage III melanosomes*
      - ▲ Found in the cytoplasm or dendrites of melanocytes
      - ▲ Tyrosinase activity becomes positive and round or oval, electron dense, deposits of melanin found on the internal filament network
      - ▲ Melanization begins at this stage
    - *Stage IV melanosomes*
      - ▲ Found in the cytoplasm or dendrites of melanocytes
      - ▲ Round or oval, electron opaque
      - ▲ Fully melanized
      - ▲ Possess melanin, no enzymatic activity
- Tyrosinase
  - Cofactor: copper (Cu^{2+})
  - Catalyzes two reactions
    - Hydroxylation of tyrosine to DOPA (dihydroxyphenylalanine)—this is the rate limiting step
    - Oxidation of DOPA to DOPAquinone

PIGMENTED LESIONS

Melasma (Fig. 9-1)

- Melasma may be caused by the presence of more biologically active melanocytes in the affected skin rather than increase in melanocytes
- Predominantly affects Fitzpatrick skin types III and IV. Genetic and hormonal influences in combination with UV radiation

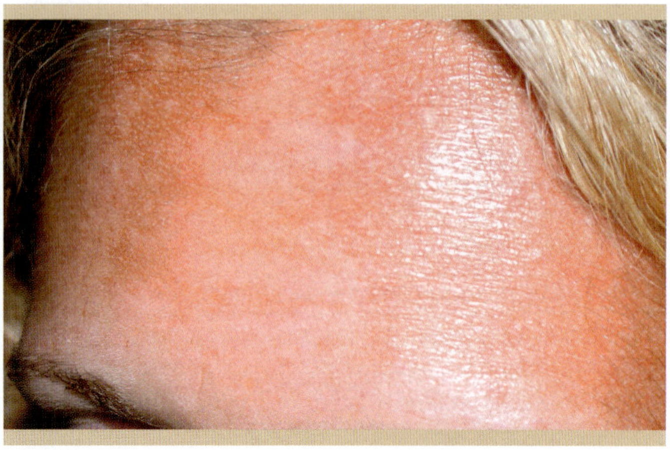

FIGURE 9-1 Melasma. (*Used with permission from Dr. Asra Ali.*)

- May be precipitated by the following: oral contraceptive pills, pregnancy, thyroid dysfunction, cosmetics, and phototoxic or photoallergic medication reaction
- Clinical findings
  - Brown reticulated hyperpigmented macules and patches, can be confluent or punctate
- Clinical subtypes
  - *Centrofacial*: forehead, cheeks, upper lip, nose, and chin
  - *Malar*: symmetrical involvement of the upper cheek area
  - *Mandibular*: ramus of the mandible
  - Depth may be epidermal, dermal, or mixed
- Diagnosis
  - Wood's light (wavelength, 340–400 nm): identifies depth of pigment; epidermal pigment enhanced, dermal pigment is not
- Treatment
  - Topical: broad spectrum sunscreen is cornerstone of therapy. Topical therapy with a triple combination agent appears to be the most clinically effective: hydroquinone, tretinoin, and topical steroid. Other commonly used, but less studied agents: azelaic acid, kojic acid, ascorbic acid, and arbutin
  - Chemical peels: glycolic acid may be the most efficacious α-hydroxy peeling agent. Should be used in combination with daily use of depigmenting agent
  - Device-based: carbon dioxide fractional ablative laser appears to be the most promising but more evidence is needed, especially in darker skin types

Becker Nevus (Fig. 9-2)

- Acquired lesion in adolescents, most commonly on scapular region
- Normal number of basal melanocytes, with increased melanin in the basal cell layer (epidermal melanotic hypermelanosis)

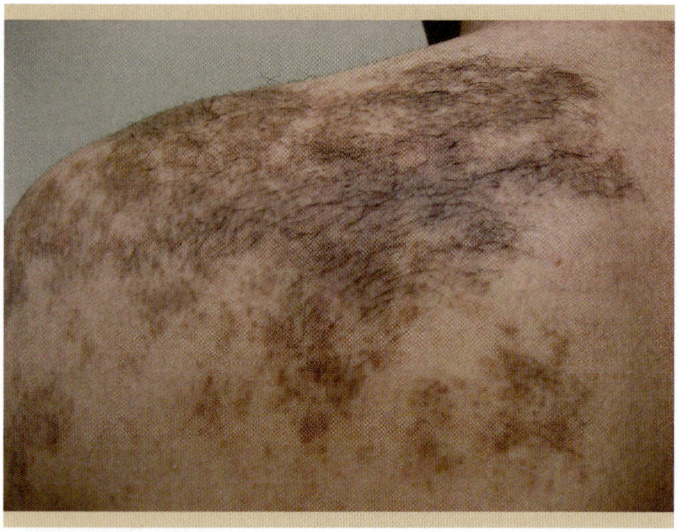

FIGURE 9-2 Becker nevus. (*Used with permission from Dr. Asra Ali.*)

- Androgen dependent—becomes more predominant in adolescence
- Clinical findings
  - Large, focal, brown, hair-bearing verrucous plaque
  - Back, shoulder, and submammary areas are common
  - No Blaschko linear pattern
  - Associated with underlying musculoskeletal abnormalities (smooth muscle hamartomas, muscular hypoplasia of the shoulder girdle) and cutaneous abnormalities (ipsilateral breast hypoplasia)
- Histology
  - Normal number of melanocytes with increased melanin pigment of basal layer, mature hair follicles with increased arrector pili muscles, thick bundles of smooth muscles
- Treatment
  - Surgical excision, laser hair removal

Congenital Nevomelanocytic Nevus (CNN) (Fig. 9-3)

- Presence of a pigmented lesion is noted at birth or soon thereafter
- Categorized by size:
  - Small (< 1.5 cm in diameter)
  - Medium (1.6–19.9 cm)
  - Large or giant (> 20 cm in adolescents and adults or comprising 5% of the body surface area or greater in infants, children, and preadolescents):
  - Lifetime risk of developing a melanoma for patients with a large CNN is 5%, approximately half occur during the first 5 years of life
- Related physical findings
  - *Leptomeningeal melanocytosis/neurocutaneous melanocytosis*: symptomatic and asymptomatic forms. Risk factors include giant pigmented nevi located

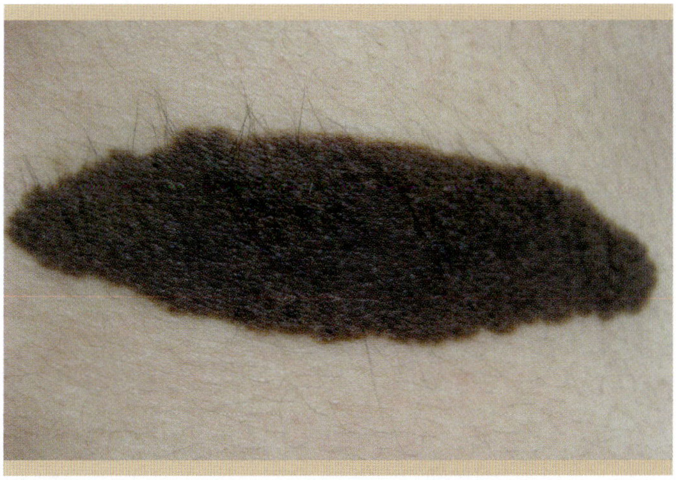

FIGURE 9-3 Congenital nevus. (*Used with permission from Dr. Asra Ali.*)

on the head, neck, or posterior midline and/or with multiple satellite lesions. May present with concurrent involvement of meninges (typically leptomeninges) and/or central nervous system (typically temporal lobes); can lead to a communicating hydrocephalus; symptoms: irritability, photophobia, papilledema, nerve palsies; diagnosis is made by contrast-enhanced MRI, most sensitive imaging method to document CNS metastases, progressive myelination after 6 months may obscure melanin signal

- Diagnosis of CNN
  - Histology: epidermal nevomelanocytes, dermal nevomelanocytes in sheets, nests, cords, and/or single cells around and within adnexal components
  - Dermoscopy: globular/cobblestone or reticular pattern
- Treatment
  - Clinical observation, lesional photography, surgical excision, and chemotherapy for metastatic disease

Spitz Nevus

- Benign, usually acquired proliferations of melanocytes
- 50% of cases occur in children younger than 10 years of age
- Usually located on the face and extremities they tend to spare the palms, soles, and mucus membranes
- B-RAF mutations are not noted; but H-RAS mutations have been identified in lesions
- Clinical findings
  - Typically solitary dome-shaped red/brown papule with a smooth surface/face; may occasionally present as widespread eruptive lesions or as grouped lesions (agminated)
  - Pigmented spindle cell nevus of Reed: variant of Spitz nevus, usually in adolescent girls; dark brown or black papule on the thigh
- Histology
  - Spitz nevus: predominantly compound, junctional and intradermal lesions may be seen; large and/or spindle-shaped melanocytes, usually in nests with artifactual clefts; periodic acid Schiff-positive and diastase resistant eosinophilic globules (Kamino bodies or colloid bodies), and dermal inflammatory cell infiltrate
  - Pigmented spindle cell nevus of Reed: melanocytes are spindle shaped, vertically oriented, can extend down eccrine ducts, and/or involve hair follicles
- Treatment
  - Excision (narrow to 5-mm margins, based on clinical factors and degree of atypia)

Blue Nevus (Fig. 9-4)

- Origin unknown
- Blue color due to Tyndall effect: preferential absorption of long wavelengths of light by melanin and the scattering of shorter wavelengths
- Clinical findings
  - Three main types of blue nevi:
    - *Common blue nevus*: blue-black papule, usually less than 10 mm in diameter, over 50% are found on the dorsal aspect of hands and feet, scalp, and buttocks
    - *Cellular blue nevus*: gray-blue solitary, larger than common blue nevus (usually 1–2 cm in diameter), usually firm smooth-surfaced papules; buttocks, the sacral region; melanoma developing in cellular blue nevi has been reported
    - *Combined*: blue nevus with a nevomelanocytic nevus; blue nevus may be either a common or cellular type with an associated overlying intradermal, compound, junctional, or Spitz nevus component
  - Malignant blue nevus (melanoma) may develop in relation to a cellular blue nevus; presents as a growing dermal nodule with or without ulceration
- Other physical findings
  - *Carney syndrome (complex)*: autosomal dominant (*PRKAR1A* gene), cardiac, cutaneous, and mucosal myxomas; lentigines, blue nevi, endocrine disorders, and testicular tumors
  - *LAMB syndrome*: lentigines, atrial myxomas, mucocutaneous myxomas, and blue nevi
  - *NAME syndrome*: nevi, atrial myxomas, myxoid tumors (myxoid neurofibromas), and ephelides
  - *Familial multiple blue nevi syndrome:* autosomal dominant, multiple lesions are present on the head and the neck, the trunk, the extremities, and the sclera, not associated with other cutaneous or systemic findings
- Histology
  - *Common:* dermal elongated, dendritic, variably pigmented melanocytes, Grenz zone usually separates the lesion from the epidermis

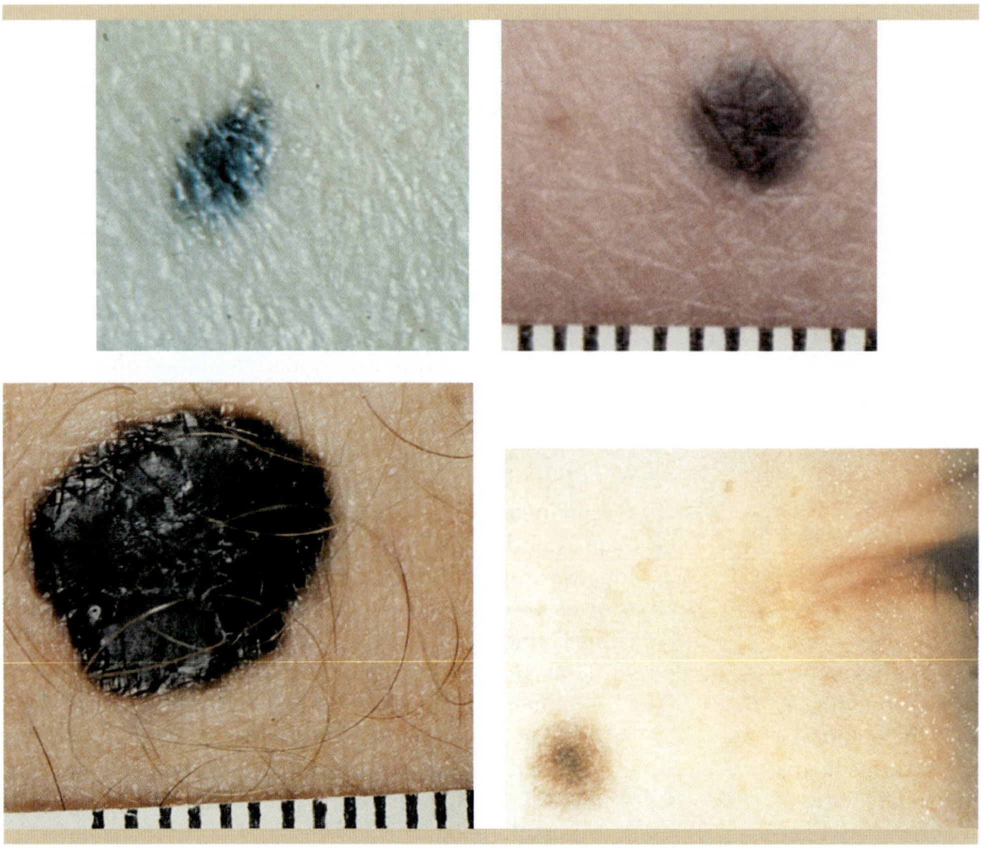

FIGURE 9-4 Blue nevus. *(Reproduced with permission from Wolff K et al: Fitzpatrick's Dermatology in General Medicine, 7th Ed. New York: McGraw-Hill, 2008.)*

- *Cellular:* two distinct cell types, dendritic melanocytes as in the common type, together with islands of plump, oval melanocytes with abundant cytoplasm, a round or oblong nucleus and central nucleolus, may extend into the subcutis with a diffuse or nested pattern
- *Combined:* macrophages with melanin, single dendritic melanocytes at the dermoepidermal junction with intraepidermal prolongations
- *Epithelioid blue nevus*: majority of large- to medium-sized pigmented cells that are globular and polygonal (epithelioid), and a minority of cells that are spindled and dendritic
- Treatment
  - Observation for stable lesions, excision, and histologic evaluation for changing lesions

Café-au-Lait Macules (Fig. 9-5)

- Discrete, evenly pigmented, pale brown macules, smooth or irregular margins
- Appear at or soon after birth and may enlarge in size
- Isolated lesions occur in up to 20% of the population
- Increased melanin in basal keratinocytes (epidermal melanotic hypermelanosis)
- Associated diseases
  - Neurofibromatosis type 1 (CALM are seen in 95% of patients), mutations in the *NF1* gene encoding neurofibromin protein
  - CALM are also seen in McCune-Albright syndrome, tuberous sclerosis, Fanconi anemia (mental retardation, aplastic anemia, and risk for malignancy), Silver-Russell syndrome; Legius, Cowden, Bloom, Watson, and Westerhof syndromes; multiple endocrine neoplasia type I and IIb; Banyan-Riley-Ruvalcaba and Maffucci syndromes

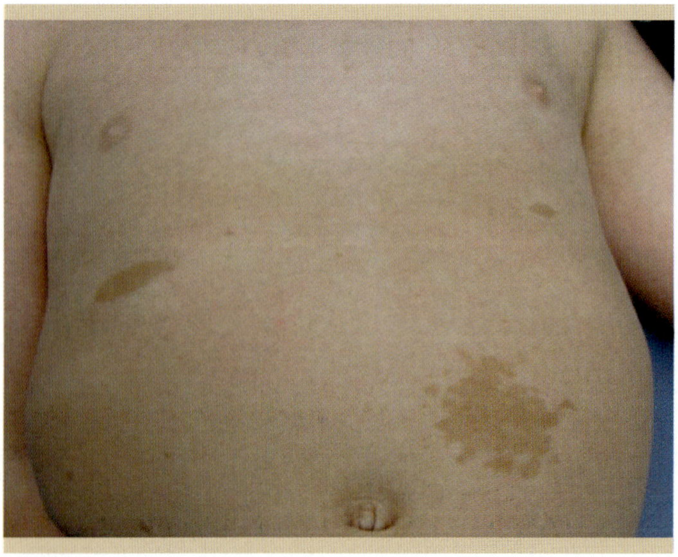

FIGURE 9-5 Café-au-lait macules. *(Used with permission from Dr. Jason Miller.)*

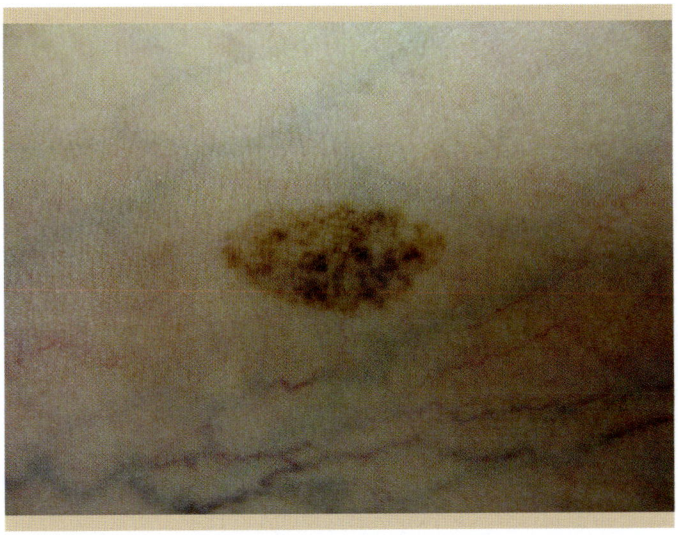

FIGURE 9-6 Nevus Spilus. (*Used with permission from Dr. Jason Miller.*)

- McCune-Albright syndrome (Albright syndrome): sporadic, *GNAS1* gene mutation (stimulates G protein, which increases cAMP), large café-au-lait macule with a jagged "coast of Maine" border, precocious puberty, polyostotic fibrous dysplasia (pseudocysts of long bones and base of skull), recurrent fractures, limb-length discrepancies, and endocrinopathies, normal life span
- Treatment of CALM: not necessary, although can consider Q-switched laser (Nd:YAG, ruby, and erbium:YAG laser) or intense pulsed light to lighten lesion, with variable response

Nevus Spilus (Fig. 9-6)

- Presents during late infancy or early childhood
- Clinical findings
  - Circumscribed, lightly pigmented patch with darkly pigmented, speckled nevomelanocytic macules or papules
- Histology
  - Increased number of melanocytes in the tan background; flat dark areas resemble a lentigo with increased melanocytic hyperplasia or melanocytic dysplasia, collection of nevus cells are seen in the dark papular areas (can have junctional nevus, epithelioid and/or spindle cell nevi, or blue nevi)
  - Risk of malignant transformation, clinical dermatoscopic monitoring is advised

Lentigo Simplex

- Acquired brown to dark variegated to uniformly colored macules
- Not induced by sun exposure and may occur anywhere on the skin
- Associated with the following syndromes
  - *Peutz-Jeghers syndrome* (see Chapter 32): autosomal dominant, oral pigmentation, and benign gastrointestinal polyps
  - *LEOPARD syndrome*: lentigines, electrocardiographic conduction defects, ocular hypertelorism, pulmonary stenosis, abnormal genitalia, retardation of growth, and deafness
  - *LAMB syndrome*: lentigines, atrial myxomas, mucocutaneous myxomas, and blue nevi
  - *Laugier-Hunziker syndrome*: oral pigmentation, nail hyperpigmentation, and absence of intestinal polyps or systemic abnormalities
- Histology
  - Mild acanthosis and basilar hyperpigmentation with melanocyte proliferation
- Treatment
  - Cryosurgery: melanocytes freeze at −4°C to −7°C, laser (Q-switched laser, intense pulsed light), tretinoin cream and hydroquinone, chemical peels

Cronkhite-Canada Syndrome

- Occurs sporadically
- Most patients are older than age 50 at the time of presentation
- Clinical findings
  - Patchy alopecia, circumscribed hypermelanosis with lentigo-like macules on extremities, and nail dystrophy
  - Sessile or semipedunculated polyps in the colon but also in the stomach and small intestine with malignant potential
- Histology
  - Increase in melanin within the basal layer without the melanocyte proliferation

Solar Lentigo

- Slowly increase in number and in size with increased ultraviolet light exposure
- Acquired lesions on sun-exposed skin, most commonly seen in Fitzpatrick skin types I–III
- Lesions are light brown; ink spot lentigo: black in color
- Histology
  - Elongated epidermal rete ridges with club-shaped extensions; increased number of epidermal melanocytes (no nesting)

Ephelides (Freckles)

- Occur on sun-exposed areas; common on central face and noted in early childhood
- Lesions appear in the summer months, may fade when sun exposure is decreased; may persist throughout life
- Light brown macules; color of the lesions tends to deepen after sun exposure
- Histology
  - Increased melanin deposition in the basal layer

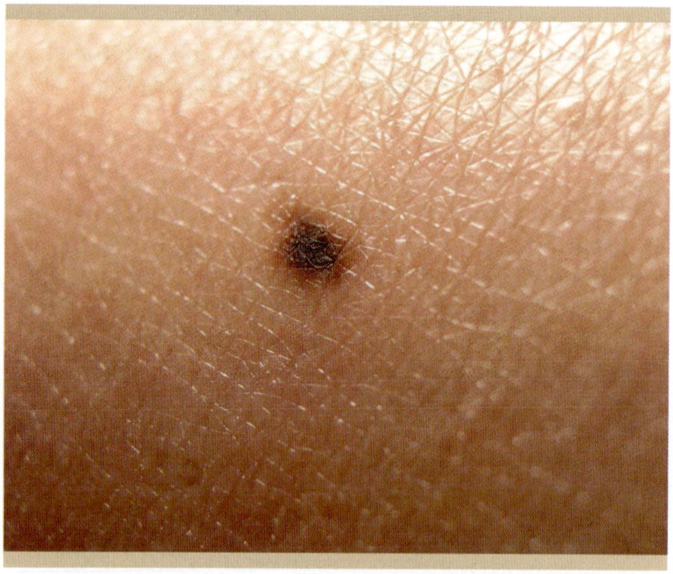

FIGURE 9-7 Junctional nevus. (*Used with permission from Dr. Asra Ali.*)

Nevocellular Nevus

- Benign neoplasms that are acquired after birth and composed of nests of melanocytes
- Stimulated by exposure to ultraviolet light, prevalence varies according to ethnicity—higher number of nevi in lighter skinned individuals
- Types of nevi
  - *Junctional nevi (Fig. 9-7)*: brown to brown/black macules, melanocytes are located at epidermal-dermal junction
  - *Compound nevi*: papules, tan to light brown, melanocytes in dermis and at epidermal-dermal junction
  - *Intradermal nevi*: papules display no melanin, melanocytes in dermis
  - *Halo nevi*: occurs when nevus is attacked by immune cells; overall prevalence rate of 0.9%; usually occurs before age of 20 years; pink or brown central nevomelanocytic nevus surrounded by a symmetric round or oval halo of depigmented skin; may present with single or multiple lesions; when associated with melanoma, the central lesions usually appears atypical
- Histology
  - *Junctional nevus*: nevomelancyte nucleus is pale staining and appears vacuolated; it is similar in size to epidermal melnanocytes, cells have pale staining cytoplasm and are arranged in nests; the cells are separated from the normal epidermis by a space caused by retraction artifact
  - *Intradermal nevus*: cells progressively decreased in size from the epidermis to reticular dermis; grenz zone (area free of nevomelanocytes) may be present
  - *Balloon cell nevus*: histologic diagnosis; foam cells are present among the nevomelanocytes
  - *Recurrent melanocytic nevus* (pseudomelanoma): due to incomplete removal of a benign nevomelanocytic nevus; melanocytic hyperplasia, lentiginous pattern, atypia may be present. Presence of dermal scar
  - *Halo nevus*: central nevomelanocytes, dermal lyphocytic (mainly T cell) infiltrate and depigmented zone devoid of epidermal melnaocytes

Dysplastic or Atypical Nevi

- No consensus on terminology
- Originally known as Clark's nevi: overlapping features with common nevi and melanoma, two of three characteristics (1) variable pigmentation, (2) irregular and asymmetric outline, and (3) having indistinct borders
- Histology
  - Major criteria: (1) basilar proliferation of atypical melanocytes which must extend at least three rete ridges or "pegs" beyond the dermal component and (2) organization of this proliferation in a lentiginous or epithelioid-cell pattern
  - Minor criteria: (1) the presence of lamellar fibrosis or concentric eosinophilic fibrosis, (2) neovascularization, (3) an inflammatory response, and (4) the fusion of rete ridges
- Proportion of cutaneous melanomas that originate from dysplastic nevi relative to those that arise from apparently normal skin and from other melanocytic nevi is not known
- Harbor mutations in BRAF comparable to common nevi, exhibit alterations in p16 or p53 expression, but Ras mutations are rare

Familial Atypical Multiple Mole and Melanoma (FAMMM) Syndrome

- Also known as the dysplastic nevus syndrome; autosomal dominant; germline mutations in the CDKN2A tumor-suppressor gene, including p16 (INK4alpha) and p14 (ARF); increased risk for developing melanoma and other malignant neoplasms (ie, pancreatic cancer)
- Presence of the following features: (1) occurrence of malignant melanoma in one or more first- or second-degree relatives, (2) presence of numerous (often > 50) melanocytic nevi, some of which are clinically atypical, (3) many of the associated nevi show certain histologic features and have an elevated lifetime risk for the development of melanoma
- Histology
  - Single melanocytes, elongation of rete ridges, with cytologic atypia of melanocytes and enlarged, hyperchromatic nuclei
  - Bridging: melanocytes aggregate into variably sized nests, which fuse with adjacent rete ridges
  - Dermal fibroplasia: lamellar and concentric, lymphocytic infiltrate
  - Shouldering: junctional component extends beyond the last dermal nest

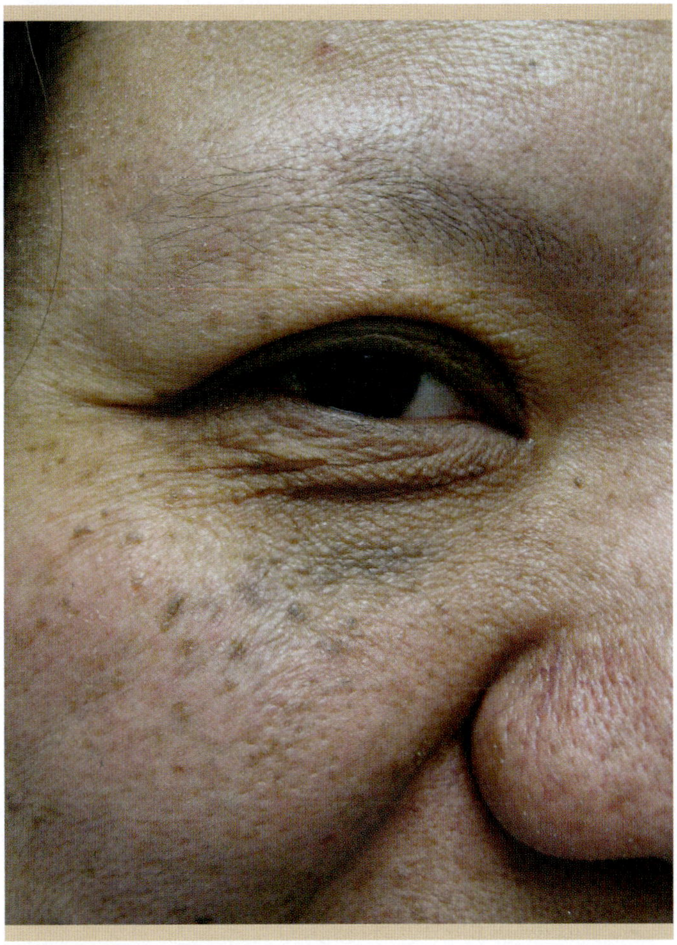

FIGURE 9-8 Nevus of Ota. (*Used with permission from Dr. Jason Miller.*)

Nevus of Ota (Nevus Fuscocaeruleus Ophthalmomaxillaris) (Fig. 9-8)

- Melanocytes that have not migrated completely from the neural crest to the epidermis during the embryonic stage
- Asian population most commonly affected, usually congenital
- Malignant melanoma has been reported to develop in a nevus of Ota
- Clinical findings
  - Blue to gray speckled macules or patches
  - Unilateral (90%). Can be bilateral. (Hori nevus: acquired bilateral blue/gray macules, no mucosal involvement)
  - Forehead, temple, malar area, or periorbital skin (Branches of V1 and V2); mucosal involvement is possible and may involve the sclera, conjunctiva (oculodermal melanocytosis) and tympanic membrane; increased risk of glaucoma (10%)
- Histology
  - Dendritic melanocytes are present and surrounded by fibrous sheaths; dermal melanophages, 5 types based on the locations of the dermal melanocytes, which are (1) superficial, (2) superficial dominant, (3) diffuse, (4) deep dominant, and (5) deep
- Treatment
  - Q-switched: alexandrite, Nd:YAG, and ruby lasers
- Prognosis
  - If untreated, lesions remain for life

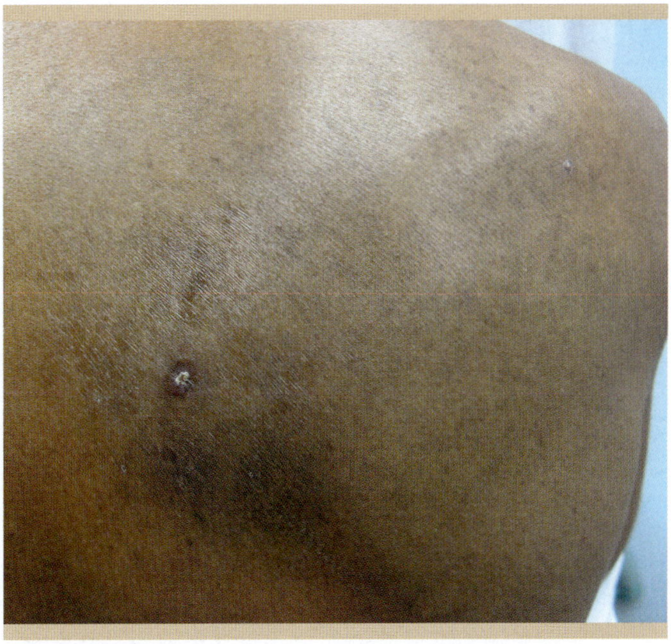

FIGURE 9-9 Nevus of Ito. (*Used with permission from Dr. Jason Miller.*)

Nevus of Ito (Nevus Fuscocaeruleus Acromiodeltoideus) (Fig. 9-9)

- Congenital, blue to gray speckled macules or patches, lesions are present over the shoulder girdle region
- May appear simultaneously with nevus of Ota
- Histology, treatment, and prognosis is similar to nevus of Ota

Congenital Dermal Melanosis (CDM) [Mongolian Spot]

- Common in Asian, African, and Hispanic persons. Rarely seen in Whites
- Entrapment of melanocytes in the dermis during their migration from the neural crest into the epidermis
- Clinical findings: blue-gray macules (due to Tyndall effect), most commonly seen on lumbosacral skin, buttocks; other areas include thorax, abdomen, arms, legs, and shoulders
- Histology
  - Dermal spindle-shaped melanocytes with fully melanized melanosomes; usually oriented parallel to the epidermis

- Prognosis
  - Regression during childhood is the typical course, but they can persist

Dowling-Degos Disease (DDD/Reticulate Pigmented Anomaly of the Flexures)

- Autosomal dominant, mutation of the keratin 5 gene on chromosome 12q
- Clinical findings
  - Reticular, macular hyperpigmentation
  - Affects axillae, groin, and other flexural areas
  - Comedo-like lesions and pitted acneiform scars near angle of mouth, neck, and back
  - *Galli-Galli disease (GGD):* acantholytic variant of Dowling-Degos disease, clinically indistinguishable from DDD. Some GGD cases described also with KRT5 mutations.
- Histology
  - Acanthosis, irregular elongation of thin branching rete ridges with a concentration of melanin at the tips, no increase in melanocytes, but increase in melanosomes
- Treatment
  - Topical Steroids, Tacrolimus, Tretinoin, or Erbium YAG laser
- Prognosis
  - Slowly progressive but not life threatening

Other Reticulated Hyperpigmentation Disorders

Confluent and Reticulated Papillomatosis of Gougerot and Carteauad (CRP)

- Grayish blue plaques with peripheral reticulated pattern may be a chronic condition
- Favors neck and upper trunk
- Treatment: antimycotic agents, tretinoin, and antimicrobial agents (i.e., minocycline and erythromycin)

Erythema Ab Igne

- Net like pigment pattern due to chronic exposure to heat (heating pads, laptops, and furniture with built in heaters)
  - Treatment: removing causative exposure, ND:YAG, and alexandrite lasers

Dyskeratosis Congenita

- Usually XLR but sometimes autosomal dominant or recessive
- DKC1 (dyskerin)—telomerase defect
- Reticulate hyperpigmentation, nail dystrophy, premalignant leukoplakia, and epiphora (continuous lacrimation)

Naegeli-Franceschetti-Jadassohn Syndrome

- Autosomal dominant—keratin 14
- Reticulate hyperpigmentation starts at age 2 and fades over time
- Hypohidrosis, heat intolerance, dental abnormalities, PPK, and absence of dermatoglyphics

Dermatopathia Pigmentosa Reticularis

- Autosomal dominant—keratin 14
- Persistent truncal reticulated pigment; nonscarring alopecia; onychodystrophy; absent dermatoglyphics with punctuate keratoderma in some

Reticulate Acropigmentation of Kitamura

- Autosomal dominant
- Atrophic, reticulate hyperpigmentation (without hypopigmentation) pigment over dorsal hands and feet, which spreads to remainder of body; sometimes palmar pits

HYPOPIGMENTED LESIONS (TABLE 9-1)

Nevus Depigmentosus

- Occurs sporadically, congenital condition
- Normal melanocyte count, decreased number of melanosomes in keratinocytes, reduced dopa activity, underdeveloped dendrites, and defect in melanosome transfer (melanin remains in melanocytes instead of transferring to keratinocytes)
- Clinical findings
  - Nonprogressive, unilateral, well circumscribed irregular, oval, or round hypopigmented macular lesion
- Diagnosis
  - *Wood's lamp*: off-white accentuation without fluorescence
  - *Dermoscopy*: reticulate pigmented spots

Nevus Anemicus (Fig. 9-10)

- Appears at birth in early childhood
- Defect at motor end plate of smooth muscle effector cells of blood vessels

TABLE 9-1 Hypopigmented Diseases and Defects

Disease	Defect
Albinism	Decreased melanin synthesis
Nevus depigmentosus	Melanosome transfer
Menkes kinky hair	Decreased tyrosinase activity
Cross syndrome	Decreased number of melanocytes
Tuberous sclerosis	Decreased number of melanocytes, decreased melanin synthesis, and decreased melanosome size
Vogt-Koyanagi-Harada	Decreased melanocytes

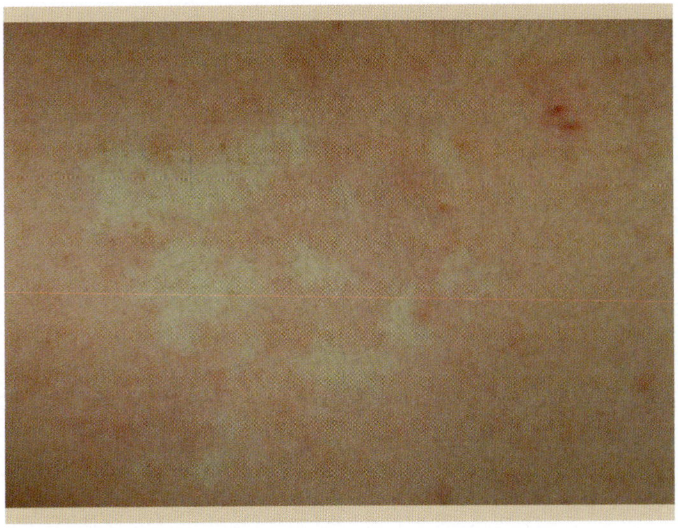

FIGURE 9-10 Nevus anemicus. (*Used with permission from Dr. Asra Ali.*)

- Focal area of blood vessel that have increased sensitivity to catecholamines; vessels are persistently vasoconstricted resulting in an area of cutaneous blanching
- Clinical findings
  - Well-defined, hypopigmented, irregularly shaped, confluent macules forming a patch, most common on trunk; stroking the adjacent skin causes it to become erythematous, while the lesion remains pale in color
- Diagnosis:
  - *Diascopy*: obliterates border due to pressure blanching the surrounding skin
  - *Wood's lamp*: no accentuation
  - *Histology*: normal epidermis, dermis, no changes in vasculature

Pityriasis Alba (Fig. 9-11)

- Melanocytes decreased in number with fewer and small melanosomes
- Commonly affects children
- Characterized as a mild form of atopic dermatitis
- Clinical findings:
  - Pale pink/light brown macules with indistinct margins, powdery scale: more apparent on darker skinned patients
- Treatment:
  - Topical steroids, emollients

Ash-Leaf Macules (See Chapter 32)

- Initial expression of tuberous sclerosis (seen in 90% of patients with TSC)
- Normal or decreased number of melanocytes with underdeveloped dendrites, and small, poorly melanized melanosomes

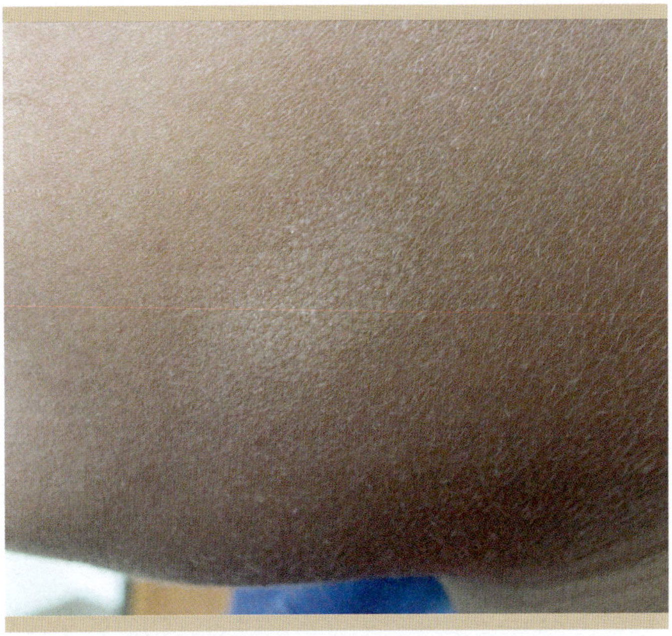

FIGURE 9-11 Pityriasis alba. (*Used with permission from Dr. Asra Ali.*)

- Clinical findings:
  - Oval hypopigmented macules, posterior trunk, upper and lower extremities
- Histology
  - Normal number of melanocytes. Melanosomes are decreased in numbers, size, and melanization

Idiopathic Guttate Hypomelanosis (Fig. 9-12)

- Common, acquired, and discrete hypomelanosis
- Usually on extremities of sun-exposed skin

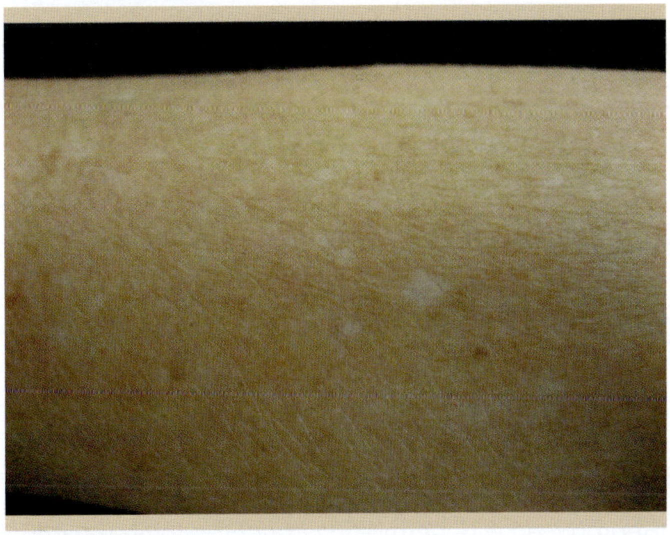

FIGURE 9-12 Idiopathic guttate hypomelanosis. (*Used with permission from Dr. Asra Ali.*)

- Incidence increases with age
- Clinical findings
  - Discrete, well-circumscribed, porcelain white round macules
- Histology
  - Flattening of the dermal-epidermal junction, moderate to marked reduction of melanin granules and melanocytes in the basal layer, epidermal atrophy, and hyperkeratosis
- Treatment
  - Cryotherapy, superficial abrasion, topical retinoids, and narrow-band UVB

Futcher Lines (Voigt Lines) (Fig. 9-13)

- Pigmentary demarcation lines
- Abrupt transitions from deeply pigmented skin to lighter-pigmented skin

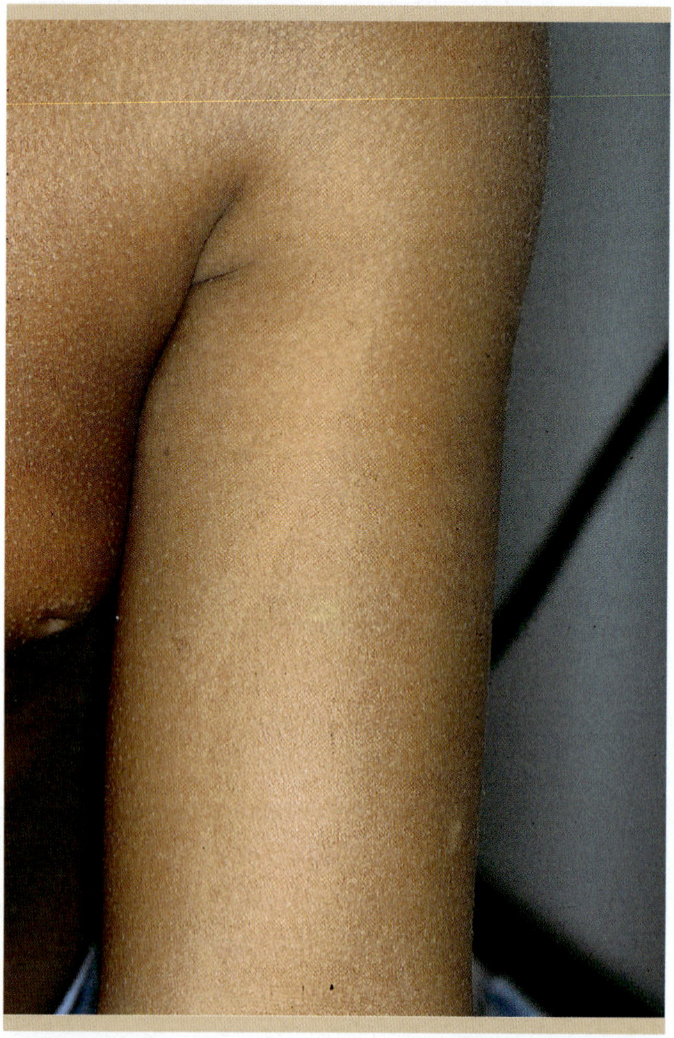

FIGURE 9-13 Futcher lines (Voigt lines). *(Reproduced with permission from Freedberg IM et al: Fitzpatrick's Dermatology in General Medicine, 6th Ed. New York: McGraw-Hill; 2003.)*

- Often present at birth tend to darken with time
- More common in black population and becomes visible during the first 6 months of life, or may be apparent at birth becoming more noticeable with age or during pregnancy
- Classification:
  - Based on location of lines of demarcation
    a. Lateral aspects of upper anterior portion of the arms across pectoral area
    b. Posteromedial portion of the lower limbs
    c. Vertical hypopigmented line in the presternal and parasternal areas
    d. Posteromedial area of the spine
    e. Bilateral aspect of the chest, marking from the mid-third of the clavicle to the periareolar skin

HYPOMELANOSIS SYNDROMES

Vogt-Koyanagi-Harada (VKH) Syndrome (Uveomeningitic Syndrome)

- T-cell mediated autoimmune disorder; the autoimmune response might be triggered by an infectious agent in a genetically susceptible individual
- Clinical findings
  - Progression occurs in the following phases:
    - *Prodrome*: fever, malaise, headache, nausea, and vomiting
    - *Meningocephalic*: meningeal symptoms with headache, meningismus, seizures, muscle weakness, or paralysis
    - *Ophthalmic and auditory stage*: posterior uveitis, photophobia, altered visual acuity, eye pain, retinal detachment, cataracts, glaucoma, dysacusis, deafness, and tinnitus (50%)
    - *Poliosis stage* (90%): symmetric vitiligo, white eyelashes and brows, alopecia
- Laboratory studies:
  - Cerebrospinal fluid: pleocytosis
- Treatment
  - High dose corticosteroids, cyclosporine, cyclophosphamide, chlorambucil, and azathioprine

Oculocutaneous Albinism (OCA)

- Autosomal recessive disorders by either a complete lack or a reduction of melanin biosynthesis in melanocytes; resulting in hypopigmentation of the hair, skin, and eyes
- The various types of OCA are caused by mutations in different genes (Table 9-2)

Oculocutaneous Albinism IA (OCA1)

- Autosomal recessive
- Mutated tyrosinase (*TYR*) gene, chromosome 11q
- Complete loss of tyrosinase function; no pigmented lesions develop on patient's skin

TABLE 9-2 Types of Oculocutaneous Albinism (OCA)

Gene	Gene product	Disease name
TYR	Tyrosinase (TYR)	OCA1, OCA1A, OCA1B *(Yellow alb.)*
OCA2	OCA2/P	OCA2 *(Brown OCA in Africans)*
TYRP1	Tyrosinase-related protein 1 (*TYRP1/TRP-1*)	OCA3 (*Rufous OCA)*
SLC45A2	Membrane-associated transporter protein/ Solute carrier family 45 member 2 (MATP/SLC45A2)	OCA4

- Melanosomes are normal
- Clinical findings
  - Complete absence of melanin in skin, hair, and eyes; "Albino" phenotype; white hair and skin, pink irides that turn blue-gray over time, decreased visual acuity, photophobia

Oculocutaneous Albinism IB

- Mutated tyrosinase (*TYR*) gene, with some tyrosinase function
- Clinical findings
  - Develop varying pigment with age, hair with pheomelanin (spherical yellow melanosomes) resulting in light yellow to brown hair color, irides can turn light tan or brown, pigmented lesions can develop (nevi, freckles, and lentigines)
  - *Temperature sensitive variant*: melanin synthesis in cooler areas of the body (i.e., extremities), but not warmer areas (> 35°C)

Oculocutaneous Albinism II (OCA2)

- Autosomal recessive, tyrosinase positive
- "Brown" OCA
- Mutation in the OCA2 gene (previously P gene) (OCA2 protein is needed for melanosomes biogenesis and as a membrane transport protein); chromosome 15
- Most common OCA worldwide
- Clinical findings
  - Hair pigment present at birth (different from OCA I), yellow to blond at birth owing to pheomelanin, irides blue-gray, skin is creamy white at birth, does not tan, and does not develop further pigment, pigmented nevi may develop
  - Brown OCA type (variant of OCA2): seen in African/African-American populations; skin and hair are lighter brown, irides gray to tan at birth; over time, hair and irides may darken, but skin remains the same
- Syndromes associated with OCA2 gene mutations: Prader-Willi and Angelman Syndrome. These syndromes involve deletion of the region of long arm of chromosome 15 (15q), which contains a portion of the OCA2/P Gene
  - *Prader-Willi syndrome*
    - Deletion of long arm of paternal chromosome 15 (imprinting)
    - Developmental syndrome
      - ▲ Clinical findings
        - △ Neonatal hypotonia, hyperphagia and obesity, hypogonadism, small hands and feet, mental retardation, skin hypopigmented, and no ocular albinism
  - *Angelman*
    - Deletion in OCA2 gene on maternal chromosome 15 (imprinting)
      - ▲ Clinical findings:
        - △ Light skin and hair, iris translucency, reduced retinal pigment, severe mental retardation, ataxic movements, and inappropriate laughter

Oculocutaneous Albinism III (OCA3)

- Autosomal recessive
- Mutation in tyrosinase-related protein 1 (*TYRP1*) on chromosome 9
- Acts as a dihydroxyindole-2 carboxylic acid (CDHICA); oxidase needed in the eumelanin pathway
- Common in South Africa, can present as rufous/red OCA or brown OCA
- Clinical findings
  - Red to brownish skin, red hair, and hazel to brown eyes

Oculocutaneous Albinism IV (OCA4)

- Defect in membrane-associated transporter protein/solute carrier family 45 member 2 (MATP/SLC45A2) on chromosome 5
- Clinical
  - Similar to OCA II

Hermansky-Pudlak Syndrome (HPS)

- Autosomal recessive; etiology has been related to defects in 9 genes: *HPS1, HPS2* (*AP3B1*), *HPS3, HPS4, HPS5, HPS6, HPS7* (DTNBP1), HPS8 (BLOC1S3), and HPS9 (PLDN)
- *HPS-1* and *HPS-4* patients get pulmonary fibrosis and granulomatous colitis
- Lysosomal membrane defect with abnormal formation of intracellular vesicles; results in accumulation of ceroid lipofuscin in macrophages in lung and gastrointestinal tract

- Characterized by oculocutaneous albinism and prolonged bleeding due, respectively, to the malformation of melanosomes and platelet-dense granules
- Tyrosinase positive
- Clinical findings
    - *Skin*: pigment dilution; skin color varies from white to light brown, pigmented nevi, and ecchymosis
    - *Hair*: cream to red/brown
    - *Eyes*: lack of retinal pigment, decreased pigment of irides, photophobia, nystagmus, decreased visual acuity, and strabismus
    - *Hematologic*: epistaxis, gingival bleeding, and prolonged bleeding
    - *Lymphohistiocytic*: ceroid (chromolipid) deposition in macrophages
    - *Lung*: pulmonary fibrosis
    - *Gastrointestinal*: granulomatous colitis (15% of patients)
    - *Cardiac*: cardiomyopathy
- Diagnosis
    - Prothrombin time/partial thromboplastin time (PT/PTT)
    - Platelet count
    - Pulmonary function test, chest x-ray, and colonoscopy if symptomatic
- Treatment
    - Avoid aspirin and other blood thinners, DDAVP, platelet and red blood cell transfusions as clinically necessary; granulomatous colitis: steroids, TNF-α inhibitors

Chediak-Higashi Syndrome

- Autosomal recessive
- Lysosomal transport protein (LYST/CHS1) gene defect, vesicular trafficking defect
- Incomplete oculocutaneous albinism
- Decreased chemotaxis of neutrophils, decreased antibody-dependent cellular cytotoxicity, presence of giant peroxidase-positive lysosomal granules in peripheral blood granulocytes; results in severe infections
- Clinical findings
    - Childhood CHS: accelerated phase: early onset with fever, anemia, and neutropenia
    - Adolescent CHS: severe infections in early childhood, no accelerated phase
    - Adult CHS: mild form, develop progressive and fatal neurologic dysfunction in middle age
    - *Eyes*: ocular hypopigmentation causes photophobia, nystagmus, and strabismus
    - *Hair*: silvery sheen
    - *Skin*: pale, deep ulcerations, petechiae, bruising, and gingival bleeding
    - *Neurologic*: weakness, ataxia, sensory deficits, and progressive neurodegeneration
    - *Lymphoma*: "accelerated phase" precipitated by viruses (e.g., Epstein-Barr virus); widespread infiltration of viscera
    - *Other*: hepatosplenomegaly, lymphadenopathy, pancytopenia, pseudomembrane, and sloughing of the buccal mucosa
- Laboratory findings
    - Giant intracellular granules in circulating neutrophils, melanocytes, neurons, and renal tubular cells
    - Granules form secondary to delayed disorder of lysosomal enzymes from cells
- Treatment
    - Bone marrow (or stem cell) transplant, acyclovir, interleukin, gamma globulin, vincristine, prednisone, and prophylactic antibiotics
- Course
    - Death at about 6 year old secondary to infection, lymphoma-like accelerated phase

Griscelli Syndrome

- Autosomal recessive; etiology has been related to defects in 3 genes: GS1 (MYO5A), GS2 (RAB27A), and GS3 (MLPH)
- Affects melanosome transport, not maturation
- Clinical findings
    - Mild skin hypopigmentation, silvery-gray hair, immunological impairment (lymphohistiocytosis), defects in the central nervous system (common in GS1, not GS2)
- Laboratory findings
    - Uneven pigment clumping in hair shaft

Alezzandrini Syndrome

- Etiology unknown, possibly due to an autoimmune process destroying melanocytes
- Clinical findings
    - Facial vitiligo, poliosis, hyperacusis, unilateral tapetoretinal (retinal pigmented epithelia) degeneration

Vitiligo (Fig. 9-14)

- Multifactorial etiology, related to both genetic and nongenetic factors, of melanocyte destruction:
    - Autoimmune hypothesis: due to defects in humoral and cellular immunity
    - Neural theory: elevated levels of some neurotransmitters and catecholamine degrading enzymes injure melanocytes
    - Oxidant stress: accumulation of free radicals is cytotoxic to melanocytes and inhibit tyrosinase
    - Autocytotoxic theory: cytotoxic precursors to melanin synthesis accumulate in melanocytes, causing cell death
- Associated with autoimmune conditions: thyroid disease (Hashimoto thyroiditis, Graves disease), diabetes mellitus, pernicious anemia, systemic lupus erythematosus, alopecia areata, Addison disease, psoriasis and multiple endocrinopathy syndrome
- Clinical findings
    - Progressive, depigmented, sharply circumscribed macules or patches

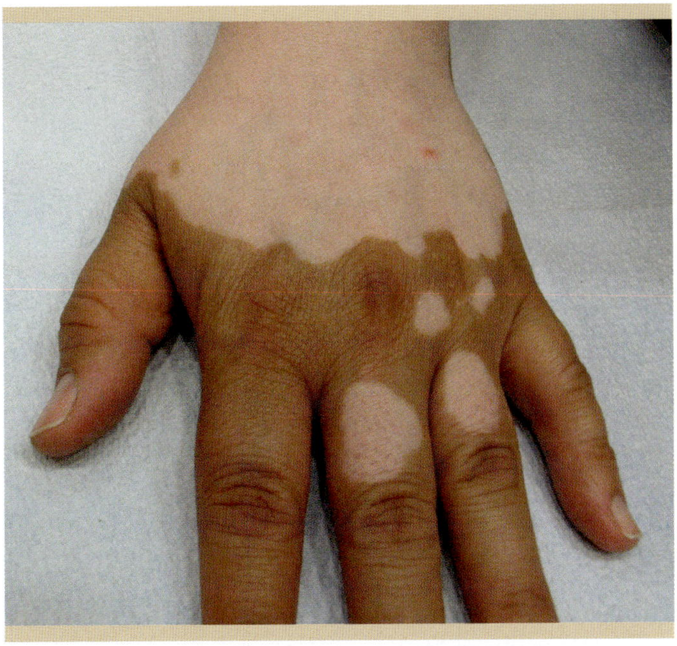

FIGURE 9-14 Vitiligo. (*Used with permission from Dr. Asra Ali.*)

- Poliosis = leukotrichia = whiteness of hair
- Canities = premature graying of hair (37% of patients)

- Clinical classification
  - *Localized*: focal (one area of the body affected), unilateral (localized in a unilateral body region, with a dermatomeric distribution), mucosal (mucous membranes are solely affected)
  - *Generalized*: acrofacial (distal fingers and periorificial affected), vulgaris (widely distributed scattered patches), mixed: acrofacial and vulgaris or segmental and acrofacial and/or vulgaris
  - *Universal*: complete or nearly complete depigmentation
  - Mixed: segmental followed by the development of generalized lesions
- Diagnosis
  - *Wood's lamp*: bright white or blue white
  - *Histology*: absence of melanocyte and melanin in the affected area; occasional lymphocytic infiltrate along advancing margins in early lesions
- Treatment
  - Narrow-band ultraviolet B, topical steroids, oral or topical psoralen plus UV-A (PUVA), topical calcineurin inhibitors, surgery: punch grafts, minigrafts, suction blister grafts, and melanocyte/keratinocyte suspension grafts

Piebaldism

- Autosomal dominant
- *C-KIT* mutation on chromosome 4, protooncogene, tyrosine kinase transmembrane cellular receptor for mast/stem cell growth factor
- Present at birth, does not progress
- Clinical findings
  - *Cutaneous*: depigmented patches midforehead, extremities; pigmented islands present
  - *Hair*: white forelock (80–90% of patients)
  - *Neurologic*: mental retardation, cerebellar ataxia, and deafness (combination is called Woolf syndrome)

Waardenburg Syndrome

- Autosomal dominant
- Defect in neural crest migration, absent melanocytes
- Four subtypes (I to IV)
  - Type I: autosomal dominant, *PAX3* (paired box) gene; transcription factor
  - Type II: autosomal dominant, *MITF* (microphthalmia-associated transcription factor) gene, chromosome 3; SLUG gene
  - Type III (Klein-Waardenburg syndrome): autosomal dominant, *PAX3* (paired box) gene, transcription factor
  - Type IV (Shah-Waardenburg syndrome): autosomal recessive, *EDN3* (endothelin receptor), EDNRB, G-protein coupled receptor; Autosomal dominant, *SOX10* (sex determining region) gene
- Diagnostic criteria are listed in Table 9-3
  - Clinical findings
  - *Skin*: depigmentation
  - *Hair*: white forelock at birth (80%), synophrys (70%)
  - *Oral*: caries

TABLE 9-3 Diagnostic Criteria for Waardenburg Syndrome

Major criteria	Congenital sensorineural hearing loss
	Pigmentary disturbances of iris; complete heterochromia iridis, partial or segmental heterochromia iridis, hypoplastic blue iridis
	White forelock
	Dystopia canthorum
	Affected first degree relative
Minor criteria	Congential leukoderma: several areas of hypopigmentation
	Synohyrys
	Broad and high nasal root
	Hypoplasia of ala nasi
	Premature graying of hair

    - *Eyes*: heterochromia, dystopia canthorum, lateral displacement of medial canthi with normal interpupillary distance; inner/outer canthi > 0.6
    - *Nose*: broad nasal root
    - *Ears*: congenital sensorineural deafness (75% of type I)
    - *Gastrointestinal*: Hirschsprung disease in type IV
- Symptoms additional to main symptoms:
    - Type I: dystopia canthorum, heterochromia irides, and sensorineural deafness
    - Type II: same as type I, but no dystopia canthorum
    - Type III: same as type I, but also have musculoskeletal, limb abnormalities (hypoplasia, contracture of elbows, fingers)
    - Type IV: same as type I, but also have Hirschsprung disease

QUIZ

Questions

1. A 40-year-old woman presents with a history of fever, seizures, photophobia, and poliosis of her eyebrows. The most likely explanation is:

    A. Antibody-mediated autoimmune disorder similar to Lupus
    B. T-cell mediated autoimmune disorder
    C. Genetic abnormality in lysosomal trafficking
    D. PAX3 mutation
    E. Cocaine use

2. Which type of oculocutaneous albinism presents with mahogany, red-brown colored skin?

    A. OCA1A
    B. OCA1B
    C. OCA2
    D. OCA3
    E. OCA4

3. Axillary reticular hyperpigmentation with increased melanosomes is related to a mutation in which gene:

    A. KRT5
    B. P gene
    C. HPS3
    D. SLC45A
    E. Laminin 332

4. A 14-year-old patient presents with numerous ephelides, blue nevi, cutaneous myxomas and a history of endocrine abnormalities. Which gene mutation has been associated with this disease?

    A. GNAS
    B. Hamartin
    C. FLT3
    D. PRKAR1A
    E. FGFR3

5. Spitz nevi have been associated with genetic abnormalities in which of the following?

    A. BRAF
    B. Rb
    C. H-RAS
    D. p53
    E. PTCH

6. A 3-month-old infant presents with a 25 × 21 cm deeply pigmented patch over the central upper back, present since birth. Which is the most sensitive imaging study to identify potential neurocutaneous melanosis?

    A. Contrast CT
    B. Cranial Ultrasound
    C. PET CT
    D. Contrast MRI
    E. Noncontrast MRI

7. Which of the following gene mutations has been associated with both an increase in inner canthal distance and gastrointestinal nerve plexus dysfunction?

    A. SOX1O
    B. PAX3
    C. MITF
    D. endothelin 2
    E. c-kit

8. An 8-month-old child presents with a silver sheen to her hair, seizures, hepatosplenomegaly, lymphadenopathy, pancytopenia, recurrent *Staph aureus* skin infections, and enlarged granules noted within neutrophils on peripheral smear. Which of the following gene defects is most likely to be identified?

    A. c-kit
    B. LYST
    C. PAX3
    D. HPS1
    E. RAB27a

9. A 35-year-old woman, presents with moderate centrofacial hyperpigmentation that enhances upon Woods lamp fluorescence. This pigmentation was initially noted during her last pregnancy (2 years ago), but no treatment has yet been initiated. Which of the following would be the most appropriate initial treatment regimen?

    A. Sunscreen and topical tretinoin
    B. Sunscreen, and combination topical tretinoin, topical hydroquinone, and desonide
    C. Intense pulsed light
    D. Sunscreen, topical hydroquinone, and topical steroids
    E. Topical hydroquinone

10. Which of the following ions is necessary for the proper function of the enzyme tyrosinase?
    A. Ca^{2+}
    B. Mg^{2+}
    C. Fe^{2+}
    D. Fe^{3+}
    E. Cu^{2+}

Answers

1. B. Vogt-Koynagi-Harada is a T-cell mediated autoimmune disorder that may be related to molecular mimicry following infection. Stages include a prodrome, ophthalmic and auditory stage, and poliosis stage.
2. D. Oculocutaneous albinism type 3 presents with a mahogany, red-brown coloration of the skin. Mutations are found in the *TYRP1* gene (Tyrosinase-related protein 1).
3. A. Dowling-Degos has been associated with KRT 5 mutations. It is characterized clinically by reticulate hyperpigmentation in the flexures and comedo-like lesions with pitted scars. Galli-Galli disease is the acantholytic variant of this disease.
4. D. Carney complex consists of an autosomal dominant syndrome featuring lentigines, blue nevi, endocrine disorders, testicular tumors, and myxomatous masses of the heart, skin, and breasts. Mutations in the PRKAR1A have been identified.
5. C. Spitz nevi have been associated with mutation in the H-RAS gene and with duplications of chromosome 15. They do not have mutations in BRAF, which are seen in common nevi and melanoma.
6. D. A contrast-enhanced MRI is the most sensitive imaging study to identify melanosis or melanoma metastasis in the central nervous system. Clinical signs and symptoms may include irritability, photophobia, seizures, and hydrocephalus.
7. A. Waardenburg syndrome type IV consists of dystopia canthorum and Hirschsprung disease, likely due to neural crest developmental abnormalities. Associated mutations include SOX1O and endothelin-3 genes. Types I–III do not develop Hirschsprung disease. c-kit mutations are found in Piebaldism where, although Hirschsprung disease has been rarely reported, no dystopia canthorum would be noted.
8. B. Chediak-Higashi syndrome consists of an autosomal recessive mutation in the LYST gene resulting in abnormal microtubule-associated lysosomal trafficking. Features include hair with a silver sheen, pigmented nevi, infections (staph aureus of the skin and pneumonia), ecchymoses, lymphoma (accelerated phase), neurologic degeneration, and pancytopenia. Neutrophils will characteristically show giant granules on smear.
9. B. The combination of topical hydroquinone, tretinoin, and a topical steroid is the first-line treatment of melasama. Broad-spectrum sunscreen should be used by patients several times a day. Topical hydroquinone and topical tretinoin are both FDA category C during pregnancy.
10. E. Copper is a necessary cofactor for the function of tyrosinase, an enzyme that catalyzes the hydroxylation of tyrosine to dopa and the oxidation of dopa to dopaquinone.

REFERENCES

Bukhari IA: Effective treatment of Futcher's lines with Q-switched alexandrite laser. *J Cosmet Dermatol* 2005;4(1)27–28.

Czajkowski R, Placek W, Drewa G, Czajkowska A, Uchanska G: FAMMM syndrome: pathogenesis and management. *Dermatol Surg* 2004;30(2 Pt 2):291–296.

da Silva FT, Damico FM, Marin ML, Goldberg AC, Hirata CE, Takiuti PH, Olivalves E, Yamamoto JH. Revised diagnostic criteria for vogt-koyanagi-harada disease: considerations on the different disease categories. *Am J Ophthalmol.* 2009 Feb;147(2):339-345.

Duffy K, Grossman D: The dysplastic nevus: from historical perspective to management in the modern era: part I and II. Historical, histological, and clinical aspects. *J Am Acad Dermatol* 2012; 67(1):1.e1–e16.

El Shabrawi-Caelen L, Rütten A, Kerl H: The expanding spectrum of Galli-Galli disease. *J Am Acad Dermatol* 2007;56 (5 Suppl):S86–S91.

Fang W, Yang P: Vogt-koyanagi-harada syndrome. *Curr Eye Res* 2008;33(7)517–523.

Goldsmith LA et al. *Fitzpatrick's Dermatology in General Medicine*, 8th Ed. New York: McGraw-Hill; 2012.

Grønskov K, Ek J, Brondum-Nielsen K: Oculocutaneous albinism. *Orphanet J Rare Dis* 2007;2:43.

Happle R: The group of epidermal nevus syndromes Parts I and II. Well defined phenotypes. *J Am Acad Dermatol* 2010 Jul;63(1):1–22.

Huizing M, Gahl WA: Disorders of vesicles of lysosomal lineage: the Hermansky-Pudlak syndromes. *Curr Mol Med* 2002;2(5)451–467.

Huizing M, Helip-Wooley A, Westbroek W, Gunay-Aygun M, Gahl WA: Disorders of lysosome-related organelle biogenesis: clinical and molecular genetics. *Annual Review of Genomics & Human Genetics* 2008;9:359–386.

Ibrahimi OA, Alikhan A, Eisen DB: Congenital melanocytic nevi: where are we now? Part I and II. Clinical presentation, epidemiology, pathogenesis, histology, malignant transformation, and neurocutaneous melanosis. *J Am Acad Dermatol* 2012 Oct;67(4):495.e1–e17.

Kaplan J, De Domenico I, Ward DM: Chediak-Higashi syndrome. *Curr Opin Hematol* 2008;15(1)22–29.

Kim SK, Kang HY, Lee ES, Kim YC: Clinical and histopathologic characteristics of nevus depigmentosus. *J Am Acad Dermatol* 2006;55(3)423–428.

Knoell KA, Nelson KC, Patterson JW: Familial multiple blue nevi. *J Am Acad Dermatol* 1998;39(2 Pt 2):322–325.

Luo S, Sepehr A, Tsao H. Spitz nevi and other Spitzoid lesions part I and II. Natural history and management. *J Am Acad Dermatol* 2011 Dec;65(6):1087–1092.

Magnain C. Elias M., Frigerio J.M. Skin color modeling using the radiative transfer equation solved by the auxiliary function method: inverse problem. *Journal of the Optical Society of America, A, Optics, Image Science, & Vision* 2008 Jul;25(7):1737–1743.

McKee PH et al. *McKee's Pathology of the Skin: With Clinical Correlations*, 4th Ed. Saunders; 2012.

Oetting WS, King RA: Molecular basis of oculocutaneous albinism. *J Invest Dermatol* 1994;103(5 Suppl):131S–136S.

Price HN, Schaffer JV: Congenital melanocytic nevi-when to worry and how to treat: Facts and controversies. *Clinics in Dermatology* 2010;28(3)293–302.

Richards KA, Fukai K, Oiso N, Paller AS: A novel KIT mutation results in piebaldism with progressive depigmentation. *J Am Acad Dermatol* 2001;44(2)288–292.

Schaffer JV: Pigmented lesions in children: when to worry. *Curr Opin Pediatr* 2007;19(4)430–440.

Schaffer JV, Orlow SJ, Lazova R, Bolognia JL: Speckled lentiginous nevus: within the spectrum of congenital melanocytic nevi. *Arch Dermatol* 2001 Feb;137(2):172–178.

Shah KN: The diagnostic and clinical significance of cafe-au-lait macules. [Review] *Pediatric Clinics of North America* 2010 Oct;57(5):1131–1153.

Sheth VM, Pandya AG: Melasma: a comprehensive update: part I and II. *J Am Acad Dermatol* 2011 Oct;65(4):699–714.

Sitaram A and Marks MS: Mechanisms of protein delivery to melanosomes in pigment cells. *Physiology (Bethesda) April* 2012;27:85–99.

Sommer L: Generation of melanocytes from neural crest cells. [Review] *Pigment Cell & Melanoma Research* 2011 Jun;24(3):411–421.

Tachibana M, Kobayashi Y, Matsushima Y: Mouse models for four types of Waardenburg syndrome. *Pigment Cell Res* 2003;16(5)448–454.

Tagra S, Talwar AK, Walia RL, Sidhu P: Waardenburg syndrome. *Indian J Dermatol Venereol Leprol* 2006;72(4):326.

Tripp JM, Kopf AW, Marghoob AA, Bart RS: Management of dysplastic nevi: a survey of fellows of the American Academy of Dermatology. *J Am Acad Dermatol* 2002;46(5)674–682.

Ward DM, Shiflett SL, Kaplan J: Chediak-Higashi syndrome: a clinical and molecular view of a rare lysosomal storage disorder. *Curr Mol Med* 2002;2(5)469–477.

Wick MR, Patterson JW: Cutaneous melanocytic lesions: selected problem areas. *Am J Clin Pathol* 2005;124 Suppl: S52–S83.

Wu YH, Lin YC: Generalized Dowling-Degos disease. *J Am Acad Dermatol* 2007;57(2)327–334.

Yaghoobi R, Omidian M, Bagherani N: Vitiligo: A review of the published work. *J Dermatol* 2011;38(5)419–431.

Yashiro M, Kobayashi H, Kubo N, Nishiguchi Y, Wakasa K, Hirakawa K: Cronkhite-Canada syndrome containing colon cancer and serrated adenoma lesions. *Digestion* 2004;69(1):57–62.

CHAPTER 10

DISORDERS OF FAT

HUNG DOAN
MARIGDALIA K. RAMIREZ-FORT
RYAN J GERTZ
ANDREW J. THOMPSON
FARHAN KHAN
STEPHEN K. TYRING

NEOPLASMS OF THE SUBCUTANEOUS FAT

Lipoma

- Most common soft tissue tumor, usually present in adults over the age of 30 years
- Wide anatomic distribution, with relative sparing of the head, hands, and feet
- Usually solitary, but 5% of patients have multiple lipomas, often in those with a lipomatosis or a multisystem syndrome
- Two-thirds of lipomas have chromosomal abnormalities; translocations between 12q13-15 and several other chromosomes are most common
- Clinical features: benign, asymptomatic; soft, and mobile subcutaneous nodule with a normal overlying epidermis
- Histology
    - Circumscribed nodule surrounded by a thin fibrous capsule
    - Lobules of mature adipocytes divided by fibrous septa containing capillary-sized vessels; adipocytes have eccentrically placed nuclei (Fig 10-1A,B)
    - Absent mitotic figures
    - Microscopically may be indistinguishable from the surrounding adipose tissue
- Histologic variants
    - Angiolipoma
        - Clinical features: occurs predominantly in men; presents as a small painful nodule, often on the forearm of young adults
        - Histology: well-circumscribed and encapsulated admixture of mature adipocytes and capillary-sized vessels which contain fibrin microthrombi; histologic presentation has a large degree of variability (Fig 10-2A,B)
- Pleomorphic lipoma
    - Clinical features: occurs predominantly in middle-aged men, located on posterior neck, upper back, and shoulders
    - Histology: circumscribed; admixture of bizarre multinucleate giant cells (floret cells) and normal adipocytes
- Spindle cell lipoma
    - Clinical features: occurs predominantly in middle aged men, located on posterior neck, upper back, and shoulders
    - Histology: circumscribed; admixture of bland-appearing spindle cells and normal adipocytes with variable myxocollagenous matrix stroma, containing rope-like collagen fibers (Fig 10-3)
    - Absent mitotic activity
- Adenolipoma
    - Clinical features: most commonly located on the proximal limbs
    - Histology: admixture of mature adipocytes with eccrine sweat glands
- Intramuscular lipoma
    - Composed of mature adipocytes, located within skeletal muscle; no cytologic atypia
    - Infiltrating type has higher local recurrence rate than other types of lipomas and requires more extensive tissue resection
- Fibrolipoma: lipomas with increased fibrous tissue; no cytologic atypia
- Sclerotic lipoma
    - Clinical features: more common in distal extremities

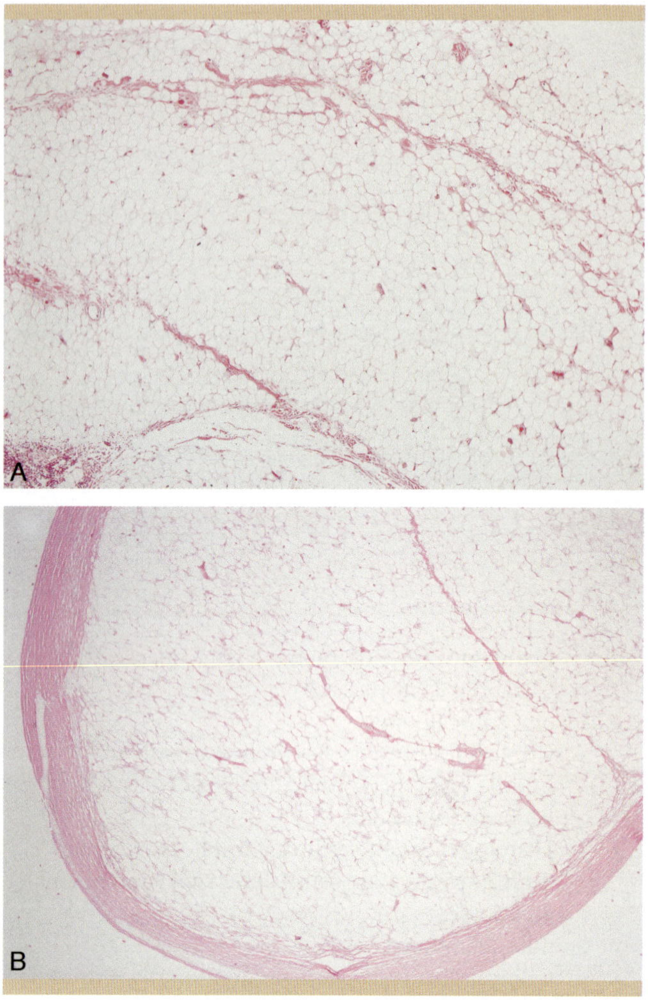

FIGURE 10-1 A and B: lipoma composed of benign adipocytes with single, large lipid vacuoles (A) and an encapsulated form (B).

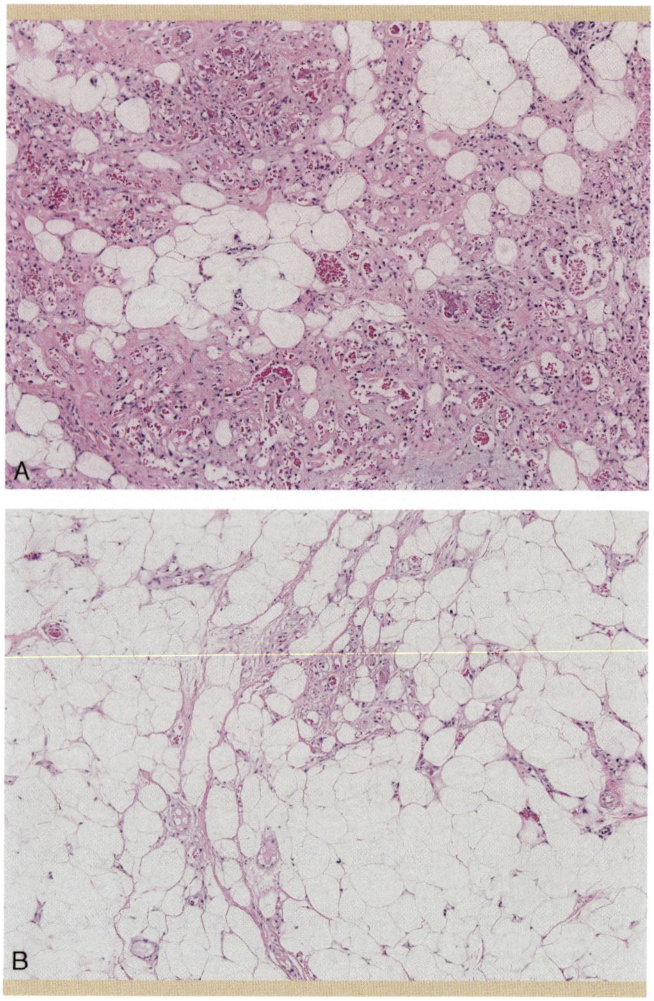

FIGURE 10-2 A and B: angiolipoma with variable degree of vascular components.

- Histology: well-circumscribed nodules, bland spindled and stellate cells, few adipocytes embedded in a collagenous to myxocollagenous stroma
  - Myxolipoma: lipoma with prominent myxoid stroma
  - Infarcted lipoma: necrotic adipocytes surrounded by multinucleate giant cells, lymphocytes, and extravasated erythrocytes
- Other types of lipomatous tumors
  - Chondroid lipoma
    - Clinical features
      - ▲ Benign tumor, occurs predominantly in females
      - ▲ Most common on proximal extremities and limb girdle
      - ▲ Involves deep subcutaneous tissue, fascia, and skeletal muscle
    - Histology:
      - ▲ Encapsulated tumor, containing nests and cords of lipoblasts with variable nuclei but no atypia; found within a chondroid matrix that can be hyalinized
      - ▲ Cells contain periodic acid–Schiff-positive glycogen
      - ▲ Alcian blue stains the matrix
      - ▲ These tumors are highly vascular
  - Myolipoma/lipoleiomyoma
    - Clinical features: occurs in deep soft tissue of abdomen and retroperitoneum; yellow-white cut surface; often presents as a palpable mass
    - Histology: admixture of mature adipocytes and smooth muscle cells, no atypia

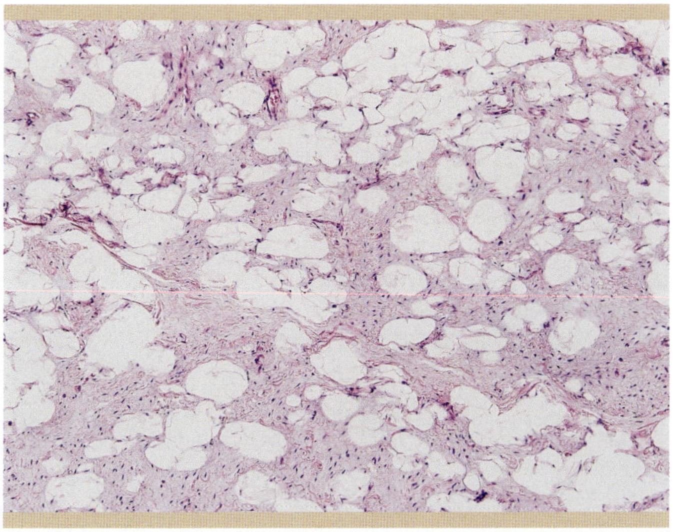

FIGURE 10-3 Spindle cell lipoma with bland spindle cells grouped along rope-like fibers of collagen in-between adipocytes.

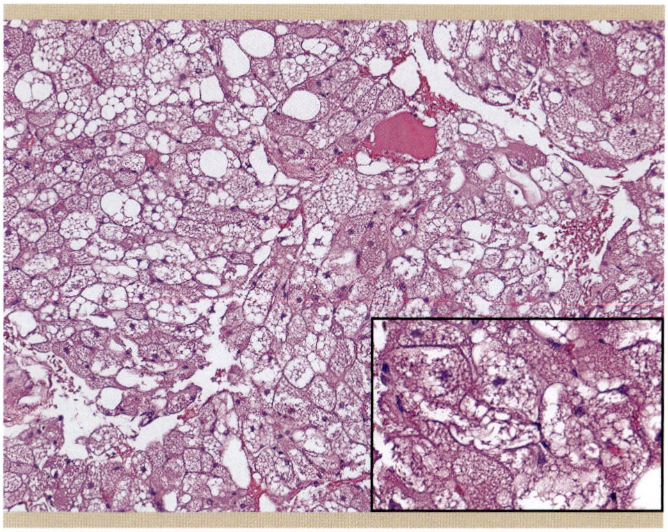

FIGURE 10-4 Hibernoma with adipocytes containing numerous, small lipid vacuoles and central, small nuclei (mulberry cells).

- Angiomyolipoma/angiolipoleiomyoma
  - Clinical features: most commonly located in kidney and are associated with tuberous sclerosis; these tumors are positive for HMB-45
  - Histology: convoluted thick-walled blood vessels, adipocytes, smooth muscle cells
- Cutaneous angiomyolipoma:
  - Clinical features: benign, slow growing and asymptomatic tumors; typically not associated with tuberous sclerosis, and are negative for HMB-45
  - Histology: convoluted thick-walled blood vessels, adipocytes, smooth muscle cells
- Hibernoma
  - Clinical features
    - ▲ Presents in a wide age distribution
    - ▲ Benign tumor derived from brown fat; typically found on the thighs, between scapula, head, neck, and chest
    - ▲ Painless, mobile, soft, solitary, deep red-brown in color
    - ▲ Structural rearrangements of chromosomes 11q13 and 11q21
  - Histology: pronounced lobulation, multivacuolated adipocytes with centrally placed nuclei (mulberry cells), eosinophilic cytoplasm (Fig 10-4)
- Lipoblastoma/lipoblastomatosis
  - Clinical features
    - ▲ Predominant in infants and children younger than 5 years of age
    - ▲ Painless, solitary, well-circumscribed, subcutaneous mass; trunk, extremities, head, and neck
    - ▲ If there is infiltration into skeletal muscle, it is termed as lipoblastomatosis
  - Histology
    - ▲ Lobulated, fibrovascular septa composed of an admixture of mature and immature adipocytes with larger nuclei and multiple lipid vacuoles (lipoblasts) (Fig 10-5)
    - ▲ Lipoblasts in different stages of development: univacuolated, bivacuolated, and multivacuolated forms

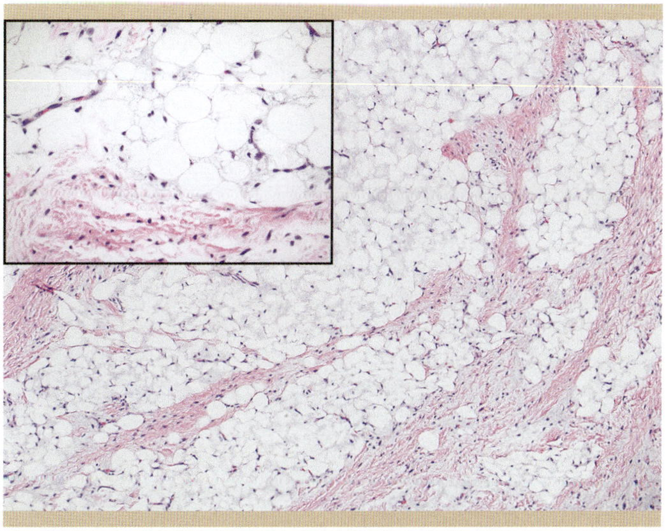

FIGURE 10-5 Lipoblastoma, note the more prominent fibrous septae, plexiform capillaries, and benign lipoblasts; lipoblasts tend to localize along septae (insert) and show variable degrees of maturity but have benign appearing nuclei.

  - ▲ Histology closely resembles myxoid liposarcoma which is exceptionally rare in patients younger than 10 years of age; lipoblastoma tends to be more lobulated and lacks the focal atypia seen in myxoid liposarcoma
- Liposarcoma
  - Clinical features
    - ▲ Soft tissue malignancy, peak incidence in sixth decade, most common in extremities, arises *de novo*
    - ▲ Commonly presents as an enlarging painless mass
    - ▲ Wide spectrum of behavior that depends on histology and location
  - Histology: all forms contain lipoblasts
    - ▲ Myxoid: most common variant, atypical lipoblasts with angulated nuclei that may be only focally present in a myxoid matrix; plexiform capillary network (chicken wire); associated t(12;16) translocation (Fig 10-6)
    - ▲ Well-differentiated (also known as atypical lipomatous tumor): mature fat with variable number of lipoblasts; scattered atypical cells with irregularly shaped hyperchromatic nuclei; only metastasizes if dedifferentiated
    - ▲ Pleomorphic: contain giant lipoblasts and is categorized with two subtypes
      - △ Common form with few bizarre giant lipoblasts that distinguish it from malignant fibrous histiocytoma (Fig 10-7)
      - △ Rare form with giant lipoblasts containing multiple cytoplasmic lipid droplets

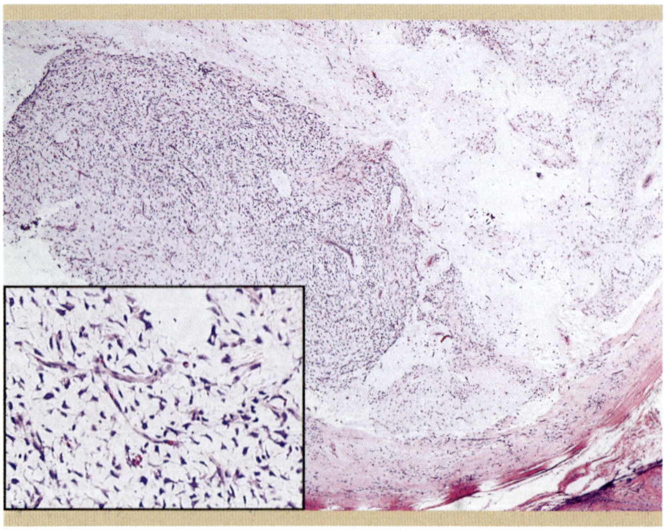

FIGURE 10-6 Myxoid liposarcoma with lipoblasts with angulated nuclei in a myxoid background.

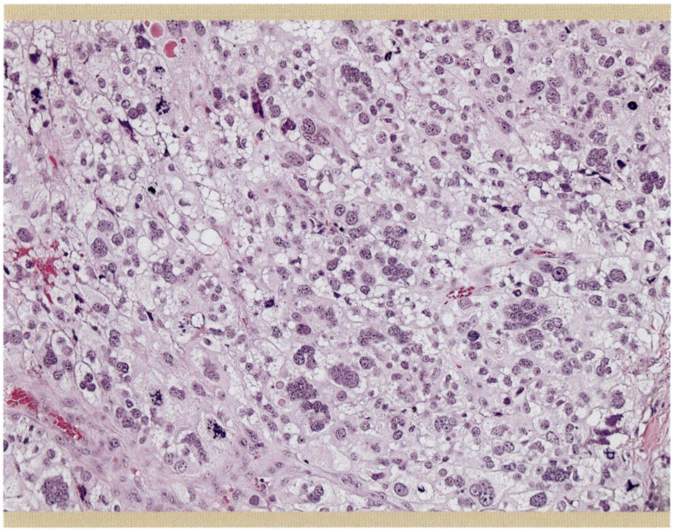

FIGURE 10-7 Pleomorphic liposarcoma with giant, multinucleated bizarre cells and frequent atypical mitotic figures.

Syndromes

- Dercum disease (adiposis dolorosa)
  - Abnormal overgrowth of adipose tissue
  - Multiple painful nodules due to compression of adjacent nerves; arms, trunk, and periarticular soft tissue
  - Typically involves the arms and trunk
  - Postmenopausal women, obese, associated with depression
  - Histology: unencapsulated and diffuse adipose tissue infiltrating into preexisting structures
- Madelung disease/benign symmetric lipomatosis
  - Middle-aged men, (usually alcoholics)
  - Fat deposits in head, neck ("horse collar"), and shoulder girdle
  - Associated with mutations in mitochondrial tRNA lysine synthase gene
  - Patients may also have peripheral neuropathy, hyperuricemia, and decreased glucose tolerance
- Familial lipomatosis
  - Autosomal dominant, most common in the third decade of life
  - Multiple discrete lipomas, mobile, encapsulated on the forearms and thighs
- Congenital lipomatosis
  - First few months of life
  - Large, subcutaneous fatty masses on chest, with extension into skeletal muscle
  - Manifests in Proteus syndrome (autosomal recessive, partial gigantism, hemihypertrophy, hemangiomas, and lymphangiomas)

- Bannayan-Zonana syndrome (Bannayan-Riley Ruvalcaba syndrome)
  - Autosomal dominant, multiple lipomas, multiple acrochordons, hemangiomas, pigmented macules on the penis, macrocephaly and delayed speech
  - Mutations in the tumor suppressor gene *PTEN*
  - Treatment is with surgical excision and liposuction

LIPODYSTROPHY

- Heterogeneous group of disorders; genetic or acquired involving a paucity or complete absence of fat
- Lipodystrophy refers to redistribution of fat
- Lipoatrophy refers to selective loss of fat
- Occurs secondary to clinical syndromes, inclusive of: metabolic syndrome, insulin resistance, hyperinsulinemia, diabetes mellitus, acanthosis nigricans, cardiovascular disease, hepatic steatosis, and polycystic ovarian disease
- Histology
  - Dependent on the type of lipodystrophy
  - Histological subsets:
    - Absence of inflammatory cells, absence of adipocytes or small adipocytes embedded in hyaline or myxoid connective tissue, numerous small blood vessels (Fig 10-8)
    - Inflammation within small fat lobules; lymphocytes, foamy histiocytes, plasma cells, normal sized adipocytes, and normal vasculature

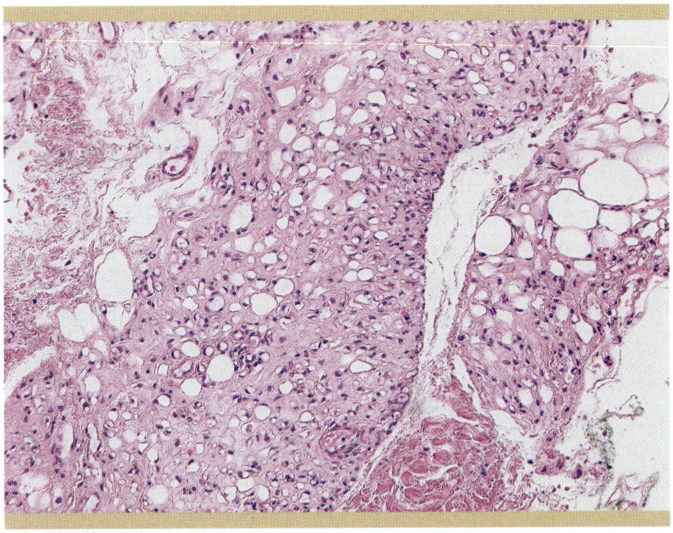

FIGURE 10-8 Lipoatrophy showing atrophic adipocytes separated by hyaline material; there are numerous small blood vessels and an absence of inflammatory cells.

Genetic Lipodystrophies

Autosomal Recessive

- Congenital generalized lipodystrophy (CGL; Berardinelli-Seip syndrome)
  - General clinical features
    - Complete absence of fat tissue; infants have a characteristic muscular appearance at birth
    - Infants have a voracious appetite, accelerated linear growth, and advanced bone age
    - Types 3 and 4 (discussed below) involve fat located in the bone marrow
    - Acanthosis nigricans occurs later in childhood; children also develop abdominal distention due to hepatomegaly
    - Other features include acromegaly, precocious puberty, and hypertrophic cardiomyopathy
  - Clinical features (listed by subcategory)
    - CGL type 1
      - ▲ *AGPAT2* (1-acylglycerol-3-phosphate O-acyltransferase 2) mutations, located on chromosome 9q34
      - ▲ Enzyme important for synthesis of triglyercerides
    - CGL type 2
      - ▲ *BSCL2* (Berardinelli-Seip congenital lipodystrophy 2/seipin gene) mutations, located on chromosome 11q13
      - ▲ Involved in lipid droplet formation
      - ▲ Cardiomyopathy and abnormal EKG (note: other forms have a normal EKG)
      - ▲ Mild mental retardation
    - CGL type 3
      - ▲ *CAV1* (caveolin 1 gene) located on chromosome 7q31
      - ▲ Important for formation of caveolae which is abundant in adipocytes
    - CGL type 4
      - ▲ *PTRF* (polymerase I and transcript release factor) on chromosome 17q21
      - ▲ Involved in biogenesis of caveolae
      - ▲ Associated with congenital pyloric stenosis, atlantoaxial instability, prolonged QT interval, and sudden death
- Lipodystrophy associated with mandibuloacral dysplasia (MAD)
  - Clinical features
    - Premature aging, mandibular and clavicular hypoplasia (bird-like facies), alopecia, acroosteolysis, mottled cutaneous pigmentation, and short stature
    - Partial lipodystrophy (type A pattern): *LMNA* (lamin A/C) mutations; loss of fat in arms and legs exclusively
    - Generalized lipodystrophy (type B pattern): *ZMPSTE24* (zinc metalloproteinase) mutations

- Lipodystrophy associated with SHORT syndrome (short stature, hyperextensibility, hernia, ocular depression, Reiger anomaly, and teething delay)
- Lipodystrophy associated with neonatal progeroid syndrome

Autosomal Dominant Disorders

- Familial partial lipodystrophy (FPL)
  - Clinical subcategories:
    - Dunnigan variety (FPLD): most common form
      - *LMNA* (lamin A/C) mutations alter plasma leptin concentration
      - Patients have normal fat distribution during childhood; however, during puberty there is loss of subcutaneous fat from arms and legs, and later from the chest and abdomen; excess fat may accumulate in face and neck
      - Associated with early onset of diabetes mellitus, severe hypertriglyceridemia and acute pancreatitis
    - FPL associated with *PPARG* (peroxisome proliferator-activated receptor γ) mutations: this form typically has loss of subcutaneous fat from arms, legs, and face
    - FPL associated with *AKT2* (v-AKT murine thymoma oncogene homolog 2) mutations
  - Treatment for lipodystrophy: oral hypoglycemic drugs or insulin; low-fat diet and exercise

Other Varieties

- Lipodystrophy associated with Hutchinson-Gilford progeria syndrome
  - Failure to thrive, delayed growth, short in stature, below average weight, accelerated aging, delayed dentition, skin appears wrinkled and aged-looking, and alopecia
  - Death occurs by age 13
- Pubertal-onset generalized lipodystrophy due to LMNA mutations
- Acquired generalized lipodystrophy (AGL) (Lawrence syndrome)
  - Most common in white women
  - Decreased fat on face, arms, and legs; presents during childhood or adolescence
  - 1/3 have preceding autoimmune disease or infection, 25% have preceding panniculitis
  - May present in the setting of cirrhosis, insulin-resistant diabetes mellitus, hyperinsulinemia, acanthosis nigricans, hypertriglyceridemia, and low serum levels of high-density lipoprotein cholesterol
- Acquired partial lipodystrophy (PL) (Barraquer-Simons syndrome)
  - Clinical features
    - More common in females; often preceded by a febrile illness
    - Associated with C3 nephritic factor; most have low levels of C3
    - During infancy or puberty there is loss of subcutaneous fat that begins on the face and spreads downward with sparing of lower extremities; increased fat in hips and legs
    - Most patients do not have glucose metabolism abnormalities; 20% have mesangiocapillary glomerulonephritis
  - Histology: decreased or absence of subcutaneous fat cells
  - Treatment: kidney transplant for uremia
- HIV-associated lipodystrophy
  - Associated with highly active antiretroviral therapy (HAART), occurs 2 months to 2 years after initiation of HAART; most often associated with stavudine and zidovudine
  - Clinical features: decreased subcutaneous fat on face, upper and lower extremities; increased subcutaneous fat on abdomen, posterior neck and upper back ("buffalo hump"), and breasts
  - Laboratory findings: insulin resistance, increased triglycerides
  - Treatment: change HAART medication (change medication class or within a class) autologous fat injections for facial lipoatrophy, fillers in patients without adequate fat reserves, liposuction of upper back, recombinant human growth hormone (rhGH), metformin
- Other lipodystrophies/lipoatrophy
  - Prior inflammatory processes involving the subcutis: lupus profundus, morphea, or panniculitis
  - Iatrogenic causes: subcutaneous injections of corticosteroids, insulin, or methotrexate
  - Subtypes of idiopathic lipoatrophies:
    - Annular lipoatrophy of the ankles
      - Clinical features: pseudosclerotic band surrounds ankles; may be preceded by inflammatory panniculitis and persistent pain; may be associated with local arthritis
      - Histology: diffuse lobular lymphohistiocytic panniculitis with fat necrosis; no evidence of vasculitis or connective tissue disease
    - Lipoatrophia semicircularis: semicircular depressions on the anterior aspects of the thighs, related to repeated microtraumas
    - Lipodystrophia centrifugalis abdominalis infantilis:
      - Clinical features
        - Affects Asian children younger than 3 years of age; acquired, localized lipodystrophy; loss of abdominal fat
        - Red and scaly skin around the area of abdominal lipoatrophy; regional lymphadenopathy; benign process, half of patients spontaneously recover after several years
      - Histology: decreased subcutaneous fat with infiltration by lymphocytes and histiocytes in the depressed area

PANNICULITIS

Septal (With Vasculitis)

- Leukocytoclastic vasculitis
  - Inflammation of postcapillary venules in the superficial plexus
  - Clinical feature: can present as subcutaneous erythematous nodules
  - Histology
    - Endothelial cell necrosis, fibrin deposition, and neutrophilic infiltrate within vessel walls
    - Septal thickening involving vessels of superficial plexus, but sparing of dermal vessels
    - No inflammatory infiltrate of adjacent fat lobules
- Superficial thrombophlebitis
  - Clinical features
    - Linear tract, tender erythematous subcutaneous nodules on the lower extremities
    - Migratory associated with underlying malignancy (Trousseau sign)
- Cutaneous polyarteritis nodosa
  - Distinguished from *systemic* polyarteritis nodosa by absence of systemic involvement
  - Overlap of 10 to 15% of patients
  - Clinical features
    - Bilateral erythematous nodules or livedo reticularis of lower extremities
    - Ulceration—protracted disease
    - Systemic—purpuric papules
    - Good prognosis
  - Histology: septal inflammation of medium-sized arteries and arterioles of subcutaneous fat

Septal (Without Vasculitis)

- Erythema nodosum
  - Most common nonvasculitic panniculitis
  - Etiology: summarized in Table 10-1, *Streptococcal* (in children), sarcoidosis, drugs, chronic inflammation (ulcerative colitis), and malignancy
  - Commonly affects women 3 to 5 times more often than men
  - Clinical features:
    - Sudden onset of bilateral painful subcutaneous nodules of lower extremities (knees, shins, and ankles)
    - Associated symptoms: arthralgias, fever, malaise, headache, and abdominal pain
    - Erythema contusiformis: characteristic progression of erythema to green or yellow discoloration, resembling a healing contusion
    - Chronic variant (EN migrans): unilateral lower extremity
    - Lesions last 3 to 6 weeks, recurrence is not uncommon
  - Histology:
    - Lymphocytic inflammation along septal and periseptal adipose tissue with relative paucity in center of lobule (Fig 10-9)
    - Prominent giant cells infiltrate along septae
  - Treatment: treat the underlying condition, cessation of potential causative medications, analgesia with aspirin or NSAIDs, potassium iodide and rarely systemic corticosteroids
- Necrobiosis lipoidica
  - Bilateral inflammatory plaques involving the subcutis
  - Associated with diabetes mellitus
  - Progress over years, rarely painful
  - Clinical features: red-brown papules coalescing to a form yellow plaques with central atrophy; plaques have an erythematous and distinct border with radial enlargement
  - Histology:
    - Frequently shows thickening of septae and plasma cells at the junction between the deep dermis and subcutaneous adipose tissue
    - Rarely can have lipomembranous fat necrosis
    - Characterized by deep dermal granulomatous inflammation with sclerosis, collagen degeneration, and palisading histiocytes
  - Treatment: intralesional steroids, oral aspirin with dipyridamole or pentoxifylline
- Necrobiotic xanthogranuloma
  - Clinical features:
    - Well-demarcated yellow-to-violaceous indurated plaques, occur periorbitally
    - Tendency towards ulceration
    - Associated with IgG κ-type monoclonal gammopathy; seen in multiple myeloma patients
  - Histology:
    - Usually a dermal lesion that can extend into the subcutis
    - Palisading granulomatous panniculitis with abundant histiocytes, giant cells, lymphocytes, hyaline necrobiosis, and cholesterol clefts
  - Treatment: treat underlying condition (paraproteinemia), melphalan, prednisolone, and plasmapheresis
- Rheumatoid nodule
  - Clinical features
    - Occurs in up to 20% of patients with rheumatoid arthritis
    - Typically presents proximal to the elbow or finger joints
    - Firm, fixed subcutaneous nodules
  - Histology: palisading granulomas composed of histiocytes with a center containing eosinophilic granules or fibrin
  - Surgical resection is indicated if the lesion becomes ulcerated or is painful

TABLE 10-1 Etiologic Factors in Erythema Nodosum

Infections		Drugs	Malignancy	Misc
Bacterial	Viral infections	Sulfonamides	Hodgkin disease	Sarcoidosis
Streptococcal infections	Infectious mononucleosis	Bromides	Non-Hodgkin lymphoma	Ulcerative colitis
Tuberculosis	Hepatitis B	Iodides	Leukemia	Colon diverticulosis
Yersinia infections	Milker nodules	Oral contraceptives	Sarcoma	Crohn disease
Salmonella infections	Orf	Minocycline	Renal carcinoma	Behçet syndrome
Campylobacter infections	Herpes simplex	Gold salts	Postradiotherapy for pelvic carcinoma	Reiter syndrome
Brucellosis	Measles	Penicillin		Sweet syndrome
Tularemia	Cytomegalovirus infections	Salicylates		Pregnancy
Atypical mycobacterial infections	Fungal infections	Chlorothiazides		Takayasu arteritis
Chancroid	Dermatophytes	Phenytoin		IgA nephropathy
Meningococcemia	Blastomycosis	Aminopyrine		Chronic active hepatitis
Corynebacterium diphtheriae infections	Histoplasmosis	Arsphenamine		Granulomatous mastitis
Cat-scratch disease	Coccidioidomycosis	Hepatitis B vaccine		Vogt-Koyanagi disease
Propionibacterium acnes	Sporotrichosis	Nitrofurantoin		Sjögren syndrome
Shigella infections	Aspergillosis	Pyritinol		
Gonorrhea		D-Penicillamine		
Syphilis		Thalidomide		
Leptospirosis		Isotretinoin		
Q fever		Interleukin 2		
Lymphogranuloma venereum				
Chlamydia psittaci infections				
Mycoplasma pneumoniae infections				

Requena L, Yus ES.: Panniculitis. Part I. Mostly septal panniculitis. *J Am Acad Dermatol* 2001 Aug;45(2):163–183.

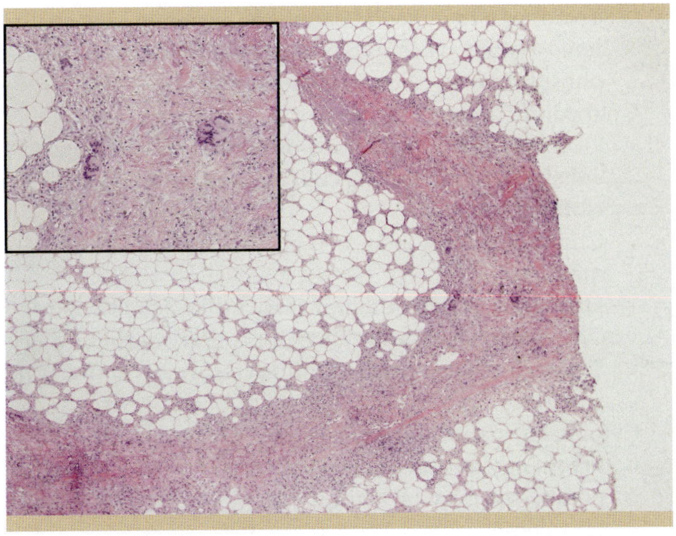

FIGURE 10-9 Erythema nodosum with classic septal panniculitis harboring giant cells (insert).

- Scleroderma (subcutaneous morphea, morphea profunda)
  - Clinical features
    - Extension of scleroderma into subcutaneous fat, sometimes presents only with subcutaneous involvement
    - Indurated plaques or nodules, can progress or resolve with atrophy and residual hyperpigmentation
  - Histology:
    - Thickened and hyalinized collagen bundles with lymphocytic infiltration around small blood vessels, most prominently around the junction of the deep dermis and subcutaneous adipose tissue, with sparing of the upper dermis
    - Subcutaneous tissue has hyalinization
    - Sweat glands are displaced to the mid dermis with diminished number of sebaceous glands and hair follicles; mucin deposition in the deep dermis
  - Treatment: intralesional steroids, penicillamine
- Subcutaneous granuloma annulare
  - Granuloma annulare variant occurring in subcutis
  - Clinical features
    - Found often on head, hands, buttocks, and anterior lower extremity
    - Occurs commonly in children and young adults
    - 25% of the time coexists with classic granuloma annulare
  - Histology: palisading granulomas composed of histiocytes with a center containing mucin

Lobular (With Vasculitis)

- Erythema nodosum leprosum
  - Vasculitis from immune complex deposition in lepromatous leprosy patients (type 2 reaction)
  - Clinical features
    - Erythematous and violaceous nodules involving extremities
    - Lesions involve deep dermis and variably subcutis, can regress or progress to purulent open ulcers
  - Histopathology
    - Neutrophilic lobular panniculitis
    - Leukocytoclastic vasculitis
    - May have foamy macrophages
    - Immunofluorescence shows complement and IgG immune complex deposition
  - Treatment: thalidomide, clofazimine, minocycline, and prednisone
- Lucio phenomenon
  - Rare variant of type 2 reaction in lepromatous leprosy (previously denoted type 3 reaction)
  - Clinical features: diffuse hemorrhagic necrotizing ulcers that occur with diffuse nonnodular lepromatous leprosy patients
  - Histology
    - Necrotizing vasculitis of the small vessels with foamy histiocytes that contain numerous acid-fast bacilli
    - Endothelial proliferation with obliteration of vascular lumen
- Nodular vasculitis (erythema induratum of Bazin)
  - Most common form of lobular panniculitis
  - Clinical features
    - Chronic tender erythematous subcutaneous nodules on posterior lower extremities
    - Violaceous, cold, nontender, and tend to ulcerate
    - Usually occur in middle-aged women
    - Associated with *Mycobacterium tuberculosis*
  - Histology
    - Lobular panniculitis fat necrosis
    - Infiltration with histiocytes and giant cells
    - Vasculitis with lymphocytes and granulomatous inflammation with endothelial swelling, edema, and sclerosis of the walls
  - Treatment: treat *M. tuberculosis* if present, potassium iodide, compression for venous insufficiency, NSAIDS for pain
- Crohn disease
  - Chronic inflammatory disease of gastrointestinal tract
  - Clinical features:
    - Cutaneous component includes erythema nodosum, pyoderma gangrenosum, and erythema multiforme
    - Abscesses, sinuses, tracts, and fistulas of genital and perianal areas
  - Histology: subcutaneous granulomas that can have necrosis

Lobular (Without Vasculitis)

- A1-antitrypsin deficiency
  - Mainly lobular panniculitis with ulceration
  - A1-antitrypsin (A1AT) is produced in the liver
  - Normally inhibits trypsin, chymotrypsin, thrombin, neutrophilic neutral protease, factor VIII, pancreatic elastase, collagenase, plasmin, kallikrein, and urokinase
  - Over 90 allelic mutations lead to variants in mobility (PiMM is normal, PiS and PiZ variants are abnormally slow on electrophoresis)
  - Most common amino acid substitution: glutamic acid to lysine at position 342
  - Homozygous PiZZ allele associated with lowest serum level of A1AT
  - Low A1AT levels correlates with uncontrolled activation of inflammatory cells and damage after an insult (i.e., smoking, injury)
  - Pathophysiology: associated with direct injury in A1AT individuals and uncontrolled proteolytic degradation of tissues
  - Clinical features
    - Associated with cirrhosis, pancreatitis, *panacinar* emphysema, glomerulonephritis, vasculitis, acquired angioedema
    - Recurrent painful subcutaneous nodules that ulcerate and drain oily-yellow fluid (related to fat released from lobules)
    - Can occur on face, extremities, or trunk; mimics cellulitis; resolve with atrophic scarring
  - Histology
    - Neutrophilic lobular panniculitis, however, neutrophilic infiltrate dissects around the fat lobules
    - The neutrophilic infiltrate can characteristically track upward into dermis, splaying collagen fibers
  - Diagnosis: decreased serum A1AT levels
- Caliciphylaxis
  - Characterized by calcium deposition in small- and medium-sized vessels
  - Poor prognosis with up to 80% mortality
  - Association with chronic renal disease and elevated parathyroid hormone
  - Clinical features
    - Painful violaceous, reticulate patches and plaques (similar to livedo reticularis) evolving to necrotic nonhealing ulcers
    - Digital gangrene may require amputation
    - Extremities, thighs, and buttocks most commonly involved
  - Histology
    - Calcium deposition in small- to medium-sized vessels of reticular dermis and involved subcutaneous lobules
    - Inflammation with fat necrosis, foamy histiocytes, and intralobular calcification
  - Treatment: therapeutic parathyroidectomy; in chronic renal disease, calcium binding resins, low calcium and phosphate diet, calcium hemodialysis
- Cold panniculitis
  - Occurs in children after exposure to cold (sucking ice cubes, ice pops); during cold months with tight clothing
  - Clinical features: indurated plaques with ill-defined margins
  - Histology: lobular inflammatory infiltrate of lymphocytes and histiocytes; edema of papillary dermis
  - Treatment: avoid cold, warming (resolves within days), and loose clothing
- Cytophagic histiocytic panniculitis
  - Frequently fatal disease characterized by subcutaneous nodules that can be painful
  - Histology
    - Defined as mostly lobular inflammatory and often hemorrhagic infiltrate with histiocytes and mature T-lymphocytes
    - Characteristic "bean bag" cells composed of macrophage cytophagocytosis of erythrocytes, leukocytes, or lymphocytes
- Factitial and iatrogenic panniculitis
  - Etiology
    - Subcutaneous injection of foreign substance
    - Subcutaneous injection of drugs (meperidine, povidone, pentazosin, and vitamin K) or cosmetic substances (silicone, polymehtyl-methacrolate microspheres, and Bioplastique)
  - Histology
    - Mostly lobular panniculitis; neutrophilic infiltrate in early lesions followed by granulomatous infiltrate
    - Histopathology relates to nature of substance
      - ▲ Sclerosing lipogranuloma: paraffinoma from mineral oil injection; "swiss cheese" morphology replacing fat lobules with variably sized cavities
      - ▲ Silicone: granulomas consisting of foamy histiocytes, multinucleated giant cells surrounding impurities
- Infective panniculitis
  - Infection of lobules of fat with bacterial or fungal infiltrate
  - Common pathogens: *Streptococcus pyogenes, Staphylococcus aureus, Pseudomonas* spp, *Klebsiella, Nocardia* spp, *Brucella,* atypical mycobacteria, *Mycobacterium tuberculosis, Candida* spp, *Fusarium* spp, *Histoplasma capsulatum, Cryptococcus neoformans, Actinomyces israelii, Sporothrix schenkii, Aspergillus fumigates,* and chromomycosis
  - Primary results from direct inoculation (i.e., animal bites or scratch)
  - Secondary results from primary pulmonary disease (hematogenous or direct extension)

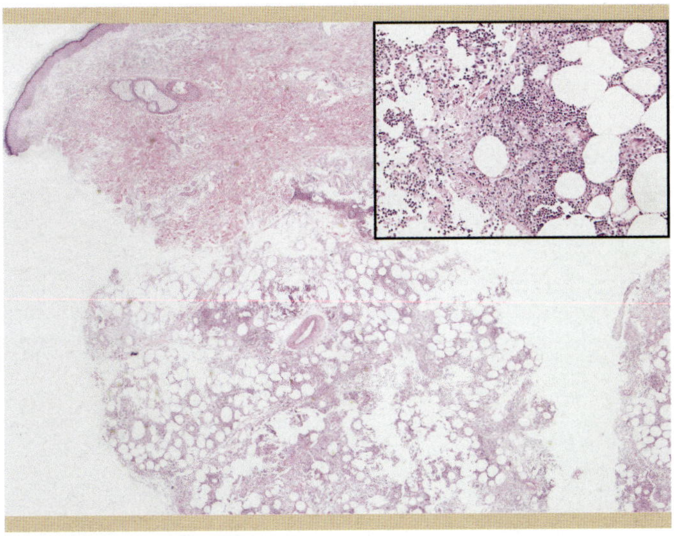

FIGURE 10-10 Neutrophilic lobular panniculitis with a pattern of inflammation consistent with bacterial etiology.

- Histology
  - Mostly lobular panniculitis without vasculitis
  - Bacterial: diffuse neutrophilic infiltrate in fat lobules with extension into dermis (Fig 10-10)
  - Fungal: extensive fibrosis in candidal panniculitis; suppurative granulomas in subcutaneous tissue
  - Secondary infection: dilated vessels containing organisms, deep reticular dermal inflammation
- Lupus panniculitis
  - Clinical variant of lupus erythematosus (LE); may precede or follow discoid or systemic LE
  - Clinical features
    - Crops of tender, deep subcutaneous nodules; involves face, scalp, trunk, breast, buttocks; rarely lower extremities
    - Lesions can appear at sites of trauma (i.e., injections); lipoatrophy after resolution
  - Histology
    - Up to 50% with epidermal and dermal changes of discoid lupus (interstitial mucin deposition, dermal-epidermal vacuolar morphology, and enlarged basement membrane)
    - Remaining have predominantly lymphocytic lobular panniculitis; hyaline fat necrosis is often evident
    - Immunofluorescence: linear deposition of IgM and C3 at dermal-epidermal junction (lupus band)
  - Treatment: systemic steroids or hydroxychloroquine
- Oxalosis
  - Primary: autosomal recessive; deficiency in 2-hydroxy-2-oxoadipate carboxylase (type 1) or D-glyceric dehydrogenase (type 2)
  - Secondary: excessive oxalate or glycolic acid (ethylene glycol poisoning, intravenous glycerol or xylitol, methoxyflurane anesthesia, pyridoxine deficiency, chronic renal failure with hemodialysis, aberrant gastrointestinal absorption)
  - Clinical features: livedo reticularis and acral gangrene (cutaneous); recurrent renal stones
  - Histology: calcium deposits and yellow-brown oxalate crystals around blood vessels in deep dermis and subcutis
  - Treatment: renal transplant; liver transplant to recover enzyme function; serum alkalinization
- Pancreatic panniculitis
  - Subcutaneous fat necrosis associated with acute or chronic pancreatitis or pancreatic disease (pseudocysts or adenocarcinoma)
  - Pathogenesis: release of lipase into bloodstream with deposition and inflammation at distant site
  - Clinical features
    - Commonly affects knees and ankles
    - Fluctuant erythematous subcutaneous nodules; often ulcerate with oily brown exudates (liquefactive fat necrosis)
  - Histology: there is saponification (with calcification) and precipitation in "ghost" adipocytes; hypocalcemia may be present
  - Resolves with resolution of pancreatic disease
- Post-steroid panniculitis
  - Occurs in children abruptly withdrawn or tapered from systemic steroids
  - Clinical features: bilateral cheek involvement; deep subcutaneous nodules forming within 1 week of steroid withdrawal
  - Histology
    - Infiltrate of foamy histiocytes and lymphocytes in fat lobules; needle-shaped clefts (fatty acid crystals which dissolved from tissue processing)
    - Mostly self-resolves, ulcerating lesions heal with atrophic scar
  - Treatment: readministration of steroids with a more gradual taper in early lesions
- Sclerema neonatorum
  - Affects severely underweight premature newborns
  - Associated with serious infections, congenital heart disease, or severe developmental defects
  - Related to high ratio of unsaturated to saturated fatty acids
  - Clinical features
    - Diffuse yellow-white indurated plaques on buttocks progressing to involve large areas of body
    - Poor prognosis, treat underlying condition
  - Histology: sparse lobular panniculitis; characteristic radial needle-shaped clefts in adipocytes and multinucleated giant cells
- Subcutaneous fat necrosis of the newborn
  - Occurs within first 2 to 3 weeks of healthy newborns

- Clinical features
  - Indurated violaceous plaques and nodules on buttocks, thighs, shoulders, and cheeks
  - Elevated ratio of unsaturated fat to saturated fat; association with hypercalcemia
- Histology: lobular panniculitis with lymphocytes, histiocytes multinucleated giant cells, radially arranged needle-shaped clefts, and calcification
- Spontaneously resolves, good prognosis
- Treatment: etidronate (for hypercalcemia)

- Sclerosing panniculitis (lipodermatosclerosis)
  - Association with chronic venous insufficiency in middle-aged women
  - Clinical features
    - Erythematous and edematous tender plaques on medial aspects of one or both lower extremities progressing to marked wood-like induration
    - Fibrosis of deep dermis leads to "inverted bottle" deformity
    - Evidence of venous stasis, ulceration, and telangiectasia of overlying skin
  - Histology
    - Stasis dermatitis (increased capillaries and venules in papillary dermis, hemosiderin deposition, and fibrosis)
    - Fully developed lesions show lobular panniculitis, atrophic fat lobules, septal thickening and fibrosis, peripheral foamy macrophages
  - Treatment: treat venous stasis (compression stockings), stanozolol
- Subcutaneous sarcoidosis
  - Associated with African-Americans and women
  - Clinical features
    - Commonly red to violaceous papules and plaques, variable onset
    - Erythema nodosum: subcutaneous nodules on lower extremities without superficial involvement, favorable outcome
    - Lupus pernio (chronic violaceous plaques involving face and nose) from chronic systemic involvement
    - Other variants: verrucous, psoriasiform, annular, or hypopigmented
  - Histology: noncaseating granulomas of fat lobules and scant lymphocytes at periphery (Fig 10-11)
  - Treatment
    - Topical or intralesional steroids for localized conditions
    - Systemic steroids for systemic involvement
    - Immune modulators and biologics may be of benefit
- Traumatic panniculitis
  - Blunt trauma, frequent in women with large breasts
  - Mammary traumatic panniculitis: indurated deep subcutaneous nodule, may have peau d'orange

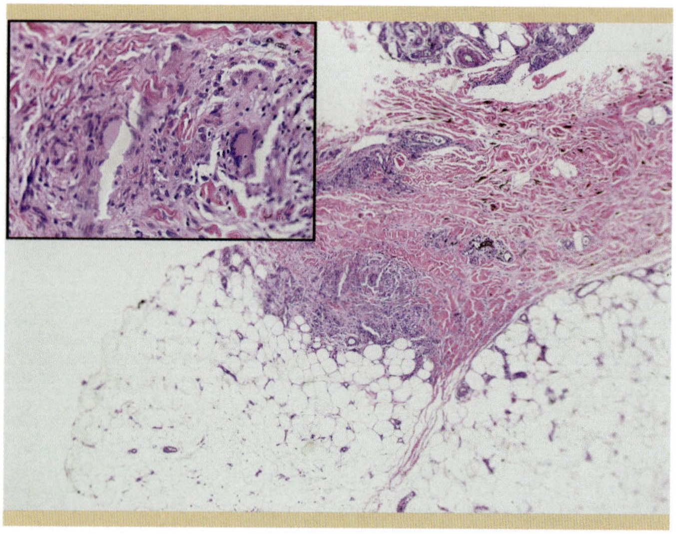

FIGURE 10-11 Subcutaneous sarcoidosis showing noncaseating granuloma at junction of deep dermis and fat lobule.

  - Histology: fat necrosis, cystic spaces within fat lobules, foamy histiocytes, fibrosis and hemorrhage may be present
- Panniculitis in dermatomyositis (DM)
  - Cutaneous manifestation of DM
  - Clinical features: nodular, indurated tender plaques
  - Histology: lobular panniculitis with intense lymphocytic and plasma cell infiltrate, necrosis and fibrosis of lobular adipocytes, calcification
  - Treatment: systemic steroids with or without methotrexate

Disorders Erroneously Considered as Specific Variants of Panniculitis

- Subcutaneous "panniculitic" lymphoma
  - High-grade lymphoma predominantly involving subcutaneous tissues, not a true panniculitis
  - Clinical features
    - Indurated plaques and nontender subcutaneous nodules mimicking panniculitis
    - Constitutional symptoms: fever, malaise, night sweats, fatigue, myalgia, weight loss, hepatosplenomegaly, serosal effusions, and pancytopenia
  - Histology
    - Subcutaneous infiltrate of pleomorphic T-lymphocytes in fat lobules; large and hyperchromatic nuclei, numerous mitoses
    - Immunohistochemistry: positive for CD2, CD3, CD5, often CD8, negative for CD4 and CD56; intense positivity for cytotoxic granular proteins granzyme B, TIA-1, and perforin
    - Evidence of EBV etiology in endemic areas (Asia)

- Weber-Christian disease
  - Classically referred to as *syndrome of lobular panniculitis without vasculitis*, systemic symptoms and involvement of visceral fat tissue
  - Early diagnoses of *Weber-Christian* disease have a more specific diagnosis
- Rothmann-Makai disease
  - Relapsing nodular panniculitis with no other symptoms
  - Obsolete term
- Lipomembranous or membranocystic panniculitis
  - Histopathologic term rather than a clinical entity
  - Cystic cavities lined by crenulated hyaline membranes, positive staining for periodic acid–Schiff and Sudan black, and elastase negative
- Eosinophilic panniculitis
  - Septal or lobular panniculitis with predominance of eosinophils
  - Nonspecific reactive process rather than a true panniculitis

QUIZ

Questions

1. A 40-year-old man presents with a tender mobile subcutaneous nodule. On biopsy, pathology shows a well-circumscribed mass containing adipocytes with a prominent vascular pattern and occasional thrombi. What is the diagnosis?

   a. Spindle cell lipoma
   b. Liposarcoma
   c. Angiolipoma
   d. Pleomorphic lipoma

2. A 55-year-old man presents with a painless, rapidly enlarging subcutaneous mass on his thigh. Wide excision revealed a delicate plexiform capillary network containing lipoblasts, and normal adipocytes in a myxoid stroma. Under immunohistochemistry the cells stain positive for S100. What other location is this tumor typically found?

   a. Head and neck
   b. Mediastinum
   c. Acral
   d. Retroperitoneum

3. A 60-year-old obese woman presents with progressive onset of multiple painful subcutaneous nodules on her trunk, neck, and upper extremities. Biopsy revealed a diffuse infiltrate of adipose tissue into adjacent nerves and muscle. What other medical condition is this associated with?

   a. Depression
   b. Hypercalcemia
   c. Metabolic alkalosis
   d. Renal tubular acidosis

4. A 38-year-old woman presents with progressive loss of subcutaneous fat on her face and torso. She denies recent changes in diet, medications, or illnesses. What labs should be checked?

   a. Protein electrophoresis
   b. Urine analysis
   c. Chest radiograph
   d. Liver function tests

5. A 22-year-old female college student presents with warm, tender erythematous subcutaneous nodules on her lower extremities bilaterally. She started oral contraceptive medications recently. What would be expected under histopathology?

   a. Dense reactive fibrosis with spindle cells
   b. Lobulation with multivacuolated adipocytes and centrally placed nuclei
   c. Eosinophilic infiltrate in a lobular panniculitis
   d. Septal inflammation with multinucleated giant cells

6. A 68-year-old woman presents with a well-demarcated yellow-brown plaque on her left cheek. Pathology reveals areas of necrobiosis with granulomatous inflammation and occasional cholesterol crystals. What is the most likely association?

   a. IgG paraproteinemia
   b. IgA paraproteinemia
   c. Non-Hodgkin lymphoma
   d. Bilateral hilar infiltrates on chest radiograph

7. A 53-year-old man from El Salvador presents with multiple violaceous painful subcutaneous nodules on his extensor surfaces and reports neuropathy and anesthesia of his upper and lower extremities. What type of reaction is this?

   a. Jarisch-Herxheimer reaction
   b. Type 1
   c. Type 2
   d. Lucio reaction

8. A 60-year-old woman on chronic hemodialysis presents with dusky reticular patches on her lower thighs bilaterally that ulcerate and form eschars. Biopsy reveals areas of calcification in the vessel walls. What abnormal laboratory finding is consistent with this condition?

a. Hyperparathyroidism
b. Hypoalbuminemia
c. Leukocytosis
d. Cyroglobulinemia

9. A 3-week-old full-term infant presents to the emergency department with erythematous, violaceous, firm nodules, and plaques involving the back and buttocks. What is the diagnosis?

a. Sclerema neonatorum
b. Erythema toxicum neonatorum
c. Subcutaneous fat necrosis of the newborn
d. Alpha-1-antitrypsin deficiency

10. A 32-year-old man presents with tender erythematous subcutaneous nodules of his lower extremities, recent fever, arthralgias and abdominal pain. He reports that he has Crohn Disease. Histology reveals septal thickening of subcutaneous fat, granulomatous changes and multinuclated giant cells. What other findings may be present?

a. Pyostomatitis vegetans
b. Posterior uveitis
c. Bilateral hilar infiltrates on chest radiograph
d. Recent usage of trimethoprim/sulfamethoxazole

Answers

1. C. The histologic description is characteristic of angiolipoma. Spindle cell lipomas contain bland-appearing spindle cells and normal adipocytes. Liposarcoma contains adipocytes and lipoblasts, and may stain for S100 (in one-third of cases). Pleomorphic lipoma contains bizarre multinuclated giant cells with normal adipocytes.
2. D. This is liposarcoma, the most common sarcoma in adults. It typically is found in the retroperitoneum, thighs, and inguinal region.
3. A. This is a description of Dercum disease (adiposis dolorosa). It classically presents in postmenopausal women and is associated with nervous system dysfunction and depression is often comorbid. Other conditions associated include obesity, dementia, confusion, weakness, and lethargy. Surgical management of lipomatosis and weight loss may help with symptoms.
4. B. This is acquired partial lipodystrophy associated with the C3 nephritic factor. This factor binds factor H, an inhibitor of C3 resulting in uncontrolled activation of C3 causing glomerulonephritis. This condition is also associated with diabetes mellitus and glucose and insulin levels should be monitored.
5. D. This is erythema nodosum, the prototypical septal panniculitis. Typical causative agents include medications (including oral contraceptive prescriptions and antibiotics) and infectious agents (*Streptococcus* most common). The causative agent should be identified (discontinue medications, determine the infectious agent, chest radiographs, etc.) and lesions typically self-resolve and can be managed conservatively with analgesics.
6. A. This is necrobiotic xanthogranuloma and is most commonly periocular with an associated IgG paraproteinemia.
7. C. This patient most likely has erythema nodosum leprosum (ENL). He presents from an endemic area, with the typical lesions of ENL and associated neuropathy seen in this type of leprosy. This is considered borderline lepromatous leprosy and is considered a type 2 reaction. Type 1 reaction is either a downgrading or resolving reaction in tuberculoid or lepromatous leprosy and presents with nonspecific macular or papular skin eruption with satellite lesions and constitutional symptoms. Jarisch-Herxheimer reaction is found after treatment of secondary syphilis resulting from release of endotoxin from spirochetes. Lucio reaction occurs specifically in individuals with leprosy from Mexico or the Caribbean and appears as large ulcerations of the lower extremities.
8. A. This is calciphylaxis, also called calcific uremic arteriolopathy, and typically occurs secondary to hyperparathyrodism from chronic hemodialysis. This is a rare but life-threatening cutaneous condition. Typically the hypercalcemia secondary to the hyperparathyroidism results in an increased calcium-phosphate product leading to calcium deposition in medium-sized blood vessels and subsequent inflammation. While no good treatments exist, hyperbaric oxygen and the calcium sequestering compound sodium thiosulfate have shown efficacy.
9. C. This is subcutaneous fat necrosis of the newborn. The distinguishing feature between this condition and sclerema neonatorum is that sclerema neonatorum is associated with preterm infants (up to 50% are premature) and the lesions rapidly spread. The lesions in subcutaneous fat necrosis of the newborn are discrete mobile plaques on the back, thighs, and cheeks. Fat necrosis and crystallization are characteristic. Erythema toxicum neonatorum is a benign erythematous eruption involving the face and trunks of newborns.
10. B. This is erythema nodosum in the setting of inflammatory bowel disease. As with other autoimmune conditions, posterior uveitis is typical and frequent ophthalmologic evaluation is necessary.

REFERENCES

Adhe V., Dongre A., Khopkar U.: A retrospective analysis of histopathology of 64 cases of lepra reactions. *Indian J Dermatol,* 2012;57:114–117.

Bassett MD et al: Deep-seated, well-differentiated lipomatous tumors of the chest wall and extremities: the role of cytogenetics in classification and prognostication. *Cancer* 2005;103(2): p. 409–416.

Brenn T. *Chapter 129. Neoplasms of Subcutaneous Fat* in *Fitzpatrick's Dermatology in General Medicine*, 8th Ed., L.A. Goldsmith, et al., ed. The McGraw-Hill Companies: New York; 2012.

Dauden E. and M.J. Onate: Calciphylaxis. *Dermatol Clin* 2008;26(4):557–568, ix.

Delgado-Jimenez Y., J. Fraga and A. Garcia-Diez: Infective panniculitis. *Dermatol Clin* 2008;26(4):471–480, vi.

Dimson O.G. and N.B. Esterly: Annular lipoatrophy of the ankles. *J Am Acad Dermatol* 2006;54(2 Suppl):S40–42.

Fraga J. and A. Garcia-Diez: Lupus erythematosus panniculitis. *Dermatol Clin* 2008;26(4):453–463, vi.

Fletcher CDM, Unni K.K., Mertens, F. *Chapter 1. Adipocytic tumours* in *World Health Organization classification of tumours. Pathology and genetics of tumors of soft tissue and bone.* IARC Press: Lyon; 2002.

Gallardo F. and R.M. Pujol: Subcutaneous panniculitic-like T-cell lymphoma and other primary cutaneous lymphomas with prominent subcutaneous tissue involvement. *Dermatol Clin* 2008;26(4):529–540, viii.

Garcia-Romero D. and F. Vanaclocha: Pancreatic panniculitis. *Dermatol Clin* 2008;26(4):465–470, vi.

Guhl G. and A. Garcia-Diez: *Subcutaneous sweet syndrome. Dermatol Clin* 2008;26(4):541–551, viii–ix.

Haimovic A. et al. Sarcoidosis: a comprehensive review and update for the dermatologist: part I. Cutaneous disease. *J Am Acad Dermatol* 2012;66(5):699 e1–e18; quiz 717–718.

Haimovic A. et al.: Sarcoidosis: a comprehensive review and update for the dermatologist: part II. Extracutaneous disease. *J Am Acad Dermatol* 2012;66(5):719 e1–e10; quiz 729–730.

Herranz P. et al.: Lipodystrophy syndromes. *Dermatol Clin* 2008;26(4):569–578, ix.

Hendrick S.J., Silverman A.K., Solomon A.R. et al.: Alpha-1 antitrypsin deficiency associated with panniculitis. *J Am Acad Dermatol* 1988;18:684–692.

Montgomery H., O'Leary P.A., Barker N.W.: Nodular vascular diseases of the legs: erythema induratum and allied conditions. *JAMA* 1945;128:335–341.

Moreno A., J. Marcoval, and J. Peyri: Traumatic panniculitis. *Dermatol Clin* 2008;26(4):481–483, vii.

Nelson L. and K.J. Stewart: Experience in the treatment of HIV-associated lipodystrophy. *J Plast Reconstr Aesthet Surg* 2008;61(4)366–371.

Pollex R.L. and R.A. Hegele: Hutchinson-Gilford progeria syndrome. *Clin Genet* 2004;66(5)375–381.

Quesada-Cortes A. et al.: Cold panniculitis. *Dermatol Clin* 2008;26(4):485–489, vii.

Requena C., O. Sanmartin, and L. Requena: Sclerosing panniculitis. *Dermatol Clin* 2008;26(4):501–504, vii.

Requena L. Normal subcutaneous fat: necrosis of adipocytes and classification of the panniculitides. *Semin Cutan Med Surg* 2007;26:66–70.

Requena L. and E.S. Yus: Erythema nodosum. *Dermatol Clin* 2008;26(4):425–438, v.

Sanmartin O., C. Requena, and L. Requena: Factitial panniculitis. *Dermatol Clin* 2008;26(4):519–527, viii.

Segura S. and L. Requena: Anatomy and histology of normal subcutaneous fat, necrosis of adipocytes, and classification of the panniculitides. *Dermatol Clin* 2008;26(4):419–424, v.

Snow J.l., Su D. *Lipomembranous (membranocystic) fat necrosis: clinicopathologic correlation of 38 cases. Am J Dermatopathol* 1996;18(2)151–155.

Su W.P., Person J.R. Morphea profunda: A new concept and a histopathologic study of 23 cases. *Am J Dermatopathol* 1981;3(3)251–260.

Torrelo A. and A. Hernandez: Panniculitis in children. *Dermatol Clin* 2008;26(4):491–500, vii.

Torabian S.Z., Fazel N., Knuttel R.: *Necrobiotic xanthogranuloma treated with chlorambucil. Dermatol Online J* 2006;12(5) [accessed November, 14 2012].

Valverde R. et al.: Alpha-1-antitrypsin deficiency panniculitis. *Dermatol Clin* 2008;26(4):447–451, vi.

Weiss S.W., Goldblum J.R. *Chapter 15. Benign lipomatous tumors* and *chapter 16. Liposarcoma* in *Enzinger and Weiss's Soft Tissue Tumors*, 5th Ed. Philadelphia: Mosby: Elsevier; 2008.

CHAPTER 11

CUTANEOUS TUMORS

JOY H. KUNISHIGE
ALEXANDER J. LAZAR

SURFACE EPITHELIAL TUMORS

Seborrheic Keratosis

- Appearance: sharply delineated, scaly or greasy, tan papules that appear "stuck on" the surface (Fig. 11-1)
- Location: upper trunk, shoulder, face, and scalp (sun-exposed areas), but can occur anywhere (except palms and soles)
- Demographics: more than 30 years
- Histology: epithelial proliferations characterized by hyperkeratosis, papillomatosis, and acanthosis, with horn pseudocysts (called "pseudo" because they connect to surface, and they have no true epithelial lining)
- Leser-Trelat syndrome: sudden onset of numerous seborrheic keratoses associated with internal malignancies, most commonly GI adenocarcinoma, breast carcinoma, and lymphoma
- Variations
  - Inverted follicular keratosis: verrucous, intradermal or "inverted" form of irritated seborrheic keratosis along a hair follicle, with prominent squamous eddies
  - Dermatosis papulosa nigra: multiple small, pedunculated, and heavily pigmented tag-like papules on the face of African-American and Afro-Caribbean patients (Fig. 11-2)
  - Stucco keratosis (keratosis alba): white-to-light brown, flat keratotic papule on dorsa of feet, ankles, hands, and forearms
  - Melanoacanthoma: deeply pigmented seborrheic keratosis in which an epidermal proliferation of large dendritic melanocytes is identified
  - Acanthosis nigricans: hyperpigmented velvety plaques on neck and axillae associated with obesity, diabetes, and endocrinopathies; histology similar to seborrheic keratosis but no acanthosis
  - Confluent and reticulated papillomatosis (CARP): multiple brown verrucous papules in reticulated pattern on inframammary or interscapular trunk during puberty; histology similar to seborrheic keratosis but no acanthosis and pityrosporum can be identified
  - Lichenoid keratosis: solitary pink to red-brown papule on forearm or upper chest; may represent inflamed lentigo, actinic keratosis, or seborrheic keratosis

Epidermal Nevus

- Appearance: yellowish-brown warty papules or plaques (Fig. 11-3)
- Location: usually trunk and extremities
- Demographics: birth or during childhood
- Characterization: congenital hamartoma (nevus) of epidermis
- Three subtypes
  - Nevus verrucosus: solitary or multiple localized lesions
  - Nevus unius lateralis: extensive unilateral linear distribution
  - Ichthyosis hystrix: extreme involvement with bilateral or generalized distribution
- Histology: hyperkeratosis, papillomatosis, acanthosis, and elongation of the rete ridges
- Syndromes
  - Epidermal nevus syndrome: skeletal, ocular, and central nervous system (CNS) abnormalities
  - Nevus comedonicus syndrome: nevus comedonicus with cutaneous, skeletal, and CNS abnormalities
- Variations
  - Nevus sebaceus: see Sebaceous Tumors
  - Linear porokeratosis: see Porokeratosis
  - Linear epidermal nevus: verrucous yellow-brown papules in a linear arrangement (systemic form follows Blaschko lines) due to heterozygous point mutation in the keratin 10 gene; histologically resembles nevus sebaceus with focal epidermolytic hyperkeratosis and lack of adnexal components
  - Nevus comedonicus: group of open comedones on face, trunk, neck, and upper extremities; keratin-filled invaginations of the epidermis

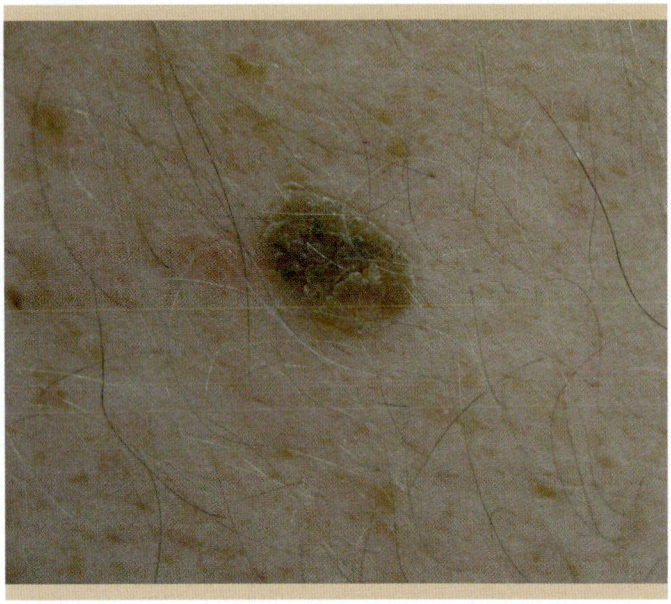

FIGURE 11-1 Seborrheic keratosis. (*Used with permission from Dr. Asra Ali.*)

Acrokeratosis Verruciformis of Hopf

- Appearance: dry, rough, skin-colored, verrucoid papules
- Location: dorsal forearms, hands, and feet
- Demographics: develops in infancy or early childhood
- Characterization: if multiple, can be associated with Darier disease
- Histology: hyperkeratosis, acanthosis, orthokeratosis, hypergranulosis, and mild papillomatosis with a "church spire" appearance

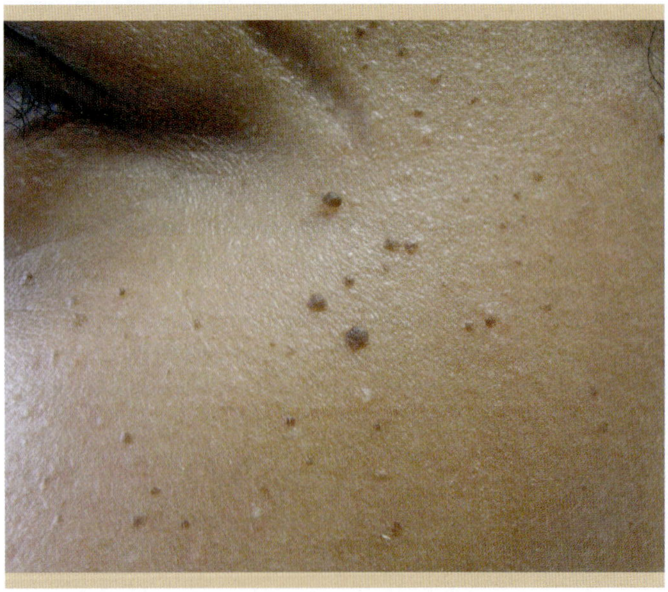

FIGURE 11-2 Dermatosis papulosa nigra. (*Used with permission from Dr. Asra Ali.*)

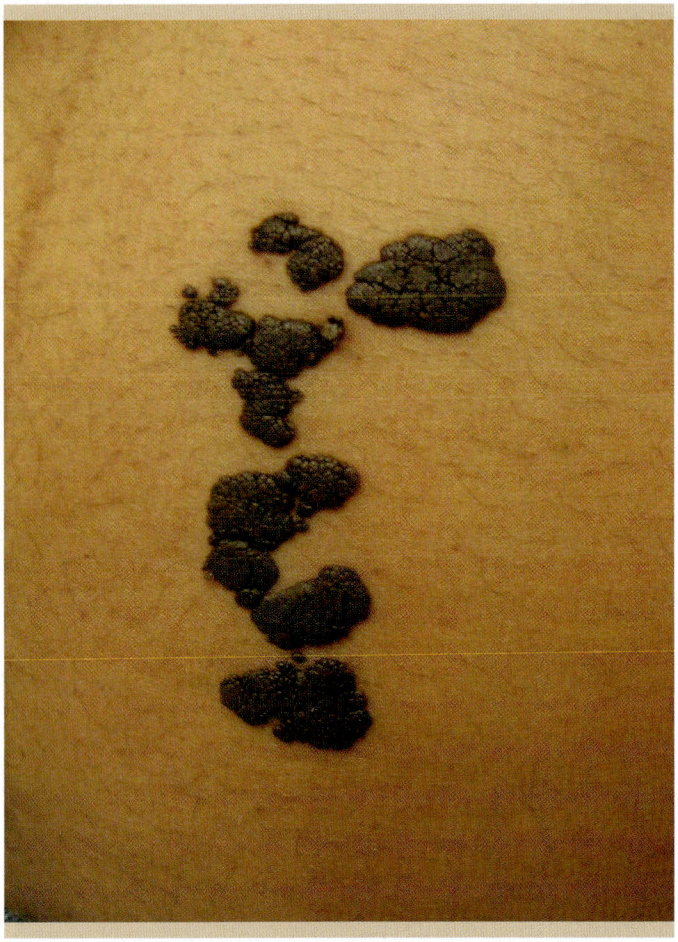

FIGURE 11-3 Epidermal nevus. (*Used with permission from Dr. Asra Ali.*)

Intraepidermal Epithelioma of Borst-Jadassohn

- Characterization: currently regarded as a recognizable histopathological pattern rather than a precise clinicopathologic entity
- Histology: nests of clonal keratinocytes in the background of a seborrheic keratosis, actinic keratosis, hidroacanthoma simplex sometimes referred to as intraepidermal eccrine poroma, or Bowen disease

Porokeratosis

- Appearance: annular hyperkeratotic papule or plaque with atrophic center and thread-like border (Fig. 11-4)
- Characterization: misnomer since no relationship to pore of eccrine duct
- Histology: cornoid lamella (column of parakeratosis over hypogranulosis and dyskeratosis that corresponds to annular ridge seen clinically)
- Variations
  - Porokeratosis of Mibelli: this prototype is a larger plaque that develops during first decade; more prominent cornoid lamella

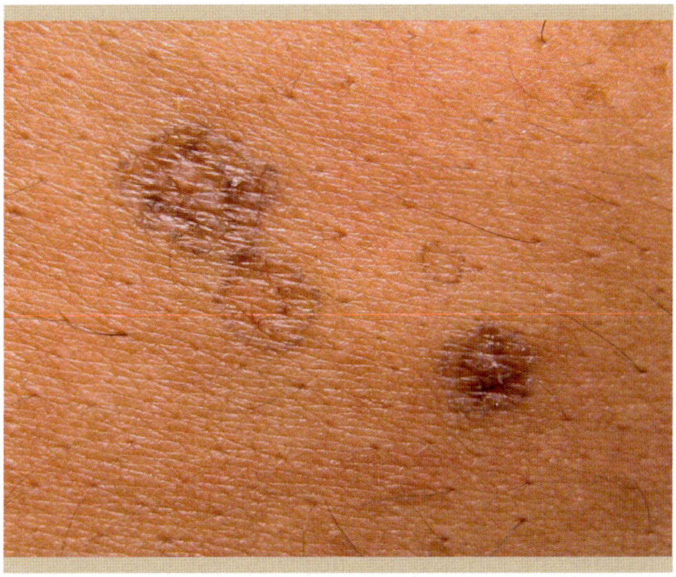

FIGURE 11-4 Porokeratosis. (*Used with permission from the Department of Dermatology, University of Texas Medical Branch at Galveston.*)

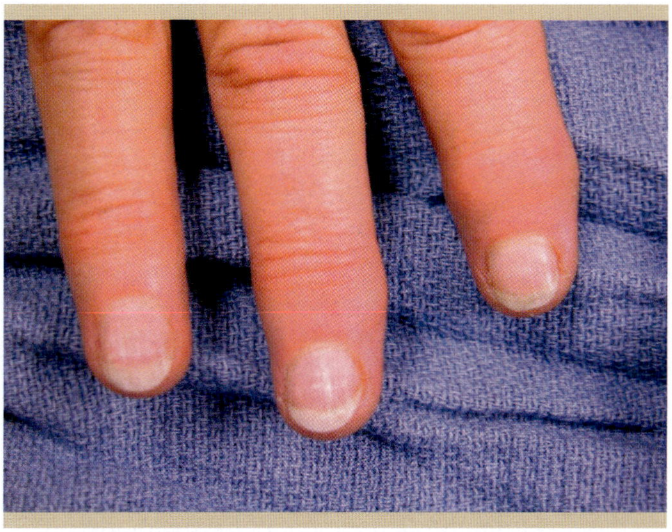

FIGURE 11-5 Mees lines. (*Used with permission from the Department of Dermatology, University of Texas Medical Branch at Galveston.*)

   - Linear porokeratosis: epidermal nevus affecting extremities and following lines of Blaschko
   - Porokeratosis punctata palmaris et plantaris: small foci that begin in young adults
   - Disseminated superficial actinic porokeratosis (DSAP): most common type presents as papules scattered over the extensor forearms and legs; this type has lowest risk for developing SCC

Warty Dyskeratoma (Isolated Dyskeratosis Follicularis)

- Appearance: umbilicated papule with keratotic plug
- Location: head, neck, or face (sun-exposed skin)
- Histology: epidermal cup-shaped invagination with focal acantholysis, dyskeratosis (corps ronds and grains), and parakeratosis

Arsenical Keratosis

- Appearance: gray, firm, hyperkeratotic papules
- Location: usually on palms, forearms, soles, trunk, and face
- Characterization
   - Arsenic impairs nucleotide excision repair and enhances proliferation of human keratinocytes; found in medications, Fowler solution, and well water
   - Can turn into squamous cell carcinoma (most commonly) or basal cell carcinoma; also associated with internal malignancies (GI adenocarcinoma)
   - Mees lines on the fingernails (Fig. 11-5)
- Histology: thick, compact hyperkeratosis, parakeratosis, and acanthosis with atypical keratinocytes; may resemble Bowen disease

Large Cell Acanthoma

- Appearance: solitary, slightly scaly papule with sharply demarcated borders
- Location: sun-exposed areas
- Characterization: thought to represent a type of actinic keratosis, but now considered by many to be an infrequent stage of solar lentigo evolution
- Histology: hyperkeratosis, keratinocytes are 2 times larger than normal without atypia, and lentiginous hyperpigmentation

Clear Cell Acanthoma (Pale Cell Acanthoma)

- Appearance: papule or nodule with well-defined borders and crust, less than 2 cm
- Location: usually anterior lower extremities
- Histology: proliferation of pale keratinocytes (periodic acid–Schiff (PAS) staining positive due to cytoplasmic accumulation of glycogen) with sharp demarcation from normal epidermis, neutrophils in epidermis, microabscesses in stratum corneum, and dilated capillaries in dermal papillae

Epidermolytic Acanthoma

- Appearance: solitary tumor arising on the trunk of older patients
- Histology: compact hyperkeratosis, papillomatosis, acanthosis, perinucleolar vacuolization of keratinocytes in stratum spinosum, hypergranulosis with large basophilic keratohyaline granules and intracytoplasmic eosinophilic bodies (epidermolytic hyperkeratosis)

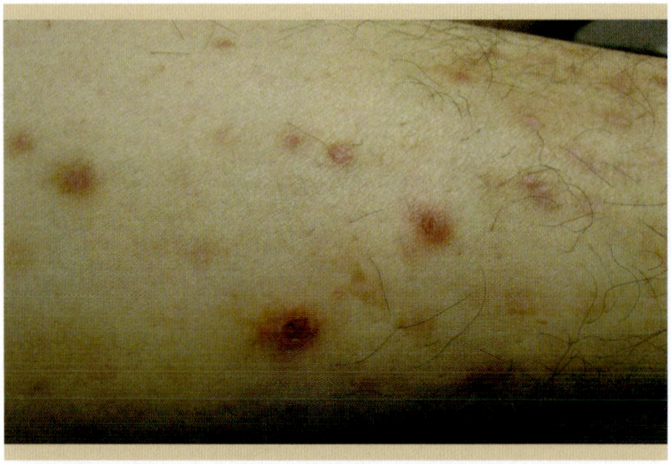

FIGURE 11-6 Prurigo nodularis. (*Used with permission from the Department of Dermatology, University of Texas Medical Branch at Galveston.*)

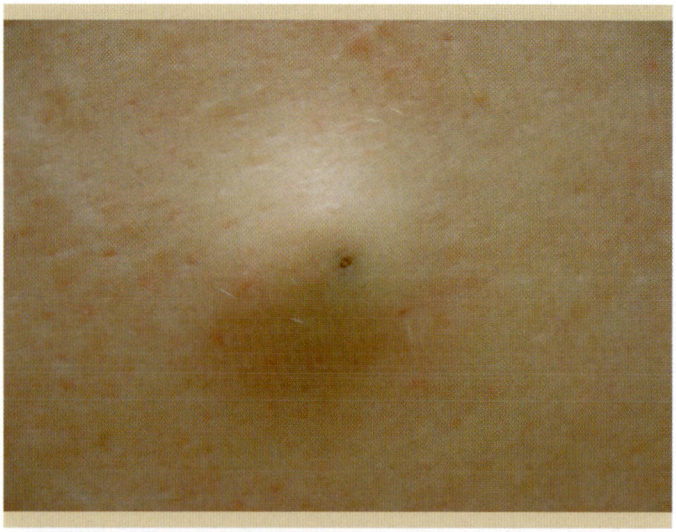

FIGURE 11-7 Epidermal inclusion cyst. (*Used with permission from Dr. Asra Ali.*)

Prurigo Nodularis

- Appearance: multiple or solitary nodules, usually symmetric with excoriations present, extremely pruritic (Fig. 11-6)
- Characterization: within the spectrum of lichen simplex
- Histology: pseudoepitheliomatous hyperplasia, hyperkeratosis, hypergranulosis, focal parakeratosis, occasional spongiosis and exocytosis of mononuclear cells, and vertical collagen between elongated rete

Acanthoma Fissuratum

- Appearance: pink or flesh-colored nodule with a central groove at sites of pressure from eyeglasses
- Location: lateral nasal bridge and retroauricular sulcus (granuloma fissuratum)
- Histology: acanthosis with broad rete ridges and central depressed area corresponding to the groove seen clinically

Chondrodermatitis Nodularis Helicis (CNH)

- Appearance: tender, skin-colored to erythematous nodule on helix or antihelix
- Characterization: thought related to sleeping on affected side, but other proposed etiologic factors include trauma or actinic damage
- Histology: Epidermal hyperplasia and ulceration over granulation, fibrosis, solar elastosis, and degenerated cartilage

CYSTS

Epidermoid Cyst (Epidermal Inclusion Cyst, Follicular Infundibular Cyst)

- Appearance: smooth dome-shaped subcutaneous nodule with or without punctum (Fig. 11-7)
- Location: face, neck, and trunk, but can occur anywhere
- Demographics: young and middle-aged adults
- Characterization: most common type of cyst of the skin
- Histology: cyst wall is squamous epithelium with granular layer similar to surface epidermis and contains lamellated keratin; cyst rupture can cause inflammatory reaction with foreign-body giant cells, lymphocytes, plasma cells, and neutrophils
- Variations
  - Milium: much smaller epidermoid cyst (1–2 mm) (Fig. 11-8)

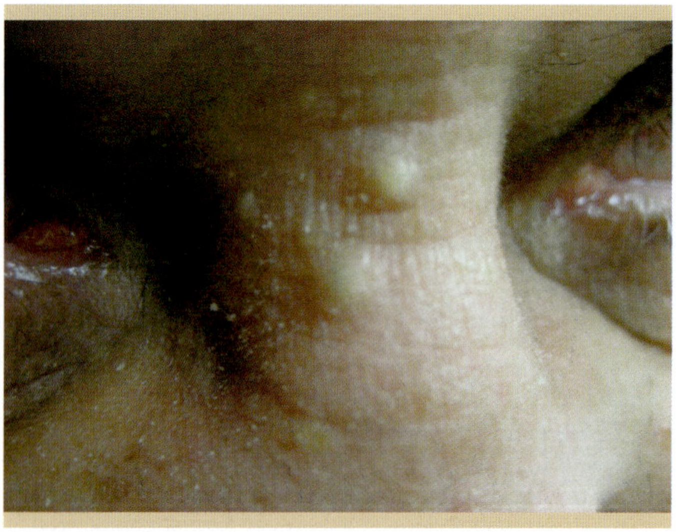

FIGURE 11-8 Milia. (*Used with permission from Dr. Asra Ali.*)

- Ear pit: preauricular pits or cysts lined by stratified squamous epithelium with a granular layer; should prompt hearing evaluation in newborns
- Proliferating epidermoid cyst: unlike proliferating trichilemmal cysts, only 20% occur on scalp; most have peripheral proliferation into surrounding dermis and may have infiltrative growth pattern

Pilar Cyst (Trichilemmal Cyst)

- Appearance: smooth, firm, mobile nodule
- Location: mostly on scalp
- Characterization: derived from the outer root sheath of the hair follicle
- Histology: cyst wall is squamous epithelium lacking a granular layer, contains compact, homogenized keratin, calcification, and cholesterol clefts common
- Variations
  - Proliferating trichilemmal cyst (see Follicular Tumors)
  - Pilomatricoma (see Follicular Tumors)

Dermoid Cyst

- Appearance: subcutaneous freely mobile cyst; occasionally fixed to periosteum
- Location: lateral upper eyelid, may have intracranial extension
- Demographics: develops in infancy or early childhood
- Characterization: hamartomatous lesion due to sequestration of epithelium along embryonal lines of closure
- Histology: cyst wall is squamous epithelium with granular layer, contains lamellated keratin and hair follicles open into the cyst
- Variation
  - Pilonidal cyst: part of the follicular inclusion tetrad that presents as inflamed, painful nodule in upper gluteal cleft; cystic space or sinus tract contains hair and keratin, and is lined with granulation tissue and inflammation

Vellus Hair Cyst

- Appearance: minute solitary cyst, or multiple on child's chest
- Histology: cyst lined by squamous epithelium with granular layer, contains lamellated keratin and vellus hair shafts; K17 staining positive but K10 staining negative
- Variation
  - Eruptive vellus hair cysts: acneiform eruption on chest that may be associated with ectodermal dysplasias, particularly pachyonychia congenital type 2

Steatocystoma

- Appearance: firm, translucent to yellow nodule that extrudes yellowish oily material
- Location: trunk, head, neck, earlobes
- Characterization: true sebaceous cyst

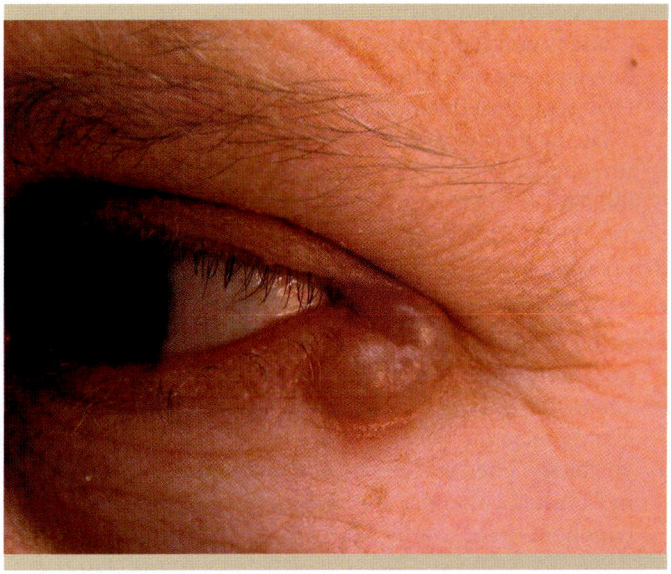

FIGURE 11-9 Hidrocystoma. (*Used with permission from the Department of Dermatology, University of Texas Medical Branch at Galveston.*)

- Histology: cyst wall embedded with flattened sebaceous glands and lined with crenulated eosinophilic cuticle of keratin instead of a granular layer; K10 and K17 staining positive
- Variant
  - Steatocystoma multiplex: autosomal dominant disorder that presents during adolescence (mutations in gene encoding keratin 17); can be associated with pachyonychia congenital type 2

Hidrocystoma (Cystadenoma)

- Appearance: solitary, translucent, bluish cyst (Fig. 11-9)
- Location: eyelid or cheek
- Histology: unilocular or multilocular dermal cyst lined by a double layer of cuboidal cells (eccrine) or apocrine decapitation

Branchial Cleft Cyst

- Appearance: smooth, painless mass
- Location: preauricular cheek, jaw, or lateral neck anterior to sternocleidomastoid muscle
- Demographics: child or young adult
- Characterization: remnant of the second branchial cleft in embryonic development
- Histology: lined by stratified squamous or respiratory (pseudostratified ciliated columnar) epithelium with goblet cells, lymphoid tissue often present

Bronchogenic Cyst

- Appearance: small, solitary, painless mass
- Location: above sternal notch

- Demographics: present at birth
- Characterization: formed from portions of foregut during development of tracheobronchial tree
- Histology: pseudostratified, cuboidal, or columnar ciliated epithelium with or without goblet cells, may be surrounded by smooth muscle, mucous glands, lymphoid follicles, or cartilage

Thyroglossal Duct Cyst

- Appearance: solitary, fluctuant, painless mass that moves with swallowing
- Location: midline neck, near hyoid bone
- Characterization: vestigial remnant of the tubular thyroid gland precursor
- Histology: lined by cuboidal, columnar, or pseudostratified ciliated columnar epithelium; thyroid follicles and lymphoid tissue nearby

Mucocele

- Appearance: translucent papule or nodule
- Location: mucosal surface of lip
- Characterization: caused by minor salivary gland trauma
- Histology: ruptured minor salivary duct or gland adjacent to cystic space filled with sialomucin (PAS positive, diastase resistant; also positive acid mucopolysaccharide stains)

Digital Mucous Cyst

- Appearance: translucent papule or nodule
- Location: dorsal proximal nail fold
- Characterization: some represent herniation of joint space
- Histology: mucin in clefts between collagen bundles under acral epidermis, positive staining with acid mucopolysaccharide stains

DUCTAL (APOCRINE/ECCRINE) TUMORS

Apocrine/Eccrine Nevus

- Appearance: hyperhidrotic patch
- Location: scalp, axilla, upper extremities, presternal, or inguinal area
- Characterization: rare hamartoma of apocrine or eccrine unit
- Histology: increased size or number of mature apocrine or eccrine glands
- Variations
  - Eccrine angiomatous hamartoma: increased number of eccrine glands with small blood vessels, nerve fibers, mucin, and fat
  - Porokeratotic eccrine ostial nevus: cornoid lamellae associated with eccrine ducts on hands and feet; some classify with epidermal nevi

Tubular Apocrine Adenoma

- Appearance: rare, slow-growing nodule with female predominance (2:1)
- Location: most often on scalp and perianal skin
- Characterization: may be on spectrum between syringocystadenoma papilliferum (apocrine) and primary eccrine adenoma (eccrine)
- Histology: well-circumscribed dermal tumor (without epidermal connection) composed of well-formed tubules; papillary projections without stroma extend into lumina

Nipple Adenoma (Erosive Adenomatosis, Florid Papillomatosis, Superficial Papillary Adenomatosis)

- Appearance: unilateral crusted papule or plaque
- Location: on the nipple; may mimic Paget disease
- Characterization: ductal hyperplasia of the lactiferous ducts
- Histology: mixture of intraductal papilloma and tubular glands with apocrine decapitation, lined by epithelial and myoepithelial cells, usually communicating with the surface epithelium; plasma cell or lymphocytic infiltrate sometimes

Hidradenoma Papilliferum

- Appearance: solitary, mobile nodule which may exhibit superficial erosion
- Location: vulvar or perianal regions
- Demographics: young or middle-aged women
- Histology: well-circumscribed, cystic tumor (usually without communication to surface) with maze-like glandular spaces, and papillary processes with apocrine differentiation

Syringocystadenoma Papilliferum

- Appearance: erythematous, warty solitary plaque, or linear arrangement of papules (Fig. 11-10)
- Location: most common on scalp
- Characterization: often found in association with nevus sebaceus (5–20%)
- Histology: epithelial-lined papillae invaginating from the overlying epidermis and lined with a double layer of cells (columnar layer with apocrine decapitation on the luminal side, and a cuboidal layer at the periphery); fibrovascular cords with plasma cells

Cylindroma

- Appearance: pink, firm, rubbery nodule; solitary or multiple coalescing into "turban tumor"
- Location: scalp, head, neck, sometimes trunk or genitalia
- Characterization: cylindroma and spiradenoma are considered part of a spectrum of more primitive sweat gland lesions; multiple cylindromas prompt consideration of Brooke-Spiegler syndrome; malignant cylindromas may develop

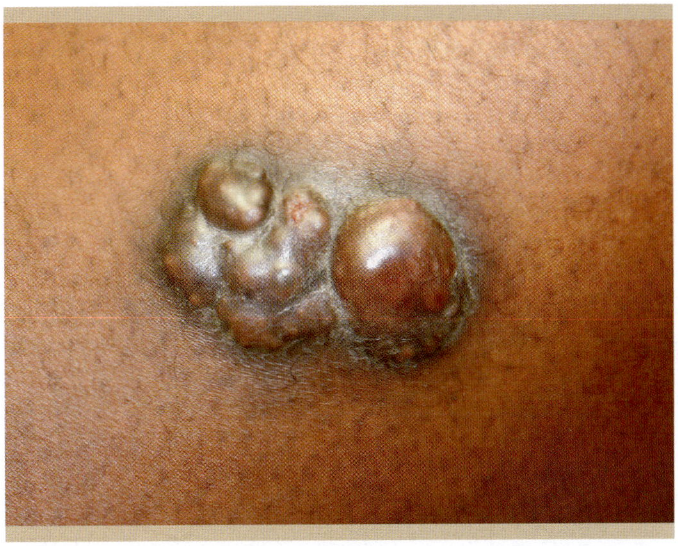

FIGURE 11-10 Syringocystadenoma papilliferum. (*Used with permission from the Department of Dermatology, University of Texas Medical Branch at Galveston.*)

- Histology: dermal tumor without connection to the overlying epidermis; multiple lobules of basaloid tumor cells surrounded by a hyaline basement membrane that fit together like pieces of a jigsaw puzzle; eosinophilic hyaline sheaths and hyaline droplets are PAS positive (composed of type IV collagen and laminin)
- Brooke-Spiegler syndrome: autosomal dominant condition (*CYLD* gene on chromosome 16q) characterized by multiple cylindromas, spiradenomas, and trichoepitheliomas

Spiradenoma

- Appearance: solitary, painful dermal nodule with bluish hue in adolescents and young adults
- Location: scalp, neck, and upper trunk
- Histology: sharply demarcated dermal nodule of "big blue balls" comprised of two cell types: peripheral dark small blue cells arranged in rosettes, and central pale large blue cells; can have overlapping features with cylindroma

Syringoma

- Appearance: usually multiple, skin-colored to tan, flat-topped small papules (Fig. 11-11)
- Location: lower eyelids and upper cheeks
- Demographics: commonly seen in females at puberty; associated with Down syndrome, Marfan syndrome, and Ehlers-Danlos syndrome
- Characterization: eccrine duct adenoma
- Histology: small ducts with elongated tails (tadpoles) embedded in a sclerotic stroma, lumens filled with PAS positive eosinophilic, amorphous debris; histologic

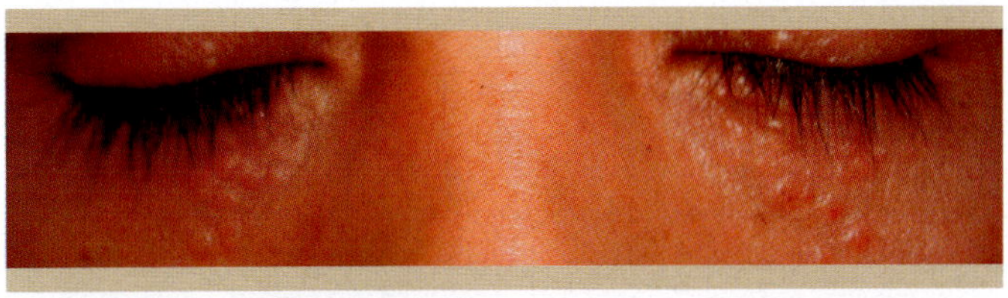

FIGURE 11-11 Syringoma. (*Used with permission from Dr. Melissa Bogle.*)

differential diagnosis includes sclerotic basal cell carcinoma, desmoplastic trichoepithelioma, and microcystic adnexal carcinoma
- Variations
  - Eruptive syringomas: large crops on anterior chest of child, present in ~18% of Down syndrome patients
  - Clear cell syringomas: associated with diabetes mellitus

Chondroid Syringoma (Mixed Tumor of the Skin)

- Appearance: solitary, skin-colored, slow growing firm nodule or cyst
- Location: head and neck
- Demographics: middle age, males > females
- Histology: clusters of tumor cells and ductal structures set in a chondroid, myxoid, and fibrous stroma; areas of ossification can be noted

Eccrine Poroma

- Appearance: painless, skin-colored, firm to rubbery, dome-shaped nodule, less than 2 cm in diameter
- Location: scalp, palm, or sole of foot
- Demographics: middle age
- Histology: solid masses of cuboidal or basaloid epithelial cells with ovoid nuclei; tumor in continuity with overlying epidermis; small sweat ducts usually present
- Variations
- Intraepidermal poroma (hidroacanthoma simplex): confined to the surface epidermis
- Juxtaepidermal poroma: broad connection to epidermis but also involving the superficial dermis
- Intradermal poroma (dermal duct tumor): tumor restricted to dermis
- Eccrine poromatosis: greater than 100 papules on palms/soles

Eccrine Acrospiroma (Nodular Hidradenoma)

- Appearance: solitary, slow-growing, painless nodule; usually less than 2 cm in diameter (Fig. 11-12)
- Location: usually on scalp, face, or trunk
- Characterization: some authors consider hidroacanthoma simplex, poroma, dermal duct tumor, and hidradenoma under the unifying term of "eccrine acrospiroma"
- Histology: well-circumscribed nests of tumor cells made up of basaloid and clear cells; sweat duct lumina present
- Variations

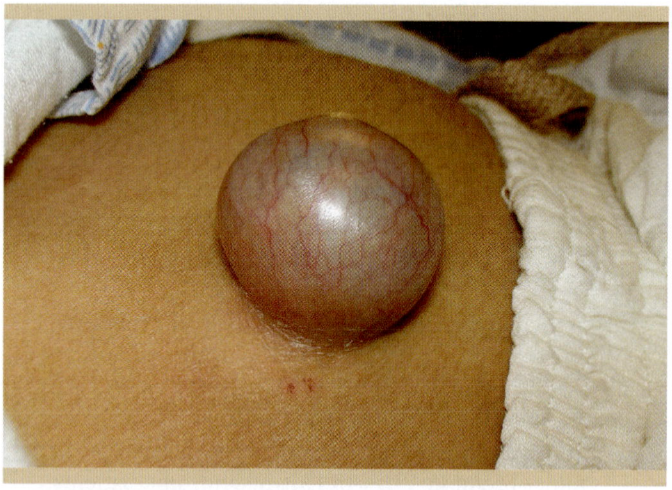

FIGURE 11-12 Eccrine acrospiroma. (*Used with permission from the Department of Dermatology, University of Texas Medical Branch at Galveston.*)

- Clear cell hidradenoma: pale or clear cells containing glycogen (PAS staining positive)
- Solid-cystic hidradenoma: common on scalp; prevalent cystic spaces plus solid areas

Malignant Sweat Gland Tumors

- Appearance: solitary, slow-growing papule or indistinct plaque
- Location: usually on upper lip, nasolabial area, or periorbital regions
- Characterization: malignant transformation of above-described adnexal tumors may be marked by rapid growth, ulceration, and bleeding
- Histology: deeply infiltrating strands of ductal cells with small lumina; pleomorphic, hyperchromatic, highly mitotic with areas of necrosis; perineural invasion common
- Variations
  - Microcystic adnexal carcinoma (sclerosing sweat duct carcinoma): indurated plaques or nodules on the upper lip, chin, nasolabial fold, nose; aggressive local invasion and indolent course
    - Histology: superficial portion contains keratinous cysts and abortive hair follicles in desmoplastic stroma; deeper portion features basaloid nests (resembling sclerosing basal cell carcinoma) and small ducts without atypia reminiscent of syringoma; perineural invasion frequently seen; epithelial membrane antigen (EMA) and carcinoembryonic antigen (CEA) staining positive
  - Primary mucinous carcinoma (adenocystic carcinoma): slow-growing, erythematous or blue nodules or plaques on head and neck, especially eyelids; middle-aged to elderly males (2:1); locally aggressive but rare metastasis
    - Histology: duct-forming tumor cells suspended in abundant pools of mucin, compartmentalized by delicate fibrous septa
  - Adenoid cystic carcinoma (ACC): slow and relentless painful plaques more than 3 cm; middle-aged to elderly women; typically originates in salivary glands but can have primary cutaneous presentation on scalp more than trunk/extremities
    - Histology: irregularly shaped aggregation of basaloid cells arranged in solid and/or sieve-like patterns (cribriform); propensity for perineural invasion; CEA and EMA positive
  - Apocrine carcinoma (Fig. 11-13): rare, solitary or multiple nodules and plaques measuring 2 to 8 cm in diameter in the axillae or anogenital area
    - Histology: infiltrating dermal or subcutaneous nonencapsulated papillary tumor with ductal, solid, or mixed pattern; apocrine secretions and cords of neoplastic cells with variable pleomorphism, abnormal mitotic activity and necrosis; CAM 5.2, CEA, and S–100 positive
  - Malignant chondroid syringoma (malignant mixed tumor): extremely rare, solitary, painful, flesh-colored, or erythematous nodule, predilection for trunk and distal extremities (foot most common); typically develops de novo and 60% metastasize
    - Histology: infiltrative growth pattern, abnormal mitoses, tumor necrosis

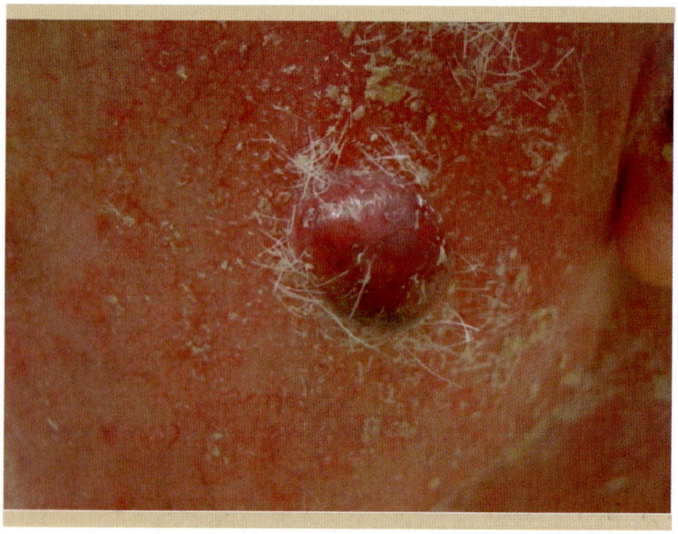

FIGURE 11-13 Apocrine adenocarcinoma. (*Used with permission from the Department of Dermatology, University of Texas Medical Branch at Galveston.*)

- Porocarcinoma: verrucoid plaque or polypoid growth in older individuals, usually on the lower extremities; about 20% metastasize
  - Histology: large islands and small, irregularly shaped nests with infiltrative borders; focal necrosis with clear cell areas, ductal structures, intracytoplasmic lumina formation, and squamous differentiation; PAS staining positive and usually diastase sensitive, cytokeratin, CEA, and EMA staining positive
- Spiradenocarcinoma: aggressive tumor, usually originates on a long-standing solitary lesion of spiradenoma on the lower extremities; local recurrences and metastasis
  - Histology: basaloid cells and occasional ductular differentiation extend into adipose; focal areas of necrosis and mononuclear reactive inflammation; low-molecular-weight cytokeratin and EMA staining positive

Paget Disease (Mammary and Extramammary)

- Appearance: patches resemble well-demarcated eczema, contact dermatitis, or Bowen disease with intense pruritus
- Location: extramammary Paget occurs in areas rich in apocrine sweat glands (groin, perianal, scrotum, or vulva)
- Demographics: elderly white women
- Characterization: nearly 100% of mammary Paget associated with intraductal breast cancer; up to 15% of extramammary Paget associated with underlying carcinoma (e.g., adnexal adenocarcinoma, colorectal, or urothelial carcinoma, etc.), underlying malignancy more common with perianal location
- Histology: Paget cells (large, vacuolated cells with a bluish cytoplasm) in the lower epidermis which spread along the rete ridges and adnexal structures; sialomucin stains with PAS and diastase, colloidal iron, and mucicarmine; Paget cells stain with EMA, CEA, cytokeratin 7
- Immunostaining sometimes helpful for excluding associated internal malignancy

FOLLICULAR TUMORS

Trichoblastoma

- Appearance: well-circumscribed papule
- Location: head and neck
- Characterization: benign proliferation with follicular germinative differentiation; term "trichoblastoma" previously referred lesions larger and deeper than classic trichoepitheliomas
- Histology: well-circumscribed dermal aggregates of epithelial, basaloid, and mesenchymal components in a fibromyxoid stroma that extend into the subcutaneous tissue; increased mitotic activity and minimal pleomorphism

Trichoepithelioma

- Appearance: smaller dome-shaped papules
- Location: usually nose or nasolabial folds
- Characterization: follicular germinative differentiation like trichoblastoma, but also superficial follicular differentiation and more stroma
- Histology: palisading basaloid cells in a dense stroma with horn cysts, calcification, and papillary mesenchymal bodies; artifactual clefting is uncommon (in contrast to basal cell carcinoma); lacks deep and infiltrating growth pattern, perineural infiltration, and ductal differentiation (in contrast to microcystic adnexal carcinoma)
- Syndromes
  - Multiple trichoepithelioma: autosomal dominant, multiple on face start at puberty
  - Brooke-Spiegler syndrome: multiple trichoepitheliomas, cylindromas, spiradenomas, and milia, with risk for basal cell adenomas and gland adenocarcinomas (see Cylindromas above)
  - Rombo syndrome: vermiculate atrophoderma, milias, hypotrichosis, vellous hair cysts, basal cell carcinomas, and peripheral vasodilatation with cyanosis
  - Bazex syndrome: follicular atrophoderma, hypotrichosis, basal cell carcinoma, and localized or generalized hypohidrosis
- Variations
  - Desmoplastic trichoepithelioma: narrower strands of tumor cells, keratinous cysts, and calcification within prominent sclerotic stroma (resembling sclerosing basal cell carcinoma but pleomorphism, palisading, and peripheral clefting are not seen); must also exclude microcystic adnexal carcinoma
  - Giant solitary trichoepithelioma: deep involvement of the reticular dermis and subcutaneous tissue most common in perianal region
  - Trichoadenoma: rare solitary tumor located on the face, up to 5 cm in size; groups of horn cysts connected by epithelial strands; cells more squamous than basaloid

Trichofolliculoma

- Appearance: papule or nodule with central depression and protruding tuft of thread-like hairs (trichoids)
- Location: face
- Histology: follicular buds with vellus hairs radiating out from cystic space (usually communicating with the surface)
- Variations
  - Sebaceous trichofolliculoma: small sebaceous elements found within the follicular units
  - Pilar sheath acanthoma: usually on the upper lip of adults; keratin-filled dilated follicular infundibulum and marked lobular epithelial proliferation without hair shafts

- Dilated pore of Winer: usually on the face or trunk; dilated open follicle filled with keratin and irregular budding of the epithelium

Fibrofolliculoma

- Appearance: multiple small dome-shaped papules
- Location: face, scalp, and upper trunk
- Histology: dilated, well-formed hair follicle with a central keratin plug and anastomosing strands of basaloid cells arising from the infundibulum; surrounded by a fibrous stroma; residual sebaceous glands are often incorporated into the lesion
- Birt-Hogg-Dube syndrome: autosomal dominant (*BHD* gene on 17p) association of multiple fibrofolliculomas, acrochordons, trichodiscomas, pulmonary disease (spontaneous pneumothorax, pulmonary cysts), and renal tumors

Trichodiscoma

- Appearance: dome-shaped papules
- Location: face, scalp, and upper trunk
- Characterization: proliferation of the hair mantle on spectrum with fibrofolliculoma
- Histology: horizontally oriented epithelial cords surrounded by prominent stroma that contains fusiform and stellate fibroblasts and thin-walled blood vessels (similar to stroma of angiofibroma)

Trichilemmoma (Tricholemmoma)

- Appearance: smooth or warty papule or papules
- Histology: endophytic epithelial lobule with peripheral basal cell palisading and thickened eosinophilic hyaline basement membrane zone; cells located toward the center are clear (increased glycogen, PAS positive)
- Cowden syndrome: autosomal dominant disorder due to dysfunctional lipid phosphatase (loss of *PTEN*, chromosome 10q) resulting in multiple facial trichilemmomas, acral keratoses, dermal fibromas, oral mucosal papillomas, and systemic malignancies such as thyroid, breast, and endometrial carcinomas
- Variations
  - Desmoplastic tricholemmoma: lobulated tumor with irregular cords that infiltrate into the dermis; infiltrating pattern may be mistaken for malignant tumor (e.g., trichilemmal carcinoma, squamous cell carcinoma, or morpheaform basal cell carcinoma)
  - Tumor of the follicular infundibulum: dermal strands of clear epithelial cells parallel to the epidermis; also considered variant of seborrheic keratosis

Pilomatricoma (Calcifying Epithelioma of Malherbe)

- Appearance: firm, deep-seated nodule with angular elevation of skin ("tent sign")
- Location: head, neck, shoulders
- Demographics: occurs at any age; more common in children and young adults
- Characterization: activating point mutation in CTNNB1 with accumulation of nuclear β-catenin
- Histology: nodule resembling cyst composed of 2 cell types: uniform basaloid cells with high mitotic activity (early lesion), and necrotic cells with eosinophilic cytoplasm and lost nucleus called "shadow cells" (older lesion); transitional areas where basal cells turn into shadow cells; calcification, ossification, keratin debris predominant in older lesions; pilomatrical features can rarely be seen in the epidermoid inclusion cysts and is believed to be pathognomic of Gardner syndrome

Proliferating Trichilemmal Cyst (Pilar Tumor)

- Appearance: rare, enlarging dermal nodule
- Location: most common on scalp
- Characterization: arises within trichilemmal cyst
- Histology: well-circumscribed nodule, but cyst wall proliferating inward with trichilemmal keratinization (no granular layer); horn pearls and squamous eddies

SEBACEOUS TUMORS

Sebaceous Hyperplasia

- Appearance: yellowish papules with central umbilication (Fig. 11-14)
- Location: face, especially forehead and nose
- Histology: increased number of enlarged sebaceous lobules grouped around a centrally located, wide sebaceous duct

Sebaceous Adenoma

- Appearance: yellow papule or nodule, less than 1 cm
- Location: usually face or scalp
- Demographics: middle-aged adults
- Histology: well-circumscribed neoplasm composed of mature sebaceous cells (sebocytes) and peripheral, smaller basaloid (germinative) cells that represent less than 50% of the total lesional cells
- Muir-Torre syndrome: autosomal dominant defect in DNA mismatch repair gene, most commonly with loss of hMSH2 or hMLH1 protein expression; one or more sebaceous neoplasms (sebaceous adenoma, sebaceoma, or rarely sebaceous carcinoma) plus one or more visceral malignancies (most commonly gastrointestinal, endometrial, or genitourinary carcinomas)

Sebaceoma

- Appearance: yellow ill-defined plaque, 1 to 3 cm
- Location: face and scalp
- Demographics: elderly female predominance (4:1)

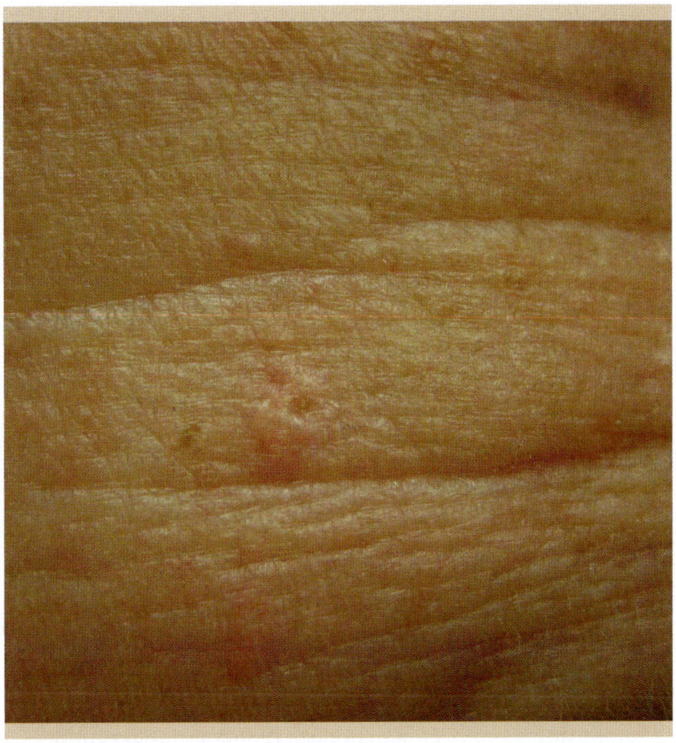

FIGURE 11-14 Sebaceous hyperplasia. (*Used with permission from Dr. Asra Ali.*)

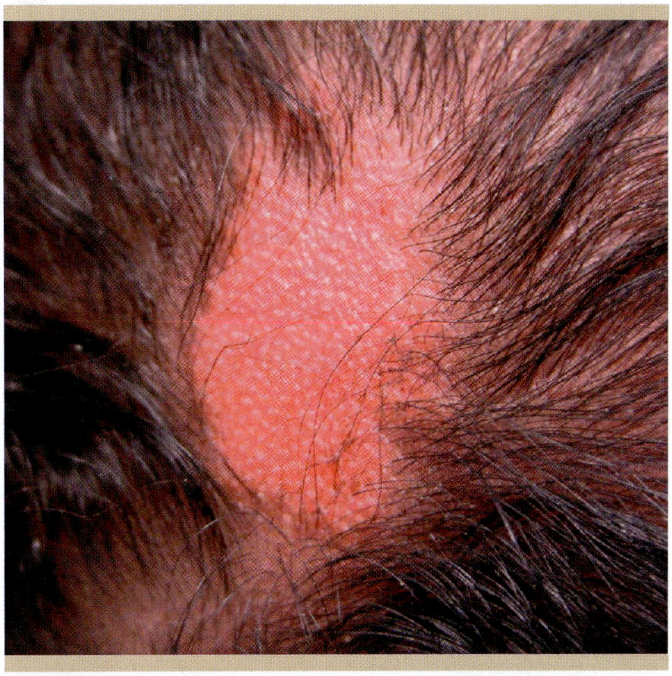

FIGURE 11-15 Nevus sebaceus. (*Used with permission from the Department of Dermatology, University of Texas Medical Branch at Galveston.*)

- Characterization: on spectrum with sebaceous adenoma, but deeper and more seboblastic (germinative) differentiation
- Histology: composed of sebocytes and smaller basaloid (germinative) cells that represent more than 50% of the total lesional cells
- Muir-Torre syndrome: see Sebaceous Adenoma above

Nevus Sebaceus of Jadassohn (Fig. 11-15)

- Appearance: 3 clinical stages
  - At birth: solitary, hairless, pinkish, yellow, orange, or tan plaque with a smooth or velvety macular surface
  - Puberty: lesion becomes verrucous and nodular; sebaceous glands enlarge and cause papillomatosis
  - Later in life: lesions may develop various types of appendageal tumors, including syringocystadenoma papilliferum (8–10%), trichoblastoma (5%), trichilemmoma (2–3%), sebaceoma (2–3%), syringoma, apocrine cystadenoma, hidradenoma, or keratoacanthoma
  - Apparently benign basaloid epithelial proliferations resembling basal cell carcinoma can be identified in 5 to 7% of cases of nevus sebaceus
  - Malignant tumors (apocrine carcinoma, basal cell carcinoma, squamous cell carcinoma) have been reported to arise in association with nevus sebaceus on occasion
- Location: face or scalp
- Histology: papillomatous and acanthotic hyperplasia, numbers of mature or nearly mature sebaceous glands are increased in the dermis, ectopic apocrine glands in the deep dermis beneath sebaceous glands, and reduced number of hair follicles
- Syndromes
  - Neurocutaneous syndrome: mental retardation, epilepsy, neurologic deficits, and rare skeletal deformities
  - Epidermal nevus syndrome (Schimmelpenning-Feuerstein-Mims syndrome, organoid nevus phakomatosis): combination of extensive sebaceous nevi with central nervous system, cardiac, ophthalmic, and skeletal muscle disorders

Sebaceous Carcinoma

- Appearance: firm, slow-growing, yellowish nodule
- Location: 75% arise in the periocular region (upper lid 2–3 times more common than lower lid), often mistaken for a chalazion, can mimic keratoconjunctivitis or blepharoconjunctivitis
- Demographics: sixth to seventh decade
- Characterization: aggressive clinical course with high recurrence rate (up to 40%); metastasis occurs in 14 to 25% of cases to lymph nodes and viscera

- Histology: infiltration of dermis by lobules composed of a mixture of small basaloid (germinative) cells and poorly differentiated sebaceous cells; marked pleomorphism, abnormal mitoses, and necrosis; pagetoid spread is seen in 40 to 80% of cases; oil red-O staining can be performed in frozen sections to highlight the sebocytes
- Muir-Torre syndrome: nonperiocular sebaceous carcinomas are much more commonly associated with the syndrome; see Sebaceous Adenoma

FIBROUS AND "FIBROHISTIOCYTIC" TUMORS

Acrochordon (Skin Tags, Fibroepithelial Polyp)

- Appearance: solitary or multiple skin-colored papules (Fig. 11-16)
- Location: neck, axilla, inguinal areas, and eyelids

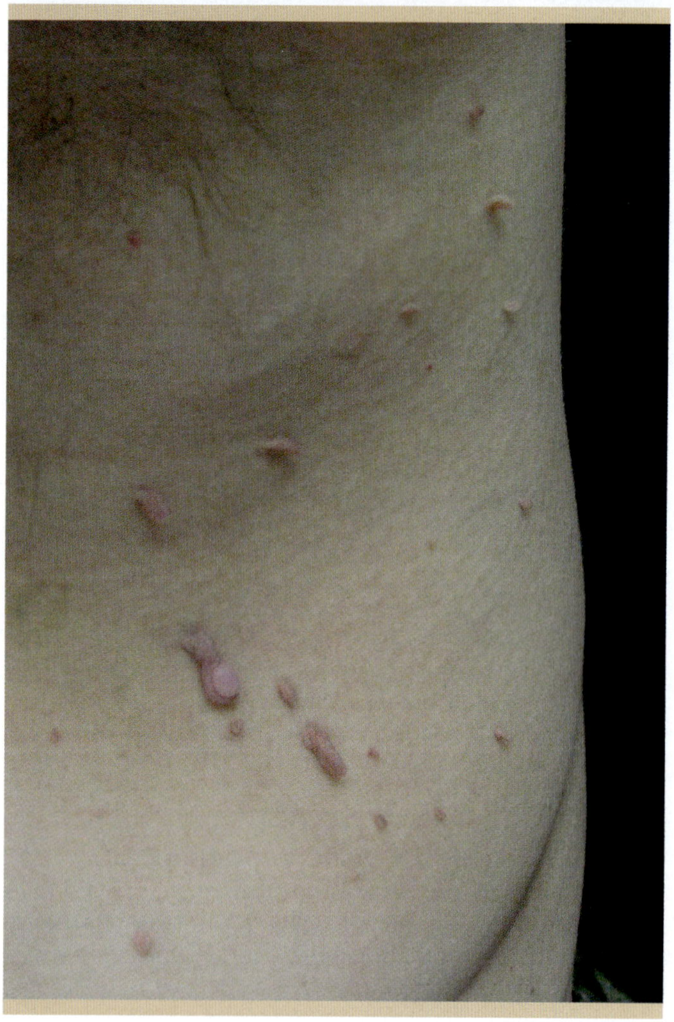

FIGURE 11-16 Acrochordon. (*Used with permission from the Department of Dermatology, University of Texas Medical Branch at Galveston.*)

- Histology: pedunculated polyp covered by epidermis with papillomatosis and acanthosis, fibrovascular stroma with fat tissue and dilated blood vessels
- Variation
    - Lipofibroma: acrochordon with large percentage of fat cells

Angiofibroma (Fibrous Papule)

- Appearance: dome-shaped skin-colored papule
- Location: nose and medial cheeks
- Histology: concentric oriented (around follicles) or perpendicular (to the epidermis) collagen fibers with stellate fibroblasts and teleangiectasias
- Syndromes
    - Tuberous sclerosis: autosomal dominant genetic linkage to chromosome 9q34 (*TSC1*) or 16p31 (*TSC2*) in families with tuberous sclerosis; two-thirds of cases are due to spontaneous mutation of *TSC2*; multiple, bilateral angiofibromas near the nasolabial folds at puberty (adenoma sebaceum), periungual fibromas, white shagreen patches, enamel teeth pits, CNS involvement (epilepsy and low intelligence), also ophthalmologic, cardiac, and pulmonary manifestations
    - Multiple endocrine neoplasia type I: familial tumor syndrome with facial angiofibromas, collagenomas, lipomas, gastrinomas, insulinomas, prolactinomas, and carcinoid tumors
- Variation
    - Pearly penile papules: angiofibromas along penile coronal sulcus

Dermatofibroma (DF), (Benign Fibrous Histiocytoma)

- Appearance: firm, pink to brown papulonodule that dimples when pinched (Fig. 11-17)
- Location: lower extremities but can be anywhere
- Histology: fibrohistiocytic proliferation entrapping thickened "keloidal" collagen at the periphery of the lesion; foamy histiocytes, multinucleated giant cells, and vessels in variable proportion are also seen; the overlying epidermis is acantholytic with tabled rete ridges and increased pigmentation of basal keratinocytes (induction phenomenon)
- Variations
    - Cellular dermatofibroma: larger with higher recurrence rate; more cellular with greater number of fibroblasts, can infiltrate fat and resemble dermatofibrosarcoma protuberans
    - Aneurysmal (hemosiderotic) dermatofibroma: large dilated blood spaces without endothelial lining and extravasated red blood cells with associated hemosiderin deposition; commonly mistaken for a vascular tumor
    - Atypical dermatofibroma (dermatofibroma with giant cells): large, atypical giant cells with pleomorphic nuclei and prominent nucleoli

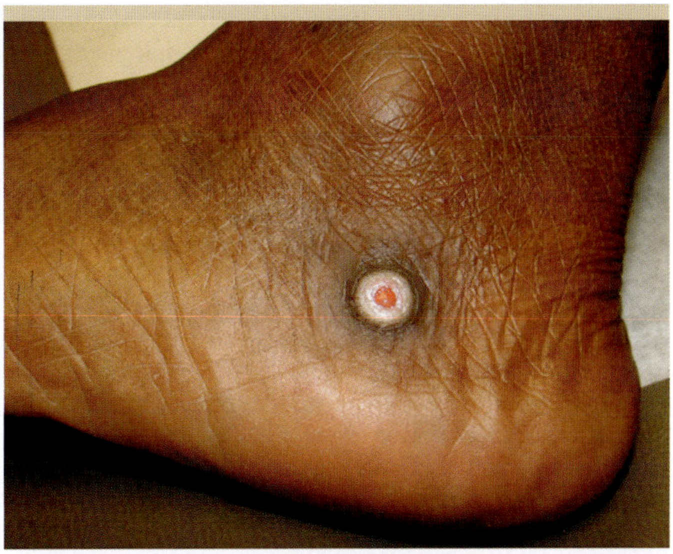

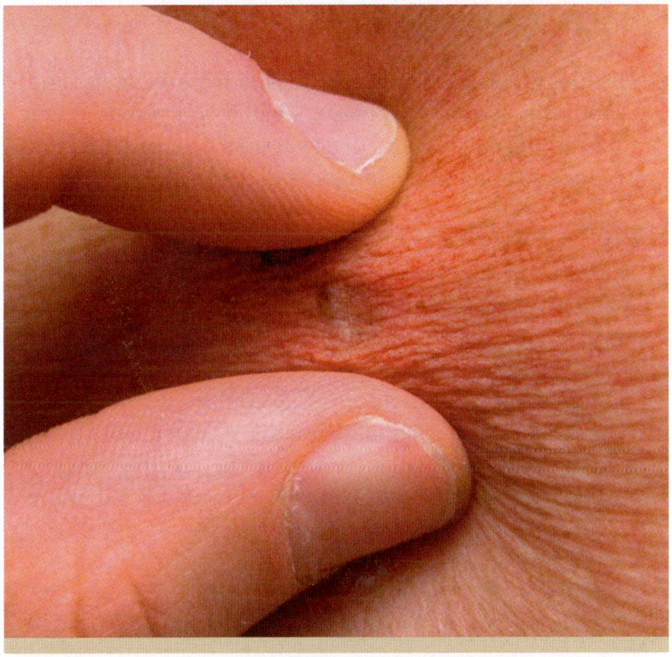

FIGURE 11-17 A. Cellular dermatofibroma. B. Dermatofibroma and dimple sign. (*Used with permission from the Department of Dermatology, University of Texas Medical Branch at Galveston.*)

- Atrophic dermatofibroma: hypocellular with atrophic epidermis and hyalinization of collagen
- Xanthomatous dermatofibroma: foamy macrophages that resemble an xanthoma, Touton giant cells sometimes
- Palisading dermatofibroma: prominent nuclear palisading, verocay-like bodies, can resemble Schwannoma
- Epithelioid cell histiocytoma: exophytic nodule or polypoid tumor with epidermal collarette, clinically resembling pyogenic granuloma or intradermal Spitz nevus; composed of epithelioid cells with abundant cytoplasm, numerous giant cells, and foamy macrophages
- Sclerotic fibroma: well-circumscribed hyalinized plywood pattern of dense collagen
- Dermatomyofibroma: shoulder of younger women; bundles of spindle cells parallel to epidermis resembling leiomyoma or dermatofibrosarcoma protuberans; actin staining positive and CD34 staining negative; probably a distinct entity

Scar

- Characterization: due to dermal and/or subcutaneous trauma or iatrogenic tissue damage
- Histology: bands of fibroblasts and dense collagen, often oriented parallel to the epidermis; granulation tissue present early with progression to collagen deposition and fibrosis
- Variations
  - Hypertrophic scar: thick, elevated scar that does not extend beyond the boundaries of the initiating injury; most frequently on the head and neck, shoulders, chest, and knees; no racial predilection (Fig. 11-18)
  - Keloid (Fig. 11-19): scar that extends beyond the boundaries of the initiating injury, more common on ear and chest of black skin; thick hyalinized bundles of eosinophilic collagen, less cellular than hypertrophic scar

Fibromatosis

- Demographics: present at birth or develops later
- Characterization: group of benign soft tissue tumors characterized by proliferation of mature fibroblasts and collagen with infiltrative growth pattern, and potential local recurrence

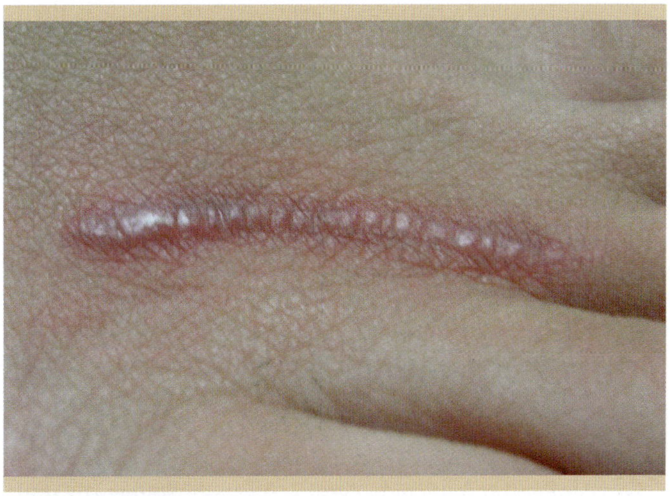

FIGURE 11-18 Hypertrophic scar. (*Used with permission from Dr. Asra Ali.*)

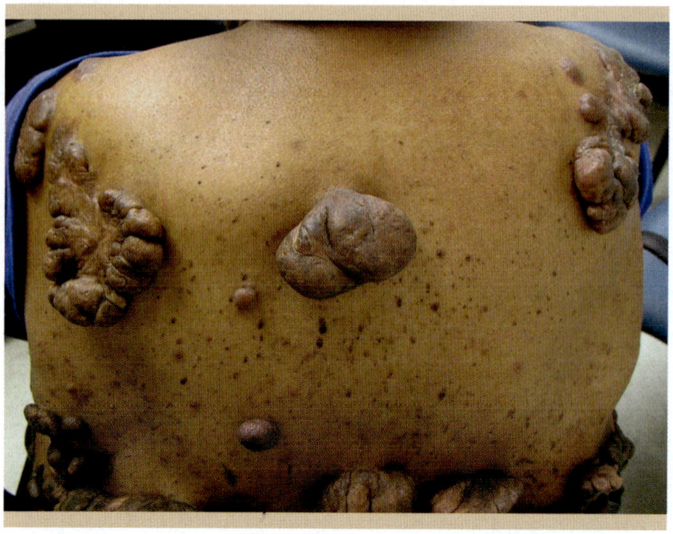

FIGURE 11-19 Keloid. (*Used with permission from the Department of Dermatology, University of Texas Medical Branch at Galveston.*)

- Histology: whorls of spindle cells; no mitoses
- Variations
  - Infantile myofibromatosis: slow-growing rubbery nodules on head at birth or infancy; if multiple, associated with visceral involvement (35% cases); surgical excision with recurrence but then spontaneous remission; spindle cells and also branching blood vessels in "staghorn" pattern
  - Congenital generalized fibromatosis: one to hundreds of nodules that may involve bone
  - Infantile digital fibromatosis (inclusion body fibromatosis, Reye tumor): rapidly growing nodules on dorsolateral digits of infant that recur but then spontaneously regress; eosinophilic intracytoplasmic inclusion bodies within the spindle cells (smooth muscle actin staining positive, Masson-trichrome positive)
  - Juvenile hyaline fibromatosis: autosomal recessive mutation of capillary morphogenesis protein 2 (*CMG2*) on chromosome 4q; slow-growing, skin-colored papules and nodules on face, scalp, and back; preceded by flexural contractures and gingival hyperplasia; irregular masses of spindle fibroblasts and deeply eosinophilic, hyalinized, collagen-like material (PAS staining positive, EM: microfilaments)
  - Palmar and plantar fibromatosis (Dupuytren contracture and Ledderhose disease): firm nodules in the distal palmar aponeurosis with progression to crippling flexion at the fourth and fifth metacarpophalangeal joints; questionable association with alcoholism
  - Penile fibromatosis (Peyronie disease): Solitary or multiple hardened plaques within tunica albuginea most common on the upper (dorsal) penis. Spectrum of symptoms from inflammation to painful curvature of the penile shaft; middle-aged to older adult men.
  - Knuckle pads: hyperkeratosis of the dorsal finger joints without significant symptoms or contracture
  - Desmoid fibromatosis: deeper fibromatosis usually only secondarily involving dermis that is associated with activating mutations in *CTNNB1*, the gene encoding β-catenin; Gardner fibroma is a variant associated with Gardner syndrome

Fibrous Hamartoma of Infancy

- Appearance: painless, skin-colored nodule on upper arm
- Demographics: frequently in boys less than 1 year old
- Characterization: may grow rapidly but benign
- Histology: triad of spindle cells in myxoid stroma, fibrous fascicles, and adipose tissue

Acquired Digital Fibrokeratoma

- Appearance: slow-growing, firm nodule or outgrowth from a digit or acral skin (Fig. 11-20)
- Histology: pedunculated papule with hyperkeratosis and acanthosis; mature fibroblasts, small blood vessels, elastic tissue in the dermis, and dense dermal collagen fibers oriented parallel to the long axis of the lesion

Angiomatoid Fibrous Histiocytoma

- Appearance: slow-growing, painless subcutaneous nodule that may or may not be accompanied by systemic symptoms, anemia, and paraproteinemia
- Location: extremities
- Demographics: children or young adults
- Characterization: originally described as a type of malignant fibrous histiocytoma with better prognosis; translocations of the *ATF* gene have been detected in the

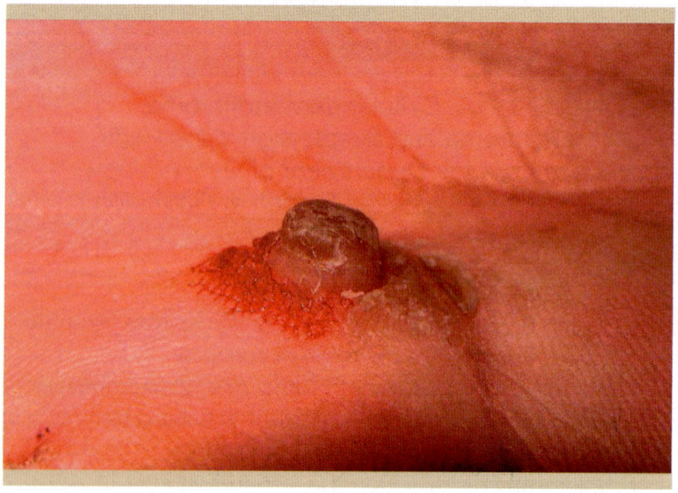

FIGURE 11-20 Acquired digital fibrokeratoma. (*Used with permission from the Department of Dermatology, University of Texas Medical Branch at Galveston.*)

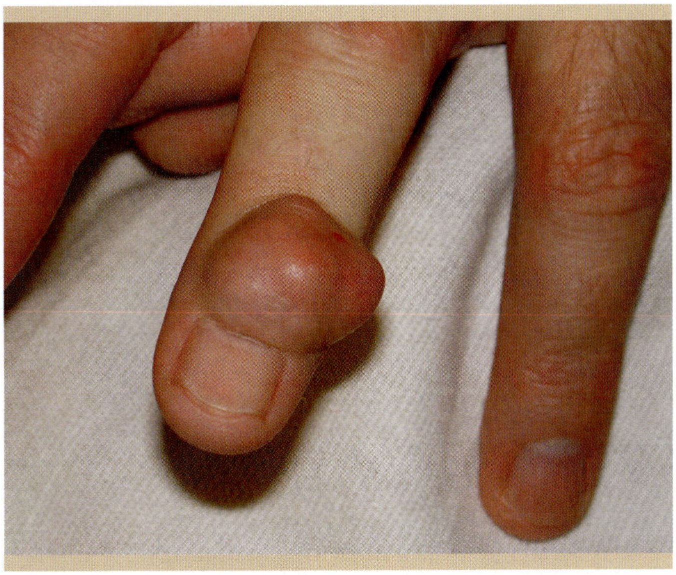

FIGURE 11-21 Giant cell tumor of tendon sheath. *(Used with permission from the Department of Dermatology, University of Texas Medical Branch at Galveston.)*

few cases published: *EWSR1-CREB1* is most common, but *FUS-ATF1*, and *EWSR1-ATF1* (most frequent genetic alteration in clear cell sarcoma) are also seen
- Histology: relatively uniform, pale, round or short spindle-shaped eosinophilic cells with ovoid vesicular nuclei, interspersed with blood-filled sinusoidal spaces and foci of hemorrhage; desmin, muscle actin (HHF-35), CD99, and CD68 immunoreactive (up to 50% of cases), smooth muscle actin is negative

Giant Cell Tumor of the Tendon Sheath

- Appearance: slow-growing, fixed nodule (Fig. 11-21)
- Location: dorsal hand or finger
- Demographics: third to fifth decade, slightly female predominance
- Characterization: most common tumor of the hand is benign; possibly a deep variant of dermatofibroma
- Histology: proliferation of fibroblasts and foamy histiocytes, multinucleated giant cells (osteoclast-like), and areas of hemorrhage with hemosiderin deposition

Atypical Fibroxanthoma (AFX)

- Appearance: locally aggressive, red plaque or nodule on sun-exposed skin
- Location: head (especially ear), neck, and dorsal hands
- Demographics: elderly
- Characterization: rarely metastasize; superficial form of malignant fibrous histiocytoma
- Histology: proliferation of bizarre spindle-shaped, foamy, and pleomorphic cells within background of dermal solar elastosis; sometimes giant cells; many atypical mitoses; CD68 and CD10 staining positive, S100 and cytokeratin staining negative

Malignant Fibrous Histiocytoma (MFH)

- Appearance: deep subcutaneous mass
- Location: extremities (especially lower)
- Demographics: most common soft-tissue sarcoma; occurs in late adult life with male predominance (2:1)
- Characterization: may originate from histiocyte, fibroblast, or undifferentiated stem cell; the superficial form (above the fascia) is associated with better survival
- Histology: proliferation of fibroblasts, histiocyte-like cells, and bizarre giant cells with severe pleomorphism that may show atypical mitoses; histologic variations include storiform-pleomorphic (most common), myxoid or myxofibrosarcoma, angiomatoid, inflammatory, and giant cell

Dermatofibrosarcoma Protuberans (DFSP) (Fig. 11-22)

- Appearance: slow-growing plaque that often progresses to a multinodular mass
- Location: trunk or proximal extremities
- Demographics: third to fourth decade
- Characterization: aggressive local invasion, frequent local recurrences, and rare metastasis to lung; t(17;22) and ring chromosomes; fusion of COL1A1 and *PDGFB* results in

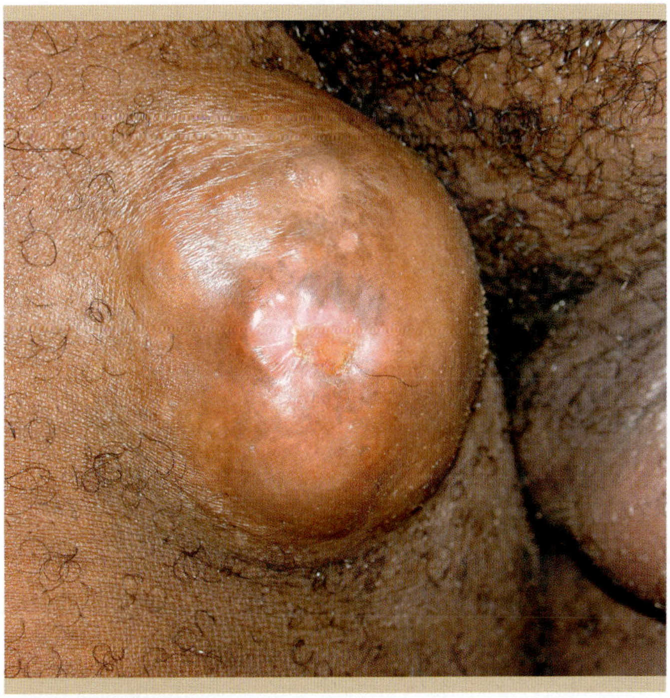

FIGURE 11-22 Dermatofibrosarcoma protuberans. *(Used with permission from the Department of Dermatology, University of Texas Medical Branch at Galveston.)*

strong overexpression of platelet-derived growth factor (PDGFβ)
- Histology: monomorphous spindle cells in storiform pattern with honeycomb-like infiltration of adipose, myxomatous areas and polymorphous cells may be present, and few mitoses; prominent CD34 positivity and Factor XIIIa negativity distinguish this from dermatofibroma
- Variations
  - Bednar tumor (pigmented DFSP): prominent deposits of melanin and dendritic melanocytes
  - Fibrosarcomatous DFSP: more cellularity, atypia, and mitoses, focal fascicular or "herringbone" pattern; represents transformation to a higher-grade tumor with ~20% metastatic rate
  - Myxoid DFSP: extensive myxoid features
  - Giant cell fibroblastoma: occurs in children on the chest wall, back, thighs; previously separate, but now with same chromosomal abnormalities as DFSP; variable myxoid, sclerotic, and sometimes dermatofibrosarcoma-like areas, cleft-like, angiomatoid pseudovascular spaces, and scattered multinucleate giant cells

SMOOTH MUSCLE TUMORS

Congenital Smooth Muscle Hamartoma

- Appearance: solitary plaque with vellus hairs, with or without a follicular pattern; diffuse skin involvement produces a "Michelin-tire baby" appearance
  - *Vermiculation*: wormlike movements upon stroking the lesion
  - Pseudo-Darier sign: stroking induces transient induration with piloerection
- Location: trunk
- Histology: marked increase of smooth muscle fibers in the dermis, grouped fibers are in bundles arranged haphazardly and are not attached to hair follicles, and basal hyperpigmentation
- Variant
  - Becker nevus: pigmented patch of increased terminal hair on shoulder or upper trunk of male adolescent; see increased hair follicles and sometimes smooth muscle on histology

Leiomyoma

- Appearance: rubbery pink to brown papulonodules, often painful
- Location: shoulder or limbs
- Demographics: young adults
- Histology: fascicles of smooth muscle, fusiform cells with longitudinal striations and thin, cigar-shaped nuclei with blunt ends; desmin and smooth muscle actin staining positive, Verhoeff-van Gieson staining positive (yellow), trichrome staining positive (pink-red)
- Variations
  - Piloleiomyoma: multiple papules on shoulder or face associated with burning sensation spontaneously or after cold, emotion, and pressure; arise from arrector pili muscle and see infiltrative pattern
  - Genital leiomyoma: painless papules on areolae or genitalia arising from mammillary, vulvar, or dartoic muscle (Dartotic leiomyoma)
  - Angioleiomyoma: benign and well-defined deep nodule arising from vascular smooth muscle, most common on lower leg; pseudoencapsulated collection of numerous blood vessels surrounded by thick walls and smooth muscle bundles

Leiomyosarcoma

- Appearance: pink to brown nodule or plaque
- Location: common on extremities
- Demographics: peak in fifth to sixth decade
- Characterization: malignant tumor of smooth muscle; negligible metastatic rate if originate from arrector pili or genital smooth muscle so confined to dermis, high metastatic rate if originate from vascular smooth muscle and located deeper
- Histology: high cellularity with pleomorphic and hyperchromatic spindle cells, high mitotic activity and occasional necrosis; desmin and smooth muscle actin immunoreactive

ADIPOSE TISSUE TUMORS

Lipoma

- Appearance: solitary or multiple elastic nodules of the subcutis (Fig. 11-23)

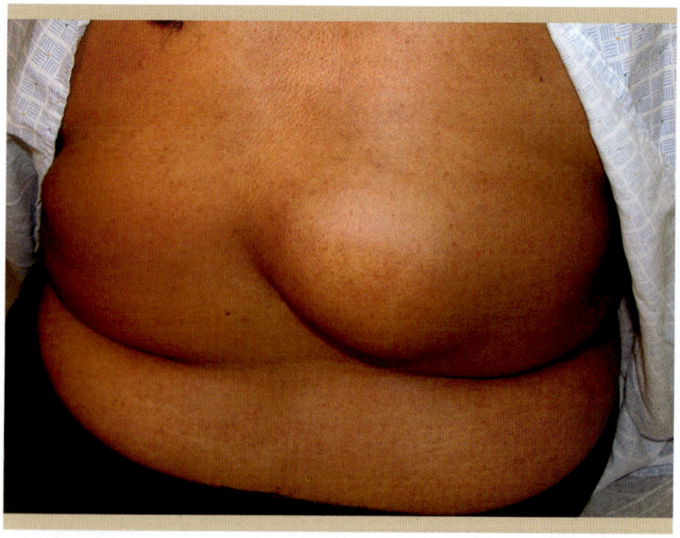

FIGURE 11-23 Lipoma. (*Used with permission from the Department of Dermatology, University of Texas Medical Branch at Galveston.*)

- Location: neck, trunk proximal extremities
- Characterization: benign tumor of mature fat; some related to *HMGA2* gene (12q) which encodes a high mobility group protein involved in regulation of transcription and/or the *LPP* gene (lipoma-preferred partner; 3q) which may be involved in cell adhesion and mobility
- Histology: well-circumscribed proliferation of mature fat; fine capsule sometimes
- Syndromes
  - Familial multiple lipomatosis: discrete, mobile lipomas on forearms and thigh
  - Proteus syndrome: overgrowth of multiple tissues and hamartomas including lipomas
  - Benign symmetric lipomatosis (Madelung disease): symmetric diffuse and infiltrative lipomas on head, neck, and shoulders; favors male alcoholics
  - Adiposis dolorosa (Dercum disease): multiple painful, circumscribed lipomas on abdomen, buttocks, and lower limbs of postmenopausal women
  - Also Gardner syndrome, Bannayan-Riley-Ruvalcaba syndrome, and Cowden disease
- Variations
  - Angiolipoma: usually seen in young adults as subcutaneous mass less than 2 cm, sometimes painful; many small blood vessels which often contain thrombi
  - Angiomyolipoma: adipose tissue present with smooth muscle and vessels in variable degree (may be a distinct entity)
  - Fibrolipoma: intermixed fibrous tissue
  - Myolipoma: smooth muscle actin and desmin staining positive
  - Infiltrating lipoma: skeletal muscle between adipocytes on lower extremities
  - Spindle cell lipoma: posterior neck or upper back; triad of mature fat cells, spindle cells, and thick "ropey" collagen; CD34 staining positive; 13q deletion that encompasses the *RB1* locus
  - Pleomorphic lipoma: posterior neck; atypical hyperchromatic multinucleated giant cells with nuclei arranged in a floret pattern (floret giant cells) that may resemble liposarcoma; forms a spectrum with spindle cell lipoma having same 13q deletion
  - Hibernoma: upper back, axilla, chest wall, or thigh of young adults; fetal adipocytes (brown fat) with central nucleus and vacuolated, granular cytoplasm; often lobulated and divided by fine fibrous septa

Liposarcoma

- Appearance: deep and rapidly enlarging mass
- Location: thigh and buttock
- Demographics: more than fifth decade
- Characterization: second most common soft tissue sarcoma after malignant fibrous histiocytoma; usually originates below subcutis, from deep soft tissue of extremities or retroperitoneum
- Histology: lipoblasts with cytoplasmic lipid-laden vacuoles that cause indentation of the hyperchromatic nucleus; variable nuclear polymorphism
- Variations
  - Atypical lipomatous tumor: term for liposarcomas originating from and restricted to the limbs were complete surgical excision is possible, denotes much lower risk for metastasis; 12q13~15 amplification including the MDM2 genes which inactivates p53
  - Well-differentiated liposarcoma: like lipoma but also occasional lipoblasts and scattered atypical cells with hyperchromatic nuclei; terminology used for retroperitoneal cases or others areas not amenable to complete surgical extirpation; 12q13~15 amplification
  - Dedifferentiated liposarcoma: areas of well-differentiated liposarcoma with adjacent nonlipogenic (dedifferentiated) component, usually with abrupt interface; dedifferentiated zones have appearance of a higher grade sarcoma with prominent mitoses; retains the 12q13~15 amplification but behaves much more aggressively
  - Myxoid liposarcoma: spindle cells in a mucinous stroma and prominent vascular pattern (branched "chicken wire" capillaries); associated with t(12;16) fusing *DDIT3* and *FUS*; on rare occasion, *EWSR1* (22q) substitutes for *FUS*
  - Round cell liposarcoma: more cellular with dense, small round hyperchromatic nuclei (variant of myxoid liposarcoma that is more aggressive, but with same translocation)
  - Pleomorphic liposarcoma: highly pleomorphic spindle cells and bizarre multinucleated multivacuolated giant cells; increased mitoses; *P53* mutations are common

Lipoblastoma

- Appearance: slow-growing subcutaneous mass
- Location: extremities, head, neck, and trunk
- Demographics: infancy and childhood (< 3 years old)
- Histology: lipoblasts, mature adipocytes, and prelipoblasts in a lobular pattern and separated by a loose fibrous septa; may resemble well-differentiated liposarcoma but found in young children; 8q breakpoints leading to activation of the proto-oncogene pleomorphic adenoma gene 1 (*PLAG1*)

Nevus Lipomatosus Superficialis

- Appearance: multiple soft, yellow to skin-colored papules; large lesions along skin folds may create "Michelin-tire baby" appearance
- Location: hip or buttock
- Demographics: newborn to adolescent
- Histology: lobules of mature adipose tissue in the superficial dermis

NEURAL TUMORS

Neuroma

- Appearance: skin-colored papules or nodules, often painful
- Histology: normal appearing or hyperplastic nerve bundles surrounded by fibrotic stroma; S-100 protein and myelin basic protein staining positive
- Multiple mucosal neuroma syndrome (multiple endocrine neoplasm, MEN type IIb or III): autosomal dominant association of multiple mucosal neuromas (lip, tongue, and eyelid), pheocromocytoma, and medullary carcinoma of the thyroid; MEN IIb is associated with mutations in the *RET* gene
- Variations
    - Traumatic or amputation neuroma: traumata sites of trauma or surgical wound; on neonates lateral palm, it may represent amputation in utero of supernumerary digit
    - Palisaded encapsulated neuroma (PEN): solitary firm papule on adult face; well-circumscribed but not truly encapsulated, palisading not as common as name implies, nor is the lesion truly encapsulated
    - Morton neuroma: usually found between toes; not a true neuroma, but represents a degenerative response to chronic low-grade tissue damage

Neurofibroma

- Appearance: soft papule or polypoid nodule
- Histology: fusiform, fine, often wavy spindle cells and fine collagenous fibers; sometimes compact, loose or even myxoid; S-100 protein staining positive
- Syndromes
    - Neurofibromatosis type I (NF1, von Recklinghausen disease, or Peripheral Neurofibromatosis): autosomal dominant mutation of a gene on chromosome 17q causing defect in neurofibromin protein (encoded by the *NF1* gene), a negative regulator of the Ras oncogene; café-au-lait macules, freckling of axilla or groin (Crowe sign), optic gliomas, iris hamartomas, and distinctive osseous lesions (e.g., sphenoid dysplasia and thinning of long bone cortex)
    - Neurofibromatosis type II (NF2, Bilateral Acoustic NF, or Multiple Inherited Schwannomas, Meningiomas, and Ependymomas [MISME syndrome]): autosomal dominant mutation of a gene on chromosome 22 causing a defect in the merlin tumor suppressor protein resulting in bilateral masses on eighth cranial nerve, schwannomas, meningiomas, gliomas, ependymomas, and juvenile posterior subcapsular lenticular opacity (juvenile cortical cataract)
- Variations
    - Plexiform neurofibroma: involves an entire large nerve with its branches that presents as "bag of worms" on palpation; virtually pathognomonic of neurofibromatosis 1 (NF1)
    - Diffuse neurofibroma: occurs on head, neck, and trunk of children and young adults as thick plaque of infiltrating neurofibromatous tissue; 20 to 30% of cases associated with NF1

Schwannoma (Neurilemmoma)

- Appearance: solitary or multiple papules or nodules, sometimes painful
- Histology: encapsulated subcutaneous nodule; proliferation of Schwann cells with elongated nuclei and blunted ends in 2 often intermixed histologic patterns (Antoni A and B)
- Antoni A: cells form loose fascicles with nuclei aligned in parallel arrays (Verocay bodies); S-100 protein positive
- Antoni B: less cellular areas that are sometimes myxoid and edematous

Dermal Nerve Sheath Myxoma (Neurothekeoma)

- Appearance: raised soft papule and nodule
- Location: usually face or upper extremities
- Demographics: middle-aged adults (females more common)
- Characterization: nerve sheath proliferations can be classified as classic myxoid (true nerve sheath myxoma) or cellular (cellular neurothekeoma); these represent distinct and separate entities (see below)
- Histology: well-defined, lobulated dermal mass with lobules of spindle and epithelioid cells in myxoid matrix, separated by thin fibrous septa; sparse mitotic activity; S-100 protein positive

Cellular Neurothekeoma

- Appearance: pink or brown papulonodule up to 3 cm
- Location: head, neck, and upper trunk
- Demographics: children and young adults (females more common)
- Characterization: immature tumor of uncertain differentiation
- Histology: poorly circumscribed fascicles of epithelioid and spindle cells; S-100 protein negative, but reactive for NKI-C3 and possibly protein gene product 9.5 (PGP 9.5)

Granular Cell Tumor

- Appearance: small papule or nodule
- Location: frequent on oral mucosa (especially tongue), trunk, arms, or anywhere on skin
- Demographics: third to sixth decade
- Histology: pseudoepitheliomatous hyperplasia over round cells with brightly eosinophilic, granular cytoplasm and pustulo-ovoid bodies (phagolysosomes that are PAS positive); also S-100 protein positive

Merkel Cell Carcinoma (Neuroendocrine Carcinoma of the Skin, Trabecular Carcinoma)

- Appearance: rapidly growing nodules
- Location: photo-damaged skin of head and neck
- Demographics: elderly
- Characterization: aggressive tumor with high metastatic potential, see Chapter 12
- Histology: strands, trabeculae, and nests of undifferentiated tumor cells with scant cytoplasm, round to oval nuclei with fine chromatin, and inconspicuous nucleolus (histologically similar to small cell carcinoma of the lung); CK20 and Cam 5.2 staining positive in paranuclear dot-like pattern; neuron-specific enolase (NSE), synaptophysin, and chromogranin staining positive; S-100 protein, CEA, and leukocyte common antigen (LCA) staining negative; thyroid transcription factor (TTF) staining negative (positive in small cell carcinoma of lung)

OTHER TUMORS

Osteoma Cutis (Cutaneous Ossification)

- Appearance: dermal or subcutaneous white papule or nodule
- Histology: spicules of bone in the dermis or subcutaneous tissue with cement lines, osteocytes, osteoblasts, and multinucleated osteoclasts
- Albright hereditary osteodystrophy: short stature, obesity, round face, mental weakness, and cutaneous ossifications of the dermis and fat; characterized by a lack of renal responsiveness to parathyroid hormone; dermal ossification also seen in plate like osteoma cutis and miliary osteomas of the face

Supernumerary Digit

- Appearance: congenital skin-colored papule
- Location: hands, feet; usually near the fifth finger
- Histology: dome-shaped, fibrous stroma with many nerves, sometimes cartilage or bone

Accessory Tragus

- Appearance: asymptomatic congenital papule (Fig. 11-24)
- Location: preauricular cheek or neck
- Histology: pedunculated shape with connective tissue, fat, and sometimes cartilage; many vellus hair follicles

Accessory Nipple (Supernumerary Nipple)

- Appearance: congenital pigmented or skin-colored macule, or umbilicated papule (Fig. 11-25)
- Location: embryonic milk line
- Histology: epidermis present over central pilosebaceous structure, dermis contains smooth muscle bundles, and mammary glands/ducts; identical to regular nipple

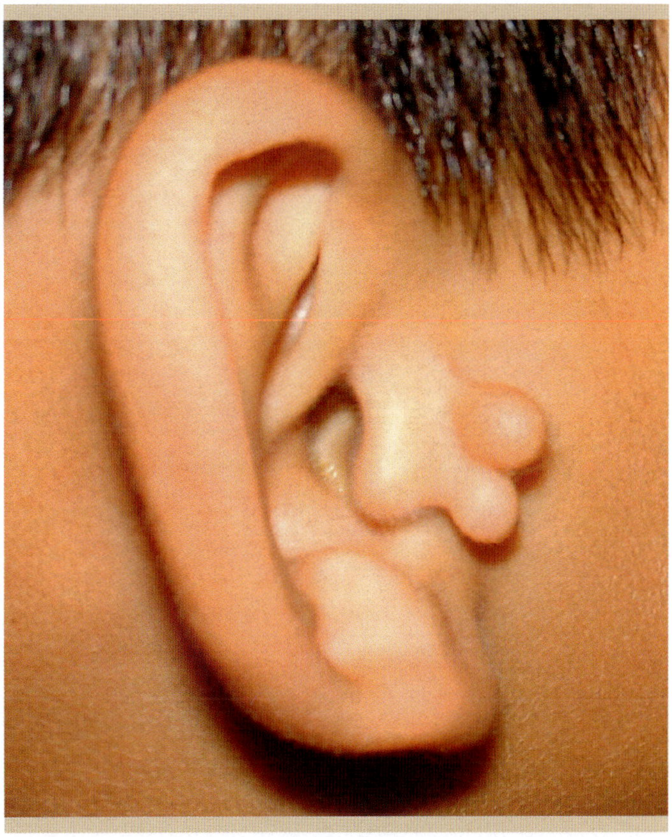

FIGURE 11-24 Accessory tragus. (*Used with permission from the Department of Dermatology, University of Texas Medical Branch at Galveston.*)

Primitive Non-Neural Granular Cell Tumor

- Appearance: exophytic, polypoid papule to nodule
- Location: variety of sites
- Demographics: wide age range
- Histology: this rare tumor consists of oval- to spindle-shaped cells with prominent granular cytoplasm; CD68 staining focally positive, NKI-C3 (nonspecific marker of lysosomes) staining diffusely positive, S-100 protein staining negative and is thus unrelated to the classic granular cell tumor described above

Cutaneous Metastases

- Appearance: very firm, painless dermal papule or nodule that may ulcerate
- Location: generally near primary malignancy
- Characterization: the most common malignancies to metastasize to the skin are listed below; though common, prostate cancer very rarely metastasizes to skin
- Histology: similar to primary cancer or slightly dedifferentiated
- Variations
    - Breast metastases: may present as carcinoma erysipeloides (sharply demarcated red plaque), carcinoma

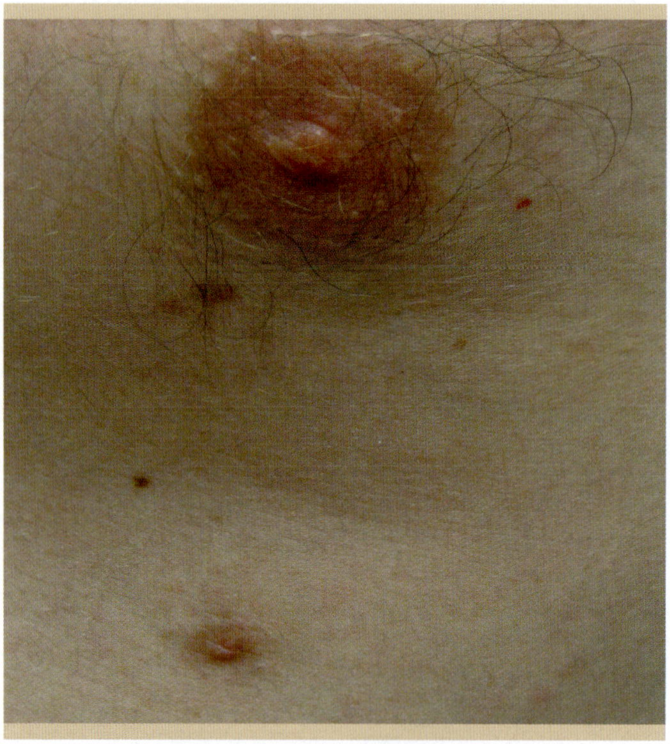

FIGURE 11-25 Accessory nipple (*Used with permission from the Department of Dermatology, University of Texas Medical Branch at Galveston.*)

telangiectoides (red papules and telangiectasias), or carcinoma en cuirasse (dusky indurated plaque with peau d'orange surface); histologically see tumor cells and small glands in lymphatics, in capillaries, or in single-file pattern between collagen bundles
- Melanoma and squamous cell carcinoma metastases: black or skin-colored dermal nodules near previous malignancy; histology shows similar pathology but without connection to epidermis
- Lung metastases: pink nodules on chest wall; see dense small cell infiltration in small cell carcinoma; TTF stains positive in small cell carcinoma (but not in Merkel cell carcinoma)
- Colon metastases: dermal nodules on abdominal wall (Sister Mary Joseph nodule on umbilicus originally reported with gastric carcinoma); adenocarcinomas may display gland formation and signet rings histologically
- Renal cell carcinoma metastases: though an uncommon adenocarcinoma, 7% metastasize to skin; prominent vascular appearance clinically and microscopically notable

QUIZ

Questions

1. Which of the following is not associated with diabetes?

   A. Xanthomas
   B. Syringomas
   C. Dermatofibromas
   D. Lipomas
   E. Rubeosis

2. Which of the following is not associated with steatocystomas?

   A. Hidrotic ectodermal dysplasia
   B. Anhidrotic ectodermal dysplasia
   C. Pachonychia congenita (type 1)
   D. Pachonychia congenita (type 2)
   E. All are associated

3. A patient presents with multiple firm, rubbery pink nodules on the face, some are coalescing into a plaque covering the scalp. Which is the most likely gene defect?

   A. *BRAF*
   B. *CYLD*
   C. *NF1*
   D. *NFKB*
   E. *P53*

4. Which is not a feature of microcystic adnexal carcinoma?

   A. Subtle clinical presentation
   B. Large plaque on nose or upper lip
   C. Biphasic histologic appearance
   D. Perineural involvement
   E. Marked cytologic atypia

5. A patient presents with brightly erythematous eczematous patches on the perineal skin. Biopsy shows large bluish cells in the epidermis that are EMA, CEA, and cytokeratin 7 positive. Which immunostaining profile would be most suspicious for internal malignancy?

   A. CK20 (−), GCFDP-15 (−)
   B. CK20 (−), GCFDP-15 (+)
   C. CK20 (+), GCFDP-15 (−)
   D. CK20 (+), GCFDP-15 (+)
   E. S100 (+)

6. Which of the following is associated with Muir-Torre syndrome?

   A. Clear cell syringoma
   B. Acrokeratosis verruciformis of Hopf
   C. Syringocystadenoma papilliferum
   D. Fibrofolliculoma
   E. Sebaceous adenoma

7. Translocation of platelet-derived growth factor (PDGF) B-chain and the collagen 1A1 promoter is a therapeutic target for which tumor?

   A. Keloidal scars
   B. Atypical fibroxanthoma
   C. Dermatofibrosarcoma protuberans
   D. Sebaceous carcinoma
   E. Merkel cell carcinoma

8. A patient with multiple leiomyomas should be screened with which of the following examinations?

   A. CT scan of the chest
   B. Retinal examination
   C. Mammogram
   D. Renal ultrasound
   E. Colonoscopy

9. Which is the most common tumor arising in association with nevus sebaceus of Jadassohn?

   A. Basal cell carcinoma
   B. Apocrine carcinoma
   C. Sebaceous carcinoma
   D. Syringocystadenoma papilliferum
   E. Sebaceoma

10. In a patient with neurofibromatosis, which of the following would develop last?

   A. Plexiform neurofibroma
   B. Café au lait macules
   C. Intertriginous freckling
   D. Optic gliomas
   E. Cutaneous neurofibromas

Answers

1. C. Diabetes is associated with eruptive xanthomas, clear cell syringomas, lipomas, and rubeosis (flushed appearance improved by dietary diabetic control). Multiple eruptive dermatofibromas have been reported in patients with systemic lupus erythematous, atopic dermatitis, and immunosuppression.

2. C. Pachyonychia congenital type 1 (Jadassohn-Lewandowsky) is an ectodermal dysplasia characterized by nail dystrophy, follicular hyperkeratosis, and angular cheilitis. It is distinguished from pachyonychia congenital type 2 (Jackson-Lawler) at puberty, when type 2 patients develop steatocystoma multiplex and eruptive vellus hair cysts.

3. B. Multiple cylindromas and some coalescing into a large plaque covering the scalp (turban tumor) is a characteristic of Brooke-Spiegler syndrome (familial cylindromatosis). Both this Multiple Familial Trichoepitheliomas are autosomal dominant disorders of the *CYLD* gene (chromosome 16q), which encodes a deubiquitinating enzyme.

4. E. The lack of cytologic atypia sometimes makes differentiation from desmoplastic trochiepithelioma difficult. Infiltrative plaques on the midface tend to be larger than they appear clinically, histologically appears as basaloid strands in the upper dermis but as ductal structures in the deeper dermis, and frequently have perineural involvement.

5. C. This profile favors endodermal origin and underlying visceral malignancy. CK20 (−) and GCFDP-15 (+) favors cutaneous origin, so there may be an underlying adnexal adenocarcinoma or no underlying malignancy. S100 (+) is seen in melanoma in situ, which would not stain with EMA, CEA, or CK7.

6. E. Muir-Torre syndrome is an autosomal dominant cancer-predisposing condition defined by one or more sebaceous neoplasms (sebaceous adenoma, sebaceous epithelioma, or rarely sebaceous carcinoma) and one or more visceral malignancies, including colon cancer. Patients and first-degree relatives should undergo screening colonoscopy as colon adenocarcinoma may precede development of cutaneous tumors. Acrokeratosis verruciformis of Hopf is an autosomal dominant disorder that can be associated with Darier disease. Clear cell syringoma is associated with diabetes, while syringocystadenoma papilliferum and fibrofolliculoma are seen in nevus sebaceus and Birt-Hogg-Dube syndrome, respectively.

7. C. Imatinib mesylate (Gleevec) targets the PDGF receptor (and other tyrosine kinase receptors), and has been tried in patients with dermatofibrosarcoma protuberans (DFSP)

8. D. Germline mutations in the fumarate hydratase gene (chromosome 1q) underlie multiple cutaneous and uterine leiomyomatosis syndrome (Reed syndrome), which is associated with early-onset papillary renal cell carcinoma. Fumarate hydratase is an enzyme of the mitochondrial Krebs cycle.

9. D. Various types of appendageal tumors may develop in association with nevus sebaceus of Jadassohn. They include syringocystadenoma papilliferum (8–10%), trichoblastoma (5%), and rarely trichilemmoma (2–3%), sebaceoma (2–3%), syringoma, apocrine cystadenoma, hidradenoma, or keratoacanthoma. Basaloid epithelial proliferations resembling basal cell carcinoma can be identified in 5 to 7% of cases of nevus sebaceus. Malignant tumors (apocrine carcinoma, basal cell carcinoma, squamous cell carcinoma) have been described to arise seldom in association with nevus sebaceus.

10. E. Plexiform neurofibromas are congenital; café au lait macules are congenital or appear during infancy; Lisch nodules, freckling, and optic gliomas begin during elementary school; and the multiple cutaneous neurofibromas develop at puberty.

REFERENCES

Bolognia JL et al. *Dermatology*, 2nd Ed. St. Louis: Mosby; 2008.

Calonje E et al. *McKee's Pathology of the Skin: With Clinical Correlations*, 4th Ed. Philadelphia: Elsevier-Mosby; 2012.

Goldsmith LA et al. *Fitzpatrick's Dermatology in General Medicine*, 8th Ed. New York: McGraw-Hill; 2012.

Holst VA, Junkins-Hopkins JM, Elenitsas R: Cutaneous smooth muscle neoplasms: clinical features, histologic findings, and treatment options. *J Am Acad Dermatol* 2002;46(4):477-490.

Rapini RP: *Practical Dermatopathology*. 2nd Ed. Edinburgh: Elsevier-Saunders; 2012.

Sanchez RL and Raimer SS: *Dermatopathology*. Georgetown: Landes Bioscience; 2001.

Weedon D: *Skin Pathology*, 3rd Ed. London: Churchill Livingstone; 2010.

Weiss SW, Goldblum JR: *Enzinger and Weiss's Soft Tissue Tumors*, 5th Ed. St. Louis: Mosby; 2008.

CHAPTER 12

MELANOMA AND NON-MELANOMA SKIN CANCER

SUMAIRA AASI
MICHELLE LONGMIRE

TUMOR SUPPRESSOR GENES

- Negative cancer regulators
- Cause apoptosis of DNA-damaged cells and block cell division
- Encode cell-cycle regulators, adhesion molecules, DNA repair enzymes, or signal transduction pathway molecules
- p53 most common cancer mutation, present in one-half of all human cancers; ninety percent of squamous cell carcinomas (SCCs) and in most basal cell carcinomas (BCCs) and actinic keratosis (Fig. 12-1)
- *PTCH1* member of the patched gene family that acts as a tumor suppressor in BCC.
- *CDKN2* mutation of this tumor suppressor leads to familial syndrome of pancreatic cancer and melanoma
- *ARF* functions as a melanoma tumor suppressor by inducing p53-independent senescence

Extrinsic and intrinsic apoptotic pathways

- Lead to the activation of the aspartate-specific cysteine proteases (caspases) that mediate apoptosis
- Extrinsic pathway
  - Involves engagement of particular "death" receptors that belong to the tumor necrosis factor receptor (TNF-R) family (e.g., Fas, DR5, and PERP)
  - Also causes the formation of the death-inducing signaling-complex (DISC)
- Intrinsic pathway
  - Triggered in response to DNA damage
  - Associated with mitochondrial depolarization and release of cytochrome c from the mitochondrial intermembrane space into the cytoplasm
  - Cytochrome c, apoptotic protease-activating factor 1 (APAF-1), and procaspase-9 form a complex termed the *apoptosome* (caspase-9 is activated and promotes activation of caspase-3, caspase-6, and caspase-7)
- Mutation is not the only way to inactivate tumor suppressor genes; function also can be blocked by methylation of their promoter

ONCOGENES

- Genes with growth-promoting activity
- Proto-oncogene is a normal gene that can become an oncogene due to mutations of increased expression
- Mutated gene causes cellular products to become constitutively active
- Are dominant
- If a normal gene (protooncogene) is present at a locus along with 1 mutated gene (oncogene), the abnormal product takes control
- May derive from viruses (e.g., *Src, ras, cmyc*)
- Oncogenic NRF2 mutations occur in squamous cell skin cancers
- Human Merkel cell polyomavirus (MCV or MCPyV) is an oncoprotein implicated in the progression of Merkel cell carcinoma (MCC)

CARCINOGENESIS

- Two-hit theory of Knudsen
- First: inheriting a defect in the familial form (5–10% of cancers result from germ-line mutations) or exposure to a carcinogen
- Second: ongoing exposure to the carcinogen that acts as a tumor promoter or cocarcinogen

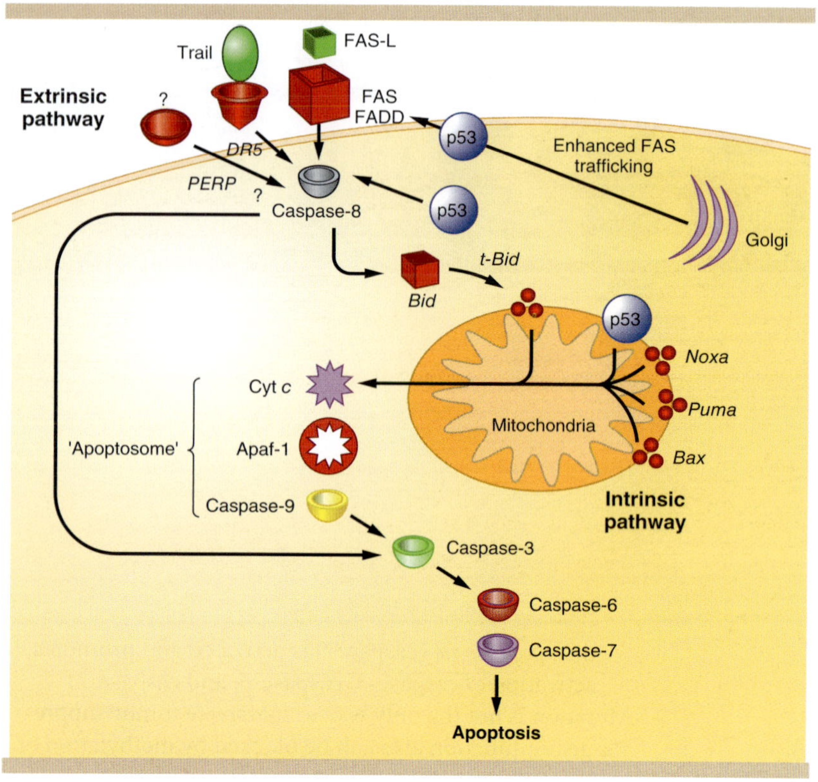

FIGURE 12-1 A model for p53-mediated apoptosis.

- Repeated assault on the DNA leads to mutations that cause the cell cycle to lose control
- Mutations from ultraviolet B (UV-B) light cause cytosine (C) to change to thymine (T)

AP-1 (ACTIVATING PROTEIN-1)

- Negative regulator for procollagen transcription; blocked by retinoids
- Collective term referring to dimeric transcription factors composed of *Jun, Fos,* or *ATF* subunits (protooncogenes)
- UV-B induces AP-1 binding to DNA at the AP-1-binding site
- AP-1 up regulates mRNA expression for gelatinase and collagenase
- AP-1 blocks collagen gene expression in dermal fibroblasts
- AP-1 proteins regulate the expression and function of cell-cycle regulators such as *p53*
- Absence of c-Jun results in elevated expression of the tumor suppressor gene *p53*
- Overexpression of c-Jun suppresses *p53*

NON-MELANOMA SKIN CANCER

Basal Cell Carcinoma

- Neoplasm derived from nonkeratinizing cells that originate in the basal cell layer
- Most common malignancy in humans
- Mutations in hedgehog pathway genes, primarily genes encoding patched homolog 1 (*PTCH1*) and smoothened homologue (*SMO*)
- Clinical and histologic subtypes
  - Nodular (Fig. 12-2)
  - Pigmented (Fig. 12-3)
  - Cystic
  - Superficial (Fig. 12-4)
  - Micronodular
  - Morpheaform/sclerosing and infiltrating
- Risk factors/etiological factors
  - Ultraviolet radiation
  - Other radiation: x-rays and Grenz rays

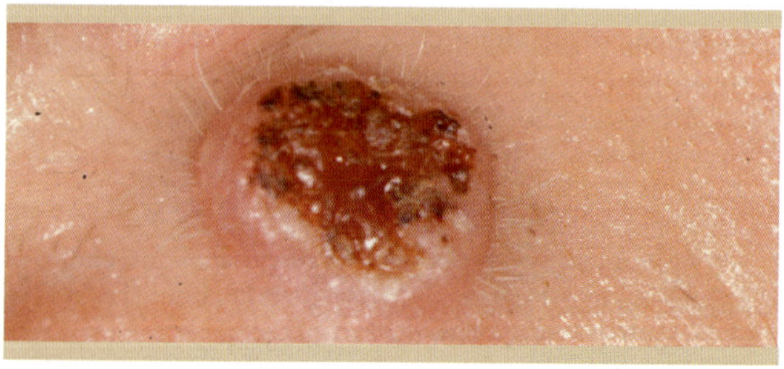

FIGURE 12-2 Basal cell carcinoma. *(Used with permission from Dr. Adelaide Hebert.)*

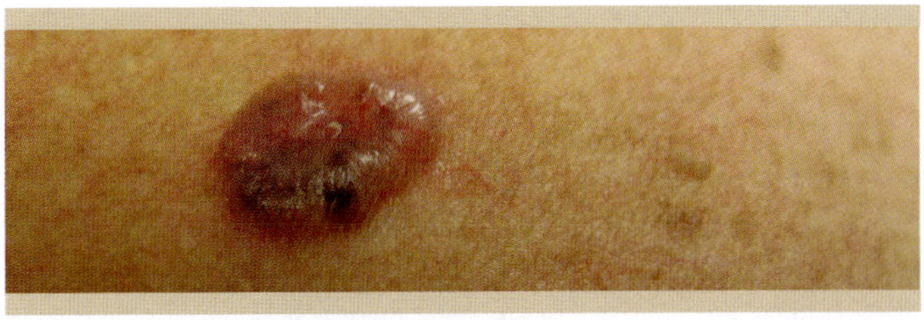

FIGURE 12-3 Pigmented basal cell carcinoma. (*Used with permission from Dr. Asra Ali.*)

- Arsenic exposure
- Xeroderma pigmentosum
- Nevoid BCC syndrome (also known as basal cell carcinoma nevus syndrome [BCCNS] or Gorlin syndrome)
  - Autosomal dominant; abnormalities in the *patched* (*PTCH*) gene, chromosome 9
  - 1 in 60,000 to 120,000
  - Complete penetrance with variable expressivity
  - Starts at an early age (starting at age 20 or earlier)
  - Characteristic facies: broad nasal root, frontal bossing, hypertelorism
  - Multiple BCCs
  - Opacity and cataract or glaucoma
  - Odontogenic keratocysts
  - Palmoplantar pitting
  - Intracranial calcification; calcification of the falx
  - Bifid ribs
  - Various tumors: medulloblastomas, meningioma, fetal rhabdomyoma, ameloblastoma, and ovarian fibromas

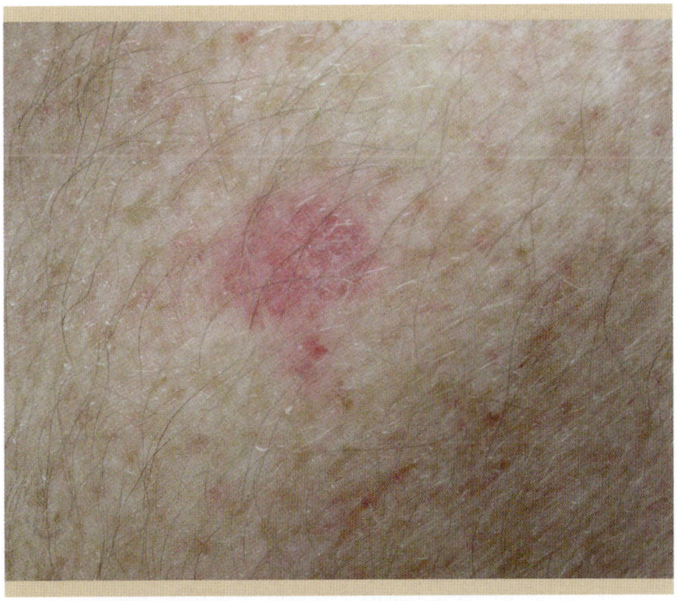

FIGURE 12-4 Superficial basal cell carcinoma. (*Used with permission from Dr. Asra Ali.*)

- Bazex-Dupre-Christol syndrome
  - X-linked dominant
  - Follicular atrophoderma ("ice pick" marks, especially on dorsal hands)
  - Multiple BCCs: face, neck, and the upper part of the trunk
  - Local anhidrosis/hypohidrosis
  - Hypotrichosis
  - Respiratory tract or digestive tract carcinomas
- Rombo syndrome
  - Autosomal dominant
  - Milia
  - Hypertrichosis
  - Trichoepitheliomas
  - Peripheral vasodilation
- Course
  - Incidence of new NMSC after initial skin cancer diagnosis
  - About 35% at 3 years
  - About 50% at 5 years
- Staging
  - TNM classification
  - Stage 0: Tis, N0, M0
  - Stage I: T1, N0, M0
  - Stage II: T2, N0, M0; T3, N0, M0
  - Stage III: T4, N0, M0; any T, N1, M0
  - Stage IV: any T, any N, M1
- Low-risk tumors
  - Borders are well defined; primary tumor; nonimmunosuppressed; nodular or superficial subtype
  - Trunk and extremities: less than 2 cm
  - Cheek/forehead/scalp/neck: less than 1 cm
- High risk tumors
  - Aggressive histology: recurrent, micronodular, metatypical, sclerosing/morpheaform, infiltrative, or perineural
  - Recurrent, immunosuppressed, BCCNS, ill-defined borders, setting of irradiated skin
  - Trunk and extremities: greater than 2 cm
  - Cheek/forehead/scalp/neck: greater than or equal to 1 cm
  - Mask areas of face (central face [nose, periorbital, cutaneous and mucosal lips, chin], periauricular, temple)
- Dermoscopy
  - arborizing (treelike) telangiectasia
  - large blue/gray ovoid nests
  - ulceration
  - multiple blue/gray globules
  - maple-leaflike areas, and spoke-wheel areas
- Treatment
  - Electrodesiccation and curettage
  - Cryotherapy
  - Imiquimod cream
  - Photodynamic therapy (PDT)

- Radiation therapy: nonsurgical candidates, debilitated patients
- Excision
- Mohs micrographic surgery
- Intralesional interferon
- Hedgehog inhibitors are orally active small molecule that target hedgehog pathway for locally advanced or metastatic BCC
- Regular use of sunscreens has been shown to prevent the development of further AK and invasive SCC in immunocompromised organ transplant recipient
- Oral celecoxib treatment inhibits BCC carcinogenesis

Squamous Cell Carcinoma In Situ [Bowen Disease (BD)]

- Malignant tumor of keratinocytes (Fig. 12-5)
- Neoplastic process limited to the epidermis
- Vulvar BD associated with increased risk of uterine, cervical, and vaginal cancer, possibly due to HPV infection
- Erythroplasia of Querat (EQ)
  - Occurs on mucosal surfaces of penis in uncircumcised males
  - Coinfection with HPV subtypes 8, 16, 39, 51
  - Progresses to invasive SCC in approximately 10%
  - Preventive measures: circumcision and hygiene

Leukoplakia

- Most common precancerous lesion of oral mucosa
- White plaque on oral mucosa that cannot be rubbed off
- Potential to become oral SCC
- Risk factors: tobacco, alcohol, HPV

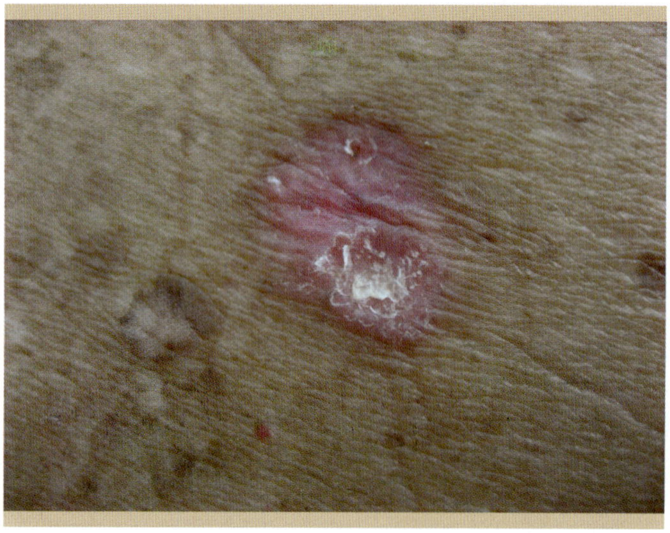

FIGURE 12-5 Bowen disease. (*Used with permission from Dr. Asra Ali.*)

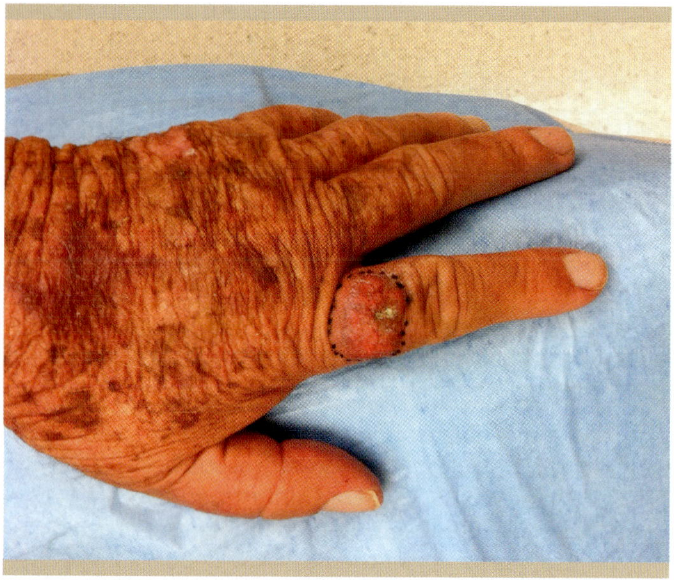

FIGURE 12-6 Squamous cell carcinoma.

Erythroplakia

- Red macule or patch of oral mucosa
- Least common but greatest potential to become oral SCC
- Treatment: complete excision or Mohs surgery

Squamous Cell Carcinoma

- Second most common form of skin cancer *(Fig. 12-6)*
- Malignant tumor of keratinocytes
- Predisposing conditions
  - Immunosuppression (especially solid-organ transplant recipients, chronic lymphocytic lymphoma, human immunodeficiency virus [HIV] infection)
  - Psoralen and ultraviolet A light (> 300 treatments)
  - Chemical carcinogens (tar, soot, arsenic)
  - Smoking
  - Genetic syndromes (i.e., xeroderma pigmentosum)
  - Chronic inflammatory conditions (i.e., discoid lupus erythematosus, erosive oral lichen planus, morphea, lichen sclerosus)
  - Chronic infections (i.e., osteomyelitis)
  - Chronic scarring conditions (i.e., burn scars, chronic ulcers, thermal injury, irradiated skin [ionizing radiation])
  - Periungual SCC—often associated with HPV 16
- Keratoacanthoma (Fig. 12-7)
  - Well-differentiated SCC
  - Solitary, rapidly growing, dome-shaped papulonodule with a central, horn-filled, craterlike depression
- Verrucous carcinoma
  - Rare, indolent form of SCC that presents as an exophytic verrucous tumor
  - Oral cavity (oral florid papillomatosis)
  - Foot (epithelioma cuniculatum)
  - Genitals (giant condyloma of Buschke and Lowenstein)

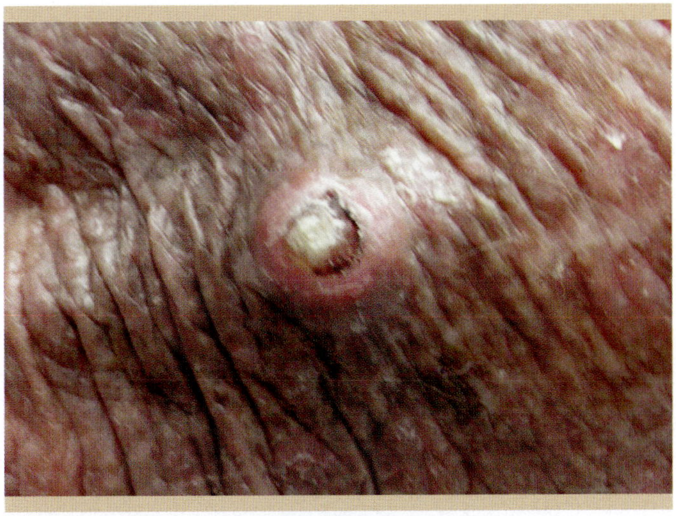

FIGURE 12-7 Keratoacanthoma. (*Used with permission from Dr. Asra Ali.*)

- High-risk SCCs and metastatic rate
  - Metastasis to primary or first echelon draining lymph nodes
  - Size: greater than 2 cm
  - External ear: 11%
  - Lip: 10 to 14%
  - Histologic risk factors: depth more than 4 mm or Clark level IV, poorly differentiated or spindle-cell type, lack of inflammatory infiltration
  - Organ transplant patient metastatic rate is 18 to 36 times that of the general population
  - Perineural invasion: 35%; local recurrence rate as high as 47%
- Marjolin ulcer
  - SCC arising in a chronic site of inflammation: old burn scar or a draining sinus tract
- Treatment
  - Small, low-risk lesions in nonsurgical candidates
  - Cryosurgery
  - Electrodesiccation and curettage
  - Photodynamic therapy (PDT)
  - Topical therapy (imiquimod, fluorouracil)
- Standard treatment
  - Excision
  - Mohs micrographic surgery
  - Radiation
- Patients with regional disease
  - Focused neck dissection
  - Superficial parotidectomy
  - Adjuvant radiation therapy
  - Primary radiation if inoperable tumor
  - Five-year survival for patients with metastases 26.8%

MELANOMA

- Accounts for 4% of all skin cancer; accounts for 79% of deaths related to skin cancer
- More than 50% of cases are believed to arise de novo
- Approximately 10 to 20% of all patients with melanoma have a family history of melanoma
- Risk factors for cutaneous melanoma
  - Dysplastic nevi in familial melanoma
  - Greater than 50 nevi 2 mm or greater in diameter
  - One family member with melanoma
  - Previous history of melanoma
  - History of acute, severe, blistering sunburns
  - Freckling
- Clinical types
  - Superficial spreading (Fig. 12-8): most common type (70%)
  - Lentigo maligna (Fig. 12-9): 10% of all melanomas
  - Acral lentiginous melanoma (ALM)
    - Approximately 2 to 8% of melanoma in Caucasians
    - Approximately 29 to 72% of melanoma in dark-skinned individuals
  - Amelanotic melanoma: less than 2% of melanomas
  - Mucosal: approximately 3%
  - Nodular: 10 to 15% (Fig. 12-10)
  - Subungual melanoma (Fig. 12-11)
- Genes implicated in the development of melanoma
  - Cyclin-dependent kinase inhibitor 2A (CDKN2A) resides on chromosome 9p
    - Cell-cycle regulatory gene
    - Protein target: inhibitor of cyclin-dependent kinase 4 (CDK4)
    - Encodes 2 distinct gene products that are regulators of cell division cycle

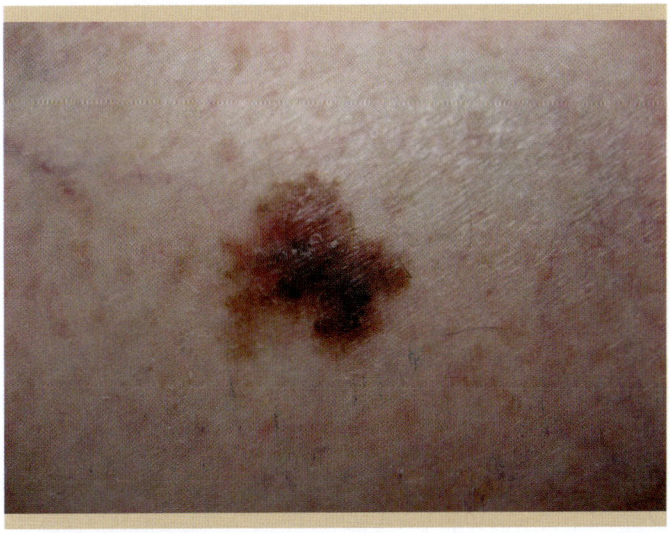

FIGURE 12-8 Superficial spreading melanoma. (*Used with permission from Dr. Asra Ali.*)

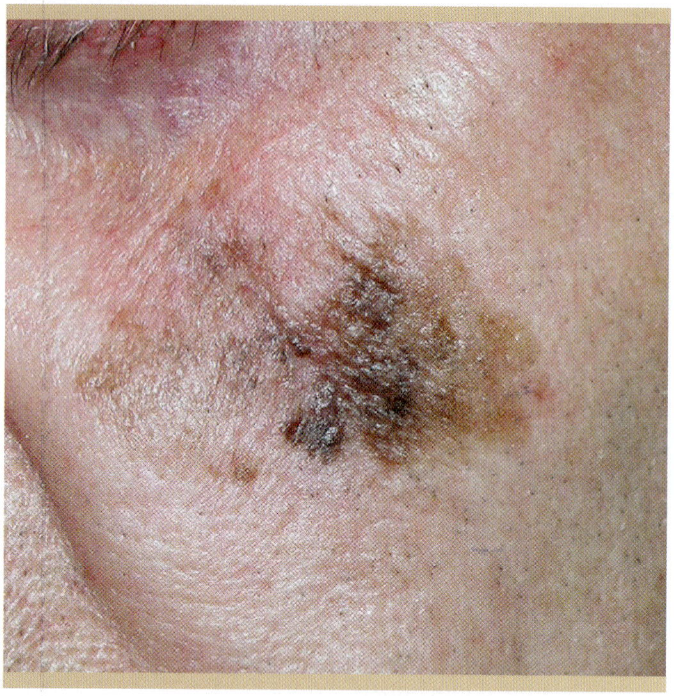

FIGURE 12-9 Lentigo maligna. (*Reproduced with permission from Wolff, et al.* Fitzpatrick's Dermatology in General Medicine, *7th Ed. © 2008. New York: McGraw-Hill; 2008.*)

- p16(INK4a): INK4 proteins inhibit complexes formed by the cell cycle kinases CDK4 and CDK6 and the D-type cyclins
- p19 (ARF): acts on the p53 pathway

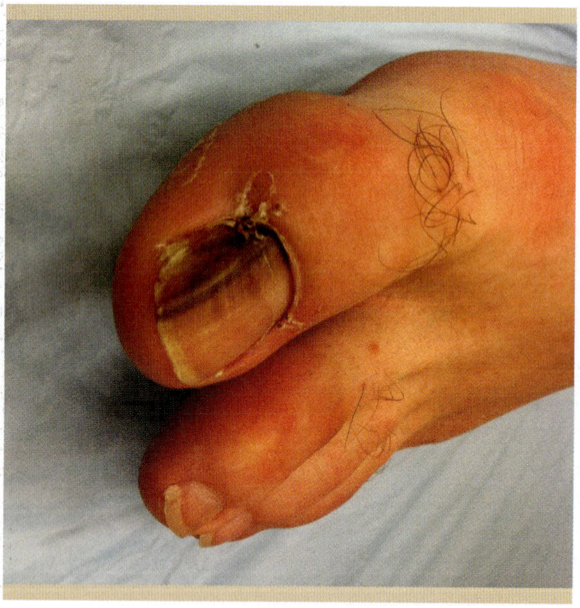

FIGURE 12-10 Melanoma arising in the nail bed of a young male.

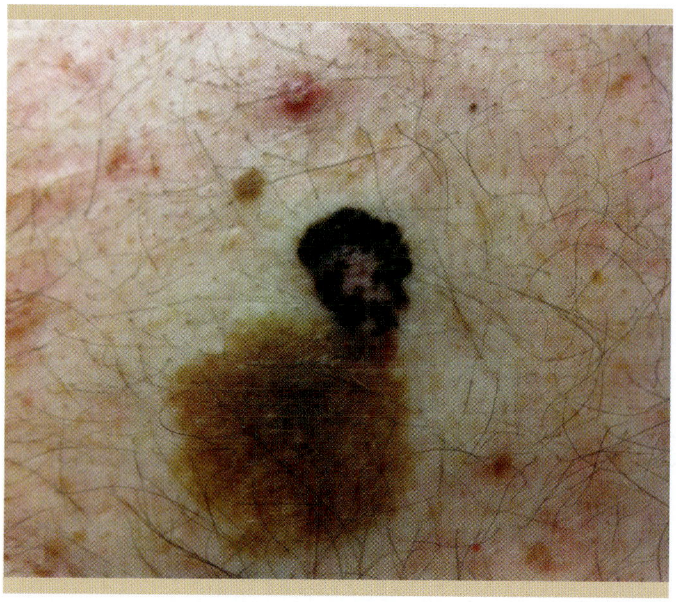

FIGURE 12-11 Melanoma arising in a congenital nevus.

- BRAF somatic missense mutations occur in approximately 66% of melanoma
- Prognosis
  - Ulceration, Breslow depth, and tumor thickness, important histologic determinants
  - Breslow depth: measured vertically in millimeters from the top of the granular layer (or base of superficial ulceration) to the deepest point of tumor involvement
- Immunohistochemical staining
  - Homatropine methylbromide 45 (HMB-45)
    - Spindle cell and desmoplastic variants fail to react with HMB-45
    - Shown to react with other neural crest-derived tumors and occasionally with adenocarcinomas and other neoplasms
    - Specificity for detecting melanoma is 96.9%
  - S-100: specificity of 70%
  - Microphthalmia transcription factor (Mitf): nuclear transcription factor critical for melanocyte development and survival
  - Tyrosinase: enzyme involved in the early stages of melanin production
  - Melan-A (or MART-1)
  - Ki67: Proliferating cell nuclear antigen
- AJCC TNM classification and staging
  - T classification
    - T1: less than or equal to 1.0 mm
      - ▲ a: without ulceration
      - ▲ b: with ulceration or level IV or V
    - T2: 1.01 to 2.0 mm
      - ▲ a: without ulceration
      - ▲ b: with ulceration

- T3: 2.01 to 4.0 mm
  - a: without ulceration
  - b: with ulceration
- T4: greater than 4.0 mm
  - a: without ulceration
  - b: with ulceration
- N classification
  - N1: 1 lymph node
    - a: micrometastasis
    - b: macrometastasis
  - N2: 2 to 3 lymph nodes
    - a: micrometastasis
    - b: macrometastasis
    - c: in-transit metastasis(-es)/satellite(s) without metastatic lymph nodes
  - N3: 4 or greater metastatic lymph nodes, matted lymph nodes, or combinations of in-transit metastasis(-es)/satellite(s) and metastatic lymph nodes
- M classification
  - M1: distant skin, subcutaneous, or lymph node metastasis
  - M2: lung metastasis
  - M3: all other visceral or any distant metastasis with elevated LD14
- Treatment: wide local excision
  - Tumors less than or equal to 1 mm depth: 1 cm margin
  - Tumors 1 to 4 mm in depth: 2 to 3 cm margins
- Lymph node management
  - Overall survival rates: Delayed lymph node dissection was not statistically significant compared with immediate node dissection
  - Sentinel lymph node (SLN) biopsy/lymphatic mapping
  - Absence of clinically palpable nodes
  - Thicker melanomas (≥ 1 mm in depth)
  - Determines presence of micrometastasis; if positive SLN, then therapeutic lymph node dissection proceeds
  - Lymphoscintigraphy: preoperative radiographic mapping and vital blue dye injection around the primary melanoma or biopsy scar; isosulfan blue dye plus sulfur-colloid-labeled technetium isotope increases accuracy of finding sentinel node
  - Performed at the time of wide local excision or re-excision
  - Identifies and removes the initial draining regional node(s)
  - Yields prognostic information but no evidence SLN; removal improves survival (current studies ongoing)
- Risk of primary tumor recurrence
  - Desmoplastic subtype
  - Positive microscopic margins
  - Recurrent disease
  - Thick primary lesions with ulceration or satellitosis
- High risk of nodal relapse
  - Extracapsular extension
  - Involvement of 4 or more lymph nodes
  - Lymph nodes measuring at least 3 cm
  - Cervical lymph node location
  - Recurrent disease
- Ipilimumab
  - Fully human antibody that binds to CTLA-4, a molecule on cytotoxic T cells. Blockage of CTLA-4 leads to a sustained active immune response against malignant cells
  - Ipilimumab, with or without a gp100 peptide vaccine improved overall survival in patients with previously treated metastatic melanoma
  - Ipilimumab in combination with dacarbazine, as compared with dacarbazine plus placebo, improved overall survival in patients with previously untreated metastatic melanoma
- Vemurafenib
  - BRAF enzyme inhibitor that leads to apoptosis of melanoma cells
  - Only effective in patients with V600 BRAF mutation
  - Treatment of metastatic melanoma with Vemurafenib in patients with tumors that carry the V600E BRAF mutation resulted in complete or partial tumor regression in the majority of patients
- Interferon alpha (IFN-α)
  - Approved by the Food and Drug Administration (FDA) for treatment of melanoma
  - Adjuvant treatment after excision in patients who are free of disease but are at high risk for recurrence: stages IIB and III
  - For primary tumors more than 4 mm depth and regional nodal disease
  - Binds to cell surface receptors, interacting with specific gene sites in both normal and neoplastic cells
  - Modulates the expression of host natural killer cells, T cells, monocytes, dendritic cells, and class I and II major histocompatibility (MHC) antigens in both neoplastic and nonneoplastic host tissues
  - Shown to have a growth-inhibitory effect when added to tumor cells in vitro
  - Eleven percent increase (26–37%) in survival rates at 5 years in the IFN-α treatment group compared with the observation arm
  - Interleukin 2 (IL-2): indirectly causes tumor cell lysis by proliferating and activating cytotoxic T-lymphocytes
- Dacarbazine (DTIC)
  - Approved by FDA for treatment of melanoma
  - Response rate of 10 to 20%
  - Combination therapy
  - Cisplatin, vinblastine, and DTIC (CVD) regimen
  - Cisplatin, DTIC, carmustine, and tamoxifen

- Radiation
  - Adjuvant treatment of regional node metastasis with extracapsular extension
  - Palliative treatment of distant metastatic disease: bone or brain
  - Factors predicting response to treatment:
    - Good performance status
    - Soft-tissue disease or only a few visceral metastases
    - Age younger than 65 years
    - No prior chemotherapy
    - Normal hepatic and renal function
    - Normal complete blood count (CBC)
    - Absence of central nervous system (CNS) metastases
- Melanoma vaccines
  - Active immunization: elicits specific or nonspecific reactivity against a tumor antigen by stimulating the patient's own immune system
  - Passive immunization: administration of antitumor antibodies or cells against a tumor antigen
  - Autologous (killed cell and recombinant types): heat shock protein extracts purified from autologous tumor cells also have been shown to have antitumor reactivity
  - Allogeneic
    - Generated using established stable cultured cell lines derived from tumors previously obtained from patients
    - Shed from tumor
    - Antigen-directed or genetically engineered
    - Polyvalent or univalent
  - Whole-cell preparations: immunizing with diverse antigens that are present on the tumor surface without knowing the exact antigen(s)
  - Gangliosides: tumor antigens that are created synthetically: GM2
  - Peptides/proteins
    - Direct loading of peptide fragments onto APCs
    - Antigenic epitopes responsible for eliciting an antitumor response consist of small peptide fragments
  - Dendritic cell vaccines
    - Recombinant viral and bacterial vaccines
    - Direct transduction
  - Cytokine and growth factor modulation
    - IL-2, interferons (IFN-α, IFN-β, IFN-γ), GMCSF, and TNF
    - Allow sustained local release of cytokines to enhance a potent local inflammatory response
  - DNA and RNA vaccines
    - Induce activation of APCs, which then present antigens to T cells
- In patients with advanced melanoma, response rate was higher and progression-free survival longer in patients receiving Gp100 peptide vaccination and IL-2 than with IL-2 alone.

Merkel Cell Carcinoma (MCC)

- MCPyV may be a contributing factor in MCC
- Neuroendocrine carcinoma of the skin
- Mortality rate is approximately 25%
- Most frequent sites: head, neck region, and extremities
- Located in or near the basal layer of the epidermis
- Clinical
  - Painless, indurated, solitary dermal nodule, slightly erythematous to deeply violaceous color
  - Three histologic features have prognostic significance: tumor thickness (depth of tumor invasion), the presence of LVI, and tumor growth pattern
  - Regional lymph nodes at presentation: 10 to 45%
  - Regional lymph node metastases during course of disease: 50 and 75%
  - Distant metastases: 50%
  - Common sites: lymph nodes, liver, bone, brain, lung, and skin
  - Local recurrence develops in 25 to 44% after primary tumor excision
- Histology
  - Trabecular: interconnecting strands of tumor cells in the dermis, with grouping of cells that appear as glands or neural rosettes
  - Intermediate: neoplastic cells in solid nests, most common pattern
  - Diffuse pattern: tumor cells interspersed among dermal collagen bundles
- Clinical staging
  - Stage IA: primary tumor les than or equal to 2 cm, with no evidence of spread to lymph nodes or distant sites
  - Stage IB: primary tumor greater than 2 cm, with no evidence of spread to lymph nodes or distant sites
  - Stage II: regional node involvement but no evidence of distant metastases
  - Stage III: presence of systemic metastases beyond the regional lymph nodes
- Treatment
  - Stage I
    - Wide local excision: 2-cm margins
    - Elective lymph node dissection (ELND)
      - ▲ Larger tumors, tumors with greater than 10 mitoses per high-power field, lymphatic or vascular invasion, and the small cell histologic subtypes
    - SLN biopsy
      - ▲ MCC sites with indeterminate lymphatic drainage
      - ▲ Effective in preventing short-term regional nodal recurrence
    - Adjuvant radiation therapy
      - ▲ Primary site and to the regional lymph node basin

  - ▲ Larger tumors, tumors with lymphatic invasion, tumors approaching the surgical margins of resection, and locally unresectable tumors
  - ▲ 50 Gy to the surgical bed and the draining regional lymphatics: delivered in 2-Gy fractions
- Stage II
  - Wide local excision of the primary tumor
  - Regional lymph node dissection
  - Adjuvant radiation therapy: primary site and to the regional lymph node basin
    - ▲ Larger tumors, tumors with lymphatic invasion, tumors approaching the surgical margins of resection, and locally unresectable tumors
    - ▲ 50 Gy to the surgical bed and the draining regional lymphatics: delivered in 2-Gy fractions
  - Adjuvant chemotherapy: regimens similar to patients with small-cell lung cancer
    - ▲ Cyclophosphamide, doxorubicin, and vincristine and etoposide plus cisplatin are the most commonly used regimens
    - ▲ Impact on survival uncertain
- Stage III
  - Chemotherapy: unresectable recurrent tumors
  - Regional lymph node dissection and adjuvant radiation therapy if the regional draining nodes have not been treated previously
  - Adjuvant radiation therapy: site of recurrence as well as regional lymph node beds

Dermatofibrosarcoma Protuberans

- Uncommon soft tissue neoplasm with intermediate- to low-grade malignancy (Fig. 12-12)
- Metastasis rare
- Locally aggressive tumor with a high recurrence rate
- Reciprocal translocations of chromosomes 17 and 22 t(17;22); fuse *COL1A1 PDGFB* gene
- Fusion protein is processed into functional PDGF-B and interacts with the PDGF receptor tyrosine kinase leading to the proliferation of DFSP tumor cells
- Less than 2% have metastases but patients with metastatic DFSP have very poor prognosis
- Most common on the trunk (42–72%), then proximal extremities (16–30%), rarely occurs above the neck (10–16%)
- Imatinib mesylate is indicated for the treatment of adult patients with unresectable, recurrent, and/or metastatic DFSP
- Surgical excision remains the mainstay of treatment
- Mohs is increasingly being used in surgical treatment
- Wide local excision has higher incidence of positive margin resection but local is comparable in Mohs and wide local excision

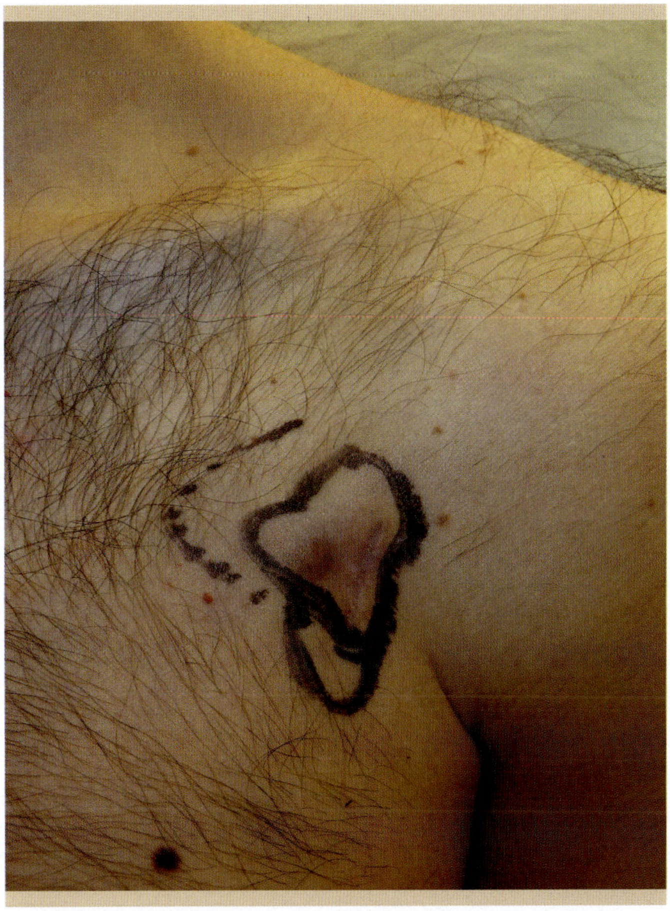

FIGURE 12-12 Dermatofibrosarcoma protuberans.

QUIZ

Questions

1. What type of virus is implicated in Merkel Cell Carcinoma?

   A. Polyomavirus
   B. Picornavirus
   C. Adenovirus
   D. Herpesvirus

2. Which mutation is associated with development of melanoma in intermittently sun-exposed skin?

   A. KIT
   B. BRAF
   C. NRAS
   D. MYC

3. Where is the most common site on the body for BCC?

   A. Nasal bridge
   B. Nasal ala
   C. Left temple
   D. Inferior orbital ridge

4. What anatomic area is associated with a higher rate of BCC development?

   A. Langer lines
   B. Lines of Blaschko
   C. Ventral, dorsal pattering lines
   D. Embryonic fusion plates

5. What cytogenetic abnormality can be found in MCC?

   A. Gene duplication of the *MYC* gene
   B. Loss of heterozygosity of chromosome 1
   C. Deletion of short arm of chromosome 5
   D. Translocation 2:13

6. What is the role of the *PTCH* gene?

   A. Activator of the hedgehog pathway
   B. Inhibitor of the hedgehog pathway
   C. Up regulator of cell division
   D. Up regulation of *BRAF*

7. A 35-year-old woman with Nevoid BCC syndrome presents with acute pelvic pain. Computer tomography reveals bilateral calcified masses in the pelvis. What is the most likely etiology of the finding?

   A. Ovarian malignancy
   B. Teratomas
   C. Benign ovarian fibromas
   D. Endometriosis

8. Which of the following may determine individual susceptibility to arsenic-induced premalignant hyperkeratoses?

   A. Individual capacity for DNA repair
   B. Individual capacity for urinary clearance of arsenic metabolites
   C. Individual capacity for UV-induced DNA damage
   D. Individual variation in p53 activity

9. Which location is associated with a higher risk of development of invasive carcinoma in Bowen disease?

   A. Face
   B. Forearm
   C. Mucous membrane
   D. Genitals
   E. Lower extremity

10. Guidelines established by the American Academy of Dermatology in 2011 do not recommend baseline tests in asymptomatic patients with the following stage of cutaneous melanoma:

    A. IA-IB
    B. IA-IIB
    C. IA-IIC
    D. IA-IIIB
    E. IA-IIIC

Answers

1. A. DNA sequences of polyomavirus (Merkel cell polyomavirus, MCV, or MCPyV) have been detected in 80% of MCC but only 16% of healthy skin. The frequent finding of clonal integration of viral DNA within the MCC genome suggests that viral infection may play a fundament role in pathogenesis of the cancer.
2. B. BRAF mutations are more common in intermittently UV-exposed skin, whereas KIT mutations are more frequently found in chronically sun-exposed skin. BRAF mutations are more commonly detected in superficial spreading melanomas and melanomas that arise on nonchronically sun-damaged skin. NRAS mutations are more common in patients with nodular melanomas and melanomas arising on chronically sun-damaged skin.
3. B. BCC most commonly occur on the head with the most frequent site being on the face specifically the nasal tip and ala which account for 70% of cases.
4. D. The anatomic distribution of BCCs correlates with embryonic fusion planes. Recent data indicate that after adjusting for surface area, BCC occurrence is greater than 4 times more likely on embryonic fusion planes.
5. B. Cytogenetic abnormalities are present in 30 to 47% of MCC. The most frequent change is loss of heterozygosity due to translocations or deletions of chromosome 1; specifically, 2 distinct regions in the most distal band 1p36 on the short arm of chromosome 1 are implicated in MCC. Similar abnormalities near this site occur in several neurocristic tumors, including melanoma, neuroblastoma, and pheochromocytoma. Other abnormalities described in MCC include losses at chromosomes 3, 13, and 22 and partial trisomy of chromosomes 1, 11, 18, and X. Unlike neuroendocrine (small cell) carcinoma of the lung, gene amplifications are rare in cutaneous MCC.
6. B. In mammals, *PTCH* is an important inhibitor in the hedgehog signaling pathway, whose downstream proteins can lead to cell proliferation. *PTCH* is frequently mutated in sporadic basal BCCs. Its wide-reaching activity accounts for the findings in patients with Nevoid BCC syndrome.
7. C. Genitourinary findings in Nevoid BCC syndrome include bilateral calcified ovarian fibromas, found in 14 to 24% of women. Ovarian fibromas are often asymptomatic and rarely become malignant.
8. A. The individual capacity of DNA repair may determine degree of chromosomal aberration, a primary determinant of susceptibility to developing arsenic-induced premalignant hyperkeratoses.
9. D. The risk of invasive carcinoma is estimated to be higher for genital Bowen disease or erythroplasia of Queyrat at 10%.

10. C. Guidelines established by the American Academy of Dermatology in 2011 do not recommend baseline tests in asymptomatic patients with stage IA-IIC cutaneous melanoma.

REFERENCES

Ballo MT, Ang KK: Radiotherapy for cutaneous malignant melanoma: rationale and indications. *Oncology* 2004;18(1): 99-107; discussion 107-10, 113-114.

Banerjee M, Sarma N, Biswas R, Roy J, Mukherjee A, Giri AK: DNA repair deficiency leads to susceptibility to develop arsenic-induced premalignant skin lesions. *Int J Cancer* Jul 15 2008; 123(2):283-287.

Bichakjian CK, Halpern AC, Johnson TM, et al. Guidelines of Care for the Management of Primary Cutaneous Melanoma. American Academy of Dermatology. http://www.aad.org/education-and-quality-care/clinical-guidelines/current-and-upcoming-guidelines. Accessed June 9, 2011.

Cox NH, Eedy DJ, Morton CA: Guidelines for management of Bowen's disease: 2006 update. *Br J Dermatol* Jan 2007;156(1):11-21.

Devitt B, Liu W, Salemi R, Wolfe R, Kelly J, Tzen CY: Clinical outcome and pathological features associated with NRAS mutation in cutaneous melanoma. *Pigment Cell Melanoma Res* Aug 2011;24(4):666-672.

Ellerhorst JA, Greene VR, Ekmekcioglu S, et al. Clinical correlates of NRAS and BRAF mutations in primary human melanoma. *Clin Cancer Res* Jan 15 2011;17(2):229-235.

Feng H, Shuda M, Chang Y, Moore PS: Clonal integration of a polyomavirus in human Merkel cell carcinoma. *Science* Feb 22 2008;319(5866):1096-1100.

Flaherty KT, Puzanov I, Kim KB, et al. Inhibition of mutated, activated BRAF in metastatic melanoma. *N Engl J Med* Aug 26 2010;363(9):809-819.

Goessling W, McKee PH, Mayer RJ: Merkel cell carcinoma. *J Clin Oncol* 2002;20(2):588-598.

Goldsmith LA et al. *Fitzpatrick's Dermatology in General Medicine*, 8th Ed. New York: McGraw-Hill; 2012.

Gollard R, Weber R, Kosty MP et al. Merkel cell carcinoma: review of 22 cases with surgical, pathologic, and therapeutic considerations. *Cancer* 2000;88(8):1842-1851.

Haag ML, Glass LF, Fenske NA: Merkel cell carcinoma: diagnosis and treatment. *Dermatol Surg* 1995;21(8):669-683.

Haigh PI, DiFronzo LA, McCready DR: Optimal excision margins for primary cutaneous melanoma: a systematic review and meta-analysis. *Can J Surg* 2003;46(6):419-426.

Han A, Chen EH, Niedt G, Sherman W, Ratner D: Neoadjuvant imatinib therapy for dermatofibrosarcoma protuberans. *Arch Dermatol* Jul 2009;145(7):792-796.

Hodi FS, O'Day SJ, McDermott DF, et al. Improved survival with ipilimumab in patients with metastatic melanoma. *N Engl J Med* Aug 19 2010;363(8):711-723.

Horwitz SM: Novel therapies for cutaneous T-cell lymphomas. *Clin Lymphoma Myeloma* 2008;8(Suppl 5):S187-S192.

Lee JH, Choi JW, Kim YS: Frequencies of BRAF and NRAS mutations are different in histologic types and sites of origin of cutaneous melanoma: a meta-analysis. *Br J Dermatol* Apr 2011;164(4):776-784.

Lemm D, Mugge LO, Mentzel T, Hoffken K: Current treatment options in dermatofibrosarcoma protuberans. *J Cancer Res Clin Oncol* May 2009;135(5):653-665.

Lui et al. Affected members of melanoma-prone families with linkage to 9p21 but lacking mutations in CDKN2A do not harbor mutations in the coding regions of either CDKN2B or p19ARF. *Genes Chromosomes Cancer* 1997;19:52-54.

Maldonado JL, Fridlyand J, Patel H, et al. Determinants of BRAF mutations in primary melanomas. *J Natl Cancer Inst* Dec 17 2003;95(24):1878-1890.

Marks ME, Kim RY, Salter MM: Radiotherapy as an adjunct in the management of Merkel cell carcinoma. *Cancer* 1990;65(1):60-64.

McArthur G: Dermatofibrosarcoma protuberans: recent clinical progress. *Ann Surg Oncol* Oct 2007;14(10):2876-2886.

McKee PH: *Pathology of the Skin: With Clinical Correlations*. London: Mosby-Wolfe; 1996.

Newman JC, Leffell DJ: Correlation of embryonic fusion planes with the anatomical distribution of basal cell carcinoma. *Dermatol Surg*. Aug 2007;33(8):957-964; discussion 965.

Nghiem P, McKee PH, Haynes HA: Merkel cell (cutaneous neuroendocrine) carcinoma, In: Sober AJ, Haluska FG, eds. *Skin Cancer*. Hamilton: BC Decker; 2001, 127-141.

Platz et al. Screening of germline mutations in the *CDK4, CDKN2C*, and *TP53* genes in familial melanoma: a clinic-based population study. *Int J Cancer* 1998;78:13-15.

Schwartz JL, Griffith KA, Lowe L, et al. Features predicting sentinel lymph node positivity in Merkel cell carcinoma. *J Clin Oncol* Mar 10 2011;29(8):1036-1041.

Schwartzentruber DJ, Lawson DH, Richards JM, et al. gp100 peptide vaccine and interleukin-2 in patients with advanced melanoma. *N Engl J Med* 2011;364:2119-2127.

Shimizu A, O'Brien KP, Sjoblom T, et al. The dermatofibrosarcoma protuberans-associated collagen type Ialpha1/platelet-derived growth factor (PDGF) B-chain fusion gene generates a transforming protein that is processed to functional PDGF-BB. *Cancer Res* Aug 1 1999;59(15):3719-3723.

Shuda M, Kwun HJ, Feng H, Chang Y, Moore PS. Human Merkel cell polyomavirus small T antigen is an oncoprotein targeting the 4E-BP1 translation regulator. *J Clin Invest* Sep 2011;121(9): 3623-3634.

Thomas JM, Newton-Bishop J, A'Hern R, et al. Excision margins in high-risk malignant melanoma. *New Engl J Med* 2004;350(8):757-766.

Von Hoff DD, LoRusso PM, Rudin CM, et al. Inhibition of the hedgehog pathway in advanced basal-cell carcinoma. *N Engl J Med* Sep 17 2009;361(12):1164-1172.

Vortmeyer AO, Merino MJ, Böni R, Liotta LA, Cavazzana A, Zhuang Z: Genetic changes associated with primary Merkel cell carcinoma. *Am J Clin Pathol* May 1998;109(5):565-570.

Walker GL et al. Mutations of the *CDKN2/p16* gene in Australian melanoma kindreds. *Hum Mol Genet* 1995;4:1845-1852.

Zuo L et al. Germline mutations in the p16 binding domain in familial melanoma. *Nature Genet* 1996;12:97-99.

CHAPTER 13

VASCULAR TUMORS AND MALFORMATIONS

DENISE W. METRY
JOHN C. BROWNING
ASRA ALI

OVERVIEW

- Vascular tumors of infancy and childhood
  - Infantile hemangioma
  - "Congenital hemangiomas" (noninvoluting, or NICH; rapidly involuting, or RICH)
  - Kaposiform hemangioendothelioma
  - Tufted angioma
  - Pyogenic granuloma
- Vascular tumors of adulthood
  - Kaposi sarcoma
  - Angiolymphoid hyperplasia with eosinophilia
  - Endovascular papillary angioendothelioma (Dabska tumor)
  - Intravascular papillary endothelial hyperplasia (Masson tumor)
  - Low-grade angiosarcomas
    - Epithelioid hemangioendothelioma
    - Spindle cell hemangioendothelioma
    - Retiform hemangioendothelioma
  - Angiosarcoma
- Vascular malformations
  - Capillary
    - Salmon patch
    - Port-wine stain
    - Cutis marmorata telangiectatica congenital
    - Phakomatosis pigmentovascularis
    - Unilateral nevoid telangiectasia
    - Angiokeratomas
  - Lymphatic: microcystic, macrocystic, or combined
  - Venous
    - Glomuvenous malformations: glomus tumors, glomangiomas, and glomangiomatosis
  - Arterial
  - See complex vascular malformation/overgrowth syndromes

VASCULAR TUMORS OF INFANCY AND CHILDHOOD

Infantile Hemangioma (IH)

- Characteristics
  - Most common tumor of infancy
  - Characterized by endothelial cell proliferation
  - Endothelial cells derived from hemangioma express vascular endothelial growth factor (VEGF-A), VEGF receptors, TIE2, and angiopoietin-2
  - GLUT-1 (glucose transporter) is an immunohistochemical stain specific for IH in all phases of growth and involution
  - Positive staining occurs *only* with IH and *not* with any other vascular tumor or malformation
  - Proliferative phase: 6 to 12 months; rarely longer
  - Involution phase: gradual over several or more years
  - Risk factors: Caucasian, female, low birth weight, multiple gestation
- Location: more than 60% occur on head or neck, most commonly midcheek, lateral upper lip, and upper eyelid
- Types
  - Superficial, deep, or combined
    - Superficial
      - ▲ Most common
      - ▲ Raised, bright-red papule, nodule, or plaque

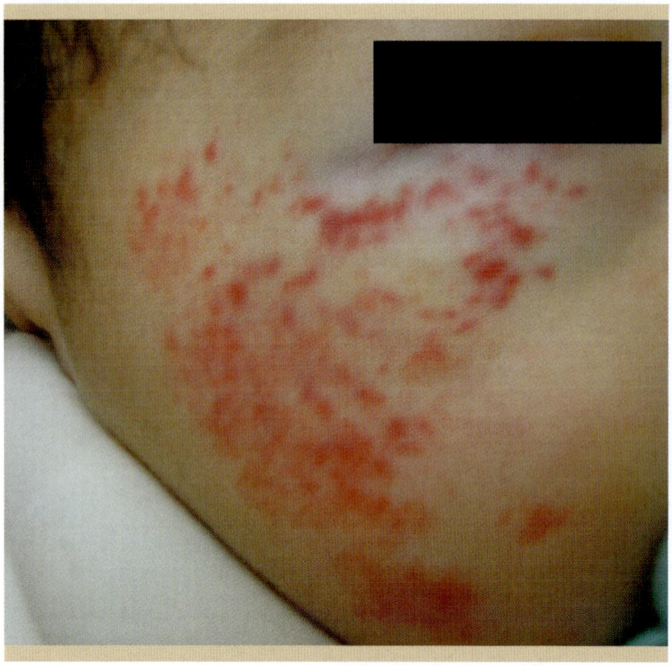

FIGURE 13-1 Combined infantile hemangioma. (*Used with permission from Dr. Denise Metry.*)

- Deep: soft, flesh-colored nodule that often has a bluish hue and/or central telangiectasias
- Combined (Fig. 13-1)

- Localized, segmental, or multiple
- Classification by morphology
  - Localized: papules or nodules that appear to arise from a single focal point and demonstrate clear spatial containment
  - Segmental (Fig. 13-2)
    - Plaque-like and show a linear and/or geographic pattern over a cutaneous territory
    - Much more likely to be complicated, require more intensive and prolonged therapy, and have a poorer overall outcome
  - Multifocal
    - Generally defined as five or more small, localized lesions
    - Multiple hemangiomas are associated with multiple births
- Complications
  - Ulceration
    - Most common in proliferative phase
    - Often leads to pain, scarring, bleeding, and secondary infection
    - Favors IH in trauma-prone sites: lip, perineum, intertriginous, posterior scalp, and back
  - Scarring
    - More common with segmental IH, localized IH of superficial, raised morphology with sharp "cliff drop" border, ulceration

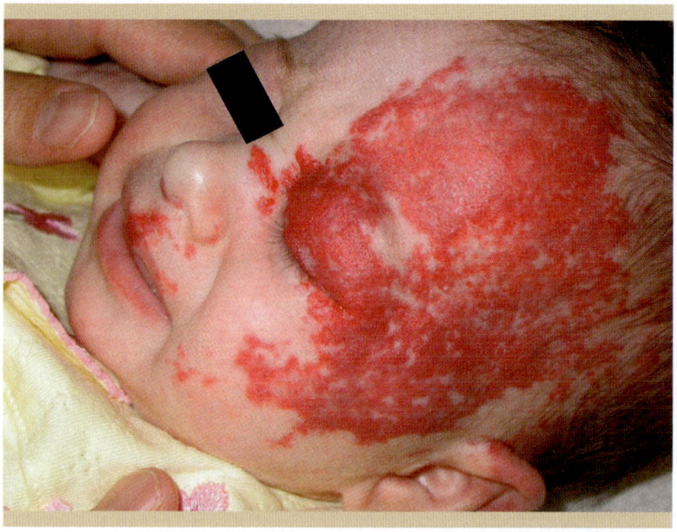

FIGURE 13-2 Segmental facial infantile hemangioma. (*Used with permission from Dr. Denise Metry.*)

    - High-risk locations: lip (especially when crossing the vermillion border), nasal tip, and ear
- Vital organ compromise
  - Visual obstruction
    - ▲ Amblyopia from stimulus deprivation or astigmatism
    - ▲ Most common when IH involves upper eyelid (Fig. 13-3)
    - ▲ Refer to ophthalmology

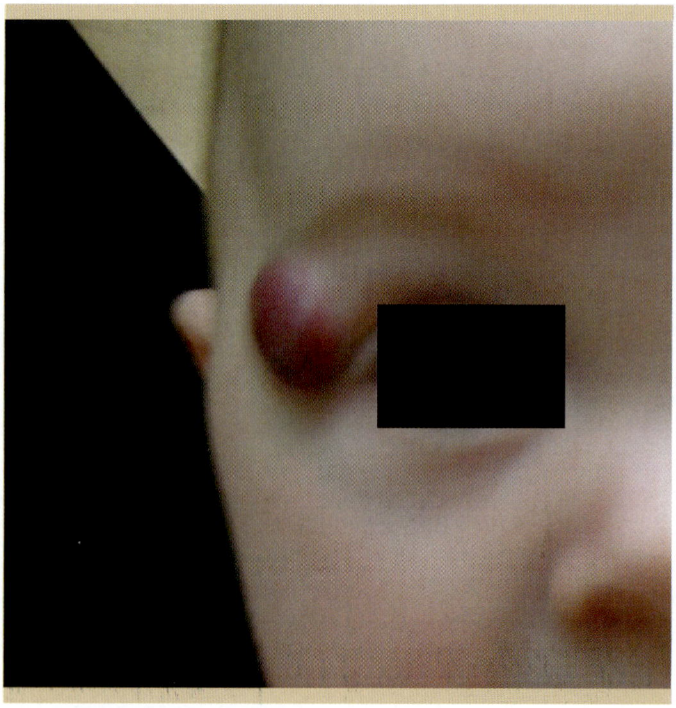

FIGURE 13-3 Segmental hemangioma. (*Used with permission from Dr. Denise Metry.*)

- Airway (especially subglottic) IH
  - ▲ Associated with segmental IH in a cervicofacial or "beard" distribution
  - ▲ Watch for development of stridor
  - ▲ Endoscopy for definitive diagnosis
- Visceral IH
  - Associated with multifocal *and* solitary segmental IH
  - Liver most worrisome site
  - Complications of multifocal and diffuse liver hemangiomas include acquired hypothyroidism due to hemangioma expression of type 3 thyronine deiodinase and macrovascular high-flow shunting that can lead to low- or high-output cardiac failure
  - Gastrointestinal IH can rarely lead to significant bleeding
  - Brain IH can very rarely lead to mass effects/neurologic sequelae
- Lumbosacral IH
  - Segmental lesions that span the midline and often are flat or telangiectatic in appearance are at highest risk
  - Risk: spinal dysraphism (especially tethered cord; supragluteal cleft deviation is an especially concerning clinical sign), LUMBAR syndrome (see below)
  - MRI best study for spinal dysraphism
- Developmental anomalies
  - PHACE syndrome
    - ▲ *P*osterior fossa (Dandy-Walker) brain malformations, *h*emangioma (segmental, usually cervicofacial), cerebrovascular *a*rterial anomalies, *c*ardiac defects/coarctation of the aorta, *e*ye anomalies
    - ▲ Sometimes referred to as PHACE(S) when ventral developmental defects such as sternal clefting and supraumbilical raphe are present
    - ▲ Structural cerebral and cerebrovascular anomalies: most common and potentially serious manifestations
    - ▲ Cerebrovascular anomalies can lead to progressive vasculopathies causing stroke in early childhood
    - ▲ Higher-risk infants for stroke have MRA findings of severe, long-segment narrowing or nonvisualization of major cerebral or cervical vessels without anatomic evidence of collateral circulation, often in the presence of concomitant cardiovascular comorbidities
    - ▲ Workup
      - △ MRI/MRA of brain and neck
      - △ Cardiac echo or MRI/MRA of chest
      - △ Eye examination
  - LUMBAR syndrome
    - ▲ *L*ower body hemangioma and other cutaneous defects, *u*rogenital anomalies, *u*lceration, *m*yelopathy, *b*ony deformities, *a*norectal malformations, *a*rterial anomalies, and *r*enal anomalies
    - ▲ Hemangiomas often "segmental" and "minimal growth" in morphology and extensive, often covering the entire limb
    - ▲ Myelopathies (including spinal dysraphism) most common extracutaneous manifestation
    - ▲ Can be considered regional variation of PHACE
- Diagnosis
  - Generally clinical
  - Surgical biopsy (±GLUT-1 staining) warranted if any suspicion for malignancy
  - Imaging studies cannot generally be relied on to distinguish a benign from malignant vascular tumor
- Treatment
  - Most common indications: ulceration, vital organ compromise, to improve the ultimate cosmetic outcome
  - Options
    - Meticulous wound care for ulceration
    - Systemic propranolol is rapidly becoming standard of care for complicated hemangiomas
    - Mechanism of action for hemangiomas under investigation
    - Side effects: hypotension, bradycardia, hypoglycemia, bronchospasm, congestive heart failure, gastrointestinal complications, sleep disturbance, cool or mottled extremities, hyperkalemia, rash or dry skin, depression, dental caries, and drug interactions due to metabolism within cytochrome P-450 system
    - Hypoglycemia may be most serious potential complication, usually related to decreased oral intake or an overnight fast
    - Mild symptoms of hypoglycemia: sweating, tremors, tachycardia, anxiety, and hunger
    - Severe symptoms of hypoglycemia: lethargy, poor feeding, seizures, apnea, hypothermia, and loss of consciousness
    - Topical beta-blocker (timolol maleate) an option for relatively small, superficial hemangiomas of minor cosmetic concern
    - Systemic glucocorticoids are an alternative to propranolol for complicated hemangiomas, or can be used in combination for severe cases
    - Side effects: cushingoid facies, personality changes, delayed skeletal growth, hypertension, and immunosuppression
      - ▲ Second-line agents:
        - △ Vincristine (vinka alkaloid chemotherapy agent)

        - Administered intravenously through a central venous catheter
        - Side effects: immunosuppression, peripheral neuropathy, constipation, jaw pain, leukopenia, and anemia
    - Interferon (20% risk of spastic diplegia in infants)
    - Excisional or laser surgery in select patients

"Congenital" Hemangiomas

- Types: noninvoluting (NICH), rapidly involuting (RICH)
    - Uncommon
    - Fully developed at birth and GLUT-1-negative
- RICH
    - Gray-violaceous tumor
    - Most common on an extremity
    - Focal hepatic "hemangiomas," which tend to be large, solitary, GLUT-1 negative tumors, have been determined the hepatic equivalent of "congenital hemangiomas" of the skin
    - Undergoes rapid involution during the first year of life with characteristic atrophy
- NICH
    - Most commonly presents on the trunk
    - Oval to round plaque with coarse, central telangiectasias, and a surrounding rim of pallor
    - Often feels warm to palpation and may have a slight bruit
    - Path is hybrid between a vascular tumor and malformation

Kaposiform Hemangioendothelioma (KHE)

- Characteristics
    - Rare
    - Histologically benign but clinically aggressive tumor
    - Clinical and histologic overlap with tufted angioma not uncommon
    - Prox-1, a lymphatic endothelial nuclear transcription factor, is expressed in both kaposiform hemangioendothelioma and tufted angioma
    - Most commonly affects children younger than 2 years and is often present at birth
    - Male-female incidence equal
    - Generally solitary
    - Favors the skin (particularly trunk, extremities) or retroperitoneum
    - Grows rapidly
    - Early on develops distinct violaceous color as a clue to underlying Kasabach-Merritt phenomenon (KMP)
    - KMP = life-threatening thrombocytopenia as a result of platelet trapping within the tumor
        - Consumption coagulopathy with very low platelet counts and low fibrinogen levels
        - Does not occur with IH

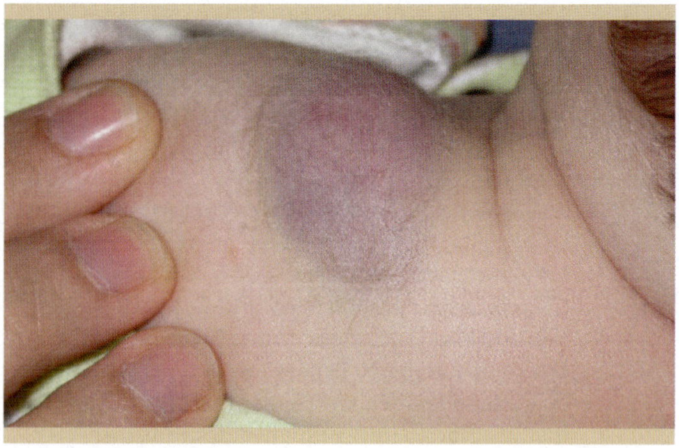

FIGURE 13-4 Tufted angioma. (*Used with permission from Dr. Denise Metry.*)

- Pathology: densely infiltrated nodules composed of spindle cells with minimal atypia and infrequent mitoses and slit-like vessels containing hemosiderin; GLUT-1-negative
- Treatment
    - Corticosteroids and/or vincristine often used as first-line therapy; sirolimus has recently shown promising results in KHE with KMP
    - Complete surgical excision if feasible
    - Heparin should be avoided as it can stimulate tumor growth and aggravate platelet trapping

Tufted Angioma (Angioblastoma of Nakagawa) (Fig. 13-4)

- Characteristics
    - Uncommon, histologically benign tumor
    - Clinical and histologic overlap with KHE not uncommmon
    - Presents during infancy or early childhood; presence at birth uncommon
    - Most common on trunk, extremities
    - Slow, lateral extension occurs over months to years
    - Spontaneous regression may uncommonly occur, especially with congenital presentations
    - Variable presentation
        - Large, darkly erythematous plaque with cobblestone surface
        - Sometimes with overlying vellus hair growth, tenderness, and sweating
        - Associated with KMP less commonly than kaposiform hemangioendothelioma
- Histology: tufts of capillaries throughout dermis, "cannonball" pattern

Pyogenic Granuloma (Fig. 13-5)

- Characteristics
    - Can be seen at any age, but majority occur during childhood

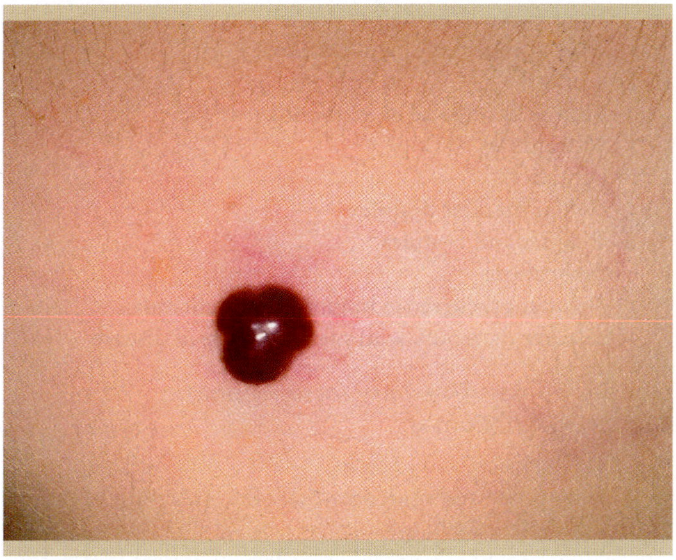

FIGURE 13-5 Pyogenic granuloma. (*Used with permission from Dr. Denise Metry.*)

- Prior history of trauma in minority
- Most common on head and neck; mucosal lesions more common in females, especially during pregnancy
- Usually presents as rapidly growing, bright-red papule or nodule
- Bleeds repeatedly and profusely; generally does not regress
- Umbilical granulomas seen in neonates have similar clinical appearance, but if persistent, may represent umbilical remnant (imaging recommended)

- Histology: well-circumscribed lobular proliferation of capillaries; possible erosion of epidermis
- Treatment
  - Depends on location/size
  - Most small lesions can be shave excised or curetted with light electrodessication to the base
  - Alternatives: excision, pulsed-dye or carbon dioxide laser, cryotherapy
- Course: recurrence more common with larger lesions

VASCULAR TUMORS OF ADULTHOOD

Kaposi Sarcoma (KS)

- Associated with human herpesvirus type 8
- Subtypes
  - Classic KS
    - Males, older than 50 years, predominant in Mediterranean and Jewish populations
    - Increased risk of lymphoreticular neoplasms
    - Violaceous macules with slow progression to plaques
    - Distal lower extremities, unilateral involvement with centripetal spread to a disseminated and multifocal pattern
    - Oral cavity and GI tract (90%); possible involvement of lung, spleen, and heart
    - Benign course owing to slow progression
  - African endemic KS
    - Black Africans, males more than females, third to fourth decades
    - In children, the disease runs a fulminant course with rapid dissemination
    - Clinicopathologic subvariants
      - ▲ Nodular: benign, similar to classic KS
      - ▲ Florid or vegetating type: nodules extend into deep dermis, subcutis, muscle, and bone
      - ▲ Infiltrative: like florid/vegetating type but more aggressive
      - ▲ Lymphadenopathic: affects children and young adults, usually confined to lymph nodes but may affect skin and mucous membranes
  - KS in iatrogenically immunocompromised patients
    - Presents in organ-transplant, autoimmune, and cancer patients
    - Discontinuation of therapy may cause regression of KS lesions
  - Epidemic HIV-associated KS
    - Oral mucosa (palate most common) is initial site of presentation in 10 to 15%
    - Early lesions appear as small pink/reddish macules or dermatofibroma-like papules
    - Extracutaneous sites: lymph nodes, gastrointestinal tract (80% of AIDS patients, usually duodenum and stomach), and lungs (bronchospasm, cough, and respiratory insufficiency)
- Histology
  - Patch stage: proliferation of spindle-shaped cells in upper dermis; neoplastic cells outline irregular, bizarre slits and clefts
  - Plaque stage: multiple dilated and angulated vascular spaces outlined by attenuated endothelium, solid cords, and fascicles of spindle cell arranged between jagged vascular channels
  - Tumor stage: spindle cells in interlacing fascicles in dermis; lack of pronounced pleomorphism and nuclear atypia, slit-like vascular spaces with extravasated red blood cells (RBCs)
- Treatment
  - Ionizing radiation
  - (Poly) chemotherapy: vinblastine or vincristine; combination with actinomycin D, adriamycin, bleomycin, and dacarbazine; liposomal encapsulated doxorubicin and daunorubicin
  - Interferon-α in combination with antiretrovirals (zidovudine)

- Topical tretinoin gel
- Topical imiquimod
- Intralesional injections of β-human chorionic gonadotropin (β-hCG)

Angiolymphoid Hyperplasia with Eosinophilia

- Characteristics
  - Occurs mainly in the West
  - Thought to be inflammatory or reactive process
- Location: head, trunk, and extremities
- Presentation
  - Peripheral eosinophilia
  - Papules or nodules
  - Young adults, females more than males
- Diagnosis/pathology
  - Irregular vessels lined by plump endothelial cells with "hobnail" appearance
  - Infiltrate of lymphocytes, histiocytes, and eosinophils

Kimura's Disease

- Characteristics
  - Occurs mainly in Asia
  - Classified as cutaneous lymphoid hyperplasia
- Location: head
- Presentation
  - Solitary or multiple nodules
  - Young to middle-aged adults
  - Almost exclusively male
  - Peripheral eosinophilia and lymphadenopathy
- Diagnosis/pathology
  - Hyperplasia of small vessels lined with plump endothelial cells within the dermis or subcutis
  - Dense infiltrates of lymphocytes, plasma cells, histiocytes, and eosinophils
  - Multiple lymphoid follicles with germinal centers

Intravascular Papillary Endothelial Hyperplasia (Masson Pseudoangiosarcoma)

- Characteristics
  - Reactive hyperplasia after intravascular thrombosis
  - As a focal change in a preexisting vascular lesion (hemangioma, pyogenic granuloma, or vascular malformation)
  - Small (<2 cm in diameter), firm, blue or purple nodule
  - Located on extremities, usually fingers
- Histology
  - Papillated vascular structures extending from the wall within vascular lumina are lined by single layer of plump endothelial cells
  - Occluded by thrombus
- Treatment: simple excision

Low-Grade Angiosarcoma

- Types
  - Endovascular papillary angioendothelioma (Dabska tumor)
  - Epithelioid hemangioendothelioma
  - Retiform hemangioendothelioma
- Location
  - Skin or soft tissue of extremities
  - Extremities > scalp
- Presentation
  - Solitary tender nodule
  - Plaques and nodules
- Complications
  - Frequent recurrence but low metastatic rate
  - Greater than 50% with metastasis die of disease

Dabska Tumor (Papillary Intralymphatic Angioendothelioma)

- Characteristics
  - Low-grade angiosarcoma that affects the skin of children
  - Slow-growing, painless, intradermal nodule that grows to 2 to 3 cm
- Laboratory studies
  - Immunoreactivity for factor VIII-related antigen, *Ulex europaeus* agglutinin I, vimentin, blood group isoantigens, and C2.1 antibody
  - Histology
    - Multiple vascular channels that interconnect
    - Lined by atypical endothelial cells; vacuolated cytoplasm, and hyperchromatic eccentric nuclei
    - Weibel-Palade bodies may be present
- Treatment: wide local excision is the treatment of choice; regional lymph node dissection if clinically necessary
- Prognosis: favorable prognosis; however, they can be locally invasive and have the potential to metastasize

Hemangioendothelioma (Epithelioid and Spindle)

- Characteristics
  - Poorly circumscribed, usually biphasic proliferation of venous or capillary vessels
  - Minimal dysplasia, few mitotic figures, and minimal differentiation toward a vascular lumen or channel
  - A third of epithelioid hemangioendotheliomas develop metastases in regional lymph nodes
  - Red/blue nodules that may be multiple and are usually superficial
  - Distal extremities (particularly the hands)
  - Second and third decades of life
- Types
  - Epithelioid hemangioendothelioma: vessels are intermixed with solid sheets of epithelioid cells
  - Spindle cell hemangioendothelioma: spindle-shaped mesenchymal cells; this can occur at any age; thought to represent a reactive vascular tumor arising in conjunction with malformed vasculature (primarily lymphatic); can be associated with Maffucci's syndrome
- Histology: slit-like vascular channels, mild extravasation of erythrocytes, and hemosiderin deposition; epithelioid

cells have abundant eosinophilic cytoplasm; spindle cell variant has bland bipolar mesenchymal fibroblast-like cells that may contain vacuoles that stain with *Ulex europaeus* and cytoplasmic factor VIII-associated antigen

- Treatment
  - Wide surgical excision
  - Greater than 50% of cases recur at the operative site or several centimeters distant

Retiform Hemangioendothelioma

- Characteristics
  - Slowly growing exophytic or plaque-like tumor is usually noted in young adults, predominantly on the lower limbs
  - May be associated with radiotherapy or chronic lymphedema
- Histology: arborizing vessels; focal solid areas composed of spindle and epithelioid; vessels lined by "hobnail" endothelial cells, prominent stromal lymphocytic infiltrate

Angiosarcoma (Fig. 13-6)

- Characteristics: subtypes
  - Idiopathic angiosarcoma
    - Elderly patients
    - Purpuric macule, plaque, nodule, or ulceration
    - Location: scalp, upper forehead
  - Lymphedema-associated angiosarcoma
    - Edematous arm of women after mastectomy on side with lymphadenectomy (Stewart-Treves syndrome)
    - Bluish plaques, nodules, and vesicles
  - Postirradiation angiosarcoma: years after radiotherapy
- Diagnosis
  - Histology
    - Irregular anastomosing vascular channels
    - Lined by hyperchromatic, pleomorphic endothelial cells; mitosis prominent
  - Immunohistochemistry: CD31, CD34, and factor VIII-related antigen are less specific

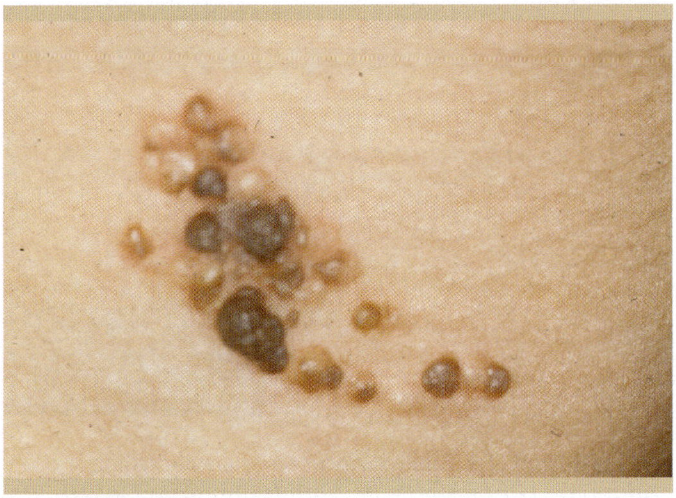

FIGURE 13-6 Angiosarcoma. (*Used with permission from Dr. Adelaide Hebert.*)

VASCULAR MALFORMATIONS

- Localized or diffuse errors of embryonic development affecting any segment of the vascular tree including arterial, venous, capillary, and/or lymphatic vessels
- Divided into 2 major categories: (1) slow-flow (capillary, lymphatic, and venous malformations) and (2) fast-flow (arteriovenous malformations and arteriovenous fistulae)
- Complex, combined vascular malformations also occur
- Affect approximately 1.2 to 1.5% of the population
- Most sporadic (nonfamilial)

Capillary

Salmon Patch (Nevus Simplex) (Fig. 13-7)

- Characteristics
  - Best classified as capillary malformation
  - Prognosis generally differs from port-wine stain
  - Thought to represent persistent fetal circulatory patterns in the skin
  - Disappears when the autonomic innervation of these vessels matures during infancy
  - Present in nearly half of all newborns
- Slow flow
- Location: nape of neck > eyelid > glabella ("angel's kiss") > nasolabial region
- Presentation
  - Pink to red patch
  - Usually fades by 1 to 2 years of age, although some lesions (especially those of the nape) may persist

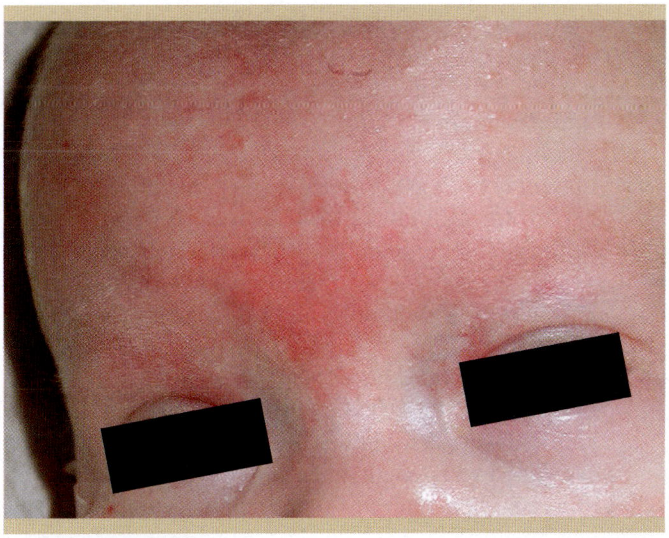

FIGURE 13-7 Nevus simplex. (*Used with permission from Dr. Denise Metry.*)

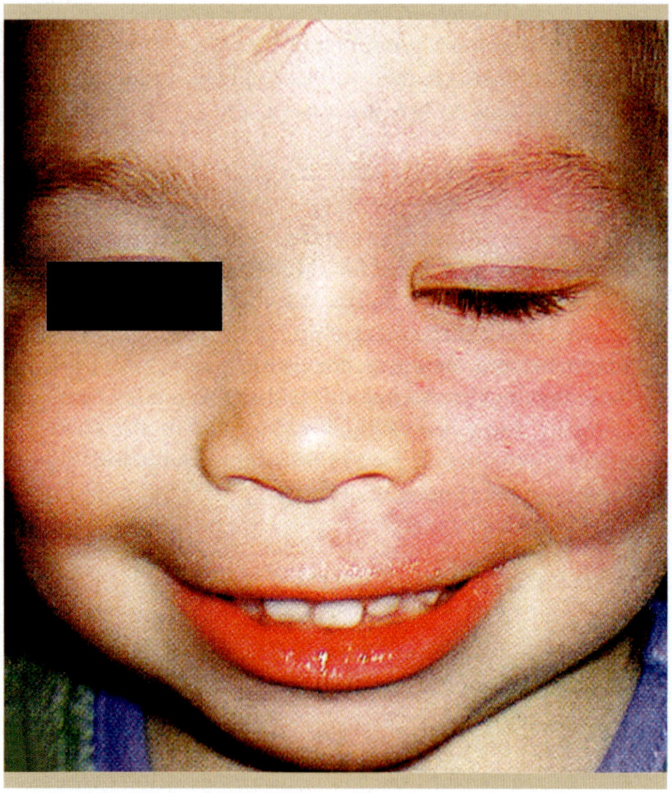

FIGURE 13-8 Port-wine stain. (*Reprinted with permission from Wolff et al. Fitzpatrick's Dermatology in General Medicine*, 7th Ed. New York: McGraw-Hill; 2008.)

Port-Wine Stain (Nevus Flammeus) (Fig. 13-8)

- Characteristics
  - Capillary malformation
  - Slow flow
  - Composed of dilated, ectatic capillary-to-venule sized vessels in the superficial dermis, with a paucity of surrounding normal nerve fibers
- Location: variable
- Presentation
  - Present at birth as erythematous patch
  - Persists throughout life
  - With age (predominantly with facial lesions), the vessels gradually dilate, leading to a dark red or deep purple color with nodules and/or pyogenic granuloma-like lesions
- Complications/associations
  - Bony and soft tissue hypertrophy, especially in the V2 and V3 facial distributions, extremity lesions may be associated with length discrepancy
  - Sturge-Weber syndrome (encephalotrigeminal angiomatosis)
    - Triad
    - Facial port-wine stain
- Usually trigeminal V1 dermatome: forehead and upper eyelid
- Approximately 10% of infants with port-wine stain in trigeminal V1 location will have Sturge-Weber syndrome
    - Ipsilateral ocular vascular anomalies: can lead to retinal detachment, glaucoma, and blindness
    - Leptomeningeal vascular anomalies: can lead to early-onset seizures
  - Midline facial stains have been associated with Beckwith-Wiedemann syndrome
- Diagnosis/pathology: dilated, mature capillaries in the superficial dermis
- Treatment
  - Flashlamp-pumped, pulsed-dye laser (585 and 595 nm)
    - Low risk of scarring
    - Multiple treatments required
    - Most patients achieve lightening but not complete clearance
    - V2 and distal extremity lesions less responsive
  - Cosmetic camouflage

Cutis Marmorata Telangiectatica Congenita (Fig. 13-9)

- Characteristics
  - Congenital, with reticulate purple network
  - Most cases occur sporadically
  - May be associated with atrophy and/or ulceration
  - Limb +/− trunk
  - Limb girth discrepancy: common; other associated anomalies probably less common

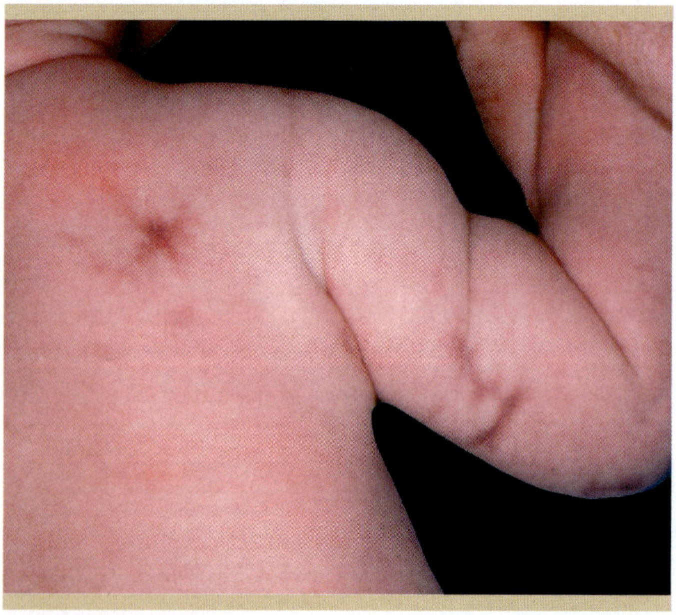

FIGURE 13-9 Cutis marmorata telangiectatica congenita. (*Reprinted with permission from Goldsmith LA et al. Fitzpatrick's Dermatology in General Medicine*, 8th Ed. New York: McGraw-Hill; 2012.)

- Diagnosis: generally clinical
- Treatment: no treatment is needed unless associated anomalies
- Erythema improves over time
- Macrocephaly-capillary malformation (formerly macrocephaly-cutis marmorata telangiectatica congenita syndrome) is a distinct entity (see vascular malformation syndromes)

Hereditary Hemorrhagic Telangiectasia (Osler-Weber-Rendu Syndrome)

- Inheritance: autosomal dominant
- Results from mutations in endoglin, activin receptor-like kinase 1 or rarely Smad4, which modulate TGF-*B* signaling in vascular endothelial cells
- Diagnosis is based on family history and the presence of 3 separate manifestations:
  1. Mucocutaneous telangiectasia (especially fingertips, lips, oral mucosa, and tongue)
  2. Spontaneous recurrent nosebleeds
  3. Visceral involvement (GI tract, pulmonary, hepatic, cerebral, and/or spinal AVM)

Phakomatosis Pigmentovascularis

- Characterized by association of capillary malformation with a melanocytic or epidermal lesion (dermal melanocytosis, nevus spilus or speckled lentiginous nevus, nevus anemicus)
- Hereditary disorder thought to be explained by the "twin spot" phenomenon

Unilateral Nevoid Telangiectasia (UNT)

- Characteristics
  - Congenital or acquired patches of superficial telangiectases in a unilateral linear distribution
  - May result from a somatic mutation during embryologic development
  - Third and fourth cervical dermatomes most common sites, thoracic dermatomes, or scattered distant sites also may be involved
  - Pathogenesis of UNT remains unknown, possibly related to hormonal causes
- Histology: dilated capillaries in the superficial dermis
- Treatment: pulsed-dye lasers

Angiokeratoma

- Characteristics
  - Slow flow
  - Capillary ectasia in the papillary dermis
  - May produce papillomatosis, acanthosis, and hyperkeratosis of the epidermis
- Types
  - Angiokeratomas of Fordyce
    - Uncommon
    - 2- to 4-mm red-to-blue domed papules with keratotic surface
    - Peak incidence after the third decade; more common in males
    - Most often on the scrotum and vulva
    - Lesions number from one to many (>100)
  - Angiokeratoma circumscriptum
    - Uncommon
    - Small red macules coalesce to form large acanthokeratotic plaques
    - Usually occurs in childhood; equally common in males and females
    - Often found on the extremities
    - Associated with vascular malformations and atrophy or hypertrophy of regional soft tissue and bone
  - Angiokeratoma corporis diffusum (Fabry disease)
    - Rare
    - X-linked inherited disorder
    - Caused by a deficiency of the lysosomal enzyme α-galactosidase
    - Unremitting deposition of neural glycosphingolipids in the lysosomes of: vascular endothelium, fibroblasts, and pericytes of the dermis, heart, kidneys, and autonomic nervous system
    - Clinical findings:
      - ▲ Skin: verrucous papules, deep red to blue-black in color, between the umbilicus and the knees, with a predilection for the scrotum, penis, lower back, thighs, hips, and buttocks
      - ▲ Ocular: corneal opacities and posterior capsular cataracts
      - ▲ Neurologic: burning, tingling paresthesias, hemiplegia, hemianesthesia, balance disorders, and personality changes
      - ▲ Extremities: chronic edema of the feet and arthritis of the distal interphalangeal joints
      - ▲ Cardiac: infiltration results in angina, myocardial infarction, mitral valve prolapse, congestive heart failure, hypertension, mitral insufficiency, and ventricular hypertrophy
      - ▲ Urinalysis: urinary maltese crosses of lipid globules
  - Angiokeratoma of Mibelli
    - Uncommon
    - Multiple 3- to 5-mm dark red papules with verrucous surface
    - Most often affects females younger than 20 years
    - Most often found on dorsa of fingers and toes; less commonly observed on elbows, knees, shoulders, and earlobes
    - Associated with recurrent chilblains and acrocyanosis
    - Autosomal dominant inheritance with variable penetrance

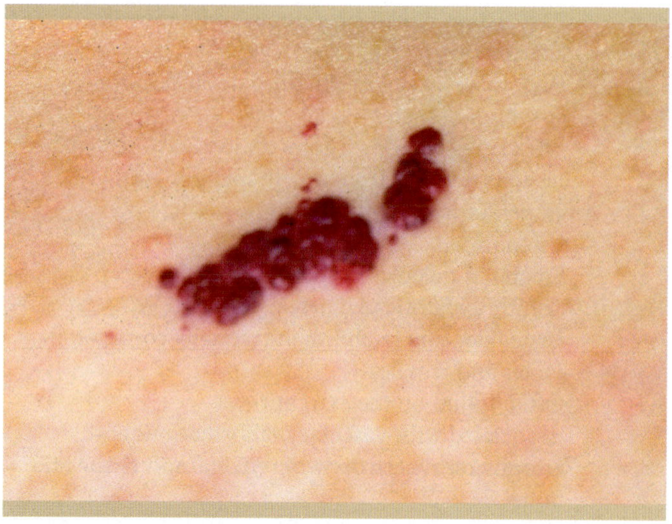

FIGURE 13-10 Solitary angiokeratoma. (*Used with permission from Dr. John Browning.*)

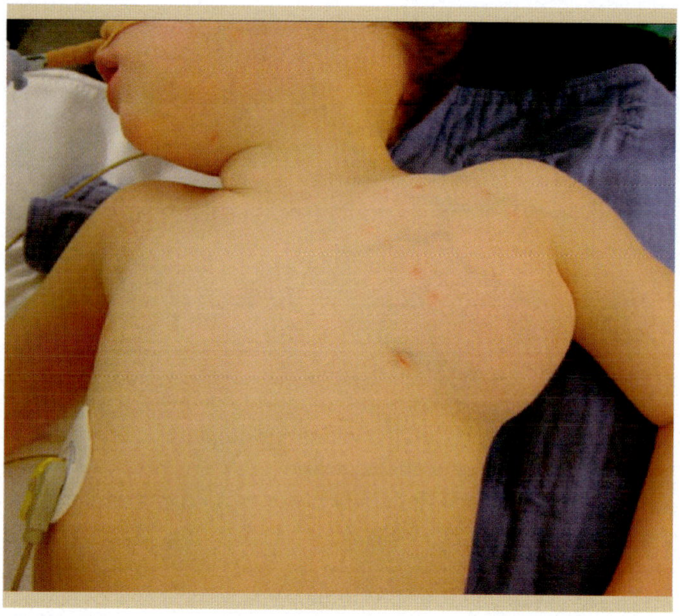

FIGURE 13-11 Lymphatic malformation. (*Reprinted with permission from Wolff et al. Fitzpatrick's Dermatology in General Medicine,* 7th Ed. New York: McGraw-Hill; 2008.)

- Solitary angiokeratoma (Fig. 13-10)
  - Most common type
  - 2- to 10-mm dark papules or plaques that keratinize and turn blue-black
  - Peak incidence during third to fourth decades of life; more common in males
  - Presents most often on the lower extremities
- Treatment
  - Either ablation or excision can be performed
  - Erbium or carbon dioxide laser to remove the hyperkeratotic-acanthotic epidermis, followed by the use of lasers that target hemoglobin
  - Cryotherapy

Lymphatic Malformation (Fig. 13-11)

- Characteristics
  - Slow flow
  - Subcategorized by vessel size: microcystic (lymphangioma circumscriptum, lymphangioma), macrocystic (cystic hygroma), or combined
- Location
  - Macrocystic
    - Compressible mass with normal overlying skin
    - Axilla/chest, cervicofacial region (most common), mediastinum, retroperitoneum, buttocks, and anogenital areas
    - Large, nuchal lesions documented on fetal ultrasound associated with an increased risk of aneuploidy, chromosomal abnormalities including Down or Turner syndrome, cardiac malformation, and perinatal death
  - Microcystic: axillary folds, shoulders, neck, proximal limbs, perineum, tongue, and floor of mouth
- Presentation
  - May become evident at birth or become so in early childhood
  - Microcystic lymphangiomas of the skin
    - Consist of grouped, clear vesicles ("frog spawn")
    - May contain blood, giving lesions a pink, purple, or black color
    - May have overlying hyperkeratosis
- Complications/associations: numerous, depending on location, but disfigurement, infection, intralesional bleeding most common
  - Progressive osteolysis, caused by diffuse soft-tissue and skeletal lymphatic malformations, is called Gorham-Stout syndrome
    - Histopathologic features show replacement of bone with vascular malformation, leading to gradual and often complete resorption of bone resulting in pathologic fractures
- Diagnosis
  - Lymphedema should be considered a type of lymphatic malformation
    - Congenital lymphedema (Milroy disease) is an autosomal dominant disorder caused by a mutant, inactive VEGFR3 receptor, and presents at birth or early in life with lower leg edema
    - Generalized lymphatic dysplasia is a rare form of edema characterized by systemic involvement such as intestinal lymphangiectasia, ascites, pleural or pericardial effusions, and pulmonary lymphangiectasia

- Diagnosis
  - Histologically composed of thin-walled vessels lined by lymphatic endothelial cells, which are immunopositive for podoplanin (D2-40) and LYVE-1
  - MRI: best means of determining lesion extent
- Treatment
  - Surgery and/or sclerotherapy: mainstay of therapy, although cure rarely achieved except with well-localized lesions
  - Sclerotherapy is most effective for macrocystic subtypes and involves entering the cavity by direct puncture, aspiration of fluid and injection of sclerosant. This causes obliteration of the lymphatic lumen by endothelial destruction with subsequent sclerosis/fibrosis; several sessions are typically required
  - Laser photocoagulation: can be temporizing measure for microcystic cutaneous lesions
  - Elastic compression stockings for extremity lesions

VENOUS MALFORMATION: GENERAL

- Characteristics: slow flow, the most common of all vascular anomalies
- Most commonly sporadic
  - Fifty percent due to loss-of-function mutation in TIE2, a receptor tyrosine kinase involved in vascular remodeling
- Location: skin, subcutaneous tissues, and mucosa
- Presentation
  - Present, though not always evident, at birth
  - Usually solitary and localized
  - Soft, deep-blue masses that are easily compressible and slowly refill on release
  - Swell with dependency or activity
  - Enlarge proportionally with the child and undergo slow expansion over time
  - Phleboliths (progressive calcifications) are a hallmark of venous malformation and a common source of localized pain
  - Pain and stiffness on morning awakening and dull aching are other common complaints
- Associated conditions
  - Familial cutaneous mucosal VM: autosomal dominant
    - One to two percent of VMs
    - Characterized by small VMs of the skin and gastrointestinal mucosa
  - Blue-rubber bleb nevus syndrome: sporadic
    - Skin (most commonly trunk, palms, and soles) and bowel VMs
    - Bowel lesions commonly lead to chronic gastrointestinal bleeding

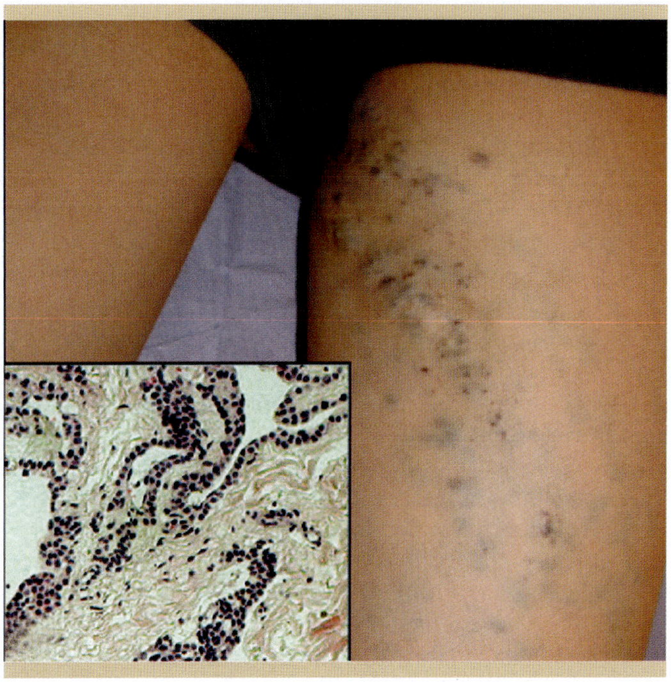

FIGURE 13-12 Superficial glomuvenous malformation on the thigh; note presence of mural glomus cells on H&E stained histologic sample. (*Reprinted with permission from Goldsmith LA et al. Fitzpatrick's Dermatology in General Medicine,* 8th Ed. New York: McGraw-Hill; 2012.)

  - Glomuvenous malformations: also known as glomus tumors, glomangiomas, or glomangiomatosis (Fig. 13-12)
    - Autosomal dominant inheritance; 5% of all VMs
    - Caused by loss-of-function mutations in glomulin, involved in vascular smooth muscle cell differentiation
    - Multiple, blue nodular dermal lesions with cobblestone-like appearance
    - Most common on extremities
    - Poorly compressible, painful
    - Surgical resection often best treatment option
  - Diagnosis
    - Histology: anomalous, dilated veins with irregularly thickened walls
    - MRI best means of determining lesion extent
  - Treatment
    - Elastic support stockings of affected extremity
    - Low-dose aspirin may be useful for painful thrombosis
    - Sclerotherapy and/or surgery reserved for lesions causing significant functional compromise, symptoms or cosmetic deformity

Arteriovenous Malformation

- Characteristics: fast flow, the most dangerous type of vascular anomaly

- Consist of disorganized arteries and veins that directly communicate (shunt)
- Most commonly sporadic
- Presentation
  - Present at birth but often remains latent until adolescence or local trauma
  - Early lesions may appear as a faint vascular stain that is often mistaken for a capillary malformation
  - Eventually manifests as a warm, pulsatile mass with draining veins, and deepening of color
  - End stage lesions: ulceration, bleeding, intractable pain, and disfigurement
  - Location: intracranial > extremities > trunk > viscera
- Associated conditions
  - Capillary malformation-AVM (CM-AVM) caused by mutations in *RASA1*
  - Includes Parkes-Weber syndrome and intracranial or extracranial AVM
- Diagnosis
  - Initial: ultrasonography with Doppler imaging
  - MR angiography (MRA) or superselective angiography for further delineation
- Treatment
  - Angiographic embolization alone or in combination with surgical excision is the mainstay of treatment
  - Treatment generally delayed until significant symptoms or endangering signs develop

Complex Vascular Malformation/Overgrowth Syndromes

Beckwith-Wiedemann Syndrome

- Inheritance: sporadic
- Clinical
  - Capillary malformation at midforehead
  - Macroglossia, exomphalos, linear earlobe creases; circular depression on helix
  - Organomegaly (big baby, big tongue, and big organs)
- Potential complications/associations
  - Malignancies: Wilms tumor, adrenal cortical carcinoma, rhabdomyosarcoma, and hepatoblastoma
  - Gastrointestinal: omphalocele and intestinal malrotation

Cloves Syndrome

- Clinical
  - Acronym for congenital lipomatous overgrowth, vascular malformation, epidermal nevi, and musculoskeletal anomalies (scoliosis, skeletal and spinal anomalies, seizures)

Klippel-Trenaunay-Weber Syndrome

- Inheritance: sporadic
- Characterized by combined capillary-lymphaticovenous malformation associated with soft-tissue and skeletal hypertrophy
  - Most commonly affects lower extremity > upper extremity > trunk
  - Overgrowth of affected limb apparent at birth or occurs within the first few months to years of life
- Diagnosis: primarily MRI and MRV
- Treatment
  - Generally conservative with compression therapy; sclerotherapy and/or surgery can be considered in select patients
  - Regular visits to clinically and radiographically assess for limb length discrepancy; if significant, refer to orthopedics

Macrocephaly-Capillary Malformation Syndrome

- Formerly known as macrocephaly-cutis marmorata telangiectatica congenita (CMTC) syndrome, but distinct entity from CMTC
- Inheritance: sporadic
- Clinical features
  - Macrocephaly, neonatal hypotonia, developmental delay, segmental overgrowth, syndactyly, asymmetry, connective tissue defects, and capillary malformations

Maffucci Syndrome

- Inheritance: sporadic
- Clinical features
  - Triad of chondrodysplasia of one or more limbs, multiple enchondromas, and vascular lesions (venous malformations and spindle cell hemangioendotheliomas)
  - Bony enchondromas lead to exostoses, recurrent fractures
  - Risk of chondrosarcoma (15–20%), angiosarcoma, fibrosarcoma, osteosarcoma, lymphangiosarcoma, and intracranial tumors

Parkes-Weber Syndrome

- Similar to Klippel-Trenaunay syndrome, but with additional component of capillary-arteriovenous malformation/fistula
- AVM clinically evident at birth
- Caused by mutations in *RASA1*

Proteus Syndrome

- Inheritance: sporadic
- Clinical
  - Disproportionate overgrowth of multiple tissues in association with various cutaneous and subcutaneous mesodermal hamartomas, including vascular malformations
  - Changes can be present at birth or develop over time
  - Striking cerebriform hyperplasia of the plantar feet
- Associated with mutations in *PTEN* tumor-suppressor gene

PTEN Hamartoma Tumor Syndrome

- Results from mutation in *PTEN*, a gene encoding a tumor suppressor protein involved in cell cycle regulation
- Mutations are responsible for 2 disorders that predispose to cancer: Bannayan-Riley-Ruvalcaba syndrome and Cowden syndrome
- Associated vascular anomalies tend to be fast-flow radiographically, but disordered growths of blood vessels, adipose tissue, and fibrous tissue histopathologically
- Clinical features of Bannayan-Riley-Ruvalcaba syndrome: macrocephaly, penile freckling, macrosomia at birth, lipomas, hamartomatous intestinal polyposis, proximal myopathy, and various degrees of developmental delay
- Clinical features of Cowden syndrome (generally identified in adulthood): range of mucocutaneous manifestations and increased risk for tumor development in the breast, thyroid, and endometrium
- Patients with fast-flow vascular malformations should undergo clinical and genetic evaluation for *PTEN* mutations

QUIZ

Questions

1. Acquired hypothyroidism is a potential complication of

   A. Kaposiform hemangioendothelioma
   B. Multiple or diffuse hepatic hemangiomas
   C. PHACE syndrome
   D. Solitary cutaneous infantile hemangioma
   E. None of these

2. A 2-month-old infant presents with a segmental, facial infantile hemangioma located in a "beard" distribution, including the lower lip. Which of the following are potential complications?

   A. Airway hemangioma
   B. Cardiovascular anomalies
   C. Cerebrovascular anomalies
   D. Ulceration
   E. All of these

3. An otherwise healthy 2-month-old infant is started on oral propranolol for a painful, ulcerated hemangioma of her perineum that has not responded adequately to standard wound care. Which of the following is the most serious potential side effect of propranolol to consider?

   A. Bronchospasm
   B. Hyperkalemia
   C. Hypoglycemia
   D. Hypothyroidism
   E. Gastrointestinal complications

4. Which of the following features help distinguish a glomuvenous malformation from classic venous malformation?

   A. Autosomal dominant inheritance
   B. Nodular, cobblestone-like appearance
   C. Pain with compression
   D. Poor compressibility
   E. All of these

5. All of the following syndromes classically include "overgrowth" EXCEPT:

   A. CLOVES
   B. Hereditary Hemorrhagic Telangiectasia (Osler-Weber-Rendu)
   C. Klippel-Trenaunay-Weber
   D. Macrocephaly-capillary malformation
   E. Proteus

6. The following are subtypes of Kaposi sarcoma (KS), EXCEPT:

   A. African endemic KS
   B. Classic KS
   C. Epidemic HIV-associated KS
   D. Asian endemic KS
   E. All of the above are subtypes

7. All of the following statements regarding classic Kaposi sarcoma are true, EXCEPT:

   A. It is more common in men than women
   B. Involvement of the upper extremities is more common than the lower extremities
   C. Ionizing radiation may be used as a form of treatment
   D. Topical imiquimod may slow progression of the disease
   E. The lungs, spleen, and heart may be involved

8. Mutations in *RASA-1* have been linked to which of the following?

   A. Capillary malformation-arteriovenous malformation syndrome
   B. Extracranial arteriovenous malformations
   C. Intracranial arteriovenous malformations
   D. Parkes-Weber syndrome
   E. All of these

9. Which of the following statements best describes Dabska tumor?

   A. A rare, low-grade angiosarcoma that often affects the skin of children
   B. Reactive hyperplasia after intravascular thrombosis
   C. An exophytic tumor in young adults, predominantly located on the lower extremities

D. A vascular tumor present at birth that undergoes rapid involution
E. A violaceous tumor associated with thrombocytopenia

10. LUMBAR syndrome is an acronym for all of the following EXCEPT:

A. Bony deformities
B. Liver hemangiomas
C. Renal anomalies
D. Spinal dysraphism
E. Urogenital anomalies

Answers

1. B. Complications of multifocal and diffuse liver hemangiomas include acquired hypothyroidism due to hemangioma expression of type III thyronine deiodinase.
2. E. Segmental hemangiomas, especially when located in trauma-prone locations such as the lip, are at higher risk of ulceration. Segmental hemangiomas of the face are also at risk for PHACE syndrome, of which cerebrovascular and cardiovascular anomalies are the most common complications. Lastly, segmental hemangiomas in a "beard" facial distribution have a known association with concomitant airway hemangioma.
3. C. Potential side effects of oral propranolol include hypotension, bradycardia, hypoglycemia, bronchospasm, congestive heart failure, gastrointestinal complications, sleep disturbance, cool or mottled extremities, hyperkalemia, rash or dry skin, depression, dental caries, and drug interactions due to metabolism within cytochrome P450 system. Of these, hypoglycemia may be most serious potential complication, usually related to decreased oral intake or an overnight fast.
4. E. Classic venous malformations are most commonly inherited sporadically, and present as soft, deep-blue, nontender masses that are easily compressible and slowly refill on release.
5. B. HHT is characterized by mucocutaneous telangiectasias, spontaneous recurrent nosebleeds, and a risk of arteriovenous malformations in the lungs, brain, and liver. Overgrowth is not a feature.
6. D. African endemic KS, classic KS, and epidemic HIV-associated KS are all subtypes of KS. Asian endemic KS is not a distinct KS subtype.
7. B. Classic KS typically affects males older than 50 years, predominant in Mediterranean and Jewish populations. These patients have increased risk of lymphoreticular neoplasms. Clinically, classic KS appears as violaceous macules with slow progression to plaques. It involves the distal lower extremities, with unilateral involvement and centripedal spread to a disseminated and multifocal pattern. The oral cavity and GI tract (90%) are commonly affected; possible involvement of lung, spleen, and heart. Classic KS has a benign course owing to slow progression.
8. E. Mutations in *RASA-1* have been linked to capillary malformation-arteriovenous malformation syndrome, intracranial and extracranial arteriovenous malformations, and Parkes-Weber syndrome.
9. A. Dabska tumor is a low-grade angiosarcoma that affects the skin of children. It is a slow-growing, painless, intradermal nodule. Dabsk tumor has immunoreactivity for factor VIII-related antigen, Ulex europaeus agglutinin I, vimentin, blood group isoantigens, and C2.1 antibody. Histologically, multiple vascular channels that interconnect are lined by atypical endothelial cells; vacuolated cytoplasm, and hyperchromatic eccentric nuclei. Weibel-Palade bodies may be present. Wide local excision is the treatment of choice; regional lymph node dissection if clinically necessary. Prognosis is favorable; however, the tumor can be locally invasive and has the potential to metastasize.
10. B. LUMBAR syndrome is an acronym for *l*ower body hemangioma and other cutaneous defects, *u*rogenital anomalies, *u*lceration, *m*yelopathy (most commonly including spinal dysraphism), *b*ony deformities, *a*norectal malformations, *a*rterial anomalies, and *r*enal anomalies. Liver hemangiomas are not a feature.

REFERENCES

Buckmiller LM: Update on hemangiomas and vascular malformations. *Curr Opin Otolaryngol Head Neck Surg* 2004 Dec;12(6):476-487.

Drolet BA, Frommelt PC, Chamlin SL, et al. Initiation and use of propranolol for infantile hemangioma: report of a consensus conference. *Pediatrics* 2013;131(1):128-140.

Fevurly DR, Fishman SJ: Vascular anomalies in pediatrics. *Surg Clin N Am* 2012;92(3):769-800.

Gampper TJ, Morgan RF: Vascular anomalies: hemangiomas. *Plast Reconstr Surg* 2002 Aug;110(2):572-585.

Goldsmith LA et al. *Fitzpatrick's Dermatology in General Medicine*, 8th Ed. New York: McGraw-Hill; 2012.

Marler JJ, Mulliken JB: Current management of hemangiomas and vascular malformations. *Clin Plast Surg* 2005 Jan; 32(1):99-116, ix.

McKee PH: *Pathology of the Skin: With Clinical Correlations*. London: Mosby-Wolfe; 1996.

Metry DW: Potential complications of segmental hemangiomas of infancy. *Sem Cut Med Surg* 2004;23(2):107-115.

Mulliken JB, Fishman SJ, Burrows PE: Vascular anomalies. *Curr Probl Surg* 2002;37(8):517-584.

Spring MA, Bentz ML: Cutaneous vascular lesions. *Clin Plast Surg* 2005 Apr;32(2):171-186.

Werner JA, Dunne AA, Lippert BM, et al. Optimal treatment of vascular birthmarks. *Am J Clin Dermatol* 2003;4(11):745-756.

CHAPTER 14

GENODERMATOSIS

NNENNA G. AGIM
JOY H. KUNISHIGE
MARZIEH THURBER
ADRIENNE M. FEASEL
ADELAIDE A. HEBERT

EPIDERMOLYSIS BULLOSA (EB)

- Disorder with the formation of bullae and erosions following mechanical trauma to the skin and mucosa
- All types of EB patients exhibit fragile skin and blisters. Scarring, nail dystrophy, milia, and scarring alopecia occur in the forms involving the lamina lucida and below
- Gene defects cause abnormalities in structural proteins of the epidermis and the epidermal-dermal junction
- Subtypes are classified based on the ultrastructural level of blisters (Table 14-1), mode of inheritance, and the clinical features
- There are four major EB types (Table 14-2) and multiple related subtypes (Table 14-3)

Diagnosis

- Transmission electron microscopy (EM): evaluation of level of skin cleavage: intraepidermal, intralamina lucida, or sublamina densa
- Immunofluorescence mapping (IFM): monoclonal antibodies, can identify the structural protein most likely mutated resulting in the different forms of EB (Table 14-4) (Fig 14-1)
- Mutational analysis: determines the mode of inheritance and the precise site(s) and type(s) of molecular mutation present (Table 14-5)

Epidermolysis Bullosa Simplex (EBS)

- Autosomal dominant (AD) (most common) or recessive
  - Targeted proteins include: keratins 5 and 14 (basal cell keratin), desmoplakin, plakophilin-1 (Table 14-6)
  - When the defect involves keratins 5 and 14, the bulla results from a split through lowest part of basal keratinocyte
- Dominant subtypes
  - Localized EBS:
    - *Weber-Cockayne type*: localized lesions on the palms and soles, hyperhidrosis, most common type of EBS (Fig 14-2)
  - Generalized EBS:
    - *Koebner type*: presents during infancy and early childhood, generalized lesions (extremities are more severely involved), palmoplantar hyperkeratosis
    - *Dowling-Meara type* (EBS herpetiformis): onset at birth, herpetiform grouped vesicles on annular erythematous base, nail dystrophy, oral mucosal involvement
  - Other subtypes:
    - *EB simplex with mottled pigmentation*: onset at birth, generalized distribution, mottled or reticulated brown pigmentation
    - *Superficial type*: disruption of the stratum granulosum
    - *Acantholytic type*: hyperkeratosis and bullae of the palms and soles
- Recessive subtypes:
  - *Muscular dystrophy type*: abnormality of plec 1 (plectin 1/intermediate filament binding protein), hemidesmosomal protein 1 (HD1/protein needed for hemidesmosome formation), causes split through lowest part of basal keratinocyte, muscular dystrophy occurs in the limb-girdle
  - *Type unrelated to muscular dystrophy*: homozygous K14 nonsense mutation
  - *Skin fragility syndrome*: abnormal plakophillin (desmosomal protein, PKP1), classified as a variant of acantholytic EB, but also considered a form of ectodermal dysplasia; formation of intraepidermal acantholysis; alopecia, palmoplantar keratoderma, painful fissures, nail dystrophy, cheilitis, hypohidrosis

TABLE 14-1 Ultrastructural Findings Among Major Types and Selected Subtypes of EB

EB Type or Subtype	Ultrastructural Site of Skin Findings	Other Ultrastructural Findings
EB simplex (EBS)		
EBS, localized	Basal layer	Split may spread to suprabasilar layer
EBS, DM	Basal layer in subnuclear cytoplasm	Dense, circumscribed clumps of keratin filaments (most commonly observed
EBS-MD	Predominantly in basal layer, above level of HD attachment plaque	Reduced integration of keratin filaments with HD
EBS-AR	Basal keratinocytes	Absent or reduced keratin filaments within basal keratinocytes
EBSS	Split usually at interface between granular and cornified cell layers	—
EBS, lethal acantholytic	Suprabasal cleavage and acantholysis	Perinuclear retraction of keratin filaments
EBS, plakophilin-1 deficiency	Midepidermal cell-cell separation	Diminutive suprabasal desmosomes; perinuclear retraction of keratin filaments
EBS-PA	Lower basal layer, above level of HD plaque	Reduced integration of keratin filaments with HD
Junctional EB (JEB)		
JEB-H	Lamina lucida	Markedly reduced or absent HD; absent SBDP
JEB-nH	Lamina lucida	HDs may be normal or reduced in size and number
JEB-PA	Lamina lucida	Small HD plaques often with attenuated SBDP
Dominant dystrophic EB (DDEB)		
DDEB, generalized	Sublamina densa	Normal or decreased numbers of AFs
DDEB-BDN	Sublamina densa	Electron-dense stellate bodies within basal layer; reduced AFs
Recessive dystrophic EB (RDEB)		
RDEB, severe generalized	Sublamina densa	Absent or rudimentary AFs
RDEB, generalized other	Sublamina densa	Reduced or rudimentary-appearing AFs
RDEB-BDN	Sublamina densa	Electron-dense stellate bodies within basal layer; reduced AFs

AF, anchoring fibril; *AR*, autosomal recessive; *BDN*, bullous dermolysis of the newborn; *DM*, Dowling-Meara; *EBSS*, EBS superficialis; *H*, Herlitz; *HD*, hemidesmosome; *MD*, muscular dystrophy; *nH*, non-Herlitz; *PA*, pyloric atresia; *SBDP*, sub-basal dense plate.

Reprinted with permission from Fine JD, Eady RA, Bauer EA, et al. The classification of inherited epidermolysis bullosa (EB): Report of the Third International Consensus Meeting on Diagnosis and Classification of EB. *J Am Acad Dermatol* 2008 Jun;58(6):931–950. Epub 2008 Apr 18.

TABLE 14-2 The Four Major EB Types

Level of Skin Cleavage	Major EB Type	Known Targeted Protein(s)
Intraepidermal ("epidermolytic")	EBS	Keratins 5 and 14; plectin; α6β4 integrin; plakophilin-1; desmoplakin
Intralamina lucida ("lamina lucidolytic")	JEB	Laminin-332 (laminin 5); type XVII collagen; α6β4 integrin
Sublamina densa ("dermolytic")	DEB	Type VII collagen
Mixed	Kindler syndrome	Kindlin-1

DEB, dystrophic EB; EBS, EB simplex; JEB, junctional EB.

Reprinted with permission from Fine JD, Eady RA, Bauer EA, et al. The classification of inherited epidermolysis bullosa (EB): Report of the Third International Consensus Meeting on Diagnosis and Classification of EB. *J Am Acad Dermatol* 2008 Jun;58(6):931–950. Epub 2008 Apr 18.

TABLE 14-3 The Major EB Subtypes

Major EB Type	Major EB Subtypes	Targeted Protein(s)
EBS	Suprabasal EBS	Plakophilin-1; desmoplakin; ? others
	Basal EBS	Keratins 5 and 14; plectin; α6β4 integrin
JEB	JEB-H	Laminin-332 (laminin-5)
	JEB, other	Laminin-332; type XVII collagen; α6β4 integrin
DEB	Dominant DEB	Type VII collagen
	Recessive DEB	Type VII collagen
Kindler syndrome	—	Kindlin-1

DEB, dystrophic EB; *EBS*, EB simplex; *JEB*, junctional EB.

Reprinted with permission from Fine JD, Eady RA, Bauer EA, et al. The classification of inherited epidermolysis bullosa (EB): Report of the Third International Consensus Meeting on Diagnosis and Classification of EB. *J Am Acad Dermatol* 2008 Jun;58(6):931–950. Epub 2008 Apr 18.

- *EBS with pyloric atresia*: (possibly AR), widespread congenital absence of skin, pyloric atresia, malformed pinnae and nasal alae; joint contractures; cryptorchidism

Junctional Epidermolysis Bullosa (JEB)

- Autosomal recessive
  - Split within lamina lucida
  - Targeted proteins include: Laminin 5, type XVII collagen, α6β4 integrin (Table 14-7)
- Two main subtypes:
  - *JEB-Herlitz*: defect of laminin-5 gene (codes for an anchoring filament glycoprotein), more severe than other subtype with associated premature death, generalized blistering, multisystem disease: eyes (corneal, conjunctival), mucosa (tracheobronchial, oral, pharyngeal, esophageal, rectal, and genitourinary [GU]); delayed puberty, exuberant granulation, pitted teeth
  - *JEB-non-Herlitz*: defect found in laminin-5 and bullous pemphigoid antigen-2 (type XVII collagen, 180 kDa), milder form of JEB; corneal erosions, teeth with pitted enamel
- *Generalized atrophic benign EB (GABEB)*: ambient temperature causes increased blistering, blisters heal with atrophy
- *Junctional epidermolysis bullosa with pyloric atresia*: AR, defect in α6β4 integrin gene; affects hemidesmosome, split within lamina lucida, pyloric atresia present at birth, rudimentary ears, GU malformations, may be associated with large areas of aplasia cutis, focal segmental glomerulosclerosis
- *JEB inversa*
  - Blisters located in intertriginous areas, presents at birth, atrophic scarring, dystrophic or absent nails, intraoral erosions; esophagus and anus may be severely involved
- *Laryngo-onycho-cutaneous syndrome* (LOC syndrome, Shabbir syndrome): AR; associated with mutations in the a3 chain of laminin-332; blisters commonly found on face and neck, onset first few months of life, hoarseness, exuberant granulation of conjunctiva and/or larynx
- *JEB, late onset (EB progressive)*
  - AR, onset young adulthood or later, hyperhidrosis, absent dermatoglyphs; affects hands, feet, elbows, and knees; nails are absent or dystrophic, intraoral erosions

TABLE 14-4 Antigenic Alterations in EB Skin

Antigen	Abnormal Staining in:	Usual Pattern of Staining
Keratin 14	EBS-AR	Absent or markedly reduced
Laminin-332 (laminin-5)	JEB-H	Absent or markedly reduced
	JEB-nH generalized	Reduced
Collagen	JEB-nH, generalized	Absent
	JEB-nH, localized	Reduced
Type VII collagen	RDEB, severe generalized	Absent or markedly reduced
	JEB-nH, localized	Reduced
Type VII collagen	RDEB, severe generalized	Absent or markedly reduced
	RDEB, generalized other	Reduced
	RDEB, inversa	Variable
	DEB-BDN (only during period of active blistering)	Granular staining within basal and suprabasal keratinocytes; absent or markedly reduced staining along DEJ
Plectin	EBS-MD	Absent or reduced
	EBS-PA	Absent or reduced
	EBS-Ogna	Reduced
α6β4 Integrin	JEB-PA	Absent or reduced
	EBS-PA	Absent or reduced
	JEB-nH	Reduced
Kindlin-1	Kindler syndrome	Absent, reduced, or normal

Reprinted with permission from Fine JD, Eady RA, Bauer EA, et al. The classification of inherited epidermolysis bullosa (EB): Report of the Third International Consensus Meeting on Diagnosis and Classification of EB. *J Am Acad Dermatol* 2008 Jun;58(6):931–950. Epub 2008 Apr 18.

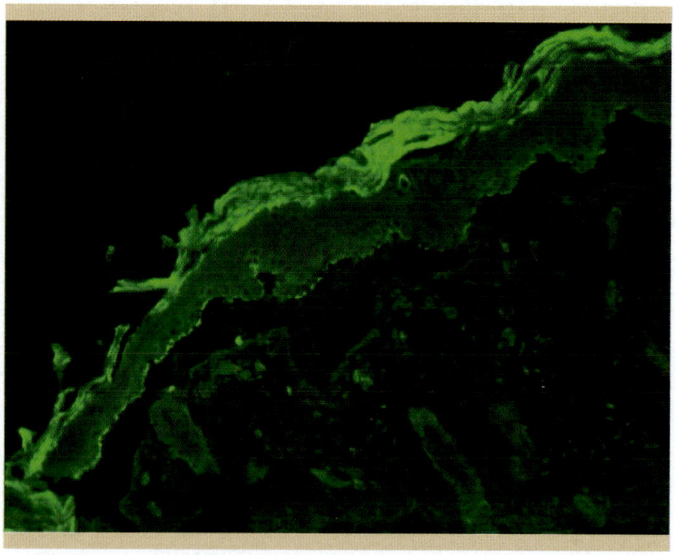

FIGURE 14-1 Epidermolysis bullosa immunomapping. *(Used with permission from Dr. Agim.)*

Epidermolysis Bullosa Dystrophica (Fig. 14-1)

- Autosomal dominant and recessive types
- Due to defects of type VII collagen found in the anchoring fibril protein and in most cases are related to *COL7A1* gene mutations (Table 14-8)

Dominant Dystrophic Epidermolysis Bullosa

- Fewer anchoring fibrils (type VII collagen)
- Subepithelial split below lamina densa
- *Generalized type (Pasini; Cockayne-Touraine)*: AD, Cockayne-Touraine: onset at birth with generalized blistering, hypertrophic lesions, acral distribution, dystrophic nails (Fig 14-3)
- *Pasini variant*: onset in infancy with more extensive blistering that heals with atrophic scars and milia; albopapuloid lesions (white papular lesions) on the trunk, intraoral lesions
- Transient bullous dermolysis of the newborn is subtype that resolves by age 1 or 2 years

Recessive Dystrophic Epidermolysis Bullosa (RDEB)

- Absent anchoring fibrils (type VII collagen)
- Subepithelial split below lamina densa
- *RDEB mitis*: involves acral areas and nails, localized form
- *Severe generalized (Hallopeau-Siemens type)*: generalized lesions and clubbing of the digits, pseudosyndactyly of fingers and toes (mitten hand deformity), flexion contractures, esophageal strictures and webs, stenosis of urethra and anal canal, phimosis, corneal scarring, squamous cell carcinoma can develop in nonhealing wounds; glomerulonephritis, renal amyloidosis; IgA nephropathy; chronic renal failure (CRF); cardiomyopathy; delayed puberty; osteoporosis most severe type (Fig 14-4)

TABLE 14-5 Mutational Analyses and Inherited EB: Summary of Findings by EB Type and Subtype

EB Type	EB Subtype	Target Gene (Protein)	Types of Mutations Known
EBS	Suprabasal	PKP1 (plakophilin-1)	Spl, Del, NS
		DSP (desmoplakin)	NS, Del
	Basal	*KRT5* (keratin-5)	MS, NS, Del, Spl
		KRT14 (keratin-14)	MS, NS, Del, Ins, Spl, in-frame del/ins
		PLEC1 (plectin)	MS, NS, Del, Ins, in-frame del/ins
		ITGA6, ITGB4 (alpha6β4 integrin)	MS, NS, Del, Ins, Spl
JEB	Herlitz	*LAMA3, LAMB3, LAMC2* (laminin-332)	NS, Del, Ins, Spl
	Other	*LAMA3, LAMB3, LAMC2* (laminin-332)	MS, NS, Del, Ins, Spl
		COL17A1 (type XVII collagen)	MS, NS, Del, Ins, Spl
DEB	Dominant	COL7A1 (type VII collagen)	MS Spl
	Recessive	COL7A1 (type VII collagen)	MS Ins Del NS Spl
Kindler syndrome		KIND1 (kindlin-1)	NS Spl Ins Del

Del, deletion; *in-frame del/ins*, in-frame deletion and insertion; *Ins*, insertion; *MS*, missense mutation; *NS*, nonsense mutation; *Spl*, splice site mutation. In many cases with recessive inheritance, two different mutations are present in one individual compound heterozygosity.

Reprinted with permission from Fine JD, Eady RA, Bauer EA, et al. The classification of inherited epidermolysis bullosa (EB): Report of the Third International Consensus Meeting on Diagnosis and Classification of EB. *J Am Acad Dermatol* 2008 Jun;58(6):931–950. Epub 2008 Apr 18.

TABLE 14-6 EBS Subtypes

Major EBS Types	EBS Subtypes*	Targeted Proteins
Suprabasal	*Lethal acantholytic EB*	Desmoplakin
	Plakophilin deficiency	Plakophilin-1
	EBS superficialis (EBSS)	?
Basal	EBS, localized (EBS-loc)†	K5, K14
	EBS, Dowling-Meara (EBS-DM)	K5, K14
	EBS, other generalized (EBS, gen-nonDM; EBS, gen-nDM)‡	K5, K14
	EBS-with mottled pigmentation (EBS-MP)	K5
	EBS with muscular dystrophy (EBS-MD)	Plectin
	EBS with pyloric atresia (EBS-PA)	Plectin; *EBS*, 6β4 integrin
	EBS, autosomal recessive (EBS-AR)	K14

EBS, EB simplex.
*Rare variants shown in italics.
†Previously called EBS, Weber-Cockayne.
‡Includes patients previously classified as having EBS-Koebner.

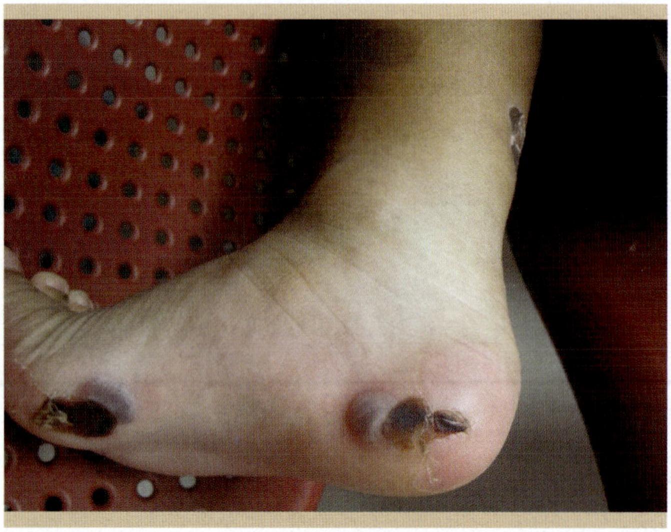

FIGURE 14-2 Epidermolysis bullosa simplex. (*Used with permission from Dr. Agim.*)

TABLE 14-7 Junctional EB Subtypes

Major JEB Subtype	Subtypes*	Targeted Proteins
JEB, Herlitz (JEB-H)	—	*Laminin* 5 (Laminin-332)
JEB, other (JEB-O)	JEB, non-Herlitz, generalized (JEB-nH gen)†	*Laminin* 5 (Laminin-332); type XVII collagen
	JEB, non-Herlitz, localized (JEB-nH loc)	Type XVII collagen
	JEB with pyloric atresia (JEB-PA)	α 6β4 Integrin
	JEB, inversa (JEB-I)	*Laminin* 5 (Laminin-332)
	JEB, late onset (JEB-lo)‡	?

*Rare variants shown in italic type.
†Formerly known as generalized atrophic benign EB (GABEB).
‡Formerly known as EB progressive.

TABLE 14-8 Dystrophic EB Subtypes

	Targeted Protein	All Subtypes*
DDEB	DDEB, generalized (DDEB-gen)	Type VII collagen
	DDEB, acral (DDEB-ac)	
	DDEB, pretibial (DDEB-Pt)	
	DDEB, pruriginosa (DDEB-Pr)	
	DDEB, nails only (DDEB-na)	
	DDEB, bullous dermolysis of the newborn (DDEB-BDN)	
DDEB	DDEB, generalized (DDEB-gen)	Type VII collagen
	DDEB, acral (DDEB-ac)	
	DDEB, pretibial (DDEB-Pt)	
	DDEB, pruriginosa (DDEB-Pr)	
	DDEB, nails only (DDEB-na)	
	DDEB, bullous dermolysis of the newborn (DDEB-BDN)	
DDEB	DDEB, generalized (DDEB-gen)	Type VII collagen

DDEB, dominant dystrophic EB; *RDEB*, recessive dystrophic EB.
*Rare variants in italic type.

- *Generalized other (non-Hallopeau-Siemens type)*: blisters present at birth, gastrointestinal (GI) abnormalities
- *RDEB inversa:* onset at birth, distribution of blistering is intertriginous, acral, lumbosacral, axial; esophageal strictures, anal strictures and fissures, oral erosions, partial fusion of the digits with contractures, females with vaginal involvement and scarring
- *RDEB centripetalis*: initial acral distribution of blisters with centripetal spread, milia, atrophic scarring, nail dystrophy

Other Dystrophic EB Subtypes

- *Acral:*
  - Dominant dystrophic EB (DDEB) or recessive dystrophic EB (RDEB) (Fig 14-5): blisters located on hands and feet, dystrophic or absent nails; develops during infancy

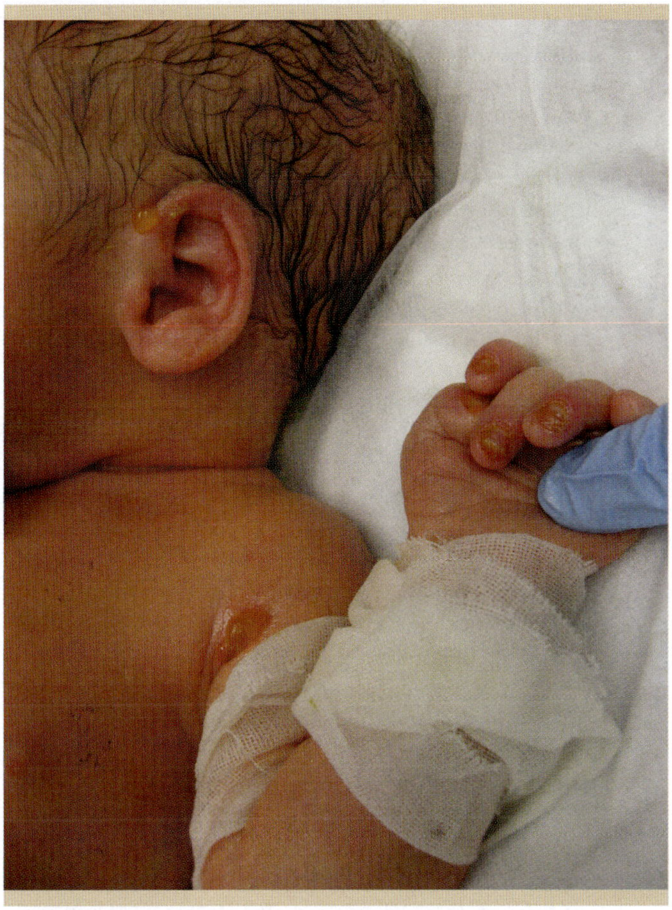

FIGURE 14-3 Junctional epidermolysis bullosa. (*Used with permission from Dr. Agim.*)

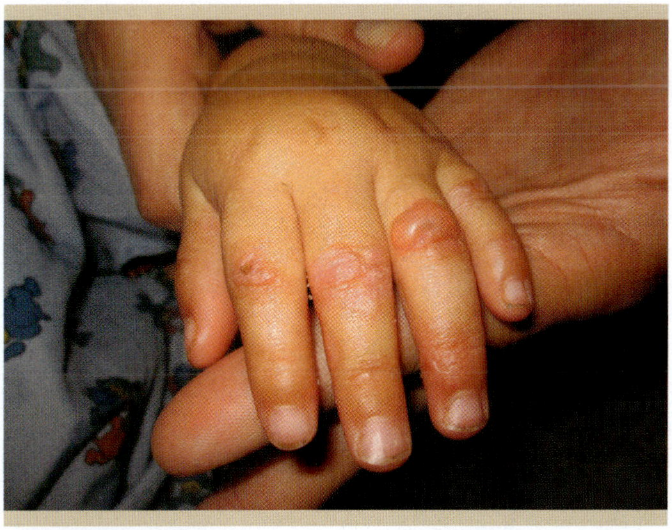

FIGURE 14-4 Dominant dystrophic EB. (*Used with permission from Dr. Agim.*)

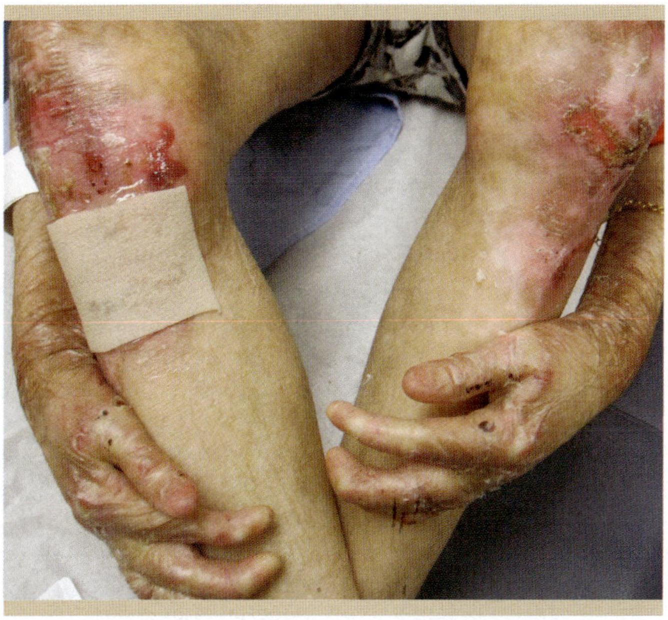

FIGURE 14-5 Recessive dystrophic EB. (*Used with permission from Dr. Agim.*)

- *Pretibial*:
  - DDEB and RDEB: blisters develop during birth or infancy, located on pretibial area, hands and feet; nails (fingers and toes), lichen planus like lesions, dystrophic or absent nails
- *DEB pruriginosa:*
  - Rare variant of DEB due to COL7A1 dominant and recessive mutations, which is characterized by severe itching and lichenoid or nodular prurigo like lesions, mainly involving the extremities
- *DDEB nails only*: onset at birth or infancy
- *Kindler syndrome:*
  - Autosomal recessive
  - Combination of features of *dystrophic epidermolysis bullosa and congenital poikilodermas* (e.g., Rothmund-Thompson)
  - Due to a mutation in the gene *KIND 1* encoding for kindlin-1: component of focal contacts in basal keratinocytes: multiple cleavage planes (intraepidermal, junctional, or sublamina densa)
  - Generalized blistering, onset at birth, poikiloderma; photosensitivity; mental retardation (rare); bone abnormalities (rare), gingival hyperplasia, cutaneous atrophy, colitis (may be severe); esophagitis, urethral strictures

Diagnosis of Epidermolysis Bullosa

- Electron microscopy on biopsy at the edge of a fresh blister, include both unblistered and blistered skin
- Immunofluorescence studies to detect abnormal protein antigens and serial monitoring of the patient

- Skin biopsy
- Upper GI series or endoscopy
- DNA mutation analysis
- Treatment: symptomatic care

DISORDERS OF PIGMENTATION

Neurofibromatosis I (Von Recklinghausen Disease)

- Autosomal dominant disease
- Defect of NF1 gene (chromosome 17q11.2) codes for neurofibromin: tumor suppressor; down-regulates activity of RAS (associated with increased cell proliferation and possible tumor formation)
- Neurofibromin, also positively regulates intracellular cyclic adenosine monophosphate (cAMP) levels, which modulate cell growth and differentiation in the brain
- Diagnosis: requires two or more of the following features:
  - Less than 6 Café-au-lait macules
    - 1.5 cm or larger in postpubertal individuals
    - 0.5 cm or larger in prepubertal individuals
  - Two or more neurofibromas or 1 plexiform neurofibroma
    - Most common tumor seen in patients with NF1
  - Axillary (Crowe sign) or inguinal freckling
  - Optic glioma: tumor of the optic pathway
  - Two or more lisch nodules: pigmented spots that are hamartomas of iris
  - Distinctive bony lesion: dysplasia of the sphenoid wing, dysplasia or thinning of long bone cortex
  - First-degree relative with NF-1
- Clinical features
  - *Café-au-lait spots (CALs):* often present at birth; flat, evenly pigmented macules or patches, may fade as patient ages, in which case, Wood's lamp may aid in diagnosis (Fig 14-6)
  - *Skinfold freckling*: usually not apparent at birth but appears in early childhood
  - *Lisch nodules* are asymptomatic, raised, pigmented hamartomas of the iris; diagnosis by slit lamp. They are present in most adult NF1 patients
  - *Discrete neurofibromas*: benign peripheral nerve sheath tumors, develop during adolescence. They are composed of a mixture of cell types including Schwann cells, fibroblasts, mast cells, and vascular elements
  - *Plexiform neurofibromas*: may diffusely involve nerve, muscle, connective tissue, vascular elements, and overlying skin. Since they can remain clinically silent for many years, diagnosis may be incidental by imaging studies or by the effects of the tumor on associated organs or structures. Congential forms may occur. Tenderness is a common complaint (Fig 14-7)
  - *Optic pathway gliomas:* typically arise in young children, second most common tumor in NF1 patients, low-grade pilocytic astrocytoma that typically arises in the optic nerve and chiasm, hypothalamus, brainstem, and/or cerebellum
  - *Increased risk of malignancy*: neurofibrosarcoma, astrocytoma, rhabdomyosarcoma, myelogenous leukemia, malignant peripheral nerve sheath tumor
  - *Other neurological complications*: macrocephaly, hydrocephalus, cognitive impairment, headaches, seizures, and cerebral ischemia
  - *Learning disabilities*: common in children with NF1, but frank mental retardation (IQ <70) is uncommon
  - *Skeletal abnormalities*: Kyphoscoliosis
  - *Endocrine disease*: (acromegaly, cretinism, hypothyroidism, hyperparathyroidism, precocious puberty)

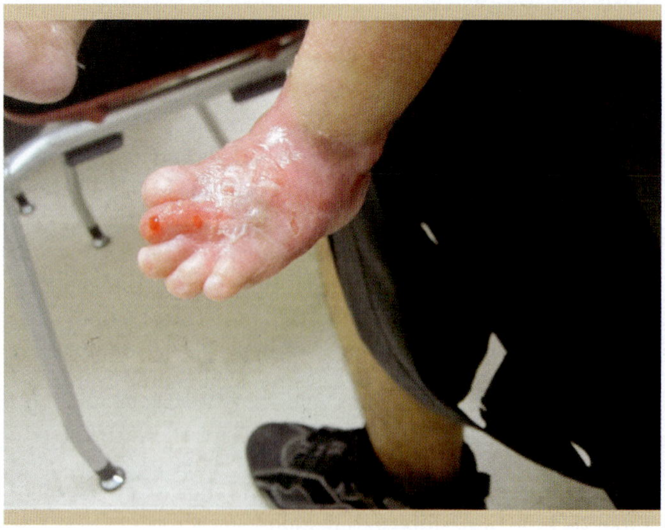

FIGURE 14-6 Recessive dystrophic EB, acral. (*Used with permission from Dr. Agim.*)

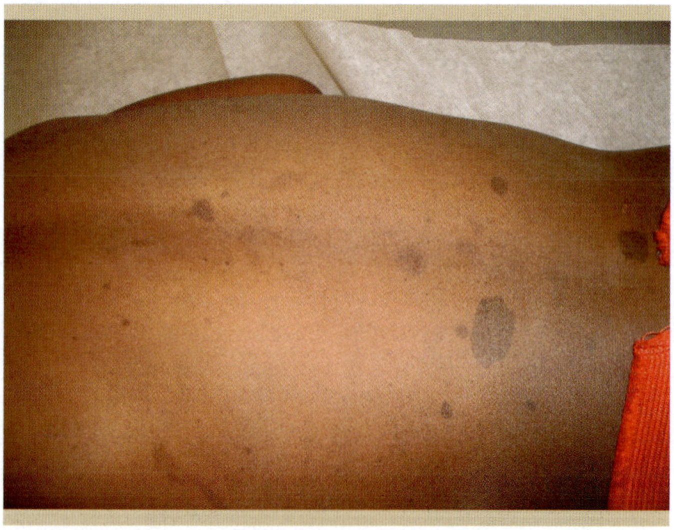

FIGURE 14-7 Café au lait macules. (*Used with permission from Dr. Agim.*)

- Variants of NF-1:
  - *Segmental or mosaic* NF1: when one of the two NF1 genes sustains a mutation during fetal development; a localized area of the developing fetus is affected
  - *Watson syndrome*: multiple café au lait spots, dull intelligence, short stature, pulmonary valvular stenosis, and only a small number of neurofibromas, and lisch nodules
  - *Neurofibromatosis-Noonan syndrome (NFNS):* children with NF1 also display the following features (similar to Noonan syndrome): pectus excavatum, hypertelorism, short stature
  - Legius syndrome: newly described syndrome with mutation in SPRED1 gene where patients have cutaneous features similar to NF-1 (café au lait macules, freckling) but fewer internal complications. Learning disability, macrocephaly, lipomas, and polydactyly may occur. Neurofibromas are unusual
- Management (Table 14-9)
  - Requires a multidisciplinary approach
  - Abnormalities on the visual examination should prompt Magnetic resonance imaging (MRI) evaluation ("screening" or "baseline" MRI evaluations, as they are not predictive)
  - Serial ophthalmologic and neurologic exams

Neurofibromatosis II (Bilateral Acoustic Neurofibromatosis)

- Autosomal dominant disease
- Defect of NF2 gene coding for schwannomin or merlin (chromosome 22q11)
- Diagnosis: requires either of the following:
  - Bilateral cranial nerve eight masses (acoustic neuromas)
  - First-degree relative with NF-2 plus either unilateral eighth nerve mass or two of the following: neurofibroma, schwannoma, optic glioma, meningioma, juvenile posterior subcapsular opacity
- Clinical
  - *Unilateral hearing loss* with or without tinnitus, dizziness, or imbalance
  - *Mononeuropathy* mainly affects the facial nerve, resulting in a Bell's-like palsy
  - *Spontaneous malignant transformation of schwannomas* to malignant peripheral nerve sheath tumours (MPNST); more than 10 times as likely to occur following radiation treatment
  - *Central Nervous System (CNS) tumors*: meningiomas, the second most common tumor in NF2 patients, occurs supratentorially in the falx and around the frontal, temporal, and parietal regions. Ependymomas and

TABLE 14-9 Age-Dependent Manifestations and Management of NF1

Age	Manifestations and Management
1–2 years	• Café-au-lait macules • Plexiform neurofibromas • Tibial dysplasias (anterolateral bowing of lower leg): may require orthopedic referral
3–5 years	• Skinfold freckling • Lisch nodules • Optic pathway gliomas: requires serial neurologic, ophthalmologic, and MRI scans once detected. Further management is warranted if there is tumor progression • Learning disabilities: requires planning with parents and teachers and early intervention if detected • Precocious puberty: requires endocrinologic and radiographic evaluation • Plexiform neurofibromas: requires regular follow-up
Late childhood and early adolescence	• Dermal neurofibromas • Plexiform neurofibromas: requires regular follow-up • Scoliosis: requires orthopedic evaluation for possible bracing and/or surgery
Lifelong	• Neurofibromas • Pain • Plexiform neurofibromas: requires regular follow-up • Malignant peripheral nerve sheath tumor (MPNST) • Other malignant neoplasms

gliomas usually located in the cervical spine or brain stem
- *Ophthalmic involvement*: cataracts, optic nerve meningiomas, and retinal harmartomas may cause visual loss
- *Cutaneous tumors*: schwannomas with occasional neurofibromas

- Diagnosis
  - MRI scan with gadolinium enhancement
  - Pathology: schwannomas, encapsulated tumors of pure Schwann cells, grow around the nerve; may contain blood vessels and have areas of sheets in intertwining fascicles (Antoni A) and looser arrangements (Antoni B). S-100 protein and vimentin positive
- Treatment
  - Management by a multidisciplinary team
  - Microsurgery and radiation treatment for patients with aggressive tumors
  - Visual and audiological testing

VASCULAR-RELATED DISORDERS

Von Hippel-Lindau Syndrome

- Autosomal dominant
- VHL gene (chromosome 3); tumor suppressor gene
- VHL gene affects the VCB-CUL2 complex, which targets a protein called hypoxia-inducible factor (HIF). HIF is involved in cell division and the formation of new blood vessels
- Presents by fourth decade
- Diagnostic criteria: (1) more than one hemangioblastoma in the CNS, (2) one CNS hemangioblastoma and visceral manifestations of VHL, or (3) one manifestation and a known family history of VHL
- Clinical findings
  - *Common tumors*: cerebellar, medullary, or spinal cord hemangioblastomas with increased intracranial pressure, spinal cord compression; retinal hemangioblastomas with visual impairment, and renal cell carcinoma (RCC)
  - *Endocrine tumors*: pheochromocytoma (usually intra-adrenal), adrenal carcinoma, pancreatic islet cell cancers
  - *Cysts*: renal and pancreatic
  - Phenotypic variability (types of presentation of VHL patients):
    - *Type 1*: retinal or CNS hemangioblastomas and RCC but not pheochromocytoma
    - *Type 2*: at least one affected individual has pheochromocytoma in the family; Type 2A: retinal and CNS hemangioblastomas are present, but rarely RCC occur; Type 2B hemangioblastomas, RCC and pheochromocytoma
  - *Other clinical features*: polycythemia secondary to increased erythropoietin, capillary malformation on head and neck, endolymphatic sac neoplasm, cardiac rhabdomyoma, hepatic cyst, adenoma, and/or angioma, carcinoid of the common bile duct, bone cysts or hemagiomas, and café-au-lait spots
- Screening and management (Table 14-10)
  - Imaging modalities: ultrasonography, computed tomography (CT), MRI, radionuclide studies, and angiography

Ataxia-Telangiectasia (Louis-Bar Syndrome)

- Autosomal recessive
- Mutation in *ATM* gene (*a*taxia-*t*elangiectasia *m*utated/located on chromosome 11q22–23); codes for protein kinase, involved in cellular responses to DNA damage and

TABLE 14-10 Screening of Patients With VHL and At-Risk Relatives (Cambridge Protocol)

Type of Patient	Recommended Screening
Affected asymptomatic patient	• Annual physical examination and urine test • Annual direct and indirect ophthalmoscopy • Annual fluorescein angiography or angiography • Annual renal ultrasonographic examination • MRI or CT scan of the brain every 3 years to age 50 years then every 5 years thereafter • Abdominal CT scanning every 3 years (more often if multiple renal cysts are present) • Annual 24-hour urine collection for vanillylmandelic acid (VMA) levels
At-risk relatives—same protocol as above with additional age based exams	• Annual direct and indirect ophthalmoscopy from age 5 years • Annual fluorescein angiography or angiography from age 10 years until age 60 years • MRI or CT scanning of the brain every 3 years from ages 15–40 years, then every 5 years until age 60 years • Abdominal CT scanning every 3 years from ages 20–65 years

cell cycle control; defective DNA repair with increased sensitivity to ionizing radiation

- Clinical findings
  - Progressive ataxia, presenting symptom when a child begins to walk; affects the extremities first and then speech; due to depletion of granular and Purkinje cells in cerebellum
  - Oculocutaneous telangiectasias by ages 3 to 6 years
  - Respiratory infections owing to decreased humoral and cellular immunity; decrease in the total number of CD4+ cells
  - Decreased development of thymus gland
  - Malignancies: 40% non-Hodgkin lymphomas, 25% leukemias, 25% (most leukaemias and lymphomas are of T-cell origin); assorted solid tumors (adenocarcinoma of the stomach, dysgerminoma, gonadoblastoma, and medulloblastoma) and 10% Hodgkin lymphomas
  - Hypogonadism
- Diagnosis (Table 14-11)
- Treatment, symptom based
  - *Basal ganglia dysfunction*: L-DOPA derivatives, dopamine agonists and, occasionally, anticholinergics
  - *Loss of balance, speech and coordination*: amantadine, fluoxetine, or buspirone
  - *Tremors*: gabapentin, clonazepam, or propranolol
  - *Hypogammaglobulinemia with antibody deficiency*: immune globulin replacement
  - *Sinopulmonary infections*: antibiotics
  - *Lymphoid hematopoietic malignancies*: chemotherapy

Hereditary Hemorrhagic Telangiectasia (HHT/Osler-Weber-Rendu Syndrome)

- Autosomal dominant
- Mutation of:
  - *HHT1* gene containing endoglin (chromosome 9q33–34); it encodes a membrane glycoprotein found onhuman vascular endothelial cells
  - *HH2* gene contains the *activin-like receptor kinase* (*ALK-1*) on chromosome 12q; it encodes transforming growth factor-β receptors
- Presents in childhood to early adulthood
- Diagnosis
  - Based on the Scientific Advisory Board of the HHT Foundation International Inc. consensus on clinical diagnostic criteria—Curaçao Criteria for HHT:
    - *Definite*: three criteria are present
    - *Possible or suspected*: 2 criteria are present
    - *Unlikely*: fewer than 2 criteria are present
- Criteria
  - Epistaxis: spontaneous, recurrent nose bleeds
  - Telangiectasias: characteristic sites—lips, oral cavity, fingers, nose
  - Visceral lesions: gastrointestinal telangiectasia (with or without bleeding), pulmonary arteriovenous malformation (AVM), hepatic AVM, cerebral AVMs, spinal AVM
  - Family history: first-degree relative with HHT according to these criteria
- Clinical findings
  - Triad of epistaxis, telangiectasia, and family history
  - Telangiectasias are common in third to fourth decade but begin erupting in childhood: face, palms, soles, conjunctiva, oral mucosa
  - Recurrent epistaxis
  - Gastrointestinal telangiectasias with hemorrhage
  - Hepatic or pulmonary AVMs: causing right-to-left shunts (most serious problem)
  - Neurologic involvement: seizures and focal neurologic symptoms
- Laboratory and imaging studies
- Complete blood count: evaluate for anemia or polycythemia
- Arterial blood gas
- MRI to check for CNS and pulmonary AVMs
- Treatment
  - Symptomatic medical and surgical care to decrease the amount of bleeding experienced by the patient

TABLE 14-11 Laboratory Evaluation of A-T Patients

Alpha-fetoprotein	Elevated
Radiation response	Hypersensitive
p53 stabilization	Defective
ATM mutations	Yes
ATM protein	Absent/detectable
ATM kinase activity	Absent
ATM signalling pathways	Defective

Proteus Syndrome

- Sporadic inheritance
- AKT1 gene mutation; PTEN in ~20%
- Formerly classified under PTEN overgrowth syndromes which include Cowden syndrome and Bannayan Riley Ruvalcaba. Some previously described Proteus patients have also been reclassified as having a variant of Cowden syndrome
- Diagnostic criteria (Table 14-12)
- Clinical findings
  - Asymmetric overgrowth of tissues and neoplasms
    - *Cutaneous involvement*: cerebriform connective tissue nevi, epidermal nevi, vascular malformations, lipomas, lipohypoplasia, and dermal hypoplasia

TABLE 14-12 Diagnostic Criteria for Proteus Syndrome

Mandatory General Criteria	Mosaic Distribution of Lesions, Progressive Course, Sporadic Occurrence
Specific criteria (A, or 2 from group B, or 3 from group C)	
Group A	Connective tissue nevus
Group B	Epidermal nevus Disproportionate overgrowth (1 or more) Limbs, skull, external auditory meatus, vertebra, viscera (spleen and/or thymus) Specific tumors before the end of the second decade (either one): bilateral ovarian cystadenomas, parotid monomorhphic adenoma
Group C	Dysregulated adipose tissue (either one): lipomas, regional absence of fat Vascular malformations (1 or more): capillary, venous, and/or lymphatic Facial phenotype: dolichocephaly, long face, low nasal bridge, wide or anteverted nares, open mouth at rest

Reprinted with permission from Nguyen D, Turner JT, Olsen C, Biesecker LG, Darling TN: Cutaneous manifestations of proteus syndrome: correlations with general clinical severity. *Arch Dermatol* 2004 Aug;140(8):947–953.

  - *Extracutaneous manifestations*: skeletal overgrowth (macrocephaly, frontal bossing), visceral overgrowth (pharyngeal or vocal cord), tumors (epibulbar dermoid of the eye, ovarian cystadenoma), pulmonary and intracranial cysts, hernias, hydrocele, and undescended or absent testes, venous and lymphatic malformations
  - AKT-1 functions in same pathway as neurofibromin
- Treatment: multidisciplinary approach

Klippel-Trenaunay Syndrome

- Sporadic inheritance
  - Triad of (1) capillary vascular malformation (port-wine stain), (2) varicose veins and/or venous malformation, and (3) soft-tissue and/or bony hypertrophy
- Clinical findings
  - Usually affects one limb; most commonly leg, then arm, and trunk
  - Capillary, venous, and lymphatic malformations
  - Soft-tissue and bony hypertrophy (Fig 14-8)

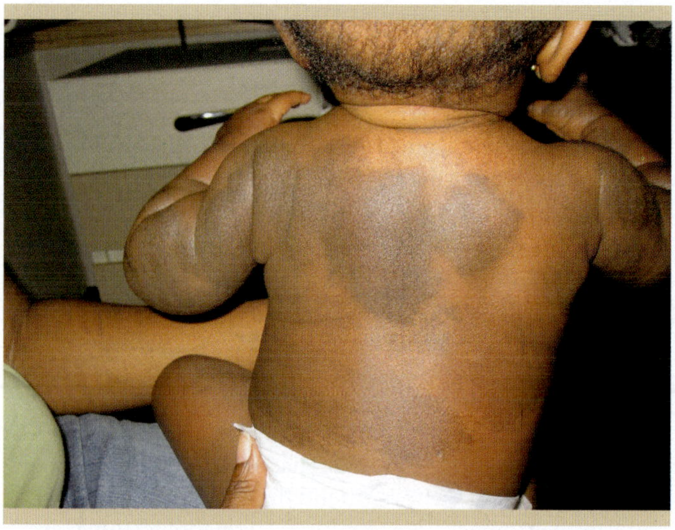

FIGURE 14-8 Congenital plexiform neurofibroma. (*Used with permission from Dr. Agim.*)

  - Other features: phleboliths, deep venous thromboses, pulmonary emboli, thrombophlebitis, cellulitis, intraosseous vascular malformations, arthritis, neuropathic pain, spina bifida, hypospadias, polydactyly, syndactyly, oligodactyly, hyperhidrosis, decalcification of involved bones
  - Parkes-Weber is a distinct vascular malformation which has AV fistulas underlying the capillary malformation with associated soft-tissue anomalies (Fig 14-9)
  - Cutaneous manifestations: chronic venous insufficiency with stasis dermatitis, lipodermatosclerosis, varicosity, atrophy blanche, corona phlebectatica, and, ultimately, breakdown of the skin with ulcerations, hypertrichosis

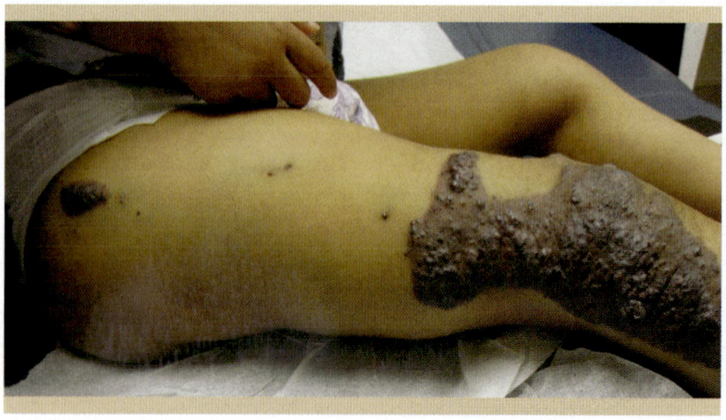

FIGURE 14-9 Klippel Trenauny with capillary and venolymphatic malformations. (*Used with permission from Dr. Agim.*)

- Treatment: compression stockings, surgical intervention, sclerotherapy, or endovascular laser ablation depending on patient's symptoms
- Cellulitis and thrombophlebitis: analgesics, elevation, antibiotics, and corticosteroids
- Limb discrepancies: shoe inserts or orthopedic surgery

Sturge-Weber Syndrome (Encephalotrigeminal Angiomatosis)

- Sporadic inheritance
- Neural crest defect
- Clinical findings
  - *Facial port-wine stain*
    - Presents at birth and is typically unilateral (85%), involving the ophthalmic (V_1), maxillary (V_2), and/or mandibular (V_3) divisions of the trigeminal nerve
    - Occurs wtih ipsilateral leptomeningeal vascular anomalies (capillary, venous, and AV malformations) and/or choroidal vascular lesions with glaucoma (unilateral)
    - Involvement of any portion of the V_1 distribution may indicate underlying neurological and/or ocular disorders
  - *Roach classification scale:*
    - Type I—both facial and leptomeningeal angiomas (LA); may have glaucoma
    - Type II—facial angioma alone (no CNS involvement); may have glaucoma
    - Type III—isolated LA; usually no glaucoma
  - Neurologic complications: seizures, psychomotor delay in infancy, headaches and migraines, hemiparesis
  - Tram-track calcification in cortex
  - Diagnostic tests
  - Head CT and MRI: diagnosis of intracranial calcifications and leptomeningeal angiomas
  - CSF analysis: elevated protein
- Treatment
  - Port-wine stains: laser (pulsed dye laser)
  - Seizures: anticonvulsants for focal
  - Headaches: NSAIDs
  - Medical or surgical control of intraocular pressure

CONNECTIVE TISSUE DISORDERS

Ehlers-Danlos Syndrome

- Connective tissue disorder characterized by skin extensibility, tissue fragility, and joint hypermobility
- Collagen V defect, less frequently tenascin-X
- Autosomal dominant
- Clinical
  - Types of Ehlers Danlos:
    - *Classical (EDS I and II)*

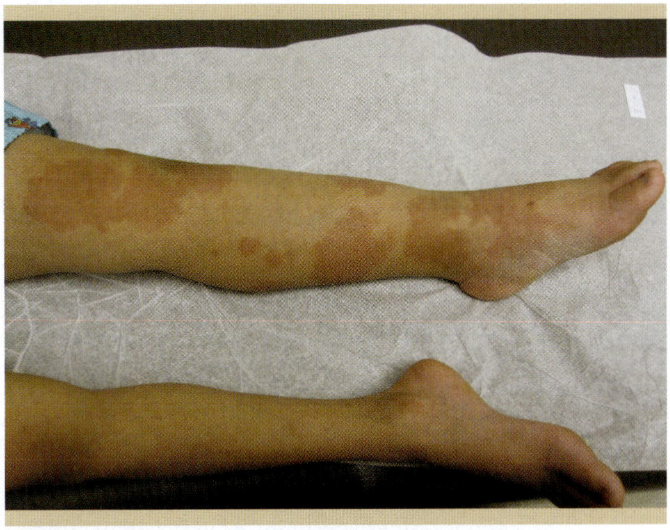

FIGURE 14-10 Parkes Weber (with AV fistulae). (*Used with permission from Dr. Agim.*)

      - AD, abnormal type V collagen (*COL5A1, COL5A2 mutations)*
        - Clinical findings: skin hyperextensibility (Fig 14-10), easy bruising, wide, atrophic scars, joint hypermobility with sprains, dislocations, muscle hypotonia, hernias
        - May have cardiac defects: mitral valve defects
        - Molluscoid pseudotumors: spongy tumors found over scars and pressure points (more common in type 1EDS)
        - Spheroids (fat-containing cysts)
    - *Hypermobility (EDS III)*
      - Autosomal dominant
      - Clinical findings: joint hypermobility with recurrent dislocations, chronic pain, mild skin hyperextensibility
        - Mitral valve prolapse
    - *Vascular (type IV, ecchymotic or arterial type)*
      - Autosomal dominant, collagen III defect (COL3A1)
      - Clinical findings: thin, translucent skin with bruising, characteristic facies (prominent eyes, small lips, pinched nose, hollow cheeks, and lobeless ears), hypermobility of small joints with dislocation, varicose veins; arterial, intestinal, and uterine rupture which may cause sudden death; keloids, molluscoid pseudotumors, pneumothorax, inguinal hernia
      - Cerebrovascular bleeding in younger patients; intracranial aneurismal rupture, spontaneous carotid-cavernous sinus fistula and cervical artery aneurysm

- *Kyphoscoliosis (type VI or ocular-scoliotic type)*
  - ▲ Autosomal recessive
  - ▲ Lysyl hydroxylase deficiency (*LH1* gene)
  - ▲ Clinical findings: generalized joint laxity with severe hypotonia, progressive scoliosis; unable to ambulate by early adulthood, scleral fragility, prone to global rupture, retinal hemorrhage and detachment, glaucoma, discolored sclera, arterial rupture, marfanoid habitus, osteopenia, and osteoporosis
  - ▲ LH can be measured in the amniotic fluid
- *Arthrochalasia (formerly VIIA and B)*
  - ▲ Autosomal dominant
  - ▲ Deficiency of proA1 or proA2 chains of collagen type I
  - ▲ Clinical findings: congenital bilateral hip dislocations, joint hypermobility with subluxations, kyphoscoliosis, mild osteopenia, skin laxity with bruising, atrophic scars, muscle hypotonia, or short stature
- *Dermatosparaxis (type VIIC)*
  - ▲ Autosomal recessive
  - ▲ N-terminal peptidase of type I collagen I (*ADAMTS2* gene)
  - ▲ Clinical findings: severe skin fragility, redundant sagging skin (resembles cutis laxa [CL]), easy bruising, large hernias, premature rupture of membranes at delivery, no impairment of wound healing
- *Other types*
  - ▲ X-linked form (formerly type V)
    - △ X-linked recessive pattern
    - △ Clinical findings: skin laxity, orthopedic abnormalities
  - ▲ Periodontal (formerly type VIII)
    - △ AD
    - △ Clinical findings: gingival inflammation and resorption with loss of permanent teeth; variable presentation of skin laxity, joint hyperextensibility, and bruising
  - ▲ X-linked cutis laxa (formerly type IX)
    - △ X-linked recessive
    - △ Clinical findings: occipital bony prominences, poor healing with scarring, intracellular copper-dependent enzymes, chronic diarrhea with orthostatic hypotension
    - △ Fibronectin (formerly type X) and benign hypermobile joint syndrome (formerly type XI)

Osteogenesis Imperfecta (OI)

- Characterized by increased bone fragility and low bone mass

TABLE 14-13 Characteristics of Osteogenesis Imperfecta (OI)

OI Subtype	Characteristics
I	Thin skin, blue sclera Lax joints, kyphosis, abnormal dentition Aortic valve disease, mitral valve prolapsed, long bone fractures, vertebral compression fractures
II	In utero fractures, limb avulsion at delivery Perinatal death common due to respiratory insufficiency following rib fractures Aortic valve disease, blue sclera
III	In utero fractures Progressive scoliosis, limb bowing, crippling deformity Blue sclera, triangular facies, short stature
IV	Fractures at birth, abnormal teeth Improvement with age

- Majority of patients (about 90%) have a mutation in *COL1A1* or *COL1A2*, the genes encoding collagen type I (found in bone)
- Patients have low trabecular bone mineral density and thin cortices, and also small, slender bones
- Mostly autosomal dominant
- Four main subtypes with different mutations resulting in varying severity of disease (Table 14-13)
- *Other subtypes*: noncollagen related defects
  - Type V: autosomal dominant (genetic defect unknown) moderate to severe bone fragility, irregular mesh-like appearance of lamellar bone
  - Type VI: autosomal recessive. Moderate to severe skeletal fragility; bone biopsy shows lamellae with fish-like appearance and excessive osteoid
  - Type VII: autosomal recessive. Rhizomelia, coxa vera, reduction is expression of cartilage-associated protein (CRTAP)
- All characterized by osseous fragility
- May develop hearing loss due to otosclerosis

Marfan Syndrome

- Autosomal dominant; mutation in fibrillin-1 (*FBN1*), chromosome 15; main component of extracellular microfibrils associated with elastin within elastic fibers
- Diagnosis: based on clinical criteria (Ghent nosology). Major and minor criteria of the following organ systems are evaluated in the patient: ocular, skeletal, integumental,

respiratory, and cardiovascular. Major criteria in two systems with involvement of a third system are needed to make an unequivocal diagnosis

- Criteria include:
  - Skeletal system (two of the components comprising the major criterion, or one component comprising the major criterion plus two of the minor criteria)
    - *Major criteria*: presence of at least four of the following manifestations: pectus carinatum, pectus excavatum requiring surgery, reduced upper to lower segment ratio or arm span to height ratio more than 1.05, positive wrist and thumb signs, scoliosis of more than 20° or spondylolisthesis, reduced extension of the elbows (<170°), medial displacement of the medial malleolus causing pes planus, protrusio acetabulae of any degree (ascertained on x-ray)
    - *Minor criteria*: pectus excavatum of moderate severity, joint hypermobility, highly arched palate with dental crowding, facial appearance (dolicocephaly, malar hypoplasia, enophthalmos, retrognathia, down-slanting palpebral fissures)
  - Ocular system (two of the minor criteria)
    - *Major criterion*: ectopia lentis
    - *Minor criteria*: abnormally flat cornea (as measured by keratometry), increased axial length of globe (as measured by ultrasound), hypoplastic iris or hypoplastic ciliary muscle causing a decreased miosis
  - Cardiovascular system (major criterion or only one of the minor criteria)
    - *Major criteria:* dilatation of the ascending aorta with or without aortic regurgitation and involving at least the sinuses of Valsalva, or dissection of the ascending aorta
    - *Minor criteria*: mitral valve prolapse with or without mitral valve regurgitation, dilatation of main pulmonary artery, in absence of valvular or peripheral pulmonic stenosis or any other obvious cause, younger than the age of 40 years, calcification of the mitral annulus below the age of 40 years, or dilatation or dissection of the descending thoracic or abdominal aorta below the age of 50 years
  - Pulmonary system (one of the minor criteria must be present)
    - *Major criteria:* none
    - *Minor criteria:* spontaneous pneumothorax, or apical blebs (ascertained by chest radiography)
  - Skin and integument (major criterion or one of the minor criteria)
    - *Major criterion:* lumbosacral dural ectasia by CT or MRI
    - *Minor criteria:* striae atrophicae (stretch marks) not associated with marked weight changes, pregnancy or repetitive stress, or recurrent or incisional herniae
  - Family history (one of the major criteria must be present)
    - *Major criteria:* having a parent, child, or sibling who meets the diagnostic criteria listed below independently, presence of a mutation in FBN1 known to cause the Marfan syndrome, or presence of a haplotype around FBN1, inherited by descent, known to be associated with unequivocally diagnosed Marfan syndrome in the family
    - *Minor criteria:* none
- Requirements for the diagnosis of Marfan syndrome
  - *For the index case*: major criteria in at least two different organ systems and involvement of a third organ system
  - *For a family member:* presence of a major criterion in the family history and one major criterion in an organ system and involvement of a second organ system
- Course: premature death secondary to cardiovascular defects
- Treatment: surgery, β-blockers

Cutis Laxa (Generalized Elastolysis)

- Categorized by mode of inheritance and phenotypes: autosomal dominant, autosomal recessive (CL type I, CL type II, and type III-de Barsy syndrome), X-linked recessive (occipital horn syndrome), or acquired
- Characterized by redundant, loose, and inelastic skin
- Genetic defects: AD-ELN gene (elastin), autosomal recessive-fibulin-5 gene (FBLN5), or X-linked recessive-ATP7A
- Acquired cases: associated with penicillin, penicillamine, complement deficiency, lupus, amyloid, erythema multiforme, contact dermatitis, and Sweet syndrome
- Clinical findings
  - *Autosomal recessive:*
    - *Cutis laxa, type I*: perinatal form, presents with pulmonary and other internal manifestations, leading to premature death
    - *Cutis laxa type II*: (also called *cutis laxa with joint laxity and developmental delay);* presents with sagging jowls, epicanthic folds, antimongoloid slant, maxillary hypoplasia, blue sclera, depressed nasal bridge, apparent ocular hypertelorism, and long philtrum, growth retardation, developmental delay, microcephaly, wrinkling of skin on the abdomen, hernia, joint laxity, and dislocation
    - *de Barsey syndrome*: rare type, associated with cutis laxa, retarded psychomotor development and corneal clouding due to degeneration of the tunica elastica of the cornea, growth retardation, may be pseudoathetoid movements
  - *Autosomal dominant*: benign course; primarily, skin involvement, infrequent systemic complications, normal life expectancy
  - *X-linked recessive*: skin laxity, skeletal and genitourinary tract abnormalities

- Histology: special elastin specific stains (Verhoeff–van Gieson and orcein) show loss, fragmentation, or both, or decreased number of elastic fibers

Pseudoxanthoma Elasticum (Grönblad–Strandberg Syndrome)

- Autosomal recessive more common than autosomal dominant
- *ABCC-6* gene, chromosome 16p; encodes multidrug resistance associated protein 6 (MRP6), which belongs to the ABC (ATP binding cassette) transmembrane transporter family of proteins
- D-Penicillamine implicated in drug-associated cases
- Progressive fragmentation and calcification of elastic fibers in skin, blood vessels, and Bruch membrane of the eye
- Clinical findings
  - Redundant intertriginous skin
  - "Plucked chicken" or "gooseflesh" appearing skin with yellow papules typically developing on the neck and may coalesce into plaques; other areas affected include antecubital and popliteal fossae, axillae, inguinal, and periumbilical areas. Mucosal membranes may also be affected. Lesions are asymptomatic
  - Affected skin may become lax and wrinkled
  - *Perforating PXE*: occurs with extrusion of calcium deposits
  - *Ocular manifestations*: angioid streaks in Bruch membrane (seen in 85% of patients): irregular, reddish-brown, or grey lines that radiate from the optic disc. They are due to degenerated and calcified elastic fibers of the retina that causes breaks in Bruch membrane. The earliest eye finding is a peau d'orange appearance (yellowish mottled pigmentation) of the retina. Other findings: colloid bodies, macular degeneration, optic nerve head drusen (whitish-yellow irregularities of the optic disc), and "owl's eyes" (paired hyperpigmented spots)
  - *Cardiovascular manifestations*
    - Claudication, hypertension, myocardial infarction (MI), cerebrovascular accident (CVA), coronary artery disease (CAD), renovascular hypertension, congestive cardiac failure, renal failure
  - *Gastrointestinal bleeds*: (seen in 10% of patients) due to calcified submucosal vessels
- Diagnostic criteria
  - *Major*: characteristic skin lesions: cobblestone lesions in flexural areas, characteristic eye findings: angioid streaks, peau d'orange retinal appearance, maculopathy, characteristic histologic findings seen with elastic tissue and calcium stains
  - *Minor*: characteristic histologic findings of nonlesional skin; family history of PXE in first-degree relatives
- *Histology*: hematoxylin-eosin stains—elastic fibers are basophilic because of the calcium deposition; fibers fragmented, swollen, and clumped in the middle and deep reticular dermis
- *Course*: decreased life span owing to cardiovascular disease
- Management: regular eye exams, cardiology assessment, laboratory tests—CBC, ferritin, serum lipids, urinalysis; aspirin for high risk patients

Tuberous Sclerosis (Bourneville Syndrome, Epiloia)

- Autosomal dominant or spontaneous mutation
- Hamartin (*TSC1,* chromosome 9q34); protein function: together with tuberin, hamartin regulates mTOR-S6K, and cell adhesion through interaction with ezrin and Rho
- Tuberin (*TSC2,* chromosome 16p13.3); protein function: together with hamartin, tuberin regulates mTOR-s6K and GTPase-activating proteins. Tuberin has a role in cell cycle
- Clinical findings
  - Triad of *epi*lepsy, *low i*ntellignce, *a*denoma sebaceum (*epiloia*) (old term, consider eliminating)
  - Epilepsy: begins during the first year of life
  - Cutaneous manifestations
    - *Hypomelanotic macules*: most common cutaneous manifestation (90–98% of patients) (Fig 14-11)
    - *Bilateral facial angiofibromas*: hamartomatous nodules of vascular and connective tissue, in a butterfly pattern over the malar eminences and nasolabial folds (80% of children)
    - *Shagreen patch*: connective tissue nevi, usually found on lumbosacral flank (Fig 14-12)
    - *Forehead fibrous plaque*: yellow-brown or flesh-colored plaque, histology shows angiofibroma
    - *Ungual fibroma*: Koenen tumor, connective tissue hamartoma, adjacent to or below nail plate

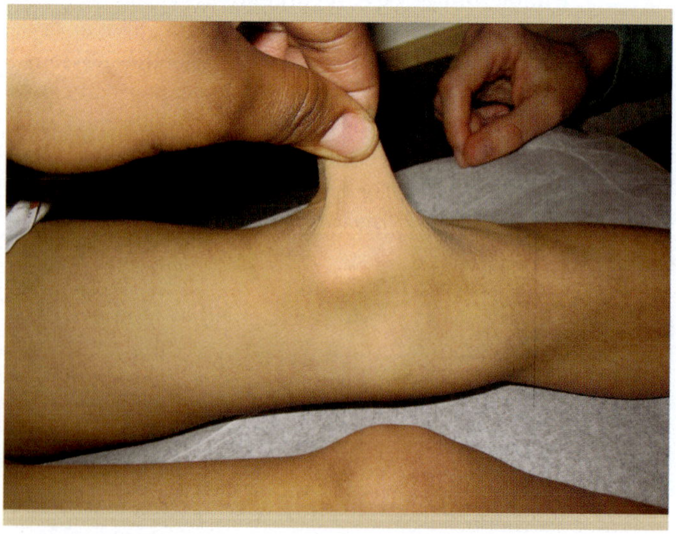

FIGURE 14-11 Ehlers Danlos. (*Used with permission from Dr. Agim.*)

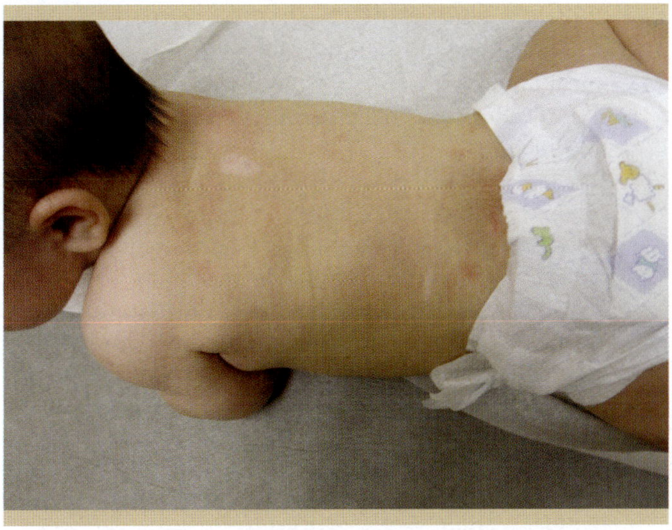

FIGURE 14-12 Ash leaf macules. (*Used with permission from Dr. Agim.*)

- Other manifestations
  - *Brain lesions*: cortical tubers (proliferation of glial and neuronal cells), subependymal nodules (hamartomas), subependymal giant-cell tumours, and white matter abnormalities
  - *Dental abnormalities*: dental pits (90% of patients)
  - *Cardiac manifestations*: rhabdomyomas, mainly located in ventricles, recede over time
  - *Renal manifestations*: bilateral angiomyolipomas (70–90% of patients), RCC, renal cysts, smooth-muscle cell carcinoma
  - *Ocular manifestations*: retinal hamartomas (40–50% of patients), mulberry lesions are composed of glial and astrocytic fibers
  - *Pulmonary manifestations*: lymphangiomyomatosis (alveolar smooth-muscle proliferation with cystic destruction of lung)
  - *Hepatic manifestations*: rare angiomyolipomas
- Diagnosis requires the presence of two major features, or one major and two minor criteria
  - Diagnostic criteria for tuberous sclerosis:
    - Major features
      - ▲ Nontraumatic ungual or periungual fibroma; Koenen tumor
      - ▲ Shagreen patch (connective tissue nevus) migration lines
      - ▲ Hypomelanotic "ashleaf" macules (three or more)
      - ▲ Facial angiofibromas or forehead plaque pits in dental enamel
      - ▲ Multiple retinal nodular hamartomas
      - ▲ Cortical tuber
      - ▲ Subependymal nodule
      - ▲ Subependymal giant-cell astrocytoma
      - ▲ Cardiac rhabdomyoma, single or multiple
      - ▲ Lymphangiomyomatosis, renal angiomyolipoma, or both
    - Minor features
      - ▲ Multiple, randomly distributed
      - ▲ Hamartomatous rectal polyps
      - ▲ Bone cysts
      - ▲ Cerebral white matter radial
      - ▲ Gingival fibromas
      - ▲ Nonrenal hamartoma
      - ▲ Retinal achromic patch
      - ▲ Confetti-like skin lesions
      - ▲ Multiple renal cysts
- Management: electroencephalography, cranial MRI, genetic testing, echocardiography, renal unltrasonography, chest CT, ophthalmic examination

Buschke-Ollendorf Syndrome (Dermatofibrosis Lenticularis)

- Autosomal dominant
- *LEMD3* gene
- Increased desmosine and elastin in skin
- Clinical findings
  - Dermatofibrosis lenticularis disseminata: symmetrical skin colored to yellowish grouped papules and nodules forming plaques; localized on the trunk: sacrolumbar region and extremities
  - Osteopoikilosis: radiopaque round or oval spots in the epiphyses and the metaphyses of the long bones, pelvis, and the bones of hands and feet, no increased fracture risk
- Histology: thickened collagen fibers in the dermis; fragmented elastic fibers
- Prognosis: normal life span

Focal Dermal Hypoplasia (Goltz Syndrome)

- X-linked dominant (lethal in males)
- Mutations in PORCN and Wnt signaling may be implicated
- Clinical findings
  - *Cutaneous anomalies*: atrophic, linear hypopigmented or hyperpigmented patches, telangiectatic streaks in Blaschko lines, fat herniations through dermal defects (focal dermal hypoplasia), papillomas on lips, perineum, axilla, absent/dystrophic fingernails, sparse, brittle hair (Fig 14-13)
  - *Skeletal anomalies*: syndactyly with "lobster claw" deformity, ectrodactyly, polydactyly, absence or hypoplasia of digits, scoliosis, skeletal asymmetry, clavicular dysplasia, spina bifida occulta, osteopatha striata (linear striations primarily in the long bones)
  - *Dental anomalies*: hypodontia, oligodontia, microdontia, enamel fragility, dysplasia, malocclusion
  - *Eye findings*: micophthalmia, bilateral coloboma of the iris, ectopia lentis, strabismus, anopthalmia

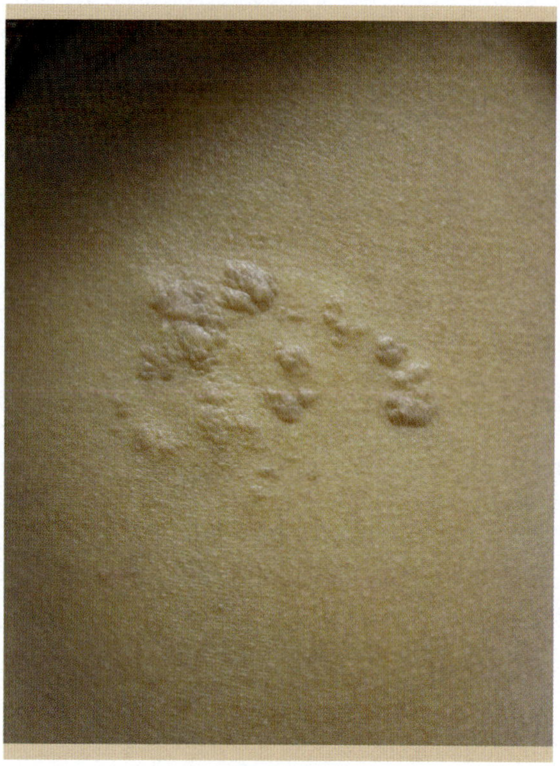

FIGURE 14-13 Goltz syndrome. (*Used with permission from Dr. Agim.*)

- *Other manifestations*: mild mental retardation, hearin defects, horse shoe kidneys, hernias: inguinal, umbilical, epigastric
- *Cardiac anomalies*: cardiac tumors, congenital heart disease (truncus arteriosus)

- Course: normal life span

Lipoid Proteinosis (Urbach-Wiethe Syndrome, Hyalinosis cutis et mucosae)

- Autosomal recessive
- ECM1
- Clinical findings
  - Dental anomalies and loss of teeth early
  - *Cutaneous manifestations*: eyelid with beaded papules (appear as a string of pearls), yellow waxy papules on skin, lips, palate, generalized skin thickening, hyperkeratosis at sites of trauma (hands, elbows, knees), pock-like or acneiform scars, infiltration of mucous memebranes (pharynx, tongue, soft palate, lips) leading to difficulty in breathing, hoarseness
  - *CNS manifestations*: temporal and hippocampal sickle or bean-shaped calcifications
- Histology: dermal deposition of diastase-resistant PAS positive hyaline material
- Treatment: CO_2 laser treatment of vocal cords and eyelid papules; etretinate, penicillamine

Aplasia Cutis Congenita

- Autosomal dominant, autosomal recessive, or sporadic
- Clinical findings
  - Localized absence of epidermis, dermis, subcutis, bone or dura
  - Well-demarcated erosions/ulcerations; 65% occur on scalp, 25% of cases are found on the trunk or limbs
  - May present as an isolated defect or be combined with congenital malformations (abnormal limbs, dysraphism, facial cleft, abnormalities of the eyes, digestive tract, heart, neurological malformations), chromosome anomalies (Down syndrome, 4 p-syndrome), or other disorders such as bullous epidermolysis and pyloric stenosis
  - Adams-Oliver syndrome (AOS): aplasia cutis most commonly of the scalp and skull, and terminal transverse limb defects, congenital heart disease
- Treatment: wound care, most lesions heal with scar formation

PREMATURE AGING AND PHOTOSENSITIVE DISORDERS

Progeria (Hutchinson-Gilford Progeria Syndrome)

- Autosomal dominant
- Lamin A defect (LMNA): produces some normal lamin A and some mutated lamin A (progerin)
- Clinical findings
  - Premature signs of aging: alopecia (including scalp and eyebrows), prominent scalp veins and forehead, classical facial features including micrognathia (small jaw), prominent eyes and a convex nasal profile (beak-like nose), and circumoral cyanosis
  - High-pitched voice
  - Loss of subcutaneous fat, muscle wasting
  - Cutaneous: mottled hyperpigmentation, sclerodermoid changes on lower extremities
  - Dystrophic teeth
  - Skeletal manifestations: frequent osteolysis, limited joint mobility (contractures), coxa valga, shortened clavicles, short stature
  - Cardiovascular and cerebrovascular diseases: myocardial ischemia and infarction as well as stroke; angina, chronic congestive heart failure, or transient ischemic attacks
- Course: premature death in teens owing to atherosclerotic complications (angina, MI, CHF, CVA)

Werner Syndrome (Progeria Adultorum, Progeria of the Adult, Pangeria)

- Autosomal recessive
- *WRN* gene (*RECQL2)* encodes DNA helicase
- Decreased growth of skin fibroblasts

- Increased urinary hyaluronic acid (abnormal glysoaminoglycan metabolism)
- Clinical findings
  - Premature aged appearance: muscle wasting, progressive alopecia, premature graying of hair, mild diabetes, cataract formation, loss of subcutaneous fat, dermal atrophy with resulting tight, shiny skin on face and extremities (scleroderma-like changes), poikiloderma, leg ulcers, soft-tissue and blood vessel calcifications, arteriosclerosis, mesenchymal tumors
  - Short stature, osteoporosis, osteoarthritis
  - Ocular: posterior subcapsular cataracts
- Course: premature death in fourth decade owing to malignancy or atherosclerosis

Acrogeria (Gottron Syndrome, Familial Acromicria)

- Autosomal recessive
- Onset occurring up to age 6 years
- Clinical findings
  - Cutaneous atrophy and subcutaneous wasting of the face and extremities
  - Hair unaffected

Rothmund-Thomson Syndrome (Poikiloderma Congenitale)

- Autosomal recessive
- *RECQL4* (RecQ DNA helicase); chromosome 8q24.3
- Onset ages of 3 to 6 months
- Clinical findings
  - Cutaneous manifestations: poikiloderma, photosensitivity, scaling, hyperkeratosis, and disturbance of hair growth
  - Other abnormalities include: cataracts, congenital bone defects, soft-tissue contractures, osteogenesis imperfecta, short stature, small skull, hypogonadism, dystrophic nails and teeth
  - Malignancies: osteosarcoma, fibrosarcoma, and nonmelanoma skin cancers

Cockayne Syndrome

- Autosomal recessive
- Type 1: CSA (also called CNK1 or excision-repair cross-complementing group 8, *ERCC8* gene); chromosome 5q12-q13
- Type 2: CSB (also called *ERCC6* gene); chromosome 10q11, 80% of cases
- Deficiency in transcription-coupled nucleotide excision repair (TC-NER)
- Increased sister chromatid exchanges
- Clinical findings
  - *Cutaneous manifestation*: photosensitive skin eruption (may affect any sun-exposed area). Pruritus, no increased risk of cutaneous or visceral malignancy
  - *Typical facies*: progeroid, with sparse, dry hair, facial lipoatrophy, large ears, and a thin nose
  - *Ocular findings*: poor pupillary dilatation, enophthalmos (due to loss of subcutaneous fat), optic nerve hypoplasia, and retinal pigmentation, "salt and pepper," retinal pigmentation, cataracts (15% of patients)
  - *Musculoskeletal, central nervous, and genitourinary systems*: kyphoscoliosis and flexion deformities of the hips, knees, and ankles; abnormal gait, developmental delay and mental retardation, microcephaly, large hands and feet
  - *Sensorineural hearing impairment*
  - *Genitourinary*: Approximately one-third of boys have undescended testes and girls frequently exhibit menstrual irregularities
  - *Cockayne syndrome I (CS-I),* classic Cockayne syndrome, symptoms begin after the first year of life, survive into adolescence and early adulthood
  - *Cockayne syndrome II (CS-II)/Pena-Shokeir type*: exhibit intrauterine growth retardation, poor postnatal growth, congenital cataracts or early structural eye abnormalities, and severe and more rapidly progressive neurologic impairment
  - CS is frequently associated with xeroderma pigmentosum (XP) and trichothiodystrophy (TTD): these disorders exhibit sensitivity to ultraviolet (UV) light and defects in NER
- Treatment: supportive: photoprotection, physical therapy, and optimizing nutrition; genetic counseling

Bloom Syndrome

- Autosomal recessive
- *BLM* gene (*RECQL3)* encodes a DNA helicase, chromosome 15
- Chromosomal instability, increased rate of sister chromatid exchange
- Increased incidence in Ashkenazi Jews
- Clinical findings
  - Onset in infancy
  - Cutaneous findings: erythema, telangiectasias in butterfly distribution, chelitis, café au lait macules
  - Short stature; characteristic facies
  - High-pitched voice, hypogonadism, infertility
  - Malignancy: 20% have leukemia, lymphoma, or colon cancer
  - Other medical problems: type 2 diabetes mellitus, chronic lung disease, immune deficiency with recurrent gastrointestinal and respiratory infections, abnormal liver function tests

Seckel Syndrome (Microcephalic Primordial Dwarfism)

- Autosomal recessive
  - Mutation of pericentrin (PCNT) gene, functions to anchor both structural and regulatory proteins in the centrosome

- Clinical findings
  - Bird-headed dwarfism: growth retardation, microcephaly, micrognathia, beak-like nose, dwarfism
  - Other manifestations: mental retardation, trident hands, skeletal defects, hypodontia, hypersplenism, premature graying

SYNDROMES WITH MALIGNANCY

Dyskeratosis Congenita (Zinsser-Engman-Cole Syndrome)

- *X-linked recessive* (xq28), gene mutation DKC1; encodes dyskerin—a nucleolar protein found in small nucleolar RNA protein complexes
- *Autosomal dominant*: milder spectrum of disease; gene mutation of human telomerase RNA component (hTERC); responsible for synthesizing telomeric DNA repeats; the mutation results in genomic instability and widespread cell death
- *Autosomal recessive*: unknown genetic mutation
- *Hoyerall-Hreidearsson syndrome*: severe variant of DC, multisystem disorder that develops in the neonatal period and infancy; severe growth retardation of perinatal onset, bone marrow failure, immunodeficiency, cerebellar hypoplasia and microcephaly
- Clinical findings
  - Triad of nail dystrophy, increased skin pigmentation, and mucosal leukoplakia
  - *Mucocutaneous features:*
    - Poikiloderma neck, face, chest and arms (90% of patients)
    - Dystrophic nails (90% of patients) with longitudinal ridging and splitting with complete nail loss
    - Mucosal leukoplakia (80% of patients): lingual mucosa, buccal mucosa, palate, and tongue (most commonly affected). Increased risk of malignancy at leukoplakia sites (35% of patients) (Fig 14-14)
    - Other findings: cutaneous atrophy, hyperhidrosis of the palms and soles, telangiectasias, cracking, fissuring, bullae formation, loss of dermal ridges, hair tufts with keratotic plugs on the limbs and keratinized basal cell papillomas, alopecia, amyloidosis
  - *Nonmucocutaneous features:*
    - Pulmonary disease (20% of patients)
    - Ophthalmic manifestations: epiphoria due to nasolacrimal duct blockage, conjunctivitis, blepharitis, pterygium formation, ectropion, strabismus, cataracts, and optic atrophy
    - Skeletal manifestations: (20% of patients): mandibular hypoplasia, osteoporosis, abnormal bone trabeculation, avascular necrosis and scoliosis

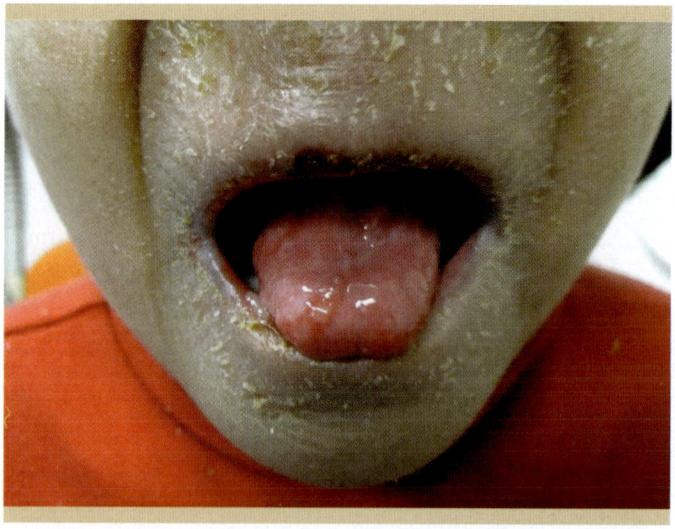

FIGURE 14-14 Dyskeratosis congenital, oral lesions. *(Used with permission from Dr. Agim.)*

    - Dental abnormalities: leukoplakia, hyperpigmentation, periodontal disease, hypocalcified teeth, taurodontism
    - Genitourinary abnormalities: hypoplastic testes, hypospadias, phimosis, urethral stenosis, horseshoe kidneys
    - Gastrointestinal abnormalities: esophageal webs causing dysphagia, hepatomegaly, cirrhosis
    - Neurological abnormalities: altered mental status, learning difficulties, peripheral neropathy
    - Other abnormalities: microcephaly, intracranial calcification, deafness, and choanal atresia. Bone marrow failure resulting in peripheral cytopenias (75% of patients develop pancytopenia, responsible for death in 70% of patients)
- Course: death in third to fourth decade due to malignancy (usually SCC), gastrointestinal bleed, or infection

Xeroderma Pigmentosa

- Multigenic, multiallelic, autosomal recessive disease
- Eight complementation groups: (XP-A to XP-G) associated with defects in NER, (XP variant form, XP-V) affects the ability to replicate DNA templates carrying unrepaired DNA damage (Table 14-14)
- Clinical findings
  - XP-A: most profound DNA repair defect with minimal repair activity and neurological symptoms commonly occurring
  - XP-C: severe skin lesions, rare neurological symptoms
  - *Ocular symptoms* (80% of patients) include photophobia, conjunctivitis, corneal vascularization, and opacification; malignant tumors may also arise
  - *Mucocutaneous manifestations* (Fig. 14-10): skin appears prematurely aged, increased incidence of

TABLE 14-14 Xeroderma Pigmentosa Features and Mutations

Complementation Group	Mutation	Features
A	XPA	Neurologic abnormalities Most common in Japan DeSanctis-Cacchione syndrome is subtype
B	ERCC3	Xeroderma pigmentosum-Cockayne syndrome complex (XP/CS)
C	XPC	Most common in USA No neurologic abnormalities
D	ERCC2	DNA helicase defect XP/CS, trichothiodystrophy (XP/TTD), cerebro-ocular-facial syndrome (COFS)
E	DDB2	Mild disease, no neurologic changes
F	ERCC4	Mild disease, no neurologic changes
G	ERCC5	Neurologic symptoms only, XP/CS
Variant	XPV POLH	No neurologic abnormalities

actinic keratosis, keratoacanthoma, squamous cell carcinoma, basal cell carcinoma, melanoma beginning in childhood; poikiloderma
  - *Neurologic manifestations*: progressive cognitive deterioration mainly in complementation groups A, D, and G: sensorineural deafness, spasticity, ataxia, hyporeflexia
  - *DeSanctis-Cacchione syndrome*: subtype mainly associated with XPA, distinguished by severe neurologic disease, dwarfism, and immature sexual development
- Prognosis: two-thirds die by third decade
- Treatment
  - Aggressive avoidance of sun exposure
  - High-dose oral isotretinoin
  - Excision of cutaneous malignancies
  - Imiquimod 5% cream, 5-fluorouracil cream
  - Skin screenings every 3 months
  - Ophthalmologic evaluation

Muir-Torre Syndrome

- Autosomal dominant disorder characterized by the combination of sebaceous gland tumors of the skin and internal malignancies
- Subtype of hereditary nonpolyposis colorectal cancer syndrome (HNPCC, also called Lynch syndrome)
- Defect in DNA mismatch repair (MMR) genes
  - Most often *MSH2* located on chromosome 2p
  - Sometimes *MLH1* located on chromosome 3p
- Presents in fifth to sixth decade
- Diagnostic criteria
  - Group A: sebaceous andenoma, sebaceous epithelioma, sebaceous carcinoma, keratoacanthoma
  - Group B: visceral malignancy
  - Group C: multiple keratoacanthomas, multiple visceral malignancies, family history of Muir-Torre syndrome
  - Diagnosis requires: criterion from group A and group B, or all three from group C
- Clinical findings
  - Cutaneous tumors: sebaceous tumors: adenomas, hyperplasia, epitheliomas, sebaceous carcinomas; may also present with keratoacanthomas
  - Internal malignancies: adenocarcinoma of the colon is most common cancer; other sites include genitourinary tract, hematologic and breast malignancies have also been reported
- Treatment: sebaceous adenoma and epithelioma—excision or cryotherapy; sebaceous carcinoma—wide excision, radiotherapy, or Mohs surgery; keratocanthoma—excision

Cowden Syndrome (Multiple Hamartoma Syndrome)

- Autosomal dominant
- PTEN defect (phosphate and tensin homolog, also called MMAC1), found on 10q23; the gene defect is also found in Bannayan-Riley-Ruvalcaba syndrome (BRRS) and Proteus-like syndrome, collectively termed PTEN overgrowth syndromes

- Presents in second to third decade
- Diagnostic criteria
  - Mucocutaneous lesions alone if
    - More than six facial papules with more than 3 trichilemmomas
    - Cutaneous facial papules and oral mucosal papillomatosis
    - Oral mucosal papillomatosis and acral keratoses
    - Six or more palmar/plantar keratoses, or
  - Two major criteria but one must include macrocephaly or Lhermitte-Duclos disease, or
  - One major and 3 minor criteria, or
  - Four minor criteria
    - *Pathognomonic criteria*: facial papules (facial trichilemmomas and papillomatous papules), acral keratoses and oral papillomatosis
    - *Major criteria:* breast cancer, thyroid cancer, macrocephaly, hamartomatous outgrowths of cerebellum (Lhermitte-Duclos disease)
    - *Minor criteria*: thyroid lesions (goiter, adenoma), hamartomatous intestinal polyps, fibrocystic disease of the breast, lipomas, fibromas, genitourinary tumors or malformations, mental retardation (IQ < 75)
- Clinical findings
  - *Mucocutaneous lesions*: facial trichilemmomas, acral keratoses, oral papillomas—found mainly on the buccal and gingival mucosa, where coalescent lesions lead to a characteristic cobblestone-like pattern; other cutaneous lesions: lipomas, xanthomas, vitiligo, neuromas, hemangiomas, lentigines, acanthosis nigricans
  - *Extracutaneous findings*
    - *Breast abnormalities*: fibrocystic breast changes, fibroadenomas
    - *Thyroid abnormalities*: (60%) goiter, benign adenoma, thyroglossal duct cyst, hyperthyroidism or hypothyroidism, thyroiditis
    - *Gastrointestinal abnormalities*: polyps have low malignant potential, diverticula, hepatic hamartomas
    - *Urogenital abnormalities*: ovarian cysts, uterine leiomyomas, hydocele and varicocele in males, hypoplastic testes, vulvar and vaginal cyts
    - *Ocular abnormalities*: cataracts, angioid streaks, myopia
    - *Nervous system abnormalities*: neuromas, neurofibromas, meningiomas
    - *Skeletal abnormalities*: adenoid facies, bone cysts, craniomegaly, high arched palate, kyphoscoliosis, pectus excavatum, rudimentary sixth digit, syndactyly
  - *Internal malignancy*: breast adenocarcinoma (at least 20% of cases); follicular thyroid adenocarcinoma (7%), endometrial cancer, adenocarcinoma of the colon, hepatocellular carcinoma
  - *Lhermitte-Duclos disease*: variant with cerebellar hamartomas and ataxia
- Diagnosis and evaluation
  - Baseline studies: thyroid function tests, thyroid scanning, complete blood count, urinalysis, mammography and chest radiography

Gardner Syndrome

- Autosomal dominant; 25% of cases occur due to spontaneous mutations
- Adenomatosis polyposis coli (APC) gene, a tumor suppressor gene; linked to 5q21-q22
- Defect also found in familial adenomatous polyposis (FAP)
- Promotes destruction of β-catenin: component of a transcription factor complex
- Clinical findings
  - *Gastrointestinal manifestations*: polyposis of colon by second to fourth decade; most develop colon or rectal cancer
  - *Skeletal manifestations*: osteomas of the skull and jaw (50% of patients), supernummerary teeth
  - *Cutaneous manifestations*: epidermoid cysts of head and neck (66% of patients), fibromas, neurofibromas, lipomas, leiomyomas, pigmented skin lesions
  - *Tumors*: desmoid, fibromas, hepatoblastoma
  - *Ocular manifestations*: congenital hypertrophy of the retinal pigment epithelium (CHRPE)
  - *Other manifestations*: papillary thyroid cancer, menigiomas, hepatoma, hepatoblastoma, fibromas, leiomyomas, lipomas, biliary and adrenal neoplasms, osteosarcoma, chondrosarcoma
- Diagnosis: DNA analysis
- Treatment: colonoscopies, prophylactic colectomy, high fiber diet, screen family members with large bowel and upper GI surveillance, as well as thyroid and possibly hepatic surveillance

Peutz-Jeghers Syndrome (Periorificial Lentiginosis) (Fig. 14-15)

- Autosomal dominant or sporadic
- *STK11* gene (serine/threonine protein kinase, *LKB1*) tumor suppressor gene; mapped to chromosome 19p13.13
- Presents in childhood
- Clinical findings
  - *Cutaneous findings*: lentigines on mucosa, periorificial skin, palms, digits; present at birth; lesions on the skin and lips often fade after puberty, while intraoral lesions persist
  - *Gastrointestinal findings*: hamartomatous polyps (more common in small intestine) may cause bleeding, pain, intussuception, obstruction; adenocarcinoma
  - *Genitourinary findings*: ovarian neoplasm—most common sex cord tumor with annular tubules (SCTAT), mucinous epithelial ovarian tumor, serous

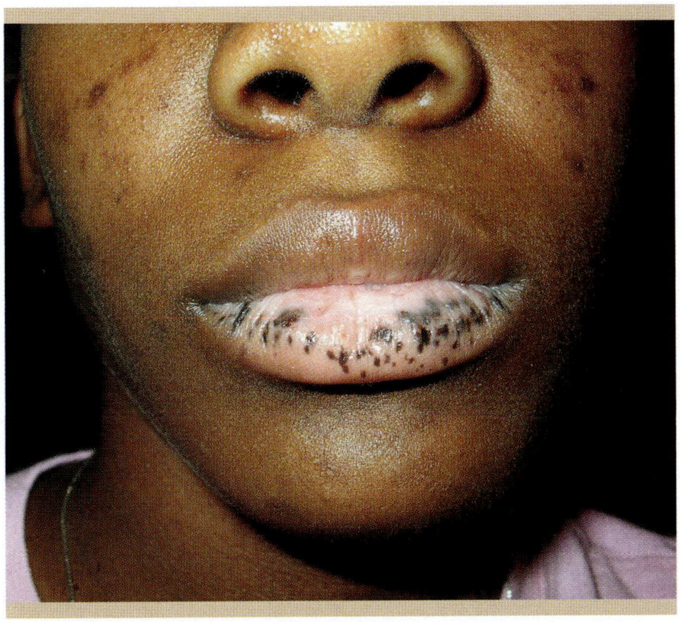

FIGURE 14-15 Peutz-Jeghers syndrome. (*Used with permission from Dr. Asra Ali.*)

tumor, and ovarian mature hamartoma; endometrial adenocarcinoma and adenoma malignum of the cervix
    - *Endocrine findings*: gynecomastia due to calcified Sertoli cell testicular tumors
    - *Other findings*: breast cancer (usually ductal), pancreatic cancer
- Diagnosis: monitor with colonoscopy, polypectomy
- Course: normal life span if malignancy detected early

Multiple Endocrine Neoplasia IIa (Sipple Syndrome)

- Autosomal dominant
- Receptor tyrosine kinase (*RET*) protooncogene; activation of *RET* protein and results in hyperplasia of target cells—such as C cells (clear large cells in a perifollicular or parafollicular location; precursor lesion for medullary thyroid carcinoma [MTC]) in the thyroid gland and chromaffin cells in adrenal glands
- Clinical findings
    - Macular or lichen amyloidosis
    - Hyperparathyroidism with parathyroid hyperplasia (20% of cases) or adenoma
    - Thyroid hyperplasia or MTC
    - Pheochromocytoma, bilateral in 70% of cases; age at onset is approximately 40 years; patients present with hypertension, sweating, palpitations and tachycardia, nausea, vomiting, polyuria, polydipsia
- Diagnosis: *RET* germline mutation testing
- Laboratory work up: calcitonin levels, urine catecholamine; plasma free and urinary fractionated metanephrines
- Imaging studies: pheochromocytomas: CT scan, MRI, metaiodo-benzylguanidine (MIBG) scanning; OctreoScan imaging, positive emission tomography (PET)
- Treatment: total thyroidectomy with radical lymph-node dissection (patients 5 years or older with *RET* mutation); pheochromocytomas: surgical excision

Multiple Endocrine Neoplasia IIb (Multiple Neuroma Syndrome)

- Autosomal dominant
- *RET* mutations; protooncogene
- Chromosomal locus 10q11
- Clinical findings
    - Mucosal neuromas may result in thickened lips, eyelid eversion
    - Medullary thyroid carcinoma; aggressive, occurs in childhood
    - Pheochromocytoma
    - Marfanoid habitus
    - Adrenomedullary hyperplasia; multifocal and often bilateral
    - Gastrointestinal ganglioneuromatosis with megacolon; constipation or diarrhea
- Laboratory work up: calcitonin levels, urine catecholamine; plasma free and urinary fractionated metanephrines
- Imaging studies: pheochromocytomas: CT scan, MRI, MIBG scanning; OctreoScan imaging, PET
- Course: normal life span with early detection and treatment of thyroid carcinoma
- Treatment: total thyroidectomy with radical lymph-node dissection (patients 5 years or older with *RET* mutation); pheochromocytomas: surgical excision

Carney Complex

- Autosomal dominant; mutations in the PRKAR1A gene; encodes the R1a regulatory subunit of protein kinase A
- The following syndromes are now included under Carney complex:
    - LAMB (lentigines, atrial myxomas, mucocutaneous myxomas, and blue nevi)
    - NAME (nevi, atrial myxoma, myxoid neurofibroma, and ephelides)
- Clinical findings: pituitary adenoma, Sertoli-cell tumors, thyroid nodules, cardiac myxomas (accounts for 7% of all cardiac myxomas)
- Cutaneous findings: skin myxomas, melanotic schwannomas, lentigines (common areas: face, trunk, lips)
- Imaging studies: echocardiography
- Treatment: surgical excision of intracardiac myxomas

DISORDERS ASSOCIATED WITH IMMUNODEFICIENCY

Wiskott-Aldrich Syndrome (WAS)

- X-linked recessive
- WAS gene, Xp11; genetic defect in Wiskott-Aldrich syndrome protein (WASp)
- Decreased sialophorin (CD43) on surface of lymphocytes
- Impaired T- and NK-cell function
- Clinical findings
  - Atopic dermatitis with secondary infection, allergies, asthma
  - Recurrent bacterial infections
  - Thrombocytopenia, petechiae, bloody diarrhea
  - Increased IgA, IgD, and IgE, but decreased IgM
- Course: death from infection, hemorrhage, or lymphoreticular malignancy
- Laboratory studies
  - serum immunoglobulin levels, complete blood cell count
- Imaging studies
  - CT: splenomegaly, rule out malignancy. Evaluation of intracranial bleeding, sinus, or pulmonary infections
- Treatment: topical steroids and moisturization for eczema, intravenous immunoglobulin and/or steroids for thrombocytopenia; bone marrow transplantation

Chronic Granulomatous Disease

- X-linked recessive, sometimes autosomal recessive
- Mutations in nicotinamide dinucleotide phosphate (NADPH) oxidase subunits (e.g., $gp91^{phox}$ subunit of cytochrome b or $p47^{phox}$)
- Deficient killing of phagocytised organisms
- Clinical findings
  - Pyodermas, perianal abscesses, and perioral ulcers
  - Pneumonia and emphyema
  - Osteomyelitis with *Serratia*
  - Hepatosplenomegaly with granulomas
  - Nitroblue tetrazolium assay abnormal (abnormal leukocytes unable to reduce dye and make blue color)
- Treatment includes interferon gamma

Hyperimmunoglobulin E Syndrome

- Autosomal dominant
- Chromosome 4q
- Increased levels of IgE
- Clinical findings
  - Eczematous rash
  - Cold abscesses with *Staphylococcus, Streptococcus,* or *Candida*
  - Sinopulmonary infections with *Staphylococcus, H. Influenza,* or fungus
  - Osteopenia with bone fractures and scoliosis
  - Retention of primary teeth and other dental anomalies
  - Job syndrome is a subgroup with hyperextensible joints

Severe Combined Immunodeficiency

- X-linked recessive, sometimes autosomal recessive
- Most have defects in γ chain of IL-2 receptor, adenosine deaminase, or JAK 3 pathway
- Impaired T-cells, may also affect NK- and B-cells
- Clinical findings
  - Absent thymus on x-ray, lack tonsillar buds
  - Recurrent infections with *Candida, Staphyloccocus,* and *Streptococcus*
  - Pneumonias with *Pneumocystis carinii*, Parainfluenza, or *Cytomegalovirus*
  - Chronic viral diarrhea, malabsorption, and failure-to-thrive
  - Graft-versus-host reaction to *in utero* maternal lymphocytes
  - Must irradiate blood products before transfusion and avoid live vaccines
  - Omenn syndrome: severe variant with failure-to-thrive, alopecia, and erythroderma; secondary to RAG 2 gene mutation

Leukocyte Adhesion Deficiency (LAD)

- Autosomal recessive
- *CD18* gene (part of an integrin)
- Impaired leukocyte mobilization
- Clinical findings
  - Gingivitis can lead to loss of teeth
  - Poor wound healing, so wounds become large ulcers
  - Delayed separation of umbilical cord
  - Differentiate this from Type II LAD which also has mental retardation and short stature; defect in GDP-fucose biosynthesis

DISORDERS WITH CHROMOSOME ABNORMALITIES

Down Syndrome (Trisomy 21)

- Mainly sporadic secondary to nondisjunction at chromosome 21
- Presents at birth
- Clinical findings
  - Single palmar crease
  - Nuchal skin folds
  - Syringomas
  - Elastosis perforans serpiginosa
  - Xerosis and lichenification with age
  - Alopecia areata
  - Flat nasal bridge, short broad neck, epicanthal folds, small mouth with protruding scrotal tongue
  - Mental retardation and seizures
  - Congenital heart disease
  - Duodenal atresia
  - Acute myelogenous leukemia
- Course: increased infant mortality secondary to congenital heart defects and neoplasms

Turner Syndrome (Gonadal Dysgenesis, Ullrich-Turner)

- Sporadic loss of one X chromosome (XO monosomy)
- Some cases demonstrate mosaicism
- Clinical findings
  - Dermatologic findings: melanocytic nevi, koilonychia, increased keloids, webbed neck
  - Low-set hairline, patchy alopecia
  - Triangular facies, short stature, shield chest with wide-set nipples, cubitus valgus
  - Primary amenorrhea, infertility
  - Mental retardation
  - Horseshoe kidneys
  - Coarctation of aorta
- Treatment: estrogen replacement, treatment of congenital anomalies

Noonan Syndrome

- Autosomal dominant
- *PTPN11* gene encoding protein tyrosine phosphatase SHP2, recently SOS1 and RAF1 mutations reported
- Clinical findings
  - Resemble Turner syndrome with short stature, webbed neck, low posterior hairline, cubitus valgus
  - Crytptorchidism
  - Cardiac malformations (pulmonic stenosis)
  - Lymphedema
  - Tendency for keloid formation
- Treatment: correction of cardiac defects

Klinefelter Syndrome

- 47,XXY
- Decreased serum testosterone
- Clinical findings
  - Hypogonadism, gynecomastia
  - Tall with low hairline
  - Sparse body hair
  - Mental retardation, psychiatric problems in one-third of patients
  - Thrombophlebitis, leg ulcers
  - Risk of gonadal tumors, breast cancer
- Treatment: testosterone replacement and wound care

QUIZ

Questions

1. Connexins 26, 30, and 31 are associated with Keratitis-Ichthyosis-Deafness syndrome, hidrotic ectodermal dysplasia, and erythrokeratoderma variabilis, respectively. What additional screening test would capture a finding allelic to any of these conditions?

   A. Eye exam
   B. Hearing test
   C. Chest radiograph
   D. Echocardiogram

2. Other than Human hair basic keratins 1 and 6, monilethrix may be caused by a mutation in which of the following?

   A. Loricrin
   B. Plakophilin
   C. Desmocollin
   D. Desmoglein IV

3. The most common malignant tumor in children is a feature of which genodermatosis?

   A. Basal cell nevus syndrome
   B. Birt Hogg Dube syndrome
   C. Cowden syndrome
   D. Muir-Torre syndrome

4. Epidermolysis bullosa with muscular dystrophy is due to a defect in:

   A. Collagen VII
   B. Plectin
   C. alpha 6 beta 4 integrin
   D. Kindlin

5. All of the following syndromes feature café au lait macules EXCEPT:

   A. Neurofibromatosis
   B. Legius syndrome
   C. Peutz Jeghers
   D. Russell Silver

6. Which primary immunodeficiency may present with a dermatomyositis like eruption following echovirus infection?

   A. Chronic granulomatous disease
   B. IgM deficiency
   C. Leukocyte adhesion deficiency
   D. X linked gammaglobulinemia

7. The PTEN gene has been implicated in all of the following conditions except:

   A. Bannayan Riley Ruvalcaba
   B. Naegeli Jadassohn Franschetti
   C. Cowden syndrome
   D. Proteus syndrome

8. In a patient with classic Ehlers-Danlos, testing for the most common mutation is negative. You suspect as an alternative candidate gene:
   A. Lysyl hydroxylase
   B. Tenascin X
   C. COL5A1/2
   D. COL1A1/2

9. Which of the following syndromes does not typically have an oral finding?
   A. Urbach-Wiethe
   B. Multiple endocrine neoplasia IIb
   C. Schimmelpenning
   D. Pachyonychia congenita

10. All of the following photosensitive disorders feature increased risk for internal malignancy except:
   A. Cockayne syndrome
   B. Rothmund-Thompson syndrome
   C. Xeroderma pigmentosa
   D. Bloom syndrome

Answers

1. B. Nonsyndromic deafness is associated with mutations in connexins 26, 30, and 31 among others. Screening by audiology in a patient or family members can assess for this finding.
2. D. Desmoglein IV has been implicated in some cases of monilethrix in addition to established reports of Hhb 1 and 6. Loricrin is implicated in Vohwinkel syndrome variants, while desmocollin and plakophilin are involved in subcorneal pustular dermatosis and Naxos syndrome, respectively.
3. A. medulloblastomas may occur in nevoid basal cell carcinoma syndrome. In addition to their characteristic cutaneous features, Birth hogg Dube is associated with renal cancer, Cowden syndrome with breast and thyroid malignancy and Muir-Torre with sebaceous and gastro-intestinal carcinoma
4. B. Plectin is mutated in EBS-MD, collagen VII is featured in dystrophic epidermolysis bullosa, alpha 6 beta 4 integrin in junctional epidermolysis bullosa or epidermolysis bullosa simplex and kindlin in Kindler syndrome.
5. C. Peutz Jeghers syndrome features mucosal lentiginosis however café au lait macules are not a distinct feature of this condition. Neurofibromatosis, Legius syndrome, and Russell Silver on the other hand have this skin finding as a diagnostic clue.
6. D. X-linked gammaglobulinemia may present with a DM-like eruption following echovirus infection. Female carriers of CGD may have discoid lupus lesions, LAD may feature delayed separation of the umbilical stump and IgM deficient patient have extensive verrucae.
7. B. NFJ is associated with a disorder of reticulate pigmentation associated with keratin 14 mutation. PTEN has been implicated in 80% of classic Cowden syndrome patients (KILLIN also described), 60% of BRRS patients, and 20% of those with Proteus. AKT1 is the newer mutation associated with Proteus syndrome.
8. B. Tenascin X has been implicated in some patients with EDS who do not have collagen V mutations, which are most commonly found in classic EDS. Collagen I is more closely associated with osteogenesis imperfecta but also EDS-arthrochalasia type and lysyl hydroxylase, encoded by the PLOD1 gene is associated with the kyphoscoliosis subtype of EDS.
9. C. Schimmelpenning syndrome is an epidermal nevus syndrome featuring extensive nevus sebaceus with potential concomitant skeletal, neurologic, and ophthalmologic dysfunction. MEN IIb may feature mucosal neuromas; pachyonychia congenital, nonmalignant oral leukokeratosis and lipoid proteinosis, mucosal infiltration (hyalinosis cutis et mucosae).
10. A. Cockayne syndrome patients do not have a significantly increased internal malignancy risk. Rothmund-Thompson is associated with SCCs and osteosarcoma, Blood syndrome with lymphoreticular and gastrointestinal malignancy and XP with ocular melanoma in addition to the myriad of skin cancers.

REFERENCES

Epidermolysis Bullosa

Bauer JW, Lanschuetzer C: Type XVII collagen gene mutations in junctional epidermolysis bullosa and prospects for gene therapy. *Clin Exp Dermatol* 2003;28(1):53-60.

Fine JD: Epidermolysis bullosa, in Bolognia JL, Jorizzo JL, Rapini RP, eds. *Dermatology*. New York: Mosby; 2003, 491-498. *J Am Acad Dermatol*. 2008 Jun;58(6):931-950.

Fine JD, Bauer EA, McGuire J, Moshell A, eds. *Epidermolysis Bullosa: clinical epidermiologic, and laboratory advances, and the findings of the National Epidermolysis Bullosa Registry*. Baltimore: Johns Hopkins University Press; 1999, 206-204.

Fine JD et al. Cancer and inherited epidermolysis bullosa: lifetable analyses of the National Epidermolysis Bullosa Registry study population, in Fine JD, Bauer EA, McGuire J, Moshell A, eds. *Epidermolysis bullosa: clinical epidermiologic, and laboratory advances, and the findings of the National Epidermolysis Bullosa Registry*. Baltimore: Johns Hopkins University Press; 1999, 175-192.

Fine JD et al. Premature death and inherited epidermolysis bullosa: contingency table and lifetable analyses of the National Epidermolysis Bullosa Registry study population, in Pai S, Marinkovich MP: Epidermolysis bullosa: new and emerging trends. *Am J Clin Dermatol* 2002;3(6):371-380.

Fine JD et al. The classification of inherited epidermolysis bullosa (EB): report of the Third International Consensus Meeting on Diagnosis and Classification of EB.

Uitto J, Pulkkinen L, McLean WH: Epidermolysis bullosa: a spectrum of clinical phenotypes explained by molecular heterogeneity. *Mol Med Today* 1997;3(10):457-465.

Disorders of Pigmentation

Barbagallo JS, Kolodzieh MS, Silverberg NB, Weinberg JM: Neurocutaneous disorders. *Dermatol Clin* 2002;20(3):547–560, viii.

Berlin AL, Paller AS, Chan LS: Incontinentia pigmenti: a review and update on the molecular basis of pathophysiology. *J Am Acad Dermatol* 2002;47(2):169–187.

Bolger WE, Ross AT: McCune-Albright syndrome: a case report and review of the literature *Int J Pediatr Otorhinolaryngol* 2002; 65(1):69–74.

Denayer E, Chmara M, Legius E et al. Legius syndrome in 14 families *Hum Mutat* 2011;32(1):E1985–E1998.

Denayer E, Descheemaeker MJ, Legius E et al. Observations on Intelligence and Behavior in 15 patients with Leguis syndrome. *Am J Med Genet C Semin Med Genet.* 2011;157(2):123–128.

Eng, Charis: PTEN: one gene, many syndromes. *Hum Mutat* 2003 Sep;22(3):183–198.

Happle R: A fresh look at incontinentia pigmenti. *Arch Dermatol* 2003;139(9):1206–1208.

Harris-Stith R, Elston DM: Tuberous sclerosis. *Cutis* 2002;69(2): 103–109.

Huizing M, Boissy RE, Gahl WA: Hermansky-Pudlak syndrome: vesicle formation from yeast to man. *Pigment Cell Res* 2002;15(6):405–419.

Krishtul A, Galadari I: Waardenburg syndrome: case report. *Int J Dermatol* 2003;42(8):651–652.

Lindhurst MJ, Sapp JC, Biesecker LG et al. A Mosaic Activating Mutation in AKT1 associated with Proteus Syndrome. *N Engl J Med.* 18;365(7):611–619. Epub 2011.

Mollaaghababa R, Pavan WJ: The importance of having your SOX on: role of SOX10 in the development of neural crest-derived melanocytes and glia. *Oncogene* 2003;22(20):3024–3034.

Muram-Zborovski TM, Stevenson DA, Rong Mao et al. SPRED1 mutations in a Neurofibromatosis Clinic *J Child Neurol.* 2010 Oct;25(10):1203–1209.

Okulicz JF, Shah RS, Schwartz RA, Janniger, CK: Oculocutaneous albinism. *J Euro Acad Dermatol Venereol* 2003;17(3):251–256.

Reynolds RM, Browning GG, Nawroz I, Campbell IW: Von Recklinghausen's neurofibromatosis: neurofibromatosis type 1. *Lancet* 2003;361(9368):1552–1554.

Shiflett SL, Kaplan J, Ward DM: Chediak-Higashi syndrome: a rare disorder of lysosomes and lysosome related organelles. *Pigment Cell Res* 2002;15(4):251–257.

Sumner K, Crockett DK, Mao R et al. The SPRED1 variants repository for Legius syndrome *G3 (Bethesda).* Nov;1(6):451–456. Epub 2011.

Syrris P, Heathcote K, Carrozzo R et al. Human piebaldism: six novel mutations of the proto-oncogene KIT. *Hum Mutat* 2002;20(3):234.

Ward DM, Shiflett SL, Kaplan J: Chediak-Higashi syndrome: a clinical and molecular view of a rare lysosomal storage disorder. *Curr Mol Med* 2002;2(5):469–477.

Zlotogorski A, Marek D, Pras E et al. An autosomal recessive form of monilethrix is caused by mutations in DSG4: clinical overlap with localized autosomal recessive hypotrichosis *Journal of Investigative Dermatology* 2006;126:1292–1296.

Disorders of Vascularization

Amitai DB, Fichman S, Merlob P et al. Cutis marmorata telangiectatica congenita: clinical findings in 85 patients. *Pediatr Dermatol* 2000;17(2):100–104.

Bedocs PM, Gould JW: Blue rubber-bleb nevus syndrome: a case report. *Cutis* 2003;71(4):315–318.

Bertucci V, Krafchik BR: What syndrome is this? Ollier disease + vascular lesions: Maffucci syndrome. *Pediatr Dermato* 1995;12(1):55–58.

Cirulli A, Liso A, D'Ovidio F et al. Vascular endothelial growth factor serum levels are elevated in patients with hereditary hemorrhagic telangiectasia. *Acta Haematol* 2003;110(1):29–32.

Di Cataldo A, Haupt R, Fabietti P, Schiliro G: Is intensive follow-up for early detection of tumors effective in children with Beckwith-Wiedemann syndrome? *Clin Genet* 1996;50(5):372–374.

Dragieva G, Stahel HU, Meyer M et al. Proteus syndrome. *Vasa* 2003;32(3):159–163.

Frevel T, Rabe H, Uckert F, Harms E: Giant cavernous haemangioma with Kasabach-Merritt syndrome: a case report and review. *Eur J Pediatr* 2002;161(5):243–246.

Hale EK: Klippel-Trenaunay syndrome. *Dermatol Online J* 2002; 8(2):13.

Jessen RT, Thompson S, Smith EB: Cobb syndrome. *Arch Dermatol* 1977;113(11):1587–1590.

Karsdorp N, Elderson A, Wittebol-Post D et al. Von Hippel-Lindau disease: new strategies in early detection and treatment. *Am J Med* 1994;97(2):158–168.

Kihiczak NI, Schwartz RA, Jozwiak S et al. Sturge-Weber syndrome. *Cutis* 2000;65(3):133–136.

Lonser RR, Glenn GM, Walther M et al. Von Hippel-Lindau disease. *Lancet* 2003;361(9374):2059–2067.

Meine JG, Schwartz RA, Janniger CK: Klippel-Trenaunay-Weber syndrome. *Cutis* 1997;60(3):127–132.

Montagu Ashley: *The Elephant Man: A Study in Human Dignity.* London: E.P. Dutton; 1971.

Paller AS: Vascular disorders. *Dermatol Clin* 1987;5(1): 239–250. Review.

Shim JH, Lee DW, Cho BK: A case of Cobb syndrome associated with lymphangioma circumscriptum. *Dermatology* 1996;193(1):45–47

Spiller JC et al. Diffuse neonatal hemangiomatosis treated successfully with interferon alfa-2a. *J Am Acad Dermatol* 1992;27(1):102–104.

Treves Sir Frederick: *The Elephant Man and Other Reminiscences.* London: Cassell and Co; 1923.

Zvulunov A, Esterly NB: Neurocutaneous syndromes associated with pigmentary skin lesions. *J Am Acad Dermatol* 1995;32(6):915–935.

Connective Tissue, Premature Aging, and Photosensitive Disorders

Andiran N, Sarikayalar F, Saraçlar M, Cağlar M: Autosomal recessive form of congenital cutis laxa: more than the clinical appearance. *Pediatr Dermatol* 2002 Sep-Oct; 19(5):412–414.

Anttinen A et al. Neurological symptoms and natural course of xeroderma pigmentosum. *Brain* 2008 Aug;131(Pt 8):1979–1989.

Badame AJ: Progeria. *Arch Dermatol* 1989;125(4):540–544. Review.

Beighton P et al. Ehlers-Danlos syndromes: revised nosology, Villefranche, 1997. Ehlers-Danlos National Foundation (USA) and Ehlers-Danlos Support Group (UK). *Am J Med Genet* 1998;77(1):31–37.

Bender MM, Potocki L, Metry DW: What syndrome is this? Cockayne syndrome. *Pediatr Dermatol* 2003 Nov-Dec;20(6):538–540.

Bergen AA, Plomp AS, Schuurman EJ et al. Mutations in ABCC6 cause pseudoxanthoma elasticum. *Nat Genet* 2000;25(2):228–231.

Blunt K, Quan V, Carr D, Paes BA: Aplasia cutis congenita: a clinical review and associated defects. *Neonatal Netw* 1992;11(7):17–27.

Byers PH: Ehlers-Danlos syndrome: recent advances and current understanding of the clinical and genetic heterogeneity. *J Invest Dermatol* 1994;103(5 Suppl):47S–52S.

Byers PH: Osteogenesis imperfecta: perspectives and opportunities. *Curr Opin Pediatr* 2000;12(6):603–609.

Casanova D, Amar E, Bardot J, Magalon G: Aplasia cutis congenita. Report on 5 family cases involving the scalp. *Eur J Pediatr Surg* 2001 Aug;11(4):280–284.

Chen L, Oshima J: Werner syndrome. *J Biomed Biotechnol* 2002; 2(2):46–54.

Cheung MS, Glorieux FH: Osteogenesis imperfecta: update on presentation and management. *Rev Endocr Metab Disord* 2008 Jun;9(2):153–160.

Curatolo P, Bombardieri R, Jozwiak S: Tuberous sclerosis. *Lancet* 2008 Aug 23;372(9639):657–668.

De Paepe A et al. Revised diagnostic criteria for the Marfan syndrome. *Am J Med Genet* 1996;62(4):417–426.

Duvic M, Lemak NA: Werner's syndrome. *Dermatol Clin* 1995;13(1):163–168.

Ehsani AH, Ghiasi M, Robati RM: Lipoid proteinosis: report of three familial cases. *Dermatol Online J* 2006 Jan 27;12(1):16.

Frieden IJ: Aplasia cutis congenita: a clinical review and proposal for classification. *J Am Acad Dermatol* 1986;14(4):646–660.

Frydman M: The Marfan syndrome. *Isr Med Assoc J* 2008 Mar;10(3):175–178.

Galadari E, Hadi S, Sabarinathan K: Hartnup disease. *Int J Dermatol* 1993;32(12):904.

Goto M: Werner's syndrome: from clinics to genetics. *Clin Exp Rheumatol* 2000;18(6):760–766.

Gupta N, Phadke SR: Cutis laxa type II and wrinkly skin syndrome: distinct phenotypes. *Pediatr Dermatol* 2006 May-Jun;23(3):225–230.

Hamada T: Lipoid proteinosis. *Clin Exp Dermatol* 2002;27(8):624–629.

Handley TP, McCaul JA, Ogden GR: Dyskeratosis congenita. *Oral Oncology* 2006 Apr;42(4):331–336.

Hardman CM, Garioch JJ, Eady RA, Fry L: Focal dermal hypoplasia: report of a case with cutaneous and skeletal manifestations. *Clin Exp Dermatol* 1998;23(6):281–285.

Harsha Vardhan BG, Muthu MS, Saraswathi K, Koteeswaran D: Bird-headed dwarf of Seckel. *J Indian Soc Pedod Prev Den* 2007;25(Suppl):S8–S9.

Kawamura A, Ochiai T, Tan-Kinoshita M, Suzuki H: Buschke-Ollendorff syndrome: three generations in a Japanese family. *Pediatr Dermatol* 2005 Mar-Apr;22(2):133–137.

Kieran MW, Gordon L, Kleinman M: New approaches to progeria. *Pediatrics* 2007 Oct;120(4):834–841.

Kim GH, Dy LC, Caldemeyer KS, Mirowski GW: Buschke-Ollendorff syndrome. *J Am Acad Dermatol* 2003;48(4):600–601.

Kocher MS, Shapiro F: Osteogenesis imperfecta. *J Am Acad Orthop Surg* 1998;6(4):225–236.

Kruk-Jeromin J, Janik J, Rykala J Aplasia cutis congenita of the scalp. Report of 16 cases. *Dermatol Surg* 1998;24(5):549–553.

Laube S, Moss C: Pseudoxanthoma elasticum. *Arch Dis Child* 2005 Jul;90(7):754–756.

Malfait F, De Paepe A: Molecular genetics in classic Ehlers-Danlos syndrome. *Am J Med Genet C Semin Med Genet* 2005 Nov 15;139C(1):17–23. Review.

Markova D, Zou Y, Ringpfeil F et al. Genetic heterogeneity of cutis laxa: a heterozygous tandem duplication within the fibulin-5 (FBLN5) gene. *Am J Hum Genet* 2003;72(4):998–1004.

Meetei AR, Sechi S, Wallisch M et al. A multiprotein nuclear complex connects Fanconi anemia and Bloom syndrome. *Mol Cell Biol* 2003;23(10):3417–3426.

Narayan S, Fleming C, Trainer AH, Craig JA: Rothmund-Thomson syndrome with myelodysplasia. *Pediatr Dermatol* 2001 May-Jun;18(3):210–212.

Ohtani T, Furukawa F: Pseudoxanthoma elasticum. *J Dermatol* 2002;29(10):615–620.

Ostler EL, Wallis CV, Sheerin AN, Faragher RG: A model for the phenotypic presentation of Werner's syndrome. *Exp Gerontol* 2002 Jan-Mar;37(2-3):285–292.

Paller AS: Wnt signaling in focal dermal hypoplasia. *Nature Genetics* 2007;39(7):820–821.

Parapia LA, Jackson C: Ehlers-Danlos syndrome—a historical review. *Br J Haematol* 2008;141(1):32–35.

Ponti G et al. Value of MLH1 and MSH2 mutations in the appearance of Muir-Torre syndrome phenotype in HNPCC patients presenting sebaceous gland tumors or keratoacanthomas. *J Invest Dermatol* 2006 Oct;126(10):2302–2307.

Poppe B, Van Limbergen H, Van Roy N et al. Chromosomal aberrations in Bloom syndrome patients with myeloid malignancies. *Cancer Genet Cytogenet* 2001;128(1):39–42.

Ringpfeil F, Pulkkinen L, Uitto J: Molecular genetics of pseudoxanthoma elasticum. *Exp Dermatol* 2001;10(4):221–228.

Riyaz N, Riyaz A, Chandran R, Rakesh SV: Focal dermal hypoplasia (Goltz syndrome). *Indian J Dermatol Venereol Leprol* 2005 Jul-Aug;71(4):279–281.

Rodriguez-Revenga L, Iranzo P, Badenas C, Puig S, Carrió A, Milà M: A novel elastin gene mutation resulting in an autosomal dominant form of cutis laxa. *Arch Dermatol* 2004 Sep;140(9):1135–1139.

Santos de Oliveira R, Barros Jucá CE, Lopes Lins-Neto A, Aparecida do Carmo Rego M, Farina J, Machado HR: Aplasia cutis congenita of the scalp: is there a better treatment strategy? *Childs Nerv Syst* 2006 Sep;22(9):1072–1079.

Sule RR, Dhumawat DJ, Gharpuray MB: Focal dermal hypoplasia. *Cutis* 1994;53(6):309–312.

Thomas ER, Shanley S, Walker L, Eeles R: Surveillance and treatment of malignancy in Bloom syndrome. *Clin Oncol (R Coll Radiol)* 2008 Jun;20(5):375–379.

Thomas WO, Moses MH, Graver RD, Galen WK: Congenital cutis laxa: a case report and review of loose skin syndromes. *Am Plast Surg* 1993;30(3):252–256.

Wang LL et al. Clinical manifestations in a cohort of 41 Rothmund-Thomson syndrome patients. *Am J Med Genet* 2001;102(1):11–17.

Yen JL, Lin SP, Chen MR, Niu DM: Clinical features of Ehlers-Danlos syndrome. *J Formos Med Assoc* 2006;105(6):475–480.

Yeowell HN, Pinnell SR: The Ehlers-Danlos syndromes. *Semin Dermatol* 1993;12(3):229–240.

Syndromes Associated With Malignancy

Braverman IM: Skin manifestations of internal malignancy. *Clin Geriatr Med* 2002;18(1):1–19.

Dokal I: Dyskeratosis congenita. *Br J Haematol* 1999;105 (Suppl 1): 11–15.

Drachtman RA, Alter BP: Dyskeratosis congenita. *Dermatol Clin* 1995;13(1):33–39.

Fassbender WJ, Krohn-Grimberghe B, Gortz B et al. Multiple endocrine neoplasia (MEN)—an overview and case report—patient with sporadic bilateral pheochromocytoma, hyperparathyroidism and marfanoid habitus. *Anticancer Res* 2000;20(6C):4877–4887.

Fistarol SK, Anliker MD, Itin PH: Cowden disease or multiple hamartoma syndrome—cutaneous clue to internal malignancy. *Eur J Dermatol* 2002;12(5):411–421.

Fotiadis C, Tsekouras DK, Antonakis P, Sfiniadakis J, Genetzakis M, Zografos GC: Gardner's syndrome: a case report and review of the literature. *World J Gastroenterol* 2005 Sep 14;11(34):5408–5411.

Gu GL, Wang SL, Wei XM, Bai L: Diagnosis and treatment of Gardner syndrome with gastric polyposis: a case report and review of the literature. *World J Gastroenterol* 2008 Apr 7;14(13):2121–2123.

Hampel H, Peltomaki P: Hereditary colorectal cancer: risk assessment and management. *Clin Genet* 2000;58(2):89–97.

Heymann WR: Peutz-Jeghers syndrome. *J Am Acad Dermatol* 2007 Sep;57(3):513–514.

Hildenbrand C, Burgdorf WH, Lautenschlager S: Cowden syndrome-diagnostic skin signs. *Dermatology* 2001;202(4):362–366.

Kitagawa S, Townsend BL, Hebert AA: Peutz-Jeghers syndrome. *Dermatol Clin* 1995;13(1):127–133.

Lehmann AR: The xeroderma pigmentosum group D (XPD) gene: one gene, two functions, three diseases. *Genes Dev* 2001;15(1):15–23.

Lim W et al. Further observations on LKB1/STK11 status and cancer risk. *Br J Cancer* 2003;89(2):308–313.

Marrone A, Mason PJ: Dyskeratosis congenita. *Cell Mol Life Sci* 2003;60(3):507–517.

Mathiak M et al. Loss of DNA mismatch repair proteins in skin tumors from patients with Muir-Torre syndrome and MSH2 or MLH1 germline mutations: establishment of immunohistochemical analysis as a screening test. *Am J Surg Pathol* 2002;26(3):338–343.

Mirowski GW, Liu AA, Parks ET, Caldemeyer KS: Nevoid basal cell carcinoma syndrome. *J Am Acad Dermatol* 2000;43(6):1092–1093.

Norgauer J et al. Xeroderma pigmentosum. *Eur J Dermatol* 2003;13(1):4–9.

Parks ET, Caldemeyer KS, Mirowski GW: Gardner syndrome. *J Am Acad Dermatol* 2001;45(6):940–942.

Schwartz RA, Torre DP: The Muir-Torre syndrome: a 25-year retrospect. *J Am Acad Dermatol* 1995 Jul;33(1):90–104.

Immunodeficiency

Bowen B et al. A review of the reported defects in the human Cl esterase inhibitor gene producing hereditary angioedema including four new mutations. *Clin Immunol* 2001;98(2):157–163.

Buckley RH: Advances in the understanding and treatment of human severe combined immunodeficiency. *Immunol Res* 2000;22(2-3):237–251.

Erlewyn-Lajeunesse MD: Hyperimmunoglobulin-E syndrome with recurrent infection: a review of current opinion and treatment. *Pediatr Allergy Immunol* 2000;11(3):133–141.

Farkas H et al. Clinical management of hereditary angio-oedema in children. *Pediatr Allergy Immunol* 2002;13(3):153–161.

Featherstone C: How does one gene cause Wiskott-Aldrich syndrome? *Lancet* 1996;348(9032):950.

Gennery AR, Cant AJ: Diagnosis of severe combined immunodeficiency. *J Clin Pathol* 2001;54(3):191–195.

Goldblatt D: Current treatment options for chronic granulomatous disease. *Expert Opin Pharmacother* 2002;3(7):857–863.

Koide M et al. Lupus erythematosus associated with C1 inhibitor deficiency. *J Dermatol* 2002;29(8):503–507.

Levy M: Disorders with Immunodeficiency, in Spitz JL, ed. *Genodermatoses: A clinical guide to genetic skin disorders*. New York: Lippincott Williams & Wilkins; 2005, 256–271.

Paller AS: Primary Immunodeficiencies, in Bolognia JL, Jorizzo JL, Rapini RP, eds. *Dermatology*. New York: Mosby; 2003, 835–852.

Shcherbina A, Candotti F, Rosen FS, Remold-O'Donnell E: High incidence of lymphomas in a subgroup of Wiskott-Aldrich syndrome patients. *Br J Haematol* 2003;121(3):529–530.

Shemer A, Weiss G, Confino Y, Trau H: The hyper-IgE syndrome. Two cases and review of the literature. *Int J Dermatol* 2001;40(10):622–628.

Thrasher AJ, Kinnon C: The Wiskott-Aldrich syndrome. *Clin Exp Immunol* 2000;120(1):2–9.

Weston WL: Cutaneous manifestations of defective host defenses. *Pediatr Clin North Am* 1977;24(2):395–407.

Chromosomal Abnormalities

Arun D, Gutmann DH: Recent advances in neurofibromatosis type. *Curr Opin Neurol* 2004 Apr;17(2):101–105.

Bertelloni S et al. Growth and puberty in Turner's syndrome. *J Pediatr Endocrinol Metab* 2003;16 (Suppl 2):307–315.

Cantani A, Gagliesi D: Rubinstein-Taybi syndrome. Review of 732 cases and analysis of the typical traits. *Eur Rev Med Pharmacol Sci* 1998;2(2):81–87.

Ch'ng S, Tan ST: Facial port-wine stains—clinical stratification and risks of neuro-ocular involvement. *J Plast Reconstr Aesthet Surg* 2008 Aug;61(8):889–893.

Comi AM: Advances in Sturge-Weber syndrome. *Curr Opin Neurol* 2006 Apr;19(2):124–128.

Daoud MS, Dahl PR, Su WP: Noonan syndrome. *Semin Dermatol* 1995;14(2):140–144.

Evans DG, Sainio M, Baser ME: Neurofibromatosis type 2. *J Med Genet* 2000 Dec;37(12):897–904.

Fine JD et al. The classification of inherited epidermolysis bullosa (EB): report of the Third International Consensus Meeting on Diagnosis and Classification of EB. *J Am Acad Dermatol* 2008 Jun;58(6):931–950. Epub 2008 Apr 18.

Frias JL, Davenport ML: Committee on Genetics and Section on Endocrinology. Health supervision for children with Turner syndrome. *Pediatrics* 2003;111(3):692–702.

Hayes A, Batshaw ML: Down syndrome. *Pediatr Clin North Am* 1993;40(3):523–535.

Hennedige AA, Quaba AA, Al-Nakib K: Sturge-Weber syndrome and dermatomal facial port-wine stains: incidence, association with glaucoma, and pulsed tunable dye laser treatment effectiveness. *Plast Reconstr Surg* 2008 Apr;121(4):1173–1180.

Herranz P et al. Rubinstein-Taybi syndrome with piebaldism. *Clin Exp Dermatol* 1994;19(2):170–172.

Lavin MF, Gueven N, Bottle S, Gatti RA: Current and potential therapeutic strategies for the treatment of ataxia-telangiectasia. *Br Med Bull* 2007;81–82:129–147. Epub 2007 Jun 23.

Lee A, Driscoll D, Gloviczki P, Clay R, Shaughnessy W, Stans A: Evaluation and management of pain in patients with Klippel-Trenaunay syndrome: a review. *Pediatrics* 2005 Mar;115(3):744–749.

Lynch TM, Gutmann DH: Neurofibromatosis 1. *Neurol Clin* 2002 Aug;20(3):841–865.

Maher ER, Bentley E, Payne SJ et al. Presymptomatic diagnosis of von Hippel-Lindau disease with flanking DNA markers. *J Med Genet* 1992 Dec;29(12):902–905.

Mitsuhashi Y, Hashimoto I: Genetic abnormalities and clinical classification of epidermolysis. *Bullosa Arch Dermatol Res* 2003;295:S29–S33.

Muneuchi J, Higashinakagawa T, Matsuoka R: Germline gain of function mutations in RAF1 cause Noonan syndrome. *Nat Genet* 2007;39(8):1013–1017.

Nguyen D, Turner JT, Olsen C, Biesecker LG, Darling TN: Cutaneous manifestations of proteus syndrome: correlations with general clinical severity. *Arch Dermatol* 2004 Aug;140(8):947–953.

Patton MA: Russell-Silver syndrome. *J Med Genet* 1988;25(8):557–560.

Perkins RM, Hoang-Xuan MT: The Russell-Silver syndrome: a case report and brief review of the literature. *Pediatr Dermatol* 2002;19(6):546–549.

Roberts AE et al. Germline gaine of function mutations in SOS1 cause Noonan syndrome. *Nat Genet* 2007;39(1):70–74.

Roizen NJ, Patterson D: Down's syndrome. *Lancet* 2003;361(9365):1281–1289.

Russell KL et al. Dominant paternal transmission of Cornelia de Lange syndrome: a new case and review of 25 previously reported familial recurrences. *Am J Med Genet* 2001;104(4):267–276.

Shimizu H et al. Epidermolysis bullosa simplex associated with muscular dystrophy: phenotype-genotype correlations and review of the literature. *J Am Acad Dermatol* 1999 Dec;41(6):950–956.

Shovlin CL et al. Diagnostic criteria for hereditary hemorrhagic telangiectasia (Rendu-Osler-Weber syndrome). *Am J Med Genet* 2000 Mar 6;91(1):66–67.

Slaugenhaupt SA, Gusella JF: Familial dysautonomia. *Curr Opin Genet Dev* 2002;12(3):307-311.

Visootsak J, Aylstock M, Graham JM Jr.: Klinefelter syndrome and its variants: an update and review for the primary pediatrician. *Clin Pediatr (Phila)* 2001;40(12):639–651.

Woodward ER, Maher ER: Von Hippel-Lindau disease and endocrine tumour susceptibility. *Endocr Relat Cancer* 2006 Jun;13(2):415–425.

CHAPTER 15

PEDIATRIC DERMATOLOGY

NNENNA G. AGIM, MD
JOHN C. BROWNING
DENISE W. METRY
ADRIENNE M. FEASEL

DISORDERS OF PIGMENTATION

Mongolian Spot (Fig. 15-1)

- Presentation
  - Blue-gray patches present at birth or early infancy
  - Usually buttocks, lumbosacral back
  - Common in black, Hispanic, and Asian races
  - Color due to Tyndall effect (scattering of light as it strikes dermal melanin)
- Course
  - Usually resolves by early to late childhood
  - Extensive Mongolian spots (dermal melanocytosis) with dorsal/ventral distribution, indistinct borders, and persistent and/or "progressive" behavior may be a sign of underlying lysosomal storage disease (most commonly GM1 gangliosidosis type 1 and Hurler disease)

Nevus of Ota (Fig. 15-2)

- Also known as oculodermal melanocytosis, nevus fuscoceruleus ophthalmomaxillaris
- Presentation
  - Unilateral bluish gray discoloration of facial skin and adjacent cornea; in darker skin blue component is less obvious
  - Affects region supplied by trigeminal nerve V_1 and V_2 ± ipsilateral sclera
  - Congenital or acquired by second decade
  - More common in black or Asian races, females
- Treatment: pigmented lesion lasers
- Course
  - Persists; both this and nevus of Ito may increase in size/intensity over time
  - Ocular involvement: risk of glaucoma, small melanoma risk

Nevus of Ito (Fig. 15-3)

- Also known as nevus fusoceruleus acromiodeltoides
- Presentation: similar to nevus of Ota but localized to unilateral shoulder, lateral neck, scapula, and/or deltoid
- Course: persists
- Treatment: pigmented lesion lasers

Mosaic Hypopigmentation (Fig. 15-4)

- Includes hypomelanosis of Ito (incontinentia pigmenti acromians), nevus depigmentosus (achromic nevus)
- Presentation
  - Benign, hypopigmented oval or round patches, bands, or swirls
  - May be localized or extensive
  - Arranged along one or more Blaschko lines
  - No preceding vesicular or inflammatory stages
  - Incidence of systemic manifestations highest with most extensive lesions
  - Most commonly central nervous system (CNS), musculoskeletal, and eyes depending on particular chromosome defect and level of mosaicism
- Course: persists

VASCULAR DISORDERS

Blueberry Muffin Baby (Fig. 15-5)

- Presentation
  - Multiple, dark blue to magenta, small, nonblanching papules and macules
  - Present at birth or by first day of life
- Etiology
  - Extramedullary hematopoiesis

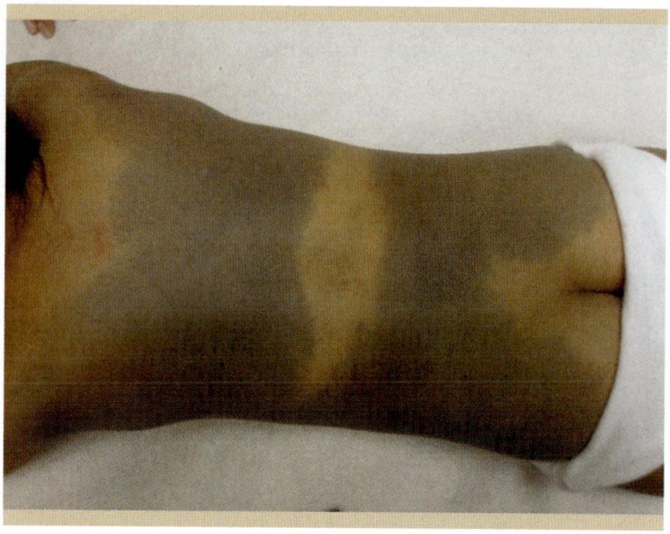

FIGURE 15-1 Dermal melanocytosis (Mongolian spot). (*Used with permission from Dr. Agim.*)

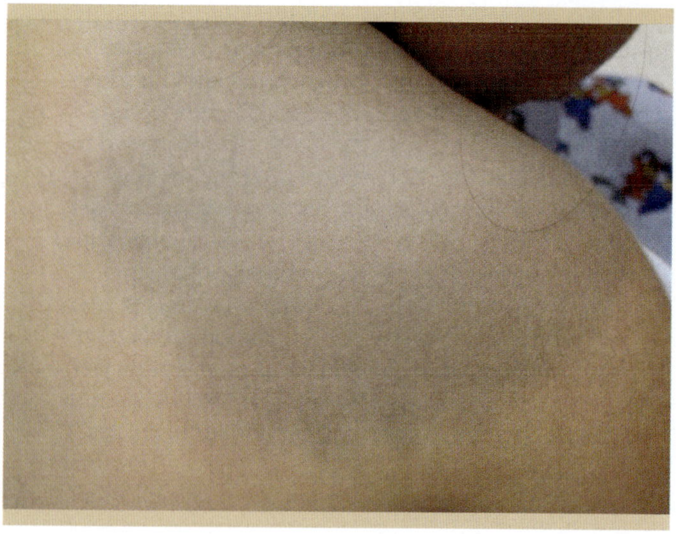

FIGURE 15-3 Nevus of Ito. (*Used with permission from Dr. Agim.*)

- Associated with congenital infections (TORCH viruses, most commonly cytomegalovirus), hemolytic disease of the newborn, hereditary spherocytosis, twin-twin transfusion syndrome
- Differential
  - Includes neoplastic-infiltrative disease (lesions typically larger, more nodular, and fewer in number)
  - Neuroblastoma, rhabdomyosarcoma, Langerhans cell histiocytosis (especially congenital self-healing histiocytosis, also known as Hashimoto-Pritzker disease), congenital leukemia (especially myelogenous)
- Course
  - Skin lesions involute spontaneously in 2 to 6 weeks
  - Evaluation may include complete blood count (CBC), viral cultures, TORCH serologies, Coombs test; skin biopsy if neoplastic infiltration suspected
- Therapy: directed toward underlying cause

Acute Hemorrhagic Edema of Infancy (Finkelstein Disease) (Fig. 15-6)

- Presentation
- Acute form of leukocytoclastic vasculitis
- Children younger than 2 years
- Often history of preceding infection
- Rapid onset
- Fever, edema, and targetoid purpuric lesions on face, ears, distal extremities

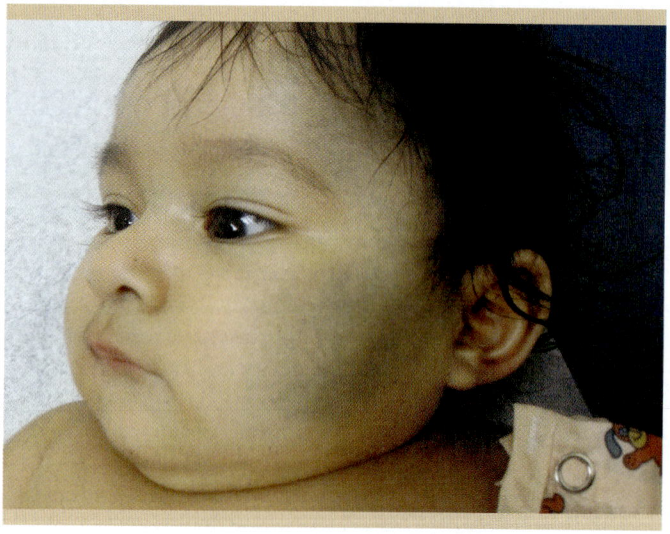

FIGURE 15-2 Nevus of Ota. (*Used with permission from Dr. Agim.*)

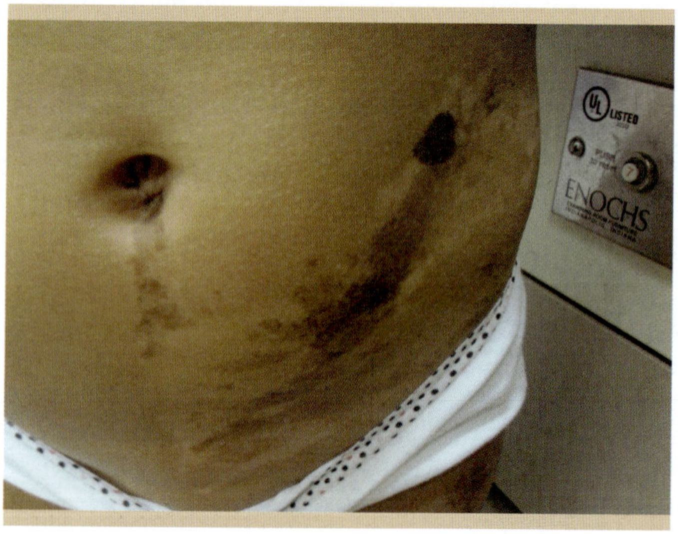

FIGURE 15-4 Cutis tricolor (mosaic hyper and hypopigmentation). (*Used with permission from Dr. Agim.*)

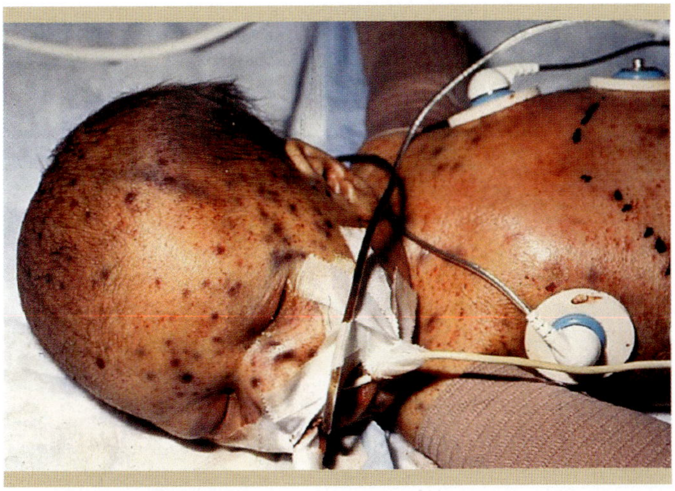

FIGURE 15-5 Blueberry muffin baby. (*Used with permission from Dr. Denise Metry.*)

- Children generally appear well despite alarming appearance of skin lesions
- Systemic symptoms: renal, joint, gastrointestinal (GI) involvement exceptional (important difference from adult Henoch-Schönlein purpura)
- Course: clinical improvement in 1 to 3 weeks

Henoch-Schönlein Purpura (Anaphylactoid Purpura) (Fig. 15-7)

- Presentation
  - Triad: characteristic skin lesions, abdominal pain, and hematuria

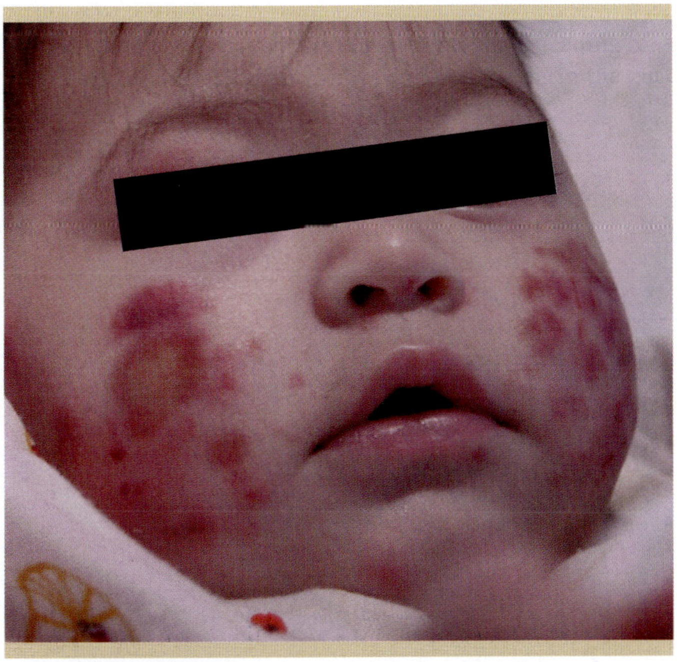

FIGURE 15-6 Acute hemorrhagic edema of infancy. (*Used with permission from Dr. Denise Metry.*)

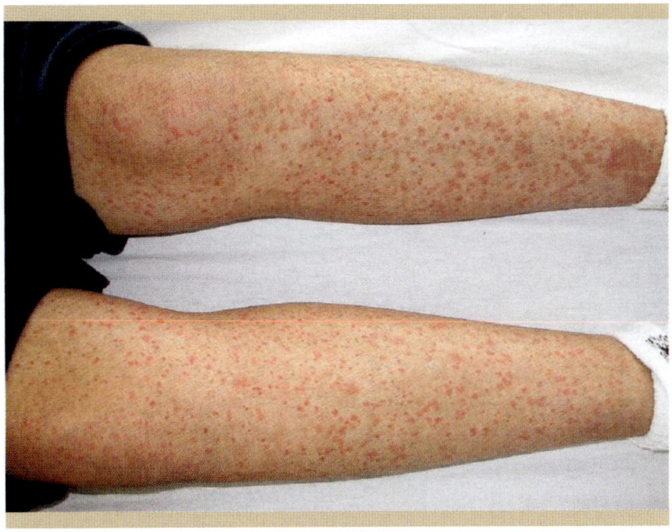

FIGURE 15-7 Henoch Schönlein purpura. (*Used with permission from Dr. Denise Metry.*)

  - Children and young adults
  - Often preceding upper respiratory infection
  - Pink or erythematous papules that become purpuric on extensor extremities, buttocks
  - Develop in crops
- Systemic signs and symptoms
  - Abdominal pain
  - Arthralgias
  - Hematuria
  - Nephritis; rare progressive glomerular disease
- Course
  - Most resolve in 6 to 16 weeks
  - May rccur
  - Severe/prolonged disease more common in older children/adolescents
  - Nephritis may manifest up to 3 years after initial onset; important to monitor urinalyses (UAs)
- Treatment: supportive care

Nevus Anemicus (Fig. 15-8)

- Presentation
  - Congenital vascular abnormality, asymptomatic
  - Most commonly occurs as a single patch of skin pallor on the trunk
  - Localized vascular hypersensitivity to catecholamines
  - Catecholamine sensitivity produces increased vasoconstriction and skin pallor
- Diagnosis
  - Diascopy: when pressure is applied to the border of the patch with a clear glass slide; the border between lesion and normal skin disappears
  - Rubbing the affected area causes erythema of the surrounding skin, but the lesion itself remains unchanged
  - Histopathology is normal
- Treatment: none

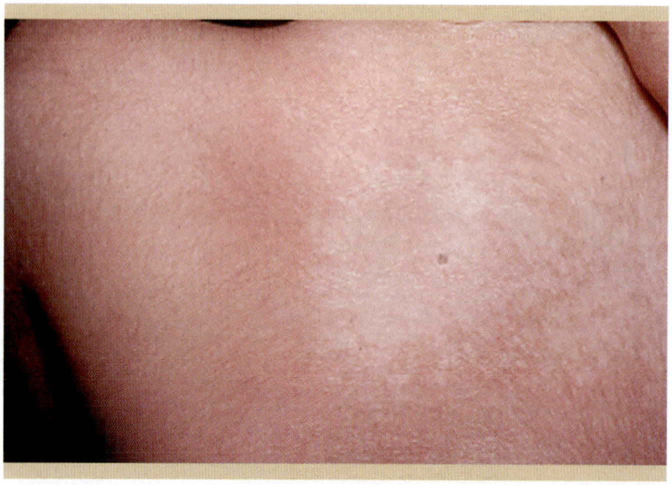

FIGURE 15-8 Nevus anemicus. (*Used with permission from Dr. Denise Metry.*)

INFECTIONS

Molluscum Contagiosum (Fig. 15-9)

- Presentation
  - Skin-colored, umbilicated papules
  - Children commonly affected
  - Contagious, with autoinoculation
- Causative organism
  - Pox virus (large DNA virus, 200–300 nm)
- Diagnosis
  - Usually clinical
  - Histology: Henderson-Patterson bodies (cytoplasmic viral inclusion bodies) on path
- Course: Individual lesions last weeks to months; total course may last several months to years
- Treatment
  - Not required because lesions will resolve spontaneously
  - Destructive options include cantharidin, curettage, cryotherapy, and topical irritants (retinoic acid, imiquimod)

Eczema Herpeticum (Kaposi Varicelliform Eruption) (Fig. 15-10)

- Presentation
  - Herpes simplex virus (HSV) infection within preexisting dermatitis (atopic dermatitis, severe seborrheic dermatitis, scabies, bullous disorders)
  - Sudden onset of grouped, uniformly sized vesicles and/or pustules that evolve into crusted erosions
  - Fever, lymphadenopathy, malaise
- Diagnosis
  - Tzanck smear
  - Biopsy
  - Rapid HSV immunofluorescence

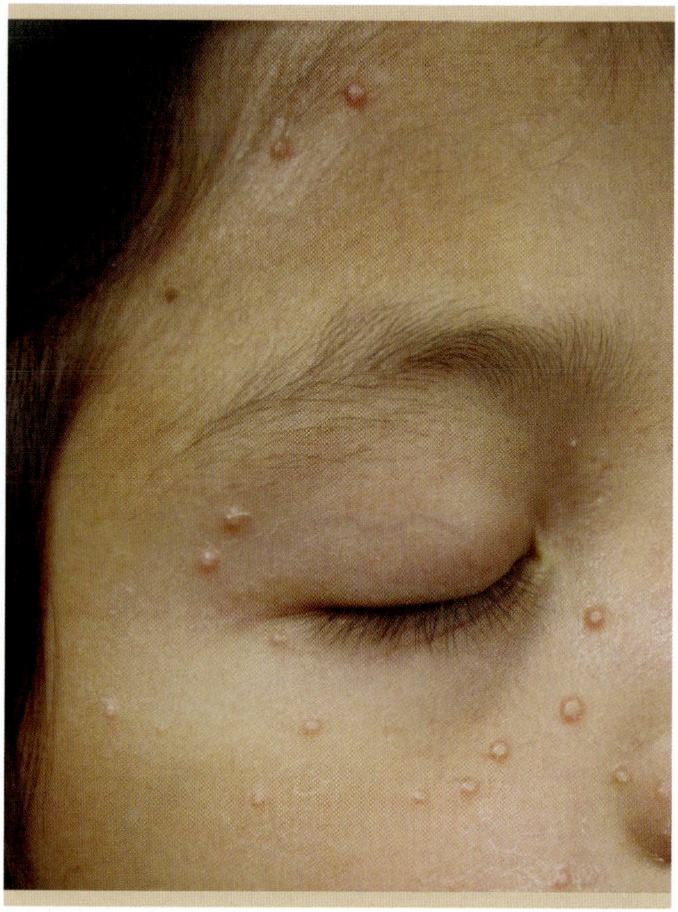

FIGURE 15-9 Molluscum contagiosum. (*Used with permission from Dr. Agim.*)

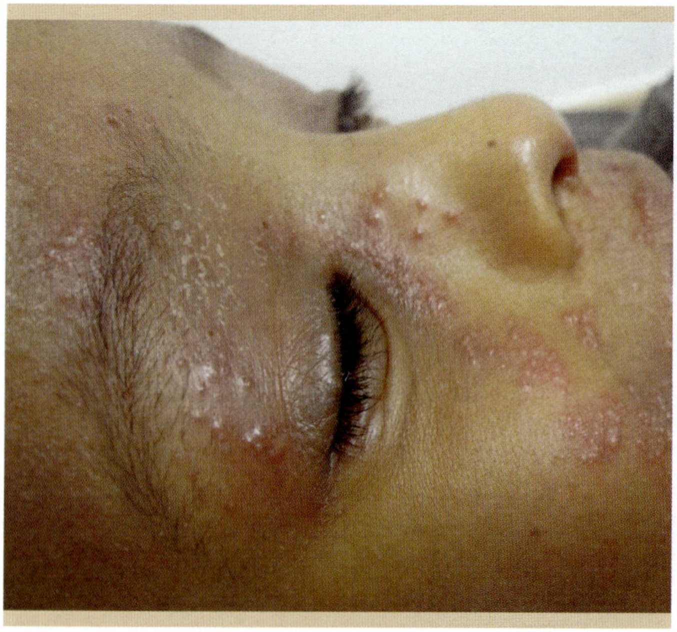

FIGURE 15-10 Eczema herpeticum. (*Used with permission from Dr. Agim.*)

- Treatment
  - First episode most serious because of risk of systemic involvement
  - Oral or intravenous acyclovir
- Prognosis
  - Estimated 20% incidence of minor recurrence

Unilateral Laterothoracic Exanthem (Asymmetric Periflexural Exanthem of Childhood) (Fig. 15-11)

- Presentation
  - Erythematous papules develop close to a flexure (typically axilla)
  - Papules coalesce and spread to involve the adjacent trunk and extremity
  - Lymphadenopathy common
  - Contralateral involvement occurs occasionally
  - Typically affects children younger than 10 years
- Causative organism
  - Etiology unknown
  - Viral cause suspected owing to high incidence of preceding upper respiratory infection or gastroenteritis
- Diagnosis
  - Mainly clinical
- Histology: lymphocytic infiltrate around eccrine ducts
- Treatment: resolves spontaneously in 2 to 6 weeks

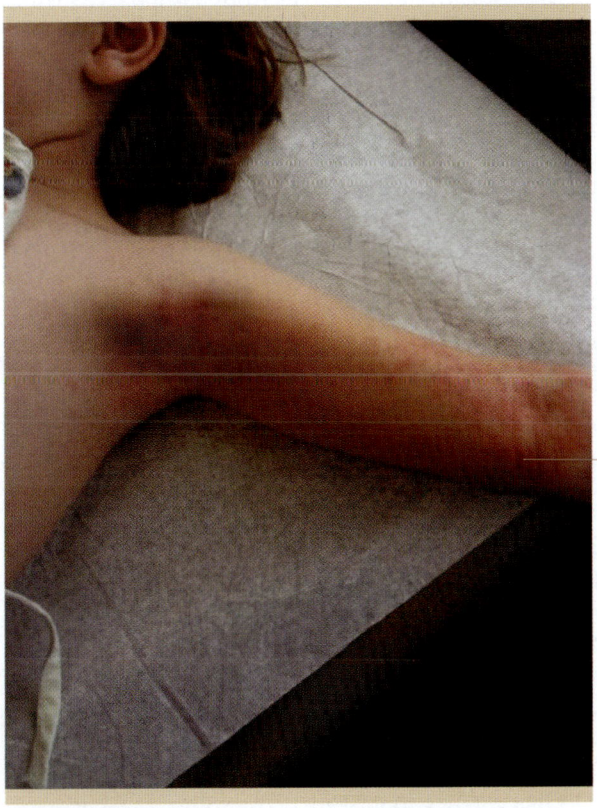

FIGURE 15-11 Unilateral laterothoracic exanthem. (*Used with permission from Dr. Agim.*)

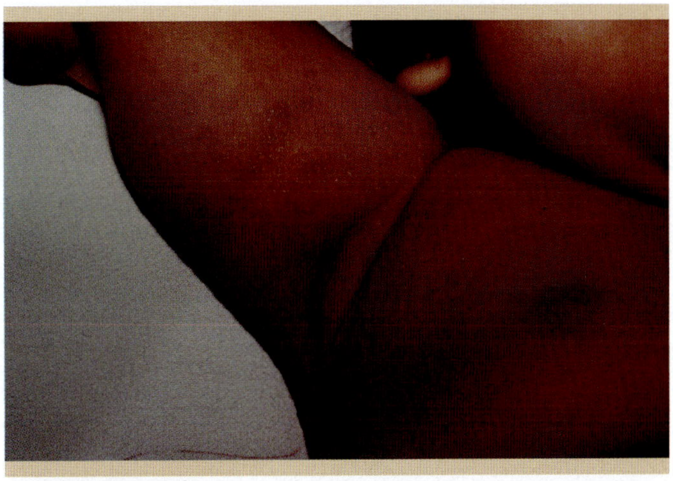

FIGURE 15-12 Scabies. (*Used with permission from Dr. Denise Metry.*)

Scabies (Fig. 15-12)

- Presentation
  - Pruritic papules, vesicles, burrows of web spaces, flexures, genitals
  - Often excoriated, impetiginized
  - Spread by close contact
  - Norwegian scabies (Fig. 15-13)
    - Heavily crusted lesions with many mites
    - Immunodeficient, debilitated patients
  - Nodular scabies (Fig. 15-14)
    - Persistent red nodules; represents hypersensitivity to mites
- Causative organism
  - Sarcoptes scabei
  - Female mite burrows and deposits eggs in stratum corneum
- Diagnosis
  - Clinical
  - Microscopic examination of mite, ova, or feces (scutula) on skin scraping
- Treatment
  - Topical 5% permethrin is treatment of choice (approved down to 2 months of age)
  - For newborn infants or pregnant/nursing women, 6 to 10% sulfur in petrolatum (permethrin is pregnancy category factor B)

Staphylococcal Scalded Skin Syndrome (Ritter Disease) (Fig. 15-15)

- Presentation
  - Acute onset of tender erythema
  - Rapid development of superficial blistering in periorificial and flexural distribution
  - Subsequent desquamation and fissuring around mouth/eyes produces classic "sad old man" face

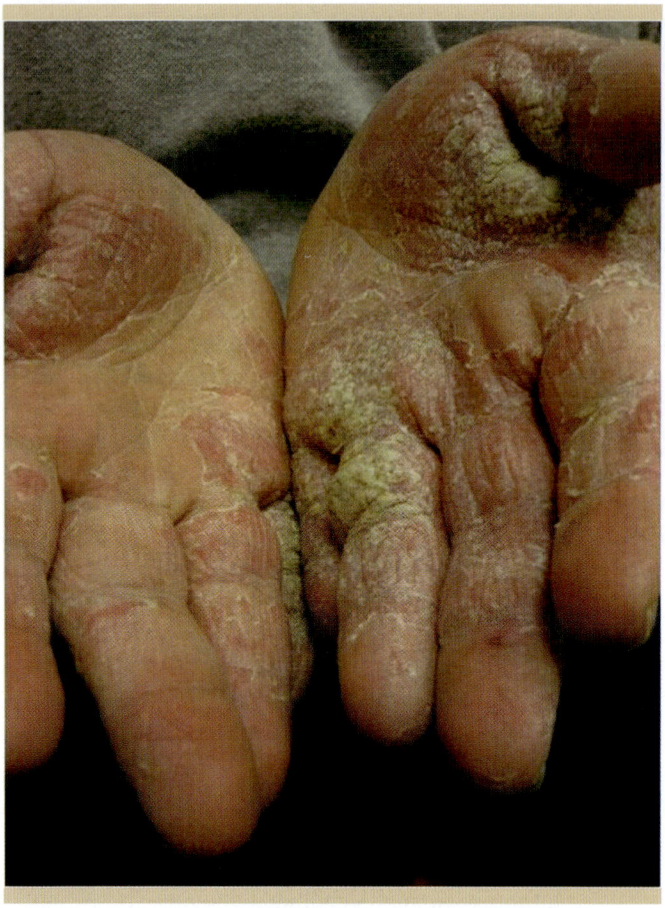

FIGURE 15-13 Norwegian scabies. (*Used with permission from Dr. Agim.*)

- Usually young children (<age 2) or adults with predisposing conditions (immunosuppression, renal impairment, overwhelming sepsis)
- Nikolsky sign present

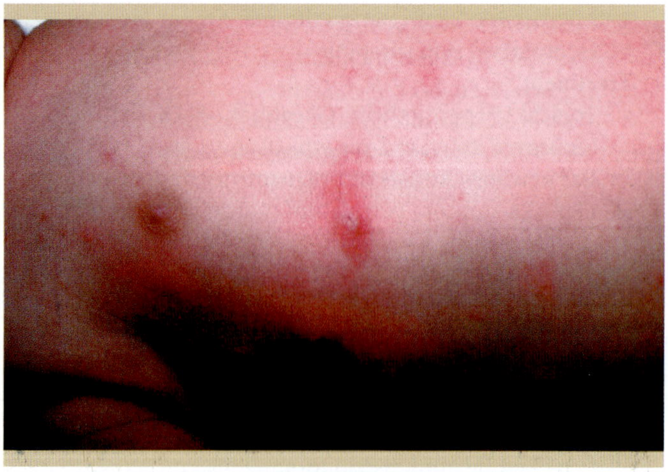

FIGURE 15-14 Nodular scabies. (*Used with permission from Dr. Denise Metry.*)

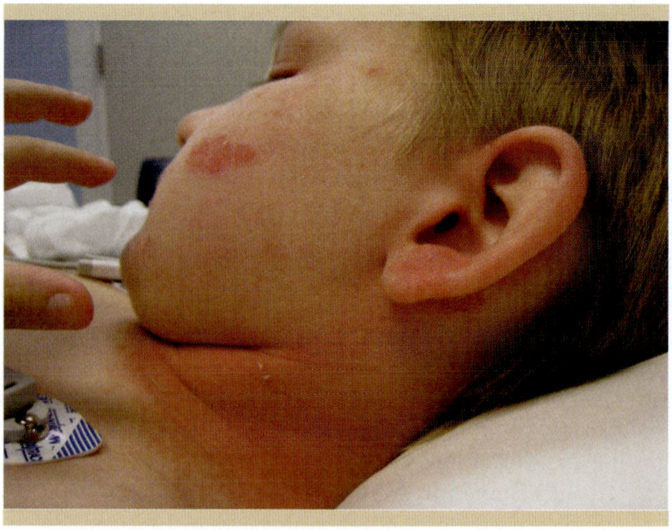

FIGURE 15-15 Staphylococcal scalded skin. (*Used with permission from Dr. Agim.*)

- Resolves without scarring but may leave dyspigmentation
- Causative organism: epidermolytic toxin of *Staphylococcus* phage group II (desmoglein 1 target)
- Diagnosis
  - May isolate *Staphylococcus* from nasopharynx (most common), blood, urine, umbilicus, conjunctivae, (not skin)
  - Histology: shows split at granular layer
- Treatment
  - Penicillinase-resistant penicillin
  - Supportive measures

DERMATOSES

Seborrheic Dermatitis ("Cradle Cap") (Fig. 15-16)

- Presentation
  - Yellowish, scaling dermatitis of scalp
  - Greasy, salmon-colored patches on face (central forehead, glabella, eyebrows, nasolabial folds), retroauricular, intertriginous areas
  - Blepharitis may be present
- Etiology: possible role of *Pityrosporum ovale (Malassezia furfur)*
- Course
  - Generally resolves by 1 year of age
  - Postinflammatory hypopigmentation characteristic of darker-skinned infants
- Treatment
  - Low-potency topical corticosteroids
  - Antiseborrheic shampoos
  - Topical antifungals

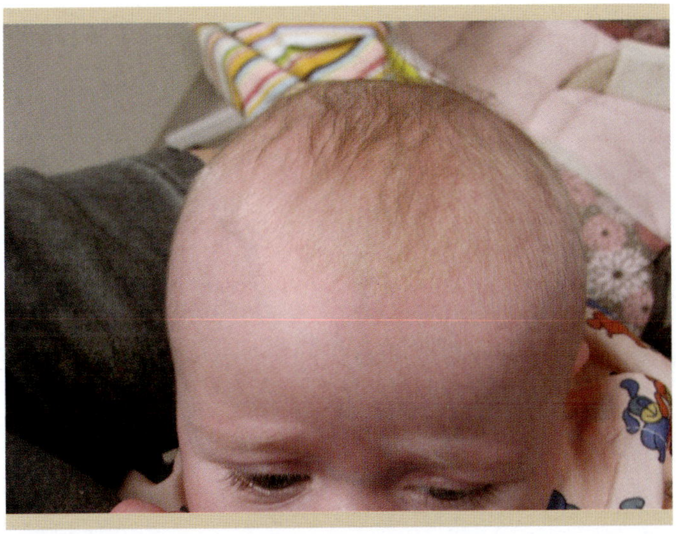

FIGURE 15-16 Seborrheic dermatitis. (*Used with permission from Dr. Agim.*)

Gianotti-Crosti Syndrome (Papular Acrodermatitis of Childhood) (Fig. 15-17)

- Presentation
  - Monomorphic papules or papulovesicles
  - Symmetrically distributed on the face, buttocks, extremities of children (generally starts on thighs/buttocks and then goes to arms and then face)
  - Lesions tend to cluster on knees and elbows
  - Usually spares the trunk
  - Lesions koebnerize
  - Constitutional symptoms: low-grade fever, lymphadenopathy, splenomegaly
- Pathology: associated with viral infections: Epstein-Barr virus (most common association in the United States), hepatitis B virus, cytomegalovirus (CMV), respiratory syncytial virus (RSV)
- Course: resolves spontaneously in 3 to 8 weeks
- Treatment: symptomatic

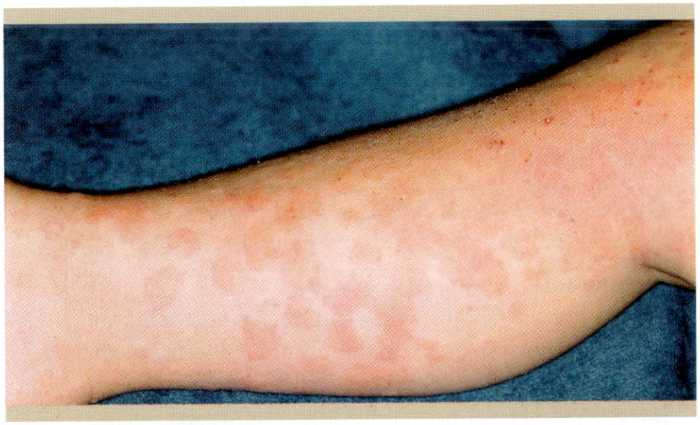

FIGURE 15-17 Gianotti Crosti. (*Used with permission from Dr. Denise Metry.*)

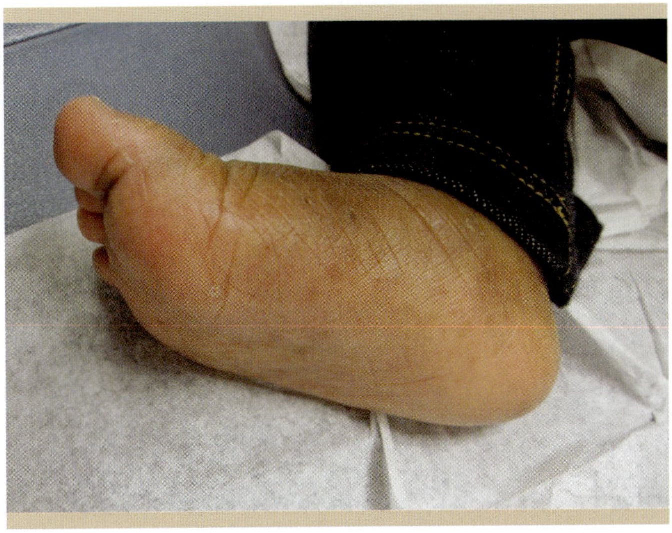

FIGURE 15-18 Acropustulosis of infancy. (*Used with permission from Dr. Agim.*)

Acropustulosis of Infancy (Infantile Acropustulosis) (Fig. 15-18)

- Presentation
  - Crops of pruritic vesiculopustules on the hands and feet of infants/young children
  - Occurs in crops every 2 to 4 weeks
  - Scabies prep negative
- Etiology: may be reactive to previous scabies exposure
- Pathology: subcorneal and intraepidermal neutrophilic abscesses
- Treatment
  - Potent topical steroids
  - Oral antihistamines
  - Oral erythromycin
  - Dapsone for exceptionally severe cases
- Course: resolves in 1 to 2 years

Transient Neonatal Pustular Melanosis (TNPM)

- Presentation
  - Very superficial vesicles, sterile pustules
  - Seen at birth in up to 4% of healthy term newborns
  - Rupture with desquamation leaves characteristic residual hyperpigmented macules generally within first 2 days of life
- Pathology: intracorneal and subcorneal neutrophilic spongiosis (few if any eosinophils)
- Treatment
  - Self-limited
  - Postinflammatory pigmentation fades in weeks to months

Erythema Toxicum Neonatorum (ETN) (Fig. 15-19)

- Presentation
  - Common; affects half of full-term newborns

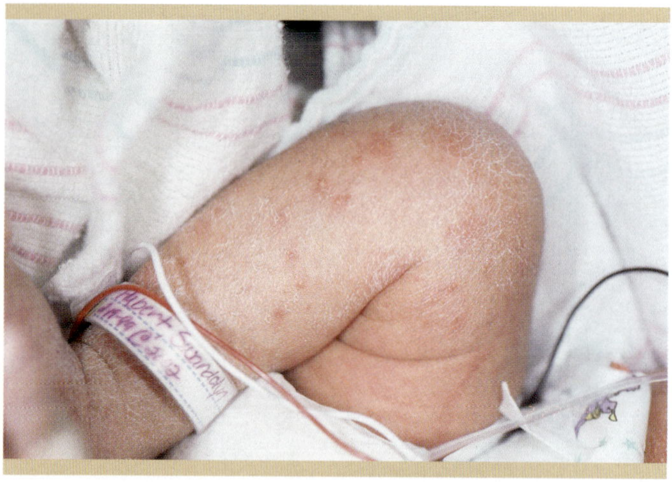

FIGURE 15-19 Erythema toxicum neonatorum. (*Used with permission from Dr. Denise Metry.*)

  - "Flea-bitten rash" of few to hundreds of erythematous macules, wheals, papules, and pustules
  - Occurs in the first 24 to 48 hours of life
  - Both TNPM and ETN almost always spare the palms and soles (important distinguishing clinical feature from congenital candidiasis)
- Histology: folliculitis with eosinophils (few neutrophils, no spongiosis)
- Treatment: resolves within 1 to 2 weeks

Lichen Striatus (Fig. 15-20)

- Presentation
  - Linear band of erythematous to skin-colored papules
  - Develops over several weeks
  - Follows Blaschko lines; nail damage if matrix involved
  - Affects children and young adults
  - Resolves within 1 to 2 years with postinflammatory hypopigmentation that improves slowly
  - Initially may be mildly pruritic
- Pathology
  - Spongiotic or lichenoid dermatitis with necrotic keratinocytes
  - Lymphocytic infiltrate around eccrine coils
- Treatment: topical anti-inflammatories may be useful for pruritus; may hasten resolution of inflammatory lesions

CUTANEOUS NEOPLASMS AND MALFORMATIONS

Epstein Pearls (Bohn Nodules)

- Presentation: white to yellow mobile papules at the hard palate (Epstein pearls) or gum margin (Bohn nodules) of newborns
- Etiology/pathology: milia

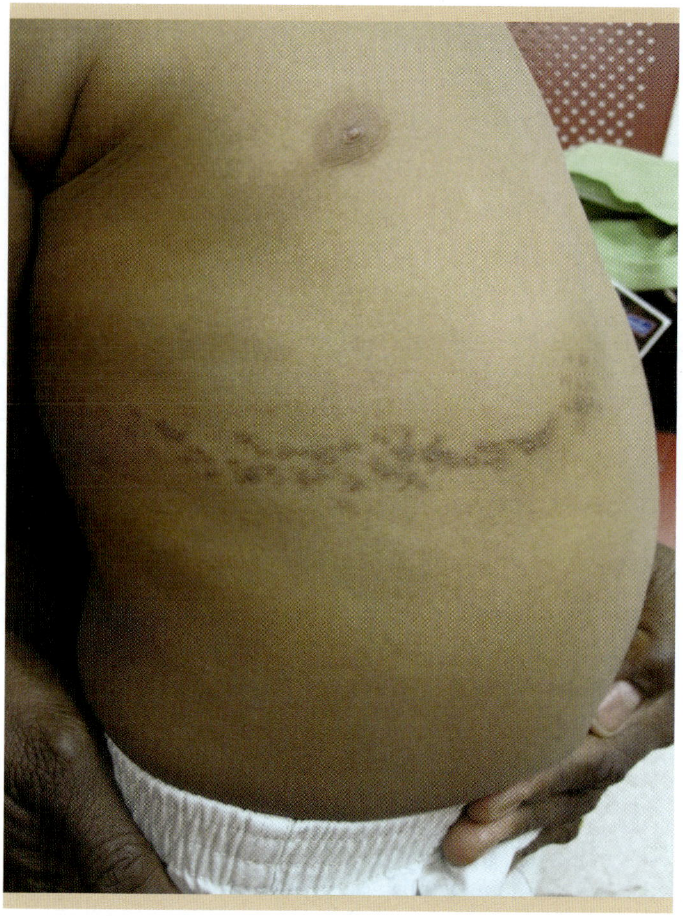

FIGURE 15-20 Lichen striatus. (*Used with permission from Dr. Agim.*)

- Treatment
  - No treatment required
  - Resolves within weeks

Pseudoverrucous Papules and Nodules (Fig. 15-21)

- Presentation: shiny, moist, flat-topped erythematous papules of diaper area or surrounding urostomy/colostomy sites
- Etiology/pathology: form of severe irritant contact dermatitis resulting from incontinence, encopresis, severe diaper dermatitis
- Treatment: protection of skin by barrier creams

Perianal (or Perineal) Pyramidal Protrusion (Fig. 15-22)

- Presentation
  - Triangular-shaped, skin-colored to erythematous nodule on the perineal median raphe, anterior to the anus
  - More than 90% of cases occur in female infants
  - Average age at presentation: 14 months
- Etiology/pathology: related to constipation, possibly lichen sclerosus et atrophicus

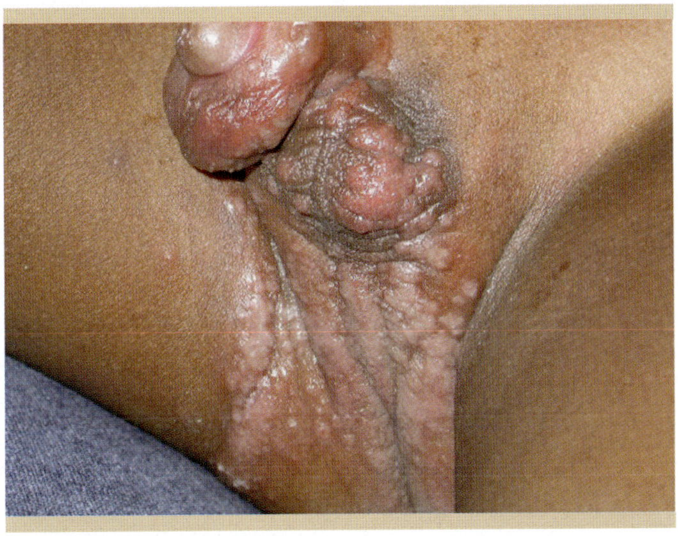

FIGURE 15-21 Pseudoverrucous papules and nodules. (*Used with permission from Dr. Denise Metry*.)

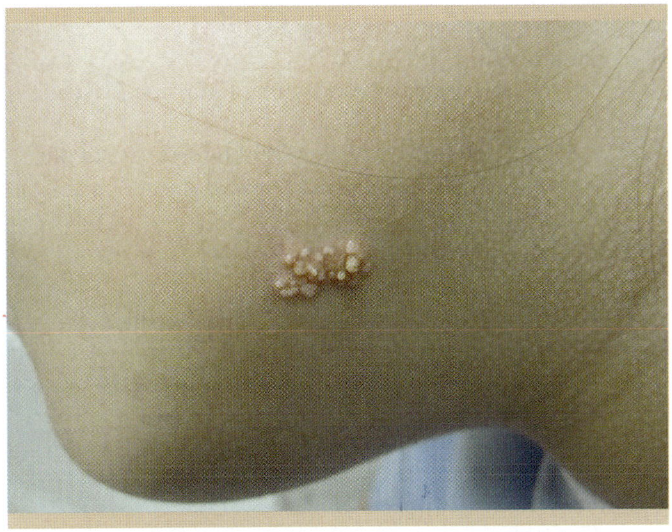

FIGURE 15-23 Nevus sebaceus of Jadassohn. (*Used with permission from Dr. Agim*.)

- Course: resolves spontaneously over several months to 1 to 2 years
- Treatment: treating associated constipation may hasten resolution

Nevus Sebaceous of Jadassohn (Fig. 15-23)

- Presentation
  - Congenital hairless, yellow to orange plaque on the scalp (usually round), face, or neck (usually linear)
  - Pebbly, velvety, or cerebriform surface, although often flat at birth
- Etiology/pathology
  - Early: increased numbers of immature sebaceous glands and hair follicles
  - Postpubertal: papillomatosis, hyperkeratosis, and hypergranulosis accompany lobules of sebaceous glands and ectopic apocrine glands
- Course/therapy
  - Prepubertal excision often considered due to low risk of secondary tumor growth later in life
  - Most commonly associated malignant neoplasm: basal cell carcinoma (BCC)
  - Most common benign neoplasm: trichoblastoma

Schimmelpenning Syndrome (Fig. 15-24)

- Presentation: large nevus sebaceus associated with ocular lesions, intracranial asses, mental retardation, seizures, skeletal, and/or pigmentary abnormalities

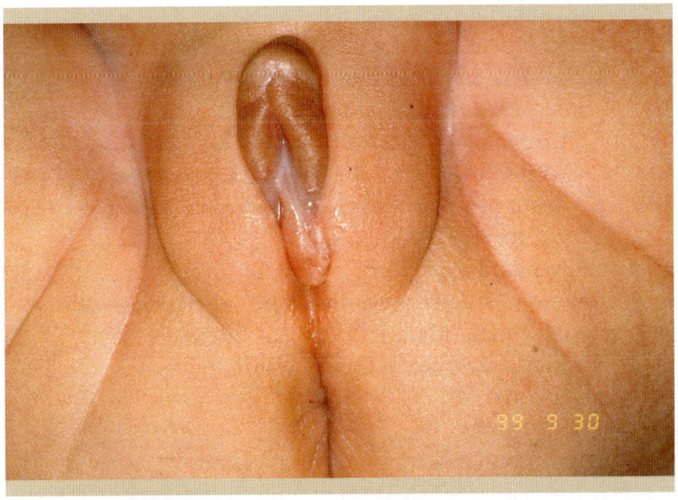

FIGURE 15-22 Perineal pyramidal protrusion. (*Used with permission from Dr. Adelaide Herbert.*)

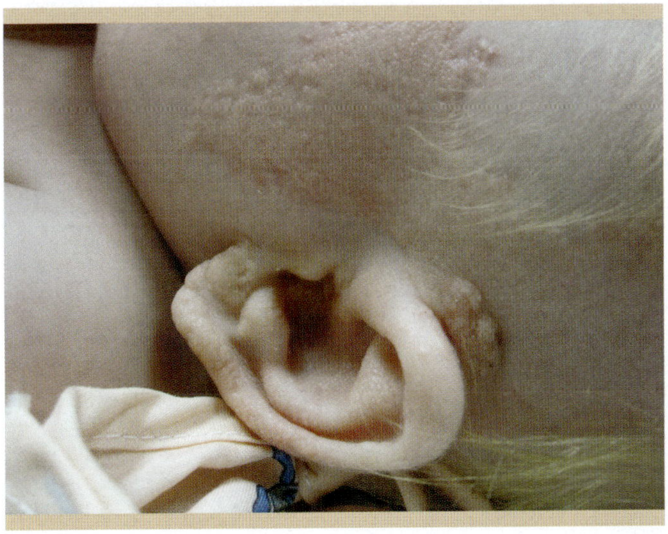

FIGURE 15-24 Schimmelpenning syndrome. (*Used with permission from Dr. Agim.*)

Linear Epidermal Nevus (Fig. 15-25)

- Presentation
  - Verrucous pink to brown papules following Blaschko lines
  - Generally presents at birth or within first year of life, sometimes later in childhood or adolescence
- Subtypes
  - Systematized epidermal nevus: extensive, bilateral lesions
  - Ichthyosis hystrix/nevus unius lateris: extensive unilateral lesions
  - Inflammatory linear verrucous epidermal nevus (ILVEN)
    - Inflammatory variant with erythema, pruritus
    - Often on an extremity or perineum in girls
- Etiology/histology
  - Hyperplasia of epidermal structures with hyperkeratosis, acanthosis, papillomatosis, some with epidermolytic hyperkeratosis
  - Accompanying parakeratosis and inflammation (with ILVEN)

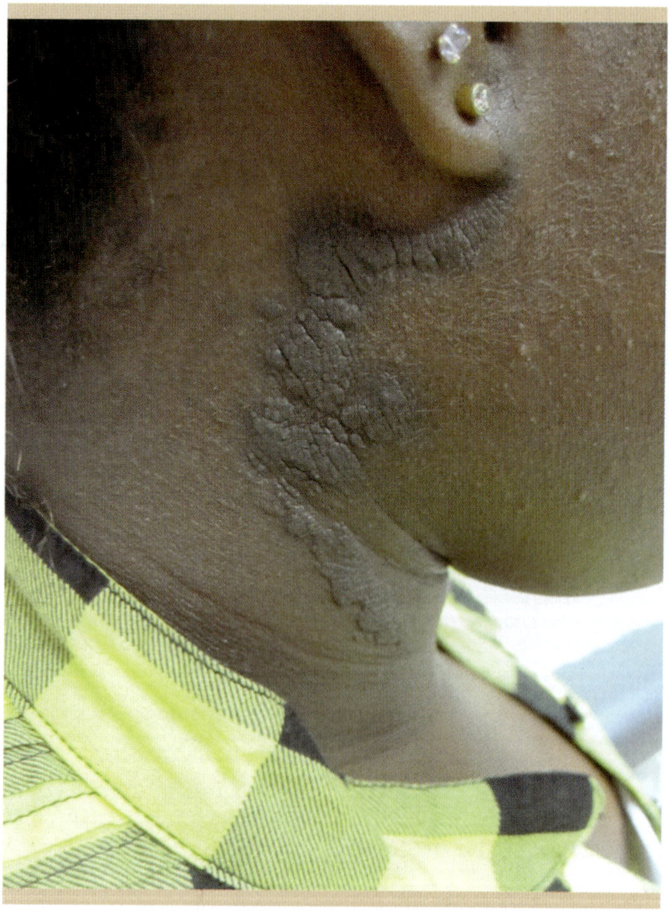

FIGURE 15-25 Linear epidermal nevus. (*Used with permission from Dr. Agim.*)

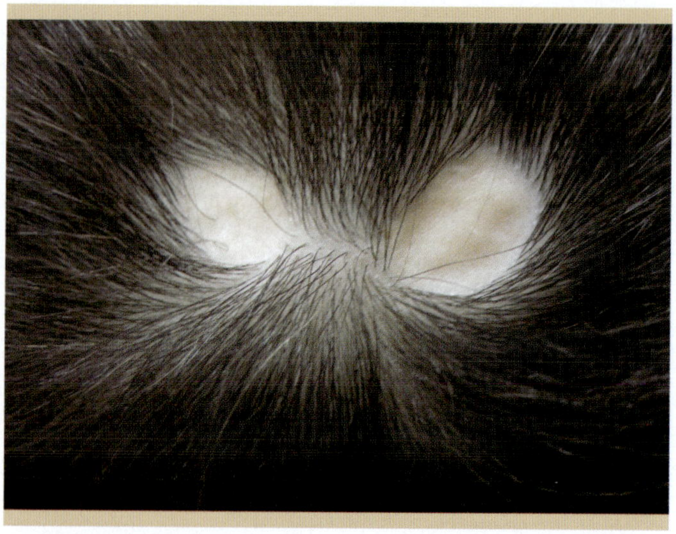

FIGURE 15-26 Aplasia cutis congenita. (*Used with permission from Dr. Agim.*)

- Course/therapy
  - Destruction by excision, laser ablation, cryotherapy, dermabrasion, chemical peels, topical retinoids
  - Recurrence is common
  - Pruritus with ILVEN often refractory to treatment

Aplasia Cutis Congenita (Fig. 15-26)

- Presentation
  - Well-demarcated ulceration or erosion often with thin, glistening membrane-like surface
  - Present at birth
  - Most commonly on vertex
  - Seventy percent solitary
  - Rare association with other developmental abnormalities
    - Irregular, large, stellate defects of the scalp associated with trisomy 13 and underlying cerebrovascular malformations
    - Large, bilateral, truncal stellate defects associated with fetus papyraceus (placental infarction after the death of a twin fetus) and gastrointestinal atresia
- Etiology/pathology
  - Sporadic or autosomal dominant inheritance with variable penetrance
  - Localized absence of the epidermis, dermis ± subcutis
- Course/therapy
  - Protection form trauma and infection
  - Most heal within several months, leaving scar
  - MRI/MRA and radiographs for large scalp defects; abdominal imaging for large truncal defects

MASTOCYTOSIS

Solitary Mastocytoma (Fig. 15-27)

- Presentation
  - One to several yellowish to brown nodule(s)
  - Presents within first 6 months of life
  - Often on trunk, upper extremities, neck
  - Darier sign: when stroked, lesion urticates
  - May develop bullae in infancy
  - Spontaneous regression over several years
  - Treatment: topical anti-inflammatories can be used for symptoms; otherwise, treatment is unnecessary

Urticaria Pigmentosa (Fig. 15-28)

- Presentation
  - Most common form of mastocytosis
  - Develops between 3 and 9 months of life
  - Persistent, pruritic red-brown-yellow macules, papules, or nodules
  - Lesions most common on the trunk
  - Positive Darier sign

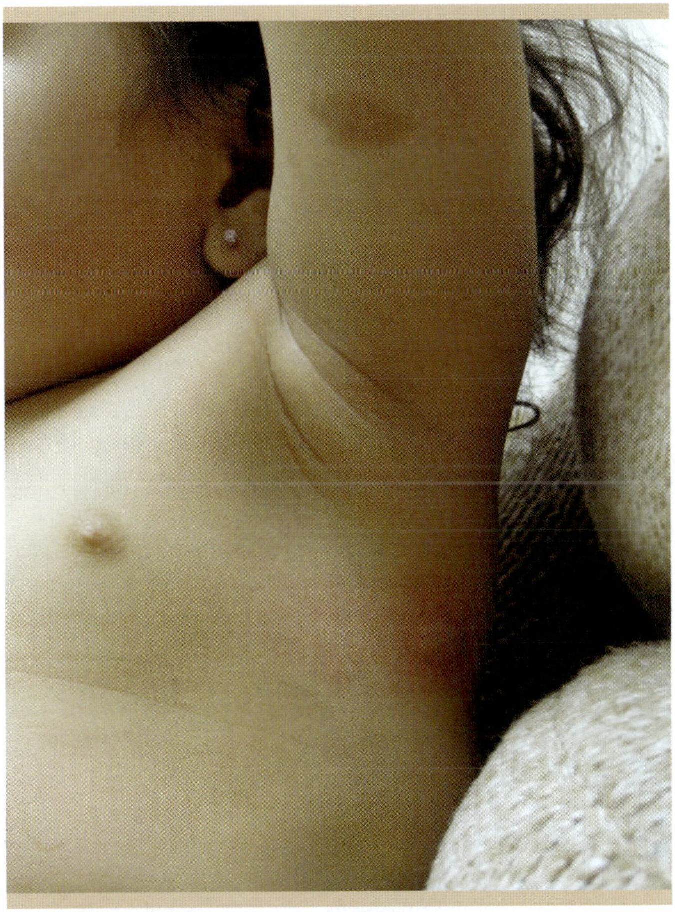

FIGURE 15-27 Cutaneous mastocytomas. (*Used with permission from Dr. Agim.*)

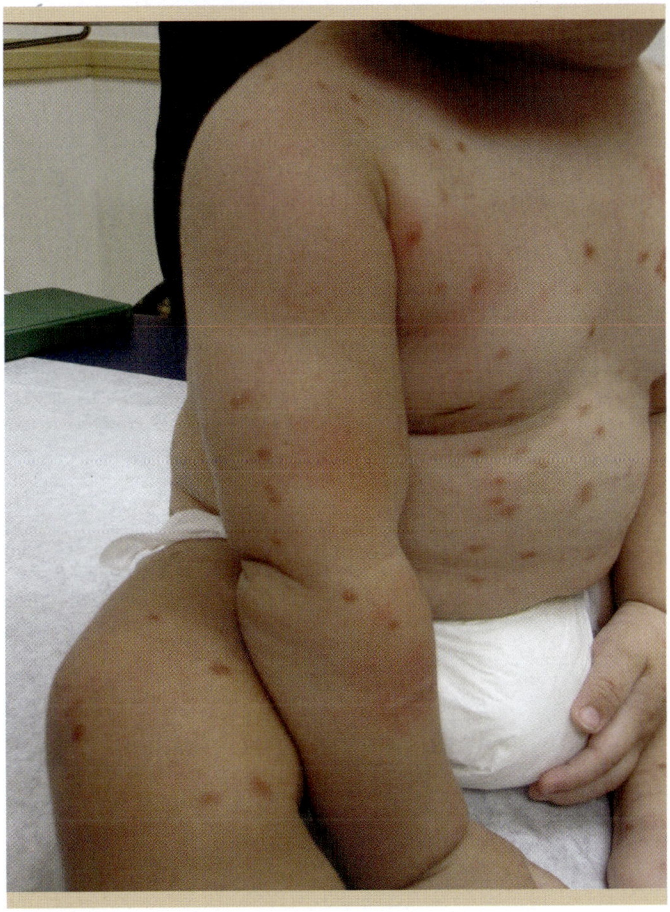

FIGURE 15-28 Urticaria pigmentosa. (*Used with permission from Dr. Agim.*)

  - Pruritus induced by rubbing, exercise, heat, mast-cell degranulators (EtOH, opiates)
- Etiology: *Hymenoptera* stings or histamine-releasing drugs may rarely cause severe symptoms, anaphylaxis
- Treatment
  - H_1 antagonists for pruritus, urticaria, flushing
  - H_2 antagonists for GI symptoms
  - Diarrhea may be controlled with cromolyn (disodium chromoglycate)
  - Calcium channel blockers may inhibit mast cell degranulation
  - Epi-Pen for patients with a history of anaphylaxis
  - Seventy percent of patients markedly improve by adolescence

Diffuse Cutaneous Mastocytosis (Fig. 15-29)

- Presentation
  - Rare
  - Presents at birth or within first few weeks of life
  - Skin diffusely infiltrated with mast cells
  - Leathery, orange-peel appearance (*peau d'orange*), especially in flexures

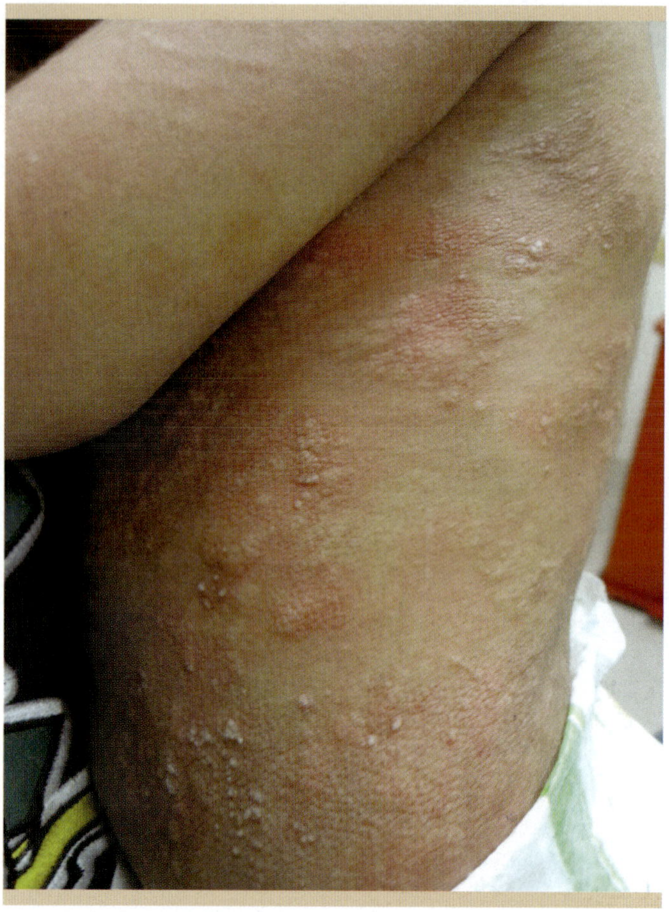

FIGURE 15-29 Diffuse cutaneous mastocytosis. (*Used with permission from Dr. Agim.*)

    - Widespread spontaneous blistering with erosions and crusts, erythroderma, pruritus
- Etiology: systemic involvement in up to 10% of children (greater in adults)

Systemic Mastocytosis

- Presentation
    - Rare mast cell accumulation in one or more organs other than the skin, especially bone marrow
    - The presence of systemic symptoms does not make the diagnosis of systemic mastocytosis
    - Invasive diagnostic procedures for
        - Patients with hematologic abnormalities
        - Persistent, localized bone pain and severe GI symptoms
        - Evidence of hepatic insufficiency
- Signs and symptoms
    - Flushing
    - Osteoporosis or sclerosis
    - Lymph node involvement
    - Hepatomegaly, splenomegaly, may have increased bleeding with heparin
    - Pancytopenia
    - Heart, kidneys, GI tract, or lung may be affected
    - Mast cell leukemia (rare) portends poor prognosis
    - Other leukemias or lymphomas may develop
- Diagnosis (of cutaneous mastocytosis)/etiology
    - Histology
        - Accumulation of mast cells in skin
        - Dense dermal aggregate of mast cells
        - Mast cells stains: Leder, toluidine blue, Giemsa
    - Mutation of c-*kit* protooncogene receptor that codes for transmembrane tyrosine kinase (also in piebaldism)
    - Serum tryptase: useful screening test for systemic mastocytosis

QUIZ

Questions

1. A 15-month-old boy with extensive dermal melanocytosis, bilateral nevi of Ota, and patchy capillary malformations (port-wine stains) should be considered to have what syndrome?

    A. Nevus unius lateralis
    B. Bilateral nevus of Ota-like macules
    C. Phakomatosis pigmentovascularis (cesioflammea)
    D. Hypermelanosis of Ito
    E. Lysosomal storage disease

2. All of the following diagnoses may present with a blueberry muffin baby, EXCEPT:

    A. Bednar tumor
    B. Hereditary spherocytosis
    C. Parvovirus B19
    D. Alveolar rhabdomyosarcoma
    E. Neuroblastoma

3. Recalcitrant innumerable molluscum and verrucae vulgaris lesions may be present in a patient in which of the following underlying diagnoses?

    A. WHIM syndrome
    B. Hypohidrotic ectodermal dysplasia with immunodeficiency
    C. Leukocyte adhesion deficiency
    D. Hyper IgD with periodic disease
    E. Naegeli-Franschetti-Jadassohn syndrome

4. The coexistence of 2 nevi such as nevus anemicus and nevus flammeus is thought to arise from the mosaic phenomenon termed:

    A. Koebnerization
    B. Post-translational methylation
    C. Chromosomal inversion
    D. Didymosis
    E. Darier sign

5. Which one of the following conditions predisposes to crusted (Norwegian) scabies?
   A. Excessive bathing
   B. Trisomy 21
   C. Exposure to pesticides
   D. Hypoglycemia
   E. Inadequate vaccination

6. This acquired blistering disorder shares the same immunologic target as that cleaved by bacterial toxins in staphylococcal scaled skin syndrome:
   A. Pemphigus vulgaris
   B. Brunsting Perry
   C. Ocular cicatricial pemphigoid
   D. Pemphigus gestationis
   E. Pemphigus foliaceus

7. The most common secondary growth seen in a nevus sebaceus is:
   A. Trichoadenoma
   B. Trichofolliculoma
   C. Trichoblastoma
   D. Fibrofolliculoma
   E. Fibroepithelioma of Pinkus

8. A 2-year-old, otherwise healthy female toddler presents with multiple scaly papules with hyperpigmented macules and collarettes of scale predominantly on the palms and soles. Treatment for scabies was ineffective. An alternative diagnosis to consider would be:
   A. Transient neonatal pustular melanosis
   B. Erythema toxicum neonatorum
   C. Acropustulosis of infancy
   D. Pustular psoriasis
   E. Dyshidrotic eczema

9. A teenaged girl returns following excision of an epidermal nevus. The pathology report indicates the presence of hyperkeratosis, papillomatosis, and vacuolization of the upper epidermis with granular degeneration. Appropriate counseling includes:
   A. Advise that this may predispose her to linear morphea
   B. Recommend adjuvant resurfacing laser treatment to prevent recurrence
   C. Review necessity for avid sun protection to avoid development of skin cancer
   D. Refer for genetic counseling due to risk of having an infant with epidermolytic hyperkeratosis
   E. Schedule vaccination against human papillomavirus (HPV)

10. In addition to causing eczema herpeticum, HSV1 may trigger erythema multiforme in susceptible individuals. Which of the following HLA types has a reported increased incidence of this phenomenon?
    A. HLA Cw6
    B. HLA DQB1*0301
    C. HLA B*5801
    D. HLA B*1502
    E. HLA B27

Answers

1. C. The constellation of extensive dermal melanocytosis in conjunction with capillary malformations (nevus flammeus) and nevus of Ota +/– nevus anemicus is seen in phakomatosis pigmentovascularis, type II. Lysosomal storage diseases may have the dermal melanocytosis without the other described features. Nevus unius lateralis is synonymous with extensive epidermal nevus. ANOLM are seen in Asian adult women and hypermelanosis of Ito does not have a vascular component.
2. A. Bednar tumors or pigmented dermatofibrosarcoma protuberans are rarely congential and usually solitary. The blueberry muffin baby presentation may occur in association with infectious (TORCH, parvovirus), neoplastic (neuroblastoma, leukemia, rhabdomyosarcoma) or other hematologic associations (spherocytosis, Blood/Rh incompatibility, myelodysplasia).
3. A. WHIM (*W*arts, *H*ypogammaglobulinemia, *I*nfection, *M*yelokathexis) syndrome is an immunodeficiency caused by mutations in *CXCR4* which may feature extensive cutaneous viral eruptions. Leukocyte adhesion deficiency features pyoderma and slow wound healing; HED ID is associated with NEMO mutation, HIDS is a periodic fever syndrome related to mevalonate kinase, and Naegeli Franschetti Jadassohn is a reticulated pigmentary disorder caused by mutations in keratin 14. None of them have this finding as a prominent symptom. Immunodeficiency should be considered in patients with overwhelming cutaneous viral infections.
4. D. Didymosis or twin spotting describes overlapping nevi of apparently differing origin. Café au lait macules and nevus depigmentosus may occur in similar fashion. Koebnerization refers to development of lesions in areas of trauma as seen in psoriasis and vitiligo. Darier sign is a diagnostic clue to mastocytosis while chromosomal inversion and post-translational methylation are genetic events that may underlie a wide variety of conditions.
5. B. Crusted (Norwegian) scabies involves massive sarcoptes mite infestation with psoriasiform to verrucous changes in skin. Predisposing factors include HIV infection, immunodeficiency due to transplant status, diabetes, trisomy 21, senility, and lepromatous leprosy. The other listed choices do not increase susceptibility.

6. E. Pemphigus vulgaris is associated with anti-desmoglein 3 antibodies. Brunsting Perry is blistering disorder of the head and neck which may involve BP 180, collagen VII, or laminin 332. Pemphigus gestationis may involve C3 deposition against BP 180 or BP 230 and ocular cicatricial pemphigoid antibodies attack α-6 β-4 integrin or laminin 332. Pemphigus foliaceus is the only one reproducibly targeting desmoglein 1.
7. C. Nevus sebaceus has been associated with a wide variety of neoplasms from trichoblastomas to basal cell or sebaceous carcinoma. Of the listed entities, trichoblastoma is most relevant and the most frequently described benign neoplasm associated with NS.
8. C. Acropustulosis of infancy is a benign relapsing and remitting palmoplantar or acral vesiculopustular eruption seen in children. It is often mistaken for scabies and some post-scabies cases have been reported. Most cases are self-limited though some may require treatment.
9. D. Epidermal nevi are considered mosaic lesions which may feature lesional mutations differing from unaffected skin. The presence of epidermolytic hyperkeratosis-like changes on the biopsy raises concern for a future fetus if she carries a germline mutation in keratins 1 or 10.
10. B. HLA- DQB1*0301 has been associated specifically with recurrent HSAV-associated erythema multiforme. B*1502 and B*5801 have been implicated in drug eruptions due to carbamazepine and allopurinol respectively. Cw6 confers increased susceptibility to early onset psoriasis while Reiter syndrome and ankylosing spondylitis may feature HLA B27

REFERENCES

Eichenfield L, Esterly N, Frieden, eds. *Textbook of Neonatal Dermatology*. Philadelphia: Saunders; 2001.

Fleet SL, Davis LS: Infantile perianal pyramidal protrusion: report of a case and review of the literature. *Pediatr Dermatol* Mar-Apr 2005;22(2):151-152.

Goldsmith LA et al. *Fitzpatrick's Dermatology in General Medicine*, 8th Ed. New York: McGraw-Hill; 2012.

Heide R, Tank B, Oranje AP: Mastocytosis in childhood. *Pediatr Dermatol* Sep-Oct 2002;19(5):375-381.

Kane KS, Lio PA, Stratigos AJ, Johnson RA: *Color Atlas & Synopsis of Pediatric Dermatology*, 2nd Ed. New York: McGraw-Hill; 2009.

McKee PH: *Pathology of the Skin: With Clinical Correlations*. London: Mosby-Wolfe; 1996.

Verbov J: *Essential Pediatric Dermatology*. Cliften, UK: Clinical Press; 1988.

Weinberg S, Prose NS, Kristal L: *Color Atlas of Pediatric Dermatology*, 3rd Ed. New York: McGraw-Hill; 1998.

CHAPTER 16

CUTANEOUS INFESTATIONS

DIRK M. ELSTON
ASRA ALI
MELISSA A. BOGLE
ALYN D. HATTER

PARASITE

- An organism that lives on or within another organism (host)
- A parasite causes harm to the host. This distinguishes parasitism from commensalism, in which the host derives no benefit but is not injured, and mutualism, where the relationship benefits both organisms
- Host, in addition to providing a steady food source, provides warmth and shelter
- Definitive host are those in which parasite becomes sexually mature and undergoes reproduction
- Reservoir hosts are those in which parasites that are pathogenic to other animals or to humans reside
- Vector are agent by which a parasite is transmitted to the host (e.g., arthropod, mollusk)

ARTHROPODA

- Bites usually result in localized, cutaneous reactions and pruritus
- Some of these organisms are medically important: fleas, lice, and ticks can transmit lethal epidemic disorders
- Many of these vector-transmitted diseases are endemic in various regions of the world
- Four classes of arthropods are of dermatologic interest and are covered in this chapter:
  - Chilopoda: including centipedes
  - Diplopoda: including millipedes
  - Insecta: including caterpillars, moths, bedbugs, lice, flies, mosquitoes, beetles, bees, wasps, hornets, fire ants, and fleas
  - Arachnida: including ticks, mites, scorpions, and spiders
- Organisms from the arthropod classes Arachnida and Insecta have a hard-jointed exoskeleton and paired, jointed legs
- Class Insecta: a group of organisms with 6 legs and 3 body segments: head, thorax, and abdomen. Includes the following orders:
  - Siphonaptera: fleas
  - Anoplura: head and body lice
  - Pthiridae: crab louse
  - Diptera: 2-winged flies, mosquitos, midges
  - Hemiptera: true bugs
  - Lepidoptera: butterflies, moths, and their caterpillars
  - Hymenoptera: ants, wasps, and bees
- Class Arachnida: a group of organisms with 8 legs and 2 body segments: cephalothorax and abdomen
  - *Ixodidae:* hard ticks
  - *Argasidae:* soft ticks
  - *Araneae:* spiders
- Centipedes and millipedes

INSECTA

Siphonaptera (Fleas)

- Wingless, laterally compressed insects with a hard, shiny integument
- The body has 3 regions: head, thorax, and abdomen
- Mouthparts are modified (paired maxillary palpi) for piercing and sucking
- Survive months without feeding
- Order *Siphonaptera* contains 2 flea families of medical importance
  - *Pulicidae:* (human, cat, dog, and bird fleas)
  - *Sarcopsylidae* (also called *Tungidae*): the sand flea
- Fleas jump, on average, about 20 cm

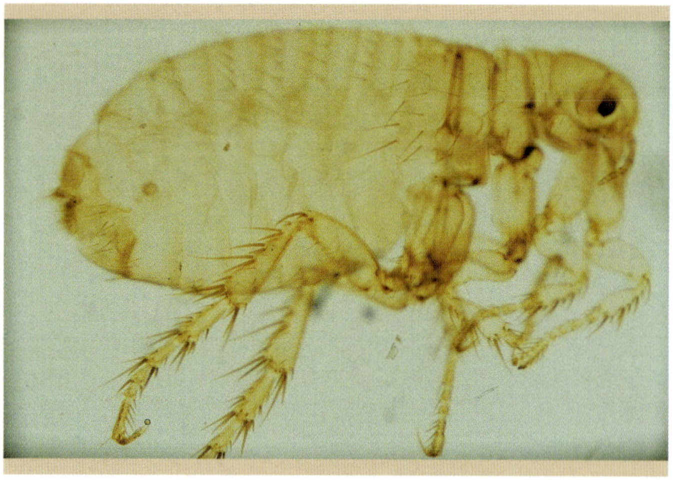

FIGURE 16-1 *Pulex irritans* (human flea).

- One flea can bite 2 to 3 times over a small area
  - Bites produce irregular, pruritic, red wheals up to 1 cm in diameter
- Patients may present with a surrounding halo with a central papule, vesicle, or bulla or with hemorrhagic macules, papules, vesicles, or bullae

1. *Pulex irritans* (human flea) (Fig. 16-1)
   - Farms, urban areas, predominant flea on dogs in portions of the Carolinas
2. *Tunga penetrans* (chigoe flea)
   - Tropical and subtropical regions of North and South America, Africa
   - Intense itching and local inflammation
   - Causes tungiasis
     - Female sand flea, which burrows into human skin at the point of contact, usually the feet
     - Head is down into the upper dermis feeding from blood vessels
     - Caudal tip of the abdomen is at the skin surface
     - Nodule (usually on the foot) that slowly enlarges over a few weeks
   - Treatment
     - Occlusive petrolatum suffocates the organism
     - Lindane, dimethyl phthalate, or dimethyl carbamate
3. *Xenopsylla cheopis* (Oriental rat flea)
   - Plague (*Yersinia pestis*)
   - Endemic (murine) typhus (*Rickettsia typhi*)
4. Cat flea (*Ctenocephalides felis*)
   - Endemic (murine) typhus (*Rickettsia felis*)

Anoplura

Pediculidae

- After attaching to the skin, these flattened, wingless insects feed on human blood and can cause intense itching
- They will die of starvation if kept off the body for more than 10 days
- They are also killed by washing in water at 53.5°C for 5 minutes
- Life span of a louse is about 30 to 45 days

1. *Pediculus humanus corporis* (body louse)
   - Up to 5 mm long
   - Vector for
     - Epidemic typhus (*Rickettsia prowazekii*)
     - Trench fever, bacillary angiomatosis, bacillary peliosis (*Bartonella quintana*)
     - Relapsing fever (*Borrelia recurrentis, Borrelia duttoni*)
   - Crowded, unsanitary conditions
   - Lives in clothing and moves to body to feed
   - Pyoderma involving areas covered by clothing, most notably the trunk, axillae, and groin; erythematous macules, papules, and wheals, as well as excoriations, also may be seen
   - Treatment: malathion 1% powder, permethrin spray
2. *Pediculus humanus capitus* (head louse) (Fig. 16-2)
   - Whitish in color and up to 3 mm long
   - Confined to the scalp
   - Lice and their eggs can withstand vigorous washing and combing
   - Nits: cementing of white eggs to the hair; usually found in the warm areas of the scalp such as behind the ears and on the posterior neck
   - Eggs hatch in approximately 7 to 9 days
   - Treatment: requires that both the adult lice and the nits be killed
   - Two treatments 1 week apart are recommended because nits hatch in 7 days

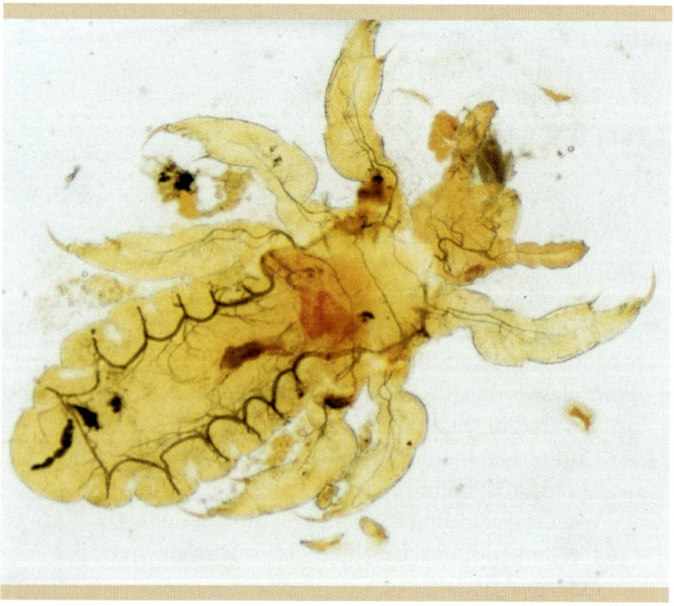

FIGURE 16-2 *Pediculus humanus capitus* (head louse).

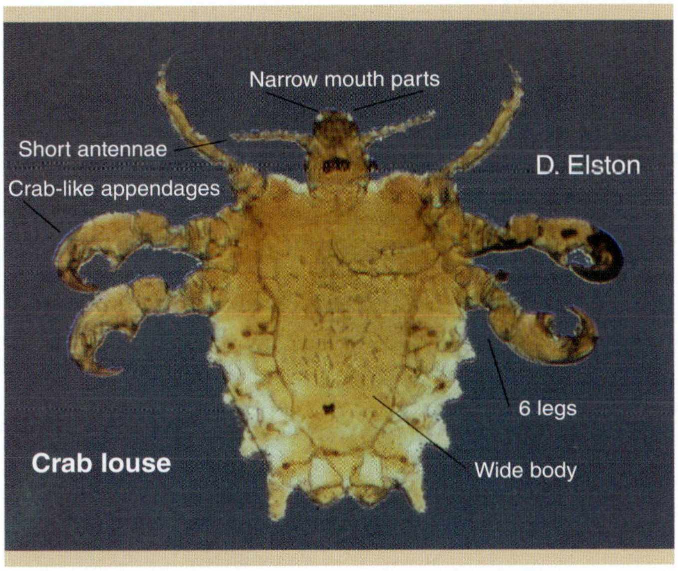

FIGURE 16-3 *Pthirus pubis* (pubic or crab louse). (*Used with permission from Dr. Dirk M. Elston.*)

- Occlusive agents that kill via asphyxiation
- Malathion lotion
- Natural pyrethrin products and synthetic pyrethroids
- Lindane, γ-benzene hexachloride
- Nits are best removed with a comb after soaking the hair in a vinegar or formic acid solution to flatten the cuticle and facilitate combing

Pthiridae

- *Pthirus pubis* (Fig. 16-3)
  - Pubic louse, crab louse
  - Short, broad body with rather stout claws on the middle and hind legs
  - Reddish brown in color
  - Often sexually transmitted
  - Rarely involves facial (eyelashes), chest, or axillary hair
  - Patients can remain asymptomatic for up to a month before pruritus develops; nits, similar to those in pediculosis capitis, are seen
  - Blue macules (maculae ceruleae) are often seen on the surrounding skin and are believed to be produced by louse saliva acting on blood products
  - Treatment: lotions or shampoos containing 1% lindane, 0.3% pyrethrins, or 5% permethrin, asphyxiating agents
  - Infestation of the eyelashes: petrolatum or fluoroscein

Diptera

- Two-winged, biting insects
- All require a blood meal at some time in their development
- Bites can manifest as immediate urticarial papules, delayed erythematous papules, or both

Flies

- Number of infectious diseases can be transmitted by biting flies
- A variety of flies commonly bite humans
- Common housefly does not bite but rather feeds on the surface of the skin
- Wound myiasis: eggs are deposited on an open wound
- Furuncular myiasis: solitary furuncle-like lesions often transferred by a mosquito vector
- Plaque myiasis: grouped boil-like lesions caused by eggs laid on wet laundry

Dermatobia Hominis (*Botfly*)

- Most common cause of furuncular myiasis
- Occurs when fly larvae (maggots) invade tissue
- Raised, erythematous papule develops at the site of the bite, most frequently on the distal extremity or scalp
- Enlarges to become an indurated nodule with a central punctum, which is the breathing hole for the larva
- Treatment
  - Surgical excision; occlussion

Sand Flies (Phlebotomus and Lutzomyia)

- Vectors for bartonellosis (*Bartonella bacilliformis*—Oroya fever, Carrion disease) and leishmaniasis
- Leishmaniasis
- *Leishmania:* protozoan infection
- *Leishmania* transform to the *promastigote* (or flagellate) form in the gut of the vector
  - Promastigote is a slender organism with a flagellum
  - After replicating, the promastigotes migrate to the sand fly's proboscis, from which they are regurgitated into the next host as the sand fly feeds
- Located within reticuloendothelial cells of infected tissues, *Leishmania* exist in an amastigote (nonflagellate) form
- Vector: sand fly (*Phlebotomus* and *Lutzomyia* species)
- Clinical
  - Cutaneous
    - Nontender, firm, red papule at bite
    - Lesion widens with central ulceration, serous crusting, and granulomas
    - Lesions may be wet or dry and become fibrotic or hyperkeratotic with healing
  - Mucocutaneous
    - Excessive tissue obstructing the nares, septal granulation, and perforation
    - Gingivitis, periodontitis, and localized lymphadenopathy
- Visceral (kala-azar/black fever)
  - Systemic infection of the liver, spleen, and bone marrow
  - *Leishmania donovani* and *Leishmania infantum*
  - Recurrent high fevers, wasting, anorexia, night sweats, diarrhea, and malaise

- Leishmaniasis recidivans
  - Occur years after a localized cutaneous lesion has healed
  - New ulcers and papules form over the edge of the old scar
- After kala-azar
  - Multiple, hypopigmented, erythematous macules
- Old World
  - *Leishmania tropica* and *Leishmania major*
  - Southwest Asia, Indian subcontinent, Mediterranean, East Africa, and republics of the former Soviet Union
  - Visceral leishmaniasis
  - Diffuse cutaneous leishmaniasis
    - *Leishmania aethiopica*
- New World
  - Throughout the Americas
  - Visceral disease
    - *Leishmania chagasi*
  - Cutaneous lesions
    - *Leishmania mexicana*
    - Solitary nodule
  - Mucocutaneous disease (espundia)
    - *Leishmania braziliensis*
    - Leishmaniasis recidivans
    - *Leishmania viannia braziliensis*
  - Diffuse cutaneous leishmaniasis
    - *Leishmania mexicana*
    - *Leishmania amazonensis*
  - Post–kala-azar leishmaniasis
    - *Leishmania donovani chagasi*
- Diagnosis
  - Culture
  - Direct agglutination test, immunofluorescence assay, or enzyme-linked immunosorbent assay (ELISA)
  - Montenegro skin test: determines delayed-type hypersensitivity reactions
- Treatment
  - Pentavalent antimony, administered intravenously or intramuscularly
  - Amphotericin B and pentamidine

Tsetse Fly (Glossina), Glossinidae Family

- Vector for African trypanosomiasis (sleeping sickness)
- Trypanosomes are ingested during a blood meal by the tsetse fly from a human reservoir, develop into epimastigotes, and are reinfected into human hosts
- Extensive antigenic variation of parasite surface glycoproteins
- West African (*Trypanosoma brucei gambiense*)
  - Slow progression
- East African (*Trypanosoma brucei rhodesiense*)
  - Rapid progression (within a week)
- Stage 1
  - Chancre
  - Hypersensitivity reaction: urticaria, pruritus, facial edema, fever, arthralgias, Winterbottom sign (posterior cervical lymphadenopathy)
  - Kerandel sign: delayed sensation to pain or a sensation of hyperesthesia
- Stage 2: central nervous system (CNS) changes
  - Headaches, behavioral changes, seizures in children
- Laboratory studies
  - Anemia, hypergammaglobulinemia, elevated erythrocyte sedimentation rate (ESR), thrombocytopenia, and hypoalbuminemia
  - Wet smear of unstained blood, bone marrow, spinal fluid, skin lesions: parasite is visualized
  - Card agglutination test for trypanosomiasis (CATT)
- Treatment
  - Early stages: suramin, pentamidine
  - CNS stage: intravenous melarsoprol B, eflornithine

Chrysops (Deer Fly)

- Vector for loaisis (see below)

Mosquitoes

- Belong to the family Culicidae
- Delicate winged insects with long proboscises and long, thin legs
- Require water to mature through the larval and pupal stages
- Can be the vector for filariasis, yellow fever, dengue fever, encephalitis, and malaria
- Cutaneous reactions to bites include urticarial wheals, delayed papules, bullous lesions, hemorrhagic necrotic lesions, excoriations, eczematous patches, and granulomatous nodules

Culex

- Vector for
  - Japanese encephalitis
  - Murray Valley encephalitis virus
  - Rift Valley fever
  - Ross River virus
  - *Sindbis* virus
  - St. Louis encephalitis (*Flaviviridae*)
  - West Nile fever: arthropathy, muscle weakness, rash
  - Filariasis *(Wuchereria bancrofti)*
  - Dirofilariasis: *Dirofilaria immitus* (dog heartworm), *Dirofilaria tenuis* (raccoons), *Dirofilaria repens* (dogs), *Dirofilaria ursi* (bears)

Anopheles

- Vector for malaria (*Plasmodium falciparum, Plasmodium malariae, Plasmodium vivax, Plasmodium ovale*)

Aedes Aegypti

- Yellow fever (*Flaviviridae*)
- Dengue

Beetles

- Blister beetles cause cutaneous injury when a potent vesicating agent, cantharidin, is released from their bodies and contacts human skin
- *Lytta vesicatoria*, also known as "Spanish fly," is the source of cantharidin
- Two species, *Epicauta vittata* (striped blister beetle) and *Epicauta pennsylvanica* (black blister beetle), are widely distributed in the United States, although more than 100 other species occur in various parts of the United States
- Blisters develop within a day and then dry up and desquamate in about a week
- Treatment: affected skin should be washed immediately with alcohol or acetone to dissolve or dilute the cantharidin

Hemiptera (True Bugs)

Cimex Lectularius (Bedbug) (Fig. 16-4)

- Feeds nocturnally on human blood
- It is 8 mm long, reddish brown, and wingless, with a greatly flattened body
- Linear arrangement of large wheals, often greater than 1 cm, which are accompanied by itching and inflammation
- Bullous eruptions can occur
- Transmission of trypasosomiasis and possibly hepatitis

Reduviid Bug (Kissing Bug, Assassin Bug)

- Vector for Chagas disease (American trypanosomiasis) caused by *Trypanosoma cruzi*
- It is 15 mm long, dark brown in color
- *Reduviid* bug ingests the trypomastigote while feeding on infected animals; it then divides and transforms in the gut of the bug into metacyclic trypomastigotes

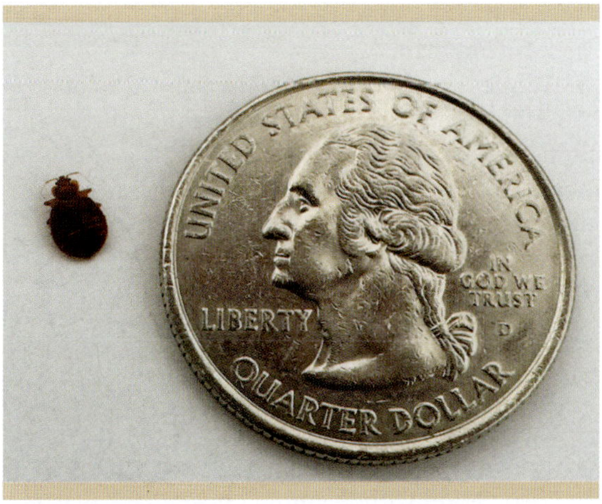

FIGURE 16-4 *Cimex lectularius* (bedbugs). (*Used with permission from Dr. Alyn D. Hatter.*)

- Bug ventures out at night to feed on exposed skin; deposit stool when biting; 80% enter through conjunctiva
- Transform into amastigotes after ingestion by macrophages; *T. cruzi* burst from the macrophages as trypomastigotes and disseminate widely to invade most human tissues
- Lymphatic spread then carries the organism to regional lymph nodes
- Chagoma: red nodule at site of bite; lasts only a few days to a couple of weeks
- Ramaña sign: bite near the eye causes unilateral periorbital conjunctivitis and edema
- Hematogenous dissemination: acute phase with fever to 104°F, vomiting, diarrhea, cough, hepatosplenomegaly, edema, myocarditis, seizures, and meningoencephalitis
- Latent phase: myocardial heart disease, with fibrosis, conduction defects
- Cardiac involvement: congestive heart failure
- Gastrointestinal (GI) system affected: dysphagia and abdominal pain, constipation secondary to megacolon (owing to destruction of the parasympathetic ganglion)
- Sequelae of myocardial damage, megacolon, megaesophagus
- Diagnosis: parasites are relatively numerous initially and easily demonstrable on peripheral blood smear
- Treatment: benzimidazole, nifurtimax

Lepidoptera (Caterpillars)

1. *Automeris io* (family Saturniidae)
   - Io moth
   - East of the Rocky Mountains from Canada to Mexico
   - Feed on deciduous (broadleaf) trees and herbaceous plants
   - Yellow-green with red and white lateral stripes
   - Urticating spines
2. *Megalopyge opercularis* (puss caterpillar, asp caterpillar) (Fig. 16-5)
   - Broad and flat
   - Dense covering of long, silky, gray to reddish brown hairs
   - Urticating spines dispersed among the hairs
3. *Sibine stimulea* (saddleback caterpillar)
   - Brown at both ends
   - Green around the middle "saddle blanket"
   - Purple-brown oval-spot "saddle"
   - Urticating spines along the sides and at the front and rear of the body
4. Hagmoth: brown with 9 pairs of variable-length lateral processes with urticating hairs
5. Buck moth
   - Purple-black with a reddish head
   - Pale-yellow dots scattered over the body with reddish to black branches
   - Stinging spines arising from tubercles

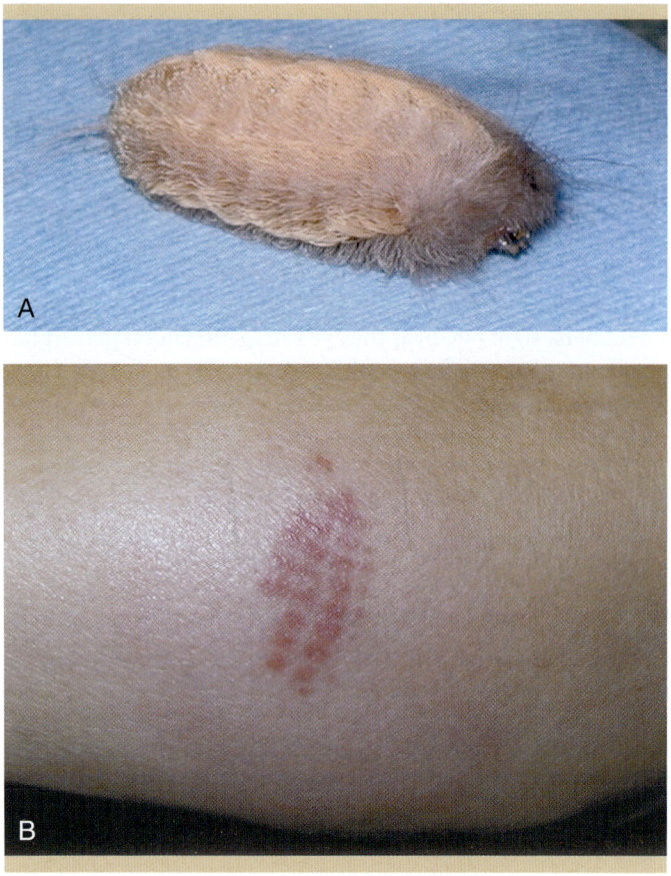

FIGURE 16-5 A: *Megalopyge opercularis* (puss caterpillar, asp caterpillar). B: Cutaneous reaction from contact with puss caterpillar. (*Reprinted from Goldsmith LA et al.* Fitzpatrick's Dermatology in General Medicine, *8th Ed. New York: McGraw-Hill; 2012, p. 2609.*)

Hymenoptera

- Known for producing a painful sting that rarely may result in anaphylaxis and death
- Reactions produced by *Hymenoptera* stings
- Local: erythema, edema, and pain at the site of the sting
- Wells syndrome, consisting of erythematous, edematous plaques composed histologically of eosinophilic granulomatous dermatitis
- Systemic toxic venom
- From multiple stings
- Constitutional symptoms
- Systemic allergic
- Immunoglobulin (Ig) E antibodies cause degranulation and the release of vasoactive substances: urticaria and angioedema
- Others: serum sickness, acute renal failure, possible Guillain-Barré syndrome

Suborder: Apocrita—Ants, Wasps, and Bees

1. Formicidae: ants
    - *Solenopsis* (fire ant)
        - Alkaloid venom contains phospholipase and hyalurinidase
        - May be red or black and live in ground colonies
        - Sting by first biting the victim with their powerful set of pincer jaws and then swiveling and stinging in a circular pattern
        - Pustules, burning itch
2. *Vespidae:* yellowjackets, hornets, paper wasps
    - Paper wasps build hives under the eaves of buildings
    - Yellow jackets are ground-nesting
    - Hornets reside in shrubs and trees
3. *Apoidea* family
    - Bumblebees and honeybees
    - Honeybees feed on flowering plants
    - Stinger contains a barb, causing it to be left on the victim along with the venom sac
    - This act eviscerates and kills the bee

ARACHNIDA

- Adult forms have 4 pairs of legs, 6-legged larvae common among ticks and mites; may cause human injury by biting, burrowing in, and feeding on skin, stinging, and delivering toxic venom
- Ticks
    - Tick-bite alopecia
        - Patchy alopecia at the site of tick attachment
        - Hair loss begins about 1 week after the tick is removed
    - Tick paralysis
        - *Dermacentor* ticks in North America
        - *Ixodes* ticks in Australia
        - Ascending flaccid paralysis
        - Symptoms usually disappear rapidly if the tick is found and removed
    - Tick-bite pyrexia
        - While the tick feeds, the host may develop fever, chills, headache, abdominal pain, and vomiting
- Natural parasites of many different animals, including mammals, birds, reptiles, and amphibians
- Vectors for numerous infectious diseases
- Two families of ticks:
    - Hard ticks (*Ixodidae*)
        - Hard chitinous dorsal shield
        - Can endure cold, humid weather
    - Soft ticks (*Argasidae*)
        - Lack a dorsal shield
        - Prefer drier environments where they live in close association with an animal host
- Most ticks fast for long periods because they cannot live on vegetable matter; blood meal is acquired mostly by chance

- Feeding is usually complete within 6 to 7 days, but the tick can remain attached to the host for an unspecified period
- Ticks require a blood meal before they can lay eggs
- Body of mites and ticks
  - Divided into 2 regions
    - Anterior: cephalothorax (or prosoma)
    - Posterior: abdomen (or opisthosoma)

Mites

Cheyletiella

- "Walking dandruff": caused by movement of mite under scales
- Live on keratin layer of small mammals (dogs, cats, rabbits)
- Pruritic dermatitis in humans who handle pets

Liponyssoides (Formerly Allodermanyssus) sanguineus

- House mouse mite
- Rickettsial pox (*Rickettsia akari*)

Ornithonyssus sylviarum

- Found in birds and domestic fowl
- Bird handlers are bitten most commonly

Dermanyssus gallinae and Ornithonyssus bursa

- Can infest domestic poultry

Dermatophagoides (Family Pyroglyphidae)

- House dust mite
- Tiny, translucent mites, generally less than 0.2 mm long
- Cause severe asthma and other allergic complaints in humans
- Humidity levels below 60% appear to support fewer mites

Family Demodicidae

Demodex Folliculorum (Fig. 16-6)

- Elongate, microscopic mites
- Live in hair follicles and sebaceous glands
- Generally asymptomatic
- May cause folliculitis
- Associated with rosacea

Harvest Mites (Family Trombidiidae)

Trombiculidae (Chigger, "Red Mite")

- Only the 6-legged larval form parasitizes other animals
- Attach to a host, feed for 2 to 3 days, molt to the nymphal stage, and then leave the host
- Skin lesions develop 3 to 24 hours later when an allergic reaction to mite saliva develops
- Pruritic red papules grouped about the waist, thighs, and legs
- Can persist for several weeks

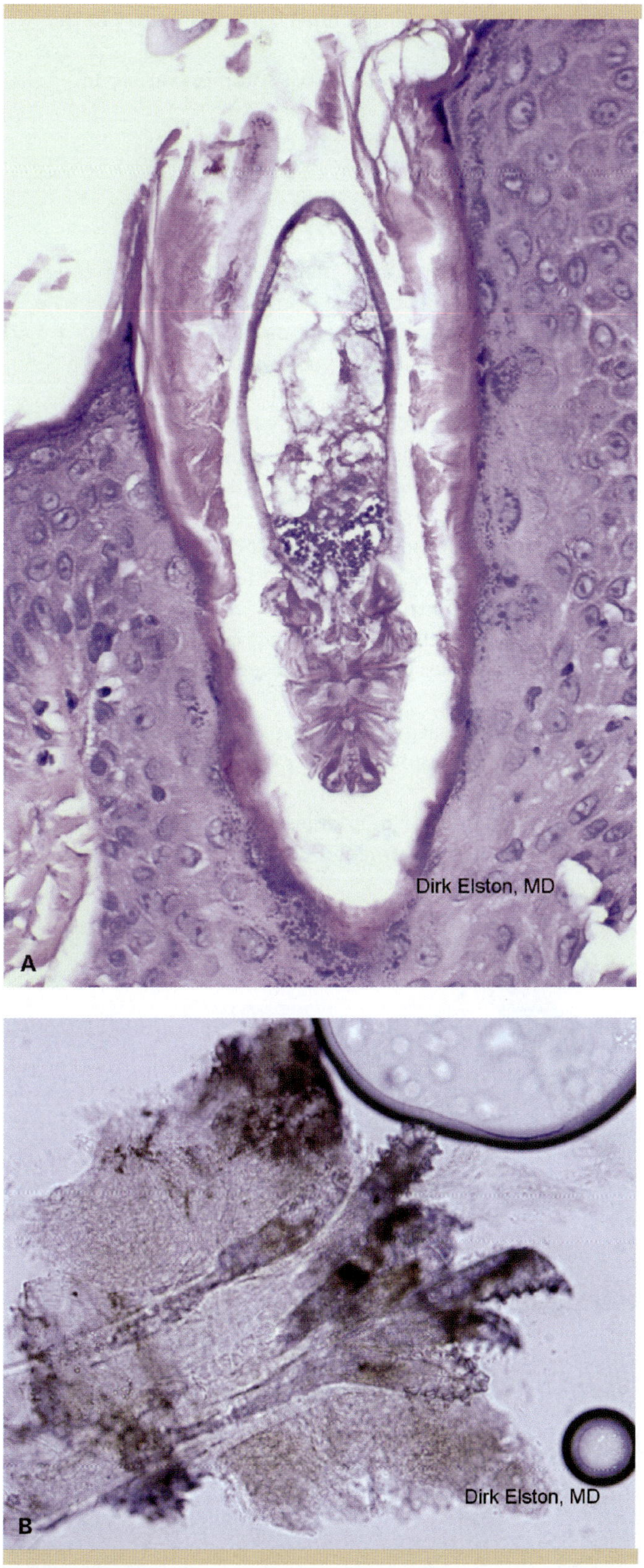

FIGURE 16-6 *Demodex folliculorum*. (*Used with permission from Dr. Dirk Elston.*)

- *Eutrombicula alfreddugesi* most common variety in the United States
- *Neotrombicula autumnalis* most common variety in Europe
- Scrub typhus (*Rickettsia tsutsugamushi*)

Scabies or Itch Mites (Family Sarcoptidae)

Sarcoptes Scabei (Fig. 16-7)

- Globular, semitranslucent mites, less than 0.3 mm long
- Adult mites copulate on the skin, after which the female will burrow, laying her eggs along the way
- Six-legged larvae hatch and take 10 to 14 days before becoming adults
- They survive off the human body for only 2 to 3 days
- Symptoms take 30 days after an immune response develops to the mites or their excrement (scybala)
- Spread by close personal contact
- Hands and wrists are affected most often
- Burrows, which are produced by the adult female mite, and erythematous papules
- In adult patients, the scalp and face are uninvolved
- Pruritus of scabies generally is severe and most noticeable at night
- Diagnosis: mites, eggs, larvae, or scybala on microscopic examination of lesional skin scrapings
- Nodular scabies
  - Erythematous, firm nodules that persist for weeks to months after treatment

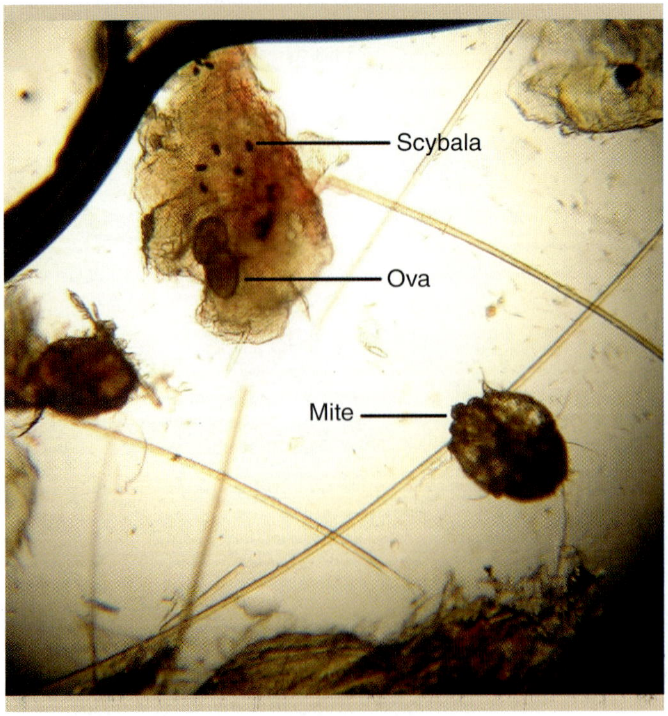

FIGURE 16-7 *Sarcoptes scabei.* (*Used with permission from Dr. Alyn D. Hatter.*)

- Crusted scabies (formerly called Norwegian scabies) scabies
  - Seen in immunocompromised or debilitated patients
  - Thick, scaling, crusted plaques that are found most commonly on the hands, feet, and scalp but may be generalized in distribution
  - Lesions contain thousands of mites
- Treatment
  - Five percent permethrin
- Lindane: avoid in young children and pregnant women owing to reports of neurotoxicity
- Approximately 5 to 10% precipitated sulfur in petrolatum
- Twenty-five percent crotamiton
- Oral ivermectin
- Nodular scabies: topical or intralesional injection of a corticosteroid

Hard or Shield Ticks (Family Ixodidae)

- Wingless arthropods
- It is 8-legged as adults, 6-legged larva
- Flattened dorsoventrally
- Often teardrop-shaped from dorsal view
- Scutum (shield) on the dorsal surface

1. *Ixodes* tick
   - *Ixodes scapularis*: eastern United States
   - *Ixodes pacificus*: in California
   - *Ixodes ricinus*: in Europe
   - Vector for
     - Lyme disease *(Borrelia burgdorferi)*
     - Babesiosis
     - Anaplasmosis
2. *Amblyomma americanum* (lone star tick) (Fig. 16-8)
   - Prominent white dot on the back of the adult female
   - Primarily found in the southern United States, although the range is expanding

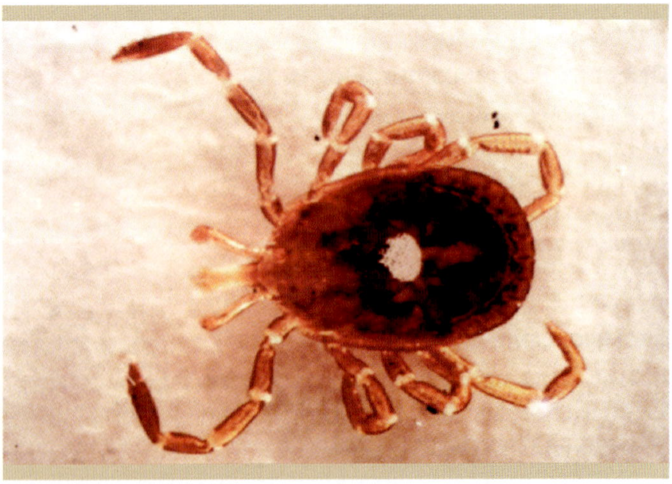

FIGURE 16-8 *Amblyomma americanum* (lone star tick). (*Reprinted with permission from Knoop et al.* Atlas of Emergency Medicine, *2nd Ed. New York: McGraw-Hill; 2002.*)

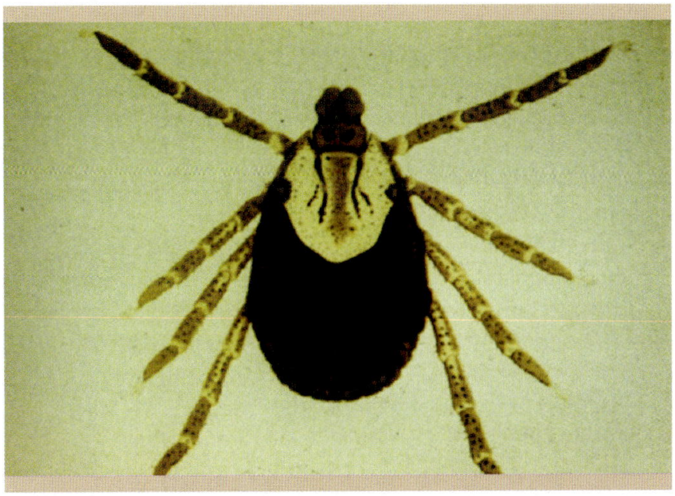

FIGURE 16-9 *Dermacentor*. (*Reprinted with permission from Knoop et al.* Atlas of Emergency Medicine, *2nd Ed. New York: McGraw-Hill; 2002.*)

- Vector for
  - Rocky Mountain spotted fever (*Rickettsia rickettsii*)
  - Ehrlichiosis (*Ehrlichia chaffeensis*)
  - Tularemia (*Francisella tularensis*)
  - Southern tick associated rash illness (STARI) (causative organism unknown)
- *Amblyomma maculatum* (Gulf Coast tick): tick paralysis

3. *Dermacentor* (Fig. 16-9)
   - Rocky Mountain spotted fever
   - Ehrlichiosis
   - Tularemia
   - Colorado tick fever
     - Causative agent, an RNA virus of the genus *Orbivirus* of the family Reoviridae
     - Limited to *Dermacentor andersoni*
   - *D. andersoni*
     - Wood tick
     - Western United States
     - Adults are generally brown but become slate gray when engorged
     - Commonly involved with tick paralysis
     - Female: dark reddish brown with a white shield covering the front third of the body
     - Male: grayish white shield area on top of the body
     - Tick paralysis
   - *Dermacentor variabilis*
     - Dog tick
     - Eastern United States
     - Tick paralysis

Soft or Leathery Ticks (Family Argasidae)

- *Ornithodoros hermsi, Ornithodoros parkeri, Ornithodoros turicata*
- Light gray and leathery in appearance
- Mouthparts are hidden underneath the body
- Transmits relapsing fever: *B. duttoni, B.recurrentis*

Araneae (Spiders)

- All spiders have a cephalothorax from which extend 8 legs and an abdomen
- A pair of jaws (chelicerae) is found at the anterior end of the cephalothorax
- Jaws terminate in sharp, chitinized fangs from which venom is ejected

Latrodectus mactans (Black Widow) (Fig. 16-10)

- Eastern and central regions of the United States
- Black with a globose abdomen that has the characteristic red hourglass-like marking on the ventral surface
- Prefer a warm, dry environment and can be found both outdoors and inside buildings
- Only the female of the species is capable of envenomating humans
- Neurotoxin (α-latrotoxin): causes release of acetylcholine and catecholamines at neuromuscular junction
- Ca^{2+}-dependent release of neurotransmitters down the concentration gradient ensues: no reuptake of the neurotransmitters
- Bite: 2 tiny red puncta; urticarial with white halo, local piloerection; little local damage
- Systemic symptoms begin within an hour, peak at 1 to 6 hours, and can last 1 to 2 days
- Severe myalgias and muscle cramping regionally and then throughout the body

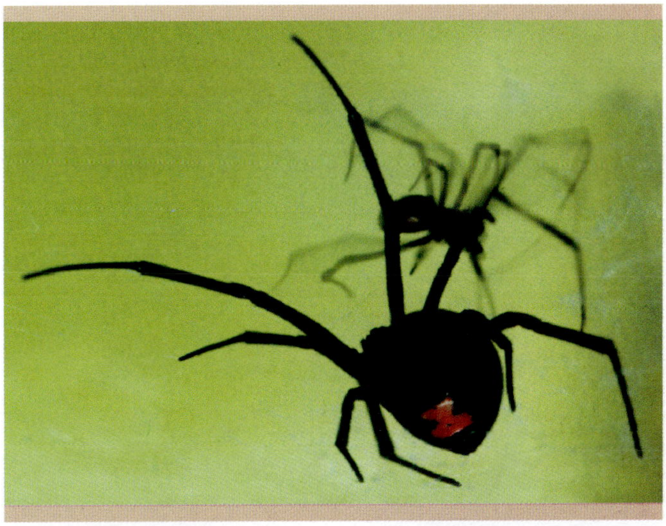

FIGURE 16-10 *Latrodectus mactans* (black widow spider). (*Reprinted with permission from Goldsmith LA et al.* Fitzpatrick's Dermatology in General Medicine, *8th Ed. New York: McGraw-Hill; 2012.*)

- Abdominal musculature is involved and may simulate an acute surgical abdomen
- Painful lymphadenopathy, hypertension, profuse sweating, nausea, and tremors
- Treatment: symptomatic—narcotics, muscle relaxants, and intravenous calcium gluconate
- Spider antivenin

Loxosceles Reclusa (Brown Recluse) (Fig. 16-11)

- Violin-like marking on dorsal aspect of the cephalothorax
- Yellow to brown cephalothorax and a tan abdomen
- From 1 to 1.5 cm in length
- South central part of the United States; they avoid daylight
- Necrotic arachnidism and disseminated intravascular coagulation
- Phospholipase (sphingomyelinase D) causes platelet aggregation, thrombosis, and massive neutrophil infiltration
- Initial bite is often painless and unnoticed by the patient; central papule and associated erythema
- Flag sign
    - Central blue-gray area due to thrombosis
    - Blanched halo from arterial spasm
    - A large surrounding area of reactive erythema
- Progression to eschar formation, dermal necrosis, and stellate ulceration
- Systemic: hematuria, anemia, constitutional symptoms, rash, cyanosis, and severe intravascular hemolysis
- Treatment
    - Tetanus toxoid
    - Rest, ice, and elevation
    - Antibiotics if superficial infection develops
    - Data are mixed concerning triamcinolone and dapsone. A delay of even 1 hour may negate any effect of dapsone

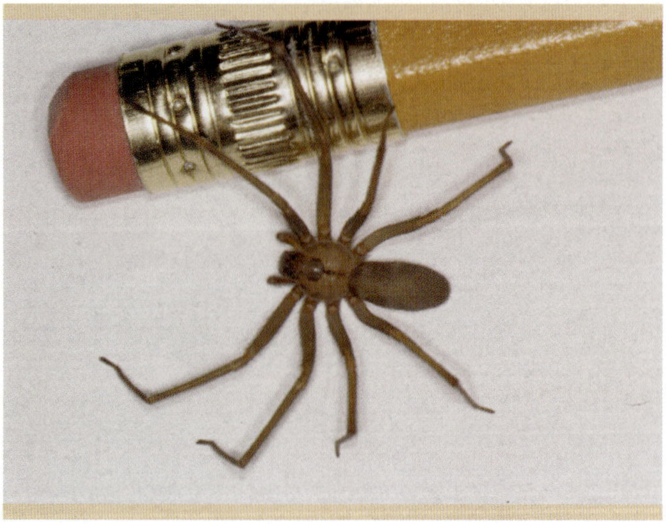

FIGURE 16-11 *Loxosceles reclusa* (brown recluse spider).

Scorpions

- Large arachnids with an elongated abdomen that terminates in a stinger
- Abdominal glands that release both neurotoxic and hemolytic venom into the stinger
- Nocturnal and hide during the daytime in dark places
- Pain and swelling at the site of sting
- Neurotoxin can result in: localized numbness, fasciculation, lacrimation, salivation, profuse sweating, urinary urgency, nausea, tongue paresthesia, restlessness, convulsions, and an increase in extraocular muscle activity
- *Centruroides sculpturatus* most toxic in United States, although it rarely results in death
- Highly dangerous scorpions include *Parabuthus*, *Uroplectes*, and *Tityus* species
- Treatment
    - Remove the stinger
    - Cool the site with ice; antivenin
    - Barbiturates or diazepam for the CNS hyperactivity
    - Atropine for cholinergic side effects of the neurotoxin

CENTIPEDES AND MILLIPEDES

American Centipedes

- Slender, segmented body that ranges in color from yellow to green to brown or black and may vary in length from 1 to 30 cm
- Nocturnal carnivores and prefer a dark, moist environment like that found under rocks and logs
- *Scutigera* species
    - Found in the eastern United States
    - Does not sting humans
- *Scolopendra* species
    - Western United States and Hawaii
    - Can inflict a painful sting
    - Immediate reaction consists of local burning pain
    - Chevron-shaped bite
    - Occasionally, local necrosis, regional lymphangitis, and lymphadenopathy
- Treatment
    - Cleanse the wound
    - Inject a local anesthetic into the wound
    - Tetanus prophylaxis
    - Systemic antihistamines

Millipedes

- Multisegmented, with a hard, often brightly colored exoskeleton
- Nocturnal vegetarians that prefer dark, moist environments
- When disturbed, some millipedes will coil into a tight spiral and then secrete a toxic liquid from repugnatorial glands located on the sides of each segment

- Causes an immediate burning sensation when it contacts human skin
- Skin then becomes yellow-brown and in 24 hours develops intense erythema and often vesiculation
- Treatment: immediate lavage of the area with alcohol or water

PROTOZOA

Cutaneous Amebiasis

- *Entamoeba histolytica*
- Humans are the major reservoir
- Clinical presentation includes an acute dysenteric form and a less symptomatic nondysenteric intestinal form
- Life cycle: cysts travel to the small intestine after ingestion from fecally contaminated food or water
- Trophozoites are released
- They reencyst and produce asymptomatic infection (resolves spontaneously within 12 months) or parasite causes symptomatic amebiasis
- Intestinal disease: acute proctocolitis (dysentery)
- Extraintestinal disease: brain and liver amebic abscesses, peritonitis, pericarditis, cutaneous lesions of amebiasis seem to be extremely rare (direct extension of intestinal disease): with painful ulcerations that may enlarge rapidly
- Diagnosis: indirect hemagglutination, immunofluorescence, and ELISAs
- Treatment: metronidazole, iodoquinol, and paromomycin

HELMINTHIC INFECTIONS

- *Helminth* is derived from the Greek word *helmins*, meaning "worm"
- Categorized as
  - Annelids (i.e., phylum Annelida, the segmented worms)
  - Nematodes (i.e., phylum Nematoda, the roundworms)
  - Platyhelminths (i.e., phylum Platyhelminthes, the flatworms)
  - Trematodes (i.e., flukes) and cestodes (i.e., tapeworms)

SOIL-MEDIATED HELMINTHIC INFECTIONS

Nematodes (Roundworms)

- Hookworm: Ancylostoma and Necator
- Strongyloidiasis
- Ascariasis
- Enterobiasis
- Trichinosis
- Dracunculiasis
- Filariasis: loiasis, onchocerciasis
- Hookworms: caused by the roundworms

Ancylostoma duodenale, Necator americanus

- Ground itch
- Life cycle: female worms, residing in the host's small intestine, release eggs that are passed in the feces
- Larvae in the soil penetrate foot and migrate to lungs through the venous system
- Larvae are then coughed up and swallowed, and they end up in the intestine and mature into adults
- Pruritic, erythematous, edematous, linear, threadlike tracts marking larval migration in the skin
- GI bleeding, iron-deficiency anemia, hypoproteinemia
- Treatment: mebendazole, albendazole

Cutaneous Larva Migrans (Creeping Eruption) (FIG. 16-12)

- *Ancylostoma braziliensis*, hookworm of wild and domestic dogs and cats
- Most common cause of cutaneous larva migrans; human is a dead-end host
- Eggs are passed from animal feces into warm, moist, sandy soil, where the larvae hatch
- Larvae penetrate skin directly but cannot penetrate basement membrane
- Larvae migrate slowly (2 cm/day) in skin, lack the ability to invade further, and complete their life cycle
- Produce raised, threadlike, serpiginous, pruritic, erythematous tracks
- Treatment: topical thiabendazole, ivermectin, albendazole

Strongyloides (Larva Currens, "Racing Larva")

- *Strongyloides stercoralis* (known as threadworm)
- Nematodes live in the small intestine
- Eggs hatch into larvae (rhabditiform), which are passed in the feces
- Larvae can penetrate skin of the host (quick migration rate of 5–10 cm/hour) and then penetrate basement membrane to affect lungs and the GI tract
- Larvae subsequently are swallowed and reach the small intestine
- Intense pruritus, purpura, serpentine urticarial streaks
- Autoinfection: transformation of noninfective larvae (rhabditiform) into infective larvae (filariform)
- Chronic strongyloidiasis
- Serpiginous wheals beginning perianally and extending to the buttocks, upper thighs, and abdomen
- Hemorrhagic pneumonia can result
- Stool for ova and parasites
- Enterotest (string test) or duodenal aspiration to examine duodenal fluid
- Blood cultures
- Enzyme immunoassay (EIA), indirect fluorescent antibody (IFA)

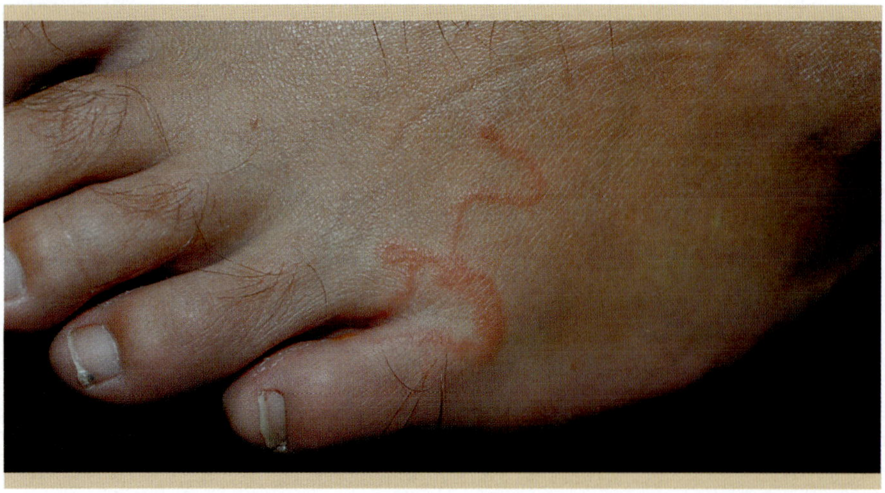

FIGURE 16-12 Cutaneous larva migrans (creeping eruption). (*Reprinted from Wolff K, Johnson RA, and Suurmond D:* Fitzpatrick's Color Atlas and Synopsis of Clinical Dermatology, *5th Ed. New York: McGraw-Hill; 2002.*)

- Chest radiograph to reveal possible patchy alveolar infiltrate
- Sputum examination
- Loefler syndrome: eosinophilia, pneumonitis
- Treatment: thiobendazole, albendazole, ivermectin

Ascariasis

- *Ascaris lumbricoides*
- Adult worms live in the small intestine; eggs are laid and then passed out in the feces
- Eggs may remain viable in soil up to 17 months
- Larvae develop within the eggs
- Eggs are ingested or inhaled from soil; larvae hatch and move to heart, lungs, and pharynx
- Swallowed larvae mature into adults in intestine
- Urticaria
- GI symptoms/obstruction
- Cough, dyspnea, asthma, and chest pain
- Stool examination for ova and parasites
- Treatment: mebendazole, pyrantel pamoate

Enterobiasis (Pinworm Disease)

- *Enterobius vermicularis*
- Most common helminth infection in industrialized countries
- After ingestion, eggs usually hatch in the duodenum within 6 hours
- Female worm migrates to the rectum after copulation and, if not expelled during defecation, migrates to the perineum (often at night)
- Pruritus ani, bruxism
- Diagnosis
  - Transparent tape is pressed against the perineum at night
- Identify eggs under the low-power lens of microscope (Fig. 16-13)
  - Treatment: pyrantel and mebendazole

Trichinosis

- *Trichinella spiralis*
- Larval cysts ingested from undercooked meat (usually pork)
- Acidity and enzymatic activity of the human digestive system disrupt the cyst, releasing large numbers of newborn larvae that penetrate the gut wall, enter the systemic circulation, and migrate to various tissues
- Larvae usually persist only in striated skeletal muscle cells, transformed into nurse cells
- Calcified cysts in muscle, elevated muscle enzymes

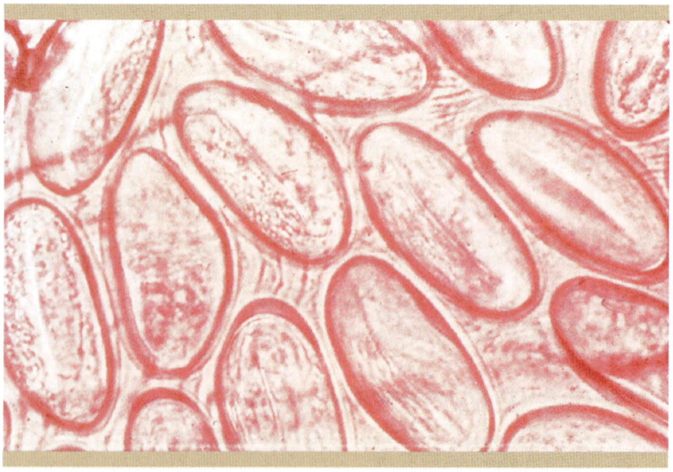

FIGURE 16-13 *Enterobius* eggs under the microscope. (*Reprinted from Freedberg IM et al.* Fitzpatrick's Dermatology in General Medicine, *6th Ed. New York: McGraw-Hill; 2003, p. 2239.*)

- Fever, myalgias, and periorbital edema (increased interstitial fluid)
- Vasculitis: splinter hemorrhages in nails and eyes
- Diagnosis
  - Enzyme immunoassay (EIA) or the bentonite flocculation (BF) test
  - Elevated creatine kinase (CK) and lactate dehydrogenase (LDH)
  - Stool examination: Charcot-Leyden crystals from eosinophils may be found in stools
- Treatment
  - Trichinosis is usually a self-limited illness
  - Prednisone
  - Mebendazole and albendazole
  - Proper cooking of meat is the most effective method to prevent infection

Dracunculiasis

- *Dracunculus medinesis*, guinea fire worm; nematode
- Ingested larvae reside in an intermediate host, a tiny freshwater crustacean or copepod
- Migrates from the GI tract to a location in the lower extremity (most commonly the foot), causing a bulla that ruptures to release the larvae back into water
- Clinical: presence of the adult worm in the subcutaneous tissue, usually lower extremity
- Constitutional symptoms
- Treatment
  - Slowly wind worm around stick
  - Metronidazole, thiabendazole may case aberrant migration of worms, and should be used with caution

Filariae

- Eight species of roundworm belonging to the family Filarioidea develop to adulthood in humans
- Larvae or microfilariae are ingested by a feeding insect vector
- Larvae are then inoculated into the vertebral host for the final stages of development
- Cutaneous group (listed below)
  - *Loa loa*
  - *Onchocerca volvulus*
  - *Mansonella streptocerca*
- Lymphatic group
  - *W. bancrofti:* causes Bancroftian filariasis
    - Genital disease: edema of scrotal skin, funiculitis, epididymitis, orchitis, and hydrocele
    - Distinctive lymphangitis of the arms or legs characterized by a unique retrograde spread or extension
    - Starting in a single node, erythematous patches of subcutaneous edema or diffuse erythema and edema develop and progress distally
    - Treatment: diethylcarbamazine, ivermectin
  - *Brugia malayi:* causes Malayan filariasis
  - *Brugia timori:* causes Timorian filariasis
    - Clinical manifestations of Malayan filariasis and Timorian filariasis:
    - Axillary or inguinal lymphadenitis, lymphangitis, and fever are common
    - Lymphatic abscesses and resulting scarring
- Body cavity group
  - *M. streptocerca*: causes streptocerciasis
  - Central and West Africa
  - Transmitted by the midge *Culicoides grahami*
  - Adult worms are found in the dermis of the patient's upper trunk
  - Microfilariae are found in the dermis and lymph nodes
  - Treatment: diethylcarbamazine
- Loiasis (*Loa loa*)
- Vector: *Chrysops* (deer fly)
- Rain forests of Central and West Africa
- Diurnal periodicity: microfilariae are found in the bloodstream in highest numbers during the day
  - Clinical manifestations
    - Transient, nontender areas of angioedema and urticaria are the major signs and symptoms
    - Calabar swellings: transient subcutaneous swellings on the extremities
    - Worm migration across conjunctiva or bridge of nose
    - Localized pain, pruritus, and urticaria
    - Arthritis, breast calcification, meningoencephalopathy, endomyocardial fibrosis, peripheral neuropathy, pleural effusions, and retinopathy
- Treatment: diethylcarbamazine
  - Mazzotti reaction: stroke or meningoencephalitis from release of dead microfilariae in blood and cerebrospinal fluid (CSF) after treatment with diethylcarbamazine (DEC); it may occur without drug therapy
- Onchocerciasis (river blindness, hanging groins, leopard skin, or sowdah)
- *O. volvulus*
- Vector: *Simulium* species of blackflies
- Tropical Africa
- Microfilariae found in the dermis, eyes, and regional lymph nodes
- Clinical manifestations
  - Pruritus, subcutaneous lumps, lymphadenitis, and blindness
  - Onchocercoma: Subcutaneous nodules common over bony prominences
  - Ocular: punctate keratitis, pannus formation, corneal fibrosis, iridocyclitis, glaucoma, choroiditis, and optic
  - "Lizard skin," "hanging skin": Fibrosis and atrophy may cause lymph nodes or portions of bowel to hang in pockets of skin
  - Hypopigmented patches in Africans ("leopard skin")

    - Hyperpigmented patches in Arabics (sowdah)
    - Facial edema/pruritus in Mexico and Guatemala (erysipela de la Costa)
- Diagnosis
    - Slit-lamp examination: microfilariae in the eye
    - Biopsy of a nodule will reveal an adult worm
- Treatment: ivermectin
- Mansonelliasis
- Vectors: midge species *Culicoides austeni* and *C. grahami*
- *M. streptocerca*
- Subcutaneous infection in humans

Toxocariasis

- Visceral larva migrans
- Caused by the roundworm of the dog and cat: *Toxocara canis* and *T. cati*
- Eggs ingested from soil; larvae penetrate bowel and lodge in organs and blood vessels
- Hemorrhage, necrosis, urticaria
- Ocular larva migrans: penetrating larva can become encysted, leading to the fomation of a large granuloma

Gnathostomiasis (Wandering Swelling, Yangtse River Edema)

- *Gnathostoma spinigerum*
- Humans eat fish that contain larvae, or larvae penetrate the skin directly
- Migrating erythematous swelling, pain, pruritus
- Treatment: surgery, ivermectin, albendazole

Trematodes (Flukes)

- Phylum Platyhelminthes contains the dorsoventrally flattened worms
- Schistosomiasis (bilharziasis)
- Life cycle
    - Eggs passed in urine (*Schistosoma haematobium*) or feces (*Schistosoma japonicum* and *Schistosoma mansoni*), hatch in water
    - From eggs, miracidia hatch into the water, where they penetrate into snails; in the snails they develop into cercariea that penetrate the host skin
    - Enter the portal venous system of the liver and travel to heart, lungs, and finally the bladder or the mesenteric vessels
- Schistosomiasis organisms (blood flukes)
    - *S. mansoni*
        - South America
        - Portal hypertension, found in large intestine and liver, eggs shed in stool
        - Location of spine on ova: lateral
    - *S. japonicum*
        - Asia
        - Portal hypertension; found in small intestine and liver; eggs shed in stool
        - Location of spine on ova: no spine
    - *S. haematobium*
        - Africa, Middle East
        - Found in bladder, pelvic/urogenital venules; eggs shed in urine
        - Location of spine on ova: apical
- Clinical
    - Cercarial dermatitis (swimmer's itch)
        - Pruritus, dermatitis
        - Skin exposure to fresh or salt water
        - Macular eruption, pruritic
        - Spares clothing-covered skin
    - Acute syndrome, Katayama fever: spiking afternoon fevers, chills, bronchitis, pneumonitis, headache, lymphadenopathy, hepatosplenomegaly, joint pain, diarrhea, urticaria, eosinophilia, leukocytosis, and an elevated erythrocyte sedimentation rate
    - Late hypersensitivity reaction: generalized urticaria, pruritus, lichenified papules, or dermatographism
- Treatment: antihistamines plus topical steroids for itch, praziquantel

Fascioliasis

- *Fasciola hepatica*
- Metacercariae on plants are ingested by sheep or humans; larvae migrate to the bile duct
- Hepatomegaly, right upper quadrant pain, jaundice, urticaria
- Treatment: surgery, bithionel, triclabendazole

CESTODA

Tape Worms

- Long, segmented worms
- Include
    - Cysticercosis
    - Echinococcosis
    - Sparganosis
    - Coenurosis
- Life cycle
    - Eggs passed from the primary host and ingested by an intermediate host, where eggs hatch
    - Larvae encyst within tissues
    - Infection of the primary host occurs by ingesting the cyst-infested flesh of the intermediate host

Cysticercosis

- *Taenia solium*
- Eggs in undercooked pork ingested and penetrate bowel to enter muscle, brain, and eyes where they develop into larvae
- Seizures, mass lesions, nodules
- Treatment: surgical excision, albendazole, praziquantel

Echinococcosis

- *Echinococcus* species (*Echinococcus granulosus*: dog; *Echinococcus multilocularis*: fox)
- Eggs from animal feces are ingested; larvae hatch and penetrate gut wall
- Hydatid cyst in the abdomen
- Treatment: surgical excision, mebendazole

Sparganosis

- *Spirometra* species
- Larvae from undercooked fish are ingested
- Enlarging subcutaneous nodule
- Treatment: surgical excision

Coenurosis

- *Taenia* species (multiceps, serialis, brauni)
- Eggs in host feces (dogs, fox, wolf)
- Ingested by herbivores (cows) and penetrate bowel to enter muscle, brain, and eyes, where they develop into larvae
- Seizures, mass lesions, subcutaneous nodules
- Treatment: surgical excision

REPTILES

Snakes

- United States: rattlesnake, cottonmouth moccasin, and copperhead (family *Crotalidae*) account for the vast majority of bites

Elapidae Family

- Coral snake
  - Round eyes
  - Red and yellow or white bands ("red on yellow kills a fellow" helps distinguish from milk snake)
  - Neurotoxic
  - Muscle fasciculations, later flaccid paralysis
- Viperidae family (pit viper)
  - Copperhead, rattlesnake, cottonmouth (water moccasin)
  - Triangular head distinct from the body
  - Elliptical "cat's eye" pupils
  - Venom with hydrolases; anticoagulant in the venom causes hemolysis and capillary leakage
  - Pain, edema, ecchymosis, vesiculation, petechiae, and tissue necrosis can develop at the site of the bite
  - Damage to vascular endothelium, hypotension

QUIZ

Questions

1. Epidemic typhus is caused by:

   A. *Rickettsia typhi*
   B. *Rickettsia felis*
   C. *Rickettsia prowazeckii*
   D. *Bartonella quintana*
   E. Both A and B

2. Body lice carry:

   A. Epidemic typhus
   B. Trench fever
   C. Relapsing fever
   D. Bacillary angiomatosis
   E. All of the above

3. Sand flies are vectors in which disease(s):

   A. Leishmaniasis
   B. Oroya fever
   C. River blindness
   D. *Loa loa*
   E. Both A and B

4. The first stage of sleeping sickness is characterized by a (an):

   A. Chancre
   B. Buboe
   C. Lymphadenitis
   D. Persistent fever
   E. Enlargement of the spleen

5. Mosquitoes are not the vector for:

   A. Filariasis
   B. Yellow fever
   C. Dengue
   D. Encephalitis
   E. Carrion disease

6. Reduviid bugs transmit:

   A. Chagas disease
   B. Leishmaniasis
   C. Dengue
   D. Malaria
   E. Sleeping sickness

7. *Amblyomma americanum* is associated with:

   A. STARI
   B. Rocky Mountain spotted fever
   C. Erlichiosis
   D. Tuleremia
   E. All of the above

8. The toxin in *loxosceles* venom thought responsible for necrosis and hemolysis is:
   A. Hyaluronidase
   B. Latrotoxin-alpha
   C. Solenopsin D
   D. Sphingomyelinase D
   E. None of the above

9. The red mite known to infest birds, reptiles, and mammals and causes a characteristic dermatitis concentrated along lines of tightly fit clothing in campers and hikers is:
   A. *Allodermanyssus sanguineus*
   B. *Cheyletiella yasguri*
   C. *Ornithonyssus sylviarum*
   D. *Trombicula alfreddugesi*
   E. *Linuche unguiculata*

10. Creeping eruption is caused by:
    A. *Ancylostoma braziliensis*
    B. *Ascaris lumbricoides*
    C. *Strongyloides stercoralis*
    D. *Enterobius vermicularis*
    E. None of the above

Answers

1. C. The causative organism in epidemic typhus is *Rickettsia prowazeckii.* The vector is *Pediculus humanus corporis* (body louse). In contrast to epidemic typhus, *Xenopsylla cheopis* has been considered the classic vector of endemic typhus which is caused by *Rickettsia typhi* and *Rickettsia felis*. Endemic typhus has emerged as more common in South Texas, where the vector is *Ctenocephalides felis* and oppossums serve as a disease reservoir.
2. E. While head and pubic lice are not clearly linked to the spread of disease, body lice are important disease vectors, especially in refugee populations. They carry epidemic typhus, trench fever, relapsing fever, and the bacillary angiomatosis organism. When transmitted by a louse, the latter organism is more likely to cause endocarditis.
3. E. Sand flies (Lutzomyia and Phlebotomus species) serve as vectors for Leishmaniasis and Oroya fever. River blindness (onchocerciasis) and *Loa loa* (loiasis) are filarial diseases carried by black flies and deer flies, respectively.
4. A. The organisms that cause sleeping sickness are related to those that cause leishmaniasis. Both produce chancriform lesions. Sleeping sickness also causes urticaria, pruritus, facial edema, fever, and arthralgias, CNS manifestations occur in the second phase of illness.
5. E. Mosquitoes cause more human morbidity and mortality than any other group of arthropods. Among the many diseases they spread are filariasis, yellow fever, dengue, and viral encephalitis. Carrion disease is caused by *Bartonella bacilliformis* and is transmitted by sand flies.
6. A. Chagas disease is transmitted by Reduviid bugs. Bedbugs may represent a secondary vector. Leishmaniasis and sleeping sickness are spread by biting flies and malaria and dengue are spread by mosquitoes.
7. E. *Amblyomma americanum*, or lone star tick, is a vector for Tuleremia, Erlichiosis, Rocky Mountain spotted fever and STARI.
8. D. Sphingomyelinase D enzymatically degrades sphingomyelin causing cell lysis, neutrophil chemotaxis, platelet aggregation and activates complement. Latrotoxin-alpha is the toxin in black widow venom. Solenopsins are piperidine alkaloid toxins found in the venom of fire ants.
9. D. *Trombicula alfreddugesi,* aka chiggers or harvester mites, are red mites found throughout North America. They cause a pruritic eruption often along elastic lines of socks, underwear, or trousers. *Allodermanyssus sanguineus* is the house mouse mite, the vector for rickettsial pox. *Cheyletiella yasguri* is the dog mite which causes walking dandruff. *O. sylviarum* is the bird mite and vector for western equine encephalitis. *Linuche unguiculata* is the box jelly, and its nematocysts are a common cause of seabather's eruption.
10. A. *Ancylostoma braziliensis* is the most common cause of cutaneous larva migrans, or creeping eruption. In contrast, *S. stercoralis* is a threadworm that migrates through the skin at a more rapid pace causing cutaneous larva currens. *Ascaris lumbricoides* is the intestinal roundworm. *Enterobius vermicularis* is the pinworm and causes pruritus ani.

REFERENCES

Buxton PK: ABC of dermatology. Insect bites and infestations. *Br Med J* 1988;296:489–491.

Centers for Disease Control: Southern Tick Associated Rash Illness. Atlanta. 2015. http://www.cdc.gov/stari/. Accessed May, 2014.

Chaudhry AZ, Longworth DL: Cutaneous manifestations of intestinal helminthic infections. *Dermatol Clin* 1989;7:275–290.

Goldsmith LA et al. *Fitzpatrick's Dermatology in General Medicine*, 8th Ed. New York: McGraw-Hill; 2012.

Mackey SL, Wagner KF: Dermatologic manifestations of parasitic diseases. *Infect Dis Clin North Am* 1994;8:713–743.

McGinley-Smith DE, Tsao SS: Dermatoses from ticks. *J Am Acad Dermatol* 2003;49:363–392.

McKee PH: *Pathology of the Skin: With Clinical Correlations*. London: Mosby-Wolfe; 1996.

Meinking TL, Burkhart CN, Burkhart CG: Changing paradigms in parasitic infections: common dermatological helminthic infections and cutaneous myiasis. *Clin Dermatol* 2003;21:407–416.

Metry DW, Hebert AA: Insect and arachnid stings, bites, infestations, and repellents. *Pediatr Ann* 2000;29(1):39–48.

Normann SA: Venomous insects and reptiles. *J Fla Med Assoc* 1996;83:183–186.

Rosen T: Caterpillar dermatitis. *Dermatol Clin* 1990;8:245–252.

Wilson DC, King LE Jr: Spiders and spider bites. *Dermatol Clin* 1990;8:277–286.

CHAPTER 17

VIRAL DISEASES

RANA MAJD MAYS
RACHEL A. GORDON
WHITNEY L. DELOZIER
NATALIA MENDOZA
STEPHEN K. TYRING

DNA VIRUSES

1. Pox viruses
2. Papillomaviruses
3. Herpes viruses
4. Parvoviruses
5. Hepadnavirus

Pox Viruses

- Large, enveloped, double-stranded, linear DNA viruses
- Belong to the Poxviridae family
- Replicate in the cytoplasm, except for the adenovirus
- Poxviruses of clinical importance include smallpox, vaccinia, monkeypox, molluscum contagiosum, orf, and milkers' nodules

MOLLUSCIPOX (MOLLUSCUM CONTAGIOSUM; MCV)

- Common, benign, self-limiting skin disease
- Generally affects pediatric age group
- Virus commonly acquired by skin-to-skin contact (nonsexual)
- Incubation period is from 2 weeks to 6 months
- Four different strains have been identified (based on restriction endonuclease digestion pattern). Two main subtypes: MCV I, responsible for the majority of infections in the United States, and MCV II (more prevalent in HIV patients); both are genital/nongenital
- Clinical
  - 3- to 6-mm erythematous or skin-colored, dome-shaped, umbilical papules distributed over the trunk and face. The lesions may persist for 6 to 8 weeks or more (Fig. 17-1)
  - In immunocompromised patients, especially HIV-infected individuals, thousands of papules distributed on the body and face. High risk of bacterial infection and treatment resistance
  - Genital papules: usually sexually transmitted, most common in adults (Fig. 17-2)
  - Positive Koebner reaction
  - Free virus cores found in all layers of epidermis
- Diagnosis
  - Clinical
  - Confirmatory biopsy in some cases. Henderson-Paterson bodies (molluscum bodies) = viral particles in infected keratinocytes, eosinophils
- Treatment
  - Resolution is often preceded by inflammation, uncomplicated lesions heal without scaring
  - Physical destruction (salicylic acid, liquid nitrogen, cantharidin, lactic acid, CO_2, trichloroacetic acid)
  - Immune modulation: imiquimod
  - Manual extrusion (curettage) of the lesions
  - Cidofovir in immunocompromised patients

SMALLPOX

- Caused by variola virus; variola minor also known as alastrim
- Serious, contagious, and sometimes fatal infectious disease
- Eradicated after a successful worldwide vaccination program
- Face-to-face contact is not required to be infected, direct contact with infected body fluids or contaminated objects
- Humans are the only natural host
- Clinical
  - Incubation 12 to 13 days, fever, malaise, backache, body aches, and exanthem that appears after 2 to 4 days
  - Two clinical forms: *Variola* major, most common and severe form with a 30% incidence of mortality (secondary to pulmonary edema from heart failure), 4 clinical

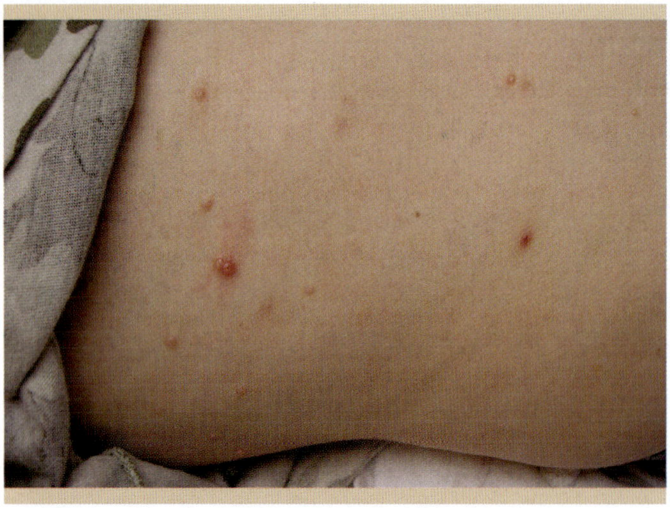

FIGURE 17-1 Molluscum contagiosum. (*Used with permission from Dr. Adelaide Hebert.*)

types: ordinary, modified (by previous vaccination), flat, and hemorrhagic; and *Variola* minor, less severe and 1% mortality

- Early rash appears as small red spots in the mouth; macules → papules → vesicles → pustules; all lesions exist in the same stage
- Complications: corneal ulceration, laryngeal lesions, encephalitis, hemorrhage

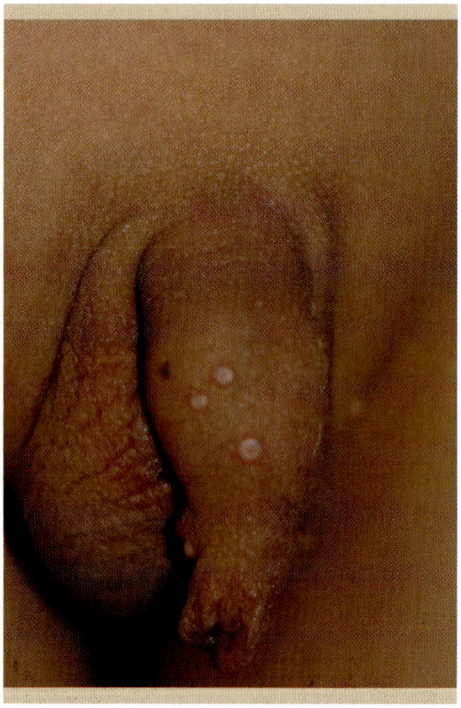

FIGURE 17-2 Molluscum contagiosum genital. (*Used with permission from Dr. Adriana Motta.*)

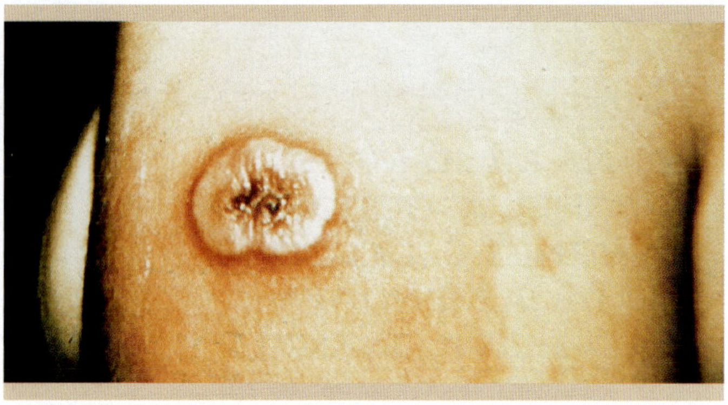

FIGURE 17-3 Vaccinia. (*Used with permission from Dr. Stephen Tyring.*)

  - Progressive vaccinia related to immunosuppression, malignancy, radiation therapy, or AIDS
- Vaccination: rare postvaccinal encephalitis and progressive vaccinia; high level immunity for 3 to 5 years and decreasing immunity thereafter
- Diagnosis
  - Clinical
  - Histology: balloon and reticular degeneration with hemorrhage inclusion bodies, polymorphonuclear cells
- Treatment
  - No antiviral treatment for smallpox; cidofovir suggested

VACCINIA (FIGS. 17-3 AND 17-4)

- Laboratory virus used to vaccinate against smallpox and monkeypox
- Infection occurs primarily in laboratory workers
- Congenital vaccinia infection of the fetus in the last trimester with cutaneous lesions (no other associated congenital abnormalities)
- Clinical
  - Vaccination reactions
    - Papule (3–4 days after vaccination)

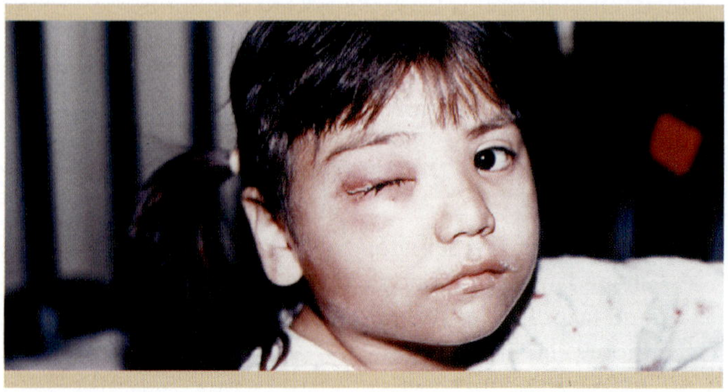

FIGURE 17-4 Vaccinia eye. (*Used with permission from Dr. Stephen Tyring.*)

- Vesicle with surrounding erythema, umbilicated (5–6 days)
  - Pustule (8–9 days) confirms successful vaccination
  - Crust (12+ days)
  - Scar (17–21 days)
- Systemic symptoms such as malaise, lymphadenopathy, myalgia, headache, chills, nausea, fatigue, and fever may appear at day 8.
- Usually self-limited except in immunocompromised individuals
- Progressive vaccinia is one of the most severe complications (life threatening) of smallpox vaccination
- Suspected when there is no evidence of normal resolution of the lesion at the vaccination site within 14 days and progression to central necrosis develops without surrounding erythema. Satellite and secondary lesions progress in the same fashion as the primary lesion
- Systemic symptoms occur late in the onset of the disease, death occurs as a result of an overwhelming toxemia, viremia, or septicemia
- Cases in young children are due to a congenital immune deficiency. Adult cases are usually due to acquired immunosuppression (HIV, cancer, immunosuppressive therapy)
- Treatment: vaccinia immune globulin (VIG) or surgical removal of massive lesions followed by VIG

Monkeypox

- Occasionally infects humans; predominantly residents of western and central Africa; vaccinia infection may confer protection
- Reported cases in the United States were related to direct contact with infected exotic or wild mammalian pets (prairie dogs)
- Clinical
  - Differs from the cases of monkeypox in Africa and the United States
  - Red erosion progresses to a white vesicle to an umbilicated pustule with a central hemorrhagic crust and satellite lesions
  - Dissemination may occur

Cowpox

- Infects cows, but more commonly seen in cats
- Cow/cat teats: sites of injury
- Lymphadenopathy, fever

Orf (Ecthyma Contagiosum, Scabby Mouth)

- Large ovoid virus, 250 × 160 nm with surface tubules, resistant to drying
- Endemic among sheep and goats, oxen; infection from animals or fomites: barn doors, troughs
- Uncommon dermatosis resulting from cutaneous infection with sheep pox virus. Sheep farmers, veterinarians mainly affected
- Clinical
  - Four to seven days incubation followed by 36-day period with 6 clinical stages: each lasts 6 days
  - Lesions progress through several stages. They occur at sites of contact with infected animals or fomites
  - Papular stage: red elevated lesion
  - Target stage: nodule with red center, white ring, red halo
  - Acute stage: weeping surface
  - Regenerative stage: thin, dry crust with black dots
  - Papillomatous stage: small papillomas over surface of lesion
  - Regressive: thick crusts heal with scarring
- Systemic symptoms include lymphangitis, lymphadenitis, malaise, and fever
- Diagnosis
  - Based on typical clinical skin lesion and a history of sheep exposure. It is confirmed by histological study with or without electron microscopy
  - Histology varies depending on the stage of the lesion. Epidermal necrosis is prominent with vacuolization of cells in the upper third of the stratum spinosum. Eosinophilic inclusion bodies in the cytoplasm and nucleus of infected cells and mixed infiltrate in the dermis
- Treatment
  - Spontaneous remission

Milkers' Nodules (Paravaccinia)

- Paravaccinia virus is a 140 × 310 nm, double-stranded DNA poxvirus
- It is resistant to desiccation, cold, and heat
- Endemic to cattle, on cow teats
- Occupational disease affects mainly milkers, farm workers, and veterinary surgeons
- Clinical
  - Incubation period varies from 4 days to weeks
  - Lesions usually found on the fingers, the hand, or the forearm
  - One single lesion or few lesions (in burned areas), 0.5 to 1.5 cm in diameter, firm, dome-shaped, movable, red or purplish red papules or nodules, some may have a target-like appearance and central ulceration may occur
  - Nodules grow slowly and are asymptomatic, systemic symptoms are not common
  - A milkers' nodule may not be clinically distinguishable from Orf lesions
  - Lesions heal without scarring
- Diagnosis
  - Based on typical clinical skin lesion and a history of cow exposure
  - Histology: similar to Orf
- Treatment
  - Usually self-limited (i.e., spontaneous resolution)

Human Papillomaviruses (HPV)

- Nonenveloped, double-stranded, circular DNA viruses with approximately 8000 base pairs
- HPV genome encodes early proteins (E1–E7) and late proteins (L1–L2)
- Proteins E6 and E7 are involved in oncogenesis. E6 inactivates the tumor suppressor protein p53 blocking cell apoptosis. E7 inactivates the Rb-family proteins inducing cell proliferation
- Clinical
  - Infect epithelia or skin or mucosa and mostly causes benign papillomas or warts
  - Most infections are transient; however, lesions may recur, persist or become latent (especially in immunocompromised individuals)
  - Main risk factor is close personal contact, the lesions spread by direct skin-to-skin or skin-to-mucosa contact. Other factors involved are the quantity of HPV in the lesion, the type of contact, the immune status of the individual, and the lesion location
  - Lesions may koebnerize
- HPV may cause genitomucosal lesions, nongenital cutaneous lesions, epidermodysplasia verruciformis (EV) and Heck disease
- Antiviral treatments exist (Interferon, imiquimod–indirect action and cidofovir), but most therapies aim to destroy the clinical lesions
- Two vaccines available

Nongenital Cutaneous Diseases (Table 17-1)

- Occur in 10% of children, peak incidence between 12 and 16 years old, adults are also affected but less commonly
- The clinical lesions can be classified as:
  - Verruca palmaris or plantaris (myrmecia or *palmoplantar wart*) (Fig. 17-5)
    - Clinical
      - ▲ "Anthill" HPV1
      - ▲ Volar aspects of palms/soles, tips of fingers/toes
      - ▲ Thick, endophytic papules with a central depression
      - ▲ Pain with pressure when walking
    - Diagnosis
      - ▲ Histology: ortho- and parakeratosis, acanthosis, and extensive papillomatosis. Rete ridges extend further into the dermis. Higher power intracytoplasmatic, eosinophilic, keratohyalin-like granules within the epithelial cell in the low stratum of malpighii
  - Verruca vulgaris (common warts)
    - HPV 1, 2, or 4
    - Clinical (Fig. 17-6)
      - ▲ Verrucous papules
      - ▲ The lesions can be hyperkeratotic, exophytic, and dome-shaped papules or nodules with punctuate black dots (thrombosed capillaries and capillary bleeding)
    - Treatment
      - ▲ Salicylic acid, 50% tricholoacetic acid, cantharidin, cryotherapy with liquid nitrogen, electrodesiccation, combination therapy using cryodestruction or surgery and imiquimod
  - Verrucae plana (flat warts) (Fig. 17-7)
    - HPV 3 or 10
    - Clinical
      - ▲ Slightly elevated flat flesh-colored papules that may be smooth or slightly hyperkeratotic
      - ▲ Located on dorsal hands, arms or face, often in a linear array
    - Treatment: retinoic acid 0.05% applied daily until desquamation occurs; mild irritation may occur,

TABLE 17-1 Nongenital Cutaneous Disease

	HPV Type
Common warts (verrucae vulgaris)	1, 2, 4, 26, 27, 29, 41, 57, 65
Plantar warts (myrmecia)	1, 2, 4, 63
Flat warts (verrucae plana)	3, 10, 27, 28, 38, 41, 49
Butcher warts (common warts of people who handle meat, poultry, and fish)	7
Mosaic warts	2, 27, 57
Ungual squamous cell carcinoma	16
Epidermodysplasia verruciformis (benign)	2, 3, 10, 12, 15, 19, 36, 46, 47, 50
Epidermodysplasia verruciformis (malignant or benign)	5, 8, 9, 10, 14, 17, 20, 21, 22, 23, 24, 25, 37, 38

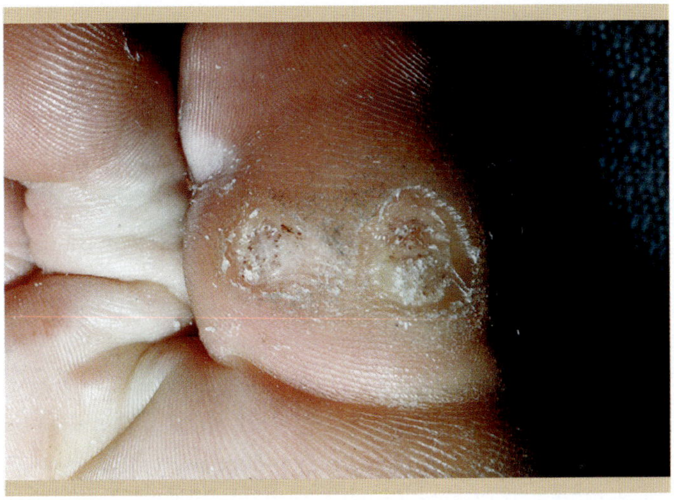

FIGURE 17-5 Plantar warts. (*Used with permission from Dr. Stephen Tyring.*)

imiquimod or a combination of the treatment options

- Butcher warts
  - HPV 7
  - Proliferative hand warts
  - Histology: same as common warts
- Epidermodysplasia verruciformis (EV)
  - Very rare chronic disease
  - Autosomal recessive pattern
  - Unique susceptibility to cutaneous infections by a group of phylogenetically related HPV types (mainly types 5 and 8)
  - Manifest at childhood
  - Clinical
    - ▲ Lesions are polymorphic, verruca plana-like, red-brown plaques

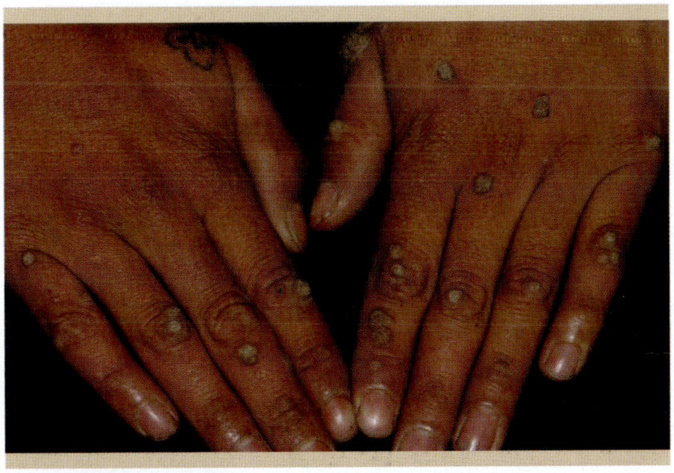

FIGURE 17-6 Verruga vulgaris. (*Used with permission from Dr. Adrian Motta.*)

FIGURE 17-7 Verruca plana (flat warts). (*Used with permission from Dr. Asra Ali.*)

    - ▲ Actinic keratoses arise after the age of 30 years and transform into bowenoid or squamous cell carcinomas (50% of patients)
  - Diagnosis
    - ▲ Clinical: confirmed by biopsy
    - ▲ Histology: stratum corneum with a basketweave apparance, uneven keratohyaline granules; large, course granules in the epidermis; koilocytes; gray cytoplasm; increase in amount of cytoplasm. Dysplasia and actinic keratoses may be evident
  - Treatment
    - ▲ No effective treatment
    - ▲ Counsel patients to protect the skin from ultraviolet radiation exposure; radiation therapy is contraindicated in EV
    - ▲ Retinoids: long-term isotretinoin has been shown to decrease number of benign lesions and slow appearance of premalignant and malignant lesions
    - ▲ Imiquimod

Anogenital Disease Associated With HPV (Table 17-2)

- HPV infection is extremely common; the United States has an annual incidence of approximately 5.5 million cases
- Risk factors include increased number of lifetime sexual partners
- HPV types involved are types 6, 11, 16, and 18

TABLE 17-2 Anogenital Diseases Associated With HPV

	HPV Type
Condyloma acuminata	6, 11, 30, 42, 43, 44, 45, 51, 52, 54
Bowenoid papulosis	16, 18, 34, 39, 42, 45
Bowen disease	16, 18, 31, 34
Giant condyloma (Buschke-Löwenstein tumors)	6, 11

- Condyloma acuminatum (anogenital warts) (Fig. 17-8)
  - Seventy-five percent of sexually active adults will have an HPV infection, most subclinical, by age 50
  - The prevalence of anogenital HPV infection peaks in women age 25 with a second peak in women older than 55 years
  - HPV 6 and HPV 11 are the most common types of anogenital HPV
  - Less commonly HPV 16, -18, -21, -22, and -55
  - Clinical
    - ▲ Flesh-colored to pink to reddish-brown, small, verrucous papules; discrete, sessile, smooth-topped papules or nodules or exophytic cauliflower-like lesions that usually are found near moist surfaces
    - ▲ Few centimeters in diameter but they may coalesce
    - ▲ Location: perianal area, crural folds, anus, rectum, urethra, vagina, cervix, labia, and vulva

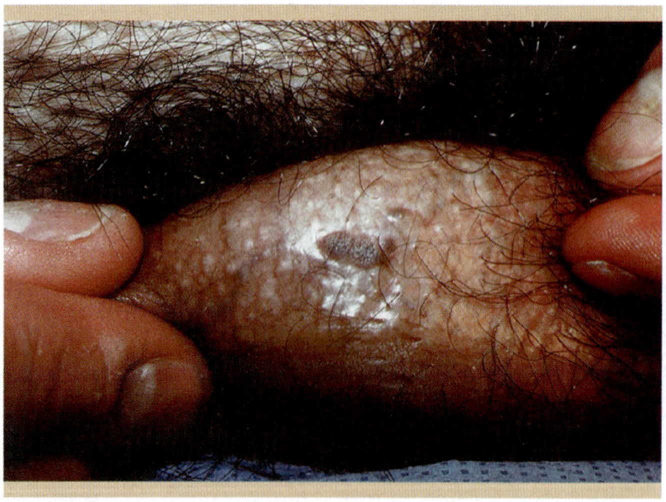

FIGURE 17-8 Anogenital disease. (*Used with permission from Dr. Stephen Tyring.*)

  - Diagnosis
    - ▲ Histology: parakeratosis (mucosa), papillomatosis, acanthosis, elongated rete ridges, occasional mitotic figures. Koilocytes: dark nuclei with dyskeratosis
  - Treatment
    - ▲ Often challenging and may require multiple visits with more than 1 treatment sometimes necessary
    - ▲ Liquid nitrogen
    - ▲ Electrocautery
    - ▲ Curettage
    - ▲ Podofilox
    - ▲ Imiquimod cream 5%
    - ▲ Use of condoms may reduce transmission
    - ▲ Topical cidofovir (not FDA approved)
    - ▲ Topical sinecatechins ointment 15%
  - Prevention
    - ▲ Two HPV vaccines: Cervarix (HPV 16 and 18) FDA approved for prevention of cervical cancer in females ages 9 to 26 and Gardasil (Merck) (HPV 6, 11, 16, 18) FDA approved for prevention of cervical cancer, vaginal cancer, vulvar cancer, and genital warts in both males and females
- Bowenoid papulosis
  - Rare manifestation of HPV infection
  - HPV 16, -18, and -33 (oncogenic)
  - Young, sexually active adults; cervix in females
  - Premalignant disease
  - Clinical
    - ▲ Red or hyperpigmented, multiple groups of well-demarcated, 2- to 3-mm papules on the external genitalia
  - Diagnosis
    - ▲ Clinically confirmed by histology
    - ▲ Histology: full-thickness dysplasia, dysplastic keratinocytes
  - Treatment
    - ▲ Cryotherapy, laser, excision, topical retinoids, 5-fluorouracil 5% solution, imiquimod 5% cream (studies show this treatment has a lower recurrence rate than other treatments)
    - ▲ Premalignant and malignant diseases. Verrucous carcinoma (giant condyloma acuminata of Buschke and Lowenstein tumor)
  - Low-grade squamous cell carcinoma
  - Infection with HPV 6, HPV 11 (types not usually associated with malignancy)
  - Clinical
    - ▲ Large exophytic tumors up to several centimeters in diameter
    - ▲ Locally invasive and destructive
    - ▲ Rarely metastasize

- Treatment
  - ▲ Local excision
- Bowen disease
  - Some cases associated with HPV
  - Clinical
  - Insidious onset, lesions have a slow rate of growth and are minimally symptomatic
  - Slightly raised plaque (sometimes misdiagnosed as eczema) with an irregular border and the surface can be fissured with adherent scales
  - Diagnosis
    - ▲ Histopathology: full thickness dysplasia of squamous epithelium
  - Treatment
    - ▲ Excision, curettage, cryosurgery, topical 5-fluorouracil and/or imiquimod
- Erythroplasia of Queyrat
  - Penile Bowen disease
  - A squamous cell carcinoma in situ
  - Located on the glans under the foreskin of the uncircumcised penis
  - Clinical
    - ▲ Red plaques with a moist surface
    - ▲ Metastasis occurs in 10 to 30%
  - Diagnosis
    - ▲ Histopathology: same as Bowen above
  - Treatment
    - ▲ Excision, curettage, cryosurgery, topical 5-fluorouracil and/or imiquimod

Nongenital Mucosal Disease (Table 17-3)

- Oral focal epithelial hyperplasia (Heck disease)
- A rare disease
- HPV types 13 and 32
- Mostly affects the aboriginal population (i.e., Native American, Greenland, etc.)
- Focal epithelial hyperplasia
- Clinical
  - It affects the labial, lingual, and buccal mucosa
  - Multiple flat-topped or dome-shaped pink-white papules, 1 to 5 mm, some lesions coalesce into plaques

TABLE 17-3 Nongenital Mucosal Disease

	HPV Type
Oral focal epithelial hyperplasia (Heck disease)	13, 32
Oral carcinoma	16, 18
Oral leukoplakia	16, 18

- Diagnosis
  - Histology: hyperplastic mucosa with thin parakeratotic stratum corneum, acanthosis, blunting and anastomosis of rete ridges, pallor of epidermal cells as a result of intracellular edema
- Treatment
  - Surgical excision
  - Cryotherapy
  - Imiquimod 5% cream
  - Sulfonamides
  - Oral vitamin A

Treatments for HPV

- Topical agents
  - Salicylic acid
    - Over-the-counter treatment
    - Removes surface keratin
  - Cantharidin
    - Dried extract of the blister beetle
    - Causes epidermal necrosis and blistering
  - Dinitrochlorobenzene (DNCB)
    - Powerful sensitizing agent
    - Induces an allergic contact dermatitis
    - Causes local inflammation and an immune response
    - Reported mutagen
  - Dibutyl squaric acid
    - Contact sensitizer
    - Unlike DNCB, it is not a mutagen and therefore may be a safer alternative
  - Trichloroacetic acid
    - Caustic compound
    - Causes immediate superficial tissue necrosis
    - Concentrations up to 80%
    - May require weekly applications
  - Podophyllotoxin
    - Derived from the roots of the Indian podophyllum plant
    - Binds to tubulin and prevents microtubule assembly
    - Genital wart treatment: application twice daily for 3 consecutive days per week for up to 4 weeks
  - Fluorouracil (5FU)
    - Used primarily to treat actinic keratoses
    - Antimetabolite: fluorinated pyrimidine
    - Active form inhibits DNA synthesis by inhibiting the normal production of thymidine
    - Effective in treating warts when used under occlusion daily for up to 1 month
    - Teratogenic
  - Imiquimod 5% cream
    - Topical cream approved for treating genital warts; used for other HPV infections
    - Anogenital warts: treat at night, 3 times a week
    - Common warts: treat nightly under occlusion

    - Palmoplantar warts: treat nightly under occlusion, alternate with a keratolytic
    - Potent stimulator of proinflammatory cytokine release
    - Works best as part of combination therapy for nonanogenital warts
  - Cidofovir
    - Nucleotide analogue of deoxycytidine monophosphate
    - Used for refractory condyloma acuminata and recurrent genital herpes
    - Cidofovir gel applied once or twice daily
    - Must be compounded
  - Tretinoin
    - Disrupts epidermal growth and differentiation, thereby reducing the bulk of the wart
- Systemic agents
  - Cimetidine
  - Type 2 histamine receptor antagonist
  - Immunomodulatory effects
  - Variable results
  - 25 to 40 mg/kg 3 times daily × 3 months
- Intralesional injections
  - Bleomycin
    - Cytotoxic polypeptide that inhibits DNA synthesis in cells and viruses
    - Side effects of bleomycin include pain with injection, local urticaria, Raynaud phenomenon, and possible tissue necrosis
    - If used periungually, bleomycin may cause nail dystrophy or nail loss
  - Interferon-α
    - Recombinant version of naturally occurring cytokine with antiviral, anticancer, and immunomodulatory effects
    - Intralesional administration is more effective than systemic administration and is associated only with mild flu-like symptoms.
    - Treatments may be required for several weeks to months before beneficial results are seen. Use for warts that are resistant to standard treatments or use in combination therapy with surgery
- *Candida* antigen
  - Stimulates the acquisition of HPV immunity
  - Its application causes trauma and inflammatory reaction
- Cryosurgery: liquid nitrogen (−196°C) is the most effective method of cryosurgery
- Lasers
  - Carbon dioxide
    - Procedure can be painful and leave scarring
    - Risk of nosocomial infection also exists in health care workers because HPV can be isolated in the plume
  - Flashlamp-pumped pulse dye laser
    - Mixed results in treating warts
    - Decreased risk of scarring and transmission of HPV in the plume smoke
    - Electrodessication and curettage
    - May be more effective than cryosurgery
    - Painful
    - More likely to scar
    - HPV can be isolated from the plume
- Surgical excision: avoid using because of the risks of scarring and recurrence (or follow with interferon)

Human Herpes Viruses (HHVs)

- Most herpes viruses measure approximately 200 nm in diameter
- Enveloped, linear, double-stranded DNA virus
- Biological features unique to herpes viruses are latency and reactivation
- Transmission: direct exposure of mucous membranes or abraded skin to the lesions or mucosal secretions of an infected individual or respiratory droplets
- Eight main types
  - HHV 1: herpes simplex virus 1 (HSV-1): herpes labialis < genitalis
  - HHV 2: herpes simplex virus 2 (HSV-2): herpes genitalis < labialis
  - HHV 3: varicella-zoster virus (VZV): chickenpox/herpes zoster
  - HHV 4: Epstein-Barr virus (EBV): mononucleosis, Gianotti Crosti, Burkitt lymphoma, oral hairy leukoplakia
  - HHV 5: cytomegalovirus (CMV): retinitis in AIDS patients
  - HHV 6: roseola infantum (exanthem subitum)
  - HHV 7: possible pityriasis rosea
  - HHV 8: Kaposi sarcoma

Herpes Simplex Virus (HSV)

- Herpes simplex virus 1 (HSV-1)
  - Belongs to the family Herpesviridae
  - Humans are the only natural reservoirs, and no vectors are involved in transmission
  - Eighty percent of US adults are infected, 85% of adults infected worldwide
  - Ninety percent orofacial, 10% genital
  - Mode of transmission is by close personal contact
  - Viral properties
    - Neurovirulence: capacity to invade and replicate in the nervous system
    - Latency
      - ▲ Establishment and maintenance of latent infection in nerve cell ganglia
      - ▲ HSV-1 infection: trigeminal ganglia are involved most commonly

- ▲ Primary infection is subclinical (90%), gingivostomatitis (10%)
- ▲ In 40% of HSV-1 seropositive persons, recurrent herpes labialis usually recur 1 to 4 times per year
- ▲ Accounts for 30% of primary but less than 5% of recurrent genital HSV
- Reactivation
  - Induced by a variety of stimuli: fever, trauma, emotional stress, sunlight, menstruation
  - Recurrent infection and peripheral shedding of HSV
  - Occurs more frequently in the perioral rather than the genital region
  - More frequent and severe in immunocompromised patients
- Clinical
  - Gingivostomatitis
    - ▲ Abrupt onset
- Children aged 6 months to 5 years
- High fever (102–104°F)
- Anorexia and listlessness
- Gingivitis is the most striking feature
- Vesicular lesions develop on the oral mucosa, tongue, and/or lips and later rupture and coalesce, leaving ulcerated plaques
- Regional lymphadenopathy
- Acute herpetic pharyngotonsillitis
- Acute disease lasts 5 to 7 days
- Viral shedding may continue for 3 weeks
  - Herpes labialis (Fig. 17-9)
    - Most common manifestation of recurrent HSV-1
    - Prodrome of pain, burning, and tingling often occurs at the site where lesions develop
    - Clinical
    - Erythematous papules develop rapidly into tiny, thin-walled, intraepidermal vesicles that become pustular and ulcerate
    - Maximum viral shedding is in the first 24 hours of the acute illness but may last 5 days
  - Diagnosis
    - Histology: acantholysis, intraepidermal vesicle, ballooning and reticular degeneration, intranuclear eosinophilic inclusion bodies, multinucleated keratinocytes (not specific)
    - Viral culture
    - Polymerase chain reaction (PCR) techniques: detection of HSV DNA
    - Immunofluorescent staining of the tissue culture cells or of smear can quickly identify HSV and can distinguish between types 1 and 2
    - Antibody testing
    - Tzanck smear: multinucleated giant cells → nucleus divides but not cell; nuclear molding; does not distinguish between HSV2 and VZV
  - Treatment: see HSV-2 below
- Herpes simplex virus 2 (HSV-2) (Figs. 17-10, 17-11, and 17-12)
  - Primary genital herpes; asymptomatic in most patients
  - Causes 70% of primary, more than 95% of recurrent genital herpes
  - Women have 45% higher risk of infection compared to men
  - Primary infection asymptomatic: 75%
  - Ninety-five percent of asymptomatic females and males actively shed virus at some point in time
  - Eighty percent of transmission is secondary to asymptomatic shedding
  - Ninety percent have recurrences
  - Clinical

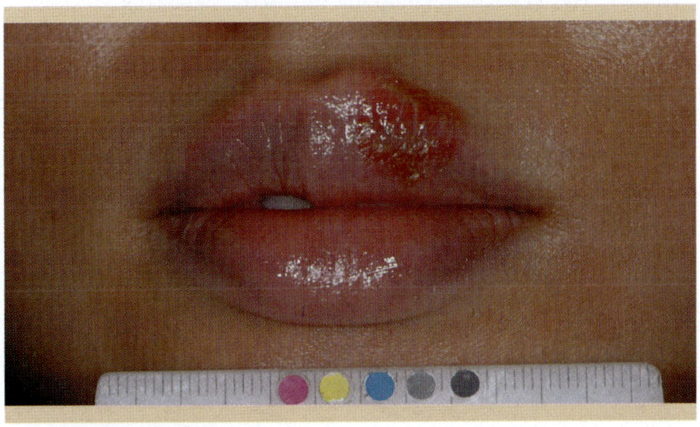

FIGURE 17-9 Herpes labialis. (*Used with permission from Dr. Stephen Tyring.*)

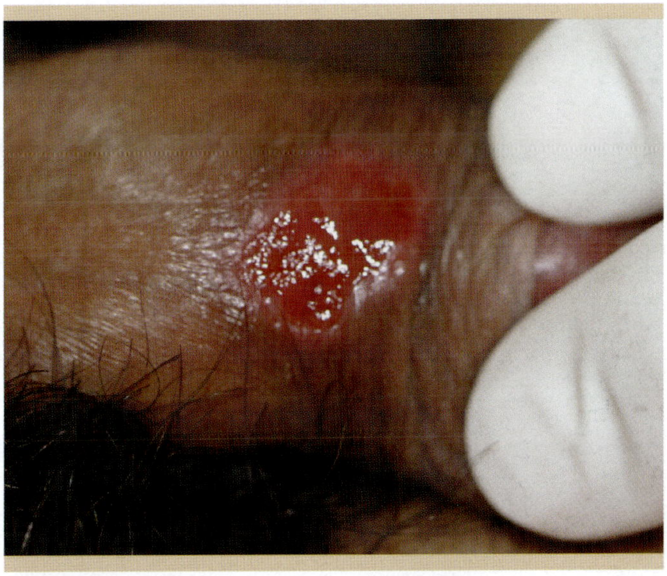

FIGURE 17-10 Primary genital herpes. (*Used with permission from Dr. Stephen Tyring.*)

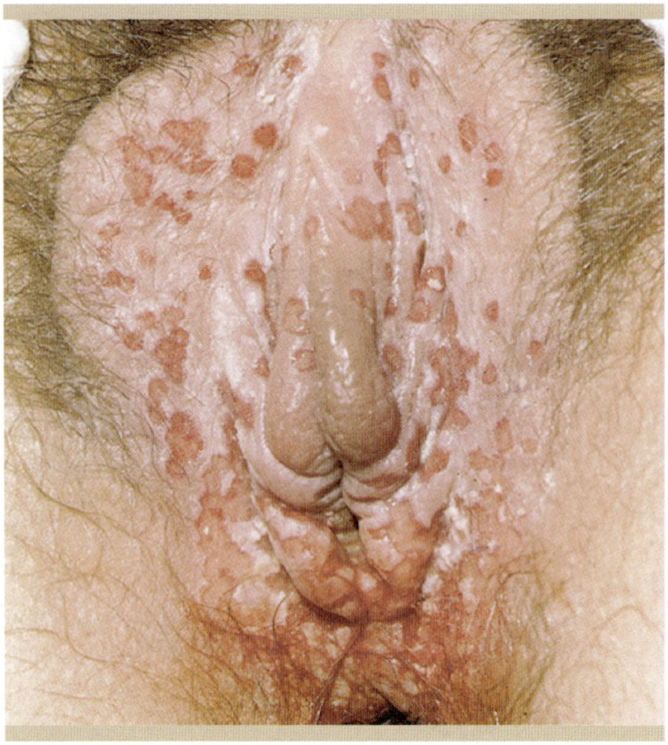

FIGURE 17-11 Genital herpes. (*Reprinted with permission from Wolff K, Johnson RA, Summond D:* Fitzpatrick's Color Atlas and Synopsis of Clinical Dermatology, *5th Ed. New York: McGraw-Hill; 2005.*)

- Incubation period is 3 to 7 days
- Cervical vesicles resulting in ulcers; can recur with or without external lesions
- Ulcerative lesions persist from 4 to 15 days
- Viral shedding lasts approximately 12 days

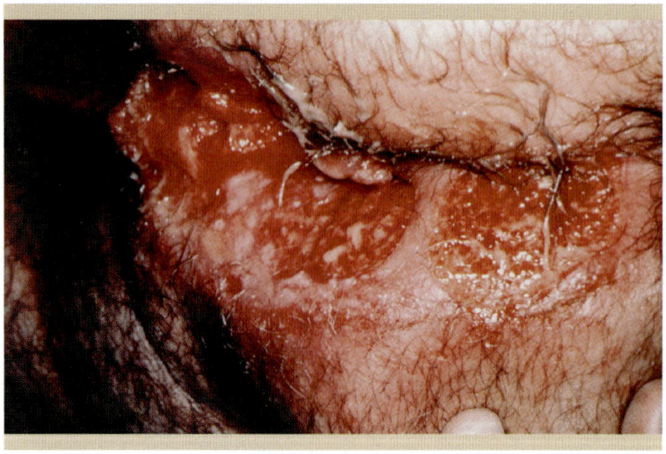

FIGURE 17-12 Herpes simplex type 2 (HSV-2). (*Used with permission from Dr. Stephen Tyring.*)

- Systemic complaints in more than 70% of primary HSV: fever, dysuria, malaise, lymphadenopathy; females greater than males
- Spread by sexual contact (1–2% days/year male, 6–8% female: asymptomatic transmission)

- Treatment
  - Acyclovir
    - ▲ First episode: 200 mg 5 times daily or 400 mg 3 times daily for 7 to 10 days
    - ▲ Recurrences: 200 mg PO 5 times daily or 400 mg 3 times daily for 5 days
    - ▲ Chronic suppressive therapy: 400 mg 2 times daily or 200 mg 3 to 5 times daily
  - Valacyclovir (Valtrex)
    - ▲ First episode: 1 g 2 times daily for 10 days
    - ▲ Recurrences: 500 mg twice daily for 3 days or 2 g 2 times daily for 1 day
    - ▲ Suppressive dosing for HSV: 500 mg to 1 g/d
  - Famciclovir (Famvir)
    - ▲ First episode: 250 mg 3 times daily for 10 days
    - ▲ Recurrences: 125 mg twice daily for 5 days or 1 g (for genital herpes) or 1.5 g once for herpes labialis)
    - ▲ Long-term suppression: 250 mg 2 times daily (70–80% effective in patients with ≥6 episodes per year)
- HSV in immunosuppressed patients
  - HIV: 95% coinfected with HSV-1/HSV-2 or both
  - Fifty-two percent of HIV infections are among people who also have HSV type 2
  - Clinical
    - Recurrent HSV may last much longer compared with immunocompetent hosts (> 30 days)
    - Chronic ulcerative HSV: persistent ulcers and erosions starting on the face or perineal region
    - Generalized acute mucocutaneous HSV: dissemination and fever after localized vesicular eruption
    - Systemic HSV: follows oral or genital lesions; areas of necrosis in the liver, adrenals, pancreas
  - Treatment of genital ulcers caused by HSV-2 with specific antivirals has been previously shown to reduce HSV-2 and HIV shedding
  - Acyclovir-resistant HSV in HIV patients (5–8%)
    - One percent cidofovir (compounded)
    - Foscarnet
      - ▲ Reversibly inhibits viral DNA polymerase
      - ▲ Does not need thymidine kinase
      - ▲ Side effects: penile ulcers, nephrotoxicity
- Other herpes manifestations
  - Herpetic whitlow
    - HSV of the fingers, occurs at or near the cuticle or at other sites associated with trauma
    - HSV-2 < HSV-1

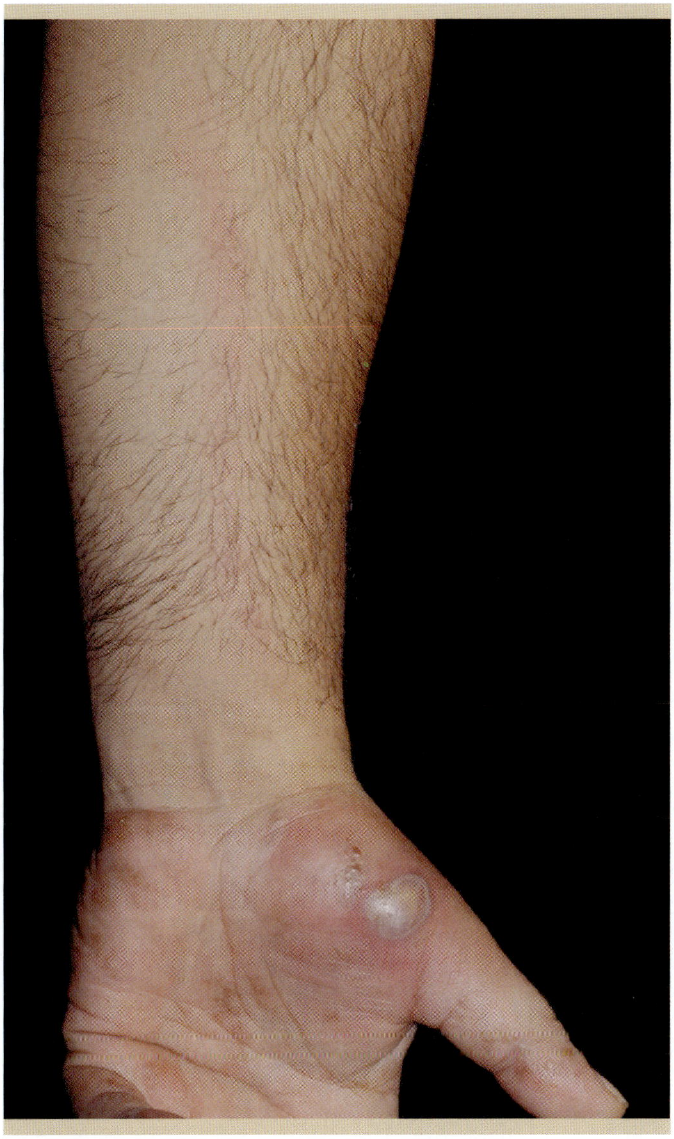

FIGURE 17-13 Herpes gladiatorum. (*Reprinted with permission from Wolff K, Johnson RA, Summond D:* Fitzpatrick's Color Atlas and Synopsis of Clinical Dermatology, *5th Ed. New York: McGraw-Hill; 2005.*)

- Herpes gladiatorum (Fig. 17-13)
  - Due to direct skin-to-skin contact among wrestlers
  - Scattered cutaneous HSV-1 lesions
- Herpes-associated erythema multiforme (EM)
  - Eighty percent of recurrent EM is thought to be associated with HSV reactivation
  - Multiple outbreaks of EM often associated with herpes reactivation
  - Pathogenesis may represent a delayed-type hypersensitivity reaction
  - Patients experience an average of 6 attacks annually, each episode lasting nearly 2 weeks
  - Self-limited

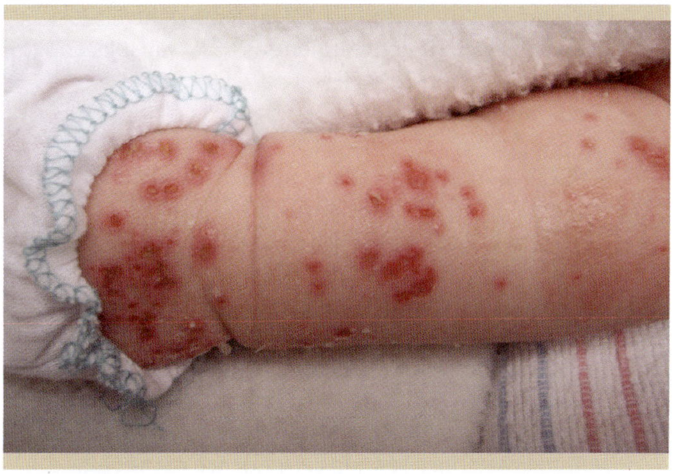

FIGURE 17-14 Eczema herpeticum. (*Used with permission from Dr. Adelaide Hebert.*)

- Herpetic keratoconjunctivitis
  - Recurrent erosions of the conjunctiva and cornea that can lead to blindness
- Lumbosacral HSV
  - Infection is typically asymptomatic but can cause sciatica
- Eczema herpeticum (Fig. 17-14)
  - Widespread HSV infection in patients with skin disorders such as atopic dermatitis, Darier disease, pemphigus, thermal burns, or Sézary syndrome
- HSV encephalitis (usually HSV-1)
  - Most common cause of sporadic encephalitis
  - Sudden onset of fever, headache, confusion, temporal lobe involvement
  - Seventy percent mortality if not treated
- Ramsay Hunt (usually VZV or HSV-1)
  - Infection of the facial nerve
  - Symptoms on the affected side typically include facial weakness and a painful herpes-type skin eruption on the pinna of the ear, and there is frequently vestibulocochlear disturbance
  - Recovery of facial movement occurs in about 50% of treated patients
- Congenital HSV
  - One in 3,500 vaginal births
- Transmission
  - Perinatal: 90%; congenital: 5 to 8%; few postnatal
  - Risk of transmission: 50% if mother has primary infection, 3 to 5% if mother has recurrent disease
  - Birth canal transmission: lesions usually on scalp, face; associated encephalitis, hepatoadrenal necrosis, pneumonia, death
  - If transmission in first 8 weeks, severe defects result

- If lesions on infant in first 10 days, mortality is 20%
- Mortality rate (if no treatment) is 65% transplacental, 80% HSV-2, and 20% HSV-1
- Treatment/prevention
  - Pregnancy
    - ▲ In infected females, initiate treatment at week 36 and continue until delivery:
      - △ Valacyclovir 1 g once daily
      - △ Famciclovir 250 mg twice daily
      - △ Acyclovir 400 mg twice or thrice daily or 200 mg 3 to 5 times daily
  - IV acyclovir for neonates: 30 mg/kg per day

- Varicella-zoster virus (human herpes virus 3 [HHV 3])
  - Approximately 98% of the adult population in the United States has serological evidence of previous infection
  - Causes chickenpox and herpes zoster
  - Chickenpox (Fig. 17-15)
    - Transmitted to others from the skin and respiratory tract
    - VZV remains dormant in sensory nerve ganglia after primary infection
    - Low-grade fever precedes skin manifestations by 1 to 2 days
    - Incubation period of about 2 weeks
    - Clinical
      - ▲ Prodromal symptoms include headache, myalgias, anorexia, nausea, and vomiting
      - ▲ Lesions: "dewdrops on a rose petal"; begin on face, scalp, trunk, with relative sparing of the extremities
    - Lesions start as red macules and pass through the stages of papule, vesicle, pustule, and eventually crust. Lesions are pruritic
    - Different stages of the rash are present simultaneously
    - Complications
      - ▲ Young immunocompetent individuals: secondary bacterial infection (*Staphylococcus aureus* or *Streptococcus pyogenes*) and scarring
      - ▲ Adults and immunocompromised patients: myelitis, large vessel granulomatous arteritis, encephalitis, varicella pneumonia, or varicella hepatitis
  - Congenital varicella syndrome
    - First 20 weeks of pregnancy: 2% risk of complications
    - Leads to intrauterine growth retardation, microcephaly, cortical atrophy, limb hypoplasia, microphthalmia, cataracts, chorioretinitis, cortical atrophy, and cutaneous scarring (areas of hypertrophic scarring with indurations and erythema located primarily on the extremities)
    - Perinatal infection occurs within 10 days of birth

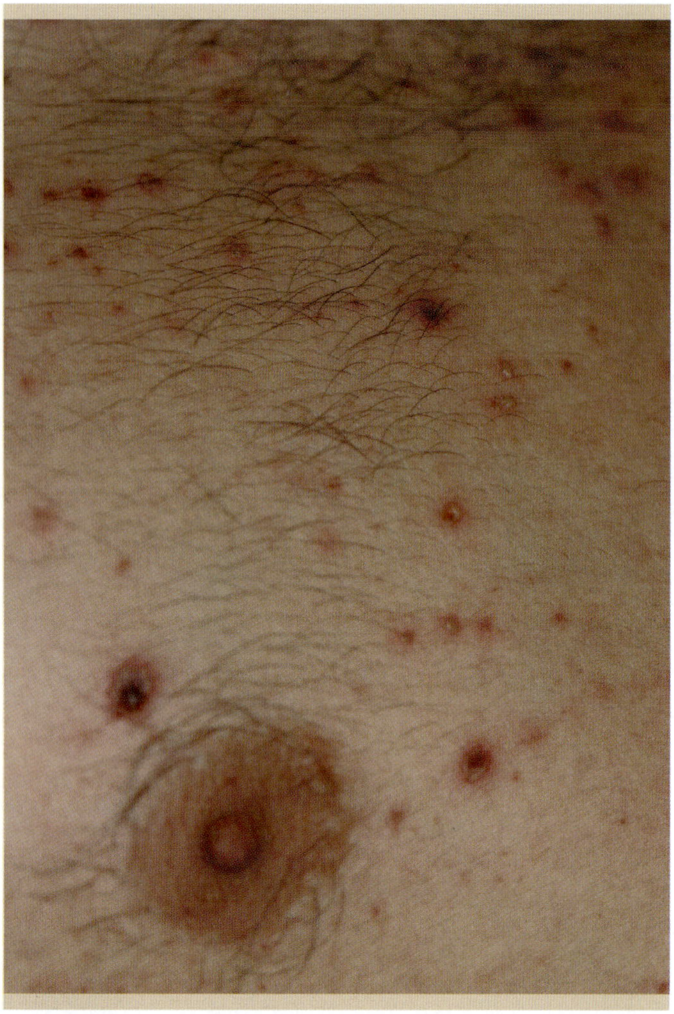

FIGURE 17-15 Chickenpox in adult. (*Used with permission from Dr. Adrian Motta.*)

    - If female gets VZV 5 days before or 2 days after delivery, the rate of mortality is 30%
  - Infantile zoster
    - Manifests within the first year
    - Maternal varicella infection after the 20th week of gestation
  - Neonatal varicella
    - Any infant with clinical or laboratory-confirmed varicella
    - Onset in the first month of life
      - ▲ Without features of varicella embryopathy
      - ▲ Infection may result from peripartum maternal infection or postnatal exposure
    - Treatment
      - ▲ Healthy children do not necessarily require acyclovir, but treatment allows them to return to school sooner
      - ▲ Acyclovir: 20 mg/kg; given orally 4 times daily for 5 to 7 days

        - Avoid aspirin to prevent Reye syndrome
        - Symptomatic care
        - Adults
            - Acyclovir, famciclovir, valacyclovir at herpes zoster doses
            - Most effective if it is started within the first 72 hours after development of vesicles
    - Varicella vaccine
        - Two doses, at 12 months and 4 to 6 years of age
        - Seroconversion: adolescents and adults have a 78% conversion rate after the first dose and 99% after the second dose
- Zoster (shingles) (Fig. 17-16)
    - Due to reactivation of latent VZV in sensory ganglion (20% incidence unless immunocompromised)
    - Incidence: 66% of cases occur in patients older than 50 years
    - Clinical
        - Rash preceded by prodrome: fever, malaise, headache, localized pain in the involved dermatome
        - Constitutional symptoms develop initially
        - Rash is in a unilateral dermatomal distribution with erythema, vesicles, pustules, and crusting
        - Contagious until crusted
        - Hutchinson sign: zoster on tip of nose (ophthalmic nerve, nasociliary division), could result in herpetic keratitis
    - Complications
        - Postherpetic neuralgia (PHN)
            - Pain following resolution of skin lesions; occurs in 10 to 15% of patients; Resolution rate is 50% by 3 months, 75% by 1 year
            - Occurs in 60% of patients older than 60 years
        - Zoster sine herpete: segmental pain without lesions
        - Ophthalmic zoster: ocular disease (20–70% of cases with V-1 Zoster), cicatricial lid retraction, ptosis, keratitis, scleritis, uveitis, secondary glaucoma, oculomotor palsies, chorioretinitis, optic neuritis, panophthalmitis
        - CNS (central nervous system) zoster: has asymptomatic cerebrospinal fluid (CSF) changes
        - Primary varicella pneumonia: 14%, higher rate in adults and immunocompromised patients
        - Reye syndrome: acute fetal encephalopathy associated with fatty degeneration of the liver, associated with aspirin treatment
        - Bacterial superinfections: usually due to *S. aureus*
        - Acute cerebellar ataxia: unsteady gait 11 to 20 days following rash

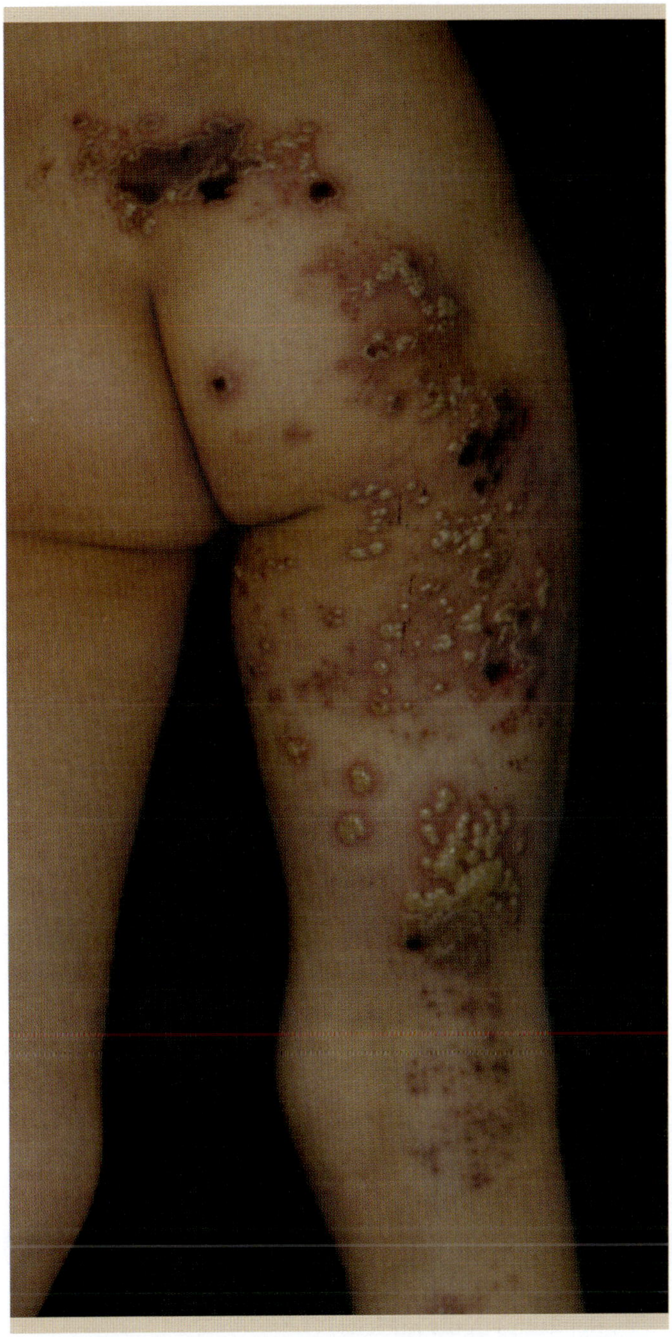

FIGURE 17-16 Zoster (shingles). (*Used with permission from Dr. Adriana Motta.*)

        - Guillian-Barré syndrome
            - Acute idiopathic polyneuritis
            - Encephalitis with headache, fever, photophobia, nausea, vomiting, and nerve palsies
            - Motor paralysis (1–5%), extension from sensory ganglion to anterior horn, first 2 to 3 weeks
            - Ramsay Hunt: facial palsy secondary to herpes-zoster infection of facial (VII) and

auditory (VIII) nerves; affects external ear, tympanic membrane; causes tinnitus, vertigo, deafness, otalgia, loss of taste
- Diagnosis
  - ▲ Nonspecific tests
    - △ Tzanck smear: multinucleated giant cells, nuclear molding
    - △ Histology: intraepidermal vesicles, balloon degeneration, reticular degeneration, inclusion bodies, margination of chromatin, vascular involvement (75% VZV)
  - ▲ Specific tests
    - △ Viral culture
    - △ PCR
  - ▲ Treatment
    - △ Acyclovir: 800 mg 5 times daily for 7 days
    - △ Valacyclovir: 1 g 3 times daily for 7 days
    - △ Famciclovir: 500 mg 3 times daily for 7 days
    - △ Pain and pruritus: analgesics, oral antipruritics, calamine lotion, cool compresses
- Treatment of PHN
  - ▲ Non-narcotic or narcotic analgesic
  - ▲ Pregabalin 50 mg 3 times daily or 75 mg twice daily
  - ▲ Gabapentin 300 to 600 mg 3 times daily
  - ▲ Gabapentin extended release recently approved (Gralise) 1800 mg daily
  - ▲ Capsaicin cream
  - ▲ Topical lidocaine gel or patch
  - ▲ Tricyclic antidepressants: (amitriptyline, maprotiline, desipramine)
  - ▲ Anticonvulsants: carbamazepine, gabapentin, pregabalin
  - ▲ Sympathetic nerve blockade
  - ▲ Steroids: methylprednisolone
  - ▲ Transcutaneous electrical stimulation
- Vaccine (Zostavax, Merck): to increase immunity in persons seropositive for VZV in order to decrease risk of zoster. FDA approved for 50 years and older

- **Epstein-Barr virus** (human herpes virus 4 [HHV 4])
  - Double-stranded DNA virus
  - Replicates in the nucleus
  - Primarily infects B-lymphocytes
  - After acute infection, EBV persists as a latent infection for life
  - Clinical
    - Infectious mononucleosis (IM)
      - ▲ Delayed primary infection with EBV
      - ▲ Young adults are typically affected and a small percentage of children and older adults contract the disease
      - ▲ Clinical
        - △ IM can be asymptomatic or have nonspecific symptoms; the incubation period varies from 4 to 6 weeks
        - △ More frequent symptoms are a triad of fever, sore throat, and lymphadenopathy (5–15%)
        - △ Rash: maculopapular (3–15% of patients)
        - △ Eighty percent of patients have rash if treated with amoxicillin or ampicillin
        - △ The resolution of the illness occurs between week 5 and 10
  - Diagnosis: see Diagnosis of EBV on p. 313
  - Treatment: supportive care, antipyretics, analgesics, topical steroids for cutaneous manifestations. Prednisone for complications such as hemolytic anemia, thrombocytopenia, or lymphadenopathy that compromises the airway
    - Gianotti-Crosti (infantile papular acrodermatitis)
      - ▲ Self-limited cutaneous response to viral infections with worldwide distribution
      - ▲ Most often in young children (between 6 months and 14 years of age)
      - ▲ Clinical
        - △ Upper respiratory syndrome
        - △ Mild systemic compromise such as low-grade fever
        - △ Inguinal and axillary lymphadenopathy and hepatosplenomegaly
        - △ Symmetric cutaneous lesions appear abruptly: exanthem with monomorphous, edematous, pink-red papules or papulovesicles, slightly pruritic and can become confluent lichenoid papules that spare the trunk
        - △ Located on cheeks, buttocks, and extensor surface of the extremities
        - △ Also associated with hepatitis B, adenovirus, CMV
        - △ Spontaneous resolution within 3 to 4 weeks
        - △ Treatment: supportive measures
    - Oral hairy leukoplakia
      - ▲ Benign EBV infection of oral mucosa epithelial cells
      - ▲ Usually associated with immunocompromised patients
      - ▲ Prevalence of the disease amongst immunocompromised patients varies between 3 and 11%
      - ▲ Secondary nonmalignant hyperplasia of epithelial cells
      - ▲ Clinical
        - △ Location: lateral and dorsolateral parts of the tongue
        - △ Flat lesion with white corrugate vertical folds or ridges that cannot be scraped off
        - △ Self-limited course with resolution within months in immunocompromised persons

- Diagnosis
  - Made clinically; confirmed with biopsy
  - Histology: hyperplasia, parakeratosis, acanthosis, and papillated epithelial surfaces. EBV detected within ballooned and nonballoned cells of the prickle cell layer and the keratinized cells of the superficial epithelium
- Kikuchi syndrome
  - Benign, self-limiting disease that resolves spontaneously within 1 to 4 months of onset
  - More common in Asia and usually affects young women in their late 20s and early 30s
  - Pathology is suggestive of hyperimmune reaction to an infectious agent causing regional lymph node enlargement
  - Clinical
    - Fever and leukopenia (50%), cervical lymphadenopathy
    - Mucocutaneous (16–40%) lesions: facial erythema, erythematous papules, plaques, nodules, cutaneous ulcers, and oral mucosal ulcers
  - Diagnosis
    - Histology: histiocytic aggregates, atypical lymphoid cells, karyorrhectic debris, and patchy necrosis
- Plasmablastic lymphoma
  - Recently discovered AIDS-related non-Hodgkin lymphoma associated with chronic EBV infection
  - Usually affects the oral cavity, especially the gingival mucosa, hard palate, and soft palate
  - Infiltrates the mucosal surface, the adjacent bone, and finally the bone marrow, which usually occurs during therapy
  - Clinical
    - Similar to Kaposi sarcoma: painful, purple-red mass in the oral cavity, usually the gingival mucosa
    - Prognosis is poor with death occurring between 1 and 24 months after diagnosis
- Burkitt lymphoma
  - Highly aggressive and poorly differentiated B-cell lymphoma with a high proliferative rate
  - EBV genome can be detected in tumor cells
  - Two types described (*i*) the endemic, or African BL (most often associated with EBV infection), and (*ii*) the sporadic
  - BL arises in the lymph nodes, nasopharyngeal mucosa, and the gastrointestinal (GI) tract
  - Cutaneous involvement is rare, only a few cases reported
  - Skin lesions include erythematous firm nodules in connection with the involved lymph node
- Nasopharyngeal carcinoma
  - Lymphoepithelial carcinoma with distinct histological types characterized by either squamous, nonkeratinizing, or undifferentiated epithelial cells
  - Prevalent disease in southern China and Southeast Asia
  - Patients have high levels of antibodies to EBV antigens
  - EBV genome is present in nasopharyngeal carcinoma cells
- Diagnosis of EBV
  - Leukocytosis
  - Lymphocytosis
  - Elevated liver function tests
  - Heterophile antibody test
    - Polyclonal secretion of antibodies by infected B cells
    - Heterophile test: nonspecific antibodies that agglutinate horse or sheep erythrocytes; heterophile antibodies may persist for 3 months after onset of illness

- Monospot test: measures acute infectious mononucleosis heterophile antibodies in a rapid qualitative fashion
- EBV serology
  - Major viral antigens
    - Latent = EBNA → EBV nuclear antigens
    - Early = EADR → early antigen, diffuse restricted
    - Late = VCA → viral capsid antigen, MA → membrane antigen
- Treatment
  - Most EBV infections are self-limited; treat symptomatically
  - Oral hairy leukoplakia: acyclovir 400 mg 5 times daily

- **Cytomegalovirus (CMV)** (human herpes virus 5 [HSV-5])
  - Enveloped double-stranded DNA virus restricted to humans
  - Transmitted through infectious secretions
  - In developing countries, 100% of the population is seropositive, and 50% in developed countries
  - Latent infection in the host occurs after infection
  - Clinical
    - Primary infection
      - Usually asymptomatic in immunocompetent subjects
      - When symptomatic, it is called CMV mononucleosis syndrome
        - Fever, fatigue and less commonly lymphadenopathy, sore throat, and organomegaly
        - One-third have a maculopapular generalized rash

- Primary infection in pregnant women
  - Occurs during the first trimester: rate of transmission is 40%
  - Most common congenital viral infection (1% of U.S. infants)
  - A threat to the fetus
  - Congenital malformations: CNS injury, sensorineural hearing loss, growth retardation, microcephaly, cerebral atrophy, periventricular calcifications, chorioretinitis, thrombocytopenia, and hepatosplenomegaly
  - Cutaneous manifestations: jaundice, purpuric macules, and papules (secondary to persistent hematopoiesis—"blueberry muffin baby")
- Immunocompromised patients
  - Retinitis, hepatitis, and colitis
  - Skin lesions: vary from vesicles to verrucous plaques, and ulcerations in the perianal area
- Complications
  - CMV pneumonia (19%)
  - Mononucleosis-like syndrome after treatment with ampicillin or amoxicillin
  - Guillain-Barré syndrome
  - Bone marrow transplant patients have highest mortality (85%) secondary to pneumonia
  - Four times higher mortality rate than for solid-organ transplant
- In pregnant women, after the first trimester, hepatitis, pneumonia, purpura, and DIC may occur
- HIV and CMV: retinitis is the most common symptom
- Diagnosis
  - Histology: vasculitis, "owl's eyes": basophilic intranuclear inclusions
  - CMV antibodies
  - Antigenemia
  - Shell vial assay
- Treatment
  - Ganciclovir: drug of choice for treatment of CMV disease
  - Valganciclovir, prodrug of ganciclovir
  - Foscarnet: treats virus that is resistant to ganciclovir and valganciclovir
  - Cidofovir: treatment of refractory CMV retinitis
  - Fomivirsen

- Human herpes virus 6 (HHV 6): roseola infantum (exanthema subitum/sixth disease) (Fig. 17-17)
  - Enveloped DNA virus
  - Spread by oropharyngeal secretions
  - Most common childhood exanthem
  - Clinical
    - Occurs most commonly in children aged 6 months to 2 years
    - Incubation: 5 to 15 days
    - Spread of infection during the febrile and viremic phase of the illness

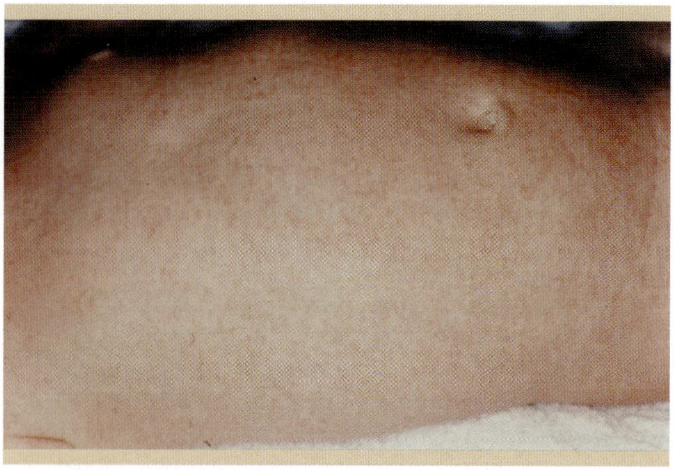

FIGURE 17-17 Roseola infantum. (*Used with permission from Dr. Stephen Tyring.*)

    - Abrupt onset with high fever (102.2–105.8°F)
    - Bulging anterior fontanelle, tonsillar and pharyngeal inflammation, tympanic injection, and lymph node enlargement
    - Fever defervesces on the fourth day, coinciding with onset of a rash
    - Rash: starts on trunk and may spread to neck and upper and lower extremities
    - Pink macules: 2 to 5 mm
    - May present with upper respiratory infection, adenopathy, CNS involvement, intussusception, thrombocytic purpura, palpebral edema (Berliner sign, "heavy eyelids") and periorbital edema and mononucleosis like (as in adults). Seizures (6–15%) during the febrile phase
    - Course: no sequelae generally observed
    - HIV + HHV 6: tropism for CD4+ cells; upregulation of CD4 expression, which is needed by the gp120 unit of HIV to infect cells
    - Bone marrow transplant patients: idiopathic bone marrow suppression secondary to virus
  - Diagnosis
    - PCR
    - Treatment
    - Symptomatic; a few case reports describe foscarnet and/or ganciclovir to be successful, but dosages are not known
- Human herpes virus 7 (HHV 7)
  - Significant homology with HHV 6
  - No clinical disease has been definitively linked to HHV 7; with questionable relationship to pityriasis rosea
  - Eighty-five percent of adults are seropositive, and most infections develop within the first 5 years of life
  - Transmitted through saliva

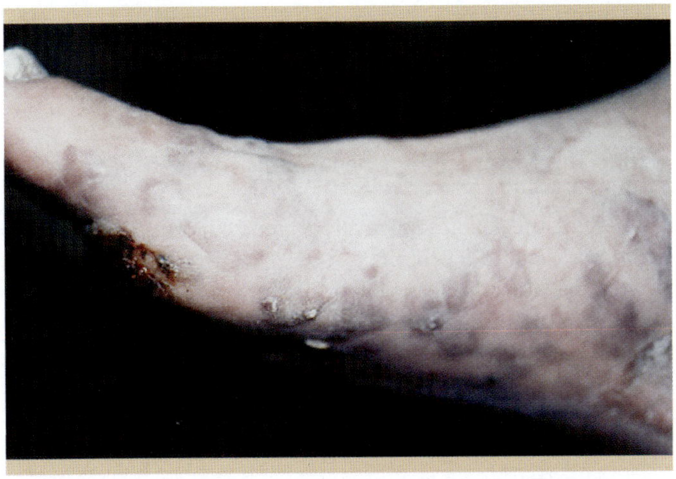

FIGURE 17-18 Kaposi sarcoma (classic). (*Used with permission from Dr. Stephen Tyring.*)

- Diagnosis
  - Serology
- Treatment
  - Symptomatic

- Human herpes virus 8 (HHV 8): Kaposi sarcoma (KS) (Figs. 17-18 and 17-19)
  - Malignancy of lymphatic endothelial cells associated with HHV 8
  - Four types
    - Endemic African KS: 50% of all childhood soft tissue tumors, usually an aggressive course
    - Epidemic AIDS-related KS: patients with advanced HIV infection
    - Immunocompromised (iatrogenic) KS: patients receiving immunosuppressive therapy; visceral involvement
    - Classic KS: sporadic and slowly progressive in 50- to 70-year-old men of Mediterranean and Eastern European background
  - Clinical
    - Brown, pink, red, or violaceous macules/patches, papules/plaques, nodules. The lesions can vary depending upon the clinical variant
    - Mucous membrane, cutaneous and visceral involvement is common (lymph nodes, GI tract, and lungs)
  - Diagnosis
    - Biopsy: spindle cells, prominent slit-like vascular spaces, and extravasated red blood cells
  - Treatment
    - Antiretroviral therapy for epidemic AIDS-related KS
    - Solitary KS lesions may be excised surgically or removed using laser surgery for patients with single lesions
    - Radiation

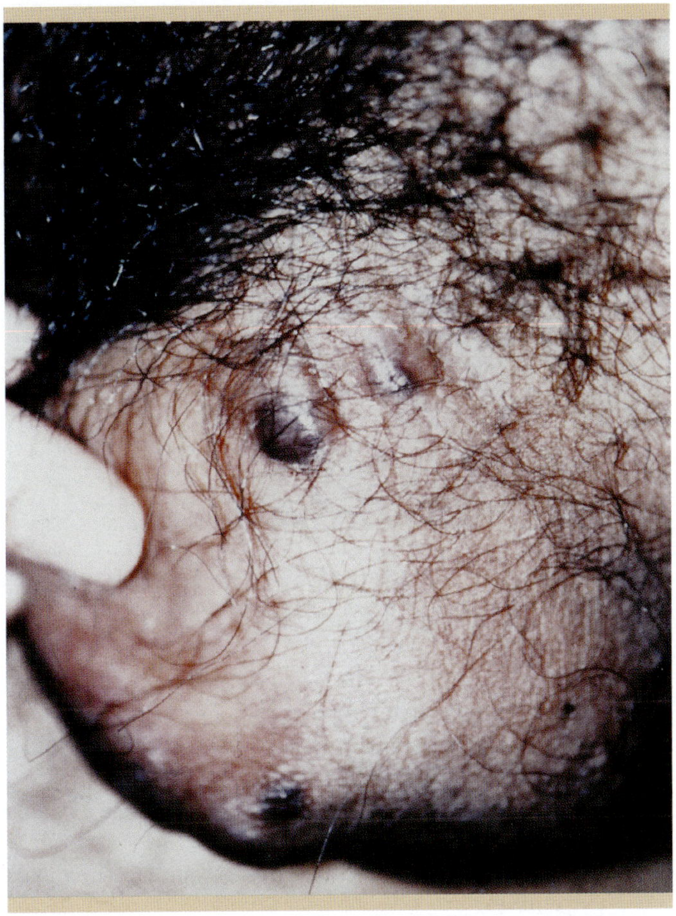

FIGURE 17-19 Kaposi sarcoma (scrotal in patient with AIDS). (*Used with permission from Dr. Stephen Tyring.*)

    - Combination of topical retinoids, intralesional vinblastine, interferon-α and chemotherapy: liposomal doxorubicin, liposomal daunorubicin, vincristine, vinblastine, bleomycin, and paclitaxel

- Herpes virus B: herpes simiae
  - Macaque herpes virus that is occasionally transmitted to humans from a bite, scratch, or open wound
  - Neurotropic: remains latent in ganglia
  - Clinical
    - In humans: initial local erythema, vesicular eruption with constitutional symptoms
    - Death secondary to encephalitis; very high mortality rate
- Treatment: nucleoside analogues (e.g., intravenous acyclovir)

Parvoviruses

PARVOVIRUS B19: "SLAPPED CHEEKS," FIFTH DISEASE, ERYTHEMA INFECTIOSUM (FIG. 17-20)

- Single-stranded DNA erythrovirus
- Tropism for rapidly dividing erythrocyte precursors

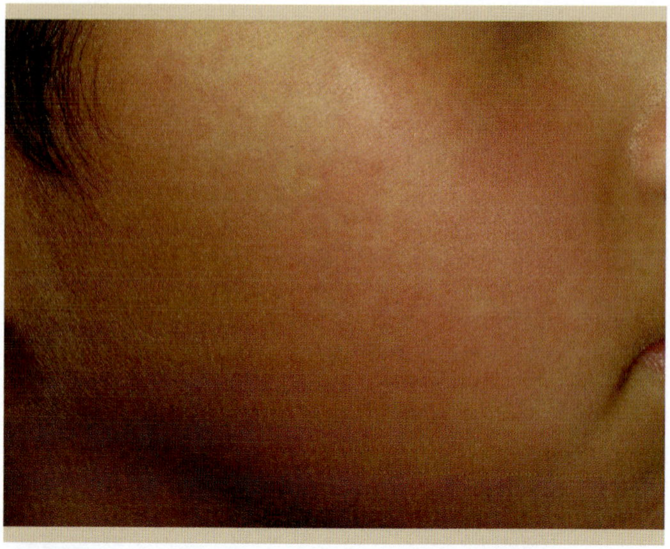

FIGURE 17-20 Parvovirus B19. ("slapped cheeks"). (*Used with permission from Dr. Stephen Tyring.*)

- Clinical
  - Twenty percent are asymptomatic
  - Headache, coryza, and low-grade fever about 2 days prior to the onset of the rash
  - Characterized by a "slapped cheek" appearance of the face on the first day
  - Erythematous, lacy macular eruption on the trunk and extremities
  - After rash fades, a lacy marble-like pattern to the skin appears: not contagious at this stage
  - Eruption can last 5 to 9 days and can recur for weeks or months with triggers such as sunlight, exercise, temperature change, bathing, and emotional stress
  - Headache, pharyngitis, fever, malaise, myalgias, arthralgias, coryza, diarrhea, nausea, cough, and conjunctivitis
  - Papular-pruritic "gloves-and-socks" syndrome: Erythematous exanthem of the hands and feet with a distinct margin at the wrist and ankle joints is present along with pain and edema
  - Complications: aplastic crisis in patients with increased red blood cell turnover, chronic anemia in immunocompromised persons, patients with chronic hemolytic anemia, fetal hydrops, sickle cell anemia, G6PD deficiency, and β-thalassemia
- Diagnosis
  - Parvovirus serology (IgM and IgG) can be determined
  - PCR
  - Complete blood count (CBC): low reticulocyte count (0–1%)
- Treatment
  - Ibuprofen or acetaminophen for fever (to prevent Reye syndrome: aspirin use is contraindicated)
  - Red blood cell (RBC) transfusions for aplastic crisis

Hepadna Viruses

Hepatitis B

- Hepadna virus
- Partially double-stranded circular DNA
- Encodes 4 overlapping open reading frames as follows:
  - S for the surface or envelope gene encoding the pre-S1, pre-S2, and S protein
  - C for the core gene, encoding for the core nucleocapsid protein and the e antigen
  - X for the X gene encoding the X protein
  - P for the polymerase gene, encoding a large protein promoting priming, RNA-dependent and DNA-dependent DNA polymerase and RNase H activities
- Transmitted sexually, perinatally, and through contact with body fluids
- Clinical
  - Incubation approximately 75 days
  - Prodromal or preicteric phase: serum sickness–like; develops in 20 to 30% of patients: arthropathy, proteinuria, hematuria
  - Icteric phase: jaundice (10 days after the appearance of constitutional symptomatology and lasts for 1 to 3 months), nausea, vomiting, and pruritus
  - Skin: urticaria/vasculitis secondary to perivascular deposition of immune complexes, hepatitis B + C3, IgM, or IgG
  - Associated conditions
    - Transient hypocomplementemia associated with urticaria
    - Polyarthritis nodosa: associated with arthralgias, fever, malaise, renal disease, nodules
    - Globulinemia: associated with chronic HBV, purpura, arthropathy, renal disease, necrotizing vasculitis, with mixed IgG and IgM
    - Others: erythema nodosum, urticaria, lichen planus, leukocytoclastic vasculitis, Gianotti-Crosti syndrome
    - Diagnosis
    - Active hepatitis B: high levels of alanine aminotransferase (ALT) and aspartate aminotransferase (AST); HBsAg (Australian antigen) and HBeAg (marker of infectivity) identified in the serum; HBcAb (IgM)
    - Chronic inactive hepatitis B: HBsAg, HBcAb of IgG type, and HBeAb also are present in the serum
    - Chronic active hepatitis B: mild to moderate elevation of the aminotransferases
- Treatment
  - Interferon-α
  - Lamivudine
  - Adefovir dipivoxil, entecavir, telbivudine, among others
  - Hepatitis B vaccine available

RNA VIRUSES

1. Picornavirus
2. Paramyxovirus
3. Togavirus
4. Flavivirus
5. Retrovirus
6. Arenavirus: Lassa fever, Argentine hemorrhagic fever, and related viruses
7. Bunyavirus: ssRNA enveloped viruses, sandfly fever virus and Hantaan virus

Picornaviruses

- Nonenveloped (naked virions)
- Size range of 20 to 25 nm
- Capsids composed of 4 different proteins
- Genome is single-stranded (ss) RNA
- Size range of 7,500 to 8,500 nucleotides
- Three major human genera
  - Rhinoviruses
  - Hepatovirus: hepatitis A virus (HAV)
  - Enteroviruses
  - Poliovirus
  - Coxsackie virus
  - Echovirus

ENTEROVIRUSES

- These are distinguished by other members of the Picornaviruses by its stability at low pH levels
  - Hand, foot, and mouth Disease (Fig. 17-21)
    - Etiology
      - ▲ Coxsackie A-16: most common
      - ▲ Enterovirus 71: causes CNS involvement
      - ▲ Primarily affects children age 3 to 10
    - Transmission (highly contagious)
      - ▲ Oral-oral
      - ▲ Oral-fecal
    - Clinical
      - ▲ Incubation period: 3 to 6 days
      - ▲ Prodrome enanthem: fever, malaise, abdominal pain
      - ▲ Oral ulcerative lesions
        - △ Location: hard palate, tongue, and buccal mucosa
        - △ Two to ten lesions develop over 5 to 10 days; vesicles on an erythematous base
      - ▲ Cutaneous lesions
        - △ Tender, elliptical, erythematous macules with a gray center, vesicles are surrounded by a red areola
        - △ Run parallel to skin lines
        - △ Few hundred lesions, peripherally distributed: hands, feet, and buttocks

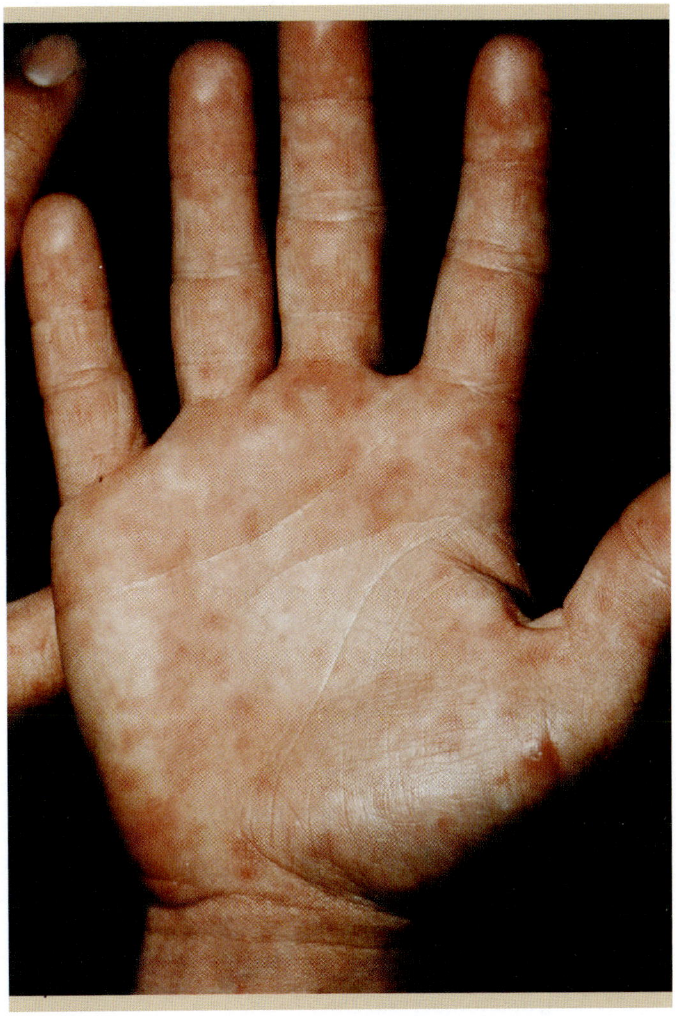

FIGURE 17-21 Hand, foot, and mouth disease. (*Used with permission from Dr. Stephen Tyring.*)

        - △ Hands < feet
        - △ Resolves spontaneously after 2 to 3 days without complications
    - Diagnosis: isolation and identification of virus in cell culture
      - ▲ Histology
        - △ Intraepidermal blister: neutrophils, monocytes, necrotic roof
        - △ Intercellular edema (reticular edema/ balloon degeneration)
        - △ Edematous dermis
        - △ Intracytoplasmic particles in a crystalline array
      - ▲ Cell culture
        - △ Detection of enterovirus RNA via PCR of blood, stool, and pharyngeal vesicles
        - △ Stool is least specific because children are able to excrete Enterovirus for up to 8 weeks in feces from a previous infection

- Treatment: symptomatic
- Herpangina
  - Transmission: fecal-oral route
  - Etiology
    - ▲ Coxsackieviruses A 1 to 10, 16, or 22
  - Clinical manifestations
    - ▲ Incubation period typically is 7 to 14 days
    - ▲ Mucus membrane lesions
    - ▲ 1 to 2 mm, gray/white papulovesicular lesions, with an erythematous surrounding
    - ▲ Location: soft palate tonsillar pillars, faucets, uvula
    - ▲ Sudden onset of fever, headache, sore throat, back/extremity pain
    - ▲ Exanthem: not distinctive in appearance for clinical diagnosis
  - Treatment: self-limited

Hepatovirus

- Hepatitis A
  - Transmission: fecal-oral route
  - Affects children and adults—commonly seen in daycare, schools, and restaurants
  - Pathogenesis
    - Viral replication within the hepatocyte's cytoplasm causes a noncytopathic infection
    - CD8 + T lymphocytes and natural killer cells that are HAV specific assist in destruction of the infected hepatocytes leading to hepatocellular injury
    - As a result, the host's immune system ultimately causes damage to the liver
  - Clinical manifestations
    - Incubation period: 2 to 7 weeks
    - Children: acute infection is self-limited
      - ▲ Symptoms include fever, malaise, vomiting, diarrhea, abdominal pain, mild hepatomegaly
      - ▲ Jaundice is seen via serological detection 1 week after onset
      - ▲ During prodrome period, there is an elevation of aminotranferase levels
    - Adults: symptomatic for several weeks up to 6 months
      - ▲ Eighty percent present with hepatomegaly
      - ▲ Seventy percent present with jaundice
      - ▲ Less then 1% progress to fulminant hepatic failure, often in patients with underlying liver disease
      - ▲ Approximately 11% of cases manifest as a transient, discrete, maculopapular, urticarial, or petechial rash
      - ▲ Rarely, persistent hepatitis A develops into a globulinemia with cutaneous vasculitis
  - Diagnosis
    - HAV RNA detection of stool, body fluids, and liver tissue
    - **GOLD STANDARD** for acute disease: serum IgM anti HAV; the antibody is positive at onset of symptoms, peaks during the convalescent phase, and stays detectable for up to 6 months after
  - Treatment: mild self-limited disease
    - Prophylactic treatment: hepatitis A vaccine now recommended for
      - ▲ All kids 12 to 23 months of age
      - ▲ All international travelers
      - ▲ Patients with chronic liver disease
      - ▲ Patients with clotting factor disorders
    - Combination vaccine for the prevention of hepatitis A and hepatitis B virus has been approved

Paramyxovirus

- Spherical
- Enveloped virus
- ssRNA

Rubeola/Measles

- Most contagious virus known
- Responsible for almost 1 million deaths worldwide
- Clinical syndromes divided into 3 categories
  - Typical
  - Modified: partially immune host, clinical signs are milder with longer incubation period
  - Atypical: infection of host previously immunized with killed virus vaccine
- Suspected case of rubeola is reportable by law for outbreak prevention
- Clinical manifestations
  - Incubation
    - Initiated with viral entry via conjunctivae or respiratory mucosa
    - Initial viremia: local replication and dissemination through lymphatic system and reticuloendothelial system
    - Experience brief respiratory symptoms, or morbilliform rash, many are asymptomatic
    - Length: 10 to 14 days
  - Prodrome
    - Second viremia occurs several days postincubation period
    - Three Cs of measles: cough, coryza, and conjunctivitis
    - Low-grade fever (101°F), malaise, anorexia
    - Length: 2 to 8 days
    - Enanthem: pathognomonic
      - ▲ Koplik spots: described as "grains of salt on a red background"
        - △ 1 to 3 mm white, gray, bluish elevations with erythematous base located on buccal and labial mucosa, adjacent to the molars
      - ▲ Appear 24 hours before exanthem

- Exanthem
  - Nonpruritic, erythematous maculopapular rash with cephalocaudal progression
  - Rash begins postauricular, progresses across face, down the trunk as upper rash fades
  - Rarely involves palms and soles
  - Erupts 5 days postprodrome, improvement of symptoms within 2 days of onset
  - Length: within 5 days, rash fades becoming nonblanching, copper-colored, followed by a fine desquamation
  - Measles is highly contagious from 4 days pre-exanthem until 4 days postexanthem
- Complications: more than 3 days postexanthema indicates a complication
  - Thrombocytopenic purpura
  - Tracheobronchitis: with involvement of upper respiratory tract
  - Otitis media and pneumonia from the secondary bacterial infection
  - Reactivation of tuberculosis: secondary to effect on cellular immunity
  - Neurological syndromes
    - Subacute sclerosing panencephalitis (SSPE): progressive degenerative disease of the CNS
      - ▲ Presents 7 to 10 years postinfection
      - ▲ Risk factor (50%): development of measles before age 2
    - Postinfectious encephalomyelitis: autoimmune-related demyelinating disease that appears within weeks of exanthem
      - ▲ Symptoms: fever, headache, seizures, confusion, coma
      - ▲ CSF analysis: pleocytosis, high protein level
- Diagnosis
  - Viral isolation in tissue culture
  - Serology
    - Standard test for confirmation: serum IgM
    - Antimeasles IgM detectable 3 days after appearance of rash, undetectable more than 30 days postexanthem
  - Hemagglutination-inhibiting antibodies: ELISA used to find antibodies from blood sample on filter paper
- Histology
  - Giant cell inclusions seen in nasopharyngeal, conjunctival, and buccal epithelial cells
  - Multinucleated giant cells
    - Warthin-Finkeldey cells: giant cells with numerous overlapping nuclei located in lymphoid tissue during prodromal stage
    - Epithelial syncytial giant cells of skin and respiratory mucosa
- Treatment
  - No antiviral agent available—recent studies show susceptibility of virus in vitro to Ribavirin
  - Second-line treatment: vitamin A (100,000–200,000 IU by mouth once daily for 2 days)
  - Isolation until 4 days after exanthem onset
- Vaccine: protective titers can last more than 16 years
  - Postexposure prophylaxis-nonimmunized infants can be vaccinated within 72 hours of exposure for protection against contraction of virus
  - Passive immunization: Immune serum globulin—given to susceptible population to prevent or modify illness if given within 6 days of exposure
  - Intramuscular injection dose: 0.25 mL/kg to 15 mL/kg (max)
  - Live vaccine is contraindicated in pregnant women
  - Anaphylactic reactions have been reported in patients with egg allergy

Togaviruses

- Enveloped
- ssRNA
  - Rubella: German measles (Fig. 17-22)
    - Affects adult and children, predominant age of infection: children 5 to 9 years old
    - Known as "3-day measles"

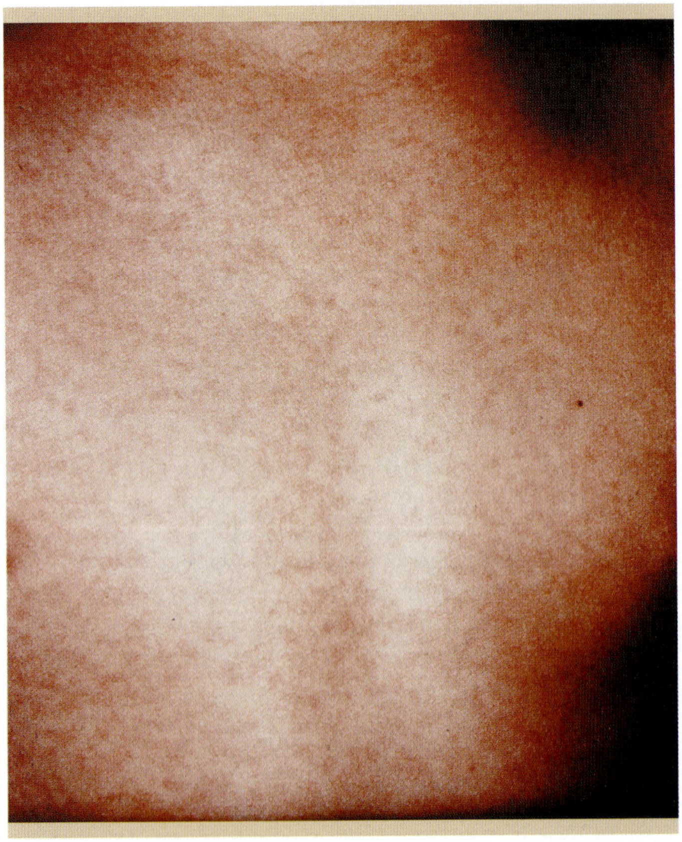

FIGURE 17-22 Rubella. (*Used with permission from Dr. Stephen Tyring.*)

- Pathogenesis
  - ▲ Virus acquired via inhalation of droplets and infection of nasopharyngeal cells
  - ▲ Replication occurs in the cytoplasm of host cells of the nasopharynx and lymph nodes
  - ▲ Hematogenous spread leads to infection of the skin and other organs. The virus is able to freely cross the placenta
  - ▲ Host sheds the virus almost 2 weeks prior to the onset of the rash, and to a lesser degree, up to a week after onset of symptoms
- Incubation period: 2 to 3 weeks
- Transmission: via droplets or direct contact with nasal secretions

• Postnatal-acquired rubella syndrome
- Clinical manifestations
  - ▲ Approximately 25 to 50% of patients can be asymptomatic; symptoms are commonly more severe in adults than children
  - ▲ Generalized tender lymphadenopathy for up to a week: involves all nodes, most striking in the suboccipital, postauricular, and posterior cervical nodes
  - ▲ Low-grade fever and malaise lasting 1 to 2 days, begins 2 weeks after initial infection
  - ▲ Enanthem: "Forchheimer spots"
    - △ Nonspecific pinpoint red macules and petechiae over the soft palate and uvula just before or along with the exanthem
  - ▲ Exanthem: erythematous maculopapular rash, progresses cephalocaudally, and may be followed by desquamation, lasts 3 to 5 days (same distribution and appearance of measles rash, with milder symptoms)
  - ▲ Myalgias and polyarthritis coincide with appearance of exanthem and can persist for a few weeks up to a month. It is most commonly found in young women
- Complications
  - ▲ Postinfectious encephalitis
  - ▲ Thrombocytopenic purpura
  - ▲ Arthritis/arthralgia

• Congenital rubella syndrome
- Affects the fetus of a pregnant woman without immunity to the virus
- Greatest hazard if fetus infected during first trimester, up to 80% suffer complications

• Clinical manifestations
- Most frequent complication if infection occurs between 2 and 8 weeks gestation
- Ophthalmologic: permanent cataracts, microphthalmia, and retinopathy
- Cardiac abnormalities: patent ductus arteriosus, pulmonary stenosis, atrial and ventricular septal defects
- Most common complication if infection occurs up to 16 weeks gestation
  - ▲ Intrauterine growth retardation
  - ▲ Sensorineural deafness
  - ▲ Neurologic: meningoencephalitis, mental retardation with behavioral disorders, large anterior fontanelle
  - ▲ Cutaneous: "blueberry muffin" purpuric skin lesion, purpura and petechiae secondary to thrombocytopenia
  - ▲ Systemic dermal extramedullary hematopoiesis

• Complications
- Spontaneous abortion (20%), stillbirth
- Premature delivery
- Panencephalitis
- Developmental endocrine abnormalities during adolescent period: hypothyroidism, diabetes mellitus, thyrotoxicosis

• Diagnosis
- Most common method: commercial enzyme immunoassay (EIA) detection of rubella-specific IgM. IgM detected 4 days after onset of rash to 8 weeks afterward
- Viral culture from nose, pharynx, blood, and urine
- Salivary antibodies to rubella
- IgG antibody to rubella virus in urine of children (up to 99% specific and sensitive)
- Fourfold increase of rubella antibody in patient serum
- Reverse transcriptase PCR detection of viral RNA prenatally, in amniotic fluid if fetus more than 15 weeks gestation

• Treatment
- Congenital rubella syndrome: no treatment available, acetaminophen for fever, and supportive care
- Postnatal rubella: no specific treatment, disease is usually self-limited
- Contact isolation in patients for 7 days after exanthem onset
- Contact isolation necessary for congenitally infected children for 1 year until cultures are negative

• Preventative measures
- MMR vaccine given in 2 doses
  - ▲ Dose #1 between 12 and 15 months of age
  - ▲ Dose #2 recommended at 4 to 6 years of age
- Contraindicated in pregnant women
- Relative contraindication in patients allergic to eggs, the immunodeficient, or immunocompromised population
- Most effective prevention of congenital rubella syndrome is immunization of nonimmune women before pregnancy or immunization immediately postpartum

Flaviviruses

- Enveloped
- ssRNA
- Flaviviruses of clinical importance: hepatitis C, yellow fever, Dengue fever, West Nile virus

Hepatitis C Virus (HCV)

- Uses an RNA-dependent RNA polymerase for viral replication which lacks proofreading ability and creates slightly mutated strands, leading to the difficulty in control of and development of a vaccine against the virus
- Transmission: percutaneous, body piercing and tattoos, inhaled cocaine, blood, sexual intercourse
- Population at risk: IV drug abusers, sexually active patients, health care workers, hemodialysis patients, blood transfusion recipients (especially before 1992)
- Incubation: 7 to 8 weeks
- Acute hepatitis C is self-limited and rarely causes hepatic failure
  - Approximately 80% of cases persist more than 6 months leading to chronic infection
- Chronic viral hepatitis is most commonly caused by HCV
  - Most patients with chronic HCV have chronic liver disease, which can progresses to cirrhosis and hepatocellular carcinoma
  - Alcohol increases the clinical severity of chronic disease
- Diseases associated with chronic hepatitis C
  - Immune complexes: skin, kidney (glomerulonephritis)
  - Sialadentitis
  - Autoimmune thrombocytopenic purpura
  - Lymphoma: increased antibodies to HCV in patients with non-Hodgkin B-cell lymphoma (20–40%)
  - Mixed cryoglobulinemia (types II and III)
  - Porphyria cutanea tarda
  - Lichen planus
  - Polyarteritis nodosa (5%)
  - Pruritus (39%)
- Clinical course
  - Usually mild with no outward signs of infection
  - Symptoms indistinguishable from other types of acute viral hepatitis
  - Fever (60%), fatigue, malaise (67%), nausea, and vomiting, anorexia
  - Jaundice (<25%)
  - Hepatomegaly
  - Dark urine (84%)
  - Mild right upper quadrant pain
  - Extrahepatic manifestation of HCV infection
    - Palmar erythema, spider nevi, asterixis, clubbing
    - Icteric sclera, temporal muscle wasting, enlarged parotid
    - Gynecomastia, scant body hair
    - Periumbilical hernia, ascities, caput medusae, abdominal bruit
    - Ankle edema
- Diagnosis
  - Bilirubin: unconjugated and conjugated can be markedly elevated
  - Alkaline phosphatase: mild elevation
  - Aminotransferases: elevated 6 to 12 weeks postexposure in acute HCV
  - Elevation of ALT levels for 6 months or more define chronic hepatitis
    - These levels fluctuate so a normal value does not indicate eradication of disease
    - AST/ALT ratio more than 1 is associated with cirrhosis in chronic HCV
  - HCV RNA becomes positive in acute cases within 8 weeks postexposure, confirmation of ongoing diseases are established via these markers
    - Hepatitis C antibody test (anti-HCV serological screening) via enzyme immunoassay test (EIA), unable to distinguish acute from chronic infection
    - Recombinant immunoblot assay—detection of antibody against 2+ antigen
      - ▲ Resolution of HCV infection is indicated by a positive immunoblot assay and 2 or more instances of undetectable HCV RNA
    - Quantitative assay to confirm HCV RNA, via PCR of the blood
      - ▲ This can help predict host response to treatment, and changes in HCV RNA levels
  - Positive results of EIA, RIBA, and PCR testing are diagnostic for active HCV infection, host should then be treated
    - If these markers persist for more than 6 months, the disease is defined as chronic liver disease
  - Positive α-fetoprotein in patients with chronic HCV may indicate hepatocellular carcinoma
- Histological findings
  - Lymphocytic infiltration, moderate degrees of inflammation and necrosis, and portal or bridging fibrosis are noted
  - Regenerative nodules are seen in patients with cirrhosis
- Treatment
  - Eradication of HCV is defined as absence of HCV RNA in serum for 6 months or more secondary to antiviral therapy
  - Antiviral therapy should be considered if:
    - Elevated ALT levels; however, up to 30% of patients with chronic HCV have normal ALT
    - Positive HCV antibody and serum HCV RNA
    - Liver biopsy shows portal or bridging fibrosis with moderate inflammation and necrosis
  - Acute HCV treatment
    - Interferon monotherapy
    - Pegylated interferon

    - Pegylated interferon + ribavarin (most effective) antiviral therapy is highly effective if given for 12 to 24 weeks
  - Chronic HCV treatment
    - Pegylated interferon + ribavirin. Weekly injections of PEG-IFN-α combined with twice daily doses of ribavirin (most effective). Two types of pegylated interferon use
      - ▲ Peg-IFN-α 2b 1.5 mcg/kg SC weekly or
      - ▲ Peg-IFN-α 2a 180 mcg SC weekly
    - Ribavirin: 400 to 600 mg taken by mouth twice daily
    - Combination therapy: treatment individualized via genotype
      - ▲ HCV genotype 1: high-dose medication for 48 weeks
      - ▲ HCV genotype 2 or 3: medication given for 24 weeks
        - △ Pegylated interferon monotherapy
        - △ Interferon monotherapy
- Combination therapy is most effective against genotype 2 and 3, leads to 80% eradication of HCV RNA
  - Treatment has a better outcome in patients older than 40 years old, absence of cirrhosis, and shorter duration of infection
  - Treatment precaution
  - Interferon therapy aggravates autoimmune disorders, and is contraindicated in patients with platelet levels less than 50,000
- Interferon therapy poses increased risk of depression and suicidal ideation and should be used with caution in certain patient populations
- Use of corticosteroids has been linked with increased mortality
- Ribavirin can induce hemolytic anemia and has strong association with birth defects and should be avoided during pregnancy

Retroviruses

- Enveloped
- ssRNA
- Use a reverse transcriptase

Human Immunodeficiency Virus (HIV)

- Estimated 1.1 million people in United States infected with HIV, affecting predominately young adults between ages 25 and 44 years
- Targets and destroys CD4+ T lymphocytes leaving the body in state of severe immunodeficiency open for opportunistic infections and malignancies
- Viral structure
  - Diploid genome: 2 molecules of RNA, p24 nucleocapsid core protein, envelope proteins: gp41 and gp120; reverse transcriptase
- Route of infection
  - HIV enters CD4 lymphocytes via adherence of envelope proteins to the cell. Reverse transcriptase converts single-stranded viral RNA to double-stranded DNA which is inserted into the hosts DNA. Virions are released and the lymphocytes are destroyed, eventually leading to an immunodeficient state
- HIV can infect CD4+ T cells, macrophages, thymic cells, astrocytes, and dendritic cells
- Stages of HIV infection
  - Viral transmission
    - Sexual activity (70%)
      - ▲ Coexistence of a sexually transmitted disease with genital ulceration has 4 times higher rate of transmission
      - ▲ Increased risk in homosexual population
  - Blood and body fluids
    - Needles
      - ▲ IV drug abusers
      - ▲ Accidental needle sticks
    - Perinatal transmission in HIV-infected women
      - ▲ Transmission has been reduced with HIV testing of pregnant women and treatment with antiretroviral drugs
      - ▲ Breastfeeding postpartum
    - Recipients of blood transfusions (especially between 1975 and 1985)
    - Organ transplantation
    - Genetics
      - ▲ Patients with a homozygous CCR5 gene mutation for a cell surface protein and coreceptor of the virus are immune to the HIV virus. Those with a heterozygous gene mutation have a slower course of disease. Patients with a CXCR1 gene mutation have a rapid progression of HIV to AIDS
  - Primary HIV infection
    - Predominant percentage of HIV infections transmitted during this time because of increased level of viremia and very nonspecific symptoms
    - Presence of acute symptoms for more than 14 days correlates with increased risk of progression to AIDS in 3 years
    - Six months postinfection: CD8 T cells allow viremia to level out and prevent further destruction of CD4 count
  - Seroconversion
    - After 4 to 10 weeks postexposure, patient will have positive HIV serology
    - Ninety-five percent of patients seroconvert within 6 months
    - Mononucleosis-like symptoms
      - ▲ Headache, retro-orbital pain, muscle aches, fever, pharyngitis, fatigue, lymphadenopathy,

weight loss, night sweats, fine morbilliform rash, and mucocutaneous ulcers
- Clinical latent period
  - Period of time with no signs of virus except lymphadenopathy
  - From seroconversion to 6 months after transmission
  - During this time there is an increased rate of viral replication and CD4 cell destruction
  - Viral load: measures rate of disease progression and antiviral therapy response in early stage of disease. Stable at 6 months, can increase very slowly without treatment
- Early symptomatic HIV infection
  - These diseases are most severe in association with the HIV infection. Cutaneous manifestations include the following:
    - ▲ Thrush
    - ▲ Oral hairy leukoplakia
    - ▲ Herpes zoster (2+ episodes)
    - ▲ Bacillary angiomatosis
- AIDS
  - Defined as a CD4+ count of less than 200 cell/mm^3
    - ▲ CD4+ count measures degree of immunosuppression
  - Also defined by diseases which have their onset in the setting of severe immunosuppresion
    - ▲ *Pneumocystis carnii* pneumonia
    - ▲ Candidiasis of the upper respiratory system
    - ▲ Kaposi sarcoma
    - ▲ *Mycobacterium avium*
    - ▲ Disseminated mycobacterium tuberculosis
    - ▲ Cytomegalovirus
    - ▲ Dementia secondary to HIV infection
    - ▲ Invasive cervical anal cancer
    - ▲ Toxoplasmosis of internal organ
    - ▲ Burkitt lymphoma
- Advanced HIV with CD4 less than 50 cell/mm^3. Patients will survive only 1 year without antiviral therapy once their disease has become so advanced

- Clinical manifestations
  - Acute retroviral syndrome: presents 4 weeks after patient infected with the virus (70% of HIV+ patients)
  - Primary symptoms (resembles symptoms of mononucleosis)
    - Headache, retro-orbital pain, muscle aches, fever, pharyngitis, fatigue, lymphadenopathy, weight loss, and a fine morbilliform rash, mucocutaneous ulcers
- Diagnosis
  - ELISA: detects antibodies in blood to virus, 3 to 7 weeks after infection (high sensitivity, moderate specificity)
  - Western blot assay: confirmatory test (low sensitivity, high specificity)
  - Viral load measured by PCR
  - Baseline testing: CD4+ cell count, chest x-ray, PPD, VDRL/RPR, serology for CMV, VZV, hepatitis, and toxoplasmosis; HIV antibody test, and HIV viral load
  - Acute HIV infection diagnosed with:
    - Positive p24 antigen
    - High viral load (> 100,000)
    - Negative serology test
    - Mild clinical symptoms
- Antiretroviral therapy (Table 17-4)
  - Without antiviral therapy, patient progresses into a stage of acquired immunodeficiency within 10 years of transmission when CD4 count reaches less than 200 cells/mm^3
  - Since development and use of highly active antiretroviral therapy (HAART), there has been a decline in the trend of newly infected HIV and AIDS patients
  - Treatment should be initiated if
    - Patient diagnosed with AIDS or has symptomatic HIV
    - CD4 count is less than 350 cells/mm^3
    - HIV RNA levels are greater than 50,000 copies/mL
  - Combination regimen
    - A non-nucleoside reverse transcriptase inhibitor + 2 nucleoside reverse transcriptase inhibitors
    - Protease inhibitor + 2 nucleoside reverse transcriptase inhibitors
    - Three nucleoside reverse transcriptase inhibitors (least effective)
  - Goal: to reduce viral load, and increase CD4 counts

TABLE 17-4 Seven Classes of Antiretroviral Drugs

Nucleoside Reverse Transcriptase Inhibitors (NRTIs)		
Drug	**Dose**	**Side Effects**
Zidovudine [Retrovir]	200 mg 3 times daily	Bone marrow suppression Myopathy
Lamivudine, 3TC [Epivir]	150 mg twice daily	Hepatitis B exacerbation Hepatomegaly with steatosis Peripheral neuropathy Rhabdomyolysis Anaphylaxis Myalgia/arthralgia Abnormal dreams
Stavudine [Zerit]	40-mg tablet twice daily	Discontinue if peripheral neuropathy occurs Hyperlactatemia Severe motor weakness Leukopenia Hepatomegaly Pancreatitis Thrombocytopenia
Didanosine [Videx]	100-mg 2 tablets twice daily	Fatal and nonfatal pancreatitis Peripheral neuropathy Lactic acidosis Anaphylactoid reactions Rhabdomyolysis Hepatotoxicity Hyperlactatemia Optic neuritis
Zalcitabine [Hivid]	Discontinued in America	
Abacavir [Ziagen]	300 mg twice daily	Fatal anaphylaxis Liver failure Renal failure Adult respiratory distress syndrome Respiratory failure Severe hypotension
Emtricitabine, FTC [Emtriva]	200-mg tablet once daily	Caution to hepatitis B patients: use can cause fatty liver Lactic acidosis Severe hepatomegaly Palmar-plantar hyper pigmentation Dyspepsia Paresthesias

(Continued)

TABLE 17-4 Seven Classes of Antiretroviral Drugs (Continued)

Nucleoside Reverse Transcriptase Inhibitors (NRTIs)		
Drug	**Dose**	**Side Effects**
Combivir	Zidovudine 300 mg Abacavir 300 mg twice daily	Zidovudine associated hematologic toxicity and myopathy Neutropenia Myositis Rhabdomyolysis Severe anemia Lactic acidosis Severe hepatomegaly Post treatment hepatitis B exacerbation
Trizivir	Zidovudine 300 mg Lamivudine 150 mg Abacavir 300 mg twice daily Has good viral suppression, should be used in cases when Efavirenz is ineffective	Not for use if weight <40 kg Fatal anaphylaxis Liver failure Renal failure Severe hypotension Adult respiratory distress syndrome Respiratory failure Lactic acidosis Rhabdomyolysis Erythema multiforme Toxic epidermal necrolysis
Atripla	Efavirenz 600 mg Emtricitabine 200 mg Tenofovir 300 mg 1 tablet at night on empty stomach	Associated with dizziness, drowsiness, impaired concentration Not recommended for patients < 18 years old. Sudden discontinuation of drug can severely exacerbate HBV infection
Epzicom	Abacavir 600 mg Lamivudine 300 mg once daily	Lactic acidosis FDA pregnancy category C Increased thirst, urination Seizures, mood changes Do not take if hypersensitivity to Abacavir
Truvada	Emtricitabine 200 mg Tenofovir 300 mg once daily on an empty stomach	Pancreatitis Lactic acidosis Severe heptomegaly with steatosis

Non-Nucleoside Reverse Transcriptase Inhibitors (NNRTIs) Commonly Seen Side Effects: Cytochrome P450 Inducers, Rash		
Drug	**Dose**	**Side Effects**
Nevirapine [Viramune]	200 mg daily × 14 days	Hepatotoxicity in women with reduced T-cell levels Fatal hypersensitivity reaction Steven-Johnson syndrome Rhabdomyolysis Granulocytopenia Angioedema Severe stomatitis
Delaviridine [Rescriptor]	200 mg 3 times daily in 3 oz water	Mild rash resolves in 3–14 days Angioedema Granulocytosis, leukopenia, pancytopenia GI bleed Cardiomyopathy Rhabdomyolysis Acute renal failure
Etravirine TMC-125 [Interlence]	100 mg 2 tablets twice daily after meals	Used for multiresistant strains, do not use in naïve patients or children Tablet must be swallowed whole with liquids Severe skin rash, extremity tingling, high blood pressure
Efavirenz [Sustiva]	600 mg at bedtime on empty stomach	CNS symptoms: confusion, depression, hallucinations, seizures, memory loss, suicidal thoughts Exfoliative dermatitis False positive marijuana drug testing Contraindicated in pregnancy

Protease Inhibitors Commonly Seen Side Effects: GI Intolerance, Cytochrome P450 Inhibitors, Metabolic Syndrome, Insulin Resistance, Truncal Obesity, and Hyperlipidemia		
Drug	**Dose**	**Side Effects**
Saquinavir [Invirase]	500 mg 2 tablets twice daily with food Given with Norvir 100 mg once daily	Hepatotoxicity Diabetes mellitus Pancreatitis Seizures Steven-Johnson syndrome Thrombocytopenia Portal hypertension Thrombophlebitis Intestinal obstruction

(Continued)

Protease Inhibitors Commonly Seen Side Effects: GI Intolerance, Cytochrome P450 Inhibitors, Metabolic Syndrome, Insulin Resistance, Truncal Obesity, and Hyperlipidemia		
Drug	**Dose**	**Side Effects**
Ritonavir [Norvir]	300 mg 2 tablets twice daily	If taken in combination with nonsedating antihistamines, sedatives hypnotics, antiarrhythmics, or ergot alkaloids—has life-threatening side effects.
Indinavir [Crixivan]	400 mg 2 tablets every 8 hours without food	Nephrolithiasis Lipodystrophy Anemia
Nelfinavir [Viracept]	750 mg 3 times daily with food	Avoid mixing with acidic food/juice Diarrhea Leukopenia Suicidal ideation Hepatitis Jaundice Don't treat pregnant patients due to ethyl methanesulfonate
Amprenavir [Agenerase]	Discontinued in the United States	
Kaletra	200 mg Lopinavir + 50 mg Ritonavir 2 tablets twice daily (used in pediatric and naïve population)	Pancreatitis Neutropenia Thrombocytopenia (peds) Exfoliative dermatitis Hemarthrosis in hemophiliacs
Fosamprenavir [Lexiva]	700 mg 2 tablets twice daily without food—for naïve patients 700 mg Fosamprenavir 2 tablets/daily + 100 Ritonvair once daily without food—for resistant patients	Increased liver enzymes Severe skin reactions Neutropenia Fat redistribution Hemolytic anemia
Tipranavir [Aptivus]	250 mg coadministered with 100 mg Ritonavir Two tablets, twice daily with food	Hypercholesterolemia, hyperlipidemia Intracranial hemorrhaging Platelet aggregation and coagulation, rash Contraindicated in: treatment naïve patients, potent CYP3A inducers, Child-Pugh class B or C
Darunavir [Prezista]	Prezista 300 mg 2 tables twice daily with food Taken with Ritonavir 100 mg 1 tablet twice daily with food for resistant patients Must be taken with Ritonavir to keep Prezista level high in blood	Severe skin rashes Neutropenia Fat redistribution Inflammation nose and throat Contains sulfa Avoid if hepatic impairment

(*Continued*)

Protease Inhibitors Commonly Seen Side Effects: GI Intolerance, Cytochrome P450 Inhibitors, Metabolic Syndrome, Insulin Resistance, Truncal Obesity, and Hyperlipidemia		
Drug	**Dose**	**Side Effects**
Atazanavir [Reyataz]	200 mg 2 tablets once daily with food (naïve patients) 300-mg Atazanavir + 100-mg Ritonavir One daily with food—for resistant patients	first or second degree AV block PR prolongation Severe hyperglycemia Neutropenia Erythema multiforme Dysuria, hematuria Jaundice Immune reconstruction syndrome Elevated CK

Nucleotide Reverse Transcriptase Inhibitors		
Drug	**Dose**	**Side Effects**
Tenofovir [Viread]	300 mg daily	Lactic acidosis Severe hepatomegaly Nephrotoxicity Hypophosphatemia Fanconi syndrome Acute renal tubular necrosis Osteomalacia with renal tubulopathy Dyspnea

Fusion Inhibitors		
Drug	**Dose**	**Side Effects**
Enfuvirtide, T-20 [Fuzeon]	90 mg subcutaneous injection twice daily for resistant strains	Injection site reactions: redness, swelling, itching Increased risk of bacterial pneumonia Glomerulonephritis Guillain-Barrè syndrome

CCR5 Coreceptor Antagonist		
Drug	**Dose**	**Side Effects**
Maraviroc [Selzentry]	300 mg twice daily only effective against CCR5-tropic HIV	Myocardial ischemia or infarction Orthostatic hypotension Hepatotoxicity Infection Malignancy

Integrase inhibitor To Be Used in Combination With Other Antiretroviral Medications		
Drug	**Dose**	**Side Effects**
Raltegravir [Isentress]	400 mg twice daily Used in multidrug-resistant strains	Diarrhea, nausea, headache Skin rash Myopathy Rhabdomyloysis Elevated levels of creatinine kinase Gastritis Myocardial infarction

QUIZ

Questions

1. A 22-year-old nursing school graduate is evaluated during preemployment physical examination for a job at a children's hospital. She has systemic lupus erythematosus, which is well controlled with prednisone, 10 mg daily. She has no recollection of chickenpox as a child; results of a varicella titer are negative.
   Which of the following is the most appropriate recommendation?

   A. No vaccination
   B. Single vaccination (shortened series), clear for work
   C. Single vaccination (shortened series), delay work for 4 weeks
   D. Two-dose vaccination series over 6 weeks, delay work for 4 weeks

2. An 18-year-old woman presents with a 3-month history of a painful, thick, endophytic papule on the sole of her right foot. She has never had the lesion treated and wants to know if it is infectious. Which one of the following HPV subtypes can be responsible for her disease?

   A. HPV 16
   B. HPV 2
   C. HPV 1
   D. HPV 1, 2, 4
   E. All of the above

3. A healthy 25-year-old sexually active man presents to your office. He is concerned about the risk of genital warts and inquires about potential options available for prevention. What is an FDA-approved preventative therapy available for this patient?

   A. No preventative therapy available
   B. HPV quadrivalent vaccine
   C. HPV vaccine against subtypes 16 and 18
   D. HPV vaccine against subtypes 6 and 11

4. You are asked to see a 35-year-old HIV+ man with a white round lesion on the lateral tongue. Biopsy reveals parakeratosis, acanthosis, and papillated epithelial surfaces. Within the keratinized cells of the superficial epithelium, you can expect to see which type of virus:

   A. Double-stranded DNA
   B. Single-stranded RNA
   C. Double-stranded RNA
   D. Single-stranded DNA
   E. None of the above

5. A 45-year-old restaurant waiter presents with acute vomiting, fever, malaise, and abdominal pain since yesterday. On examination he has hepatomegaly and jaundice. What immunoglobulin is used as the gold standard for diagnosis?

   A. Stool anti-HAV IgM
   B. Urine anti-HAV IgM
   C. Stool anti-HBV IgM
   D. Serum anti-HAV IgM

6. A 52-year-old school teacher inquires about vaccination for shingles. She has never had shingles before. What would the vaccine be beneficial toward?

   A. Significant reduction of zoster and PHN
   B. Significant reduction of zoster
   C. Complete prevention of zoster
   D. Complete prevention of zoster and PHN
   E. The vaccine is not indicated in this patient

7. A 33-week HIV+ pregnant woman was recently started on a reverse transcriptase inhibitor to decrease the risk of vertical transmission to the newborn. What is an associated adverse effect of this medication?

   A. Rhabdomyolysis
   B. Abnormal dreams
   C. Bone marrow suppression
   D. Liver failure
   E. Renal Failure

8. A 26-year-old Asian woman presents with recurrent herpes labialis. She is interested in suppressive therapy. What is/are the best recommended suppressive therapy for this patient?

   A. Acyclovir 400 mg tid
   B. Valacyclovir 500 mg 2 times daily
   C. Famciclovir 250 mg tid
   D. All of the above can be used as effective suppressive therapy

9. A newborn's examination reveals purpuric macules and papules on the entire body. He has severe microcephaly, thrombocytopenia, and hepatosplenomegaly. What is the associated diagnostic histologic finding associated with the causative agent?

   A. "Owl's eye" intranuclear inclusions
   B. Prominent spindle cells
   C. Multinucleated giant cells
   D. Parakeratosis, acanthosis, and elongated rete ridges

10. A 60-year-old woman with history of diabetes mellitus and hypertension presents with a painful erythematous vesicular rash on the left lower buttock and thigh. She has 9/10 pain and complains of trouble sleeping. What is the most appropriate treatment regimen?

   A. Antiviral only
   B. Antiviral plus gabapentin
   C. Antiviral plus gabapentin plus as needed narcotic pain medication
   D. As needed narcotic pain medication and NSAIDS
   E. Antiviral plus prednisone taper

Answers

1. D. This patient would require 2-dose vaccination with varicella. The patient is employed at a health care facility, and therefore required to have either serologic evidence of immunity to or a 2-dose vaccination series with varicella. Nonvaccination is not an option in this case given the profession of the patient and the potential risk to her patients if she were to have primary varicella infection. B and C are incorrect because varicella immunization is a 2-dose series.
2. D. The patient is presenting with a classic example of plantar wart (myrmecia). The HPV subtypes responsible for plantar warts are HPV 1, 2, 4, and 63. The HPV subtype 16 is associated with ungula squamous cell carcinoma and cervical/anogenital cancers.
3. B. The patient is interested in prevention of genital warts. Currently there are 2 FDA-approved HPV vaccines, however only one, Gardasil, is indicated for prevention of cervical cancer, anal cancer, and genital warts. Gardasil is approved for use in both males and females and is a quadrivalent vaccine. D and C are incorrect because Gardasil is aimed at protection from HPV subtypes 6, 11, 16, and 18.
4. A. The patient is presenting with oral hairy leukoplakia, which is caused by Epstein-Barr virus (EBV). EBV is a double-stranded DNA virus which replicates in the nucleus and primarily infects B-lymphocytes. After acute infection, EBV persists as a latent infection for life.
5. D. The signs and symptoms of nausea, vomiting, fever, hepatomegaly, and jaundice are compatible with acute viral hepatitis. The most likely culprit is HAV, which is transmitted via the fecal-oral route and common in restaurants, daycares, and schools. The gold standard for diagnosis of acute hepatitis A infection is serum anti-HAV IgM which is positive at onset of symptoms and stays detectable for up to 6 months after.
6. A. The herpes zoster vaccine Zostavax is FDA approved for prevention of both zoster and PHN. In clinical studies the vaccine has demonstrated significant reduction of the incidence of zoster and associated PHN. Recently the FDA expanded the indication for use in adults who are older or equal to 50 years old; therefore, the vaccine would be indicated for use in this patient.
7. C. The patient was most likely started on zidovudine, a nucleoside reverse transcriptase inhibitor (NRTI) which decreases the risk of vertical transmission in pregnant HIV+ patients. The most concerning associated adverse effect with zidovudine is bone marrow suppression.
8. B. Chronic suppressive therapy for herpes simplex infection can be achieved with any of the 3 agents. However, the correct dosage for suppression is valacyclovir 500 mg or 1 g per day. Acyclovir dosing for suppression is 400 mg 2 times daily or 200 mg tid-qid, while famciclovir dosing is 250 mg 2 times daily.
9. A. The newborn has classic signs of congenital CMV infection ("blueberry muffin baby") including purpuric macules, thrombocytopenia, hepatomegaly, and microcephaly. The histologic sign associated with CMV infected cells is "owl's eye" basophilic intranuclear inclusions. Spindle cells are associated with HHV 8; multinucleated giant cells are associated with HSV-2 and VZV; parakeratosis, acanthosis, and elongated rete ridges are associated with HPV infection.

10. C. The patient is presenting with acute herpes zoster of the S1 dermatome with severe pain. Given recent studies demonstrating a significant decrease in incidence of PHN with gabapentin and antiviral therapy, the patient should be initiated on the combination of gabapentin and antiviral therapy to decrease the likelihood of developing PHN. As needed narcotic medications should still be prescribed for acute treatment of her 9/10 pain.

REFERENCES

Ahmed AM, Madkan V, Tyring SK: Human papillomaviruses and genital disease. *Dermatol Clin* Apr 2006;24(2):157–165.

Balfour HH Jr, Kelly JM, Suarez CS: Acyclovir treatment of varicella in otherwise healthy children. *J Pediatr* 1990;116(4):633–639.

Bernstein DI, Aoki FY, Tyring SK, et al. Safety and immunogenicity of glycoprotein-D adjuvant genital herpes vaccine. *Clin Infect Dis* 2005;40:1271–1281.

Beutner KR, Tyring SK, Trofatter KF, et al. Imiquimod, a patient applied immune response modifier for the treatment of external genital warts. *Antimicrob Agents Chemother* 1998;42:789–794.

Carrasco D, Vander Straten M, Tyring SK: Treatment of anogenital warts with imiquimod 5% cream followed by surgical excision of residual lesions. *J Am Acad Dermatol* 2002;47 (4 Suppl):S212–S216.

Carrasco DA, Trizna Z, Colome-Grimmer M, et al. Verrucous herpes of the scrotum in a human immunodeficiency virus-positive man: case report and review of the literature. *JEADV* 2002;16:511–515.

Chen J, Wang L, Chen JJ, et al. Detection of antibodies to human immunodeficiency virus (HIV) that recognize conformational epitopes of glycoproteins 160 and 41 often allows for early diagnosis of HIV infection. *J Infect Dis* 2002;186(3):321–331.

Corey L, Langenberg AGM, Ashley R, et al. Recombinant glycoprotein vaccine for the prevention of genital HSV-2 acquisition: 2 double-blind, placebo-controlled trials. *JAMA* 1999;282:331–340.

Corey L, Wald A, Patel R, et al. Once-daily valacyclovir to reduce the risk of transmission of genital herpes. *N Engl J Med* 2004;350:11–20.

Dianzani F, Antonnelli G, Tyring SK, et al. The HIV RNA load in chronically infected patients circulates mainly as neutralized immune complexes. *J Infect Dis* 2002;185:1051–1054.

Fatahzadeh M, Schwartz RA: Human herpes simplex virus infections: epidemiology, pathogenesis, symptomatology, diagnosis, and management. *J Am Acad Dermatol* Nov 2007;57(5):737–763.

Fuessel Haws AL, He Q, Rady PL, et al. Nested PCR with the PGMY09/11 and GP5(+)/6(+) primer sets improves detection of HPV DNA in cervical samples. *J Virol Methods* 2004;122:87–93.

Goldsmith LA et al. *Fitzpatrick's Dermatology in General Medicine*, 8th Ed. New York: McGraw-Hill; 2012.

Gonzalez L, Gaviria AM, Sanclemente G, et al. Clinical, histopathological and virological findings in patients with focal epithelial hyperplasia from Columbia. *Int J Dermatol* 2005;44:274–279.

Horn TD, Johnson SM, Helm RM, Roberson PK: Intralesional immunotherapy of warts with mumps, Candida, and Trichophyton skin test antigens: a single-blinded, randomized, and controlled trial. *Arch Dermatol* May 2005;141(5):589–594.

Johnson SM, Roberson PK, Horn TD: Intralesional injection of mumps or Candida skin test antigens: a novel immunotherapy for warts. *Arch Dermatol* Apr 2001;137(4):451–455.

Lapolla WJ, Haitz KA, DiGiorgio CM, Magel GD, Tyring SK: Gabapentin in combination with antiviral treatment for herpes zoster patients reduces the incidence of post-herpetic neuralgia. *Archives of Dermatology* 2011;147:901–907.

McKee PH: *Pathology of the Skin: With Clinical Correlations*. London: Mosby-Wolfe; 1996.

Meadows KP, Tyring SK, Pavia AT, et al. Resolution of racalcitrant molluscum contagiosum lesions in HIV-infected patients treated with cidofovir. *Arch Dermatol* 1997;133:987–990.

Mertz GJ, Loveless MO, Levin MJ, et al. Oral famciclovir for suppression of recurrent genital herpes simplex virus infection in women. A multicenter, double blind, placebo-controlled trial. *Arch Int Med* 1997;157:343–349.

Nell P et al. Progressive vaccinia as an adverse event following exposure to vaccinia virus: case definition and guidelines of data collection, analysis, and presentation of immunization safety data. *Vaccine* Aug 1 2007;25(31):5735–5744.

Patel R, Tyring SK, Strand A, et al. Impact of suppressive antiviral therapy on the health-related quality of life of patients with recurrent genital herpes infection. *Sex Trans Inf* 1999;75:398–402.

Patera A, Ali MA, Tyring SK, et al. Polymorphisms in the genes for herpesvirus entry. *J Infect Dis* 2002;186(3):444–445.

Rady PL, Hodak E, Yen A, et al. Detection of human herpesvirus 8 DNA in Kaposi's sarcomas from iatrogenically immunosuppressed patients. *J Am Acad Dermatol* 1998;38:429–437.

Reichman RC, Oakes D, Bonnez W, et al. Treatment of condyloma acuminatum with three different α-interferon preparations administered parenterally: a double blind, placebo-controlled trial. *J Infect Dis* 1990;162:1270–1276.

Reichman RC, Oakes D, Bonnez W, et al. Treatment of condyloma acuminatum with three different interferons administered intralesionally: a multicentered, placebo-controlled trial. *Ann Intern Med* 1988;108:675–679.

Reitano M, Tyring SK, Lang W, et al. Valaciclovir for the suppression of recurrent genital HSV infection: a large scale dose range-finding study. *J Infect Dis* 1998;178:603–610.

Roncalli W, He Q, Rady PL, et al. HPV typing in Brazilian patients with epidermodysplasia verruciformis: high prevalence of EV-HPV 25. *J Cutan Med Surg* 2004;8:110–115.

Roncalli W, Neto CF, Rady PL, et al. Clinical aspects of epidermodysplasia verruciformis. *J Eur Acad Venereol* 2003;17:394–398.

Roncalli W, Rady PL, Grady J, et al. Association of p53 polymorphism with skin cancer. *Int J Dermatol* 2004;43:489–493.

Roncalli W, Rady PL, Grady J, et al. Polymorphisms of the interleukin-10 gene promotor in epidermodysplasia verruciformis patients from Brazil. *J Am Acad Dermatol* 2003;49:639–643.

Sale TA, Melski JW, Stratman EJ: Monkeypox: an epidemiologic and clinical comparison of African and US disease. *J Am Acad Dermatol* Sep 2006;55(3):478–481.

Schell B, Rosen T, Rady P, et al. Verrucous carcinoma of the foot associated with human papillomavirus type 16. *J Am Acad Dermatol* 2001;45:49–55.

Shafran SD, Tyring SK, Ashton R, et al. Once, twice, or three times daily famciclovir compared with acyclovir for the oral treatment of herpes zoster in immunocompetent adults: a randomized, multicenter, double-blind clinical trial. *J Clin Virol* 2004;29:248–253.

Spruance SL, Tyring SK, DeGregorio B, et al. A large-scale placebo-controlled, dose-ranging trial of peroral valaciclovir for episodic treatment of recurrent herpes genitalis. *Arch Int Med* 1996;156:1729–1735.

Stanberry LR, Spruance SL, Cunningham L, et al. Glycoprotein D adjuvant vaccine to prevent genital herpes. *N Engl J Med* 2002;347:1652–1661.

Sterling J, Tyring S, eds. *Human Papillomaviruses*. New York: Oxford; 2001.

Trizna Z, Evans T, Bruce S, et al. A randomized phase II study comparing four different interferon therapies in patients with recalcitrant condylomata acuminata. *Sex Trans Dis* 1998;25:361–365.

Tyring S, ed. *Antiviral Agents, Vaccines and Immunotherapies*. New York: Marcel Dekker; 2005.

Tyring S, ed. *Mucocutaneous Manifestations of Viral Diseases*. New York: Marcel Dekker; 2002.

Tyring S, Nahlik J, Cunningham A, et al. A double blind, randomized, placebo-controlled, parallel group study of oral famciclovir for the treatment of uncomplicated herpes zoster. *Ann Intern Med* 1995;123:89–96.

Tyring SK, Arany I, Stanley MA, et al. A molecular study of condylomata acuminata clearance during treatment with imiquimod: a randomized, double blind, vehicle-controlled study. *J Infect Dis* 1998;178:551–555.

Tyring SK, Belanger R, Bezwoda W, et al. A randomized, double blind trial of famciclovir versus acyclovir for the treatment of localized dermatomal herpes zoster in immunocompromised patients. *Cancer Invest* 2001;19:13–22.

Tyring SK, Beutner KR, Tucker BA, et al. Antiviral therapy for herpes zoster. *Arch Fam Med* 2000;9:863–869.

Tyring SK, Diaz-Mitoma F, Shafran SD, et al. Oral famciclovir for the suppression of recurrent genital herpes: the combined data from two randomized controlled trials. *J Cutan Med Surg* 2003;7:449–454.

Tyring SK, Douglas J, Corey L, et al. A randomized, placebo-controlled comparison of oral acyclovir and valacyclovir HCl in patients with recurrent genital herpes infections. *Arch Dermatol* 1998;134:185–191.

Tyring SK, Edwards L, Friedman DJ, et al. Safety and efficacy of 0.5% podofilox gel in the treatment of external genital and/or perianal warts: a double blind, vehicle-controlled study. *Arch Dermatol* 1998;134:33–38.

Tyring SK, Engst R, Corriveau C, et al. Famciclovir for ophthalmic zoster: A randomized acyclovir-controlled study. *Br J Ophthalmol* 2001;85:576–581.

Whitley RJ, Weiss H, Gnann Jr JW, et al. Acyclovir with and without prednisone for the treatment of herpes zoster: a randomized, placebo-controlled trial. *Ann Intern Med* 1996;125:376–383.

Yen-Moore A, Hudnall SD, Rady PL, et al. Differential expression of the HHV-8 vGCR cellular homolog gene in AIDS-associated and classic Kaposi's sarcoma: potential role of HIV-1 Tat. *Virology* 2000;267:247–251.

Zong J, Ciufo DM, Viscidi R, et al. Genotypic analysis at multiple loci across Kaposi's sarcoma herpesvirus (KSHV) DNA molecules: clustering patterns, novel variants and chimerism. *J Clin Virol* 2002;23(3):119–148.

Zong JC, Ciufo DM, Alcendor DJ, et al. High level variability in the ORF-K1 membrane protein gene at the left end of the Kaposi's sarcoma associated herpesvirus (HHV8) genome defines four major virus subtypes and multiple variants or clades in different human populations. *J Virol* 1999;73:4156–4170.

CHAPTER 18

BACTERIAL DISEASES

STEVEN MARCET
ASRA ALI
NEIL FARNSWORTH

GRAM-POSITIVE BACTERIAL DISEASES

Impetigo (Fig. 18-1)

- Superficial nonfollicular infection, due to Staphylococcus *aureus* or *group A Streptococcus,* occurs more commonly in children
- Lesions can begin as erythematous papules that evolve into a vesicle or pustule. The pustules may rupture leaving contagious honey-colored crusts
- Treatment: topical mupirocin
- Bullous impetigo is a toxin-mediated erythroderma (Fig. 18-2) is caused only by *Staphylococcus aureus* → exotoxin cleaves desmoglein 1 → separation of the epidermis at the granular layer
- Clinical (seen most frequently in newborns)
- Sharply demarcated flaccid bullae without surrounding erythema
- Treatment: dicloxacillin or first-generation cephalosporin, topical mupirocin

Ecthyma

- Differs from impetigo in that the dermis is ulcerated
- Usually caused by group A beta-hemolytic streptococci (GABHS)
- Clinical
  - Thick crusted ulcer that heals slowly and may produce a scar
  - Most commonly affects the lower extremities of children, persons with diabetes, and neglected elderly patient. Often occurs with lymphadenitis
- Histology: ulceration to dermis with bacteria, crusting and an acute inflammatory infiltrate
- Treatment: usually dicloxacillin or first-generation cephalosporin, parental antibiotics may be needed for widespread infection

Bacterial Folliculitis (Fig. 18-3)

- Most cases caused by *S. aureus*
- Superficial infection: (facial involvement is called Bockhart folliculitis): red papules/pustules, follicularly centered
- Deep infection: (facial involvement = sycosis barbae); erythematous, fluctuant nodules
- Lupoid sycosis: chronic form of sycosis barbae associated with scarring
- Treatment: topical antibiotics, systemic antibiotics may be indicated

Furuncles/Carbuncles (Fig. 18-4)

- *S. aureus* most commonly found
- Clinical
  - Deep-seated nodules around hair follicle (inflammation involves the subcutis)
  - Multiple furuncles make a carbuncle, evolve from preceding folliculitis
- Treatment: topical mupirocin and dicloxacillin; if large, then also need drainage

Abscess (Fig. 18-5)

- Cutaneous abscesses represent a collection of purulent debris in the skin
- Usually *Staphylococcus aureus* (including possibly methicillin-resistant strains)
  - Methicillin-resistant *S. aureus*: altered cell wall transpeptidase (penicillin-binding protein 2a) carried on staph chromosome cassette mecA
    - transfer by bacterial plasmids
  - *Hospital-acquired* methicillin-resistant *Staphylococcus aureus* (MRSA) usually carries mecA types I, II, and III
    - resistance to clindamycin and macrolides (inducible clindamycin resistance detectable by the "D-zone" test). *Community-acquired* MRSA commonly carries SCCmec IV

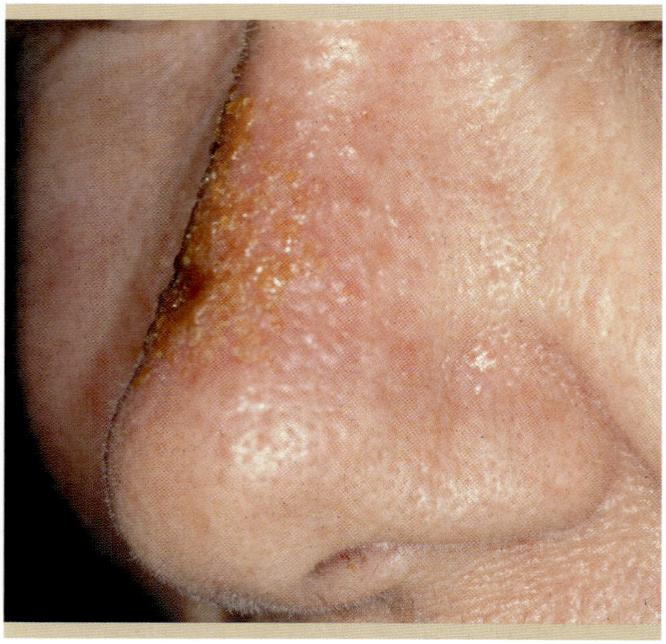

FIGURE 18-1 Impetigo. (*Used with permission from Dr. Steven Mays.*)

  - more antibiotic susceptibilities
  - MRSA usually carries an especially potent pore-forming toxin: Panton-Valentine leukocidin (via lukS/F-PV genes) → greater tissue inflammation and destruction
  - Clinical
    - Deep-seated nodules around hair follicle (inflammation involves the subcutis). Fully-formed lesions

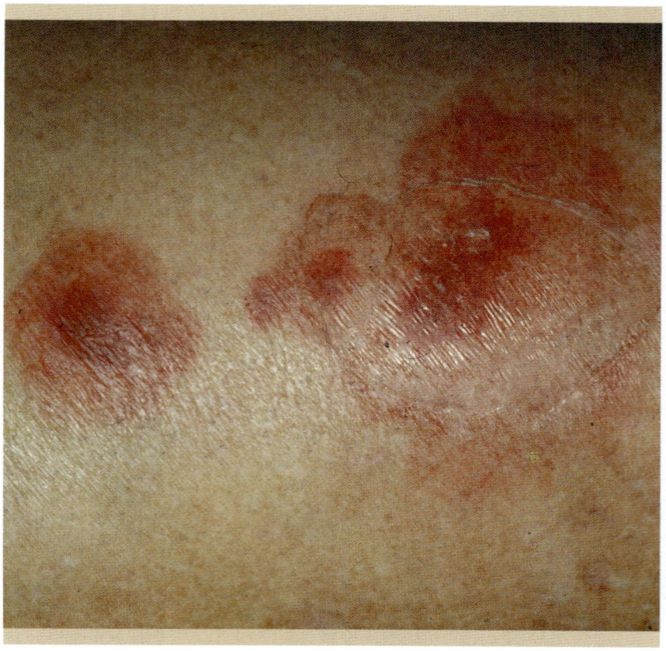

FIGURE 18-2 Bullous impetigo. (*Used with permission from Dr. Steven Mays.*)

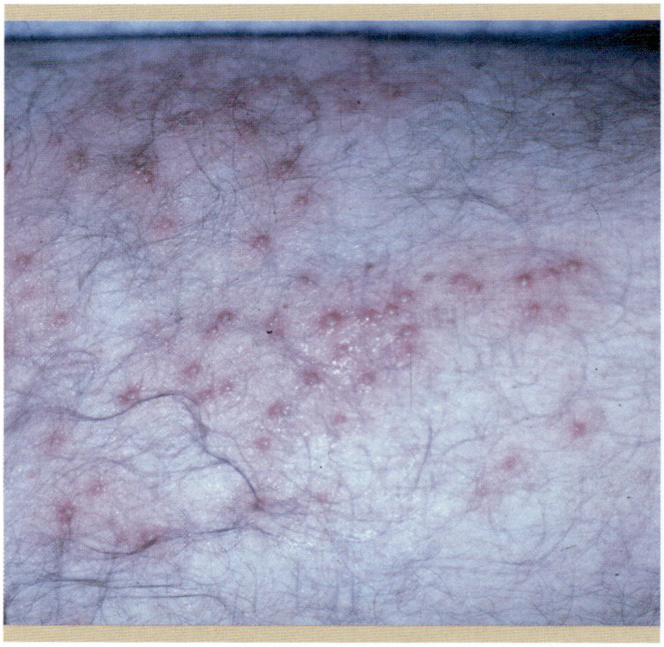

FIGURE 18-3 Folliculitis. (*Used with permission from Dr. Steven Mays.*)

are fluctuant. May be accompanied by fever, cellulitis, lymphangitis, lymphadenopathy, or leukocytosis
    - Inguinal and perineal area may involve gram-negative flora
    - Culture (useful when MRSA suspected)
- Treatment: warm compresses (to "ripen"), incision and drainage, systemic antibiotics

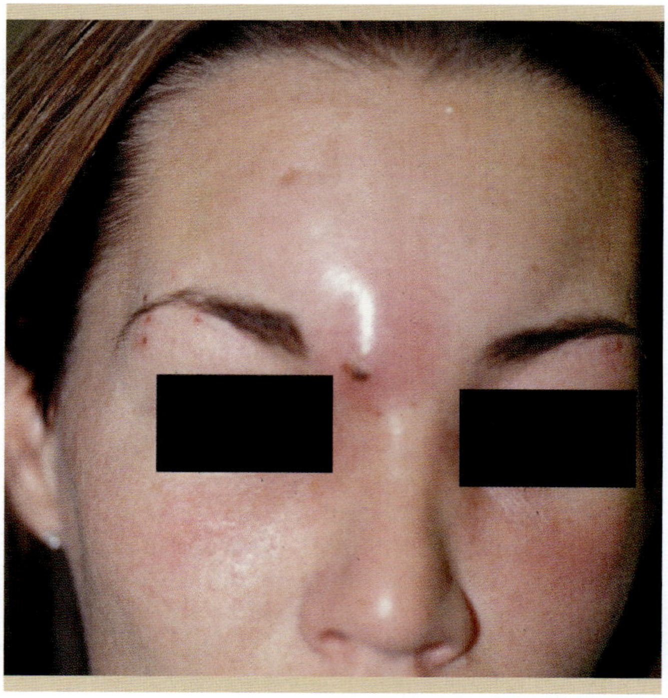

FIGURE 18-4 Furuncule. (*Used with permission from Dr. Steven Mays.*)

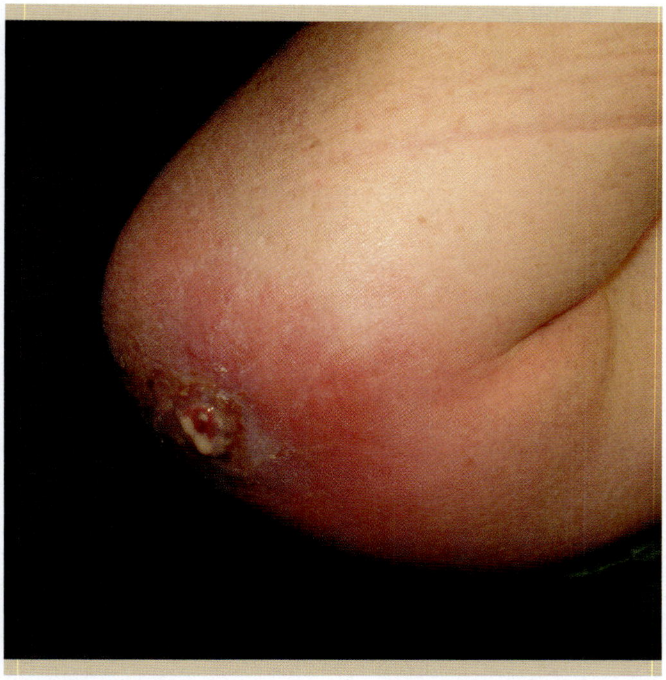

FIGURE 18-5 Abscess. (*Used with permission from Dr. Asra Ali.*)

Lymphangitis

- Infection and inflammation of the lymphatic channels
- Variety of causal bacteria—group A *Streptococcus*, *S. aureus*, even *Pasturella multocida* (cat-scratch fever)
- Clinical
  - Erythematous and irregular appearing linear streaks in the skin, extending from the primary infection site toward regional lymph nodes. Streaks may tender and warm. Can progress to bacteremia (particularly with group A *Streptococcus*)
- Diagnosis: complete blood count (leukocytosis), blood cultures (exclude bacteremia)
- Treatment: oral antibiotics with close follow-up, consider use of parenteral antibiotics in cases with systemic symptoms

Cellulitis

- Acute bacterial infection of skin and soft tissues, often follows an introduction via fissuring, laceration, puncture, or insect bite
- Vast majority of cases caused by *S. aureus, but may* rarely be caused by *Steptococcus pneumoniae* or marine vibrio species
- Clinical
  - Expanding edema, erythema, warmth, pain, tenderness. Lesions poorly circumscribed
  - Fever is common, and lymphangitis or lymphadenopathy may accompany the disease. Epidermal necrosis or disproportionate pain may indicate necrotizing fasciitis
- Treatment: mild cases treated with first-generation cephalosporins or dicloxacillin, more severe cases may be hospitalized for parenteral antibiotics

Erysipelas

- Bacterial infection of dermis with lymphatic involvement, usually by group A *Streptococcus*
- Clinical
  - Often on the legs or face. Raised, indurated erythema with a sharply-demarcated border, usually does not cross midline
- Treatment: dicloxacillin, hospitalization for the very young or debilitated

Staphylococcal Scalded-Skin Syndrome (SSSS) (Ritter Disease)

- Typically seen in children younger than 4 years of age
- Can occur in adult patients with renal insufficiency (cannot clear exotoxin)
- Exotoxins A or B; elaborated by bacteria, disseminated systemically → these toxins are serine proteases that cleave desmoglein 1 (generalized version of bullous impetigo, but in SSSS the bacteria originates from a focus of infection other than the skin)
- *S. aureus:* phage group II (types 3A, 3B, and 3C) (types 55 or 71) (exfoliative variants)
- Clinical
  - Superficial blistering (owing to disruption of the epidermal granular cell layer), sparing the mucous membranes. Periorificial and flexural accentuation may be observed
  - Nikolsky sign present (extension of a blister resulting from lateral pressure to the border of an intact blister)
- Diagnosis: frozen section tissue analysis to exclude toxic epidermal necrolysis (TEN) by level of blister formation (SSSS = subcorneal; TEN = subepidermal)
  - Cultures of bullae are typically negative, but cultures from other sites (oral/nasal cavities, throat, axillary/genital/umbilical regions, blood) may demonstrate *Staphylococcus*
  - Gram stain and/or culture from the remote infection site
- Treatment: intravenous penicillase-resistant penicillin, supportive measures
- Prognosis: mortality rate less than 4% in children, greater than 50% in immunosuppressed patients

Staphylococcal Toxic Shock Syndrome (TSS)

- Toxins produced by *S. aureus,* many that act as superantigens, lead to proinflammatory cytokine cascades involving tumor necrosis factor, interleukin-1, M protein, and interferon-γ
- Toxin-1 (TSST-1) causes most menstrual-related cases
- Many in the population have protective antibodies for these toxins and are not predisposed to the disease

- TSS may be associated with nonrayon tampons, surgical packings, and nasal packing
- Criteria for staphylococcal toxic shock syndrome:
  - Prodromal period of 2 to 3 days. Fever, hypotension
  - Skin findings: diffuse rash, occasionally patchy and erythematous, with desquamation occurring approximately 1 to 2 weeks later
  - Involvement of three or more organ systems:
    - Gastrointestinal (GI): vomiting or diarrhea
    - Muscular: myalgia, increased creatine phosphokinase level
    - Mucous membrane: vaginal, oropharyngeal, or conjunctival hyperemia
    - Renal: increased blood urea nitrogen or creatinine, urinary sediment with pyuria (without evidence of urinary tract infection)
    - Hepatic: increased total bilirubin, serum glutamic-oxaloacetic transaminase (AST, SGOT), or serum glutamic-pyruvic transaminase (ALT, SGPT)
    - Hematologic: platelets $< 100,000/mm^3$
    - Central nervous system: disorientation or alterations in consciousness without focal neurologic signs when fever and hypotension are absent
  - Labs: negative results for Rocky Mountain spotted fever, leptospirosis, measles, hepatitis B, and antinuclear antibodies. May have false-positive Venereal Disease Research Laboratory (VDRL) and Monospot testing
- Treatment: penicillinase resistant penicillin, clindamycin, intravenous γ-globulin, fluid replacement

Streptococcal Toxic Shock Syndrome

- *Streptococcus pyogenes* exotoxin A (SPEA) and *S. pyogenes* exotoxin B (SPEB): produced by GABHS
- Criteria for streptococcal TSS:
  - Isolation of group A *Streptococcus* from a normally sterile site (e.g., blood, cerebrospinal fluid [CSF], surgical wounds) or a nonsterile site (e.g., throat)
  - Hypotension (as defined earlier)
  - Involvement of 2 or more organ systems:
    - Renal: increased blood urea nitrogen or creatinine
    - Hematologic: coagulopathy
    - Hepatic: increased liver enzymes
    - Respiratory: acute respiratory distress syndrome
    - Cutaneous: tissue necrosis, (i.e., necrotizing fasciitis), erythematous/desquamating rash
- Treatment: intravenous penicillinase-resistant penicillin clindamycin, fluid therapy, and supportive measures

Blistering Distal Dactylitis

- GABHS
- Clinical:
  - Tense purulent blister of distal finger or toes, volar pad (can be confused with herpetic whitlow). Common in children and rare in adults
- Treatment: dicloxacillin or first-generation cephalosporin

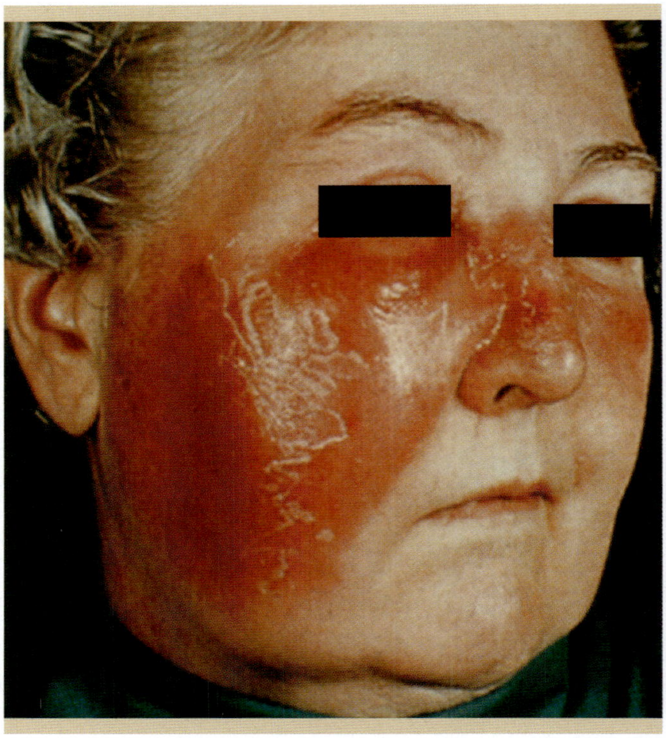

FIGURE 18-6 Erysipelas. (*Reprinted with permission from Connor DH et al. Pathology of Infectious Diseases. Stamford, CT: Appleton & Lange; 1997, p. 819.*)

Erysipelas (Fig 18-6)

- Bacterial infection of dermis with lymphatic involvement, usually by group A *Streptococcus*
- Clinical
  - Often on the legs or face. Raised, indurated erythema with a sharply-demarcated border, usually does not cross midline
- Treatment: penicllin, cephalosporins, or macrolides (azithromycin or erythromycin)

Scarlet Fever

- Toxin-producing GABHS → produces erythrogenic exotoxin
- Clinical:
  - Fever and pharyngitis → white strawberry tongue turns into red strawberry tongue after 4 days
  - Skin changes: 2 to 4 days after initiation of fever, sandpaper-like rash starting on trunk then becomes more generalized; desquamates after 4 to 5 days. Circumoral pallor
  - Pastia lines: linear petchial rash over skin folds (axillary/antecubital)
- Diagnosis: antistreptolysin O (ASO) titers
- Treatment: penicillin or erythromycin

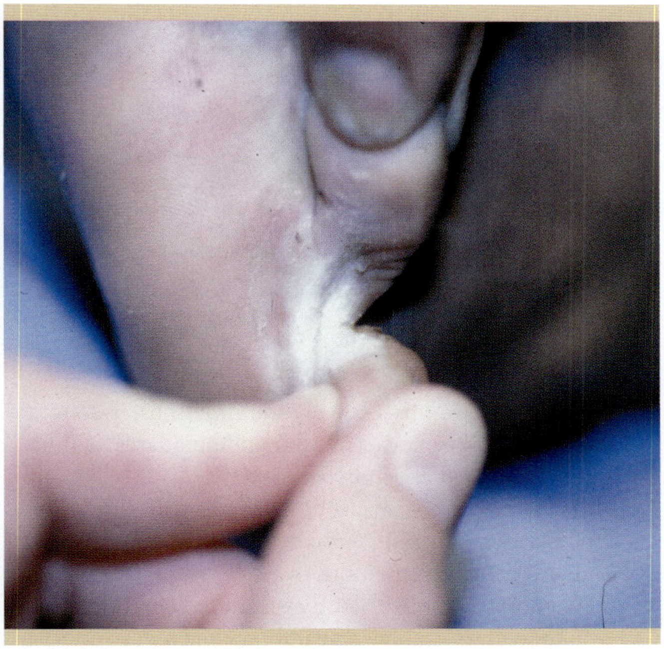

FIGURE 18-7 Erythrasma (can look like tinea between the toes). (*Used with permission from Dr. Steven Mays.*)

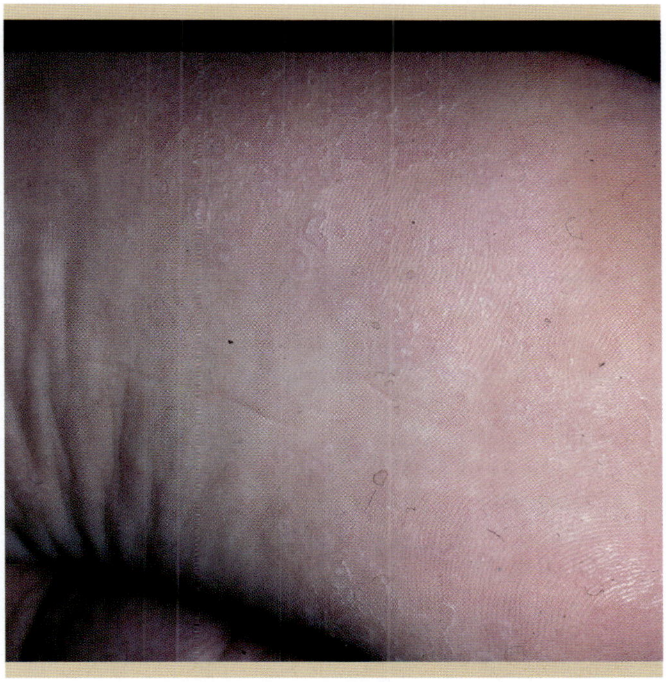

FIGURE 18-8 Pitted keratolysis. (*Used with permission from Dr. Ronald Rapini.*)

Erythrasma (Fig. 18-7)

- *Corynebacterium minutissimum* a lipophilic gram-positive aerobic diphtheroid
- Clinical:
  - Superficial infection of the intertriginous areas (axillae, groin, digital webspaces)
  - Groin/axillae show well-defined reddish brown plaques without central clearing, but it also commonly presents as white maceration between fourth and fifth webspace
- Diagnosis: fluoresce "coral red" with Wood's lamp (owing to production of coproporphyrin III by the bacteria)
- Treatment: topical erythromycin, clindamycin, miconazole, or aluminum chloride

Trichomycosis Axillaris

- *Corynebacterium tenuis* (gram-positive diphtheroid)
- Clinical:
  - White concretions on hair shaft, usually in axillae. Occasionally affects pubic hair (trichomycosis pubis). Often seen with hyperhidrosis, usually asymptomatic; however, patients may complain of malodorous sweat
- Treatment: shave affected hair; use topical clindamycin or erythromycin

Pitted Keratolysis (Fig. 18-8)

- *Kytococcus sedentarius* (previously *Micrococcus sedentarius*)
- Bacteria proliferate and produce proteinases: destroy the stratum corneum
- Clinical:
  - Shallow pits on the soles, sweaty feet, sulfur-compound by-products → malodor
- Treatment: reduce hyperhidrosis, topical clindamycin or erythromycin

Erysipeloid

- *Erysipelothrix rhusiopathiae* (gram-positive bacillus)
- Direct contact with infected meat, fish, or animal products
- Three clinical forms
  - Localized cutaneous form (erysipeloid of Rosenbach): purplish raised plaque, well demarcated on hand (common in fishermen and butchers)
  - Diffuse cutaneous form: multiple lesions appear on various parts of the body
  - Generalized or systemic infection associated with endocarditis
- Treatment: penicillin, ciprofloxacin, third-generation cephalosporin

Anthrax

- *Bacillus anthracis* (gram-positive bacillus)
- Exposure to sick animals or contaminated wool, hair, or animal hides
- Two virulence factors: (1) D-glutamyl polypeptide capsule; (2) pair of toxins: edema toxin and lethal toxin
- Clinical:
  - One- to 12-day incubation period, followed by a low-grade fever and malaise

- Pulmonary anthrax (woolsorter syndrome): 5% of anthrax cases. Due to inhalation of anthrax spores → nonspecific symptoms: low-grade fever and a nonproductive cough. Hemorrhagic mediastinal infection. Can result in septicemic anthrax. Usually fatal
  - Chest x-ray: widened mediastinum with hemorrhagic pleural effusions
- Gastrointestinal anthrax: due to ingestion of infected meat products. Mainly affects the cecum
- Cutaneous anthrax: occurs 1 to 7 days after skin exposure → "Malignant pustule": central area of coagulation necrosis (ulcer with eventual eschar), edema, and vesicles filled with bloody or clear fluid (actually *not* pustular) → ruptures to leave a black eschar and scar. Regional lymphadenopathy may persist
  - Most cases of simply zoonotically acquired cutaneous anthrax are not fatal (< 20% fatality untreated, < 1% fatality if treated)
  - Anthrax meningitis may occur after bacteremic seeding from any form of anthrax
- Diagnosis: stain exudates from ulcer with methylene blue or Giemsa; culture on blood agar: from skin, pleural fluid, CSF; serologic diagnosis (enzyme-linked immunosorbent assay [ELISA]); skin biopsy: organisms can be seen within capillaries
- Treatment: penicillin, doxycycline, quinolones; do not incise and drain secondary to dissemination
  - Postexposure prophylaxis to prevent inhalation anthrax for 60 days
  - Vaccine exists but is not readily available

Necrotizing Fasciitis ("flesh-eating bacteria")

- Life-threatening soft-tissue infection, needs urgent care and consultation
- Type I (most common): polymicrobial—*Staph, Escherichia coli, bacteroides, clostridium perfringens*
- Type II: group A *Streptococcus pyogenes* (~10%)
- Can result from trauma, chronic ulcers, surgical procedures, or occur spontaneously
- Clinical
  - In early stages, pain out of proportion to physical findings, erythema progressing to vesiculation or bullae formation → spreads from the subcutaneous tissue along the superficial and deep fascial planes → ischemia and tissue necrosis due to thrombosis → crepitus present with gas-forming aerobes
  - Septicemia; type II NF can lead to strep toxic shock syndrome
  - Fournier gangrene: localized variant of type I NF involving gentitocrural areas (usually men but can be women)
- Diagnosis: standard radiographs or computed tomography (CT) to visualize free air; deep incisional biopsy will demonstrate bacteria, thrombosis and tissue necrosis; culture; tissue biopsy; gram stain
- Treatment—Surgical debridement is paramount
  - Aerobes: (usually gram-negative organisms), ampicillin, and gentamicin
  - Anaerobes: clindamycin or metronidazole
  - Intravenous immunoglobulin

Actinomycosis

- Caused by *Actinomyces israelii,* a filamentous, anaerobic, gram-positive bacteria
- Cutaneous disease includes cervicofacial disease (lumpy jaw) or cutaneous mycetoma (Maduromycosis)
- Clinical:
  - Cervicofacial—abscess with draining sinus, usually at the angle of the jaw or in submandibular area, sulfur granules may be seen in the exudate
  - Maduromycosis—cutaneous pyoderma with characteristic purulent draining with discharged "sulfur granules" (aggregates of filamentous bacteria)
  - Diagnosis: complete blood count: mild leukocytosis; culture; gram-stained smear: branched, gram-positive filamentous rods
  - Treatment: penicillin, tetracyclines are alternatives; Maduromycosis often requires surgical intervention or even amputation

GRAM-NEGATIVE BACTERIAL DISEASES

Ecthyma Gangrenosum

- Bacteremia with skin lesions caused by *Pseudomonas aeruginosa* (gram-negative rods)
- Most often in immunocompromised patients (neutropenic or those with HIV infection)
- Clinical
  - Hemorrhagic bullae that develop into black eschars in the gluteal or perineal region (57%), extremities (30%), trunk (6%)
- Diagnosis: gram stain; blood cultures; histology: vascular necrosis with inflammatory cells and surrounding bacteria
- Treatment: penicillins, aminoglycosides, fluoroquinolones, third-generation cephalosporins, or aztreonam

Green Nail Syndrome

- *Pseudomonas aeruginosa*
- Greenish discoloration in areas of onycholysis due to pigment production: pyocyanin: blue, fluorescein: yellow/green, pyomelinin: black
- Seen in people who chronically have their hands in water
- Treatment: acetic acid solution and/or thymol 4% solution

Pseudomonas Folliculitis (hot tub folliculitis)

- *P. aeruginosa*
- Clinical:

- Exposure to whirlpools, swimming pools, and hot tubs → Pustular eruption in follicular distribution on trunk (underneath swimwear)
- Treatment: self-limited, acetic acid soaks, quinolones in severe cases

Gram-Negative Folliculitis

- *Proteus, Klebsiella, Escherichia,* and *Serratia* spp
- Complication in patients with acne vulgaris and rosacea who have received systemic antibiotics for prolonged periods of time
- Clinical
    - Acne that has not been responding to antimicrobial therapy or other therapy: 80% of patients
    - Patient's acne suddenly flares: 20% of patients
    - Superficial pustular lesions without comedones
    - Deep, nodular, and cystic lesions
- Laboratory studies: gram stain and culture
- Treatment: isotretinoin, systemic antibiotics

Otitis Externa (swimmer ear)

- Commonly due to *Pseudomonas*
- Erythema, tenderness, edema, greenish purulent discharge—topical antibiotics curative
- Malignant Otitis Externa: diabetics and immunocompromized—can be fatal, even with IV antibiotics

Gram-negative Toe Web Infection

- Superinfection of tinea by *Pseudomonas, E. coli, Proteus*
- Maceration, erythema, edema, fissuring
- Treat with vinegar-water soaks, topical phenol/gentian violet, topical/systemic antibiotics

Malakoplakia

- Commonly due to *E. coli*
- Seen mainly in immunocompromised patients
- Mainly affects genitourinary tract but may occasionally involve the skin
- Clinical
    - Yellow to pink papules, nodules, or ulcerations; draining abscesses/sinuses
    - Common areas of presentation; perianal or inguinal areas, the buttocks, and the abdominal wall
- Diagnosis:
    - Histology: foamy histiocytes with basophilic inclusions containing calcium and iron—referred to as Michaelis-Gutmann bodies (stain with von Kossa for calcium and Perls Prussian blue for iron, also stain with periodic acid–Schiff and are diastase resistant); histiocytes with fine eosinophilic cytoplasmic granules (von Hansemann cells) can also be seen
    - Culture fluid from sinuses: check for bacterial (aerobic and anaerobic), fungal, and mycobacterial pathogens
- Treatment: quinolone antibiotics and sulfonamides, excise skin lesions and drain abscesses

Rhinoscleroma

- *Klebsiella rhinoscleromatis* (gram-negative coccobacillus)
- Chronic granulomatous condition of the nose and upper respiratory tract
- Inhalation of droplets or contaminated material
- Clinical
    - Three stages:
        - rhinitic: purulent rhinorrhea
        - Proliferative : intranasal rubbery nodules or polyps; epistaxis (bloody nose)
            - ▲ Hebra nose: nasal enlargement, deformity, and destruction of the nasal cartilage
        - fibrotic: sclerosis and fibrosis with possible stenosis
- Diagnosis: culture; CT scan: soft-tissue masses of variable sizes
- Histology
    - Mikulicz cells: parasitized histiocytes
    - Silver stains (Warthin-Starry) can be used to highlight the bacteria
    - Russel body: eosinophilic bodies inside and outside plasma cells secondary to increased IgG
- Treatment: surgery combined with antibiotic therapy (tetracycline, ciprofloxacin, and rifampin)

Meningococcal Disease (Fig. 18-9)

- *Neisseria meningitides* (obligate aerobic, encapsulated gram-negative diplococcus)
- Serogroups B, C, Y, >> A, W135, X, and Z
- Transmitted from person to person via respiratory secretions
- Approximately 20 to 40% of young adults are carriers of the bacteria

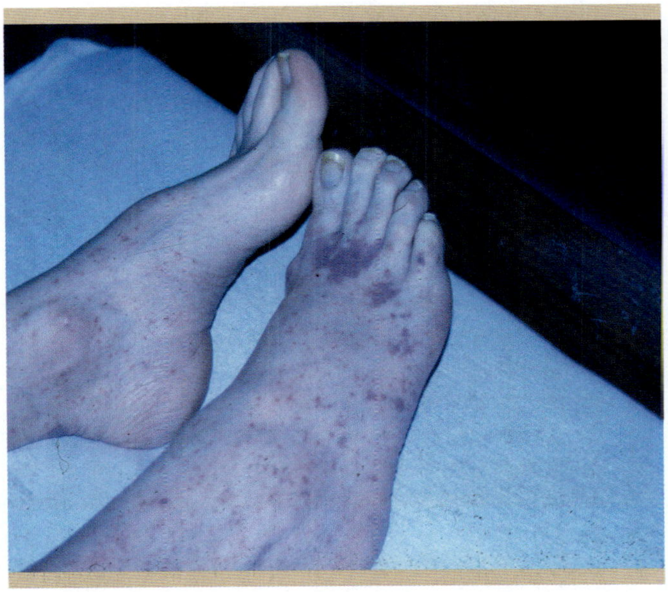

FIGURE 18-9 Meningococcal disease. (*Used with permission from Dr. Asra Ali.*)

- Persons with deficiencies of terminal complement components C5 to C9 or properdin, immunoglobulin deficiency, asplenia, and HIV infection are most susceptible
- Direct invasion of endothelial cells and indirect damage from endotoxin release
- Clinical
  - Cutaneous findings: petechiae; pustules, bullae, and hemorrhagic lesions with central necrosis; stellate purpura with a central gunmetal-gray hue
  - Fulminant meningococcemia: can present as purpura fulminans
    - Waterhouse-Friderichsen syndrome: symmetric peripheral gangrene, cyanosis, hypotension, and profound shock
  - Meningitis
    - Headache and a stiff neck; lethargy or drowsiness
  - Chronic meningococcemia: one week to as long as several months with recurrent fever and variable rash usually occurring on pressure areas or around painful joints
- Diagnosis: blood and throat cultures on blood agar; lumbar puncture; gram stain of lesional skin biopsy or aspirate specimens
  - Histology: acute vasculitis with meningcocci seen in thrombi of dermal vessels
- Prevention: a new, longer-acting, conjugated vaccine exists for types A, C, Y, and W135 that can be administered to patients 2 to 55 years of age
- Treatment: penicillin G, third-generation cephalosporin (ceftriaxone)
  - close contacts get rifampin, ciprofloxacin, or ceftriaxone

Bartonella Species

- Cat-scratch disease (CSD), oroya fever, verruga peruana, bacillary angiomatosis (BA), trench fever
- Aerobic gram-negative organisms

Cat-Scratch Disease (Benign Lymphoreticulosis)

- Mainly caused by *Bartonella henselae* (gram-negative bacillus)
- Vector: cat flea (*Ctenocephalides felis*): maintains infection in cats
- Clinical
  - Infection spread by bite or scratch from cats (particularly kittens), incubation of 3 to 12 days
  - Fever in 25 to 75% of patients
  - Constitutional symptoms: anorexia, myalgias
  - Red papules appear at the site of scratch (develops over 3–10 days)
  - Lymphadenopathy (develops 1 week to 2 months after exposure)
    - Fifty percent have involvement of a single node
    - May last 6 weeks to 2 years
  - Parinaud oculoglandular syndrome: unilateral conjunctivitis and regional lymphadenitis
  - CNS changes 1 to 2%: headaches, mental status changes, seizures, encephalitis, cerebrospinal fluid usually normal
- Diagnosis:
  - Indirect immunoflourescent antibody (IFA) for *Bartonella* (cross-reactivity between *B. henselae* and *B. quintana)*
  - Brown-Hopp tissue gram stain and Warthin-Starry silver staining show small, curved, gram-negative bacilli
  - Fourfold rise in IgG antibody levels
  - Lymph node biopsy: necrotizing granulomas
- Treatment
  - Immunosuppressed patients: azithromycin, erythromycin, doxycycline, septra, rifampin, ciprofloxacin, gentamycin
  - Immunocompetant patients: supportive care since CSD is a self-limiting disease

Bacillary Angiomatosis (Fig. 18-10)

- Etiologic agents are *B. henselae, B. quintana*
- Typically occurs in HIV (with CD4 counts < 200/μL) or in other immunocompromised patients
- Adheres to and invades red blood cells (RBCs)
- Makes an endothelial cell–stimulating factor: proliferation of both endothelial cells and blood vessels
- Clinical
  - Four cutaneous patterns
    - Erythematous papules and nodules that are nonblanching
    - Violaceous nodule (similar to Kaposi sarcoma)
    - Violaceous lichenoid plaque
    - Subcutaneous nodule that may ulcerate

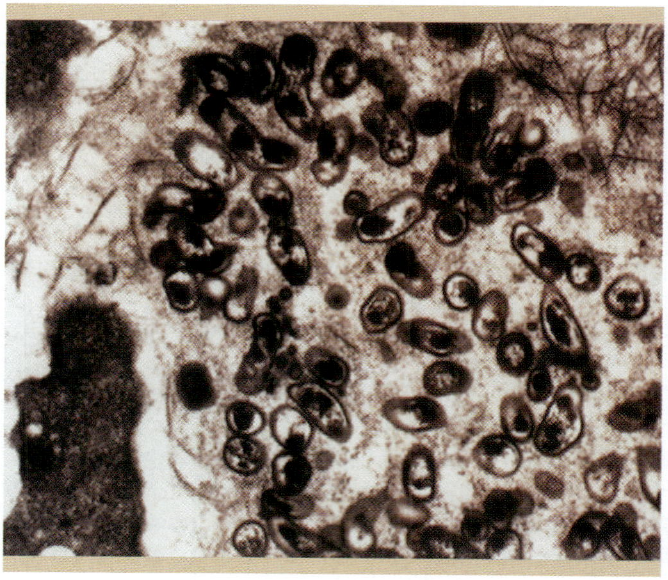

FIGURE 18-10 Bacillary angiomatosis. (*Reprinted with permission from Connor DH et al. Pathology of Infectious Diseases. Stanford, CT: Appleton & Lange; 1997, p. 408.*)

  - Other areas of the body affected by BA: brain, bone, bone marrow, lymph nodes, gastrointestinal tract, respiratory tract, spleen, and liver
  - Peliosis hepatitis: blood-filled cysts in liver of AIDS patients (occasionally are found in spleen)
    - Nausea, vomiting, diarrhea, and fever with hepatosplenomegaly
- Diagnosis:
  - Histology
    - Bacilli stain with modified Warthin-Starry stain (silver based)
    - Vascular proliferation with small vessels arranged in clusters; epithelial collarette may be observed
  - Chest x-ray and CT: pulmonary nodules
- Treatment: erythromycin and doxycycline
  - May get Jarisch-Herxheimer reaction:
    - Self-limited reaction seen after treatment of syphilis, borreliosis, brucellosis, typhoid fever, trichinellosis, leptospirosis, leprosy, Lyme disease, relapsing fever (epidemic)
    - Fever, malaise, nausea/vomiting, exacerbation of secondary rash
    - Occurs 8 hours after the first injection; resolves within 24 hours

Trench Fever

- Caused by *B. quintana* (aerobic, gram-negative bacillus)
- Incubation period of a few days to a month
- Spread by human body louse (*Pediculus humanus corporis*)
- Clinical
  - Symptoms begin with chills and fever: relapsing fever every 5 days (also can have single febrile episode occurring for 3–5 days or persistent fever lasting 2–6 weeks)
  - Headaches, neck and back pain
  - Groups of erythematous macules or papules measuring 1 cm or less
- Diagnosis: polymerase chain reaction (PCR)
- Histology: perivascular infiltrate, organisms are not visible
- Treatment: doxycycline, erythromycin

Oroya Fever (Carrion Disease) and Verruga Peruana

- Caused by *Bartonella bacilliformis*
- Vector: sand fly (*Lutzomyia verrucarum*)
- Clinical
  - Fever begins 3 to 12 weeks after bite
  - Acute form: fevers, headache, hepatsplenomegaly, hemolytic anemia (80% of RBCs infected), depressed CD4 counts
  - Chronic form: verruga peruana (Fig. 18-11)
    - Small nodules form and subsequently become larger
    - Vascular miliary, nodular and mular lesions form (resemble pyogenic granuloma)

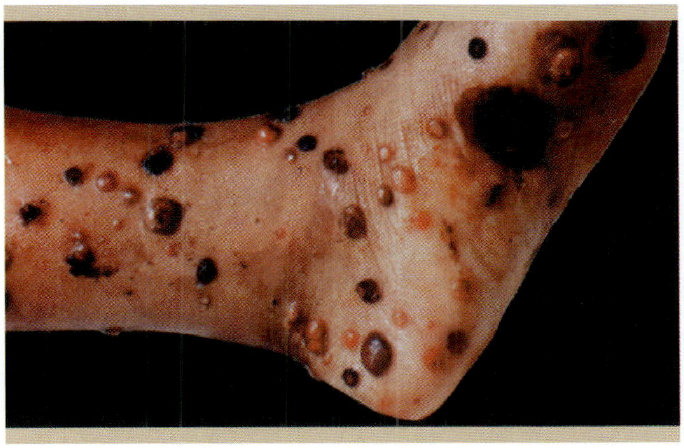

FIGURE 18-11 Verruga peruana. (*Reprinted with permission from Connor DH et al. Pathology of Infectious Diseases. Stanford, CT: Appleton & Lange; 1997, p. 434.*)

    - Can ulcerate, bleed, and heal by fibrosis over several months
    - Various stages may occur together
- Diagnosis:
  - Histology: Rocha-Lima bodies: purple cytoplasmic inclusion bodies in endothelial cells
  - Hemolytic anemia, thrombocytopenia, and elevated liver function studies
- Treatment: chloramphenicol or doxycycline

Brucellosis (Mediterranean Fever, Malta Fever, Gastric Remittent Fever, and Undulent Fever)

- *Brucella abortus, Brucella melitensis, Brucella suis,* and *Brucella canis* (aerobic gram-negative coccobacilli)
- Aerosol transmission as well as through breaks in the skin, mucous membranes, conjunctiva, and respiratory and GI tracts
- Infections are seen in occupations with direct or indirect exposures to animals, such as the meat-packing industry or from unpasteurized dairy products (goat cheese)
- Incubation is between 1 and 8 weeks
- Cell wall lipopolysaccharide (LPS): principal virulence factor that enters macrophages
- Infects organs of the reticuloendothelial system (i.e., liver, spleen, bone marrow)
- Host response results in tissue granulomas and visceral microabscesses
- Clinical
  - Acute fever, malaise, arthralgias
  - Cutaneous signs: rare granulomas, ulcerations, petechiae, purpura, and erythema nodosum
  - Other: endocarditis, sacroiliitis, meningitis, epididymo-orchitis in males
- Diagnosis:
  - Agglutination titers for anti-O-polysaccharide antibody

- Culture (bone marrow culture much more sensitive than blood culture)
- Immunoglobulin G (IgG) by ELISA
- Anemia, thrombocytopenia, pancytopenia in 6% of patients ← bone marrow biopsy showing erythrophagocytosis
- Elevated liver enzymes
- CSF reveals pleocytosis, elevated protein levels
- Echocardiogram to evaluate for endocarditis
- Treatment: doxycycline and rifampin or trimethoprim-sulfamethoxazole (TMP-SMZ) plus rifampin; drain pyogenic joint effusions or rare paraspinal abscesses

Leptospirosis (Weil Disease or Icteric Leptospirosis)

- *Leptospira interrogans* (spirochete)
- Incubation period is usually 7 to 12 days
- Infects many types of mammals: cats, dogs, cattle, pigs, squirrels, rats
- Transmitted via infected urine and then through contact with contaminated water and soil
- Over half of cases in the United States occur in Hawaii
- Clinical
  - Two distinct presentations
  - Septicemic: organism may be isolated from blood cultures, CSF, and most tissues; patients may have myalgias, weakness as well as meningitis like symptoms (headache, photophobia)
  - Immune: occurs after a few days of improvement following the septicemic stage, occurs as a result of an immune reaction to the infection
  - Subclinical meningitis with headaches, fever, petechiae
  - Cutaneous lesions: macular or maculopapular eruption with erythematous, urticarial, petechial, or desquamative lesions, jaundice (90% of patients manifest a mild anicteric form of the disease)
  - Vasculitis of capillaries: petechiae, intraparenchymal bleeding, and bleeding along serosa and mucosa
  - Organ involvement: direct hepatic injury (jaundice, hepatosplenomegaly, nausea and vomiting), alveolar capillary injury, renal tubular necrosis, myocarditis and coronary arteritis
  - CSF: ± encephalitis
- Syndromes occasionally based on species type
  - *L. autumnali*: pretibial fever (Fort Bragg fever): fevers, pretibial erythema, and ocular symptoms
  - *L. grippotyphosa*: gastrointestinal symptoms
  - *L. pomona* or *L. canicola*: aseptic meningitis:
  - *L. icterohaemorrhagiae*: jaundice (83% of patients)
- Weil syndrome: profound jaundice, renal dysfunction, hepatic necrosis, pulmonary dysfunction, and hemorrhagic diathesis
- Diagnosis
  - Serologies: microscopic agglutination test (MAT): four-fold increase
  - Indirect hemagglutination assay (IHA):
  - Dark-field microscopy of blood or rising antibodies
  - Culture: blood, CSF, urine
- Circulating antibodies may be detected or the organism may be isolated from urine; it may not be recoverable from blood or CSF
- Treatment: tetracyclines or penicillin (possible Jarisch-Herxheimer reaction)

TICK-BORNE BACTERIAL INFECTIONS

Tularemia (Ohara Disease, Deer Fly Fever)

- *Francisella tularensis* (gram-negative coccobacillus)
- Vectors: hard tick *(Dermacentor andersoni, Amblyomma americanum)* or deer fly *(Chrysops discalis)*
- Reservoir: rabbits ("rabbit fever" common in hunters)
- Incubation period of 3 to 4 days
- Clinical
  - Eight forms: depend on mode of transmission: ulceroglandular (most common), glandular, oculoglandular, oropharyngeal, pulmonary, typhoidal, meningeal, chancriform
    - Intracellular parasitism of reticuloendothelial system of humans
    - Infection common in hunters after infected animal exposure via vectors
  - Ulceroglandular (70–80% of cases)
    - Organism enters through a scratch or abrasion
    - Tender papule that ulcerates with sporotrichoid spread
    - Regional lymphadenopathy
  - Typhoidal (10–15% of cases) severe form with pneumonia, fever, myalgias
- Diagnosis: ELISA, PCR
  - blood cultures usually negative
- Treatment: aminoglycosides (streptomycin)

Lyme Disease (Fig. 18-12)

- Caused by the spirochete *Borrelia burgdorferi*
- Vector: *Ixodes* ticks (hard ticks)
- Eastern/midwestern United States: *I. scapularis and I. dammini*
- Northwestern United States: *I. pacificus*
- Europe: *I. ricinus* and *I. persulcatus*
- Clinical
  - Stage 1: early localized
    - Erythema migrans (EM) occurs in up to 80% of cases
    - Erythematous macule or papule at site of the tick bite, can have central clearing
    - Expanding figurate erythema occurs over days to weeks
    - Typically resolves in about one month

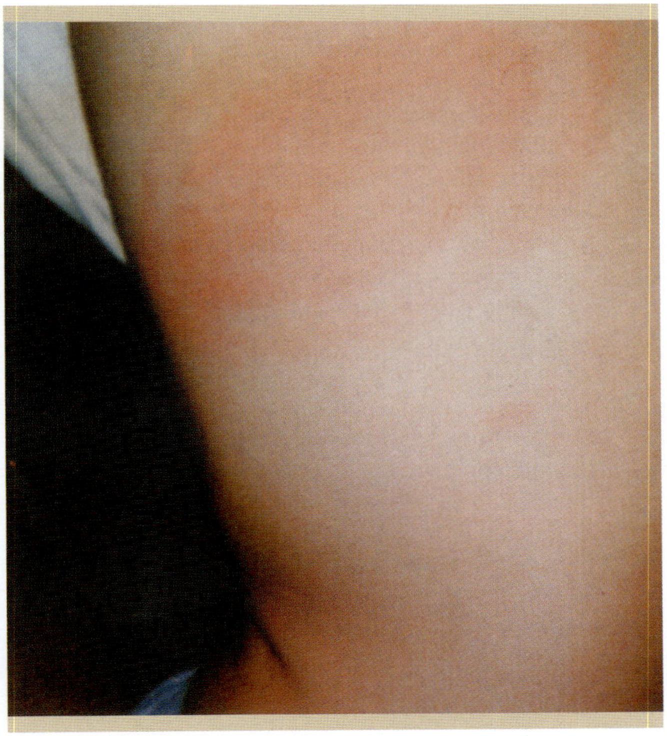

FIGURE 18-12 Lyme disease. (*Reprinted with permission from Connor DH et al. Pathology of Infectious Diseases. Stanford, CT: Appleton & Lange; 1997, p. 637.*)

- Stage 2: early disseminated disease
  - Hematogenous spread
  - Lymphocytic meningitis, cranial neuropathy, carditis (heart block, arrhythymias), and rheumatologic changes (arthralgias, oligoarthritis)
  - Borrelial lymphocytoma: bluish red nodular swelling that is almost always on the lobe of the ear or the areola of the nipple
- Stage 3: late Lyme disease
  - Acrodermatitis chronica atrophicans (ACA)
  - Twenty percent of patients have history of untreated erythema migrans
  - Develops 6 months to 10 years later
- Inflammatory phase (early): edema and erythema, usually on the distal extremities
  - Atrophic phase (late): 5 to 10% of patients develop scleroderma-like plaques
    - Loss of subcutaneous fat, with thin, atrophic, and dry skin
    - Neurologic changes (meningitis, encephalitis)
- Diagnosis
  - Antibody titer (antibodies take 4–6 weeks to develop and thus, are not usually present at the time of the rash)
  - Confirm positive ELISA antibody titers with PCR
  - False-positive results of IFA or ELISA can occur because of cross-reactivity with *Treponema pallidum*, and other spirochetal agents
  - Histology: presence of telangiectasias and cellular infiltrates of lymphocytes with admixed plasma cells; ACA demonstrates striking epidermal atrophy
- Treatment: doxycycline or amoxicillin; erythromycin for pediatric patients

Rickettsioses

- Obligate intracellular gram-negative coccobacilli
- Transmitted to humans by arthropods
- Spotted fever group
  - Rocky Mountain spotted fever
  - Rickettsial pox
  - Boutonneuse fever
- Typhus group
  - Louse-borne (epidemic) typhus
  - Brill-Zinsser disease (i.e., relapsing louse-borne typhus)
  - Murine (endemic or flea-borne) typhus
- Other rickettsial diseases
  - Tsutsugamushi disease (i.e., "scrub typhus")
  - Q fever: *Coxiella burnetii*
  - Ehrlichia

Rocky Mountain Spotted Fever

- *Rickettsia rickettsii* (obligate intracellular gram-coccobacilli)
- Disease commonly found in North Carolina and Oklahoma which account for one-third of total cases reported; other areas outside of the United States include Canada, Mexico, Central America, Colombia, and Brazil
- Vectors
  - Eastern United States: wood tick *(D. andersoni)*
  - Western United States: dog tick *(Dermacentor variabilis)*
- Clinical
  - Triad: fever, headache, and rash (1–2 weeks after tick bite)
  - Multisystem involvement is common
  - Skin lesions
    - Appear two to four days following fever
    - Blanchable macular rash that starts on extremities and spreads to trunk (centripetal)
    - Face usually spared; involvement of the scrotum or the vulva and palms/soles
    - Erythematous macules that become petechial over a few days
  - "Spotless" fever in 10% of cases
    - Desquamation occurs as the rash fades
    - Systemic findings: hepatosplenomegaly, myocarditis, thrombocytopenia, CNS involvement (confusion, lethargy, ataxia, and seizures)
  - Rumple-Leede test: multiple petechiae appear after sphygmomanometer or tourniquet

- Diagnosis
  - Elevated liver function tests
  - Blood cultures
  - Indirect fluorescent antibody
  - Direct immunofluorescence
  - Immunoperoxidase staining
  - Latex agglutination
  - Complement fixation
  - Giemsa stain
  - Lumbar puncture
  - Weil-Felix assay: agglutination of OX-strains of Proteus vulgaris with suspected rickettsia
- Treatment: tetracycline or chloramphenicol (in pediatric patients)
  - Avoid sulfa treatments; symptoms may worsen

Rickettsialpox

- Caused by *R. akari*
- Vector: rodent (house mouse) mite, *Liponyssoides sanguineus* (formerly *Allodermanyssus sanguineus*)
- Most common in boroughs of New York City (Brooklyn, Queens), found commonly in urban areas
- Incubation period is 10 to 21 days
- Clinical
  - Papular skin lesions appear at the bite site and then become vesicular with surrounding erythema → dries and forms a black eschar; no scarring
  - Sudden onset of high-grade fever and chills (3 days after skin lesions), headaches, and myalgias
  - Mild and self-limited disease which persists for about a week
- Diagnosis:
  - Cultures from blood
  - Direct fluorescent antibody test of biopsies from skin lesions
  - Indirect immunoflourescent antibody (IFA) testing
  - Complement fixation
  - Histology: mononuclear cell infiltration and necrosis of the dermis and epidermis. Perivascular inflammation with thrombi and extravasation of red blood cells
  - Giemsa stain of tissue: small coccobacillary intracellular bacteria
- Treatment: (self-limited disease); doxycycline or chloramphenicol, quinolones

Boutonneuse Fever (Mediterranean Fever)

- Causative agent is *R. conorii*
- Vector: *Rhipicephalus sanguineus* (brown dog tick)
- Incubation time of BF is usually 4 to 15 days
- Clinical
  - Fever
  - Exanthem: erythematous papules, mainly on the lower limbs
  - Tache noire (eschar, necrotic plaque) at the site of the tick bite
  - Malignant form
    - Criteria: requires two laboratory abnormalities (thrombocytopenia, increased creatinine level, hyponatremia, hypocalcemia, hypoxemia) and two clinical criteria (purpuric rash, stupor, pneumonia, bradycardia, coma, jaundice, gastrointestinal bleeding)
    - More common in patients with underlying disease or in elderly persons
    - Disease progression: acute stage is from the second to 14th day of the illness; convalescent stage starts from the 21st day
- Diagnosis:
  - Immunofluorescent antibody: direct immunofluorescence of cutaneous biopsy specimens (during active disease)
  - Culture
  - ELISA: detects antibodies to LPS of *R. conorii*
- Treatment: tetracyclines together with chloramphenicol and quinolones

Typhus Group

- Three main forms of typhus: epidemic typhus; rat-flea or endemic typhus, and scrub typhus.
- Diagnosis
  - Actual isolation and culture of *rickettsiae* are difficult
  - Serologic tests for antibodies
  - Indirect immunofluorescence assay (IFA)
  - ELISA
  - Indirect immunoperoxidase
  - Weil-Felix test
  - PCR: serum or skin biopsy
  - Complement fixation (CF)
- Treatment: doxycycline, chloramphenicol

Epidemic Typhus

- Caused by *R. prowazekii*
- Vector: human body louse (*Pediculus humanus corporis)*
- Humans are the natural reservoir
- Incubation period of 7 to 14 days
- Clinical
  - Fever, headache
  - Maculopapular rash occurs on days 4 to 7
  - Begins on the axilla and trunk and spreads peripherally
  - Can become hemorrhagic with necrosis
  - Mortality is high in untreated elderly patients
  - Brill-Zinsser disease: mild reccurence of disease: can occur months, years, or even decades after treatment

Murine Typhus (Endemic Typhus)

- Caused by *R. typhi*
- Vectors: rat or cat flea *(Xenopsylla cheopis, Ctenocephalides felis)*
- Incubation of 6 to 18 days

- Clinical
  - Erythematous macular eruption without becoming hemorrhagic or necrotic following fever

Scrub Typhus (Tsutsugamushi Fever)

- *Orientia tsutsugamushi* (formerly *Rickettsia tsutsugamushi*); it has a different cell wall structure and genetic composition than that of the rickettsiae
- Vector: trombiculid mite (larval stage of a chigger): *Leptotrombidium akamushi* and possibly *L. deliense*
- Incubation period is 5 to 20 days
- Clinical
  - Headaches, shaking chills, lymphadenopathy, conjunctival injection, fever
  - Painless papule develops at site of bite, and then a central necrosis results with formation of an eschar
  - Five to eight days after infection, dull red rash on trunk and extending to the extremities
  - Pneumonitis or encephalitis can occur; hepatosplenomegaly; regional lymphadenopathy

Ehrlichiosis

- Due to gram-negative organisms that resemble *Rickettsia*
- Human monocytic ehrlichioses (HME): *Ehrlichia chaffensis*
- Human granulocytic ehrlichiosis (HGE): *E. phagocytophilia*
- Vector:
  - HME: Lone Star tick (*Amblyoma americanum*) or wood tick (*Dermacentor variabilis*)
  - HGE: deer tick (*Ixodes persulcatus*)
- Clinical
  - Rash is rare in ehrlichiosis; however, can develop maculopapular lesions following fever
  - Rare renal failure and encephalopathy
  - Lymphadenopathy may be present
- Diagnosis:
  - Histology: characteristic morulae in the cytoplasm of leukocytes
  - Neutropenia, lymphocytopenia, or thrombocytopenia
  - Elevated immunoglobulin G (IgG) immunofluorescent antibody (IFA) *Ehrlichia* titer
- Treatment: tetracyclines; chloramphenicol is not effective in ehrlichiosis

SEXUALLY TRANSMITTED BACTERIAL INFECTIONS

Gonorrhea (Fig. 18-13)

- *Neisseria gonorrhoeae* (gram-negative intracellular aerobic diplococcus)
- Clinical
  - Men: urethritis; women: dyspareunia, bleeding or discharge

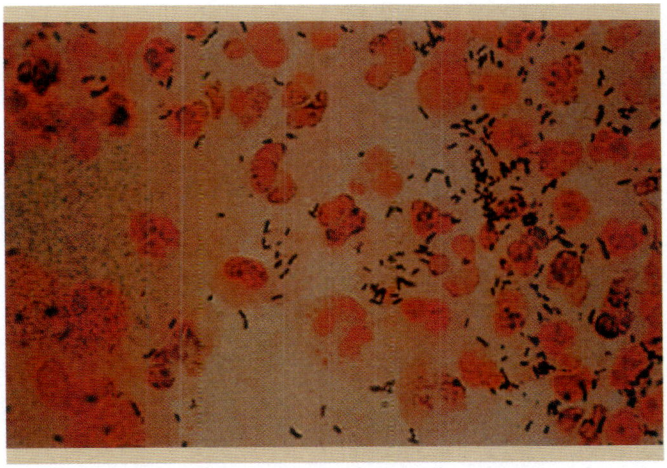

FIGURE 18-13 Gonorrhea. (*Reprinted with permission from Connor DH et al. Pathology of Infectious Diseases. Stanford, CT: Appleton & Lange; 1997, p. 686.*)

  - Neonates: bilateral conjunctivitis (ophthalmia neonatorum) after vaginal delivery from an infected mother
  - Acute perihepatitis with hepatic capsular adhesions (Fitz-Hugh-Curtis syndrome)
  - Dissemination: arthritis dermatitis syndrome (1–3% of cases)
    - Septic arthritis: knee is most common site; polyarthralgia with pain, tenderness
    - Rare gonococcal meningitis and endocarditis
  - Skin findings: maculopapular, pustular, necrotic, or vesicular lesions; face, scalp, and mouth are usually spared
- Diagnosis:
  - Culture on chocolate agar
  - Gram stain
  - Fluorescein-conjugated monoclonal antibodies, enzyme-linked immunoassays
- Treatment: ceftriaxone intramuscular, cefixime, ciprofloxacin

Granuloma Inguinale (Fig. 18-14)

- *Klebsiella granulomatis* (gram-negative rod), formerly *Calymmatobacterium granulomatosis*
- Clinical
  - Four types of skin lesions:
    - *Ulcerovegetative* (most commonly seen): painless, beefy red ulcers with clean, friable bases and distinct, raised/rolled margins; autoinoculation is common
    - *Nodular*: pruritic, soft, red nodules that ulcerate at the site of inoculation
      - ▲ Pseudobubo: nodule appears clinically as a lymph node

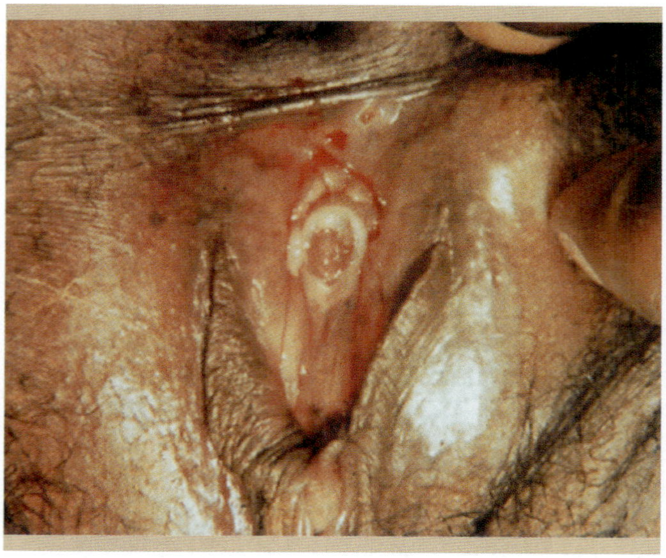

FIGURE 18-14 Granuloma inguinale. (*Reprinted with permission from Connor DH et al. Pathology of Infectious Diseases. Stanford, CT: Appleton & Lange; 1997, p. 567.*)

    - *Cicatricial*: dry ulcers that progress into scarring plaques, +/− lymphedema
  - *Hypertrophic or verrucous* (relatively rare): vegetating soft masses
- Diagnosis:
  - Culture not possible
  - Smear or biopsy with Wright, Giemsa or Warthin-Starry (silver) stain: Donovan bodies: intracytoplasmic bipolar staining, safety pin-shaped, inclusion bodies seen in histiocytes
  - Histology: acanthosis, dermis with histiocytes and plasma cells, large and vacuolated macrophages with intracellular bacilli (i.e., Donovan bodies)
- Treatment: doxycycline or trimethoprim/sulfamethoxazole

Lymphogranuloma Venereum (Fig. 18-15)

- Caused by *Chlamydia trachomatis* L1, L2 (most common), L3 serotypes
- Incubation period of 3 to 21 days
- Clinical
  - 3 stages:
    - *First stage*: small papule usually not seen, lasts 1 week, painless
    - *Second stage*: buboes (painful lymph nodes) after 2 to 6 weeks; groove sign: enlargement of the nodes above (inguinal) and below (femoral) the inguinal ligament (poupart)
    - *Third stage*: fistulas seen more often in women, proctocolitis, results in scarring/chronic lymphatic obstruction (acute rectal syndrome)

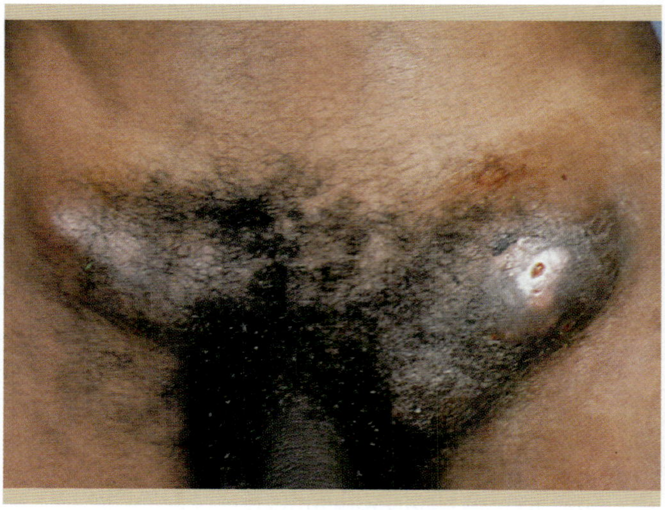

FIGURE 18-15 Lymphogranuloma venereum. (*Reprinted with permission from Goldsmith LA et al. Fitzpatrick's Dermatology in General Medicine, 8th ed. New York: McGraw-Hill; 2012, p. 2507.*)

- Diagnosis:
  - Complement fixation test with titer of 1:64
  - Culture
  - Immunofluorescent testing with monoclonal antibodies
- Treatment: doxycycline; alternative is erythromycin

Chancroid (Fig. 18-16)

- Caused by *Haemophilus ducreyi* (gram-negative bacillus)
- The bacteria secretes a cytolethal distending toxin (HdCDT): inhibits cell proliferation and induces cell death

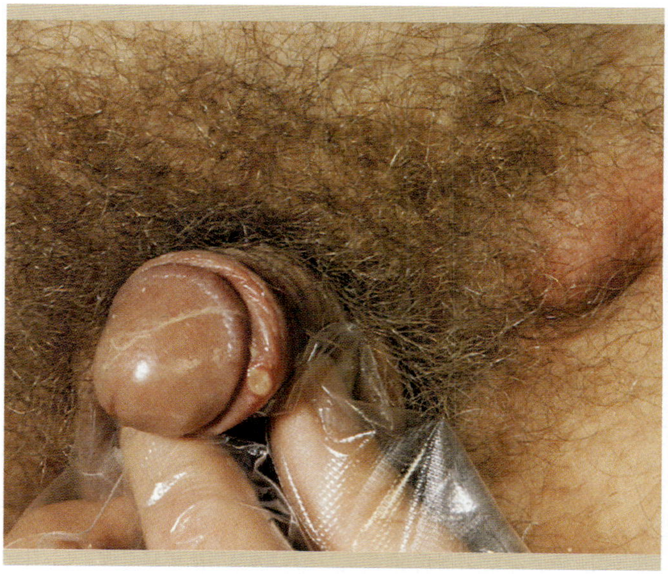

FIGURE 18-16 Chancroid. (*Reprinted with permission from Goldsmith LA et al. Fitzpatrick's Dermatology in General Medicine, 8th Ed. New York: McGraw-Hill; 2012; p. 2502.*)

- Clinical
  - Soft chancre: painful ragged punched-out ulcers, undermined borders, covered by a grayish fibrinous membrane
  - Lymph node involvement mostly unilateral and can rupture
  - Bubo: tender, fixed, inguinal lymphadenopathy
- Diagnosis
  - Gram staining: organisms in a "school-of-fish" pattern
  - Culture
  - Immunochromatography: monoclonal antibodies to the hemoglobin receptor of *H. ducreyi,* HgbA
- Treatment: azithromycin 1 g PO single dose, ceftriaxone 250 mg IM single dose, erythromycin 500 mg PO qid for 7 days, or ciprofloxacin 500 mg PO bid for 3 days; buboes should be drained

Syphilis

- Caused by *Treponema pallidum* (microaerophilic spirochete)
- Clinical
  - *Primary*
    - Occurs after incubation of approximately 3 weeks
    - Highly infectious painless chancre (ulcerated lesion with a surrounding red areola)
    - Lasts 10 to 14 days
    - Buboes: enlarged, nontender lymph nodes
  - *Secondary*
    - Occurs usually one month after chancre presents
    - Hair: alopecia ("moth eaten"), caused by papular follicular syphilids, localized patches to total alopecia
    - Mucous membrane:
      - ▲ Condyloma lata: infectious papules and small plaques develop at the mucocutaneous junctions and intertriginous areas
      - ▲ Pharyngitis
      - ▲ Mucous patches: silver-gray erosions with a red areola
    - Skin: bilaterally symmetric discrete round macules on the trunk and proximal extremities (often affecting palms and soles); can become necrotic
    - Ocular: anterior uveitis
  - *Latent syphilis*
    - Follows resolution of the secondary stage
  - Only evidence is positive serologic test for syphilis
    - Categories
      - ▲ Early latent: <1 year's duration
      - ▲ Late latent: ≥1 year's duration or of unknown duration (seroreactivity, in the absence of symptoms, greater than 2 years after inoculation)
  - *Tertiary*
    - Seroreactivity greater than 2 years with symptoms
    - Gummas: granulomas of skin and bone
    - Neurologic (neurosyphilis): may be asymptomatic or present as a subacute meningitis
      - ▲ Tabes dorsalis: demyelination of the posterior columns, dorsal roots, and dorsal root ganglia (e.g., ataxic wide-based gait and foot slap)
      - ▲ Argyll-Robertson pupil: small, irregular pupil, normal accommodation but abnormal light response (Romberg sign)
    - Cardiovascular: aortic aneursym, aortitis
  - *Congenital syphilis caused by transplacental transmission of spirochetes*
    - Early (<2 years of age)
      - ▲ Mucocutaneous changes:
        - △ Snuffles: rhinitis (nasal fluid is highly infectious)
        - △ Rhagades (Parrot lines): depressed linear scars radiating from the orifice of the mouth
        - △ Condyloma lata and mucous patches
        - △ Hepatomegaly
      - ▲ Bone changes:
        - △ Cranio tabes: reduction in mineralization of the skull, with abnormal softness of the bone
        - △ Pseudoparalysis of Parrot: child keeps limb still secondary to pain from osteochondritis
        - △ Osteochondritis: sawtooth x-ray lesion
      - ▲ Skin:
        - △ Copper-colored papulosquamous eruption, desquamative rash
        - △ Hematologic: jaundice, thrombocytopenia
    - Late (>2 years of age)
      - ▲ Interstitial keratitis: inflammation of the corneal stroma
      - ▲ Corneal opacities
      - ▲ Hutchinson teeth: peg-shaped incisors
      - ▲ Mulberry molars: poorly developed cusps
      - ▲ Saddle nose: secondary to gummatous periostitis
      - ▲ Syphilitic pemphigus congenital bullae with purulent fluid on palm
      - ▲ Bone changes:
        - △ Saber shin: anterior bowing of tibia
        - △ Frontal bossing
        - △ Higomenaki sign unilateral sternoclavicular enlargement
        - △ Bulldog jaw
        - △ Clutton joints (arthritis of both knees)
      - ▲ Recurrent arthropathy
      - ▲ Cranial nerve VIII deafness
- Diagnosis
  - Histology: often with psoriasiform and lichenoid changes and perivascular infiltration, chiefly by lymphocytes, plasma cells, and macrophages; may see spirochetes with modified Steiner or Warthin-Starry stains (silver based)

- Identification of *T. pallidum* in lesions on tissue:
  - Dark-field microscopy: immediate result
  - DFA-TP (direct fluoresence antibody test): direct fluorescent antibody *T. pallidum*, 1 to 2 days
  - immunohistochemical stains for *T. pallidum*
- *Nontreponemal serology screening*
  - VDRL test: measures IgM and IgG antibody directed against a cardiolipin lecithin-cholesterol antigen; not specific for *T. pallidum;* used to follow response to therapy (lower titers with successful treatment)
- Prozone effect:
  - May cause a false-negative reaction
  - Occurs when the reaction is overwhelmed by antibody excess and may happen in late primary or secondary syphilis
  - Should dilute the serum to at least a 1/16 dilution
- Rapid plasma reagin (RPR)
  - Develops 1 to 4 weeks after chancre
  - Fourfold decline in titer by 3 months following treatment
  - False-positive RPR results occur in 1 to 2% of the normal population
- *Treponemal tests*
  - FTA-ABS: fluorescent treponemal antibody absorption
    - ▲ Reactive 4 to 6 weeks after infection
    - ▲ Remains reactive for many years
    - ▲ Does not indicate response to therapy
    - ▲ Does not distinguish between syphilis and other treponematoses
    - ▲ Antibody (IgM and IgG) directed against *T. pallidum*
  - MHA-TP: microhemagglutination assay *T. pallidum* test
    - ▲ Remains reactive for life
    - ▲ Not recommended for monitoring reinfection or the efficacy of treatment
    - ▲ Chest x-ray for patients with tertiary syphilis to screen for aortic dilation
    - ▲ Lumbar puncture: in patients with latent syphilis, if treatment has failed or the time course of disease is unkown and if the patient is known to also have HIV
- Treatment: penicillin 2.4 million units IM
  - may have Jarisch-Herxheimer reaction (see above)

MYCOBACTERIA

Leprosy (Hansen Disease)

- Chronic granulomatous infection that affects skin and nerves
- Causative organism is *Mycobacterium leprae* (intracellular acid-fast gram-positive bacillus)
- Transmision: respiratory, human to human, armadillos, and sphagnum moss
- Humans are the primary reservoir of *M. leprae*
- Bimodal age distribution, with peaks at ages 10 to 14 years and 35 to 44 years
- Incubation: up to 5 years and may be 20 years or longer
- Clinical
  - *Neurological*
    - Acral distal symmetric anesthesia
    - Palsies of cranial nerves V and VII
    - Nerve enlargement
    - Predilection for superficial nerves (bacteria prefers lower temperatures)
    - Great auricular, ulnar, median, superficial peroneal, sural, and posterior tibial nerves (most commonly affected)
    - Anesthetic skin lesions (sensation to temperature is lost first)
  - *Cutaneous*: varies based on type of infection
    - *Ocular:* lagophthalmos (inability to close the eye/ involvement of cranial nerve [CN] VII branches), reduced corneal reflex and reduced blinking [ophthalmic branch of the trigeminal nerve (CN V2)]
  - *Classification of leprosy types*
    - Depends on the level of host cell-mediated immunity
    - TT (polar tuberculoid) ↔ BT (borderline tuberculoid) ↔ BB (borderline) ↔ BL (borderline lepromatous) ↔ LLs (subpolar lepromatous), LLp (polar lepromatous)
    - Levels are not static: patients can move through spectrum of disease through upgrading or downgrading reactions
- *Indeterminate leprosy (IL)*
  - Early form, usually no sensory loss
  - One to a few hypopigmented, macules that typically heal spontaneously
- *Tuberculoid leprosy (TT)*
  - Paucibacillary
  - Predominance of $CD4^+$ cells: cell-mediated immunity can localize infection
  - T_H1 (proinflammatory) profile: interleukin 2 (IL-2), interferon-δ (IFN-δ), and IL-12
  - Clinical
    - Erythematous large plaque with well-defined borders and atrophic center, anesthetic and anhidrotic, scalp and intertriginous areas are usually spared
    - Tender, thickened nerves
  - Histology
    - Resembles tuberculosis (TB)
    - Two histologic patterns
  - Mature epithelioid tubercles surrounded by lymphoid mantles

- Many large Langhans giant cells, fibrinoid necrosis, occasional areas of caseation necrosis, and exocytosis (associated with TT upgraded from BT)
  - Tissue may be negative for acid fast bacilli (AFB) owing to paucibacillary nature
- Prognosis: spontaneous resolution or progression to borderline leprosy

- *Borderline tuberculoid leprosy (BT)*
  - Host response is insufficient for self-cure
  - Multiple (occasionally solitary) anesthetic asymmetric annular plaques with satellite papules
  - Symmetric nerve enlargement or palsy
  - Histology: epithelioid tubercules, fewer lymphocytes than in TT; usually negative for AFB
- *Borderline leprosy (BB)*
  - Most unstable type: patients quickly upgrade or downgrade
  - Multiple annular plaques with indistinct borders compared with TT lesions; can have classic dimorphic lesions
  - Mild anesthesia
  - Histology
    - Granulomas have epithelioid differentiation; no giant cells or lymphoid mantle
    - AFB are found easily
- *Borderline lepromatous leprosy (BL)*
  - Host resistance too low to restrain bacillary proliferation
  - Destructive inflammation in nerves still occurs
  - Dimorphic lesions: annular patches with poorly marginated borders (lepromatous-like) and sharply marginated inner ones (tuberculoid-like)
  - Annular punched-out-appearing lesions also occur
  - Histology
    - Granulomas with lymphocytes and foamy macrophages
    - Nerves with inflammatory cell infiltration; bacilli and globi (*M. leprae* within multinucleate Virchow giant cells from histiocytes)
  - Patients remain in this stage, improve, or regress
- *Lepromatous leprosy (LL)*
  - Multibacillary
  - Predominance of $CD8^+$ cells
  - T_H2 (anti-inflammatory) profile: IL-4 and IL-10
  - Lack of cell-mediated immunity permits progression of the infection
  - HLA-DQ1 and TLR2 gene mutations have been associated with LL
  - Clinical (Fig. 18-17)
    - Poorly defined symmetric skin-colored plaques and nodules, begin as pale macules
    - Anhidrosis
    - Diffuse dermal infiltration
    - Leonine facies: widening of the nasal root
    - Madarosis: lateral alopecia of the eyebrows and lashes
    - Slow and progressive nerve involvement, acral distal symmetric anesthesia

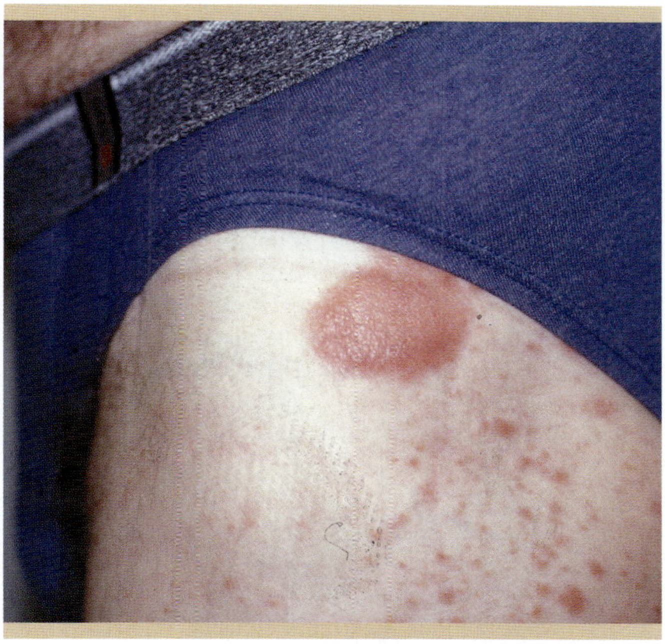

FIGURE 18-17 Lepromatous leprosy. (*Used with permission from Dr. Steven Mays.*)

    - Testicular infection: invasion of the seminiferous tubules causing sterility
    - Ocular involvement: photophobia, glaucoma, blindness
    - Oral involvement: lepromas of the hard and soft palates
    - Aseptic necrosis and osteomyelitis
  - Subpolar lepromatous (LLs): can develop reversal reactions and erythema nodosum leprosum (ENL)
  - Polar lepromatous (LLp): develops erythema nodosum leprosum
  - Histoid leprosy (HL): clinical variant of LL, occurs as a result of resistance to monotherapy; multibacillary lesion with spindle-shaped cells resembling fibrocytes without globi
  - Histology: Grenz zone (upper area of dermis is spared), foamy macrophages with globi (Virchow cells)
  - Untreated LL is progressive, it does not revert to the less severe borderline or tuberculoid types
- *Relapsing leprosy*
  - Multibacillary patients who are noncompliant or develop drug resistance
  - Early relapses (occurring within 3.5 years after stopping treatment) are probably due to insufficient treatment, and late relapses (occurring more than 3.5 years after stopping treatment) to persisting bacilli or to reinfection
  - Clinical
    - Recurrence of initial presentation
    - Florid dermatofibroma-like lesions (histoid leprosy)
    - Develop a reactional state: destructive inflammatory processes

- *Jopling's type 1 reversal reaction* (lepra reaction)
  - Delayed-type hypersensitivity reaction, leading cause of neurological impairment in patients with leprosy
  - Affects 30% of patients with borderline leprosy
  - Patients either upgrade to a more resistant state, remain unchanged, or downgrade to a less resistant state
  - Clinical
    - Abrupt conversion of previously quiescent plaques to tumid lesions and/or development of new tumid lesions in clinically normal skin
    - Dusky purple erythematous plaques
    - Iritis and lymphedema (elephantiasis graecorum)
    - Neuritis
- *Jopling's type 2 reaction* (erythema nodosum leprosum)
  - Often in LL but also in BL before, during, or after therapy
  - Clinical
    - Crops of tender bright pink nodules in clinically normal skin
    - Fever, anorexia, and malaise
    - Upper and lower extremities, facial lesions in 50%
    - Arthralgias
    - Neutrophilic leukocytosis
    - Abrupt fall in hematocrit
- *Lucio reaction*
  - Occurs in untreated diffuse lepromatous leprosy and/or relapsing leprosy
  - Seen in Mexico and the Caribbean
  - Latapi lepromatosis: diffuse nonnodular lepromatous leprosy with hemorrhagic infarcts
  - Telangiectases
  - Nasal septum perforation
  - Total alopecia of the eyebrows and lashes
  - Acral distal symmetric anesthesia
  - Crops of necrotic lesions
  - Painful ulcerations of the skin
  - Histology: ischemic necrosis secondary to endothelial parasitization by AFB; thrombosis in deep vessels
  - Treatment for Lucio reaction: rifampin
- Laboratory changes
  - Hyperglobulinemia
  - False-positive serologic test for syphilis
  - Anemia of chronic disease
  - Mild lymphopenia
  - Elevated serum lysozyme and angiotensin-converting enzyme
  - Proteinuria due to focal glomerulonephritis in ENL
  - Testicular involvement in LL males manifests as high serum follicle-stimulating hormone (FSH) and luteinizing hormone (LH) but low testosterone
  - Lepromin skin testing (Mitsuda test): intradermal injection of *M. leprae*, positive reaction occurs if a 5 mm or greater nodule appears 2 to 3 weeks following injection (usually positive in TT and BT leprosy while BB through LLp are negative)
    - Not useful in diagnosis, indicates host resistance
    - Helps in classification
- Treatment
  - Treatment may last from 6 months to 2 years. After 1 to 2 weeks of treatment, patients are considered noninfectious
  - *Paucibacillary (tuberculoid) disease*
    - Dapsone (bacteriostatic) 100 mg daily
    - Supervised rifampin (bactericidal) 600 mg monthly for 6 months
  - *Multibacillary (lepromatous) disease*
    - Dapsone 100 mg daily + supervised rifampin 600 mg monthly + clofazimine (bacteriostatic) 50 mg daily (unsupervised) and 300 mg monthly (supervised) for 2 years
    - Alternative combination of minocycline (bactericidal) 100 mg daily + rifampin 600 mg daily for 2 to 3 years, followed by monotherapy
  - *Reversal reactions*
    - Prednisone (0.5–1.0 mg/kg per day)
    - Prevents permanent nerve damage
    - Minimum of 6 months
  - *Erythema nodosum leprosum*
    - Thalidomide is the treatment of choice
    - Prednisone + clofazimine 200 mg daily

TUBERCULOSIS

- Caused by *Mycobacterium tuberculosis*
- Aerobic, intracellular, curved bacilli, acid fast
- Transmitted by airborne droplets
- Causes epithelioid granulomas with central caseation necrosis
- Clinical
  - *Multiorgan infection*
    - Pulmonary: productive cough, fever, and weight loss, hemoptysis or chest pain
    - Meningitis: headache that is either intermittent or persistent, mental status changes
    - Skeletal: spine (Pott disease), arthritis: hip or knee
    - Genitourinary: flank pain, dysuria, or frequency
    - Gastrointestinal TB: nonhealing ulcers
  - *Cutaneous TB*
    - Verrucosa cutis (prosector wart): direct inoculation → purplish or brownish-red warty growth
  - Lupus vulgaris: hematogenous spread, persistent and progressive → sharply defined reddish brown papule, plaques with a gelatinous consistency (apple-jelly color)
    - Cutis orificialis: autoinoculation into the periorificial skin and mucous membranes → yellow/red nodule on mucosa that results in ulceration
      - ▲ Patients with advanced TB; tuberculin sensitivity is strong

- Scrofuloderma
  - Direct extension of underlying TB infection of lymph nodes, bone, or joints (classically found in the neck)
  - Firm, painless lesions that eventually ulcerate with a granular base
  - Associated with pulmonary TB; Tuberculin sensitivity is strong
- Metastatic tuberculous abscess (tuberculous gumma)
  - Occurs following hematogenous spread of mycobacteria to skin in tuberculin-sensitive individuals
  - Painless, fluctuant, subcutaneous abscesses form singly or at multiple sites
- Miliary TB
  - Chronic infection; hematogenous spread from the primary infection (usually in the lungs) to other tissues
  - Small red spots that develop into ulcers and abscesses
  - Immunocompromised patients, for example, HIV, AIDS, cancer
- Tuberculid: hypersensitivity reactions to tubercle bacillus
  - Erythema induratum (Bazin disease): recurring subcutaneous nodules that may ulcerate and scar are seen in the posterior calves; tubercle bacilli are not seen; mycobacterial cultures usually are negative; histology shows a lobular panniculitis with vasculitis
  - Papulonecrotic tuberculid: crops of recurrent necrotic skin papules on knees, elbows, buttocks or lower trunk that heal with scarring after about 6 weeks
  - Lichen scrofulosorum: lichenoid eruption of small follicular papules in young persons with underlying TB

- Laboratory studies
  - Mantoux tuberculin skin test (TST): good test for latent infection; intradermal injection of 5 units (0.1 mL) of purified protein derivative (PPD); read 48 to 72 hours following injection:
    - Recent TST testing, pregnancy, or history of BCG vaccination does not contraindicate TST, but live-virus vaccination can cause a false negative, so TST should be either performed on the same day as the vaccine or 4 to 6 weeks afterward. Patients with a history of severe reaction to TST should not receive the test again
    - 5 mm or greater induration is considered positive for: immunosuppressed (HIV, transplants, anyone taking over 15 mg daily prednisone for over 1 month), close contacts to known TB cases, or patients with suggestive changes on chest x-ray
    - 10 mm or greater is positive for: healthcare workers, children under 4 years old, patients with diabetes or kidney failure, IV drug users, institutionalized patients, or recent immigrants (<5 yrs) from high-risk countries
    - 15 mm or greater is positive for patients with no known risk factors
  - Whole blood assay based on interferon-γ release (IGRA); tests for latent TB infection—more expensive, but greater specificity: prior-BCG vaccine does not cause a false positive. IGRA is a god follow-up test for patient's with a history of BCG vaccination and a positive PPD, or alternative to PPD testing altogether in this population
  - Chest radiograph: patchy or nodular upper lobe infiltrates, calcified nodules indicate old infection, small nodular lesions indicate miliary TB
  - Ziehl-Neelsen staining and culture of sputum specimens (3 consecutive days)
  - Skin biopsy: caeseating necrosis surrounded by lymphocytes, multinucleate giant cells and epitheloid macrophages (organisms may be present within)
- Treatment
  - Active disease: 4 drug regimen for 2 months: isoniazid, rifampin, pyrazinamide, and either ethambutol → followed by isoniazid and rifampin for 4 and ½ more months.
  - Rifampin, pyrazinamide, and ethambutol for the entire 6 and ½ months if patient is resistant to isoniazid
  - Second line drugs: aminoglycosides (streptomycin), quinolones (levofloxacin)
  - Carrier but no active disease: isoniazid for 9 months, or isoniazid + rifapentine for 6 months

Atypical Acid-Fast Mycobacterium (AFB)

- Acid-fast facultative saprophytes and organisms that that do not cause tuberculosis or leprosy
- Usually occur in patients that are immunocompromised
- Categorized according to their production of yellow or orange pigment and their rate of growth
- Group 1
  - Photochromogens (pigmentation on exposure to light)
  - *M. kansasii, M. marinum, M. simiae*
- Group 2
  - Scotochromogens (pigmentation formed in the dark)
  - *M. scrofulaceum, M. szulgai, M. gordonae*
- Group 3
  - Nonchromogens (no pigmentation)
  - *M. malmoense, M. xenopi, M. avium-intracellulare*
- Group 4
  - Fast growers (groups 1, 2, and 3 listed above grow slowly)
  - Grow in three to five days (e.g., *M. fortuitum, M. chelonae, M. abscessus*)

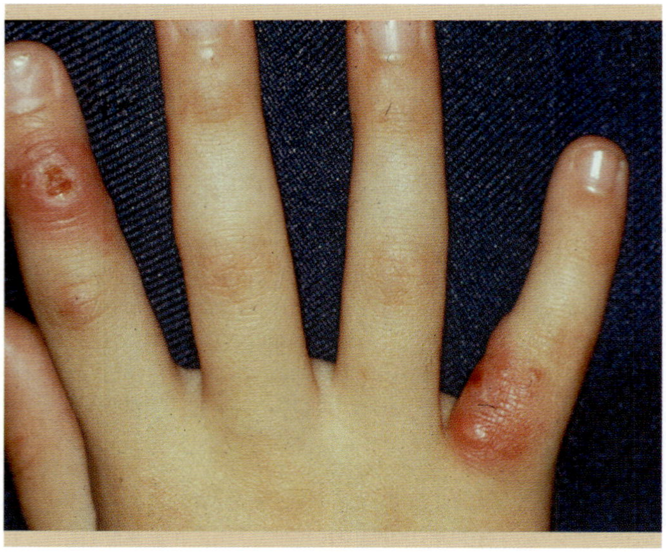

FIGURE 18-18 *M. marinum.* (Used with permission from Dr. Asra Ali.)

- Clinical
  - *M. marinum* (Fig. 18-18)
    - Clinical lesion is often called a "fish tank granuloma"
    - Infection occurs when contaminated water is exposed to traumatized skin
    - Usually an isolated nodule on the upper extremity, particulary the hand
    - Lymphangitic spread with several nodules (sporotrichoid spread)
- Treatment: minocycline, clarithromycin, physiotherapy (application of heat)
  - *M. avium-intracellulare* complex (MAC)
    - May cause lung disease in humans
    - Usually infects an immunocompromised host (patients with AIDS)
    - Skin disease rare: plaques, nodules, ulcers
  - *M. ulcerans*
    - An emerging pathogen that causes a Buruli ulcer in humans; the ulcer is deeply undermined, with scarring; lymphedema may result
    - Buruli ulcer is the third most common AFB infection worldwide (second to tuberculosis and leprosy)
    - No satisfactory antimicrobial treatment, often utilize surgery and grafting in treatment
    - Strict growth limited to fatty tissue beneath the dermis
  - *M. kansasii*
    - Pulmonary and extrapulmonary disease in humans similar to tuberculosis; cellulitis, and abscesses; disseminated or pulmonary infection are found in immunocompromised hosts, infection can result in septic arthritis
    - Difficult to treat; does not respond well to drugs
    - Grows well at 37°C
  - *M. scrofulaceum*
    - Causes scrofula (cervical adenitis)
    - Does not respond well to drugs
  - *M. fortuitum* (rapidly growing mycobacteria) (also *M. chelonae* and variety *abscessus*):
    - Causes chronic abscesses in humans
    - Primary cutaneous inoculation with possible sporotrichoid spread (linear distribution)
    - Other clinical affects include: keratitis, corneal ulcerations, osteomyelitis, lymphadenitis, and endocarditis
    - May be resistant to treatment
- Diagnosis: stain with carbolfuchsin (basic dye, red in color)
  - Tissue culture
  - Skin biopsy: suppurative granulomas (most characteristic finding) diffuse inflammation with foamy histiocytes, panniculitis, cutaneous abscesses, and necrotizing folliculitis
- Treatment: surgical drainage, debridement, and long term (>3 months) treatment with a regimen of several antibiotics used in combination: minocycline, trimethoprim, sulfamethoxazole, clarithromycin, rifampin, ethambutol

QUIZ

Questions

1. A 40-year-old patient returns to your office to have his PPD test read. You note 15 mm induration at the test site, to which the patient eagerly informs you that he was vaccinated with BCG as a child. What is an appropriate next step?

   A. Initiate 4 drug therapy for 6 months
   B. Order a chest x-ray and IGRA test
   C. Repeat the PPD in 6 weeks
   D. Repeat the PPD at another site immediately
   E. No further steps needed. The test is meaningless after BCG vaccination

2. A Hansen patient has many patches and plaques, no anesthesia, and normal facies. Six months after starting treatment with clofazamine, rifampin, and dapsone, she reports increased erythema of her existing lesions and pain in her extremities and visual disturbances. What is the appropriate action?

   A. Stop all antibiotics
   B. Add minocycline
   C. Start thalidomide
   D. Stop dapsone only
   E. Start prednisone

3. Which would you expect to find in a 1 year old with congenital syphilis?
   A. Bowed tibia
   B. Immobility of an arm
   C. Depressed nose-bridge
   D. Enlarged collar bone
   E. Deafness

4. Intracytoplasmic inclusions within endothelial cells may be seen in:
   A. Granuloma inguinale
   B. Leprosy
   C. Rhinoscleroma
   D. Verruga Peruana
   E. Malakoplakia

5. A patient presents with a draining sinus on his left mid-jaw. Pale yellow granules are visible in the discharge. What is the treatment of choice?
   A. Trimethoprim-sulfamethoxizole
   B. Dicloxacillin
   C. Azithromycin
   D. Metronidazole
   E. Penicillin

6. In which condition is *Pseudomonas* not a potential culprit?
   A. Ecthyma contagiosum
   B. Hot tub folliculitis
   C. Gram-negative toe web infection
   D. Otitis externa
   E. None of the above

7. A patient has a chronic, scaling eruption of the groin. He has tried several topical antifungals with no effect. A Wood's lamp shows coral red fluorescence. What is the pathogen?
   A. *Corynebacterium tenuis*
   B. *Kytococcus sedentarius*
   C. *Corynebacterium minutissimum*
   D. *Erysipelothrix rhusiopathiae*
   E. *Pseudomonas aeruginosa*

8. A gravely ill patient originally complaining of severe headache develops an eruption with metallic-grey irregular petechiae. Which would be appropriate chemoprophylaxis for close contacts?
   A. Penicillin G
   B. Isoniazid
   C. Cephalexin
   D. Rifampin
   E. Doxycycline

9. Necrotizing fasciitis is most commonly caused by:
   A. *Staphylococcus aureus*
   B. *Streptococcus pyogenes*
   C. *Escherichia coli*
   D. *Clostridium perfringens*
   E. Combination of the above

10. Matching exercise:

Part A—Match the following diseases with their corresponding virulence factors:

A. Staph scalded skin syndrome	1. TSST-1
B. Malignant pustule	2. Panton-Valentine leukocidin
C. Strep toxic shock syndrome	3. M-protein, erythrogenic exotoxin
D. Staph toxic shock syndrome	4. Edema factor
E. MRSA pyoderma	5. Exotoxin A, B

Part B—Match the following diseases with the corresponding vectors:

A. Tularemia	1. *Ixodes scapularis* or *pacificus*
B. Borreliosis	2. *Rhipicephalus sanguineus*
C. Scrub typhus	3. *Chrysops discalis*
D. Endemic typhus	4. *Xenopsylla cheopis*
E. Mediterranean spotted fever	5. *Leptotrombidium akamushi*

Answers

1. B. Per the CDC, remote BCG vaccination does not contraindicate TST testing. For cost reasons, it may still be preferable to use it as a screening test in this population. Follow up testing with IGRA +/− chest radiography should reveal if the test is a false-positive.
2. E. This patient has borderline leprosy and is experiencing a type 1 lepra reaction, representing an inflammatory shift toward the tuberculoid pole. Appropriate management is to continue multidrug therapy and minimize the risk of nerve and eye damage with systemic corticosteroids.
3. B. Parrot pseudoparalysis results from pain in an extremity due to syphilitic bone involvement and is a feature of early (< 2 years old) congenital syphilis. Saber shins, saddle-nose deformity, Higomenaki sign, and 8th cranial nerve deafness are classic for late congenital syphilis.
4. D. Verruga Peruana follows Oroya Fever, is caused by *B. bacilliformis*, and can have Rocha-Lima bodies within endothelial cells. Granuloma inguinale is cause by *K. granulomatis* and features Donovan bodies within histiocytes. Leprosy is caused by *M. leprae* and can have pathogen-containing globi within histiocytes (Virchow cells). Rhinoscleroma is caused by *K. rhinoscleromatis* and can show bacteria within vacuoles of histiocytes

(Mikulicz cells). Malakoplakia is usually caused by *E. coli* and features Michaelis-Gutmann bodies within histiocytes.

5. E. High-dose Penicillin G for at least 6 months is first-line treatment for cervicofacial actinomycosis. Doxycycline can be used for beta-lactam allergic patients.
6. A. Ecthyma contagiosum is caused by the Orf poxvirus. *Pseudomonas* can cause ecthyma gangrenosum.
7. C. *Corynebacterium minutissimum* causes erythrasma. It fluoresces under UVB due to production of coproporphyrin III. While susceptible to miconazole, other antifungals will commonly fail in treating this diphtheroid.
8. D. Close contacts of meningococcal patients should receive rifampin, ciprofloxacin, or ceftriaxone.
9. E. Necrotizing fasciitis (flesh-eating bacteria) is most commonly polymicrobial.
10. Part A: A-5, B-4, C-3, D-1, E-2; Part B: A-3, B-1, C-5, D-4, E-2. Tularemia is caused by *F. tularensis* and is carried by *Chrysops* deer flies, as well as *Dermacentor* and *Amblyomma* ticks. Borreliosis is carried *B. burgdorferi* which is carried by *Ixodes* ticks. Scrub typhus is caused by *O. tsutsugamushi* which is carried by *Leptotrombidium* trombunculid larvae. Endemic typhus is caused by *R. typhi* which is carried by *Xenopsylla cheopis* and *Ctenocephalides felis*. Mediterranean spotted fever is caused by *R. conorii* which is carried by *Rhipicephalus* ticks.

REFERENCES

Blume JE, Levine EG, Heymann WR: *Bacterial Diseases*, in Bolognia JL et al. *Dermatology*, London: Mosby; 2003.

CDC home page. Division of Tuberculosis Elimination. www.cdc.gov/tb. Accessed August 5, 2014.

Chian CA, Arrese JE, Pierard GE: Skin manifestations of Bartonella infections. *Int J Dermatol* 2002;41(8):461–466.

Czelusta AJ, Yen-Moore A, Evans TY, Tyring SK: Sexually transmitted diseases. *J Am Acad Dermatol* 1999;41(4):614–623.

Elston Dirk M: Community-acquired methicillin-resistant Staphylococcus aureus. *J Am Acad Dermatol* 2007;56(1):1–16.

Goldsmith LA et al. *Fitzpatrick's Dermatology in General Medicine*, 8th Ed. New York: McGraw-Hill; 2012.

McGinley-Smith DE, Tsao SS: Dermatoses from ticks. *J Am Acad Dermatol* 2002;49(3):363–392.

McKee PH: *Pathology of the Skin: With Clinical Correlations*. London: Mosby-Wolfe; 1996.

Myers SA, Sexton DJ: Dermatologic manifestations of arthropod-borne diseases. *Infect Dis Clin North Am* 1994;8(3):689–712.

Sadick NS: Current aspects of bacterial infections of the skin. *Dermatol Clin* 1997;15(2):341–349.

CHAPTER 19

FUNGAL DISEASE

WHITNEY A. HIGH

SUPERFICIAL FUNGAL INFECTIONS

Nondermatophytes: Tinea versicolor/Pityriasis versicolor (Fig. 19-1)

- Organism: *Malassezia* species (particularly *Malassezia furfur* and *Malassezia globosa*)
  - These dimorphic organisms are normal skin commensals (also known as *Pityrosporum* species), but become overgrown and assume mycelial forms to yield disease
  - Factors involved in the development of pathologic states include genetic predisposition, environmental conditions, and disorders of homeostasis
- Clinical: hypopigmented and hyperpigmented scaly plaques with fine scale upon neck, trunk, and proximal extremities; occasional an inverse forms will affect flexural areas of the body
  - Hypopigmentation is caused by elaboration of tyrosinase inhibitors
  - Hyperpigmentation is caused by enlargement of melanosomes
  - The organism uses skin oils as an energy substrate; lesions are concentrated in "sebum-rich" areas of the body
  - Occurrence prior to adrenarche is uncommon due to low sebum production
  - Lesions typically have a fine, "bran-like" scale that accentuates with skin stretching
- Diagnosis:
  - Wood's lamp: yield coppery-orange fluorescence in many cases (not all)
  - Potassium hydroxide (KOH) prep: "spaghetti and meatballs" appearance of hyphae and spores
  - Histology: round to oval yeast with short hyphae in stratum corneum
  - Culture: Sabouraud dextrose agar (SDA) with olive oil (fatty acids are required for growth); rarely utilized
- Treatment:
  - Topical management: selenium sulfide, azole and allylamine antifungals, sodium sulfacetamide, ciclopirox olamine
  - Oral management: ketoconazole, fluconazole, and itraconazole
  - Oral terbinafine: some reports describe a poor clinical response

Tinea nigra

- Organism: *Hortaea werneckii* (formerly *Exophiala werneckii* or *Phaeoannellomyces werneckii*)
  - The species is a dematiaceous (melanin-producing) yeast that inhabits the soil of tropical and subtropical climates and it has remarkable halotolerance (salt tolerance)
- Clinical:
  - Brown to black, flat, patches upon the palm or sole, caused by traumatic inoculation
  - Most often the lesions are asymptomatic, pruritus may be described on occasion
  - Classically the lesions may be confused clinically with nevi or melanoma
- Diagnosis:
  - Histology: brown, septate hyphae in the stratum corneum without a host response, accentuates with periodic acid–Schiff (PAS) or Grocott's methenamine silver (GMS), marks with Fontana-Masson stain due to melanin
  - KOH prep: branched, septate hyphae with a brown color
  - Culture: SDA, brown-black colonies (due to melanin production)
- Treatment:
  - Topical antifungals: ketoconazole, miconazole, ciclopirox olamine, terbinafine
  - Other: topical application of thiabendazole suspension has been successfully used
  - Systemic therapy: not usually required or recommended, oral itraconazole has been used successfully in some cases

Piedra

- Organism:
  - Black piedra: *Piedraia hortae*

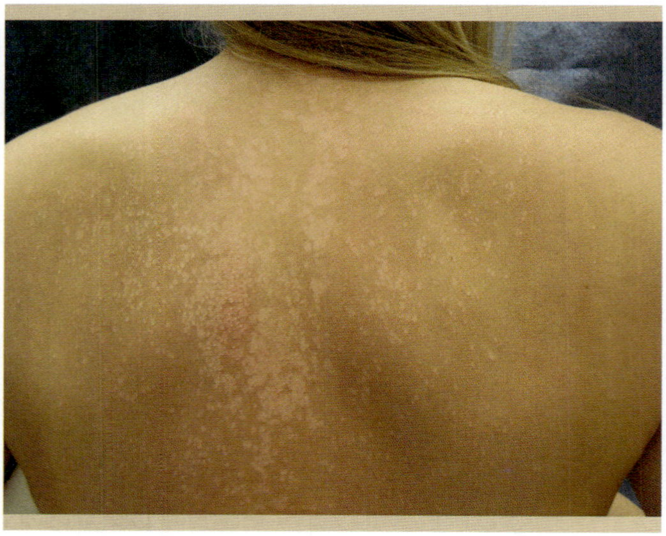

FIGURE 19-1 Tinea versicolor. (*Used with permission from Dr. Asra Ali.*)

- White piedra: *Trichosporon asahii* (formerly *Trichosporon beigelii*), sometimes also caused by *Trichosporon ovoides, Trichosporon inkin, Trichosporon mucoides, Trichosporon asteroides,* or *Trichosporon cutaneum*
- Clinical:
  - The word piedra means "stone," both conditions yield concretions of fungi that resemble stones
  - Black piedra: hard, firmly adherent, pigmented nodules upon the hair shaft of the scalp, common in tropical climates
  - White piedra: soft, less adherent, white to light-brown nodules in the beard, mustache, pubic hair, or scalp, common in temperate/semitropical climates
  - Both types of piedra lead to hair breakage and loss
- Diagnosis:
  - KOH prep of hair shaft: black piedra with tightly packed, pigmented hyphae surrounding asci, each of which contains eight ascospores; white piedra with loosely arranged, non-pigmented hyphae with blastoconidia and arthroconidia
  - Histology: BP with hyphae aligned regularly in periphery of fungal nodule, WP with hyphae less organized and with hyphae perpendicular to shaft
  - Culture: *Trichosporon* is inhibited by cycloheximide and culture requires cycloheximide-free media, growth yields wrinkled, creamy white colonies; *P. hortae* is not inhibited by cycloheximide, slow growth yields dark-brown to black colonies with a red-brown pigment on reverse
- Treatment:
  - Both forms of piedra are treated with hair shaving
  - WP is treated also with topical imidazoles, selenium sulfide, zinc pyrithione, precipitated sulfur in petrolatum, BP may be treated with oral terbinafine
  - *Trichosporon* species involved in WP can cause systemic infections in immunocompromised patients

DERMATOPHYTE INFECTIONS

- Dermatophytes are filamentous fungi that possess the enzymes necessary to use keratin as an energy substrate; these organism often infect keratinized tissue (skin, hair, and nails)
- There are three genera of dermatophytes (Tables 19-1 and 19-2)
  - Trichophyton: affects hair, nails, and skin (Table 19-3)
  - Epidermophyton: affects nails and skin
  - Microsporum: affects hair and skin
- Different species may show marked host preferences
  - Anthropophilic: affects humans
  - Zoophilic: affects animals (Table 19-4)
  - Geophilic: found in the soil
- It is common for dermatophyte infections to be referred to in the aggregate based upon the anatomic site affected (see below)

Tinea Capitis

- Clinical:
  - Dermatophyte infections of the scalp most often affect children

TABLE 19-1 Key Morphologic Criteria for Identifying Dermatophytes

Microscopic Morphology	*Epidermophyton*	*Microsporum*	*Trichophyton*
Macroconidia	Abundant, club-shaped, thick-walled, smooth, arranged in groups	Usually abundant, spindle-shaped, thick-walled, rough	Usually scarce, club-shaped, smooth, thin-walled
Microconidia	Absent	Usually scarce, elongate	Abundant, spherical, elongate, or pear shaped

TABLE 19-2 Differentiating Characteristics of Dermatophytes

Dermatophyte	Colony	Microscopic	Characteristics
Trichophyton rubrum	Fluffy white; red on reverse (no diffusion) (see Fig. 19-6)	Smooth, regular-shaped microconidia; "birds on a wire"; thin-walled microconidia	Urease (−) Hair perforation (−)
Trichophyton mentagrophytes var. *mentagrophytes* (zoophilic)	Tan, granular, brown-red color on reverse	Grapelike clusters of microconidia and spiral hyphae (see Fig. 19-7)	Urease (+) Hair perforation (+) (+) Hair invasion: large spore ectothrix
Trichophyton mentagrophytes var. *interdigitale*	Cream fluffy; reverse yellow/brown	Few pyriform microconidia	(+) Hair invasion, large spore ectothrix; (+) Hair penetration, urease positive
Microsporum gypseum (geophilic)	Cinnamon, flat powdery with brown reverse color	Thin-walled rough macroconidia, less than 6 septa, cucumber-z shaped	(+) Hair invasion: large spore ectothrix, hair fluorescence: none or dull green
Microsporum canis	White fluffy to yellowish with radiating edge, reverse yellow	Rough, canoe-shaped macroconidia; pointed tip ("snout") with at least 6 septa*	Grows on polished rice (+) hair invasion small spore ectothrix; green fluorescence
Microsporum audouinii	Downy beige; salmon pink on reverse	Microconidia and macroconidia rarely present	Does not grow on polished rice (+) Hair invasion: small spore ectothrix (yellow/green)
Trichophyton tonsurans	Brown, yellow, white suedelike; reddish brown on reverse	Smooth balloon-shaped macroconidia (rare); teardrop-shaped microconidia with varying sizes and arrangement	(+) Hair invasion, requires thiamin
Trichophyton schoenleinii	Cream-colored, cerebriform, (glaborous), heaped	Antler-shaped hyphae (favic chandeliers)	(+) Hair invasion: fluorescence green causes scutula
Trichophyton verrucosum	Cream wrinkled, heaped; cream color on reverse	Smooth-walled macroconidia (rare) with "tails"	(+) Hair invasion: large spore ectothrix, requires thiamin and/or inositol
Tricholosporum violaceum	Glaborous, wrinkled; reverse violet red	Microconidia and macroconidia not present	(+) Hair invasion: endothrix, requires thiamine
Trichophyton concentricum	White glaborous; white color reverse	Microconidia and macroconidia not present; narrow branching hyphae	Causes tinea imbricata: "tokelau"
Epidermophyton floccosum	Flat, granular, khaki color front and reverse	Large, thin club-shaped macroconidia	Produces chlamydoconidia
Microsporum nanum	Tan granular; beige color reverse	Rough-walled two-celled macroconidia ("pig snout")	(+) Hair invasion, large spore ectothrix, no fluorescence

*Note: *Epidermophyton* are smooth-walled

TABLE 19-3 Nutritional Requirements of *Tricophyton* Species

Nutritional Requirement	Species
Thiamine	*Trichophyton tonsurans,* Tricholosporum *violaceum, Trichophyton verrucosum,* some *Trichophyton concentricum*
Histidine	*Trichophyton megninii*
Niacin	*Trichophyton equinum*
Inositol and thiamine	*Trichophyton verrucosum*

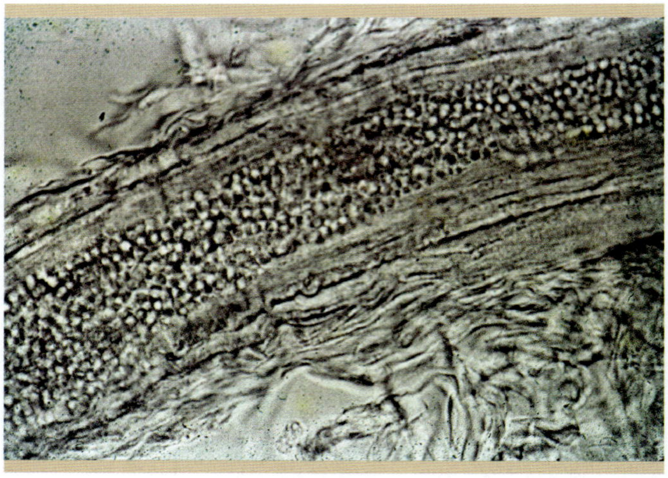

FIGURE 19-2 Endothrix. (*Used with permission from Dr. Mark LaRocco.*)

- Dermatophyte infections result in alopecia and pruritus
- Occipital lymphadenopathy may be observed
- The inflammatory process, if vigorous, may lead to scarring and permanent hair loss
- Tinea capitis may be subclassified as endothrix, ectothrix, or favus infections

- Endothrix infection (growth and sporulation within hair shaft) (Fig. 19-2 and Table 19-5)
  - *Trichophyton tonsurans*: #1 cause of tinea capitis (Fig. 19-3) in the United States; creates a "black dot" clinical presentation as the weakened hair shafts break at the skin surface yielding a comedo-like appearance; degree of in inflammation may vary
  - *Tricholosporum violaceum:* more common in Europe, North Africa, and Middle East, South Asia
  - Endothrix infections do not fluoresce

TABLE 19-4 Zoophilic Dermatophytes

Dermatophyte	Natural Hosts
Microsporum gallinae	Chickens/other birds
Microsporum nanum	Pigs (snouts)
Microsporum canis	Cats, dogs, horses
Trichophyton verrucosum	Cattle, sheep, horses
Trichophyton equinum	Horses
Trichophyton simii	Monkeys, chickens
Trichophyton mentagrophytes var. *mentagrophytes*	Cats, dogs, rabbits

- Ectothrix infection (growth and sporulation around hair shaft) (Table 19-6)
  - *Microsporum canis*: zoophilic, may cause localized outbreaks, may be acquired from dogs and cats (affected pet fur fluoresces a green color); has a bright canary yellow color on reverse in culture
  - *Microsporum audouinii*: anthropophilic, causes epidemic tinea capitis, previously most common cause of tinea capitis
  - Also *Microsporum distortum, Microsporum ferrugineum, Microsporum gypseum, Microsporum nanum,* and *Trichophyton verrucosum*
- Diagnosis:
  - Wood's lamp: many ectothrix species fluoresce; a gnomonic for ectothrix species that fluoresce is **C**ats **A**nd **D**og **F**ight & **G**rowl: *M.* ***c****anis, M.* ***a****udouinii, M.* ***d****istortum, M.* ***f****errugineum* & *M.* ***g****ypseum*)
  - KOH prep of hair shaft: broken stubs are best for examination and may be removed with forceps, by gentle rubbing with a moist gauze pad, or with a sterile toothbrush or the end of a glass slide to harvest affected hairs, broke hair stubs, and scale

TABLE 19-5 Endothrix Species

Trichophyton tonsurans
Trichophyton schoenleinii
Trichophyton soudanense
Trichophyton gourvilli
Trichophyton yaounde
Tricholosporum *violaceum*

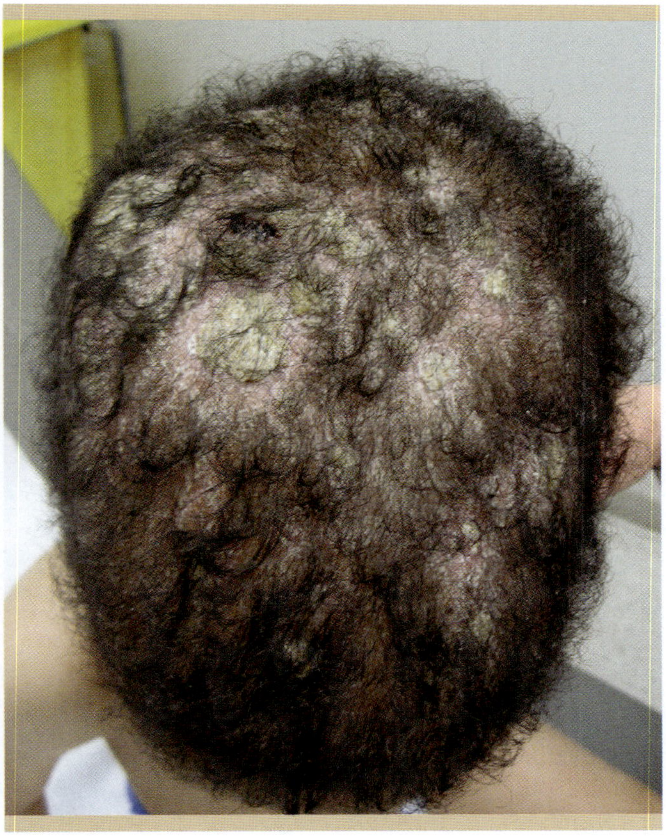

FIGURE 19-3 Tinea capitis. (*Used with permission from Dr. Jason Miller.*)

- Histology: may show fungus in the hair shaft (endothrix), or surrounding the hair shaft (ectothrix); highlight with GMS or PAS/D
- Culture: provides speciation of the organism; results may be delayed weeks
- Treatment:
  - Oral griseofulvin is effective therapy, it is often used in children due to a long safety record, but treatment courses are long (typically 6–8 weeks)
  - Newer oral antifungal medications include itraconazole, terbinafine, and fluconazole

TABLE 19-6 Ectothrix that Fluoresce

Name	Color
Microsporum distortum	Yellow/green
Microsporum audouinii	Yellow/green
Microsporum canis	Yellow/green
Microsporum ferrugineum	Yellow/green

Note: *Trichophyton schoenleinii* (favic type); causes blue/green fluorescence

  - Terbinafine may be slightly less effective for *Microsporum* species
  - Topical medications are not appropriate for tinea infections, but selenium sulfide or ketoconazole shampoo be an adjuvant agent that reduces shedding of viable spores

Tinea Favosa (Favus)

- Caused by *Trichophyton schoenleinii*; less commonly *T. violaceum* and *M. gypseum*
- Favus is a pattern of tinea that is caused by the formation of air spaces within the infected hair caused by the autolysis of hyphae
- Clinical:
  - The condition often begins in childhood and may be present for decades; patients present with scutula (yellow, cup-shaped crusting) that surrounds the hair shaft; later stages result in permanent loss of hair and scarring
- Diagnosis
  - Wood's lamp: dull green fluorescence may be observed
  - KOH prep: linear arrangement of hyphae along longitudinal axis of hair shaft, bubbling of KOH through the air spaces between hyphae
  - Culture: yields classic "brain" shaped, deeply folded and convoluted colonies with characteristic antler-shaped hyphae on microscopic examination ("favic chandeliers")
- Treatment:
  - Griseofulvin (although the course may be prolonged)
  - In vitro studies suggest the organism may be sensitive to terbinafine, itraconazole, and fluconazole

Kerion

- A severe inflammatory reaction seen in tinea capitis; may lead to scarring/permanent alopecia
- Deep-seated, boggy, erythematous areas characterized by a severe acute inflammatory infiltrate; surface culture may mislead due to bacterial overgrowth
- Usually caused by *Trichophyton* species (except for *Trichophyton rubrum*, which is an uncommon cause)
- Because of the risk of permanent scarring alopecia, and in addition to oral antifungals, some dermatologists may coadminister oral steroids to lessen the inflammatory process

Tinea Barbae and Tinea Faciei

- Tinea barbae is dermatophyte infection involving terminal facial hair; historically seen in ranchers, farmers, animal handlers (i.e., from zoophilic species acquired from cattle, dogs, etc.)
- Tinea faciei is a dermatophyte infection involving nonterminal facial hair (children/women)
- Tinea barbae/faciei both may be caused by both zoophilic and anthropophilic dermatophytes

- Most commonly caused by *T. verrucosum* (cattle); may also be caused by *Trichophyton mentagrophytes var granulosum*, *M. canis*, *T. schoenleinii*, and *Trichophyton megninii*
- Clinical: (three common forms)
  - Mild superficial type (resembles bacterial folliculitis)
  - Inflammatory deep-pustular type (kerion-like)
  - Circinate/spreading type (peripheral vesiculopustular border with central scaling)
- Diagnosis:
  - KOH prep: hyphae with or without arthroconidia
- Treatment:
  - Nonterminal hair involved: trial of topical antifungals (azoles, allylamines, etc.)
  - Terminal hair involved: oral antifungals (griseofulvin, terbinafine, and itraconazole)

Tinea Corporis

- Classically called "ring worm" by lay persons
- Caused by *T. rubrum* (most common cause), *M. canis* (seen in children), *T. mentagrophytes*, and *T. tonsurans* (seen in children with coexisting tinea capitis)
- Zoophilic fungi, such as *T. verrucosum* or *T. mentagrophytes*, may cause more inflammatory reactions
- Clinical:
  - Scaly, erythematous, annular plaques, with active borders and central clearing
  - The "active" edge may contain scale-crust, papules, or vesicles (Fig. 19-4)
  - Bullous tinea corporis is a form caused by *T. rubrum*
  - Majocchi granuloma (Fig. 19-5) is an inflammatory response similar to a kerion of the scalp, there is deep involvement of hair follicles with granulomatous plaques and folliculocentric pustules

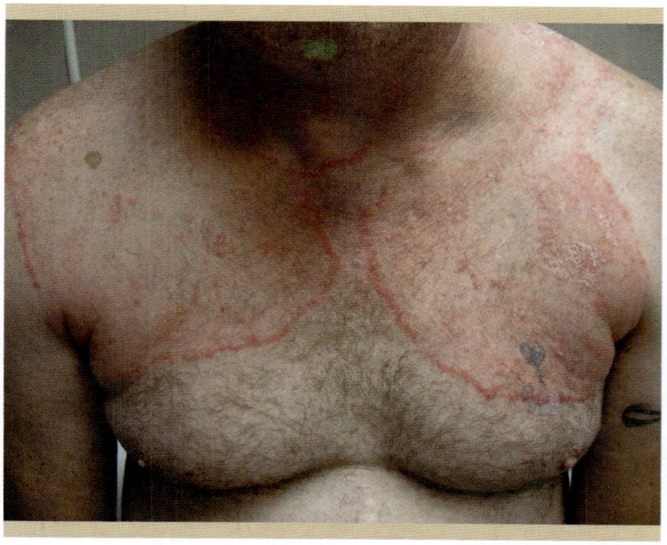

FIGURE 19-4 Tinea corporis. (*Used with permission from Dr. Jason Miller.*)

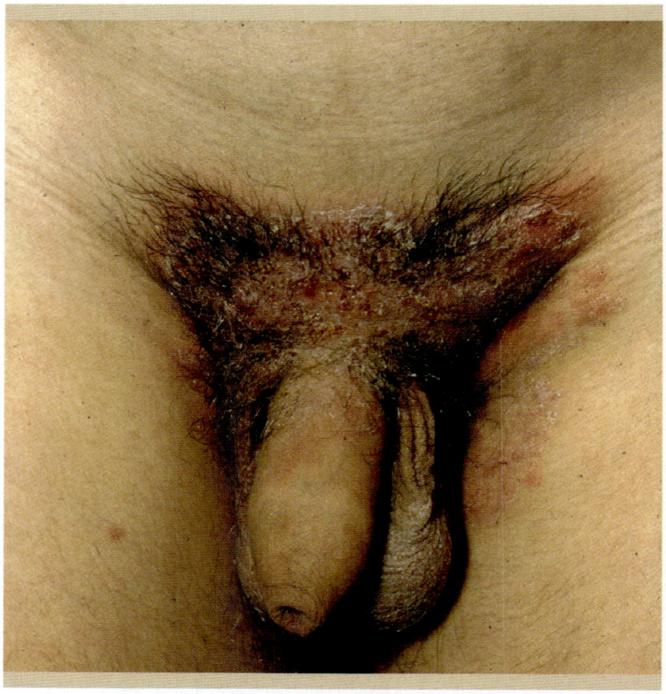

FIGURE 19-5 Majocchi granuloma. (*From Wolff K et al.* Fitzpatrick's Color Atlas & Synopsis of Clinical Dermatology, *5th Ed. New York: McGraw-Hill; 2005, p. 715.*)

  - Tinea corporis gladiatorum is any dermatophyte infection spread by direct contact between wrestlers; lesions usually occur upon the head, neck, and arms
  - Tinea imbricata (or Tokelau) is rare tropical form, seen chiefly in the South Pacific and caused by *Trichophyton concentricum*, which yields polycyclic and geographic shapes
- Diagnosis:
  - KOH prep: examination of skin scrapings reveal numerous septate branching hyphae (Fig. 19-6), hyphae may be accentuated by the addition of chlorazol E
  - Histology: septate hyphae within the stratum corneum (tinea corporis), and within the deeper extents of hair shafts with inflammation (Majocchi granuloma)
- Treatment:
  - Always consider both the body surface area (BSA) involved and the presence of terminal hair in selecting management
  - Topical antifungals: azoles, allylamines, etc. (for low BSA, no terminal hair involved)
  - Oral antifungals: terbinafine, itraconazole, and fluconazole (higher BSA, terminal hair involved/Majocchi granuloma)

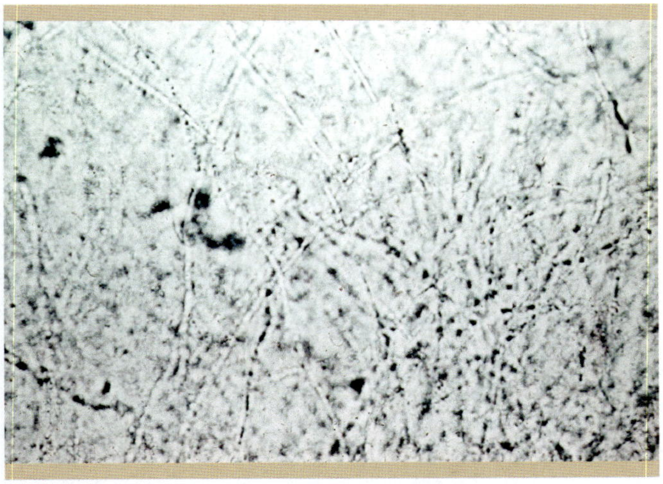

FIGURE 19-6 KOH examination of hyphae. (*Used with permission from Dr. Mark LaRocco.*)

Tinea Cruris

- More common among men, and often affects persons living in close quarters (e.g., military barracks, sporting teams, prisoners, institutionalized persons, etc.)
- Often due to *Epidermophyton floccosum* (Fig. 19-7) or *T. rubrum* (Fig. 19-8)
- Clinical:
  - Pruritic and erythematous plaques with active edge and central clearing
  - Often involves the inguinal creases and medial thighs; may also involve the buttocks, gluteal creased and waist
  - Typically spares the penis and scrotum (differs from the pattern of candidiasis)
  - Must be distinguished from candidiasis, erythrasma, and seborrheic and irritant/allergic contact dermatitis

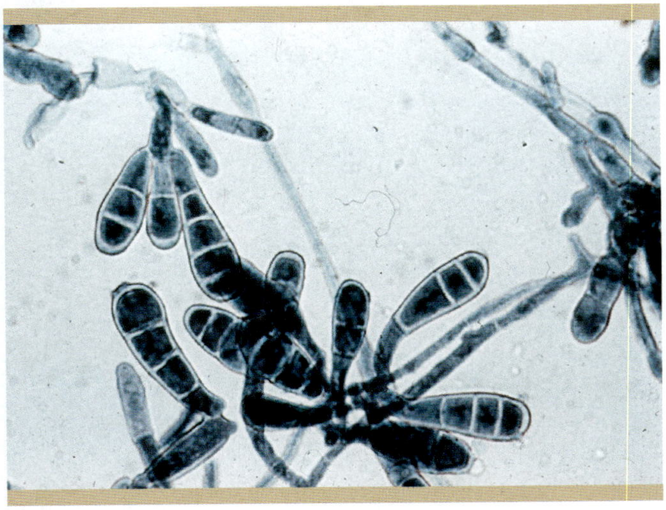

FIGURE 19-7 *Epidermophyton floccosum.* (*Used with permission from Dr. Mark LaRocco.*)

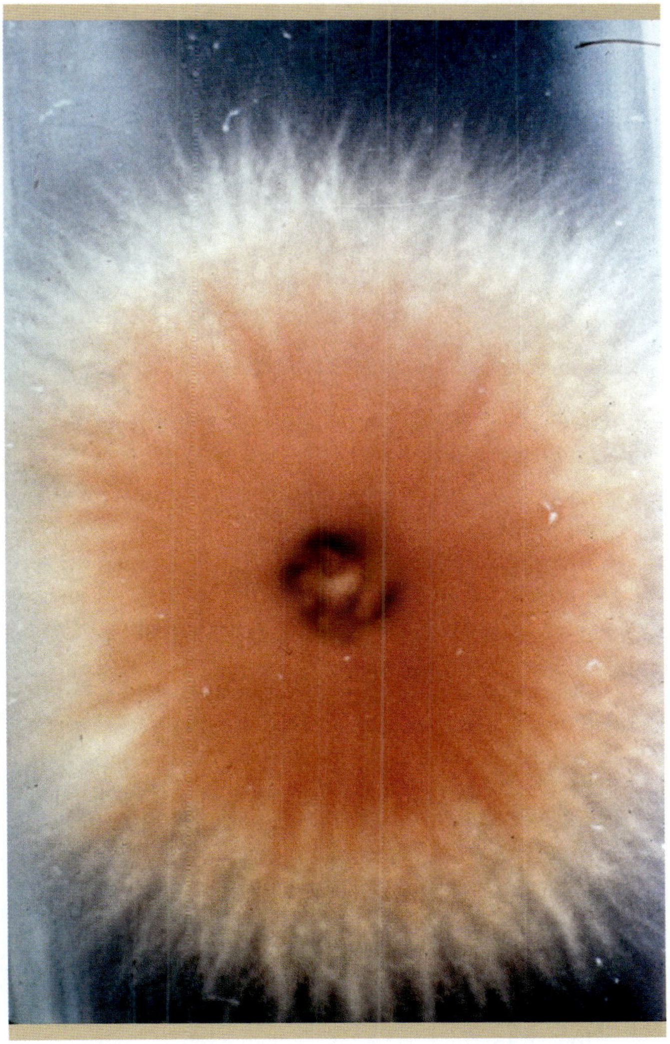

FIGURE 19-8 *Tinea rubrum.* (*Used with permission from Dr. Mark LaRocco.*)

- Diagnosis:
  - See tinea corporis above
  - Wood's lamp may be used to exclude erythrasma (which fluoresces a "coral red")
- Treatment:
  - Topical antifungals: azoles, allylamines, and ciclopirox olamine; advance to systemic agents for failures; remember that topical antifungals may also be irritants
  - Oral antifungals: terbinafine, itraconazole, and fluconazole
  - For patients with coexisting tinea pedis it may be useful to put socks on before underwear in the morning, to avoid cross-contamination

Tinea Pedis

- The most common fungal infection of all mankind; a direct consequence of footwear

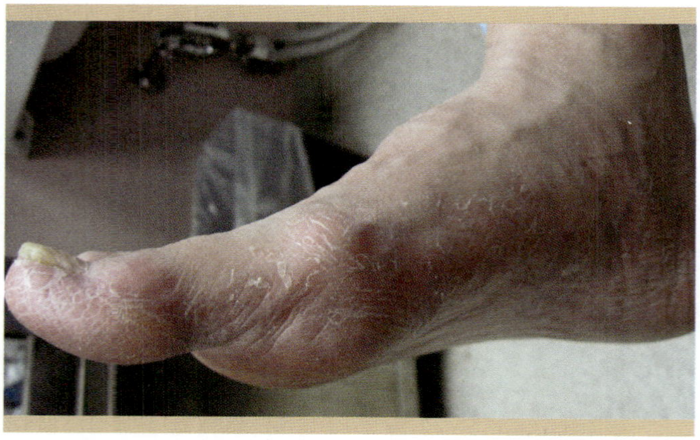

FIGURE 19-9 Tinea pedis. Chronic hypertrophic. (*Used with permission from Dr. Jason Miller.*)

- Clinical: (multiple forms)
  - Interdigital: white, macerated plaques between the toes (often between the fourth and fifth digits); commonly due to *T. rubrum*, *T. mentagrophytes* var. *interdigitale*, and *E. floccosum*
  - "Moccasin" (Fig. 19-9): well demarcated erythema with diffuse "chalk-like" scaling of the soles, with some extension upon the of sides feet; commonly due to *T. rubrum*
  - Bullous (Fig. 19-10): creates bullae upon the instep or anterior plantar surface of the foot; may be associated with dermatophytid reaction, often caused by *T. mentagrophytes* var. *mentagrophytes* (Fig. 19-11)
  - Ulcerative: ulcers and erosions in the web spaces, often with secondary bacterial infection, usually occurs in immunocompromised and/or diabetic patients
- Treatment:
  - Topical antifungals: azoles, allylamines, benzylamines; recurrence of tinea pedis is most often due to discontinuance of the medication by the patient after symptoms abate, but before the full course of therapy is completed

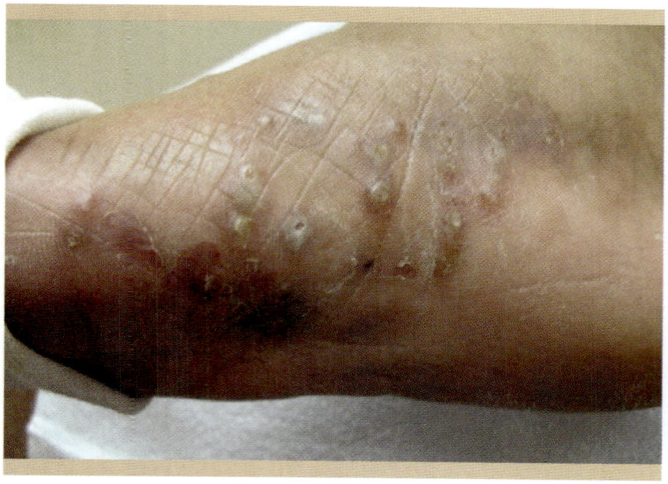

FIGURE 19-10 Tinea pedis. Vesicular bullous type. (*Used with permission from Dr. Asra Ali.*)

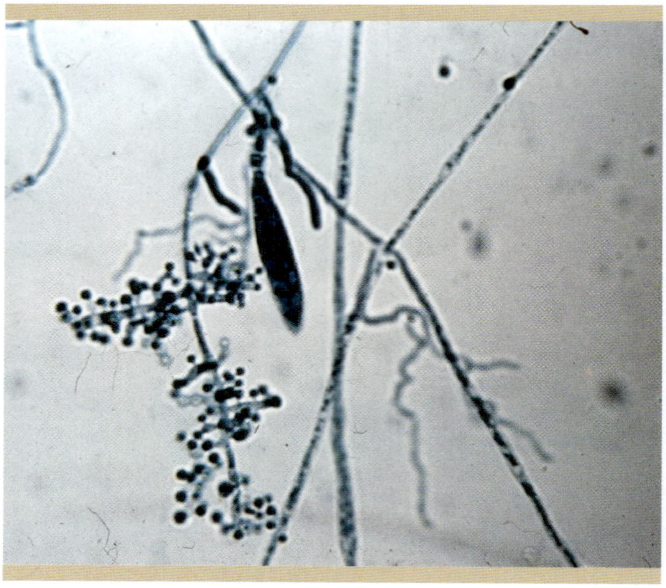

FIGURE 19-11 *Tinea mentagrophytes var. mentagrophytes.* (*Used with permission from Dr. Mark LaRocco.*)

  - Systemic antifungals: terbinafine, itraconazole, and fluconazole; useful for chronic "moccasin" type, or bullous tinea pedis
  - Other: keep feet cool and dry, keratolytics may be used with topical antifungals; also drying foot powders (+/− with antifungals) and rotating of shoes

Tinea Manuum (Fig. 19-12)

- An uncommon form of tinea overall
- Commonly caused by *T. rubrum* (a common cause of tinea pedis as well)

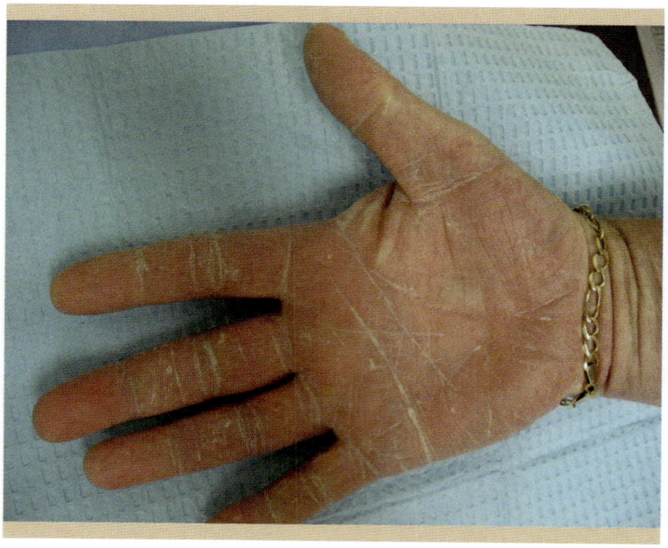

FIGURE 19-12 Tinea manuum. (*Used with permission from Dr. Jason Miller.*)

- Clinical:
  - Scaly, erythematous patches, pruritic
  - When associated with tinea pedis, it may affect just one hand (the so-called "one hand, two foot syndrome")
  - Differential diagnosis includes dihydrotic dermatitis, palmoplantar psoriasis, irritant/allergic contact dermatitis, idiopathic palmoplantar peeling
- Treatment:
  - Similar to tinea pedis

Onychomycosis

- Onychomycosis refers to *any* fungal infection of the nail
- Tinea unguium refers more specifically to nail infections caused by dermatophytes
- Nondermatophyte species causing onychomycosis include *Aspergillus* spp., *Scopulariopsis brevicaulis*, *Acremonium* spp., *Fusarium solani*, and *Chaetomium globosum*
- Fungal infection that affects the toenails (common) or the fingernails (less common)
- Toenail infection in particular affects about 10% of the population; the incidence is increasing, particularly among the elderly
- Clinical: (five main types)
  - Distal/lateral subungual
    - Occurs at free nail edge
    - Thickened nail plate and yellow discoloration, subungual debris, and onycholysis (Fig. 19-13)
    - Most commonly caused by *T. rubrum* (a common cause of tinea pedis)
  - Proximal subungual
    - Affects proximal nail plate, presents with white discoloration
    - Associated with HIV and other immunocompromised states

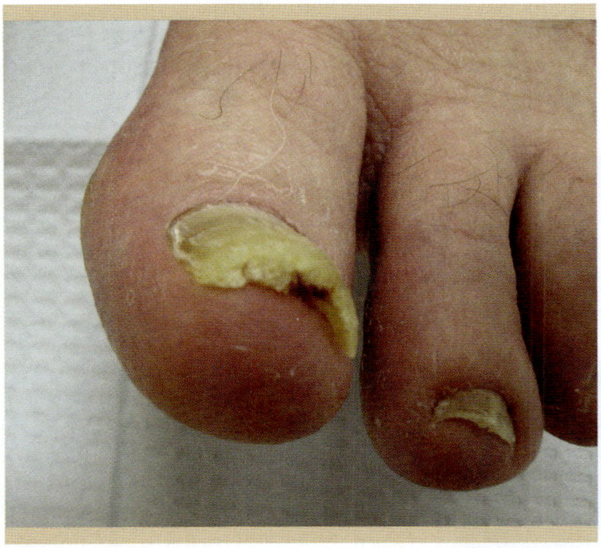

FIGURE 19-13 Onychomycosis. Distal subungual. (*Used with permission from Dr. Asra Ali.*)

  - White superficial onychomycosis (WSO)
    - Occurs on the toenail surface with white powdery patches on the nail plate
    - The nail is rough
    - *T. mentagrophytes* (adults), *T. rubrum* (children)
  - Endonyx
    - White discoloration of the nail plate, no subungual debris or onycholysis
  - Candidal nail infection
    - Paronychia and/or onycholysis of toenails and/or fingernails
    - Often with a bulbous appearance to the affected digit(s)
    - Most commonly caused by *Candida albicans*
- Diagnosis:
  - KOH prep: direct microscopy may be negative in up to 10% of cases
  - Culture: culture may be negative in up to 30% of cases; because of nondermatophyte causes the specimen should be grown on two types of media
  - Histology: while sample dependent, with a representative clipping, it has been considered to have optimal sensitivity; PAS or GMS is used to visualize fungi
  - PCR: a nested PCR assay using species-specific primer pairs based on the 28S ribosomal RNA gene exists to detect dermatophytes and nondermatophytes
- Treatment:
  - Oral antifungals: necessary in most circumstances (itraconazole and terbinafine)
  - Topical antifungals: not generally effective due to poor penetrance of the nail plate; the exception is ciclopirox olamine lacquer, but the cure rate is lower than oral therapy
  - Laser: Nd:YAG and diode, there is a paucity of evidence-based data on efficacy
  - Surgery: surgical nail avulsion; chemical removal with more than 40% urea compound
  - Combination therapy (oral, topical, surgical) may increase efficacy and decrease cost

Id Reaction (Dermatophytid reaction)

- Autoeczematization; the occurrence of a dermatophyte infection that leads to a more generalized cutaneous reaction due to the inflammatory response of the host
- Clinical:
  - Occurs at a distant site from the fungal infection
  - Dermatophytid reactions are devoid of organisms, and immunologic in etiology
  - Often presents as a vesicular dermatitis of the hands and feet
  - May evolve into a generalized scaling and eczematoid condition
- Treatment:
  - Goal is to treat the underlying dermatophyte infection, leading to resolution of the autoeczematous state

- Recurrences are common if the dermatophyte infection is inadequately treated
- Symptomatic care prior to resolution may include corticosteroids, wet compresses, antihistamines, etc.

DIMORPHIC FUNGI

- Medically relevant fungi that assume either a yeast form or mycelial form depending upon temperature
  - 35°C to 37°C: fungus grow as yeasts (parasitic phase)
  - 25°C: fungus grows as mycelial (mold/environmental form)
- Important memory gnomonic is:
  - Some: sporotrichosis
  - Can: coccidiomycosis
  - Have: histoplasmosis
  - Both: blastomycosis
  - Phases: paracoccidiomycosis

Sporotrichosis

- Caused by *Sporothrix schenckii*, a dimorphic fungus present worldwide upon decaying vegetation (e.g., wood splinters, plant thorns, sphagnum moss)
- Acquired by traumatic implantation (classic presentation was as "rose gardener disease")
- Infection spreads centripetally by lymphatic vessels (origin of the term "sporotrichoid spread")
- Clinical: (cutaneous forms)
  - Fixed cutaneous form
    - Single inoculation site with scaly, acneiform, verrucous, or ulcerative nodule; possibly with local lymphadenopathy
  - Lymphocutaneous form (Fig. 19-14)
    - Ulcerative nodules on extremities, sporotrichoid spread along lymphatics
  - Disseminated disease
    - Occurs in immunocompromised patients; may cause pulmonary lesions, septic arthritis/synovitis, mucosal lesions, pyelonephritis, orchitis, mastitis, meningitis, osseous infection, etc.
- Diagnosis:
  - Histology: inflammation and pseudoepitheliomatous hyperplasia; sparse and rare cigar-shaped yeast; extracellular asteroid bodies may be present (yeast surrounded by refractile eosinophilic halo)
  - Culture: gold standard; growth inhibited by cycloheximide; at 37°C culture yields creamy, white-tan colonies in 7 days, colonies turn brown-black in center with age
    - Yeast phase at 37°C (Fig. 19-15): elongated, cigar-shaped yeasts; rarely seen in histologic sections of tissue
    - Mold/mycelial phase at 25°C (Fig. 19-16): septate hyphae, delicate conidiophores bearing pyriform (pear-shaped) conidia in rosette clusters
- Treatment:
  - Lymphocutaneous disease: itraconazole, terbinafine, saturated solution of potassium iodide (SSKI)
  - Disseminated infection: amphotericin B (AMB)

Coccidioidomycosis (San Joaquin Valley Fever)

- Caused by *Coccidioides immitis*, a dimorphic fungus present as a saprophyte in the Lower Sonoran desert life zone; it is found in the southwestern United States
- *Coccidioides posadasii* is another species common to the southwestern United States, Mexico, and some part of South America
- The two organisms are closely related and it is thought that the clinical manifestations of infection with either organism are essentially identical
- The infection is acquired via inhalation of characteristic "boxcar-like" arthrospores, and disease is seen in humans, dogs, and horses
- Clinical:
  - The infection begins in the lungs
  - Most cases (~60%) are asymptomatic, some (~35%) present as flu-like illness with fever, chest pain, and arthralgia

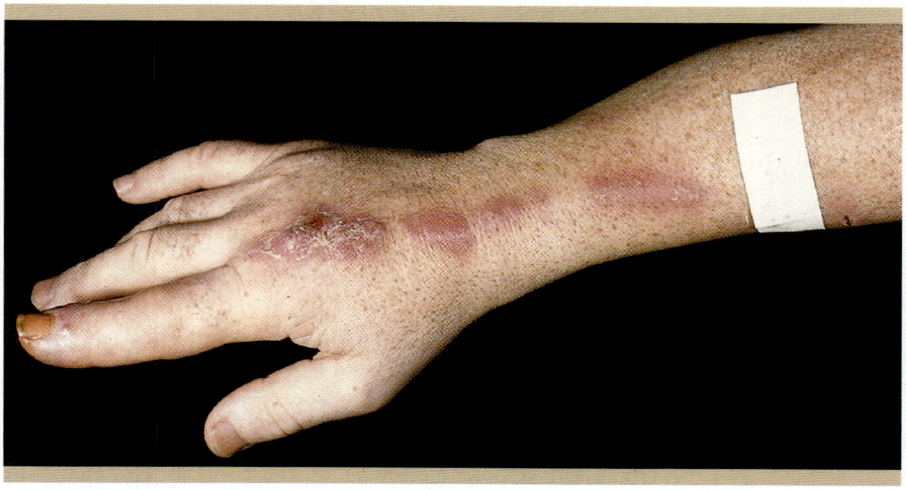

FIGURE 19-14 Sporotrichosis: Lymphocutaneous form. (*From Wolff K, Johnson RA;* Fitzpatrick's Color Atlas & Synopsis of Clinical Dermatology, *6th Ed. New York: McGraw-Hill; 2009, p. 745.*)

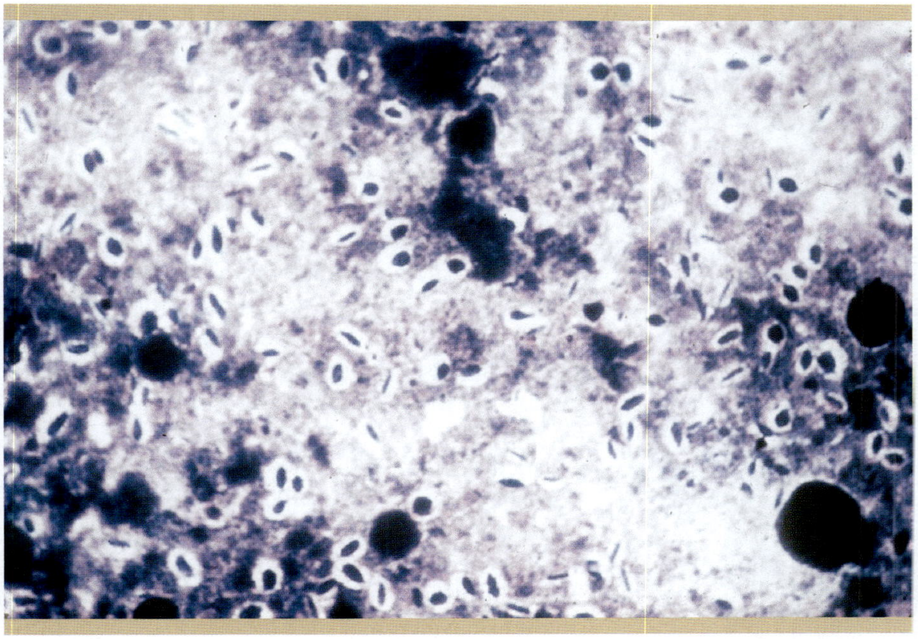

FIGURE 19-15 *Sporothrix schenckii* yeast. (*Used with permission from Dr. Mark LaRocco.*)

- Extrapulmonary dissemination is rare (<5%), but it may involve the central nervous system, skin, and pericardium
- Disseminated disease is more common in Mexicans, blacks, Filipinos, and pregnant women
- Cutaneous disease may be due to organisms in the skin or due to reactive states
  - Organism specific lesions: single or multiple papules, nodules, verrucous plaques, abscesses, pustules, sinus tracts, and/or ulceration
  - Reactive lesions associated: erythema nodosum, erythema multiforme, Sweet syndrome, interstitial granulomatous dermatitis
- Diagnosis:
  - Serology: quantitative and qualitative techniques exist
  - Histology: pseudocarcinomatous hyperplasia, dermal/subcutaneous inflammation with eosinophils, large spherules (~10–80 μm) with endospores (2–5 μm) (Fig. 19-17)
  - Culture: white to tan fluffy colony matures in 5 to 10 days; highly infectious to lab personnel who can accidentally inhale the barrel-shaped arthroconidia (Fig. 19-18)
  - Imaging: chest x-ray with characteristic "egg-shell" pulmonary cavities, pneumonia, pulmonary nodules, hilar or mediastinal lymphadenopathy, pleural effusions

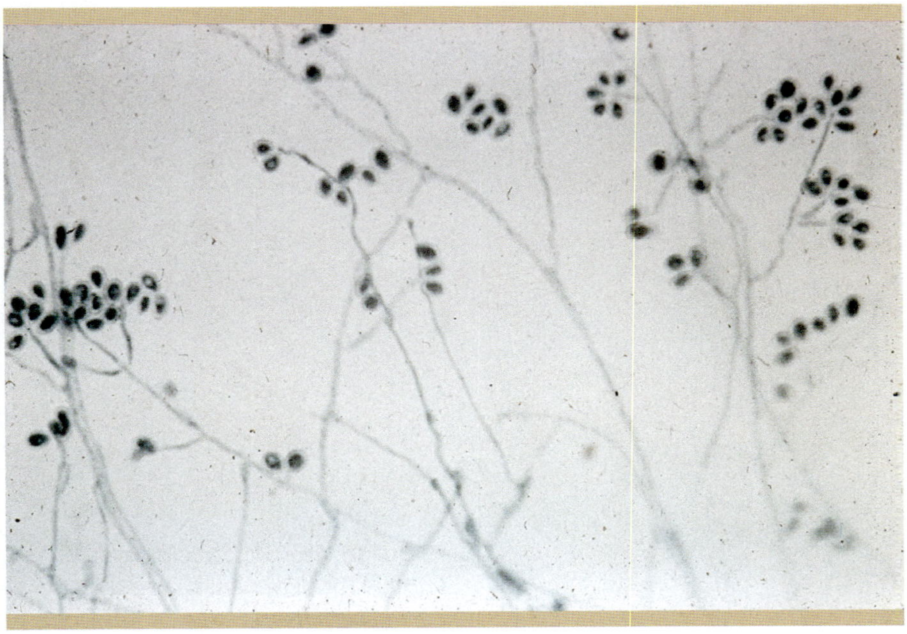

FIGURE 19-16 *Sporothrix schenckii* mold. (*Used with permission from Dr. Mark LaRocco.*)

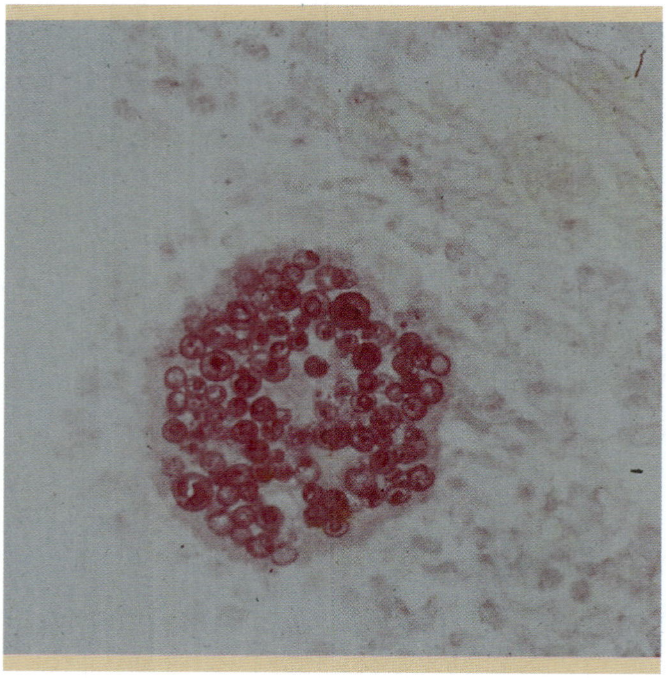

FIGURE 19-17 *Coccidioides immitis* tissue. (*Used with permission from Dr. Mark LaRocco.*)

- Treatment:
  - Asymptomatic or limited pulmonary disease in an immunocompetent person requires no treatment
  - Extrapulmonary disease and immunosuppressed patients may be treated with itraconazole, fluconazole, or AMB

Histoplasmosis (Darling Disease)

- Classic disease is caused by *Histoplasmosis capsulatum* var. *capsulatum*
- Associated with soil contaminated by bird droppings, or with bat guano from caves (i.e., spelunker disease)
- In the United States, the disease is endemic to the Mississippi and Ohio River valleys
- Clinical:
  - Acute pulmonary disease: 90% of cases are asymptomatic; in some cases there may be a self-limited illness with fever, chills, dry cough, pneumonia; only 5% develop dermatologic symptoms (erythema multiforme and erythema nodosum)
  - Disseminated histoplasmosis: develops in immunosuppressed patients; including those with immunosuppression due to use of tumor necrosis factor (TNF-α) inhibitors
    - Patients present with fever, malaise, anorexia, and weight loss
    - Hepatosplenomegaly, lymphadenopathy, pallor and petechiae (with pancytopenia)
    - May be present; Addison disease may result from adrenal involvement
    - Cutaneous lesions may include ulcers of the skin or mucous membranes, nodules, or molluscum-like papules
- African histoplasmosis is caused by *H. capsulatum* var. *duboisii* and this disease may also involve the lung, lymph nodes, bone, and skin
- Diagnosis:
  - Culture (at 25°C): white cottony colony after 2 to 4 weeks of incubation (Fig. 19-19); colonies consist of septate hyphae and tuberculated macroconidia (Fig. 19-20)
  - Histology (at 37°C): parasitized histiocytes with small (4–6 μm) oval yeast (Fig. 19-21); yeast accentuate with PAS/D or GMS stains

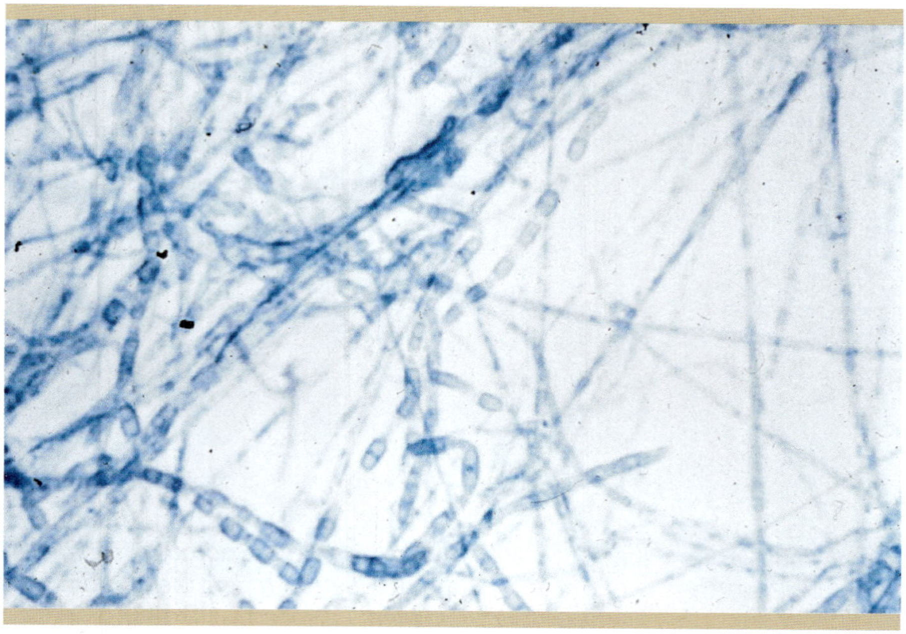

FIGURE 19-18 *Coccidioides immitis* mold phase. (*Used with permission from Dr. Mark LaRocco.*)

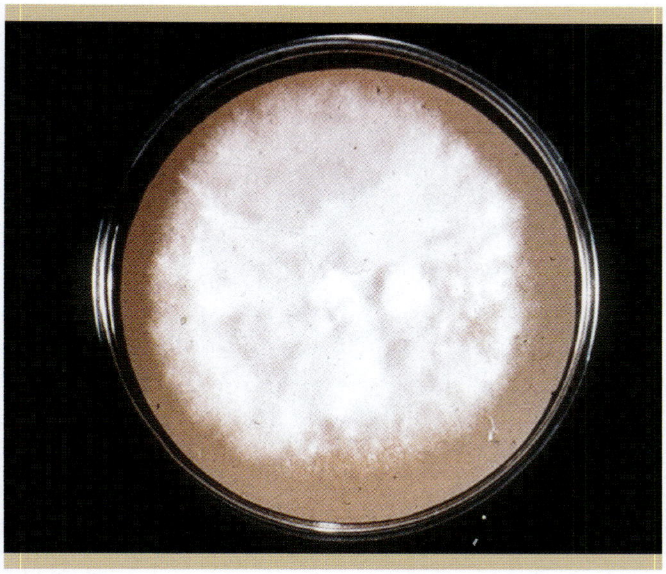

FIGURE 19-19 *Histoplasma* colony. (*Used with permission from Dr. Mark LaRocco.*)

  - Laboratory studies: elevated alkaline phosphatase levels, C-reactive protein levels, lactate dehydrogenase levels, and ferritin; pancytopenia due to bone marrow involvement
- Treatment:
  - None necessary for asymptomatic patients or for those with mild pulmonary disease and a normal immune system
  - Moderate disease may be treated with itraconazole, fluconazole (second line)
  - Extrapulmonary/disseminated infection in immunocompromised host treated with AMB

Blastomycosis (Gilchrist Disease)

- Caused by *Blastomyces dermatitidis*, a fungus endemic in the Mississippi River valley, Great Lakes region, and southeastern United States
- The disease is a problem for humans, but also for dogs; it has been associated with the wet soil of beaver dams and with aerosolization of soil in prairie-dog relocation projects
- The disease is caused by inhalation, with few cases (<20%) resulting in dissemination
- Disseminated disease often affects the skin, but may also involve the bones, prostate, genitourinary organs, or meninges and brain
- Clinical:
  - Cutaneous lesions include papulopustular lesions, nodules and abscesses, verrucous granulomas of the hands, face, and mucocutaneous areas, and cribriform scars
  - Inoculation blastomycosis is a rare and mild form of cutaneous disease in lab workers
- Diagnosis:
  - Culture (at 25°C): white colonies grow in 3 to 4 weeks; septate hyphae are present
  - Histology (at 37°C): thick-walled yeast (8–20 μm) with broad-based buds (Fig. 19-22)
  - KOH prep: broad-based buds can also be visualized by this means as well
- Treatment:
  - Itraconazole, AMB

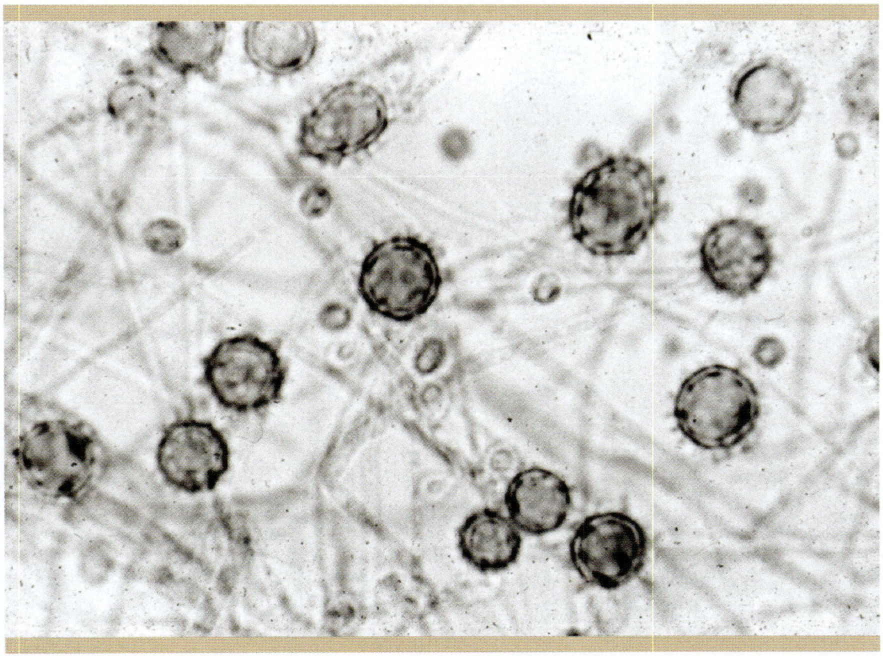

FIGURE 19-20 *Histoplasmosis capsulatum*, mold phase. (*Used with permission from Dr. Mark LaRocco.*)

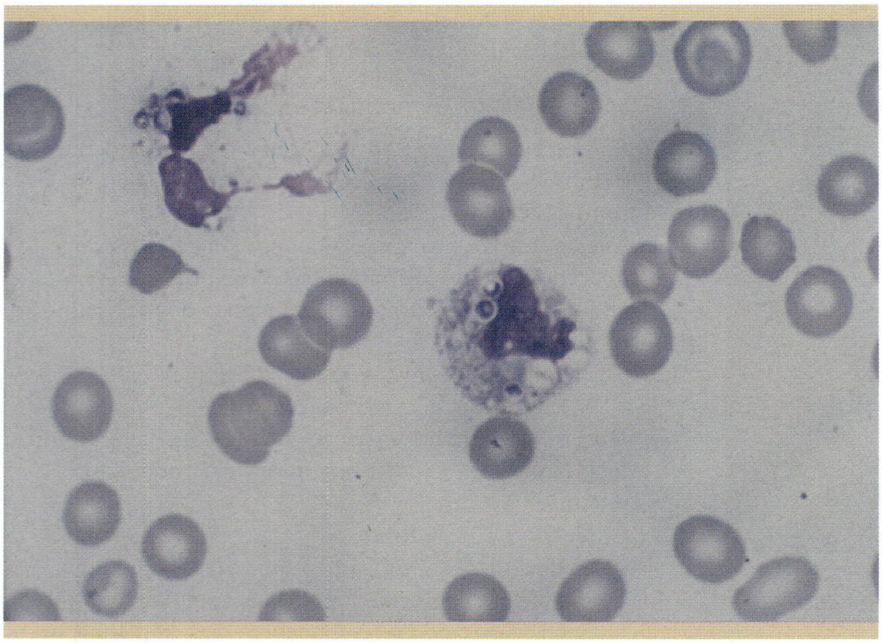

FIGURE 19-21 *Histoplasmosis capsulatum*, yeast phase within histiocytes in peripheral blood. (*Used with permission from Dr. Mark LaRocco.*)

Paracoccidioidomycosis (South American Blastomycosis)

- Caused by *Paracoccidioides brasiliensis* or *Paracoccidioides lutzii,* thermally dimorphic fungi found in South and Central America (most notably Brazil, Argentina, Colombia, and Venezuela)
- Most cases are caused by inhalation of conidia or mycelial fragments; rarely the disease may be caused by an inoculation event, particularly among those who chew on twigs to clean teeth
- *Paracoccidioides* have receptors that bind estrogen and prevent transformation of the tissue-invading yeast form; it is thought this explains the preponderance of cases among men (8:1)
- Clinical: (two common forms)
  - Juvenile form: fever, weight loss, and malaise; lymphadenopathy and hepatosplenomegaly; multiple skin lesions; mucous membrane and respiratory symptoms are unusual

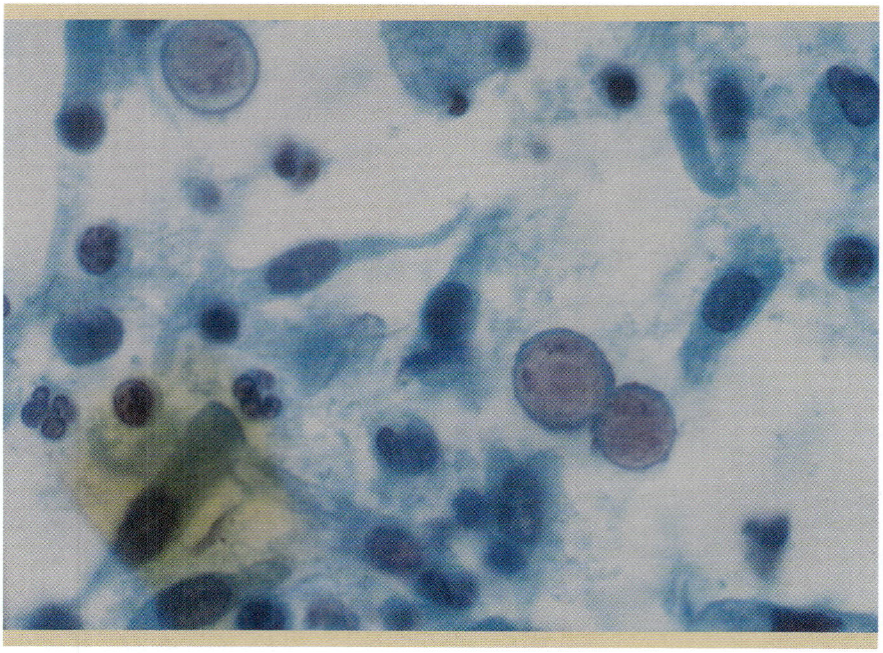

FIGURE 19-22 *Blastomyces dermatitidis*, yeast phase in tissue. (*Used with permission from Dr. Mark LaRocco.*)

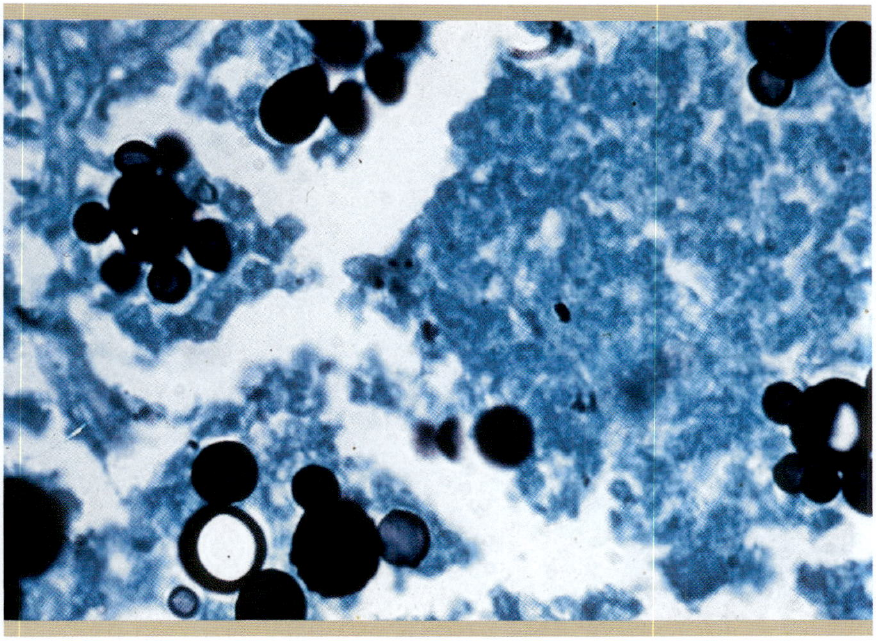

FIGURE 19-23 *Paracoccidioides brasiliensis,* yeast phase in tissue. (*Used with permission from Dr. Mark LaRocco.*)

- Adult form: primary lung infection with cough/dyspnea; fever, malaise, weight loss
  - Mucous membrane involvement (in 50% of patients), mulberry-like oral lesions (Aguiar-Pupo stomatitis), mandibular/cervical lymphadenopathy
  - Cutaneous lesions from hematologic dissemination (in 25% of patients) with crusted papules, ulcers, nodules, plaques, and verrucous lesions
  - Chronic adult form (in 33% of patients) pulmonary fibrosis or emphysematous change that can lead to pulmonary hypertension and cor pulmonale
- Diagnosis:
  - Culture (at 25°C): white to tan colony, growth in 2 to 4 weeks; the colony has septate hyphae and oval microconidia indistinguishable from *B. dermatitidis*
  - Histology (at 37°C): thin-walled yeast with narrow points of attachment between the buds and mother cells, yielding a classic "mariner's wheel" configuration (Fig. 19-23)
  - KOH prep: classic "mariner's wheel" may be visualized by this means as well
- Treatment:
  - Itraconazole (drug of choice), ketoconazole, fluconazole, AMB, TMP/SMX (trimethoprim/sulfamethoxazole) and sulfadiazine
  - Use of ketoconazole, TMP/SMX and sulfadiazine, are due to cost considerations in Central/South America, where the disease is endemic

SUBCUTANEOUS MYCOSES

- Pathogen, involves dermis, subcutaneous tissues, muscle, and fascia
- Mainly occur in the tropical and subtropical environs; fungi are usually implanted from environmental sources such as plants or soil

Chromoblastomycosis

- Localized, chronic infection of skin/subcutis caused by pigmented (dematiaceous) fungi
- Causative organisms include *Fonsecaea pedrosii, Fonsecaea pedrosii compactum, Cladophialophora carrionii, Rhinocladiella aquaspersa, Phialophora verrucosa,* and *Wangiella dermatitidis*
- Common in agricultural workers; acquired by inoculation from soil or decaying wood
- Clinical:
  - Painless, slow-growing, verrucous plaque, often with a stippling of pustules
  - Spread by direct extension
  - Localized lymphedema can occur
- Diagnosis:
  - Histology: pseudoepitheliomatous hyperplasia with inflammation; in the areas of neutrophils there are often "sclerotic cells" (also known as Medlar bodies, "copper penny" bodies) that are thick-walled and pigmented fungal elements (Fig. 19-24)
  - KOH prep: transepidermal elimination of intracellular and clumped "sclerotic cells" with single or double septum, and visible pigmentation
  - Culture: folded gray-green to black colonies
- Treatment:
  - Surgical excision and even cryotherapy has been utilized along with antifungal medications
  - Oral antifungals include itraconazole, terbinafine, and IV AMB

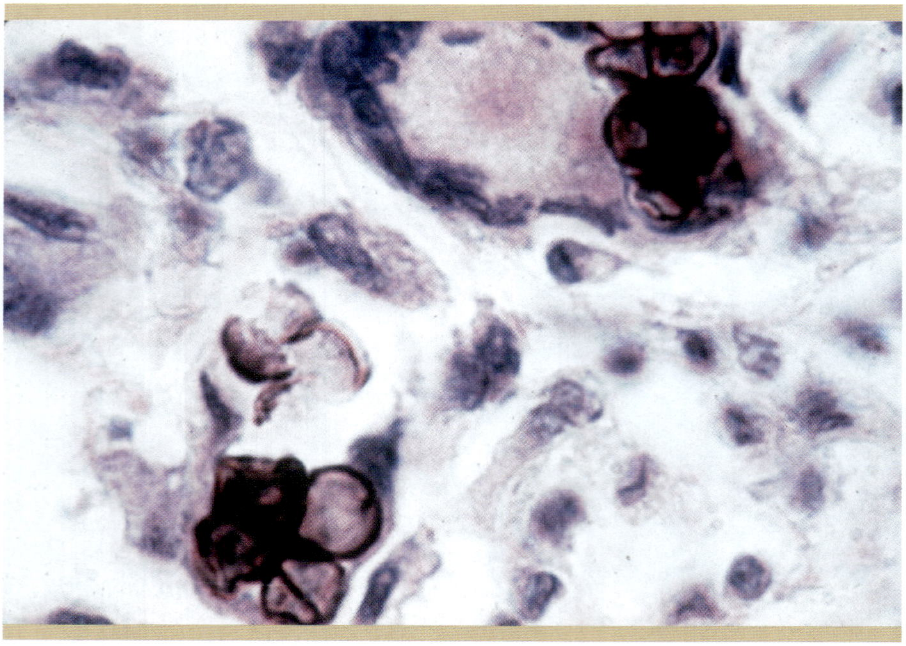

FIGURE 19-24 Chromo blastomycosis. (*Used with permission from Dr. Mark LaRocco.*)

Subcutaneous Phaeohyphomycosis

- Dematiaceous (pigmented) fungi that cause subcutaneous inflammatory cysts
- Causative organisms include *Exophiala jeanselmei, W. dermatitidis, Alternaria* spp., *Bipolaris* spp., *Curvularia* spp., *Phialophora* spp. and *Exserohilum* spp.
- The disease classically presents in carpenters and wood workers that accidentally inoculate themselves with the organism via splinters
- Clinical:
  - Indolent, painless, subcutaneous nodule; possibly with drainage
  - Local progression and extension may occur rapid in immunocompromised persons
- Diagnosis:
  - Histology: branched, spectate, hyphae with variable degrees of pigmentation; fungi are located in the cyst wall, associated with macrophages/granulomatous inflammation
  - Culture: dark leathery or wooly colonies
- Treatment:
  - Typically surgery is utilized plus or minus antifungals (itraconazole)

Mycetoma (Madura Foot, Maduromycosis)

- Caused by traumatic implantation of bacteria (actinomycetomas) or fungi (eumycetomas)
- Infections extrude characteristic "grains," comprised of the infectious microorganism; subclassification is premised upon gross examination of grains for color and texture (Table 19-7)
- Clinical:
  - Lesions most often involve the foot (due to ease of inoculation)
  - The infection involves the subcutaneous tissue, fascia, and sometimes, even the bone
  - Painless subcutaneous nodules enlarge and coalesce; fistulas and sinus tracts with purulent exudates and extrusion of grains develop; bone may be destroyed (Fig. 19-25)
- Diagnosis
  - Histology: neutrophilic inflammatory infiltrates surround filamentous fungal or bacterial grains; the size and shape of the grains aids in classification (Fig. 19-26)
  - Culture: etiologic agents are identified according to their microscopic and macroscopic features
  - Serology: enzyme-linked immunosorbent assay (ELISA) and immunodiffusion
- Treatment:
  - Actinomycetomas: trimethoprim/sulfamethoxazole plus rifampin or dapsone and streptomycin; amikacin or imipenem for recalcitrant *Nocardia* infections
  - Eumycetoma: surgical excision; oral ketoconazole, itraconazole, terbinafine, and intravenous AMB have been used with limited success; voriconazole and posaconazole have been proposed, but drug cost is an issue in endemic areas

Lobomycosis (Keloidal Blastomycosis or Lobo Disease)

- Caused by a *Lacazia loboi* (previously *Loboa loboi*), a fungus found in the Amazon basin
- Disease affects chiefly humans and dolphins (interspecies transfer has been described)

TABLE 19-7 Identification of *Mycetoma* Microcolonies

Organism	Color of Grain
Eumycetomes	
Madurella mycetomatis (hard)	Dark brown/black
Magnaporthe grisea	
Leptosphaeria senegalensis	
Pyrenochaeta romeroi	
Scedosporium apiospermum	White/yellow
Acremonium or *Fusarium* species	
Aspergillus nidulans	
Actinomycetomas	
Actinomadura madurae (soft)	White/yellow
Streptomyces somaliensis(hard)	Yellow
A. pelletieri (hard)	Red
Nocardia brasiliensis(soft)	White/requires direct microscopy to visualize
Nocardia otitidiscaviarum	

Hay RJ: Fungal infections. *Clin Dermatol.* 2006 May–Jun; 24(3):201–212.

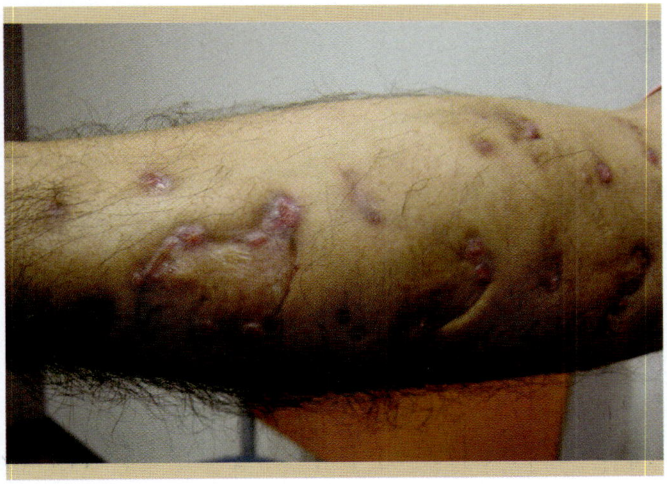

FIGURE 19-25 Actinomycetoma. (*Used with permission from Dr. Jason Miller.*)

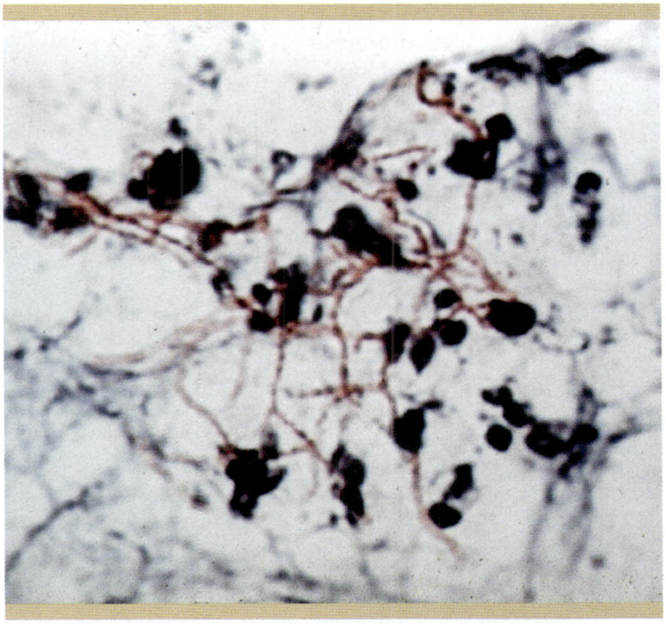

FIGURE 19-26 *Nocardia.* (*Used with permission from Dr. Mark LaRocco.*)

- Clinical:
  - Develops at sites of trauma
  - Slow-growing verrucous and keloidal nodules are common
  - Often affects the pinna of the ear, or the upper and lower extremities
  - Except for occasional lymphadenopathy, systemic symptoms are lacking
  - Squamous cell carcinoma may arise in chronic lesions
- Diagnosis:
  - Histology: acanthotic epidermis with parakeratosis, dermal fibrosis with inflammation; lemon-shaped, thick-walled, yeast (9–12 μm) joined in a chains; the overall appearance (with fibrosis and the lemon-shaped yeast) is likened to that of a "sieve"; intracellular asteroid bodies comprised of lipid myelin may occur
- Treatment:
  - Surgical excision
  - Clofazimine

Systemic Mycoses

- Infections that involve deep structures and spread through hematogenous routes to other areas of the body (skin and mucosa)
- Two forms exist: opportunistic mycoses and endemic respiratory mycoses

Opportunistic Mycoses

Candidiasis

- Candidiasis represents a heterogeneous group of infections including systemic, mucocutaneous, and vulvovaginal infections; risk factors exist for various candidal infections (Table 19-8)

TABLE 19-8 Risk Factors for Developing Candidiasis

Adults	Neonates and Children
Prolonged length of stay in an ICU	In addition to the adult risk factors:
High acute physiology and chronic health evaluation	Prematurity
II score (e.g., > 20)	Low Apgar score
Renal failure	Congenital malformations
Hemodialysis	
Broad-spectrum antibiotics	
Central venous catheter	
Parenteral nutrition	
Immunosuppressive drugs	
Cancer and chemotherapy	
Severe acute pancreatitis	
Candida colonization at multiple sites	
Surgery	

Pappas PG: Invasive candidiasis. *Infect Dis Clin North Am.* 2006 Sep;20(3):485–506.

- *Candida* spp. are thin-walled yeast (3–6 μm) that reproduce by budding
- Fifteen species exist, but the most significant human pathogens include *Candida albicans, Candida glabrata, Candida tropicalis, Candida parapsilosis, and Candida krusei*
- While *C. albicans* is a normal skin commensal, pathologic states may derive from: (1) overgrowth/colonization, (2) breakdown of normal barrier function of skin/mucosa, or (3) immune dysfunction
- Clinical:
  - Local disease
    - Oral candidiasis (thrush): creamy, white plaques of the tongue and oral mucosa; removed by scraping
    - Perleche: affect the oral commissures with scale, erythema, and fissures
    - Candidal esophagitis: seen in immunosuppressed patients (an AIDS-defining illness); dysphagia, chest pain, nausea, vomiting
    - Vulvovaginal candidiasis: erythematous mucosa with a thick, white discharge, pruritus; predisposing factors include immunosuppression, antibiotics, contraceptive devices, elevated estrogen (pregnancy)
    - Cutaneous candidiasis: bright red, "beefy" erythema, satellite pustules; often occurs in moist intertriginous areas or with occlusion
    - Erosio interdigitalis blastomycetica: macerated interdigital web space (commonly between the third and fourth fingers) of persons with chronically wet hands
    - Candidal folliculitis: pustules and nodules in hair-bearing areas; mainly seen in immunocompromised persons and among intravenous drug user
    - Candidal balanitis: erythema of the glans and/or prepuce, with pruritus and discomfort; eroded white papules and white discharge; may spread to buttocks and/or scrotum; more common in uncircumcised men
    - Candidal intertrigo: occurs skin folds; bright erythema with erosions, maceration, and satellite pustules (Fig. 19-27)
    - Candidal paronychia: loss of cuticle with erythema and scaling, may cause nail dystrophy; more common among those with chronically wet hands (bartender, etc.)
    - Candida diaper dermatitis: exacerbated by moisture under diapers, bright erythema, macerated patches, satellite pustules (Fig. 19-28)
    - Perianal candidiasis: skin maceration and pruritus are frequent with frequent extension to the perineum
  - Chronic/disseminated disease
    - Chronic mucocutaneous candidiasis: disorder of patients with T-cell dysfunction, may be related to autoimmune polyendocrinopathy-candidosis-ectodermal dystrophy (APECED) syndrome; results

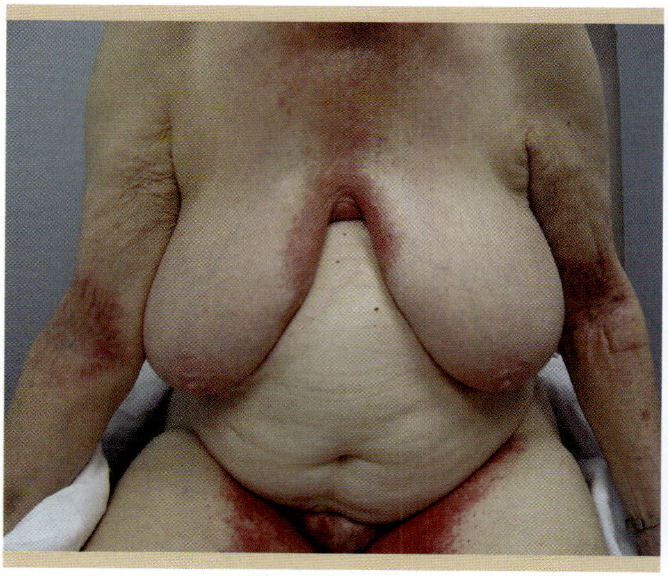

FIGURE 19-27 Candidiasis. (*Used with permission from Dr. Jason Miller.*)

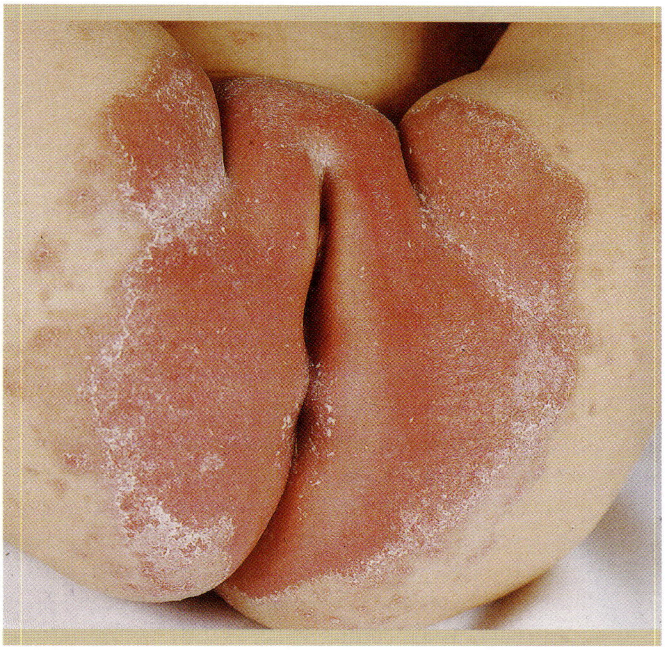

FIGURE 19-28 *Candida* diaper. (*From Wolff K, Johnson RA:* Fitzpatrick's Color Atlas & Synopsis of Clinical Dermatology, *6th Ed. New York: McGraw-Hill; 2009, p. 723.*)

in chronic candida infection of the skin, mucous membranes, hair, and nails; recalcitrant to treatment
    - Acute disseminated candidiasis: erythematous or hemorrhagic palpable rash occurs mostly among neutropenic patients
    - Chronic disseminated candidiasis: low-grade fever, right upper quadrant pain, the a palpable hepatomegaly/splenomegaly, elevated serum alkaline phosphatase; also occurs among neutropenic patients
    - Congenital candidiasis: begins in the first 24 hours of life; may have transient respiratory distress; associated with chorioamnionitis
    - Endocarditis: develops mainly in patients with a chronic indwelling catheter, also found in intravenous drug abusers; usually due to *C. tropicalis* and *C. parapsilosis*
    - Vertebral osteomyelitis: usually affects lumbosacral vertebral disks and vertebral bodies; chronic progressive localized back pain
    - Candidal endophthalmitis: retinal lesions associated with untreated candidemia
- Diagnosis:
    - KOH prep: yeast forms and pseudohyphae are present; differs from true septate hyphae of dermatophyte infections (Fig. 19-29)
    - Histology: PAS/D or GMS stains highlight yeast, and in certain ailments, vertically oriented pseudohyphae in the stratum corneum of the skin

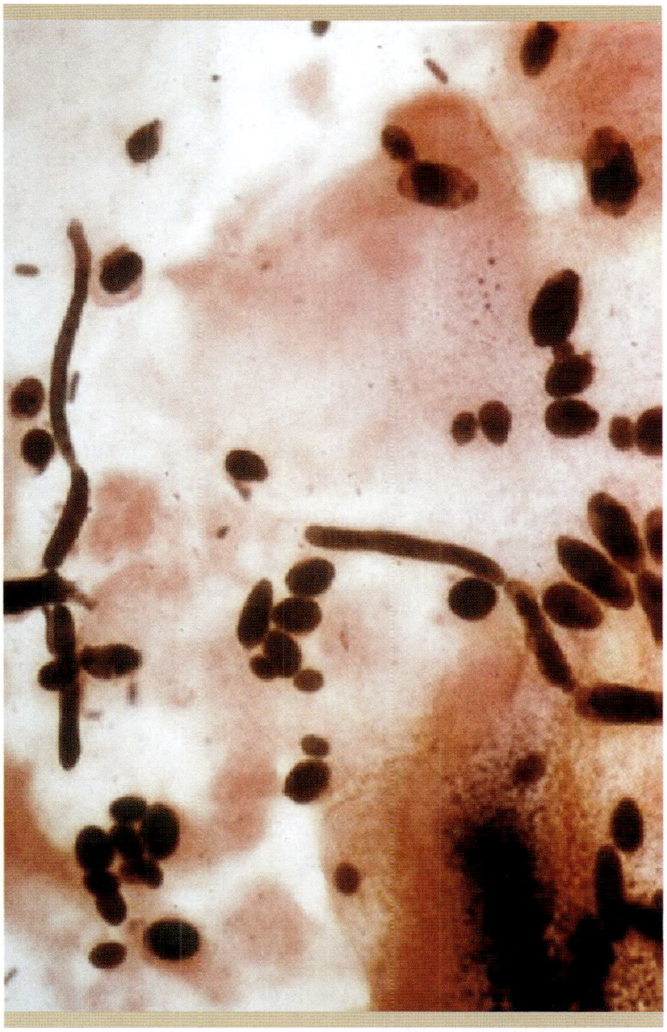

FIGURE 19-29 *Candida albicans,* microscopic view. (*Used with permission from Dr. Mark LaRocco.*)

    - Culture: white and creamy colonies grown on Sabouraud dextrose agar after 24 to 48 hours of incubation at 35°C (Fig. 19-30); grown on cornmeal agar results in characteristic chlamydospore formation
    - 1,3 β-glucan (Fungitell) assay: serologic test with high sensitivity and specificity; used for invasive candida infections only
- Treatment
    - Uncomplicated cutaneous/mucocutaneous disease: topical nystatin, topical azoles, oral troches, probiotics etc.
    - Invasive/disseminated disease: AMB, liposomal AMB, fluconazole, voriconazole, caspofungin

Cryptococcosis

- *Cryptococcus neoformans* is an encapsulated fungus that causes a systemic infection that sometimes involves the skin (10–15% of cases)

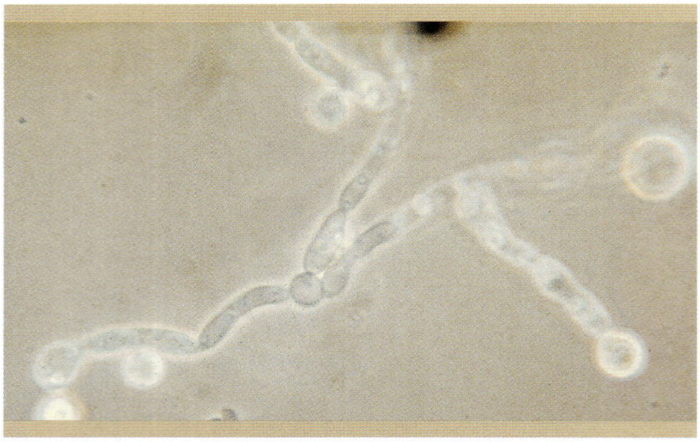

FIGURE 19-30 *Candida albicans* colony. (*From Wolff K et al.* Fitzpatrick's Color Atlas & Synopsis of Clinical Dermatology, *5th Ed. New York: McGraw-Hill; 2005, p. 717.*)

- Variants of include: *C. neoformans* var. *neoformans* (serotypes A and D) and *C. neoformans* var. *gattii* (serotypes B and C); strains of serotype D are more likely to result in skin lesions
- Either variant can cause disease, but var. *neoformans* more often affects immunocompromised persons (HIV/AIDS), while var. *gattii* more often affects immunocompetent persons
- *Cryptococcus* is found worldwide and it has been recovered from pigeon excreta, from wild and pet birds, and from soil, dust, and human skin; var. *gatti* is associated with eucalyptus
- In HIV/AIDS cryptococcus infection is typically seen when the CD4 count is less than 50 to 100 cells/μL
- Clinical:
  - Respiratory route of entry, but primary infection is usually subclinical; there may be hematogenous spread to lungs, bones, and viscera
  - Cryptococcus has a predilection for the central nervous system
  - Skin is involved in only 10 to 15% of cases, but yields widespread papules, acneiform or molluscum-like lesions of the face, and subcutaneous abscesses that may ulcerate
- Diagnosis:
  - Latex agglutination test: a sensitive and specific method for testing serum, cerebrospinal fluid, and urine
  - ELISA testing is both sensitive and specific for blood or cerebrospinal fluid, and it is capable of detecting the antigen earlier and at a lower concentration than other tests
  - Histology: infections may be gelatinous with numerous yeasts and little inflammation or granulomatous with fewer organisms and more marked inflammation; the yeast is oval and pleomorphic (4–8 μm), with a mucous capsule that appears as a washed-out halo (Fig. 19-31); the yeast marks with PAS/D or GMS, but the capsule marks with mucicarmine, colloidal iron, or Alcian blue
  - Culture: a slimy mucoid colony grown on Sabouraud agar at 37°C
- Treatment:
  - AMB, amphotericin B + 5-fluorocytosine, fluconazole

Cutaneous Aspergillosis

- A ubiquitous mold, found in most environments
- Cutaneous forms aspergillosis is most often caused by:
  - *Aspergillus flavus:* common primary cutaneous pathogen; affects intravenous sites in immunosuppressed patients

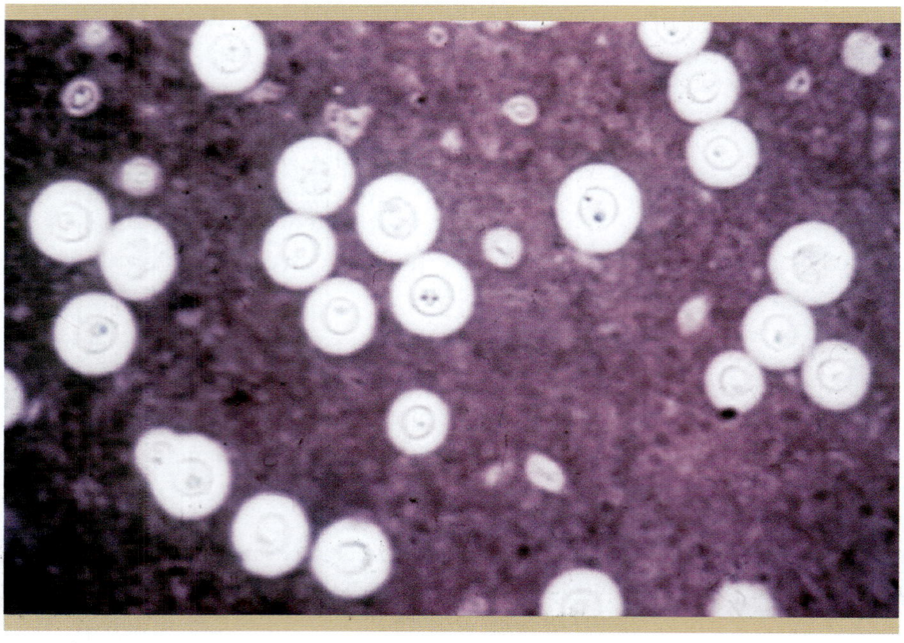

FIGURE 19-31 *Cryptococcus neoformans*, India ink preparation. (*Used with permission from Dr. Mark LaRocco.*)

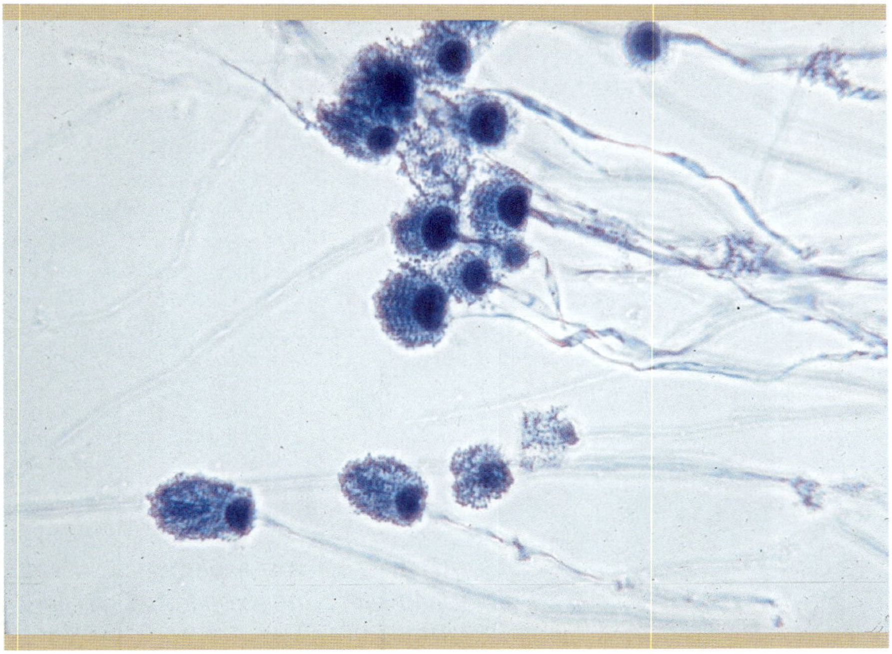

FIGURE 19-32 Aspergillus, microscopic view. (*Used with permission from Dr. Mark LaRocco.*)

  - *Aspergillus fumigatus:* most common pathogen overall, primarily affecting the lung
  - *Aspergillus niger:* associated with burn wounds
  - Rare cases of skin disease have been associated with *Aspergillus terreus* and *Aspergillus ustus*
- Clinical:
  - Aspergillosis usually begins as a pulmonary infection caused by inhalation of spores, but in the immunocompromised hematogenous dissemination may occur
  - Skin lesions occur in 5 to 10% of patients with disseminated aspergillosis
  - Skin lesions of disseminated aspergillosis may include single or multiple erythematous or violaceous papules, often with a central necrosis or an eschar
  - Primary cutaneous aspergillosis may occur with implantation of the at the site of intravenous access, particularly those covered with occlusive dressings
  - *Aspergillus* spp. are a frequent contaminant of nail cultures of dystrophic nails, but occasionally it may cause onychomycosis
  - burn wounds may be colonized by *Aspergillus* spp.
- Diagnosis:
  - Culture: rapid growth (1–3 days) of monomorphic molds at 25°C; conidiophores produce chains of conidia; different species have different conidial color, size, and spatial arrangements (Figs. 19-32 and 19-33)
  - Histology: septate hyphae with 45-degree ("acute") angle branching (Fig. 19-34); often located invading vessels walls; accentuate with PAS/D and GMS
  - Serologic tests: galactomannan test for invasive disease is available
- Treatment
  - Invasive disease: AMB, itraconazole, voriconazole, caspofungin

Zygomycosis (Mucormycosis)

- "Zygomycosis" is an older term that refers to opportunistic infections caused by fungi of the orders Mucorales and Entomophthorales
  - Mucorales: contains *Rhizopus* (most common), *Mucor, Rhizomucor, Absidia, Cunninghamella, Saksenaea, Apophysomyces, Cokeromyces, and Mortierella*
  - Entomophthorales: contains *Conidiobolus* and *Basidiobolus*
  - Species from the order Mucorales represent the dominant clinical condition, for this reason some prefer using the term "mucormycosis," rather than zygomycosis

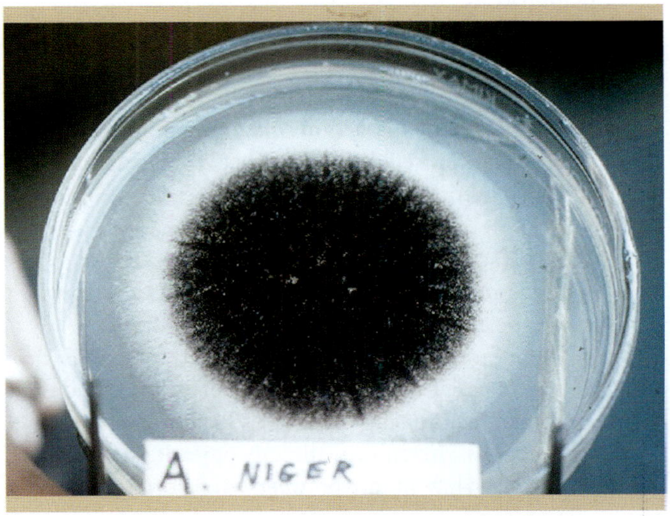

FIGURE 19-33 Aspergillus colony. (*Used with permission from Dr. Mark LaRocco.*)

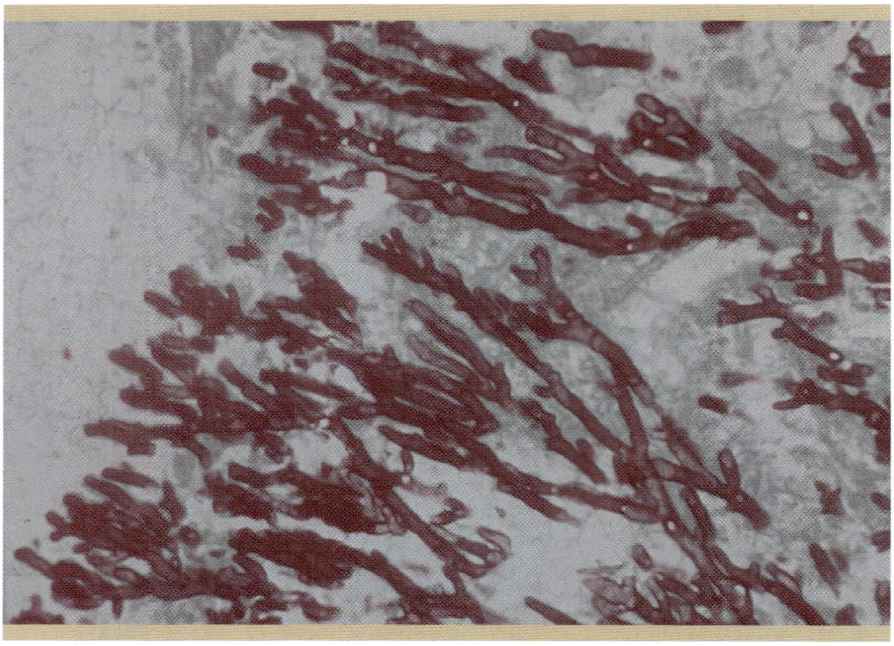

FIGURE 19-34 *Aspergillus in tissue. (Used with permission from Dr. Mark LaRocco.)*

- Clinical:
  - Zygomycoses are acute, rapidly developing, and often fatal infections (in some series the fatality rate is around 80%
  - Mucocutaneous disease (most often without any cutaneous stigmata) occurs in ketoacidotic diabetics, or those with leukemia, lymphoma, AIDS, burns, chronic renal failure, malnourishment, or iatrogenic immunosuppression
  - About 50% of primary cutaneous zygomycosis occurs in immunocompetent patients, often after trauma or as a result of contaminated surgical dressings
  - Five major clinical forms (rhinocerebral, pulmonary, cutaneous, gastrointestinal, and disseminated) all demonstrate vasculotropism that leads to infarction, gangrene, and the formation of black, necrotic, purulent debris
  - Cutaneous involvement, whether by traumatic implantation or by hematologenous dissemination, produces skin ulceration, cellulitis-like or ecthyma gangrenosum-like lesions, and necrotic abscesses
- Diagnosis:
  - Culture (at 25°C): on standard fungal media there is rapid growth (within 1–2 days) of a white cottony mold; the colony turns dark on sporulation
    - Differentiation of *Rhizopus*, *Absidia*, and *Mucor* spp. is based upon the presence of rhizoids and the spatial relationship of rhizoids to sporangia
    - *Rhizopus*: rhizoids are directly opposite sporangia
    - *Absidia*: rhizoids are between two sporangia (internodal)
    - *Mucor*: no rhizoids are present
  - Histology: broad, hyaline, ribbon-like hyphae that are not visibly septate; branching occurs at 90-degree angles ("obtuse"); asexual reproduction by production of sporangia and sporangiospores
- Treatment:
  - Combinations of surgical debridement and liposomal preparations of AMB are often employed with varying success
  - Itraconazole, posaconazole, and caspofungin have been employed for select organisms under certain circumstances

Penicilliosis

- Caused by *Penicillium marneffei*, a fungus that is endemic to Southeast Asia; the bamboo rat is a reservoir of infection in Asia; the fungus causes disease chiefly among HIV/AIDS patients, including the immunocompromised traveler
- While a dimorphic fungus, *P. marneffei* is not often discussed with other dermatologically relevant dimorphic fungi because of its geographic constraints and opportunistic qualities (Table 19-9)

TABLE 19-9 List of Dimorphic Fungii

Coccidioides immitis
Histoplasma capsulatum and *H. duboisii*
Blastomyces dermatitidis
Paracoccidiodes brasiliensis
Sporothrix schenckii
Penicillium marneffei

- Clinical:
  - The fungus is likely acquired via inhalation, leading to primary pulmonary disease
  - Dissemination in the immunocompromised leads to weight loss, hepatomegaly, umbilicated ("molluscum-like") facial lesions, and occasional skin/mucosal necrosis
  - Prominent lymphadenopathy may occur with disseminated disease
- Diagnosis:
  - Culture (at 25°C): yields a flat green colony with diffusible red pigment; the fungus has characteristic conidiophores common to *Penicillium* spp.; conversion to yeast occurs on brain heart infusion (BHI) at 37°C, and this conversion is necessary to diagnose *P. marneffei*
  - Histology: intracellular yeast in histiocytes that are divided by a centrally located transverse septum ("cross wall"); distinguishes *P. marneffei* from *H. capsulatum*
- Treatment:
  - Severe/disseminated disease is treated with AMB followed by itraconazole
  - Mild disease may be treated with oral itraconazole
  - Preliminary data suggest that voriconazole may also be
  - Long-term suppressive therapy is usually required to prevent relapse

FUSARIUM

- *Fusarium* is a family of ubiquitous fungi found in the soil, air, and on plants; the most common species are *F. solani, Fusarium oxysporum, and Fusarium chlamydosporum*
- *Fusarium* spp. may cause a broad spectrum of infections in humans, including superficial, locally invasive, and disseminated infections
- Superficial and localized forms occurs in immunocompetent patients; invasive and disseminated disease affects chiefly immunocompromised patients (particularly those with significant neutropenia or severe T-cell immunodeficiencies); burn patients are also at risk
- Clinical:
  - Infection begins after trauma or with ingestion of contaminated food
  - Various disease manifestations include venous catheter infection, septic arthritis, keratitis, endophthalmitis, endocarditis, peritonitis, and fungemia (dissemination)
  - Localized cutaneous lesions may present as a cellulitis at sites of skin breakdown caused by trauma/burns, or even as simple onychomycosis
  - Patients with disseminated disease may develop multiple, painful erythematous papulonodular lesions; lesions often manifest central necrosis, yielding an ecthyma gangrenosum-like appearance
  - A clue to disseminated fusarium infection may be the occurrence of a refractory fever in a neutropenic patient with multiple skin lesions and a positive fungal blood culture
  - About one-third of the patients with disseminated fusarium infection presented with skin lesions in different stages of evolution (papules, nodules, and necrotic lesions)
- Diagnosis:
  - Culture: colonies grow quickly; colonies may be either pale or brightly colored, and may or may not have a cottony aerial mycelium (species dependent); microscopic examination of the colonies reveals sickle-shaped ("banana-shaped," or "canoe-shaped"), multiseptate macroconidia (differs substantially from *Aspergillus* spp.)
- Treatment:
  - The organism is resistant to many antifungals, including itraconazole, fluconazole, and echinocandins (caspofungin, micafungin, anidulafungin)
  - AMB and voriconazole are the most often employed agents, posaconazole has sometimes been used

OTHER

Rhinosporidiosis

- Caused by *Rhinosporidium seeberi*, now considered to be an aquatic protozoan (new class: Mesomycetozoa); previously widely considered a fungus, it is often discussed with other fungi
- However, there continue to be divergent views on the subject, with some parties still contending that *R. seeberi* is either a cyanobacterium or a lower aquatic fungus
- Endemic to India, Sri Lanka, South America, and Africa; contact with contaminated water results in infection via traumatic inoculation; disease may affect humans, cattle, cats/dogs, goats, horses/mules, parrots, and ducks/swans
- Clinical:
  - The infection is limited to mucosal epithelium; the nose/nasopharynx is involved in ~70% of persons; the conjunctiva/lacrimal apparatus is involved in ~15%
  - Nasal disease may present with obstruction, epistaxis, rhinorrhea, postnasal drip and cough, or a foreign-body sensation
  - Eye disease is asymptomatic early on, increased tearing, photophobia, redness, and secondary infection may occur with time
  - Skin lesions present as verrucous papillomas
- Diagnosis:
  - Histology: granulomatous inflammation with characteristic thick-walled, large sporangium (usually 300–350 μm) that contain tens of thousands of sporangiospores
- Treatment:
  - Surgical excision (recurrence is common)
  - Adjunctive AMB; long courses of dapsone were anecdotally effective

Protothecosis

- Caused by *Prototheca wickerhamii,* an achloric algae present in stagnant water
- Ubiquitous in distribution, it is thought to infect humans through contact with contaminated water (or possibly contaminated soil); importantly, person-to-person transmission does not occur
- The organism is of low virulence; most persons infected are immunosuppressed; use of glucocorticoids (in any form) is a risk factor for protothecosis
- Clinical:
  - Cutaneous lesions are the most common forms of infection
  - Cases present ill-defined plaque or nodule that may have a verrucous surface
  - In healthy persons the infection most often remains confined to the site of inoculation; disseminated disease and even fatal disease can occur in the immunocompromised
  - Olecranon bursitis is a classic presentation of protothecosis
  - Tenosynovitis was reported from a contaminated sclerosing agent for varicosities
- Diagnosis
  - Histology: the diagnostic finding is a classic "morula" that consists of a specialized sporangia with a central endospore surrounded by a corona of molded endospores forming a soccer ball- or berry-like shape
  - Culture: the species grows readily upon Sabouraud media at room temperature, yielding smooth, white-to-beige colonies within 48 hours; inhibited by cycloheximide
- Treatment:
  - Protothecosis can be difficult to eradicate
  - Surgical intervention is utilized, often in combination with pharmacologic therapy
  - Successful treatment of localized disease has been described with AMB, ketoconazole, itraconazole, fluconazole, and voriconazole
  - Local physiotherapy (heating pads) may be utilized as an adjunct as well

QUIZ

Questions

1. Which of the following is not a dimorphic fungal organism?

   A. *Blastomyces dermatitidis*
   B. *Cryptococcus neoformans*
   C. *Histoplasmosis capsulatum*
   D. *Penicillium marneffei*
   E. *Sporothrix schenckii*

2. Which fungus produces characteristic barrel-shaped arthroconidia that are easily aerosolized, and of particular exposure-danger to laboratory workers?

   A. *Blastomyces dermatitidis*
   B. *Coccidiomycosis immitis*
   C. *Histoplasmosis capsulatum*
   D. *Paracoccidioides brasiliensis*
   E. *Sporothrix schenckii*

3. What dermatophyte is a common cause of tinea cruris, but does not cause tinea capitis?

   A. *Epidermophyton floccosum*
   B. *Microsporum audouinii*
   C. *Microsporum canis*
   D. *Trichophyton rubrum*
   E. *Trichophyton tonsurans*

4. Which organism may cause extracellular asteroid bodies, with yeast surrounded by brightly eosinophilic spicules?

   A. *Blastomyces dermatitidis*
   B. *Coccidiomycosis immitis*
   C. *Histoplasmosis capsulatum*
   D. *Paracoccidioides brasiliensis*
   E. *Sporothrix schenckii*

5. A biopsy demonstrates interconnected, lemon-shaped yeast, of about 9 μm in diameter, which are enmeshed within thickened collagen bundles. The best diagnosis is:

   A. *Aspergillus flavus*
   B. *Exophiala jeanselmei*
   C. *Fonsecaea pedrosii*
   D. *Lacazia loboi*
   E. *Piedraia hortae*

6. A healthy patient presents with a macular pigmented lesion upon the sole. In addition to a pigmented process, the differential diagnosis includes infection with which fungus?

   A. *Aspergillus flavus*
   B. *Exophiala jeanselmei*
   C. *Fonsecaea pedrosii*
   D. *Hortaea werneckii*
   E. *Piedraia hortae*

7. A neutropenic patient undergoing chemotherapy presents with skin lesions, a persistent fever, and a positive fungal culture that yields multiseptate, sickle-shaped macroconidia. The most likely organism involved in the infection is:

   A. *Aspergillus flavus*
   B. *Blastomyces dermatitidis*
   C. *Cryptococcus neoformans*

D. *Fusarium solani*
E. *Penicillium marneffei*

8. Which of the following drugs is most often employed to treat fusarium infections?

A. Caspofungin
B. Fluconazole
C. Itraconazole
D. Nystatin
E. Voriconazole

9. Which infection produces small, pigmented sclerotic cells or Medlar bodies in tissue?

A. Blastomycosis
B. Chromoblastomycosis
C. Coccidiomycosis
D. Cryptococcosis
E. Piedra

10. Bullous tinea pedis is associated with which dermatophyte species?

A. *Epidermophyton floccosum*
B. *Trichophyton concentricum*
C. *Trichophyton mentagrophytes*
D. *Trichophyton rubrum*
E. *Trichophyton tonsurans*

11. In tissue, which fungus forms small, 2 to 5 μm intracellular yeast entrapped within histiocytes?

A. *Blastomyces dermatitidis*
B. *Coccidiomycosis immitis*
C. *Histoplasmosis capsulatum*
D. *Paracoccidioides brasiliensis*
E. *Sporothrix schenckii*

12. Microscopic examination from a dimorphic fungal colony revealed large thick-walled yeast with broad-based bud. What is the best diagnosis?

A. Blastomycosis
B. Coccidioidomycosis
C. Cryptococcosis
D. Histoplasmosis
E. Sporotrichosis

Answers

1. B. *Cryptococcus neoformans* is not a dimorphic fungus. It produces only a yeast form and causes systemic disease in immunocompromised persons. The remainder of the species, including *Penicillium marneffei*, is dimorphic species.
2. B. *Coccidioides immitis* is a fungus that produces barrel-shaped arthroconidia with alternating empty spaces that are easily spread through aerosolization. Once inhaled arthroconidia transform into spherules containing endospores. Therefore, cultures forming arthroconidia may be dangerous to lab personnel. The disease flourishes in the Lower Sonoran Desert life zone of the southwestern United States. Latex particle agglutination and immunodiffusion test are positive in 90% of cases in early phase of the disease.
3. A. *Epidermophyton floccosum* is a common cause tinea cruris, but it does not cause tinea capitis. The most common cause of tinea capitis in the United States is *Trichophyton tonsurans.*
4. E. *Sporothrix schenckii* is a dimorphic organism, which in tissue forms rare cigar-shaped yeast. The yeast may be encrusted by eosinophilic material yielding an extracellular "asteroid body." This extracellular form of an asteroid body differs from that of *Lacazia loboi*, the causative species of lobomycosis, which forms intracellular asteroid bodies within histiocytes.
5. D. *Lacazia loboi* is the causative species of lobomycosis, a rare fungal infection common to the Amazon basin of South America. In tissue, the organism forms lemon-shaped yeast, of about 9 μm in size, which appear interconnected, like children's "pop-blocks." The infection ultimately yields a cytokine milieu that creates slow-growing, fibrotic, and keloidal lesions.
6. D. *Hortaea werneckii* (formerly *Exophiala werneckii* or *Phaeoannellomyces werneckii*) is a dematiaceous (melanin-producing) yeast with remarkable halotolerance, and in humans, it often produces a relatively asymptomatic infection with pigmented near macules upon the palm and sole that may be confused with a pigmented lesion, including melanoma.
7. D. Neutropenic patients are particularly susceptible to fungal infections, including aspergillosis, caused by *Aspergillus* species, and fusariosis, caused by *Fusarium* species. While the diseases may present in similar fashion, only *Fusarium* species produce sickle-shaped or "canoe-shaped" macroconidia in culture, and this is a key diagnostic difference.
8. E. *Fusarium* species, like *Lacazia loboi*, is notoriously resistant to many antifungal agents, including fluconazole, itraconazole, and all echinocandins, including caspofungin. Nystatin is not absorbed from the gastrointestinal tract, and would not be an appropriate agent for a systemic infection. Cases of fusariosis are usually treated with either voriconazole or amphotericin B.
9. B. Chromoblastomycosis is a fungal infection seen chiefly in the rural works in tropical and subtropical climes. It is caused by traumatic inoculation and in tissue it yields characteristic pigmented, "chestnut-brown," thick-walled sclerotic cells or Medlar bodies. These bodies are usually located in small pockets of neutrophils within a larger granulomatous process.
10. A. Vesiculobullous tinea pedis is most often caused by *T. mentegrophytes*. The eruptions occur typically upon

the forefoot or the instep area. This form of tinea pedis is also responsible for the dermatophytid reactions. During primary infection a brisk T-cell response develops, which produces an allergic reaction to the fungus, yielding the clinical presentation.

11. C. Histoplasmosis is a fungal illness caused by *Histoplasmosis capsulatum*, a yeast that presents as intracellular organisms (usually 2–5 μm in diameter) within histiocytes. This differs from *Penicillium marneffei* that produces yeast in histiocytes that are divided by a centrally located transverse septum ("cross wall"). Histoplasmosis may, however, be confused with leishmaniasis as well, but *Leishmania* species have a kinetoplast, which fungi do not possess.
12. A. In tissue, *Blastomyces dermatitidis* forms extracellular yeast with broad based buds. This is differs from: *Paracoccidioides braziliensis,* which yields a "Mariner's wheel" of narrow necked buds; *Coccidioides immitis*, which yields spherules with endospores; *Cryptococcus neoformans*, which has pleomorphic yeast with a thick gelatinous capsule; *Sporothrix schenckii*, which yields extracellular asteroid bodies; *Lacazia loboi*, which yields lemon-shaped yeast arranged in chains with fibrosis; and *Penicillium marneffei*, which yields intracellular yeast with a tranverse septum (a "cross-wall").

REFERENCES

Alyr Maibach HI: *Atlas of Infections of the Skin*. New York: Churchill Livingstone; 1999.

DiCaudo DJ: Coccidioidomycosis: a review and update. *J Am Acad Dermatol* 2006;55(6):929–942.

Edwards S: Balanitis and balanoposthitis: a review. *Genitourin Med* 1996;72(3):155–159.

Elewski BE: *Cutaneous Fungal Infections*, 2nd Ed. Marden, MA: Blackwell; 1998.

Goldsmith LA et al. *Fitzpatrick's Dermatology in General Medicine*, 8th Ed. New York: McGraw-Hill; 2012.

Hay RJ: Fusarium infections of the skin. *Curr Opin Infect Dis* 2007;20(2):115–117.

Janniger CK, Schwartz RA, Szepietowski JC, Reich A: Intertrigo and common secondary skin infections. *Am Fam Physician* 2005;72(5):833–838.

Kauffman CA: Endemic mycoses: blastomycosis, histoplasmosis, and sporotrichosis. *Infect Dis Clin North Am* 2006;20(3):645–662.

Kauffman CA: Histoplasmosis: a clinical and laboratory update. *Clin Microbiol Rev* 2007;20(1):115–132.

Kyle AA, Dahl MV: Topical therapy for fungal infections. *Am J Clin Dermatol* 2004;5(6):443–451.

Lass-Flörl C, Mayr A: Human protothecosis. *Clin Microbiol Rev* 2007;20(2):230–242.

Loo DS: Cutaneous fungal infections in the elderly. *Dermatol Clin* 2004;22(1):33–50.

Lupi O, Tyring SK, McGinnis MR: Tropical dermatology: fungal tropical diseases. *J Am Acad Dermatol* 2005; 53(6):931–951.

McKee PH: *Pathology of the Skin: With Clinical Correlations*. London: Mosby-Wolfe; 1996.

Pappas PG: Invasive candidiasis. *Infect Dis Clin North Am* 2006;20(3):485–506.

Ribes JA, Vanover-Sams CL, Baker DJ: Zygomycetes in human disease. *Clin Microbiol Rev* 2000;13(2):236–301.

Vander Straten MR, Hossain MA, Ghannoum M: Cutaneous infections dermatophytosis, onychomycosis, and tinea versicolor. *Infect Dis Clin North Am* 2003;17(1):87–112.

CHAPTER 20

NUTRITION-RELATED DISEASES

MARIGDALIA K. RAMIREZ-FORT
RIVA Z. ROBINSON
RYAN J. GERTZ
HUNG DOAN
JOSEPH CONSTANTINO
FARHAN KHAN
STEPHEN K. TYRING

DISORDERS OF CALORIC INTAKE

Obesity

- Multifactorial disease of excess body fat affecting any age group
  - Endogenous: endocrine illness
    - Hypothyroid, polycystic ovarian syndrome, adrenal hyperandrogenism, imbalance of ghrelin, and leptin
  - Exogenous: positive energy balance is stored as adipose tissue
    - Excess calories, sedentary lifestyle, minimal exercise
- Clinical manifestations
  - Systemic
    - Obesity in central areas, mammary region, buttocks
    - Obesity in limbs, greater in upper arms and thighs; genu varum due to weight-bearing
  - Cutaneous
    - Acrochordon: increases with severity of obesity, associated with Type 2 diabetes mellitus
    - Striae distensae: "stretch marks"
    - Keratosis pilaris: up to 21% of obese patients
    - Plantar hyperkeratosis: due to increased foot girth and weight bearing
    - Adiposis dolorosa (Dercum disease): rare, in postmenopausal obese women
      - ▲ Multiple symmetric painful lipomas sparing head/neck; commonly on trunk and lower extremities
  - Metabolic alterations
    - Acanthosis nigricans: insulin resistance, correlates with subsequent development of Type 2 diabetes mellitus if untreated
    - Polycystic ovarian syndrome (PCOS): infertility, dysmennorhea, insulin resistance, cystic ovaries on ultrasound
    - Hyperandrogenism secondary to metabolic dysregulation
- Diagnosis: obesity defined as BMI more than 30, or greater than 95% for age and gender
- Treatment
  - Lifestyle and dietary modification: exercise and low-calorie diet
  - Social support: family, friends, provider–patient contact
  - Medications should be used with caution: phentermine, bHCG injections, orlistat
  - Surgical: gastric bypass, or gastric outlet surgeries; necessitate monitoring for nutritional deficiencies, especially B_{12}

Anorexia Nervosa and Bulimia

- Undernourishment due to abnormal patterns of food consumption and/or purging to achieve thinness; related to underlying psychiatric distburances
- Most common in adolescent females
- Clinical manifestations
  - Cutaneous: xerosis, pruritus, lower limb edema, Russell sign (knuckle calluses due to chronic self-induced vomiting)
  - Hair: thinning and increased fragility
  - Oral: gingivitis, tooth enamel erosion, parotid gland enlargement
- Treatment
  - Cognitive behavioral therapy

- Selective serotonin reuptake inhibitors
- Hospitalization with parenteral nutrition in severe circumstances

Protein Energy Malnutrition: Undernutrtion, Marasmus, and Kwashiorkor (Fig. 20-1A,B)

- Undernutrition: all encompassing term for nutritional and caloric deficiencies
  - Related to socioeconomic status and availability of nutrients in local region
  - Favors opportunistic infections: reduced cellular immunity, phagocytic function, adaptive immunity (decreased antibody production)
  - Secondary: from HIV, pneumonia, tuberculosis, and malaria

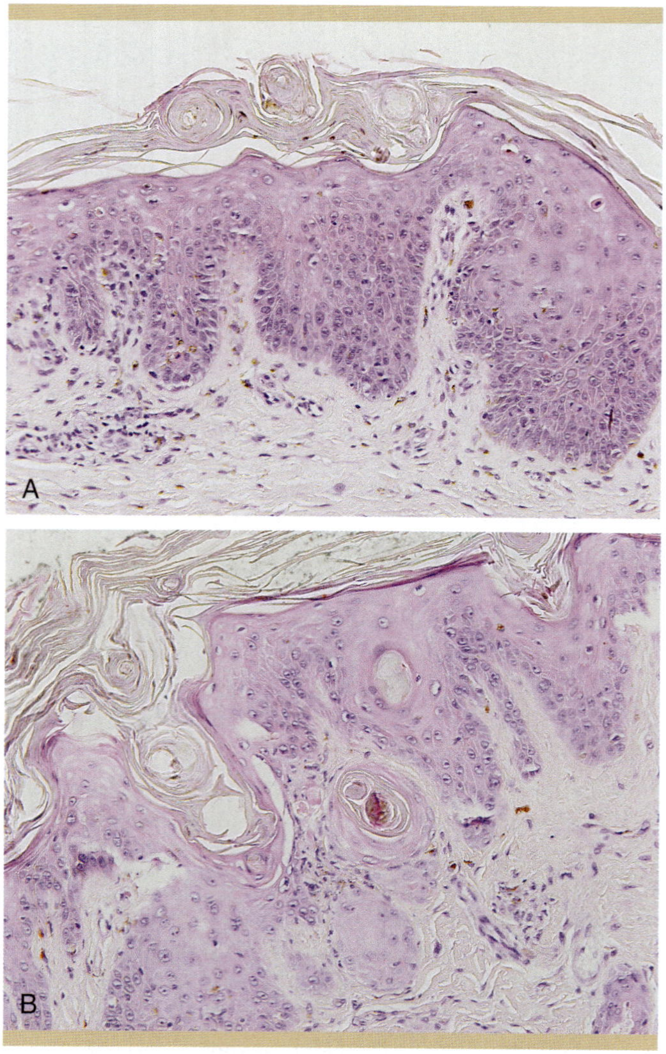

FIGURE 20-1 A, B Kwashiorkor with psoriasiform hyperplasia, hyperkeratosis, and hyperpigmentation. *(Used with permission from Jack Longley, MD, University of Wisconsin.)*

  - Diagnosis: investigate possible infectious etiologies, anemia, nutritional deficiencies (metals, vitamins, etc.)
    - Urinalysis (UA) (infection), blood smear (malaria), PPD, fecal occult blood, parasites, or ova
- Marasmus: "adapted" starvation from global nutrition deficiency
  - Occurs in developing countries: decreased intake of all macronutrients; rare in developed countries
  - Primary causes: congenital defects (difficulty feeding, degluttition), failure to thrive (neglect, inability to nurse), alcoholism, eating disorders
  - Secondary: lack of nutrient availability, low socioeconomic status, early and incorrect use of infant formula (not enough calories are given)
  - Clinical manifestations
    - Constitutional: emaciated, growth deficiency, muscular atrophy
    - Systemic involvement: hypotension, hypoglycmeia, hypothermia, constipation (in infants), anemia
    - Cutaneous: loss of turgor, thinning of skin, xerosis, loss of elasticity
  - Diagnosis: typically on history and physical examination
  - Treatment: inpatient setting, reestablish hydration and electrolyte status
    - Carefully administer early nutrition by mouth (intestinal villi need to be reestablished); risk of refeeding hypophosphatemia
    - Start at 50 kcal/kg/d and water at 125 to 150 mL/kg/d (protein accounts for 10–12%)
    - Micronutrient supplementation: single dose vitamin A 5,000 IU, iron 1 to 3 mg/d, zinc 1 mg/d
- Kwashiorkor: considered "nonadapted" starvation; traditionally considered a decrease in protein intake with adequate consumption of other macronutrients
  - New theory: kwashiorkor results from physiologic stress of acute or chronic illness increasing demands for protein in a preexisting state of starvation
  - Seen in both the developed and developing world
  - Leads to high plasma insulin at the expense of liver-derived albumin (low reserve of amino acids), decreasing plasma oncotic pressure
  - Clinical manifestations
    - Systemic
      - ▲ Weakness, especially in extremities
      - ▲ Pallor, cyanotic extremities
      - ▲ Abdominal distension: secondary to hypoalbuminemia and liver infiltration from fatty acid synthesis
    - Cutaneous: edema, pellagra-like dermatitis, areas of confluent hyperkeratosis ("flaky paint"), hyperpigmentation with scale in flexural areas
    - Hair: dry, brittle, sparse; "flag sign"—alternating segments of normal pigmentation and depigmentation along hair shaft

  - Nails: brittle and soft
  - Mucosa: cheilosis, xerophthalmia, vulvovaginitis
- Histology
  - Variable with features likely representing a combination of vitamin and mineral deficiencies
  - Psoriasiform hyperplasia with hyperkeratosis, epidermal hyperpigmentation; alternate areas with atrophy and variably shortened and flattened rete; hypogranulosis
  - Dermal edema (secondary to low albumin)
- Diagnosis: history of dietary changes (food aversion), vegeterianism, milk substitutes (rice milk, dairy creamer), dilute formula; physical examination
- Treatment: slow introduction of diet such as milk meals with nutritional supplements (i.e., zinc, magnesium, selenium, copper, multivitamins)
  - Monitor and treat electrolye imbalance

Essential Fatty Acid (EFA) Deficiency

- Unsaturated fatty acids the body cannot make: linoleic, linolenic, and arachidonic acid
- Function: select cellular absorption, prostaglandin precursor, energy storage, lamellar granule formation, cellular integrity (including immune cells)
- Etiology
  - Chronic poor absorption (i.e., short intestine syndrome)
  - Oral food formulas and total parenteral nutrition deficient in EFA
- Clinical manifestations
  - Systemic features
    - Growth failure, increased risk for infection, thrombocytopenia, anemia, hepatosplenomegaly, and neurological alterations (associated omega-3 deficiency)
  - Cutaneous
    - Xerotic, leathery skin with underlying erythema
    - Faint truncal desquamation
    - Eczema of nasolabial folds and eyebrows, extending to face and neck
    - Intertriginous erosions
    - Impaired wound healing
- Histology
  - Fissured stratum corneum on microscopy
  - Hyperkeratosis, parakeratosis, widening of intercellular spaces in stratum spinosum with disruption of intercellular junctions
  - Aberrant morphology of keratinosomes
- Diagnosis: elevated plasma eicosatrienoic acid; decreased linoleic, arachidonic acids
- Treatment: Essential fatty acid replacement, i.e., fish oil, flaxseed

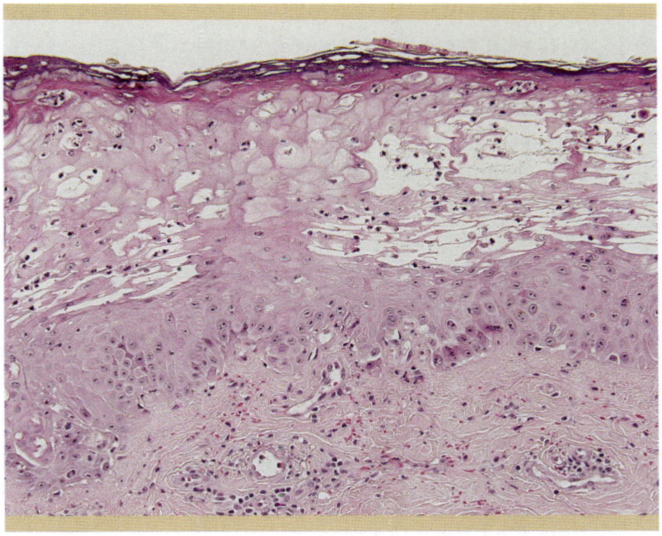

FIGURE 20-2 Necrolytic migratory erythema (Glucagonoma syndrome) with abrupt necrosis of upper epidermal layer with neutrophilic exocytosis and pustule formation. (*Used with permission from Jack Longley, MD, University of Wisconsin.*)

Necrolytic Migratory Erythema (NME) (Fig. 20-2)

- Rare cutaneous eruption characteristic of patients with glucagonoma (pancreatic α-cell neuroendocrine tumor) though it is seen in other ailments, including intestinal malabsorption, cirrhosis, and malignancy as the so-called "pseudoglucagonoma"
- Etiology may be multifactorial including nutritional deficiencies of zinc, amino acids, or essential fatty acids as well as increased inflammatory mediators
- Clinical manifestations
  - Systemic features
    - Glucose intolerance, anemia, diarrhea, malaise, weight loss, hypercoagulability, and neuropsychiatric features
  - Cutaneous
    - Cyclic presentation of initial erythema with bullous progression and subsequent crusting; crust heals with hyperpigmentation
    - Highly pruritic with painful annular plaques
    - Distribution generally includes areas of regular trauma, including buttocks, lower extremities, groin, and perineum (below the belt) as well as periorificial involvement with angular cheilitis, glossitis, and stomatitis
    - High degree of overlap with acrodermatitis enteropathica (congenital zinc metabolism defect)
- Histology
  - Parakeratosis with loss of granular cell layer, necrosis, and separation of the upper epidermis

- The upper epidermis reveals neutrophils and keratinocytes with vacuolization and dyskeratosis
- Closely resembles histology of pellagra and acrodermatitis enteropathica

- Diagnosis
  - There is no specific set of criteria
  - NME is often recognized late in the disease course in the context of glucagonoma
  - Suspect NME in the context of characteristic mucocutaneous rash and glucose intolerance (75–95% of patients are diabetic) or intestinal malabsorption, cirrhosis, or suspected malignancy
  - Serum glucagon levels can be markedly elevated in cases of glucagonoma (>500 pg/mL), and a level over 1000 pg/mL is virtually diagnostic of glucagonoma

VITAMIN ALTERATIONS

(**Fat- Soluble Vitamins (A, D, E, K):** easily accumulate to toxic levels with prolonged, excessive supplementation

Vitamin A (Retinol) Deficiency (Fig. 20-3)

- Major functions: vision, tissue differentiation, cellular membrane stability, resistance to infection
- Found in colostrum, milk, animal fats and liver, vegetables
- Etiology
  - Weaned infants
  - Chronic intestinal disturbances, that is, fat malabsorption: Crohn disease, celiac disease, cystic fibrosis, cholestatic liver disease

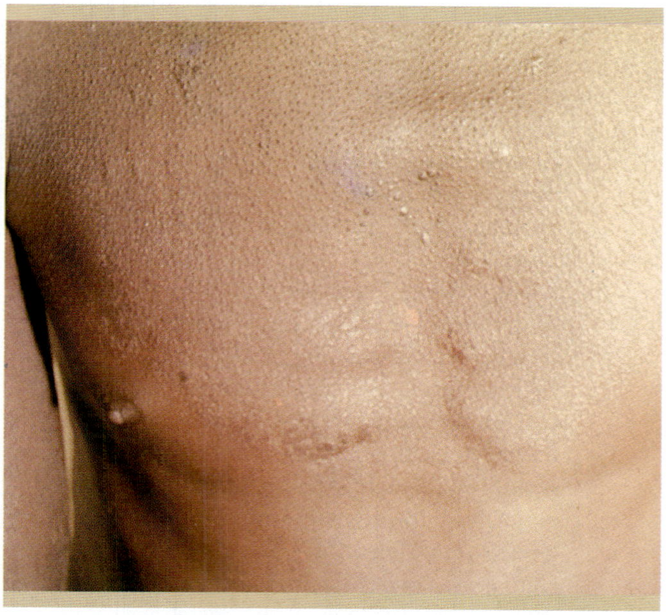

FIGURE 20-3 Vitamin A deficiency. (*Reprinted with permission from Goldsmith LA et al.* Fitzpatrick's Dermatology in General Medicine, *8th Ed. New York: McGraw-Hill; 2012, p. 1505.*)

- Clinical manifestations
  - Cutaneous findings
    - Phrynoderma ("toad skin"): follicular hyperkeratosis of extensor surfaces of the limbs, trunk, and buttocks
    - Generalized xerosis with exfoliation
    - Vaginal epithelium may become like the skin
  - Ocular findings
    - Nocturnal blindness (nyctalopia)
    - Xerophthalmia
    - Bitot spots (xerotic silver-gray plaques in the bulbar conjunctiva)
    - Keratomalacia
  - Others: growth failure, mental retardation, increased susceptibility to measles, epithelial metaplasia of the urinary tract leading to pyuria and hematuria
- Histology
  - Epithelial proliferation of basal cells and hyperkeratosis
  - Phrynoderma: follicular hyperkeratosis with keratin plugging
  - Sebaceous gland atrophy
- Diagnosis
  - Serum vitamin A level
  - Examination of ocular lesions and vaginal epithelium
- Treatment
  - Dosing based on severity of ophthalmic involvement
  - 100,000 to 300,000 IU oral vitamin A daily until resolution of symptoms and normalization of serum level
- Other pharmacologic uses of vitamin A
  - Acne/rosacea: topical tretinoin, tazarotene, and adapalene creams/gels function by decreasing keratinization; oral isotretinoin at 0.5 to 2.0 mg/kg/d blocks sebaceous gland activity and *Propinobacterium acnes* proliferation, alters keratinization, and decreases inflammation
  - Psoriasis: hyperkeratosis diminished by acitretin at 25 to 50 mg/d, with maintenance doses of 25 to 50 mg/d
  - Photoaging: sustained daily use of tretinoin cream 0.05% reduces photodamage
  - Measles prophylaxis: 200,000 IU daily for 2 days

Hypervitaminosis A

- Acute toxicity in infants ingesting more than 100,000 mcg of vitamin A or adults consuming polar bear or bearded seal liver
- Chronic supplementation greater than 25,000 IU daily for weeks or a month
- Clinical manifestations
  - Acute manifestations
    - Increased intracranial pressure: diplopia, papillary edema, paralysis of cranial nerves
    - Marked cutaneous desquamation
  - Chronic manifestations
    - Systemic: lethargy, anorexia, weight loss

  - Cutaneous: xerosis, associated with pruritus and desquamation
  - Hair: dryness, alopecia
  - Mucosal: cheilitis, gingival discoloration
  - Skeletal: bone pain, fracture
- Carotenoderma
  - Results from excessive ingestions of carotenoids, resolves with diet change
  - Yellow-orange skin, most prominent in areas of high sebaceous gland density (nasolabial folds, forehead, axilla, groin) and thickest stratum corneum (palms and soles)

Vitamin D Deficiency

- Two significant forms: D_2 and D_3
  - Vitamin D_2 (calciferol) is found mainly in fish liver oils
  - Vitamin D_3 (cholecalciferol) is naturally present in the human skin in a provitamin form (5-dihydrotachylsterol) that is photochemically activated by ultraviolet light; 3 times more potent than D_2
- Calcitriol (1,25-dihydroxycholecalciferol) is the active metabolite
  - Promotes absorption of calcium and phosphorus from the intestine
  - Increases reabsorption of phosphate in the kidney
  - Acts on bone to release calcium and phosphate
- Etiology
  - Inadequate diet
  - Lack of sunlight and excessive use of sunscreens; dark-skinned individuals
  - Malabsorptive states, i.e., celiac disease, steatorrhea, cystic fibrosis
  - Use of phenytoins or phenobarbital, which interferes with metabolism
- Clinical manifestations
  - Cutaneous: rarely alopecia
  - Bone abnormalities: osteomalacia in adults, rickets in children
    - Rickets: initial thickening of wrists and ankles; then develop bowing of long bones, rachitic rosary along chest, skull thickening, hypotonia
- Emerging data that deficiency may increase risk for several cancers, including breast, colon, prostate
- Diagnosis: total serum/plasma 25-hydroxy vitamin D less than 20 ng/mL
- Treatment: 20,000 IU D_3 or 50,000 IU D_2 PO once/week × 8 weeks; reassess: if 25-hydroxy vitamin D still less than 30 ng/mL, continue another 8 weeks; add 1 g daily oral calcium if concomitantly deficient
  - In excess (>50,000 IU/d orally): nausea, vomiting, weakness, nephrolithiasis, hypercalcemia
  - No cutaneous manifestations of excess
- Other pharmacologic uses of vitamin D
  - Psoriasis: calcipotriene ointment, a vitamin D_3 analog, decreases the size and scaling of plaques without adversely affecting calcium metabolism

Vitamin E (Tocopherol) Deficiency

- Functions as antioxidant and mediator of cellular homeostasis
- Impedes vitamin K–dependent clotting (mechanism not understood)
- Deficiency rare as vitamin E adequately supplied by regular diet
- Food sources include wheat, vegetable oils, dry fruits, greens, and seeds
- Risk factors: fat malabsorption (cystic fibrosis, pancreatic insufficiency, biliary or hepatic disease) and restricted diet
- Clinical manifestations
  - No major mucocutaneous findings
  - Spinocerebellar ataxia
  - Myopathy
  - Retinitis pigmentosa, ophthalmoplegia, ptosis
- Diagnosis: serum ratio of α-tocopherol to lipid less than 0.8 mg/g and/or erythrocyte hemolysis greater than 10% in hydrogen peroxide
- Treatment: 600 IU PO twice daily
  - In excess, may cause petechiae and ecchymoses
- Other pharmacologic uses of vitamin E
  - Wound healing: role controversial; studies show no improvement in scar appearance with topical vitamin E; contact dermatitis common
  - Immune function: oral α-tocopherol acetate 800 mg/d boosts cell-mediated immunity; decreased incidence of infection and cancer in studies of elderly

Vitamin K Deficiency

- Plays a vital role in the production of coagulation proteins (vitamin K_1); also important for bone mineralization (vitamin K_2)
- Vitamin K_1 found in green leafy vegetables and meat; vitamin K_2 produced by bacteria in the gut
- At risk groups newborns in the first 2 weeks of life, fat malabsorptive states, broad spectrum antibiotics, liver disease, megadoses of vitamin A or E, medications (cholestyramine, colestipol, orlistat, vitamin K epoxide reductase inhibitors)
- Clinical manifestations: secondary to decrease in vitamin K–dependent clotting factors II, VII, IX, and X
  - Systemic: hemorrhagic disease of the newborn; hemorrhagic diathesis if severe hypoprothrombinemia
  - Cutaneous: ecchymosis and purpura
- Diagnosis
  - Elevated serum prothrombin time (PT) and activated partial thromboplastin time (aPTT); 50% reduction in plasma prothrombin
- Treatment: oral or intramuscular vitamin K_1: 2 mg for children, 5 to 10 mg for adults; risk of anaphylaxis with intravenous form
  - Infants: 0.5 to 1 mg sc or IM given routinely at birth

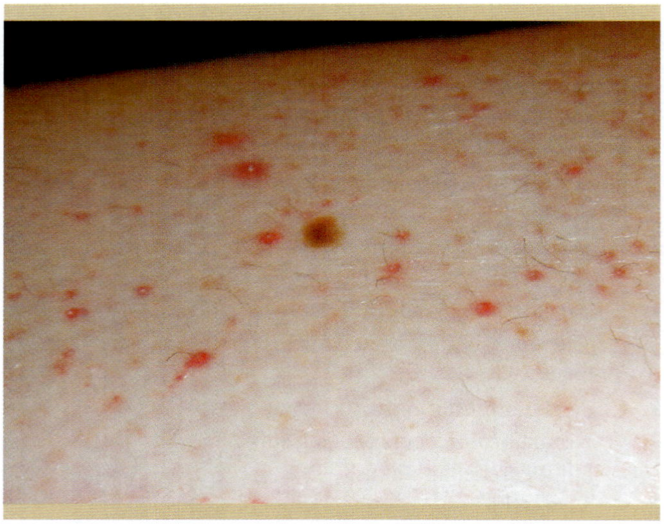

FIGURE 20-4 Vitamin C (ascorbic acid) deficiency. (*Reprinted with permission from Goldsmith LA et al.* Fitzpatrick's Dermatology in General Medicine, *8th Ed. New York: McGraw-Hill; 2012, p. 1516.*)

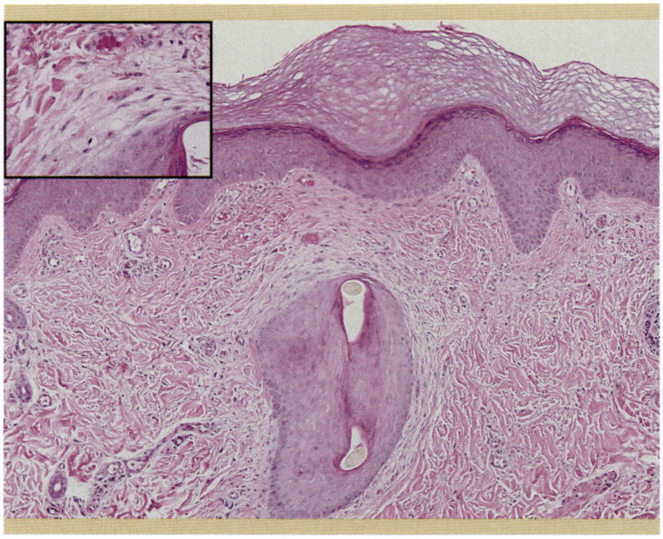

FIGURE 20-5 Vitamin C deficiency characteristically has follicular hyperkeratosis with classic coiled hairs and dermal erythrocyte extravasation. (*Used with permission from Jack Longley, MD, University of Wisconsin.*)

- Acute crisis: fresh frozen plasma
- No systemic or cutaneous signs of excess; may have injection site reaction

Water-Soluble Vitamins (Vitamin C and B-Vitamins): less likely to cause toxicity, but may have adverse side effects in high doses

Vitamin C (Ascorbic Acid) Deficiency (Figs. 20-4 and 20-5)

- Deficiency in vitamin C causes scurvy
- Major functions
  - Antioxidant protection of DNA and the eyes
  - Cellular secretion of procollagen (cofactor for prolyl hydroxylase)
  - Fatty acid metabolism
  - Iron absorption
- Etiology
  - Ascorbic acid is absorbed in the intestine by active transport.
  - Areas with poor access to fresh fruit and children age 6 to 24 months are susceptible
  - Primary deficiency: elderly, alcoholics, people on restrictive diets, and sailors
- Clinical manifestations
  - Symptoms develop 1 to 3 months after severe or total vitamin C deficiency
  - Children present with vague insidious symptoms of irritability, tachypnea, digestive alterations, anorexia
  - The 4 "Hs" of scurvy
    - *Hemorrhagic signs:* perifollicular hemorrhage (characteristically in adults), hemorrhagic gingivitis (typically above the upper incisors), epistaxis, half-moon hemorrhages along the distal nail bed, hemarthroses, subperiosteal hemorrhage (felt in the distal femur on physical examination), hematuria, melena, ocular or subdural hemorrhage
    - *Hyperkeratosis of hair follicles*: corkscrew hairs (transversely flat and curled)
    - *Hypochondriasis: cortical thinni*ng, which is sometimes desc*ribed as a "penc*il-point cortex," scorbutic rosary (resulting from abnormalities at the costochondral junction), associated pain resulting in pseudoparalysis and a typical "frog-like position"
    - *Hematologic abnormalities:* anemia due to impaired iron absorption
  - Other findings: Sjögren syndrome, malaise, lethargy, bone pain, myalgia, delayed wound healing, depression, and facial acne preceding changes in body hair
- Histology
  - Follicular hyperkeratosis and perifollicular erythrocyte extravasation
  - Classic coiled hairs in dilated follicles
- Diagnosis: based on the clinical picture, radiologic findings and patient history; laboratory tests typically unsatisfactory
  - Differential diagnosis
    - Rheumatic fever: rare in children younger than 2 years
    - Syphilis: presents with pseudoparalysis at earlier age than scurvy-related type and usually is associated with other specific signs

- Treatment
  - Acute cases may resolve with daily administration of 90 to 120 mL citrus fruit; ideal treatment is ascorbic acid dose of 100 to 120 mg or more daily
  - Prophylaxis: formula-fed infants: 35 mg of ascorbic acid daily; breast-feeding mothers: 100 mg/d; adults and children: 45 to 60 mg/d.
  - In excess of 2,000 mg/d, osmotic diarrhea and nephrolithiasis may result
    - No mucocutaneous manifestations of excess
- Other pharmacologic uses of vitamin C
  - Photoaging: in studies, 10% solution L-ascorbic acid applied topically decreased UVA-induced skin damage
  - Wound healing: role is controversial; studies show no benefit of supplemental vitamin C in healthy subjects, though subjects with existing deficiency may benefit

Vitamin B_1 (Thiamine) Deficiency

- Deficiency known as beri beri
- Found in yeast, cereals, liver, meat, eggs, and vegetables
- Thiamine pyrophosphate functions as a coenzyme in glucose and amino acid metabolism, synthesis of neurotransmitters
- Primary deficiency: seen in strict polished rice diet ("tea and toast" diet)
- Secondary deficiency: much more common
  - Alcohol-related liver disease
  - Increased depletion: hyperthyroidism, pregnancy, lactation, diarrhea, dialysis, diuretic use
- Clinical manifestations
  - Systemic: anorexia, weakness, constipation
  - Cutaneous: glossitis, edema
  - Neurologic
    - Peripheral neuropathy: "dry" beri beri
    - Mental confusion and confabulation-Korsakoff syndrome
    - Gait ataxia: Wernicke encephalopathy
  - Cardiovascular: congestive heart failure, cardiomegaly, edema—"wet" beri beri
- Diagnosis: response to thiamine replacement, whole blood or erythrocyte transketolase activity may be obtained
- Treatment: administer with meals—200 mg/d for cardiovascular involvement; 100 mg/d in peripheral neuropathy; 150 mg/d in alcoholism

Vitamin B_2 (Riboflavin) Deficiency

- Function: cofactor for flavin adenine dinucleotide (FAD)-dependent metabolism
- Rarely seen as an isolated deficiency; associated with other nutritional deficiencies
- Found in milk, cheese, liver, meat, fish, bread, eggs, and cereals
- Deficiency may be due to decreased intake, increased transit, or decreased uptake
  - Decreased intake: anorexia nervosa
  - Increased transit: infectious colitis, enteritis, lactose intolerance
  - Decreased uptake: celiac disease, bowel resection, G6PD deficiency, tropical sprue
- Clinical manifestations
  - Oro-oculo-genital syndrome (not specific to riboflavin deficiency)
    - Oral changes: angular stomatitis, atrophic glossitis
    - Ocular changes: blepharoconjunctivitis
    - Genital dermatoses: often present earliest; patchy scaling erythema or fine powdery desquamation progressing to lichenification in scrotum of men or vulva of women
  - Cutaneous: seborrheic-like scaling of nasolabial folds, ears, eyelids, mouth
  - Others: anemia, neurologic disfunction, photophobia, lacrimation, conjunctivitis
- Diagnosis: erythrocyte glutathione reductase level
- Treatment: no consensus, therapeutic doses start at 25 mg/d to prevent cataracts, mixed formulations of riboflavin contain 50 mg or 100 mg, treat daily until resolution

Vitamin B_3 (Niacin/Nicotinic Acid) Deficiency

- Deficiency known as pellagra
- Derivative of tryptophan, obtained from diet or synthesized *de novo*
  - Deficiency may either be from a niacin or tryptophan deficiency
  - Functions as coenzyme in the form of nicotinamide adenine dinucleotide (NAD) and NAD phosphate, which participate in a variety of redox reactions
- Found in animal proteins, bran, peanuts, legumes, seeds
- Risk factors
  - Primary (inadequate intake): poor B_3 or protein intake, unprocessed maize, restrictive diets
  - Secondary (inadequate absorption or conversion)
    - Crohn disease, GI surgery, intestinal parasites, chronic alcoholism
    - Medications: 6-mercaptopurine, sulfapyridine, 5-fluorouracil, phenobarbitol, ethionamide, pyrazinamide, hydantoins, isoniazid therapy (causes deficiency of pyridoxine, which is required for conversion of tryptophan to niacin)
    - Carcinoid syndrome: tryptophan diverted to serotonin
    - Hartnup disease (autosomal recessive): inborn error of tryptophan metabolism; decreased uptake and increased excretion of tryptophan
    - HIV
- Clinical manifestations
  - Pellagra: "Three Ds"—dermatitis, dementia, diarrhea
    - Four types of dermatitis
      - ▲ Photosensitivity: symmetric scaling dermatitis of sun-exposed face, dorsum of arms, and

chest; involvement of posterior neck and V of chest (Casal necklace)
    - ▲ Seborrheic-like dermatitis on the face
    - ▲ Perineal lesions
    - ▲ Thickening and pigmentation over bony prominences
  - Neurologic
    - ▲ Dementia
    - ▲ Peripheral neuropathy and dysesthesias secondary to patchy demyelinization
  - Gastrointestinal (GI) tract
    - ▲ Acute inflammation of small intestine and colon
    - ▲ Atrophic glossitis and cheilitis
- Histology closely matches that seen in NME and acrodermatitis enteropathica
- Diagnosis
  - Made in part by response to niacin supplementation
  - Urinary *N*-methylnicotinamide and 2-pyridone best measure niacin status
- Treatment: nicotinamide 100 mg PO q6h for several days or until resolution of major acute symptoms, followed by 50 mg PO q8-12h until all skin lesions heal
  - Excessive supplementation: flushing, xerosis, pruritus, acanthosis nigricans

Pyridoxine (Vitamin B_6) Deficiency

- Cofactor in the form of pyridoxine pyrophosphate, cofactor for synthesis of thiamine from serotonin
- Needed for amino acid metabolism, synthesis of niacin, prostaglandins, and neurotransmitters
- Isolated deficiency is rare, occurs with other vitamin deficiencies
- Found in vegetables, green leafy vegetables, beans, nuts, bananas, and cereals
- Primary deficiency: alcoholics, limited diets (TPN, elderly)
- Secondary
  - Medications: cycloserine, hydralazine, isoniazid, D-penicillamine, pyrazinamide
  - Uremia, cirrhosis, inflammatory bowel disease
- Clinical manifestations
  - Systemic: may cause all findings seen in niacin deficiency because pyridoxine is a cofactor for niacin production; see pellagra under section Vitamin B_3 (Niacin/Nicotinic Acid) Deficiency for more details
  - Cutaneous: nonspecific seborrheic dermatitis on face, neck, and perineum
  - Mucosal involvement: glossitis and angular stomatitis
  - Neurologic: peripheral neuropathy, seizures, depression, confusion
  - GI: anorexia, nausea, vomiting
  - Anemia
- Diagnosis: decreased serum levels of pyridoxine-5-phosphate
- Treatment: supplementation of pyridoxine 20 to 100 mg/d orally or 100 mg/d parenterally in adults
  - With prolonged daily use greater than 200 mg, photosensitivity, sensory neuropathy, and loss of proprioception may develop

Biotin (B_7) Deficiency

- Functions as a cofactor for carboxylases in carbon dioxide metabolism
- Found in liver, egg yolks; also produced by intestinal bacteria
- Deficiency occurs in shortened gut, parenteral nutrition, malabsorption syndromes (i.e., celiac disease), excessive consumption of uncooked egg white, alcoholism, and fatty acid oxidation diseases
- Prolonged use of anticonvulsants can reduce intestinal uptake, especially phenytoin, primidone, and carbamazepine
- Two rare inherited syndromes: both may be fatal if therapy not initiated early
  - Holocarboxylase synthetase deficiency (neonatal type)
  - Biotinidase deficiency (infantile type)
- Clinical manifestations
  - Cutaneous: scaling eczematoid and xerotic lesions on arms, legs, and feet; fragile nails, perioral and genital erosions, cheilosis, waxy pallor to face, alopecia
  - Neurologic findings: depression, lethargy, hallucinations, limb paresthesias
  - Others: conjunctivitis, muscle pain
- Diagnosis: urine organic acid analysis may be performed
- Treatment: for adults (acquired form), 60 mg/d; for inherited forms, 10 to 40 mg/d PO/IV/IM; adjust dose depending on severity of deficiency and response to therapy

Folic Acid (B9) Deficiency

- Tetrahydrofolate involved in single carbon transfers for amino acid, purine, and pyrimidine biosynthesis
- Found in liver, meat, milk, dried beans, and green leafy vegetables
- Supplementation in pregnancy advised to avoid neural tube defects
- Primary deficiency: poor nutrition (alcoholism, elderly, restricted diet), excessive milk boiling, goat's milk diet
- Secondary causes
  - Impaired absorption (celiac disease)
  - Increased requirement (pregnancy, etc)
  - Drugs: methotrexate, trimethoprim, oral contraceptives, pyrimethamine, phenobarbital, and phenytoin
  - Concomitant B_{12} deficiency
  - Destruction of folate by superoxide (by-product of alcohol metabolism)
- Clinical manifestations
  - Systemic: macrocytic, megaloblastic anemia with hypersegmented neutrophils

- Cutaneous: hyperpigmentation, most notable in sun-exposed areas
- Oral: glossitis, cheilitis

- Diagnosis: serum folate, must also rule out associated B_{12} deficiency
- Treatment: folic acid 1 to 5mg/d

Vitamin B_{12} (Cyanocobalamin) Deficiency

- Cofactor in tetrahydrofolate and methylmalonic acid (MMA) metabolism
  - Essential cofactor for pyrimidine biosynthesis (via tetrahydrofolate)
  - Neuropathy due to defect in MMA metabolism and production of myelin
- By-product of bacterial metabolism and found only in animal tissues (i.e., red meats, liver, eggs, etc.) but not greens or vegetables
- Ingested cyanocobalamin/hydroxycobalamin binds to intrinsic factor produced by gastric parietal cells and is absorbed in the terminal ileum
- Deficiency leads to pernicious anemia: usually related to poor absorption states
  - Achlorhydria: decreased IF from parietal cells (which also produce chloride)
  - Terminal ileum disease (Crohn, short bowel syndrome, bowel resection)
  - Contaminated fish: *Diphyllobothrium latum* tapeworm consumes dietary B_{12}
  - Pancreatic disorders
  - Celiac disease: blunt villi poorly absorb IF
- Deficiency develops slowly (ranges from 3–6 years) since body stores are large
- Clinical manifestations
  - Cutaneous: symmetric hyperpigmentation of sun-exposed and flexural areas, dark nails
  - Oral: glossitis ("beefy red tongue"), atrophy of filiform papillae
  - Neuropathy: demyelination of posterior columns (loss of proprioception and vibration sense), tingling/numbness in extremities, cognitive changes, and in extreme cases paralysis
  - Megaloblastic anemia
  - May occur with alopecia areata and vitiligo as autoimmune disease
- Diagnosis
  - Decreased serum B_{12} level
  - Test for pernicious anemia by measuring antibodies against IF
  - Schilling test: used to test for malabsorptive states
- Treatment: parenteral cyanocobalamin 1,000 mcg IM 2 times/week for 2 weeks, then 1,000 mcg/wk IM/SC for 5 weeks, then 100 to 1,000 mcg IM/SC once monthly

MINERAL ALTERATIONS

Zinc Deficiency (Fig. 20-6)

- One of most important minerals; essential to the normal function of all cells
- Enhances wound healing, may protect against UV damage
- Sources include breast milk, nuts, whole grains, green leafy vegetables, shellfish
- Two types: genetic or acquired
  - Genetic (autosomal recessive): acrodermatitis enteropathica (AE)
    - Defective intestinal zinc transporter SLC39A4 inhibits zinc absorption
    - Clinical signs occur 1 to 2 weeks after weaning from breast
  - Acquired
    - Alcoholics
    - Complication of malabsorption
    - Inflammatory bowel disease, jejunoileal bypass
- Clinical manifestations
  - Triad of diarrhea, depression, and dermatitis seen in only 20%
  - Systemic: failure to thrive, short stature, poor wound healing
  - Cutaneous: erosive (occasionally vesiculobullous) dermatitis with periorificial and acral distribution; frequent candida and staphylococci infections
  - Oral: cheilitis, stomatitis
  - Others: photophobia, conjunctivitis, alopecia
- Histology
  - Plaques have epidermal changes including confluent parakeratosis with dyskeratosis, psoriasiform hyperplasia, and hypogranulosis; vacuolar changes in the keratinocytes (paleness) in the upper epidermis

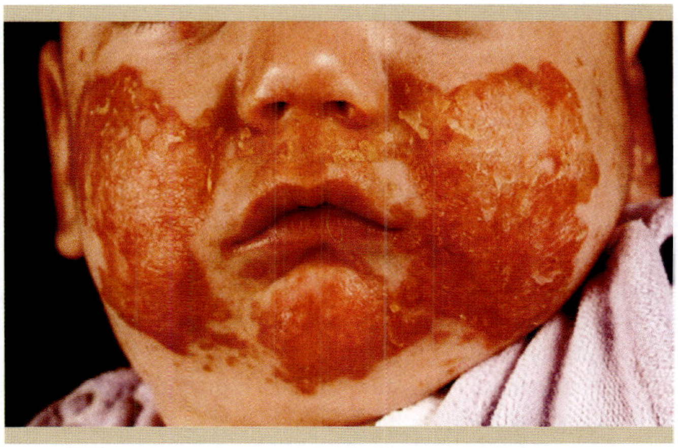

FIGURE 20-6 Acrodermatitis enteropathica. (*Reprinted with permission from Wolff, K et al.* Fitzpatrick's Color Atlas and Synopsis of Clinical Dermatology, *6th Ed. New York: McGraw-Hill; 2009.*)

- Superficial dermis can have tortuous, dilated capillaries
- Histopathology closely matches that seen in pellagra and NME
- Diagnosis: low plasma or hair levels of zinc, low serum alkaline phosphatase level
- Treatment
  - Zinc gluconate or sulfate: 3 mg/kg/day orally for AE; 1 to 3 mg/kg/d orally or 300 to 1000 μg/kg/d intravenously for acquired form
  - Warm compresses and petrolatum applied to areas of weeping or crusted dermatitis may enhance reepithelialization when used with zinc replacement

Iron Deficiency

- Function: heme and collagen synthesis; redox reactions, peroxidase, catalase, cytochromes
- Found in animal products as well as whole grains, legumes
- Chronic blood loss and poor intake are most common causes of iron deficiency
  - At-risk populations include menstruating females, people with GI bleeds, and infants on cow's milk formula
- Clinical manifestations
  - Cutaneous: generalized pruritus
  - Oral: atrophic glossitis, cheilitis
  - Hair: dry, fragile, split hair shaft; heterochromia; telogen effluvium
  - Nails: longitudinally ridged, brittle nails (early finally), with development of koilonychias (spoon-shaped deformity of the fingernails/toenails)
  - GI: anorexia, Plummer-Vinson syndrome (dysphagia from postcricoid esophageal webs), and splenomegaly with severe anemia
- Diagnosis: microcytic anemia with low serum iron, ferritin, and high transferrin
- Treatment: iron sulfate 325 mg 3 times a day

Iron Excess: Hemochromatosis

- Primary overload: hereditary hemochromatosis; mutation of HFE gene
- Secondary overload: acute toxicity after a single large dose of iron; or chronically owing to excessive accumulation of iron from diet, blood transfusions, or both
- Systemic: early symptoms include severe fatigue, impotence, arthralgia; later development of diabetes mellitus and cirrhosis
- Cutaneous: skin bronzing, ichthyosis-like changes
- Diagnosis
  - Fixed transferrin saturation elevation without other causes of iron overload
  - Serum ferritin greater than 200 μg/L in premenopausal women and 300 μg/lL in men and postmenopausal women indicates primary iron overload
  - Genetic testing for 2HFE gene mutations C282Y and H63D
- Treatment
  - Weekly therapeutic phlebotomy of 500-mL whole blood (equivalent to approximately 200- to 250-mg iron)
  - Deferoxamine mesylate (Desferal) drug of choice used in primary and secondary iron overload syndromes

Copper Deficiency

- Cofactor for the metalloenzymes, tyrosinase (melanin production), and lysyl oxidase (collagen cross-linking)
- Also involved in iron transport, free radical detoxification, and redox reactions
- Copper is bound to ceruloplasmin in bloodstream
- Found in fish, oysters, grains, liver, eggs
- Deficiency is rare, associated with other nutritional deficiencies
- Nutritional causes: malnutrition, malabsorption (celiac disease, cystic fibrosis, short bowel syndrome), unsupplemented parenteral nutrition, excessive intake of antacids, zinc, or iron (displaces copper from transporters), strictly cow's milk diet
  - Clinical manifestations
    - Cutaneous: skin and hair hypopigmentation
    - Skeletal: osteoporosis, fractures, flaring of anterior ribs
    - Neurologic: symmetric sensory loss and motor weakness of upper and lower extremities; optic motor defect and vision loss if untreated
    - Microcytic anemia, neutropenia, decreased ceruloplasmin
  - Diagnosis: neutropenia is earliest and most common indicator of deficiency
  - Treatment: copper supplementation to prevent progression, neurologic recovery is not guaranteed
- Genetic: Menkes disease (X-linked recessive); "kinky hair disease"
  - Defect in *MNK* (also called *ATP7A*) gene, a copper transporting P-type ATPase found in all tissues except liver
  - Symptoms manifest at 2 to 3 months of age: triad of neurologic degeneration, characteristic hair, and failure to thrive
    - Cutaneous: pale skin, soft, inelastic, hypopigmented skin at nape of neck, axilla, and trunk, follicular hyperkeratosis
    - "Cherubic" appearance with depressed nasal bridge, ptosis, decreased facial movement
    - Loss of developmental milestones by 2 to 3 months
    - Hair: pili torti (180-degree twists of hair), segmental shaft narrowing (monilethrix), periodic beading of hair shaft (trichorrhexis nodosa)
    - Lethargy, hypotonia, hypothermia, seizures, mental retardation, osseus alteration, anemia
  - Biochemical phenotype: (1) impaired copper absorption leads to low levels of copper in plasma, liver,

and brain, (2) reduced function of copper-dependent metalloproteases, and (3) paradoxical accumulation of copper in other tissues (i.e., duodenum, kidney, spleen, pancreas, skeletal muscle, placenta)
  - Diagnosis: clinical features, low copper and ceruloplasmin, decreased copper in cultured fibroblasts
  - Treatment with copper; histidine treatment early in disease has shown some success

Selenium Deficiency

- Vital enzyme component of thyroid hormone metabolism and glutathione peroxidase
- Sources include seafood, chicken, egg yolks, grains
- Deficiency most common in geographic areas with low soil selenium content, that is, Keshan disease in parts of China (fatal cardiomyopathy with associated pseudoalbinism, correctable with selenium supplementation)
- Deficiency with malabsorption, protein-restricted diets, and unsupplemented TPN
- Clinical manifestations
  - Cutaneous manifestations: hair/skin hypopigmentation, xerosis, leukonychia
- Diagnosis: low plasma selenium and decreased glutathione peroxidase activity
- Treatment: 100 to 200 μg/d until resolution of symptoms
  - Toxicity: oral supplementation greater than 200 μg/d or selenium sulfide shampoo use on large areas of eroded/ulcerated skin
    - Findings: dermatitis, alopecia, abnormal nails, and garlic odor breath

QUIZ

Questions

1. All of the following are skin findings associated with obesity EXCEPT:

   A. Acrochordons
   B. Acanthosis nigricans
   C. Keratosis pilaris
   D. Seborrheic dermatitis
   E. Plantar hyperkeratosis

2. A thin adolescent female presenting with xerosis, pruritus, hair thinning, and parotid gland enlargement should be treated with which of the following:

   A. Cognitive behavioral therapy
   B. Selective serotonin reuptake inhibitors
   C. Biotin
   D. A and B
   E. All of the above

3. Which of the following is an essential fatty acid:

   A. Oleic acid
   B. Palmitic acid
   C. Linoleic acid
   D. Ergosterol
   E. Cholesterol

4. Beri beri is due to a deficiency in which of the following vitamins?

   A. Vitamin A
   B. Vitamin B_1
   C. Vitamin E
   D. Vitamin C
   E. Vitamin B_2

5. Deficiency of the vitamin that functions as a cofactor for flavin adenine dinucleotide (FAD)-dependent energy metabolism may lead to which of the following conditions?

   A. Scurvy
   B. Carcinoid syndrome
   C. Pellagra
   D. Oro-oculo-genital syndrome
   E. Rickets

6. Vitamin B_{12} can be obtained from which food source?

   A. Carrots
   B. Spinach
   C. White rice
   D. Chicken breast
   E. Corn

7. An infant fed exclusively goat's milk may develop which of the following findings:

   A. Macrocytic, megaloblastic anemia with hypersegmented neutrophils
   B. Hyperpigmentation in sun-exposed areas
   C. Glossitis
   D. Cheilitis
   E. All of the above

8. Hyperkeratosis of hair follicles, hypochondriasis, and delayed wound healing is indicative of:

   A. Vitamin A toxicity
   B. Vitamin C deficiency
   C. Vitamin B_1 deficiency
   D. Vitamin B_6 deficiency
   E. Folic acid deficiency

9. Cherubic facies, kinky hair, neurologic degeneration, and failure to thrive may be associated with a deficiency of which of the following:

   A. Copper
   B. Iron
   C. Selenium
   D. Vitamin A
   E. Vitamin D

10. Which of the following is the appropriate treatment for acrodermatitis enteropathica?

    A. Iron sulfate
    B. Copper histidine
    C. Zinc gluconate
    D. Deferoxamine mesylate
    E. Pyridoxine

Answers

1. D. Seborrheic dermatitis is not associated with obesity. Acanthosis nigricans and acrochordons are indicators of development of Type 2 diabetes mellitus, and their incidence increases with the severity of obesity. Keratosis pilaris can be seen in up to 21% of obese patients. Plantar hyperkeratosis occurs in response to increased foot girth and weight bearing.
2. D. Cognitive behavioral therapy and SSRIs are mainstays of the treatment of anorexia nervosa and bulimia, as these eating disorders are related to an underlying psychiatric disturbance. In severe cases, it may be necessary to hospitalize the patient and administer parenteral nutrition.
3. C. Linoleic acid is an essential fatty acid, which provides cellular integrity along with energy storage. Essential fatty acids must be obtained from one's diet as the body is unable to synthesize them.
4. B. Vitamin B_1 (thiamine) deficiency causes beri beri. Findings may include congestive heart failure, cardiomegaly, and edema ("wet" beri beri) or peripheral neuropathy ("dry" beri beri).
5. D. Oro-oculo-genital syndrome is associated with a deficiency of riboflavin, a cofactor for FAD-dependent metabolism. This condition is characterized by angular stomatitis, atrophic glossitis, blepharoconjunctivitis, and genital erythema, desquamation, and lichenification.
6. D. Vitamin B_{12} (cyanocobalamin) is a by-product of bacterial metabolism and is only found in animal tissues.
7. E. The infant is suffering from folate deficiency because goat's milk lacks this micronutrient. Folate deficiency is associated with macrocytic, megaloblastic anemia with hypersegmented neutrophils, hyperpigmentation of sun exposed areas, glossitis, and cheilitis.
8. B. Vitamin C (ascorbic acid) functions as an antioxidant and component of collagen synthesis (cofactor for prolyl hydroxylase). Deficiency in vitamin C causes scurvy. The 4 "Hs" of scurvy include hemorrhagic signs, hyperkeratosis of hair follicles, hypochondriasis, and hematologic abnormalities.
9. A. A genetic defect in copper transport, Menkes disease manifests at 2 to 3 months of age as a triad of neurologic degeneration, kinky hair, and failure to thrive. Patients have a cherubic appearance with depressed nasal bridge, ptosis, and decreased facial movement.
10. C. Zinc gluconate is the treatment for acrodermatitis enteropathica, an autosomal recessive defect in intestinal zinc transporters. It presents in infants 1 to 2 weeks after weaning from breast milk with diarrhea, erosive dermatitis with a periorificial and acral distribution, stomatitis, failure to thrive, and poor wound healing.

REFERENCES

Bleasel NR, Stapleton KM, Lee MS, Sullivan J: Vitamin A deficiency phrynoderma: Due to malabsorption and inadequate diet. *J Am Acad Dermatol* 1999;41(2):322–324.

Bolognia JL et al. *Dermatology*, 3rd Ed. New York: Mosby; 2012.

Eledrisi MS: Vitamin A Toxicity. Emedicine (accessed May 26, 2008) OMIM (accessed May 26, 2008).

Goldsmith LA et al. *Fitzpatrick's Dermatology in General Medicine*, 8th Ed. New York: McGraw-hill; 2012.

Gonzalez JR, Botet MV, Sanchez JL: The histopathology of acrodermatitis enteropathica. *Am J Dermatopath* 1982;4(4):303–311.

Hegyi J, Schwartz RA, Hegyi V: Pellagra: dermatitis, dementia, and diarrhea. *Int J Dermatol* 2004;43(1):1–5.

Highton, A, Quell, J. Calcipotriene ointment 0.005% for psoriasis: A safety and efficacy study. *J Am Acad Dermatol* 1995;32:67–72.

Hirschmann JV, Raugi GJ: Adult scurvy. *J Am Acad Dermatol* 1999;41(6):895–906; quiz 907–910. Review.

Jiang WG, Eynard AR, Mansel RE: The pathology of essential fatty acid deficiency: is it cell adhesion mediated? *Med Hypoth* 2000;55(3):257–262.

Keller, KL, Fenske, NA: Uses of vitamins A, C, E and related compounds in dermatology: a review. *J Am Acad Dermatol* 1998; 39(4):611–625.

MacDonald A, Forsyth A: Nutritional deficiencies and the skin. *Clin Exp Dermatol* 2005;30(4):388–390.

McKee PH: *Pathology of the Skin: With Clinical Correlations*. London: Mosby-Wolfe; 1996.

Montgomery H: Nutritional and vitamin deficiency. In: *Dermatopathology*, Vol. 1. New York: Harper and Row; 1967.

Mullans E, Cohen R: Iatrogenic NME: a case report and review of nonglucagonoma-associated NME. *J Am Acad Dermatol* 1998;38:866–873.

Perafan-Riveros C, Franca LF, Alves AC, Sanches JA Jr: Acrodermatitis enteropathica: case report and review of the literature. *Pediatr Dermatol* 2002;19(5):426–431. Review.

Price NM: Vitamin C deficiency. *Cutis* 1980;26(4):375–377.

Pujol RM, Wang CY, el-Azhary RA, Su WP, Gibson LE, Schroeter AL: Necrolytic migratory erythema: clinicopathologic study of 13 cases. *Int J Dermatol* 2004;43(1):12.

Rangam CM, Bhagwat AG, Gupta JC: Cutaneous lesions in kwashiorkor. A histopathological and histochemical study. *Ind J Med Res* 1962;50(2):184–190.

Sfeir HE: Hemochromatosis. Emedicine (accessed May 26, 2008).

Sheehy TW: *Vitamin Deficiency and Toxicity*. Garden Grove, CA: Medcom, Inc.; 1985.

Tang V: Vitamin D and related disorders. Emedicine (accessed May 26, 2008).

Tierney EP, Badger J: Etiology and pathogenesis of necrolytic migratory erythema: review of the literature. *MedGenMed* 2004;6(3):4 (online publication, September 10, 2004).

Walker WA, Watkins JB, Duggan C: *Nutrition in Pediatrics*, 3rd Ed. Hamilton, London: BC Decker Inc.; 2003.

Wermers RA, Fatourechi V, Wynne AG, Kvols LK, Lloyd RV: The glucagonoma syndrome. Clinical and pathologic features in 21 patients. *Medicine* 1996;75(2):53.

CHAPTER 21

CUTANEOUS FINDINGS RELATED TO PREGNANCY

RONALD P. RAPINI

COMMON SKIN CHANGES RELATED TO PREGNANCY

- Hyperpigmentation of nipples, external genitalia
- Linea nigra: midline pigmentary demarcation line on abdomen
- Melasma: ill-defined pigmentation of cheeks, forehead
- Striae: start reddish, become whitish, redness may be improved faster by pulsed dye laser, but otherwise that and other treatments unproven to have long-term benefit
- Vascular lesions: varicosities, pyogenic granuloma
- Increased or changing nevi, melanoma: unclear if truly increased over controls
- Telogen effluvium typically starts 3 months after delivery

PRURITUS GRAVIDARUM

- This is itching without rash (up to 14% of all pregnancies)
- Potential intrahepatic cholestasis of pregnancy should be investigated in these patients, but this occurs in only 1 to 2% of all pregnancies, clinical jaundice in only 0.02% of pregnancies
- Elevated liver function tests and serum bile acid levels may occur
- Elevated glutathione S-transferase alpha (GSTA), a specific marker of hepatocellular integrity, identifies women with intrahepatic cholestasis and distinguishes them from those with benign pruritus gravidarum
- Reported increases in rates of premature delivery and perinatal mortality appear to be restricted to those in whom frank clinical jaundice develops
- Recurs in 50% of pregnancies
- Treatment: phenobarbital, cholestyramine, (ursodeoxycholic acid controversial but advocated by some)

PRURITIC URTICARIAL PAPULES AND PLAQUES OF PREGNANCY (PUPPP), POLYMORPHOUS ERUPTION OF PREGNANCY (PEP) (FIG. 21-1)

- The term PUPPP seems to be preferred in the United States and PEP in Europe
- Polymorphous eruption with papules, plaques, urticarial lesions
- The most common of the pregnancy rashes (0.6% of all pregnancies)
- Onset in abdominal striae is common, then commonly spreads to abdomen, buttocks, thighs
- Spongiosis may occur and cause confusion with pemphigoid gestationis, then immunofluorescence biopsy may be needed, since pemphigoid gestationis possibly may cause increased fetal morbidity or mortality, unlike PUPPP
- Intensely pruritic, like most of these pregnancy rashes
- Primagravids mostly, does not recur with subsequent pregnancies
- Increased incidence of twins, rapid maternal weight gain
- Usually third trimester
- Biopsy not very specific: perivascular lymphocytes with eosinophils, edema, sometimes with spongiosis or parakeratosis

PEMPHIGOID GESTATIONIS (HERPES GESTATIONIS) (FIG. 21-2)

- The term pemphigoid gestationis is preferred by many because "herpes gestationis" causes confusion with herpes virus infection and its implications
- Onset second or third trimester
- Papules, urticarial plaques, vesicles, bullae

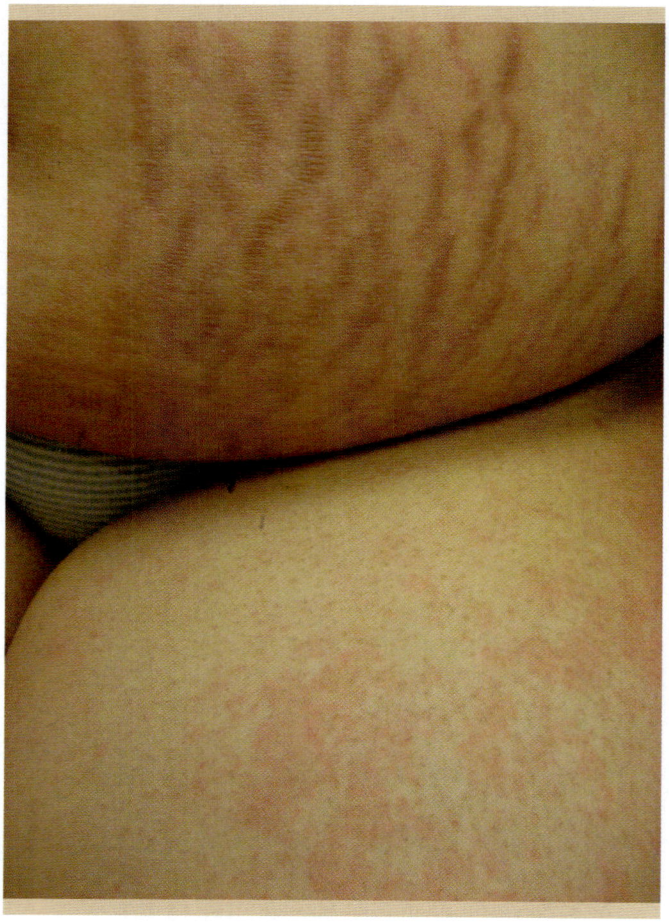

FIGURE 21-1 Pruritic urticarial papules and plaques of pregnancy (PUPPP). Note accentuation of rash in striae. (*Used with permission from Dr. Ronald Rapini.*)

- Often develops around umbilicus and extremities, later spreading to trunk, palms, and soles. Usually spares face and mucous membranes
- Autoimmune disease similar to bullous pemphigoid (but linear C3 more often seen at dermal-epidermal junction zone than IgG). In both diseases the linear band is found in the epidermal side (roof) of the subepidermal blister
- Increased HLA-DR3, DR4, B8
- Circulating IgG4 autoantibodies in the blood are called herpes gestationis factor, avidly fixes complement to basement membrane zone of epidermis, and can cross the placenta causing disease in newborns
- Target antigen is most often the NC16a domain of 180kDa protein associated with basal keratinocyte hemidesmosomes (collagen XVII, formerly called bullous pemphigoid antigen 2). Bullous pemphigoid patients may have the same target antigen, but almost always have a second target: dystonin (DST), a 230 kDa protein formerly designated BP antigen 1. The latter antigen is less commonly found in pemphigoid gestationis

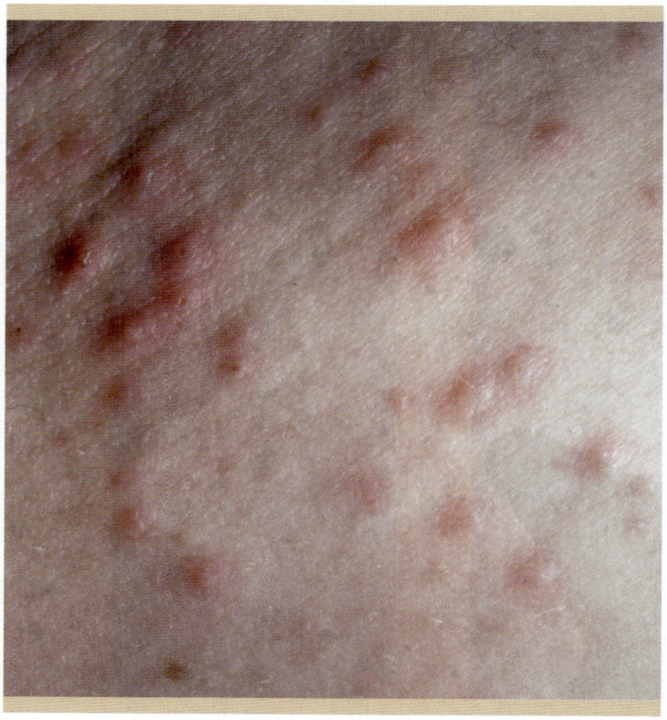

FIGURE 21-2 Pemphigoid gestationis. Papules and vesicles in this case. (*Used with permission from Dr. Ronald Rapini.*)

- Maternal health not affected, but there may be increased fetal morbidity, small infant size. Less than 5% of infants have skin lesions, these spontaneously resolve

ATOPIC ERUPTION OF PREGNANCY (PRURIGO GESTATIONIS)

- Often atopic diathesis
- Excoriated papules predominant
- Onset usually in second or third trimester
- No adverse maternal or fetal effects
- A variant known as papular dermatitis of Spangler is probably not a real entity: marked elevation of 24-hour urinary human gonadotropin (hCG) and decreased plasma estriol and cortisol was supposedly associated with fetal complications

PUSTULAR PSORIASIS OF PREGNANCY (IMPETIGO HERPETIFORMIS) (FIG. 21-3)

- Often no previous history of psoriasis
- Rarest of the pregnancy rashes mentioned here
- Papules, scaly plaques, pustules coalescing into lakes of pus

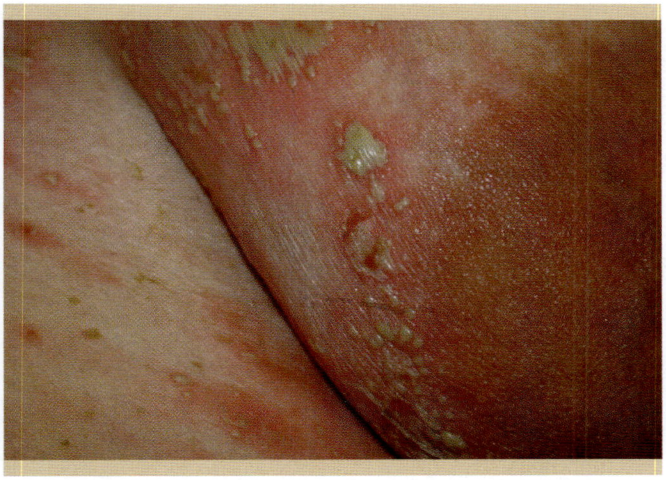

FIGURE 21-3 Impetigo herpetiformis. Pustules are predominant. (*Used with permission from Dr. Asra Ali.*)

- Favors thighs, groin, trunk, extremities. Spares face, hands, feet
- Constitutional signs: fever, chills, nausea, vomiting, diarrhea, fatigue
- Leukocytosis, secondary hypoalbuminemia, hypocalcemia, tetany
- Often recurs in subsequent pregnancies, menses, oral contraceptives
- Increased morbidity of fetus possibly from placental insufficiency

DISTINGUISHING POINTS

- All rashes are most common in third trimester, but pemphigoid gestationis may occur in the second or third, and impetigo herpetiformis may occur in any trimester
- Pemphigoid gestationis is the only one with immunofluorescence findings
- Pemphigoid gestationis is the most likely one to recur in subsequent pregnancies
- The 3 supposed increased fetal morbidity–mortality are pemphigoid gestationis, pruritus gravidarum (if cholestasis), and impetigo herpetiformis
- Most of these rashes, regardless of type, tend to resolve after delivery of the baby.
- All are treated with antihistamines (diphenhydramine is the most popular since it is FDA pregnancy class B). Cetirizine, cyproheptadine, and loratadine are also class B. Topical corticosteroids are often used but are class C. Prednisone is reserved for more serious cases, class B later in pregnancy

QUIZ

Questions

1. Match the condition with an important common finding:

a. Pemphigoid gestationis	A. Elevated GSTA
b. Pruritus gravidarum	B. Collagen XVII antibodies
c. PUPPP	C. Leukocytosis
d. Prurigo gestationis	D. Accentuation in striae
e. Impetigo herpetiformis	E. Associated with atopy

2. The rarest of the following conditions is:

   A. Pemphigoid gestationis
   B. Impetigo herpetiformis
   C. PUPPP
   D. Prurigo gestationis
   E. Atopic eruption of pregnancy

3. Tetany is most likely to be a feature of:

   A. Pemphigoid gestationis
   B. Impetigo herpetiformis
   C. Papular dermatitis of pregnancy
   D. Pruritus gravidarum
   E. Pruritic urticarial papules and plaques of pregnancy

4. Which of the following most characteristically develops around the umbilicus?

   A. Pemphigoid gestationis
   B. Impetigo herpetiformis
   C. Papular dermatitis of pregnancy
   D. Pruritus gravidarum
   E. Pruritic urticarial papules and plaques of pregnancy

5. Phenobarbital and cholestyramine are most commonly used to treat which condition?

   A. Pemphigoid gestationis
   B. Impetigo herpetiformis
   C. Atopic eruption of pregnancy
   D. Pruritus gravidarum
   E. Pruritic urticarial papules and plaques of pregnancy

6. Direct immunofluorescence is most likely to demonstrate which protein in a linear band at the dermal-epidermal junction zone in pemphigoid gestationis?

   A. IgG
   B. IgM
   C. IgA
   D. IgE
   E. C3

7. Regarding pregnancy skin findings, which problem typically starts about 3 months after delivery?

   A. Melasma
   B. Anagen effluvium
   C. Telogen effluvium
   D. Hyperpigmentation
   E. Telangiectasia

8. The rash most likely to recur in subsequent pregnancies is:

   A. Pruritus gravidarum
   B. Impetigo herpetiformis
   C. Atopic eruption of pregnancy
   D. Pemphigoid gestationis
   E. Pruritic urticarial papules and plaques of pregnancy

9. Linea nigra typically occurs on the:

   A. Nose
   B. Arms
   C. Legs
   D. Eyes
   E. Abdomen

10. Herpes gestationis factor consists of:

   A. IgG
   B. IgM
   C. IgA
   D. IgE
   E. C3

Answers

1. a.B; b.A; c.D; d.E; e.C. The 180kDa protein associated with basal keratinocyte hemidesmosomes in pemphigoid gestationis is collagen XVII, formerly called bullous pemphigoid antigen 2. Glutathione S-transferase alpha (GSTA) is elevated in women with intrahepatic cholestasis, and is a marker of hepatocellular problems in a subset of patients with pruritus gravidarum. PUPPP mainly affects first pregnancies and the rash is often accentuated in the striae. Prurigo gestationis is now often called atopic eruption of pregnancy. Leukocytosis is common in impetigo herpetiformis, which may mimic an infection.
2. B. Impetigo herpetiformis is the rarest of the pregnancy rashes. PUPPP is the most common pregnancy rash, which is fortunate since it has no known fetal complications.
3. B. Patients with impetigo herpetiformis may develop secondary hypoalbuminemia and hypocalcemia which can result in tetany.
4. A. Pemphigoid gestationis often develops around the umbilicus.
5. D. Pruritus gravidarum is often treated with phenobarbital and cholestyramine.
6. E. Linear C3 is found more often at dermal-epidermal junction zone in pemphigoid gestationis compared with the immunoglobulins.
7. C. Telogen effluvium usually starts 3 months after delivery and is self-limited.
8. D. Pemphigoid gestationis is the rash most likely one to recur in subsequent pregnancies.
9. E. The midline abdomen is the site for linea nigra.
10. A. Herpes gestationis factor, IgG4, avidly fixes complement to basement membrane zone of the epidermis.

REFERENCES

Ambros-Rudolph CM et al. The specific dermatoses of pregnancy revisited and reclassified: results of a retrospective two-center study on 505 pregnant patients. *J Am Acad Dermatol* 2006;54:395.

Black MM et al. *Obstetric and Gynecologic Dermatology*, 3rd Ed. London: Mosby; 2008.

Rapini RP: The skin and pregnancy. In: Creasy RK, ed. *Maternal Fetal Medicine*, 7th Ed. Philadelphia: Elsevier-Saunders; 2013.

CHAPTER 22

RHEUMATOLOGIC DISEASES

ASRA ALI
CAROLYN A. BANGERT

CONNECTIVE TISSUE DISEASES

- Group of systemic autoimmune diseases
- Screening
  - Antinuclear antibody (ANA): performed using indirect immunofluorescence (IF)
  - Varying concentrations of patient serum are incubated with a tissue substrate (usually human epithelial tumor line HEp-2), and any autoantibodies to nuclear antigens present in the serum bind to the substrate
  - A fluoresceinated antibody is added, and the tissue is observed under fluorescent microscopy to check for a specific staining pattern
    - Results reported as
      - ▲ Titer: level of antinuclear antibodies significant enough to be defined as a positive ANA. The standard definition is the titer exceeding that found in 95% of normal individuals (5% of normal individuals can be ANA-positive, with titers usually ≤1:320 and a speckled or homogeneous pattern)
      - ▲ Pattern: corresponds to the presence of a specific antibody. A certain pattern may indicate the presence of various rheumatologic diseases
      - ▲ A positive ANA is seen in
        - △ Systemic lupus erythematosus (SLE): 99%
        - △ Systemic sclerosis (SSc) patients: 97%
        - △ Dermatomyositis (DM) patients: 40 to 80%
- ANA patterns and their corresponding antibodies
  - Homogeneous pattern (Fig. 22-1): complete nuclear fluorescence; specific for SLE
    - Double-stranded DNA (dsDNA) or native DNA: 70% SLE, associated with lupus nephritis
    - Histone: 50 to 70% SLE; also the antibody found in drug-induced SLE (*but not in drug-induced subacute cutaneous lupus erythematosus*)
  - Rim pattern: fluorescence at edges of nucleus, anti-DNA, antihistone and antilaminin antibodies: SLE (most specific) but also may be seen in chronic active hepatitis
  - Speckled pattern (Fig. 22-2):
    - SS-A/Ro: 30 to 40% SLE; often with subacute cutaneous lupus erythematosus (SCLE), drug-induced SCLE, and neonatal LE; also seen in Sjögren syndrome (SS), DM
    - SS-B/La: 15% SLE often with SCLE, drug-induced SCLE, neonatal LE
    - Antiribonucleoprotein (RNP): 30% SLE; associated with mixed connective tissue disease (MCTD)
    - Anti-Smith (Sm): 20 to 30% SLE; very specific
- Extractable nuclear antigens (ENAs)
  - Soluble cytoplasmic and nuclear components that are bound by autoantibodies
  - Antibodies include Ro, La, Sm, RNP, Scl-70, and Jo-1
  - ENA-4 test
    - Identifies Ro, La, RNP, and Sm
    - Used to diagnose SLE, MCTD, and SS
  - Nucleolar pattern (homogeneous, speckled, or clumpy staining of nucleolus)
    - RNA polymerase I (RNA pol 1): 4 to 23% SSc
    - U3-RNP/fibrillarin: SSc
    - Topoisomerase I (Scl-70): 22 to 40% of SSc, associated with diffuse SSc
    - PM-Scl: SSc-polymyositis overlap
  - Centromere pattern (antibodies to kinetochore proteins)
    - Approximately 22 to 36% of SSc patients
    - Approximately 60 to 90% of limited SSc patients (e.g., CREST syndrome [calcinosis, Raynaud phenomenon, esophageal dysmotility, sclerodactyly, telangiectasia])

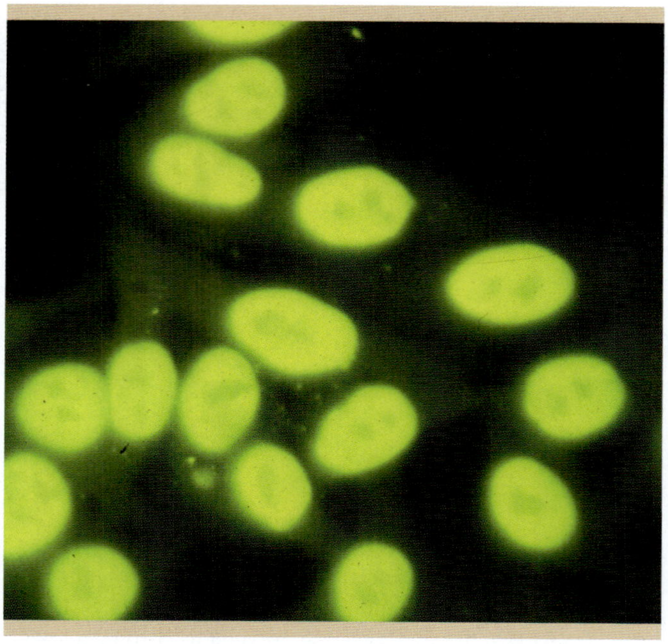

FIGURE 22-1 Homogeneous pattern. (*Used with permission from Dr. Robert Jordon.*)

Lupus Erythematosus

- Autoimmune disorder with a spectrum of presentations; may be cutaneous and/or systemic
- Cutaneous lupus subsets
  - Acute cutaneous lupus erythematosus (ACLE)
  - Subacute cutaneous lupus erythematosus (SCLE)

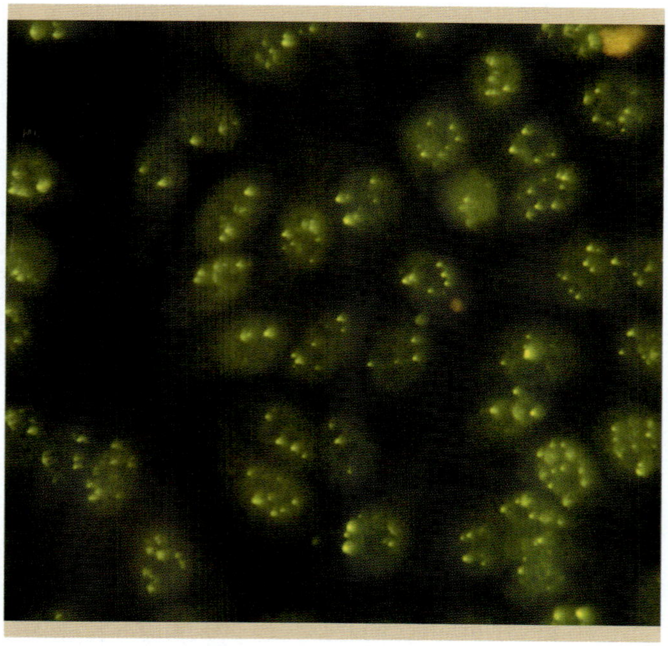

FIGURE 22-2 Speckled pattern. (*Used with permission from Dr. Robert Jordon.*)

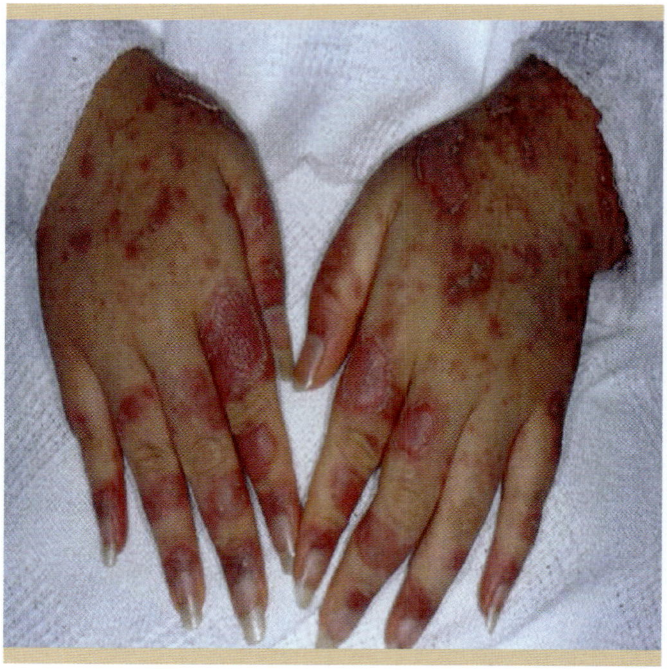

FIGURE 22-3 Acute cutaneous lupus erythematosus. (*Used with permission from Dr. Melissa Costner.*)

  - Chronic cutaneous lupus erythematosus (CCLE)
  - Systemic lupus erythematosus (SLE)
- ACLE: most specific for SLE (Fig. 22-3)
  - Localized ACLE (malar rash): occurs in 20 to 60% of SLE patients
    - Lasts from days to weeks
    - Violaceous erythematous patches or plaques over the malar eminences, may involve entire face with sparing of the nasolabial folds and palpebral eyelids (vs. DM)
    - May heal with dyspigmentation or poikiloderma, but does not scar
    - Often is painful or pruritic
    - Associated with sun exposure; systemic disease flaring is common
    - Histologic findings: focal liquefactive degeneration of the basal cell layer; perivascular and periadnexal lymphocytes
    - Immunohistology (Fig. 22-4): IgG and C3 along dermal-epidermal junction in a continuous granular or linear bandlike array (lupus band: lesional or nonlesional)
  - Generalized ACLE: characterized by erythematous macular or papular scaling, with or without edema; crusting and bullae can be present; spares the knuckles when it involves the hands (vs. DM, which involves the knuckles)

Systemic Lupus Erythematosus (SLE)

- Multisystem autoimmune disorder
- Found commonly in women of child-bearing age

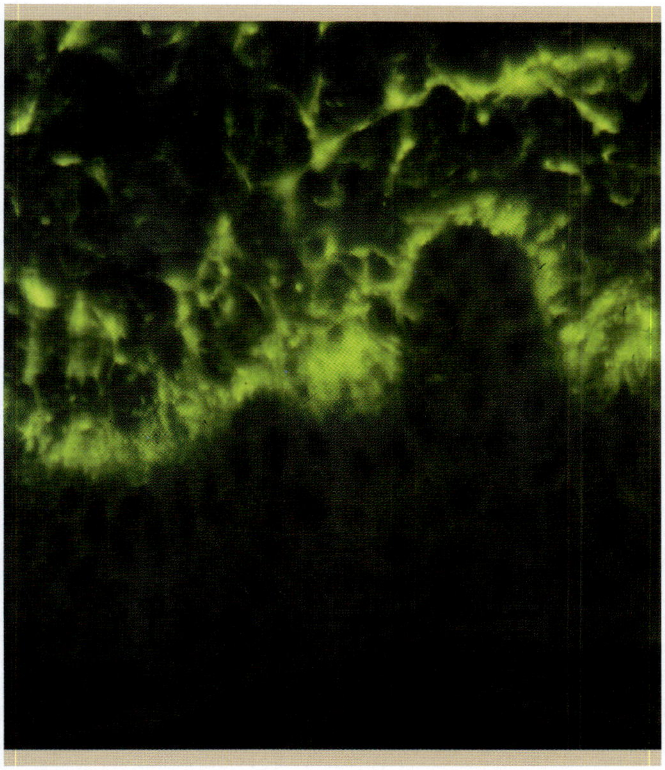

FIGURE 22-4 Immunohistology of systemic lupus erythematosus. (*Used with permission from Dr. Robert Jordon.*)

- Associated with human leukocyte antigen (HLA): DR-2 and DR-3
- Diagnostic criteria for SLE: see Table 22-1
- Other associated manifestations of lupus that may be associated with disease flares
  - Constitutional symptoms: fever, malaise, weight changes, arthralgias
  - Skin
    - Leukocytoclastic vasculitis (LCV)
    - Urticaria, urticarial vasculitis (including hypocomplementemic urticarial vasculitis)
    - Livedo reticularis: especially in patients with antiphospholipid (aPL) antibodies
    - Raynaud phenomenon (20–30% of patients)
    - Alopecia: patchy or generalized, nonscarring, similar to telogen effluvium; "lupus hairs" = whispy short hairs at anterior frontal hairline
  - Neurologic
    - Headache
    - Stroke, transient ischemic attacks (may be related to aPL antibodies)
    - Myelopathy
  - Abdominal pain: related to peritonitis, mesenteric vasculitis, and/or bowel infarction
  - Libman-sacks endocarditis, accelerated cardiovascular disease with angina
  - History of recurrent spontaneous abortions may indicate the presence of aPL antibodies
  - Laboratory tests
    - Antiphospholipid antibodies: anticardiolipin immunoglobulin G or immunoglobulin M, or lupus anticoagulant; associated with livedo reticularis, arterial and venous thrombosis without vasculitis or active SLE, and increased incidence of fetal wastage
    - Anti-dsDNA: high specificity; sensitivity is 70%, levels may correlate with disease activity (particularly with SLE nephritis)
    - Anti-Smith: highly specific for SLE, sensitivity is 30 to 40%
    - Anti-SSA (Ro) or anti-SSB (La): 15% in SLE patients; associated with neonatal lupus, SCLE, photosensitivity, low WBCs
    - Antiribosomal P: possibly with neuropsychiatric SLE
    - Anti-RNP: may be found in patients with MCTD with overlap SLE
    - Coombs test: anemia with antibodies on red blood cells
    - Antihistone: drug-induced systemic lupus erythematosus (DISLE) (*not* drug-induced cutaneous lupus erythematosus)
  - Other immunologic changes (not part of the criteria)
    - Complement deficiency: C3, C4, and C1q; low complement levels associated with flaring of systemic disease
  - Other diagnostic tests
    - Erythrocyte sedimentation rate (ESR) and or C-reactive protein (CRP): elevation in these markers of inflammation
    - Complete blood count: checks hemolytic anemia with reticulocytosis, leukopenia, lymphopenia, or thrombocytopenia
    - Urinalysis: checks proteinuria, cellular casts
    - Magnetic resonance imaging: evaluates vasculitis, stroke
    - Computed tomography: assesses pneumonitis
    - Renal biopsy: evaluates presence and type of glomerulonephritis
    - Skin biopsy: dermal-epidermal junction with lymphocytes and vacuolar change at the basal cell layer
  - Treatment: see Table 22-2

Drug-Induced Lupus Erythematosus (DILE)

- Autoantibody profile varies from classic SLE; no renal or CNS involvement; malar and discoid lesions uncommon
- Associated with antihistone antibodies (AHAs) and antinuclear antibodies commonly; not as common: anti-SS

TABLE 22-1 Classification of Systemic Lupus Erythematosus (Must, Meet 4 of 11 Criteria)

1. Malar rash	Fixed macular/papular erythema of malar eminences, spares nasolabial fold
2. Discoid rash	Erythematous plaques with adherent keratotic scaling and follicular plugging; atrophy/scarring in older lesions
3. Photosensitivity	Skin rash as the result of an unusual reaction to sunlight, either by patient or physician observation
4. Oral ulcers	Oral or nasopharyngeal, usually painless, observed by a physician
5. Arthritis	Nonerosive arthritis of 2 or more peripheral joints; tenderness, swelling, effusion
6. Serositis	a. Pleuritis: convincing h/o pleuritic pain/rub or pleural effusion, OR b. Pericarditis: by ECG, rub, pericardial effusion
7. Renal disorder	a. Persistent proteinuria, OR b. Cellular casts (RBC, Hg, granular, tubular, mixed)
8. Neurologic disorder	a. Seizures (without drug/metabolic disorder), OR b. Psychosis (without drug/metabolic disorder)
9. Hematologic disorder	a. Hemolytic anemia with reticulocytosis, OR b. Leukopenia <4,000 on 2 or more occasions, OR c. Lymphopenia <1,500 on 2 or more occasions, OR d. Thrombocytopenia <100,000
10. Immunologic disorder	a. Anti-DNA, OR b. Anti-Sm, OR c. +aPL: 1) abnormal IgG/IgM anticardiolipin Ab, 2) + lupus anticoagulant, OR 3) false-positive VDRL
11. Antinuclear antibody	Abnormal ANA by immunofluorescence or an equivalent assay in the absence of drugs

- Associated with HLA-DR4
- Patients who are slow acetylators have a higher incidence of DILE
- Can appear in up to one-fifth of patients with SLE
- Patients have 1 or more clinical symptoms of SLE (noninflammatory joint pain [90% of patients])
- Etiologic agents
  - Antiarrhythmics: procainamide and quinidine
  - Antibiotics: minocycline, rifampin, and voriconazole
  - Antitubercular: isoniazid
  - Antifungal: griseofulvin
  - Anticonvulsants: valproate, ethosuximide, carbamazepine, phenytoin, and hydantoins
  - Hormonal therapy: leuprolide acetate and oral contraceptives
  - Antihypertensives: hydralazine, methyldopa, diltiazem, and captopril
  - Anti-inflammatory: D-penicillamine and sulfasalazine and TNF-inhibitors
  - Antipsychotic: chlorpromazine
  - Cholesterol-lowering agents: lovastatin, simvastatin, and gemfibrozil
  - Antimalarial: hydroxychloroquine
  - Others: glyburide, gold salts, interferon, amiodarone, and docetaxel
- Laboratory tests
  - Positive ANA in 95%
  - AHAs in more than 75%, homogenous pattern (50–70% of patients with classic SLE)
  - Drugs not associated with AHA are minocycline and TNF-inhibitors
  - Drugs with homogenous pattern: procainamide, isoniazid, timolol, hydralazine, and phenytoin
  - In contrast, drug-induced subacute cutaneous lupus erythematosus has a speckled pattern (anti-SSA/Ro), see SCLE section below
  - Complement levels normal
- Treatment: not needed; symptoms usually clear within weeks of stopping the implicated drug

Subacute Cutaneous Lupus Erythematosus (SCLE)

- Associated with HLA-B8, HLA-DR3, HLA-DRw52, and HLA-DQ1

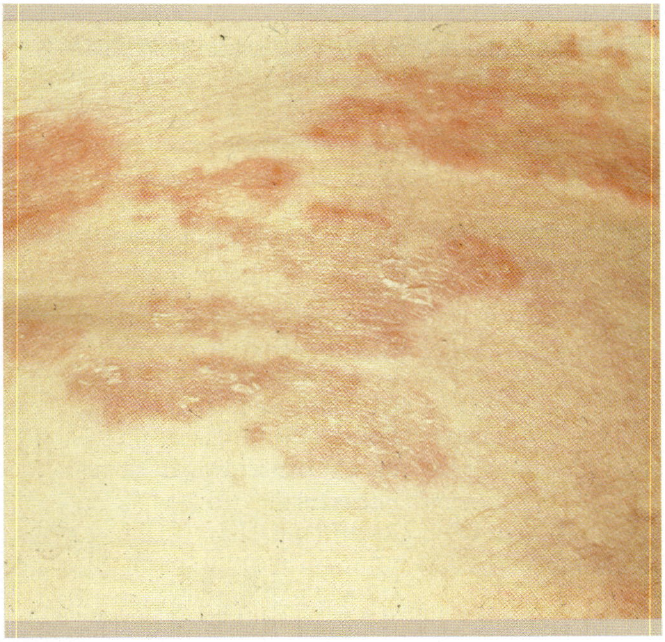

FIGURE 22-5 Subacute cutaneous lupus erythematosus. (*Used with permission from Dr. Robert Jordon.*)

- Usually occurs in Caucasian females; seen in 9 to 27% of patients with SLE
- Clinical (Fig. 22-5)
  - Begins as erythematous papules or plaques
  - Annular lesions or scaling plaques (psoriasiform or lichenoid), usually on sun-exposed areas of the body but can be generalized
  - Knuckles are usually spared when lesions occur on the hands (vs. DM, which involves the knuckles)
  - Photosensitivity to UVB, UVA, and rarely visible light
  - Waxing and waning course; may heal with transient hypopigmentation or even permanent leukoderma
- 50% of patients meet the ACR criteria for SLE (most commonly: arthritis, leukopenia, positive ANA, and photosensitivity)
- Only 10 to 20% of patients develop severe SLE (e.g., nephritis, CNS disease)
- Drug-induced SCLE: most commonly hydrochlorothiazide, calcium channel blockers, angiotensin-converting enzyme inhibitors, griseofulvin, terbinafine, and tumor necrosis factor antagonists
- Laboratory tests
  - ANA
  - Anti-Ro (SS-A) in 70%, anti-La (SS-B) in 30%
  - May be associated with rheumatoid factor positivity, hypocomplementemia, and an elevated ESR
- Positive lupus band test: complement and/or immunoglobulin along dermal-epidermal junction
- Histology: similar to ACLE
- Treatment: see Table 22-2

Chronic Cutaneous Lupus Erythematosus (CCLE)/ Discoid Lupus Erythematosus (DLE)

- Chronic, scarring, and photosensitive disease
- Occurs in 15 to 30% of patients with SLE; 5 to 20% of patients with DLE progress to SLE
- Female to male ratio: 3:1
- Clinical
  - Begins as erythematous papules or plaques
  - Progresses to plaques with follicular plugging, scale, central hypopigmentation, and peripheral hyperpigmentation
  - Localized: head and neck affected, usually with asymmetrical lesions on the face, ears, and scalp (Fig. 22-6)
  - Widespread: symmetric involvement of the trunk and extremities, more often progresses to SLE compared to localized disease
  - Lesions resolve with permanent scarring, including scarring alopecia
  - Less photosensitive than other forms
  - May involve mucous membranes
- Laboratory
  - ANA + : 20%
  - Anti-Ro (SS-A): 1 to 3%

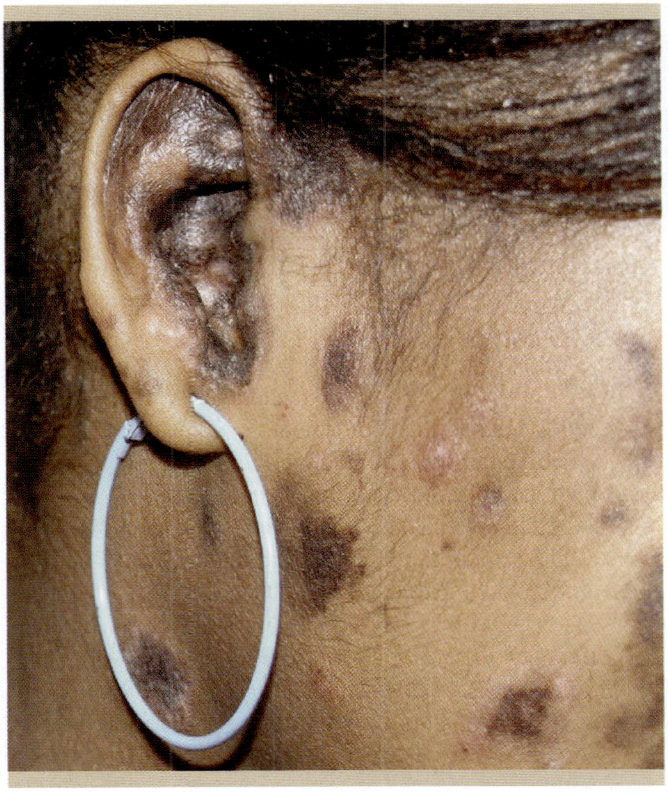

FIGURE 22-6 Chronic cutaneous lupus erythematosus (CCLE). (*Used with permission from University of Texas Houston Medical School, Dermatology Resident Teaching Collection.*)

TABLE 22-2 Treatment of Cutaneous and Systemic Lupus

	Treatment	Type	Indication
Prevention	Sun protection Smoking cessation	Clothing, UVA/UVB sunscreen, avoidance —	All CLE/SLE pts Tobacco worsens CLE/SLE, decreases efficacy of antimalarials
Topical	Corticosteroids IL corticosteroids Calcineurin inhibitors	High potency 2.5–10 mg/mL Tacrolimus, pimecrolimus	All CLE DLE, other CLE Facial/eyelid CLE
Antimalarials	Hydroxychloroquine (HCQ, plaquenil) Chloroquine (CQ) Quinacrine (QC)	Alone or + QC Alone or + QC Combine with HCQ or CQ	CLE, arthralgias, prevent SLE flares Recalcitrant CLE or HCQ intolerance Recalcitrant CLE
Immunosuppressives	Azathioprine (AZA, Imuran) Mycophenolate mofetil (MMF, CellCept) Methotrexate (MTX) Cyclophosphamide (CYC, Cytoxan) Corticosteroids	— — — — IV methylprednisolone, PO prednisone	SLE or recalcitrant CLE SLE or recalcitrant CLE Recalcitrant CLE Significant nephritis, CNS SLE Severe SLE, severe flaring CLE
Others	Thalidomide Oral retinoids	— Acitretin, isotretinoin	Recalcitrant CLE; avoid in aPL + pts (increased risk of thrombosis) Recalcitrant CLE

- Histology: similar to ACLE/SCLE, but with more marked periappendageal involvement and follicular plugging
- Direct immunofluorescence (DIF): 90% of patients on lesional skin
- Treatment of cutaneous and systemic lupus: see Table 22-2

Cutaneous Lupus Erythematosus Variants

- Tumid lupus erythematosus (TLE)
  - May be a variant of CCLE or SCLE
  - Low incidence of SLE
  - Nonscaling edematous, erythematous, insect-bite-like papules, usually in a photodistribution
  - Very photosensitive
  - Histology shows mucin and interstitial lymphocytic infiltrate with no epidermal involvement
  - Treatment: antimalarials
- Bullous systemic lupus erythematosus (BSLE)
  - Subepidermal blistering disease that is seen in patients with SLE
  - *Three types*
    - Lupus-specific bullous lupus: for example, bullous ACLE (including TEN-like ACLE), bullous SCLE, bullous CCLE; DIF may show lupus band; responds to traditional CLE treatment
    - Neutrophilic bullous lupus: resembles dermatitis herpetiformis; neutrophils at DEJ; granular IgG, IgA, IgM, and C3 at DEJ on DIF; responds well to dapsone
    - EBA-like bullous lupus: antibodies to type VII collagen; noninflammatory bullae at sites of friction; linear IgG, C3 at DEJ; recalcitrant to treatment
- Lupus erythematosus panniculitis/profundus (LEP) (Fig. 22-7)
  - Primarily affects deep dermis (profundus only) and subcutaneous fat (profundus and panniculitis)
  - Occurs in SLE and CCLE patients, or as an isolated phenomenon
  - Clinical
    - Chronic recurrent course
    - Tender, firm, subcutaneous nodules, often heal with prominent fat atrophy
    - Most commonly on proximal extremities, trunk, breasts, buttocks, and face (vs. erythema nodosum, which involves the calves)
  - Histology: dermal perivascular and periappendageal lymphocytic inflammation that extends into the subcutaneous fat; lobular panniculitis with lymphocytes, lymphoid nodules with germinal centers, plasma cells,

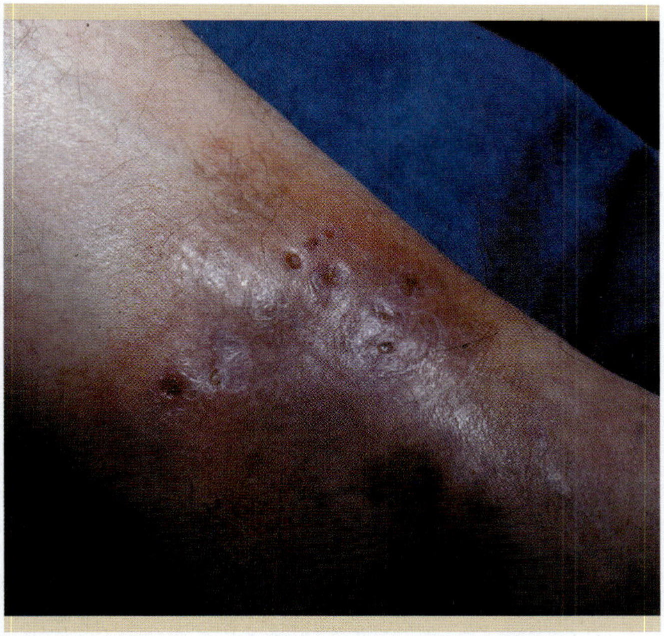

FIGURE 22-7 Lupus erythematosus panniculitis (LEP). *(Used with permission from Dr. Robert Jordon.)*

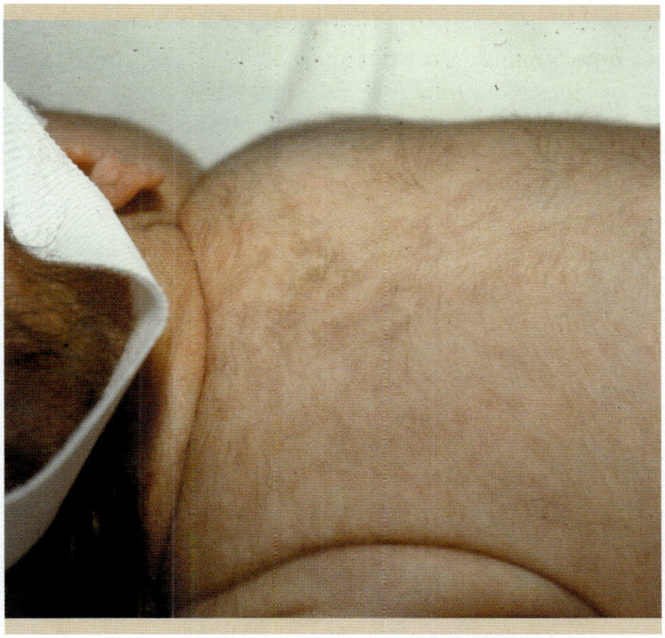

FIGURE 22-8 Neonatal lupus erythematosus (NLE). *(Used with permission from Dr. Robert Jordon.)*

and histiocytes; hyalinized fat necrosis possible epidermal atrophy and hydropic degeneration of the basal cell layer
- Treatment: similar to other forms of cutaneous LE

- Hypertrophic discoid lupus erythematosus
  - Rare variant of DLE with markedly hyperkeratotic or verrucous lesions
  - Often seen on the extensor extremities and face
  - Mimics squamous cell carcinoma, clinically and histologically
- Chilblain lupus erythematosus (CHLE)
  - Red-purple papules and plaques on the distal fingers, toes, heels, elbows, knees, and nose precipitated by cold
  - Lesions develop scale and frequently scar
  - Usually occurs in patients with DLE
- Neonatal lupus erythematosus (NLE)
  - Caused by mother's antibodies (anti-Ro [95%], anti-La, or U1-RNP) in the fetus
  - Mothers are usually asymptomatic at the time of childbirth, but may have numerous autoimmune conditions (i.e., SLE, Sjögren syndrome)
  - Maternal HLA-B8 and HLA-DR3
  - Affects 1 to 5% of infants with positive maternal anti-Ro antibodies
  - Mothers with an infant with NLE have a 25% incidence of having a subsequent affected child
  - Ro52 protein cardiac 5-HT4 serotoninergic receptor affected by maternal autoantibodies resulting in inhibition of serotonin-activated L-type calcium currents (Ica-L)
  - Clinical (Fig. 22-8)
    - Cutaneous SCLE-like lesions in 50% with well-demarcated, annular, erythematous, scaling plaques; frequently periorbital ("owl-eye")
      - Photosensitive, with lesions on the scalp, neck, and face
      - Present at birth in 66% of infants, 33% develop lesions within the first 2 to 5 months of life
    - Congenital heart block (15–30%): complete heart block requires a pacemaker; patients may develop heart failure
    - Intrauterine monitoring in mothers with Ro/La antibodies
    - Hepatosplenomegaly may occur
    - Hematologic changes: leukopenia, thrombocytopenia, anemia
    - All findings except cardiac resolve in 6 months with clearance of maternal antibodies
  - Laboratory tests
    - ANA
    - Maternal and neonatal anti-Ro, anti-La, anti-U1-RNP, anti-dsDNA
    - CBC, LFTs
    - Neonatal electrocardiography, echocardiography, fetal heart monitoring
    - Histology: hyperkeratosis, vacuolar degeneration of basal cell layer
    - IF: granular IgG at the dermal-epidermal junction
  - Treatment
    - Photoprotection
    - Mild topical steroids
    - Congestive heart failure: early placement of a pacemaker

Antiphospholipid Syndrome (APS)

- Autoimmune disorder of unknown etiology characterized by increased thrombosis and/or increased incidence of spontaneous abortions. Subgroups of APS patients—those with and those without the presence of other risk factors for arterial or venous thrombosis
- Diagnosis of APS requires the presence of 1 clinical criterion and 1 laboratory criterion
- Clinical criteria
  - Vascular thrombosis
    - Arterial thrombosis
    - Venous thrombosis
    - Small vessel thrombosis of any organ/tissue confirmed by Doppler
  - Pregnancy morbidity
    - Spontaneous abortion of a normal fetus at or after the 10th week of gestation
    - Premature birth of normal neonate at or before 34th week of gestation due to severe preeclampsia, eclampsia, or placental insufficiency
    - Three or more unexplained consecutive miscarriages before 10 weeks of gestation
- Laboratory criteria (2 or more occasions 6 weeks or more apart)
  - IgG, IgM, or anticardiolipin (aCL) antibody in medium or high titer
  - Anti-β 2 glycoprotein
  - Lupus anticoagulant
- Other clinical findings (not included as part of criteria)
  - Cutaneous findings: superficial phlebitis, leg ulcers, distal ischemia, cutaneous necrosis (noninflammatory retiform purpura), blue toe syndrome; see Fig. 22-9
  - Neurologic: transient ischemic attack, ischemic stroke, chorea, seizures, dementia, transverse myelitis, encephalopathy, migraines, pseudotumor cerebri, cerebral venous thrombosis, mononeuritis multiplex
  - Cardiac: myocardial infarction, valvular vegetations, intracardiac thrombi, atherosclerosis
  - Renal: renal vein/artery thrombosis, renal infarction, acute renal failure, proteinuria, hematuria, nephritic syndrome
  - Gastrointestinal: Budd-Chiari syndrome, hepatic/gallbladder/intestinal/splenic infarction, pancreatitis, ascites, esophageal perforation, ischemic colitis
  - Venous thrombosis: extremities/adrenal/hepatic/mesenteric/splenic vein/vena cava thrombosis
  - Endocrine: adrenal/testicular/pituitary infarction
  - Obstetric complications: spontaneous abortion, intrauterine growth retardation, hemolytic anemia, elevated liver enzymes, thrombocytopenia
  - Hematologic: thrombocytopenia, hemolytic anemia, hemolytic-uremic syndrome, thrombotic thrombocytopenic purpura
  - Ophthalmic: retinal vein/artery thrombosis, amaurosis fugax (temporary loss of vision in 1 eye caused by decreased blood flow [ischemia] to the retina)

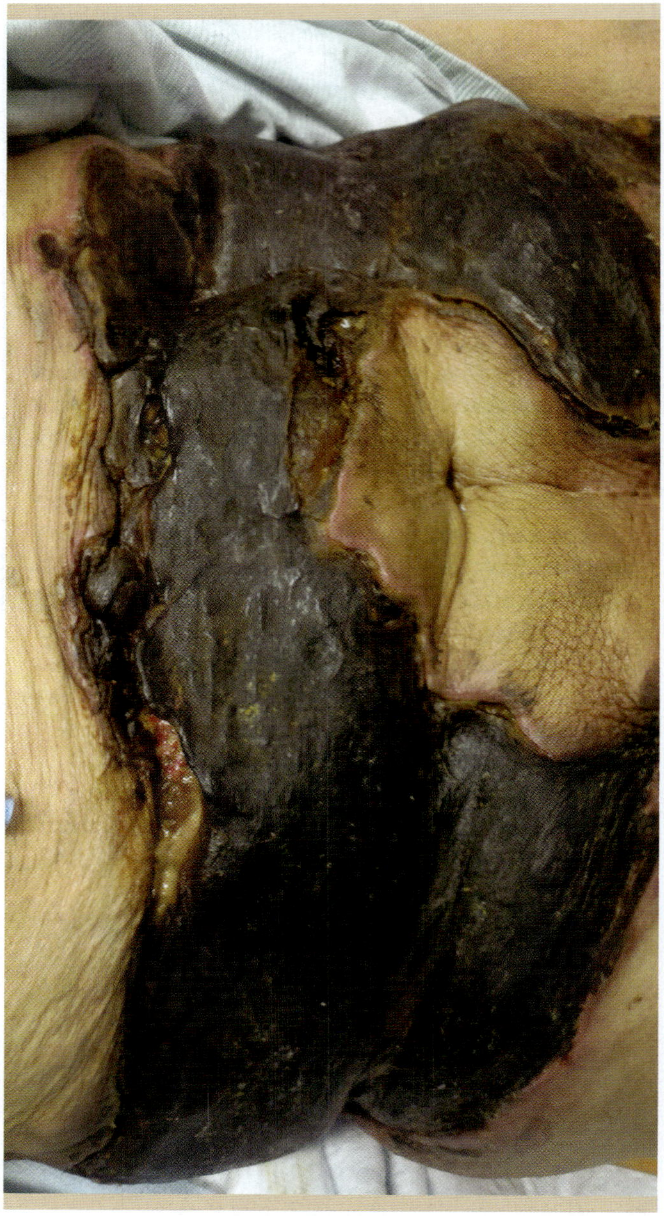

FIGURE 22-9 Antiphospholipid antibody syndrome-induced retiform purpura. (*Used with permission from Dr. Laura Lester.*)

  - SNAP syndrome: clinical manifestations of APS, without the presence of antibodies
- Conditions associated with the presence of aPL antibodies
  - Autoimmune diseases: SLE, Sjögren syndrome, rheumatoid arthritis
  - Infections: syphilis, hepatitis C, human immunodeficiency virus, malaria, leprosy, parvovirus B19, cytomegalovirus
  - Medications: procainamide, quinidine, propanolol, hydralazine, phenytoin, chlorpromazine, interferon-α, quinine, amoxicillin, sulfadoxine/pyrimethamine (fansidar), and cocaine
- HLA associated with aPL antibodies: *DRw53, DR7, DR4*

- Catastrophic antiphospholipid syndrome (CAPS): acute onset; criteria include evidence of involvement of 3 or more organ systems, and/or tissue development of manifestations simultaneously or in less than 1 week, confirmation by histopathology of small-vessel occlusion in at least 1 organ/tissue laboratory confirmation of the presence of aPL (lupus anticoagulant and/or aCL and/or anti–B-2-GP I)
- Laboratory studies: (presence of antibodies on 2 or more occasions at least 12 weeks apart)
  - Antiphospholipid (aPL) antibodies
  - Anticardiolipin (aCL) antibodies
  - Anti-β 2 glycoprotein I antibodies
  - Other antibodies to phosphatidylserine, phosphatidylthreonine (membrane phospholipids)
  - Activated partial thromboplastin time (aPTT)
  - Lupus anticoagulant (LA) test such as dilute Russell viper venom time (DRVVT)
  - False-positive serologic test result for syphilis
  - Complete blood cell count (thrombocytopenia, Coombs-positive hemolytic anemia)
  - Proteinuria and renal insufficiency from thrombotic microangiopathy
  - Approximately 45% of patients have a positive ANA
  - Ultrasound (evaluate for DVT); CT or MRI of chest (evaluate for pulmonary embolism), brain (evaluate for cerebral vascular accident), abdomen (evaluate for Budd-Chiari syndrome)
- Treatment
  - Following thrombosis: anticoagulation with intravenous heparin, followed by warfarin, heparin or low-molecular-weight (LMW) heparin
  - Recurrent spontaneous abortions: treated with subcutaneous heparin 7,500 to 12,000 units twice daily along with aspirin 81 mg daily
  - Thrombocytopenia: prednisone

Sjögren Syndrome (SS)

- Autoimmune disease that mainly affects the exocrine glands
- HLA-DR3 and HLA-DR52 in patients with primary SS
- Primary SS has xerophthalmia and xerostomia only
- Secondary SS has xerophthalmia and xerostomia and occurs with rheumatoid arthritis, SLE, SSc, DM, and MCTD
- SS criteria
  - Presence of 4 out of 6 criteria, as long as either the histopathology or serology is positive
    - Ocular symptoms of dryness
    - Oral symptoms of dryness
    - Ocular signs: a positive result for at least 1 of the following 2 tests:
      - ▲ Schirmer test
      - ▲ Rose Bengal score or other ocular dye score
    - Histopathology: focal lymphocytic sialoadenitis, with a focus score of 1 per 4 mm^2 of glandular tissue
    - Salivary gland involvement: a positive result for at least 1 of the following diagnostic tests:
      - ▲ Unstimulated whole salivary flow (<1.5 mL in 15 minutes)
      - ▲ Parotid sialography showing the presence of diffuse sialectasias, without evidence of obstruction in the major ducts
      - ▲ Salivary scintigraphy showing delayed uptake, reduced concentration, and/or delayed excretion of tracer
    - Autoantibodies: presence in the serum of the following autoantibodies: Ro(SSA) or La(SSB) antigens, or both
- Clinical findings
  - Keratoconjunctivitis sicca: xerophthalmia
  - Bilateral parotid swelling (most common sign in children)
  - Unstimulated salivary flow less than 1.5 mL/min
  - Positive Schirmer test showing decreased tear film for eyes
  - Xerostomia (Fig. 22-10): signs of reduced salivary flow, associated with angular chelitis, dental caries, oral candidiasis with resulting erythema and atrophy of the dorsum of the tongue or a white, cheesy curd that bleeds when wiped off
  - Extraglandular symptoms
    - Hepatitis (13%): also increased incidence of primary biliary cirrhosis
    - Arthritis (42%)
- Laboratory studies
  - Anti-Ro/SS-A (90%) ± anti-La/SS-B (70%)

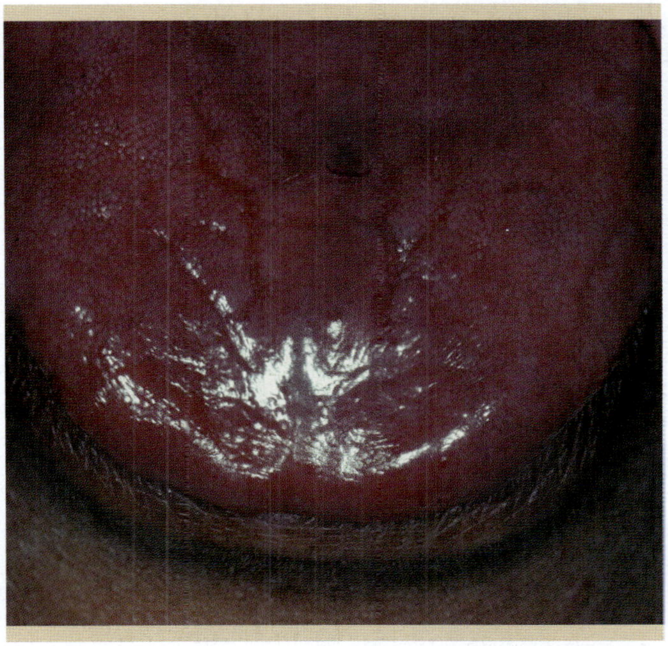

FIGURE 22-10 Sjögren syndrome (SS). *(Used with permission from Dr. Bela B. Toth.)*

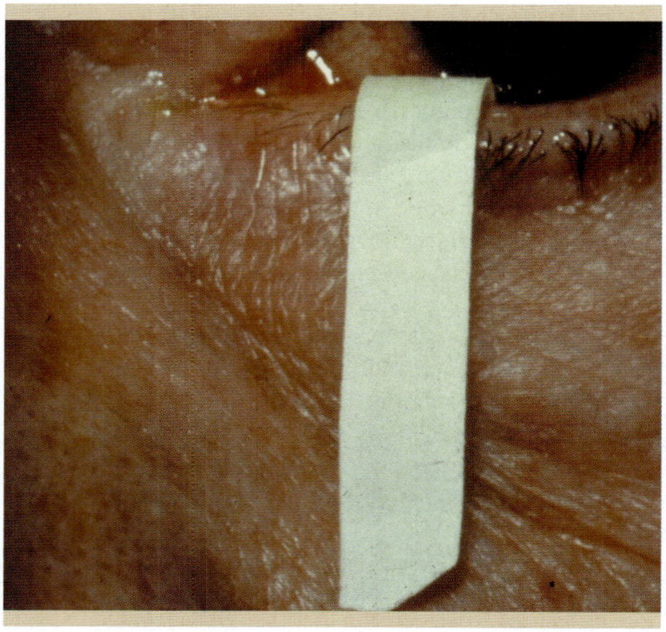

FIGURE 22-11 Positive Schirmer test. (*Used with permission from Dr. Robert Jordon.*)

- Rheumatoid factor
- Antithyroglobulin antibodies (25%)
- B-lymphocyte infiltration (20–25%) and CD4 + T-cell infiltration (70–80%) localized in the salivary glands
- Positive Schirmer test (Fig. 22-11): measures lacrimation response in the eye; filter paper strip placed in lower conjunctival sac and the wetting length achieved in 5 minutes is measured; greater than 8 mm in 5 minutes is abnormal

- Histopathology (minor salivary gland): mononuclear inflammatory infiltrates, interstitial fibrosis, and acinar atrophy
- Treatment: symptom control; no curative agent exists
  - Topical cyclosporine A (Restasis): 0.05 to 0.1% ophthalmic drops
  - Pilocarpine HCl (Salagen): 5-mg tablets, cholinergic agonist
  - Cevimeline HCl (Evozac): 30-mg tablets, cholinergic agonist binding to muscarinic receptors
  - Plaquenil (hydroxychloroquine)

MIXED CONNECTIVE TISSUE DISEASE (MCTD)

- Disease syndrome with overlapping features of SSc, SLE, and polymyositis
- Associated with HLA-DR4 or HLA-DQB1
- Controversy exists as to whether MCTD constitutes a distinct clinical entity
- Alarcon-Segovia and Villareal classification
  - Serologic criterion is a positive anti-RNP at a titer of 1:1600 or higher
  - Clinical criteria; presence of at least 3 of the following:
    - Edema of the hands
    - Raynaud phenomenon
    - Acrosclerosis
    - Synovitis
    - Myositis (laboratory or biopsy diagnosis)
- Kusukawa diagnostic criteria for MCTD
- Requirement for diagnosis: at least 1 *common symptom*, with positive U1-RNP antibodies and 1 or more findings in at least 2 of the 3 categories: A, B, and C from the *mixed findings* list
- *Common symptoms*
  - Raynaud phenomenon
  - Swollen fingers or hands
  - Presence of anti-U1-RNP
- *Mixed findings*
  - SLE-like
    - Polyarthritis
    - Pericarditis/pleuritis
    - Lymphadenopathy
    - Facial erythema
    - Leukopenia/thrombocytopenia
  - Scleroderma-like
    - Sclerodactyly
    - Pulmonary fibrosis
    - Esophageal dysmotility
  - Polymyositis-like
    - Muscle weakness
    - High creatine kinase (CK)
    - Electromyogram (EMG)
- Other clinical features
  - Arthralgias in 60%
  - Sclerodactyly
  - Interstitial lung disease, pulmonary hypertension (most common cause of death)
  - Abnormal nailfold capillaries (50%)
  - Palpable purpura (25%)
  - Vascular disturbances may lead to peripheral gangrene/leg ulcers
  - Dysphagia and dysfunction of esophageal motility
- Laboratory studies
  - CBC
  - Muscle enzymes: CK, aldolase, aspartate aminotransferase (AST), alanine aminotransferase (ALT), and lactate dehydrogenase (LDH)
  - Anti-RNP, anti-Smith, anti-Ro(SSA), anti-La(SSB), anti-Scl-70, phospholipids, anticardiolipin, and histone, complement: C3, C4
  - High-titer ANA in a speckled pattern
  - Antibodies against U1: 70-kDa small nuclear ribonucleoprotein (snRNP) at titer more than 1:1,600

- Histology: myositis
- Other tests: chest x-ray, barium swallow (evaluate esophageal motility)
- Echocardiography: (evaluate myocardial function and pulmonary artery pressure)
- Treatment
  - Corticosteroids, HCQ, CYC, AZA, MTX

Dermatomyositis (DM)

- Idiopathic inflammatory myopathy with characteristic cutaneous lesions with or without muscle inflammation and weakness
- Diagnostic criteria (3 criteria plus the rash)
  - Symmetrical muscle weakness: limb girdle muscles and anterior neck flexors (absent in amyopathic DM [ADM] and hypomyopathic DM [HDM])
  - Muscle biopsy: evidence of muscle fiber necrosis, inflammatory exudate, often perivascular (absent in ADM)
  - Elevated muscle enzymes: CPK, aldolase, LDH (absent in ADM)
  - EMG triad: small polyphasic action potentials, positive sharp waves and insertional irritability, and bizarre high frequency repetitive discharges (absent in ADM)
  - Cutaneous changes: Gottron papules/sign, heliotrope rash with periorbital edema, scaly photodistributed dermatitis
- Classification
  - Adult DM
    - Classic DM
    - Classic DM with malignancy
    - Classic DM with associated connective tissue disease
    - Clinically amyopathic DM (CADM)
      - ADM/DM sine myositis: no clinical or laboratory evidence of myositis for 6 months without treatment
      - HDM: no clinical evidence of myositis, but laboratory evidence of subclinical disease
  - Polymyositis (PM), similar clinical feature to DM: inflammatory myopathy with symmetric muscle weakness
  - Juvenile DM (JDM)
    - Classic JDM
    - Clinically amyopathic JDM
- Clinical
  - Cutaneous findings
    - Occurs 2 to 3 months prior to muscle weakness
    - Primary lesion: pruritic erythematous-violaceous patches and plaques with or without scale. Poikiloderma may be present. Lesions frequently involve scalp, anterior/posterior neck, photoexposed areas and extremities, but can involve any body area

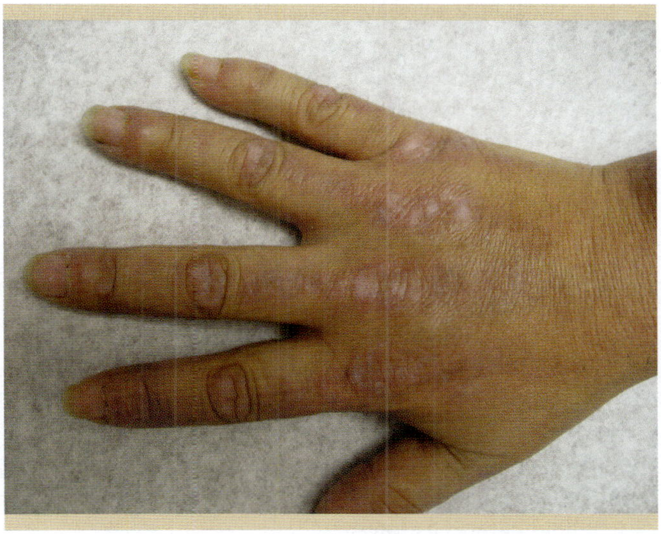

FIGURE 22-12 Dermatomyositis Gottron papules, nailfold capillary changes, and cuticular dystrophy.

    - *Heliotrope rash*: periorbital, symmetric, violaceous patches with or without edema
    - *Gottron papules*: violaceous papules overlying the following joints of the dorsal hands: metacarpophalangeal, distal interphalangeal, and/or proximal interphalangeal; most sensitive/specific feature along with Gottron sign (see Fig. 22-12)
    - *Gottron sign*: violaceous symmetric macular erythema over bony prominences of hands and elsewhere (e.g., elbows, knees, medial malleoli)
    - *Tendon streaking*: linear violaceous erythema along extensor tendons of hands/feet
    - *Nailfold capillary changes*: correlated with disease severity, capillary telangiectasia, infarcts, capillary loop dropout (whitish areas of avascularity—not seen in LE), Samitz sign cuticular dystrophy
    - *V-sign*: macular erythema and poikiloderma of V-area of neck and chest
    - *Shawl sign*: macular erythema and poikiloderma of upper back and shoulders
    - *Holster sign*: erythematous patches/plaques on bilateral hips
    - *Malar rash*: erythema of the central face but unlike ACLE, usually does not spare nasolabial folds
    - *Mechanics hands*: hyperkeratosis of the palmar and lateral surfaces of the fingers, associated with interstitial lung disease
    - *Calcinosis cutis*: cutaneous calcium deposition, usually in areas of trauma, associated with increased disease activity, JDM, 10% of adult DM
  - Extracutaneous findings
    - Proximal symmetric muscle weakness (shoulder and limb girdle)

- Dysphagia/dysphonia (esophageal/pharyngeal involvement)
- Pulmonary disease
  - ▲ Restrictive lung disease from respiratory muscle weakness
  - ▲ Interstitial lung disease: in 25 to 65% of patients, can be rapidly progressive and fatal, a leading cause of mortality, common in CADM
- Synovitis
- Raynaud phenomenon
- Cardiac disease: rare ECG changes, arrhythmias, cardiomyopathy

- JDM
  - Similar cutaneous features of classic DM in patients younger than 18 years
  - Other clinical features
    - *Vasculopathic lesions* (SQ nodules, digital ulcers) poorer prognosis
    - *Calcinosis cutis*: occurs on bony prominences; 40% of children
    - *Acquired lipodystrophy* (prevalence of 10–40%), generalized, partial, or focal, late complication of JDM, associated with more severe, chronic disease and with other disease sequelae such as calcinosis, insulin resistance, diabetes, and hypertriglyceridemia
    - *Cardiac*: Asymptomatic cardiac conduction delays or right bundle branch block (up to 50% of patients)
  - Thrombospondin-1, a mediator of angiogenesis, is increased in patients with JDM
- DM associated with malignancy
  - Reported rate of malignancy in adults varies widely: 13 to 25%; there is no reported increased risk in JDM patients
  - May precede, coincide with, or follow the diagnosis of DM
  - Risk remains elevated for 3 to 5 years following diagnosis
  - Presence of malignancy represents a major indicator of poor prognosis in DM
  - Association between a rapid onset of the disease and malignancy
  - Relative risk for ovarian cancer in female patients is 16.7
  - Reported association with the following malignancies: breast (adenocarcinoma most common), gastrointestinal, ovarian, lung
- Drug-induced DM: statins, hydroxyurea, penicillamine
- Poor prognosis associated with progressive disease, dysphagia, extensive cutaneous lesions on the trunk, cardiac issues, longer duration of symptoms before diagnosis, initiation of therapy after 24 months of muscle weakness, older age, *malignancy, progressive disease*, and *interstitial lung disease*
- Diagnosis
- *Myositis-specific antibodies* (not seen in other CTD patients)
  - Mi-2: nuclear helicase, 5% of PM/DM, 15 to 20% of DM
    - Associated with classic DM, V/shawl sign, cuticular dystrophy
    - Good prognosis
  - *Antisynthetase antibodies*
    - Antibodies to aminoacyl-tRNA synthetases, cytoplasmic antigens
    - Jo-1 (5–20% DM/PM), EJ, OJ, PL-12, PL-7 antibodies
    - Associated with antisynthetase syndrome
      - ▲ Mechanic's hands
      - ▲ Myositis (may or may not have cutaneous DM)
      - ▲ Interstitial lung disease
      - ▲ Synovitis
      - ▲ Raynaud phenomenon
      - ▲ Patients often refractory to treatment
  - *Annexin XI* (56-kDa): most sensitive for JDM
  - *Anti-CADM-140 or MDA-5*: found in 50% of CADM patients, associated with rapidly progressive ILD
  - *Anti-p155/140*: malignancy-associated DM
  - Anti-signal recognition protein (SRP): associated with severe polymyositis
  - *Other antibodies* (myositis-associated, not DM-specific)
    - *ANA*: positive in 60 to 80%, more commonly positive in CADM
    - SS-A/Ro
    - *Anti-PM-Scl* (seen in overlap of DM/PM and scleroderma)
    - *Anti-Ku* (seen in overlap of DM and with scleroderma and/or SLE)
- Laboratory studies
  - Elevation of the following: creatine kinase level (most sensitive for myositis), aldolase, AST, ALT, and LDH
  - Elevated ESR
  - Muscle studies: EMG shows a myopathic pattern, muscle biopsy, MRI
  - Histology: epithelial vacuolar changes with lymphocytic infiltrate at the dermal-epidermal junction, identical to findings of CLE
  - DIF: C5b-9 deposition at DEJ and perivascularly
  - Malignancy workup in all patients with localizing symptoms and patients older than 40 years at presentation and annually
  - Endoscopic studies of the upper and lower gastrointestinal tract should be done according to the patient's age
- Treatment
  - Systemic corticosteroids for muscle involvement

- Steroid-sparing agents for maintenance, cutaneous DM: MTX, AZA, cyclosporine (CSA), MMF; antimalarials as adjuncts for mild skin disease
- IV immunoglobulin (IVIG): for severe and refractory disease, pulmonary disease
- Cyclophosphamide: for interstitial lung disease
- Biologics: rituximab, tumor necrosis factor inhibitors (etanercept)
- Topical steroids, tacrolimus, photoprotection: for skin disease

Systemic Sclerosis (SSc)

- Multisystemic connective tissue disease with excessive collagen deposition and vasomotor disturbances
- Associated with HLA-B8, HLA-DR5, HLA-DR3, HLA-DR52, and HLA-DQB2
- Pathophysiology also associated with genetic, environmental, vascular, and autoimmune factors
- Five forms of SSc: diffuse systemic sclerosis (dSSc), limited systemic sclerosis (lSSc), transitory form (dSSc/lSSc), systemic scleroderma sine scleroderma, and malignant scleroderma
- Other factors associated with SSc pathophysiology
  - Environment-related
  - *Criteria for diagnosis of adult SSc*: diagnosis when 1 major and 2 minor criteria are present
    - Major features include centrally located skin sclerosis that affects the arms, face, and/or neck
    - Minor features include sclerodactyly, erosions, atrophy of the fingertips, and bilateral lung fibrosis
- Clinical findings
  - Mucocutaneous findings
  - *Cutaneous sclerosis*: progresses through 3 phases
    - Edematous phase: fingers with edema ("puffy phase")
    - Indurated or sclerotic phase: thickened tight skin, hair loss, and decreased sweating; begins acrally and on face/neck, proximal spread, sclerodactyly: fingertip tapering, loss of fingerpad pulp, pitted scars, digital ulcers (35%), and loss of mobility (Fig. 22-13)
    - Atrophic or late phase: dermis is firmly adherent to underlying subcutaneous fat
  - *Salt-and-pepper dyspigmentation*: vitiligo-like depigmentation with perifollicular pigment
  - *Skin ulceration*: digital tip ulcers (secondary to ischemia); ulcers over the bony prominences (attributable to contractures)
  - *Calcinosis cutis*: subcutaneous and/or intracutaneous calcinosis (Fig. 22-14)
  - *Nailfold capillary changes*: capillary loop dilation alternating with loop dropout; occur in 90% of patients
  - *Ocular symptoms*: dry eyes, blepharitis, retinal hemorrhages (with renal crisis)
  - *Oral symptoms*: xerostomia, dental decay

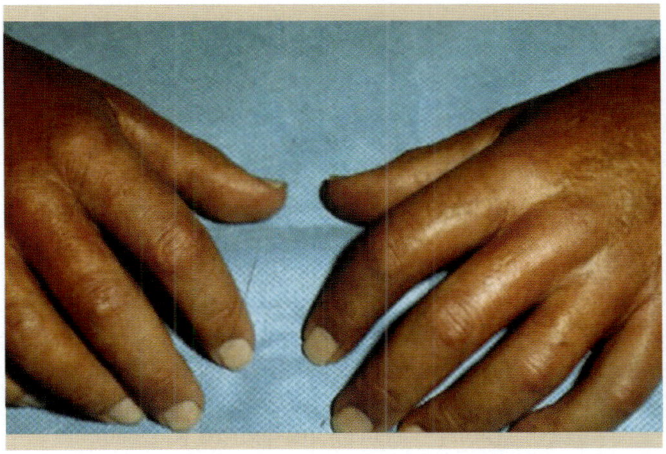

FIGURE 22-13 Sclerodactyly. (*Used with permission from Dr. Melissa Costner.*)

  - *Raynaud phenomenon*
    - Paroxysmal vasospasm of digits in response to cold exposure or emotional stress
    - Endothelial injury results in intimal hyperplasia and fibrosis
    - Ninety-five percent of SSc patients
    - Three pathogenic mechanisms: vasoconstriction, ischemia, and reperfusion (white-blue-red appearance of the skin)
    - Typically the first clinical and most common sign of SSc, may precede the disease by 5 to 10 years
    - Types of Raynaud: primary: acral color changes are the only clinical signs without any other symptom

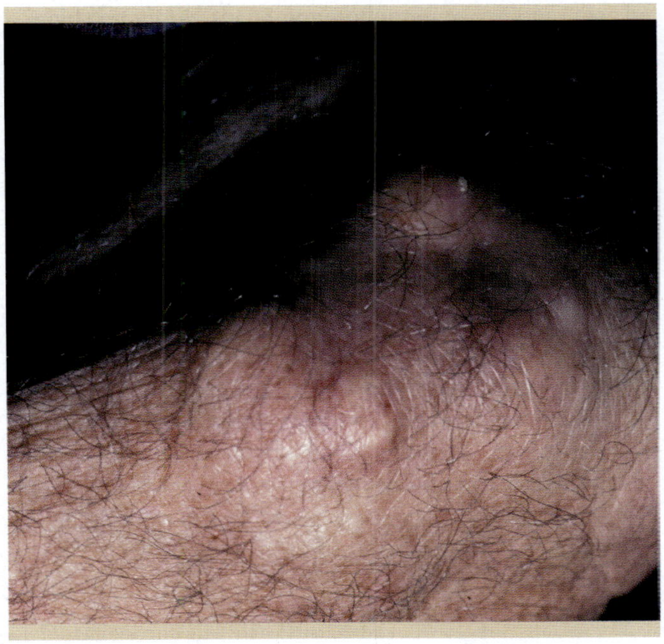

FIGURE 22-14 Calcinosis cutis. (*Used with permission from Dr. Robert Jordon.*)

and disease; secondary: color changes are associated with clinical symptoms or signs of systemic disease
- Musculoskeletal
  - *Muscle weakness*: scleroderma myopathy (proximal muscle weakness) and sclerodermatomyositis (true overlap between scleroderma and polymyositis with severe muscle weakness and elevated CPK and abnormal EMG)
  - *Arthritis*: symmetric polyarthralgia and joint stiffness (with or without gross synovitis)
  - *Tendon fibrosis*: may result in myalgia, joint pain, immobility, contractures, and fibrinous tenosynovitis with friction rub
- Gastrointestinal tract (affects 75–90% of patients)
  - *Esophageal dysmotility*
    - ▲ Ninety percent of patients, occurs in early disease, secondary to smooth muscle fibrosis
    - ▲ May lead to gastroesophageal reflux disease with symptoms of heartburn, dysphagia, and resulting in complications of Barrett esophagus and esophagitis (may cause esophageal stricture)
  - *Gastric vascular ectasia* may lead to gastroparesis
  - *Small intestinal muscle fibrosis* may lead to functional ileus (pseudoobstruction); bacterial overgrowth may cause malabsorbtion and diarrhea
  - *Colonic signs and symptoms*: megacolon, constipation, and diverticula
- Pulmonary disease: 70% of SSc patients; main cause of mortality
  - *Pulmonary interstitial fibrosis*: occurs in early disease, most commonly with diffuse SSc
  - *Pulmonary artery hypertension (PAH)*: 10 to 15% of patients, occurs later in the course of the disease, 3 types: severe isolated PAH without significant fibrosis (common in lSSc), PAH with fibrosis (common in dSSc), and lastly an indolent PAH
- Renal
  - *Scleroderma renal crisis (SRC)*, usually in dSSc (18% of patients): hypertension and oliguric renal failure; usually seen with early, rapidly progressive dSSc
  - Associated with RNA-polymerase III antibodies
- Cardiac
  - Myocardial fibrosis (<5% of dSSC), congestive heart failure, myocarditis, pericarditis, ventricular arrhythmias
- Genitourinary
  - Erectile dysfunction (12–60%)
  - Dyspareunia

- Clinical features of the 2 most common forms
  - Diffuse cutaneous systemic sclerosis (dcSSc)
    - Associated with topoisomerase I (Scl-70) in 30%
    - Quick progression of sclerosis of proximal limbs and trunk
    - Associated with pulmonary interstitial fibrosis in 30 to 60%, scleroderma renal crisis
  - Limited systemic sclerosis (lSSc)
    - Also known as CREST (*c*alcinosis, *R*aynaud, *e*sophageal dysmotility, *s*clerodactyly, *t*elangiectasia)
    - Anticentromere antibodies in 40 to 50%
    - Sclerosis confined to face, neck, and extremities distal to elbows/knees
    - Slowly progressive and indolent
    - Late phase
      - ▲ Calcinosis cutis: calcium apatite crystals found in tissue
      - ▲ Matte-like telangiectasia: can also occur with dSSc
      - ▲ PAH: leading cause of death in lSSc
  - Juvenile systemic sclerosis
    - Children younger than 16 years account for less than 5% of all cases of SSc
    - Fourfold more frequent in girls
    - Raynaud phenomenon (RP) is the first sign of the disease in 70% of patients
    - Classification criteria for JSSc: replaces previous adult classification criteria
    - Sensitivity of 90%, a specificity of 96%
    - Patient, younger than 16 years, with 1 major and at least 2 of the 20 minor criteria
- *Major criterion*: proximal sclerosis/induration of skin
- *Minor criteria*:
  - Skin: sclerodactyly
  - Vascular: Raynaud phenomenon, nailfold capillary abnormalities, digital tip ulcers
  - Gastrointestinal: dysphagia, gastroesophageal reflux
  - Renal: renal crisis, new-onset arterial hypertension
  - Cardiac: arrhythmias, heart failure
  - Respiratory: pulmonary fibrosis (high-resolution computed tomography/radiograph), diffusing lung capacity for carbon monoxide, pulmonary hypertension
  - Musculoskeletal: tendon friction rubs, arthritis, myositis
  - Neurologic: neuropathy, carpal tunnel syndrome
  - Serology: antinuclear antibodies, SSc-selective autoantibodies (anticentromere, antitopoisomerase I, antifibrillarin, anti-PM-Scl, antifibrillin, or anti-RNA polymerase I or III)
  - Scleroderma-like disorders: see Table 22-3
- Laboratory studies
  - Autoantibodies
    - *ANA*: 97% of patients; 81 to 97% in JSSc, most commonly speckled, nucleolar, centromere
    - *Topoisomerase I*: by immunodiffusion, 9 to 20% of adult patients, 20 to 34% in JSSc; associated with diffuse cutaneous involvement, increased mortality rate, due to ventricular failure secondary to ILD
    - *Centromere*: 20 to 30% of patients, most commonly found with lSSc; associated with a higher risk for calcinosis and ischemic digital loss, lower frequency of ILD, increased risk of PAH

TABLE 22-3 Scleroderma-Like Disorders

Localized scleroderma	Morphea
Increased mucin deposition	Scleromyxedema, scleredema, nephrogenic systemic fibrosis
Disorders with gammaglobulinemia	Scleromyxedema, POEMS syndrome, myeloma with scleroderma-like changes
Disorders with eosinophilia	Eosinophilic fasciitis, eosinophilia-myalgia syndrome, toxic oil syndrome
Disorders with endocrine/biochemical disorders	Insulin and non-insulin-dependent diabetes (IDDM, NIDDM), carcinoid, porphyria, phenylketonuria, nephrogenic systemic fibrosis, chronic graft-versus-host disease
Chemically-induced	Eosinophilia-myalgia syndrome, toxic oil syndrome, polyvinyl-chloride disease, organic solvents, epoxy resins exposure
Iatrogenic/drug-induced	Bleomycin, injections of pentazocine, progestin, vitamin B_{12}, vitamin K, cocaine, D-penicillamine, peplomycin, interferon-β1a, tegafur-uracil, paclitaxel, methysergide, gemcitabine, physical injury (trauma, vibration stress, radiation)
Genetic disorders	Inherited progeroid syndromes (Werner syndrome), heterogeneous group of hereditary disorders with skin thickening (melorheostosis, stiff skin syndrome, porphyria, phenylketonuria), or tight skin (restrictive dermopathy, scleroatrophic Huriez syndrome)

    - *Fibrillarin (U3-RNP)*: less than 10% of patients with SSc, associated with diffuse cutaneous disease
    - *RNA Polymerases (I-III)*: specific for SSc, 20% of patients, associated with diffuse cutaneous involvement and SSc-related renal crisis (III), greater mortality
    - *PM-Scl* (2% of patients with scleroderma): found in patients with myositis, scleroderma, and the polymyositis-scleroderma overlap syndrome (myositis, Raynaud phenomenon, arthritis, and ILD)
    - *Anti-Th/To*: 2 to 5% of patients with SSc and are associated with milder skin and systemic involvement, except for more severe pulmonary fibrosis
    - *Anti-Ku antibodies*: scleroderma-myositis overlap syndromes and a wide spectrum of rheumatic diseases
    - *Antiphospholipid (aPL) antibodies*: 20 to 25% of patients, increased frequency of pregnancy losses; anticardiolipin (aCL) antibodies: thrombosis and pulmonary hypertension
    - *Anti-U1-RNP*: 8% of patients, less cutaneous and renal involvement and favorable response to corticosteroids
    - *Anti-Ro antibodies*: Less than 35% of patients, association of SSc with Sjögren syndrome up to 20%
- Imaging studies
    - Chest radiograph: fibrosis of the lower areas of the lungs
    - Bone radiography: generalized osteopenia
    - Doppler echocardiography: left- and right-sided heart diseases
    - Pulmonary function test
    - Cine esophagram: evaluates esophageal hypomotility
    - Esophagogastroduodenoscopy: identifies erosive esophagitis, superinfection, Barrett esophagus, ulceration, and malignant transformation
    - Small bowel series: identifies characteristic hypomotility
- Histologic findings
    - Appendageal atrophy: marked mucopoly-saccharide, glycoprotein, and compact collagen (types I and III) deposition in the dermis; subintimal proliferation of small arteries and arterioles
- Treatment
    - Pulmonary: vaccinations (prophylactic influenza and *Streptococcus pneumonia),* cyclophosphamide for ILD; prostacyclin (epoprostenol and treprostinil), endothelin-1 antagonist (bosentan), and phosphodiesterase type-5 inhibitor (sildenafil) for PAH
    - Cardiac: nonsteroidal anti-inflammatory drugs or low-dose corticosteroids for pericarditis, high-dose corticosteroids for myocarditis. Digitalis and diuretics are also used
    - Renal: ACE inhibitors, dialysis, renal transplant; scleroderma renal crisis: IV captopril
    - Raynaud, digital ulcers: calcium channel blockers (nifedipine), topical nitropaste, phosphodiesterase type 5 inhibitor (sildenafil), ACE inhibitors

- Musculoskeletal: NSAIDs
- Skin disease: UVA1 phototherapy, antifibrotic agents (e.g., D-penicillamine, interferon-α, and interferon-γ); low-dose prednisone (avoid >15 mg/d as it can cause scleroderma renal crisis); MTX; MMF
- Gastrointestinal tract involvement: proton pump inhibitors (e.g., omeprazole), H_2 blockers, cisapride, and metoclopramide, endoscopic dilation, sclerotherapy for ecstatic vessels, broad spectrum antibiotics for bacterial overgrowth
- Other systemic treatments: cyclophosphamide, methotrexate, chlorambucil, 5-fluorouracil, stem cell transplantation

Localized Scleroderma (Morphea)

- Idiopathic fibrosis of the skin and adjacent structures
- Prognosis is good. Associated SSc is rare; lesions tend to regress spontaneously over 3 to 5 years, usually with residual pigmentary and atrophic changes
- Subtypes: plaque, generalized, bullous, linear, deep, and morphea-lichen sclerosus overlap (with overlying or concomitant lesions of LS)
- Etiology
  - Role of autoimmunity in the pathogenesis of morphea
  - Autoimmune conditions associated with morphea: Hashimoto thyroiditis, vitiligo, SLE, and Type 1 diabetes mellitus
  - Cytokines and growth factors released by endothelial and inflammatory cells (TH2 activation) result in fibroblast proliferation and increased deposition of extracellular matrix
  - Factors involved in promoting fibrosis in morphea: transforming growth factor-β (TGF-β), connective tissue growth factor (CTGF), IL-1, IL-4, IL-6, endothelin-1, and tissue inhibitor of metalloproteinase-1.2 T
- Clinical findings
  - Excessive collagen deposition with thickening and induration of the skin and subcutaneous tissue
  - May begin with signs of inflammation, such as erythema and warmth
  - Usually asymptomatic, but may complain of pain or pruritus
  - Surface becomes smooth and shiny, lilac-colored
  - Usually progresses over 3 to 5 years, then regresses, with skin softening and some residual atrophy/hyperpigmentation
- Types of morphea
  - *Plaque-type*
    - Most common in adults, occurs in more than 50% of cases of morphea
    - Indurated plaques 1 to 30 cm in diameter, may have an associated violaceous border (Fig. 22-15)
    - Lesions progressively become indurated, with a lilac or yellow hue and then heal with atrophy and hyperpigmentation

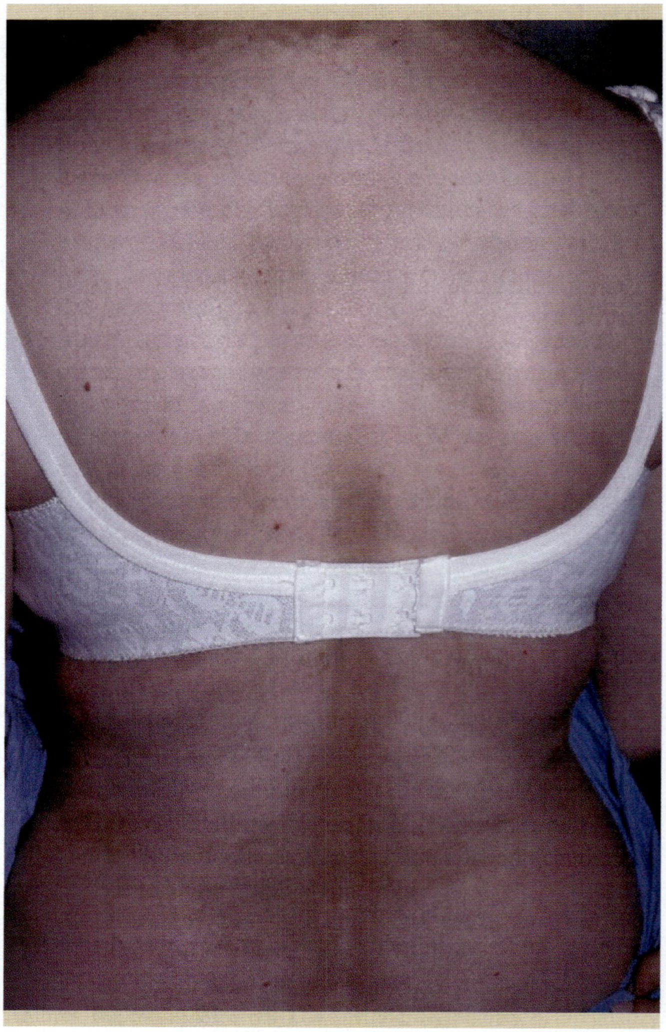

FIGURE 22-15 Plaque morphea. (*Used with permission from University of Texas Houston Medical School, Dermatology Resident Teaching Collection.*)

    - Trunk involved more commonly than extremities
    - Variants: guttate, keloidal (nodular), atrophoderma of Pasini and Pierini
    - *Linear morphea*
      - ▲ Accounts for approximately 20% of all cases; comprises up to 65% of cases of juvenile morphea
      - ▲ Linear plaques that become confluent and extend longitudinally, can impair mobility of an entire limb, can involve muscle/fascia/tendons, can impair joint mobility, can involve 1 limb, or can affect the ipsilateral trunk and other limb, but generally remains unilateral
        - △ *En coup de sabre*: affects frontoparietal scalp and paramedian forehead; rarely, may extend deeply; ocular complications such as eyelid lesions, exophthalmos, uveitis,

episcleritis, xerophthalmia, papilledema, and glaucoma (up to 15% of cases); neurologic involvement with resulting seizures peripheral neuropathy, encephalitis, central nervous system vasculitis, vascular malformations, and/or strokes
    - *Progressive facial hemiatrophy* (Parry-Romberg syndrome): variant of linear morphea with progressive hemifacial atrophy; primary lesion occurs in the subcutaneous tissue, muscle, and bone (Fig. 22-16)
- *Generalized morphea*: 13% of patients with morphea; coalescence of individual plaques or the development of multiple lesions in more than 2 anatomical sites; diffuse morphea: progression to involve widespread areas of the body (does not involve digits, unlike SSc)
- *Nodular or keloid morphea*: sclerotic papules and plaques that resemble keloid scars
- *Guttate morphea*: multiple small, usually superficial papules
- *Atrophoderma of Pasini and Pierini*: possibly an end-stage form of plaque-type morphea; dermal/fat atrophy of trunk or proximal extremities with depressed plaques with a blue-brown, gray, or violaceous hue with a sharp cut-off and deep indentation
- *Deep morphea (morphea profunda)*: involves deep dermis, subcutaneous tissue, fascia, muscle, and bone, may calcify
- Variants
  - *Subcutaneous* morphea: mainly subcutaneous involvement with rapid onset of symmetric sclerotic bound-down lesions and ill-defined borders

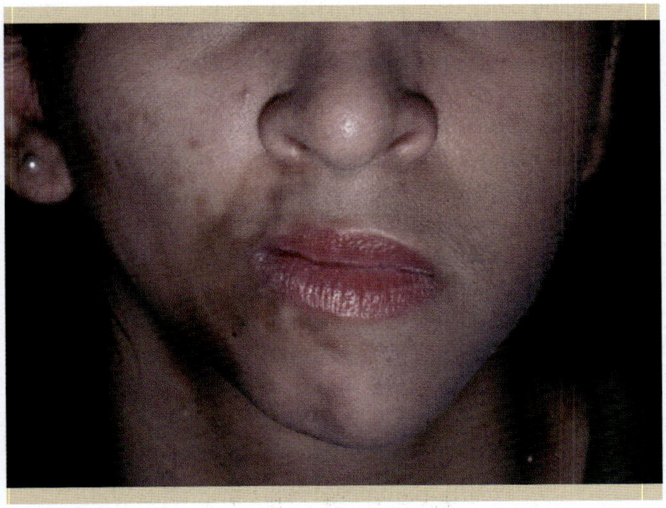

FIGURE 22-16 Parry-Romberg syndrome. (*Used with permission from University of Texas Houston Medical School, Dermatology Resident Teaching Collection.*)

    - *Morphea profunda*: all skin layers with diffuse, taut, bound-down sclerosis
    - *Eosinophilic fasciitis* (or Shulman syndrome): see "Eosinophilic Fasciitis (EF, Shulman Syndrome)" section below
    - *Disabling pansclerotic morphea of children*: poor prognosis, diffuse full-thickness sclerosis of the trunk, face, and extremities, sparing the fingertips and toes, affects the deep subcutaneous tissue, fascia, muscle, and bone
  - *Bullous morphea*: tense subepidermal bullae may occur in plaques of morphea on the extremities, trunk, face, or neck and may be superficial or extend into the dermis
- Laboratory studies
  - *ANA*
    - Positive in 40% of plaque-type or generalized morphea
    - Positive in 67% of linear morphea
  - *Anti-single-stranded DNA*: 50% of morphea patients, especially correlates with linear morphea
  - Antihistone antibodies (AHAs): 35% morphea patients
  - *Antifibrillarin antibodies*: 30% morphea patients
  - *Rheumatoid factor (RF)*: 60% of patients
  - *Polyclonal hypergammaglobulinemia*: 50% of patients
  - Antitopoisomerase II: 76% in morphea patients
  - *Complete blood count*: in patients with eosinophilic fasciitis
  - *Neurologic and ophthalmologic examinations*: patients with morphea involving the face
- Histology (*early lesions*): dense inflammatory infiltrate composed of lymphocytes, macrophages, plasma cells; *late lesions*: thickened, hyalinized collagen bundles
- Treatment
  - Topical or intralesional corticosteroids
  - Calcipotriene (vitamin D analog)
  - UVA1 phototherapy
  - Imiquimod 5% cream
  - Generalized, linear, and deep morphea: systemic corticosteroids, antimalarials, MTX, MMF
  - Physical therapy for linear morphea

Eosinophilic Fasciitis (EF, Shulman Syndrome)

- Disorder characterized by peripheral eosinophilia and fasciitis
- Scleroderma-like induration of the skin, differs from PSS since it usually spares the fingers, hands, and face and does not present with Raynaud's syndrome
- Belongs to the subtype of deep localized scleroderma or deep morphea
- Cause is unknown; however, it has been reported in association with vigorous exercise, drugs, borreliosis, arthropod bites, and trauma
- Increased expression of genes for transforming growth factor-β (TGF-β) and extracellular matrix proteins in fibroblasts

- Clinical findings
    - Sudden onset of tender, edematous, and erythematous extremities associated with weakness and muscle pain with limited motility
    - Fascial involvement can lead to contractures (75%) and separation of muscle groups by a line of demarcation (groove sign)
    - Veins may appear depressed (sunken veins)
    - Rippling of the skin and a peau d'orange change often develops
    - Associated with severe cramps, distal sensorimotor neuropathy, mononeuritis multiplex, cognitive symptoms
    - Cardiopulmonary features: pneumonitis, respiratory muscle dysfunction, pulmonary hypertension
- Differential diagnosis
- Eosinophilia-myalgia syndrome: when EF is accompanied by muscle weakness; however, in eosinophilia-myalgia syndrome there are muscle pains, polyneuropathy or pulmonary disease, and a history of L-tryptophan intake (some cases of EF are reported after L-tryptophan ingestion, suggesting an overlap in the pathogenesis)
- Scleroderma, SSc, and mixed connective tissue disorder: typical findings of these diseases include sclerodactyly, Raynaud phenomenon, and the presence of antinuclear antibodies not found in EF
- Laboratory signs
    - Peripheral blood eosinophilia (64% of patients)
    - Hypergammaglobulinemia (75% of patients)
    - ESR (50–70%)
- Histologic findings: inflammation, edema, thickening, and sclerosis of the fascia; presence of lymphocytes, plasma cells, histiocytes, and eosinophils, similar to scleroderma
- Imaging studies: ultrasound and magnetic resonance imaging in order to detect thickened fascia
- Treatment
    - Prednisone, hydroxyzine, hydroxychloroquine, photochemotherapy, and cyclophosphamide
    - Course
        - Spontaneous remission can occur
        - Ten percent of patients develop aplastic anemia

Cryoglobulinemia

- Cryoglobulins: plasma immunoglobulins or immunoglobulin-containing complexes that precipitate on exposure to cold and redissolve on warming
    - Types of cryoglobulins
        - *Type I*: (10–15%) monoclonal immunoglobulin, usually IgM or IgG
            - ▲ Associated with plasma cell dyscrasias/lymphoproliferative disorders
            - ▲ Clinically indistinguishable from those with Waldenström macroglobulinemia, multiple myeloma, immunocytoma, or chronic lymphocytic leukemia
            - ▲ Clinical findings
                - △ Associated with signs of peripheral vessel occlusion
                - △ Patients may present with clinical manifestations related to hyperviscosity syndrome, purpura lesions, livedo reticularis acrocyanosis, Raynaud phenomenon, ulcers, and gangrene
        - Mixed cryoglobulinemia (MC)
            - ▲ Etiological role of HCV in most cases of types II and III cryoglobulinemia
                - △ *Type II*: (50–60%) monoclonal IgM (rarely IgA or IgG that has rheumatoid factor [RF] activity and binds to polyclonal immunoglobulins [usually IgGs])
                - △ *Type III*: (25–30%) polyclonal IgM that has rheumatoid factor (RF) activity and binds to polyclonal immunoglobulins (usually IgGs)
            - ▲ Clinical
                - △ Typical triad: purpura, weakness, arthralgias
                - △ Multisystem organ involvement including chronic hepatitis, membranoproliferative glomerulonephitis, peripheral neuropathy due to LCV of small and medium-sized vessels
                - △ Proposed criteria for the classification of MC
                    - *Major* (serologies): mixed cryoglobulins, low C4; pathology: LCV
                    - *Minor* (serologies): rheumatoid factor +, HCV+, HBV+; pathology: clonal B-cell infiltrates (liver-bone marrow)
                - △ *"Definite" mixed cryoglobulinemia syndrome*
                    - Serum mixed cryoglobulins (±low C4) + purpura + LCV
                    - Serum mixed cryoglobulins (±low C4) + 2 minor clinical symptoms + 2 minor serological/pathological findings
                - △ *"Incomplete" or "possible" mixed cryoglobulinemia syndrome*
                    - Mixed cryoglobulins or low C4 + 1 minor clinical symptom + 1 minor serological ± pathological finding
                    - Purpura and/or LCV + 1 minor clinical symptom + 1 minor serological ± pathological finding
                    - Two minor clinical symptoms + 2 minor serological ± pathological findings
                - △ *"Essential" or "secondary" mixed cryoglobulinemia syndrome*
                - △ Absence or presence of well-known disorders (infections, immunological, neoplastic)

- Clinical findings
  - Palpable purpura (55–100%): higher in types II and III, intermittent, begins on legs
  - Raynaud's phenomenon: 33% of patients
  - Vasculitis: secondary to vascular deposition of circulating immunocomplexes
  - Arthralgias and arthritis in the proximal interphalangeal (PIP) joints, metacarpophalangeal (MCP) joints, knees, and ankles (73%)
  - Renal immune-complex disease: 33% of patients, IF demonstrates immunoglobulin and C3 deposits in the glomerulus (cryoglobulinemic glomerulonephritis)
  - Peripheral sensorimotor polyneuropathy with painful paresthesias, most commonly in types II and III
  - Systemic autoimmune disease: connective tissue diseases are seen in patients with types II and III; mainly primary SS and SLE
  - Liver involvement: high incidence of HCV in MC patients, increased enzymes, hepatomegaly, chronic hepatitis, steatosis, cirrhosis or hepatocellular carcinoma, liver failure leading to death (25%)
  - See Table 22-4 for clinical conditions that may be associated with cryoglobulinemia

TABLE 22-4 Clinical Conditions That May Be Associated With Cryoglobulinemia

Infections	
Viral	Epstein-Barr virus, cytomegalovirus, hepatitis A virus, hepatitis B virus, hepatitis C virus, HIV
Bacterial	Lyme disease, syphilis, lepromatous leprosy, Q fever, poststreptococcal nephritis, subacute bacterial endocarditis
Fungal	Coccidioidomycosis
Parasitic	Kala azar, toxoplasmosis, echinococcosis, malaria, schistosomiasis, trypanosomiasis
Hematologic Diseases	**Autoimmune Diseases**
Non-Hodgkin lymphoma	Sjögren syndrome
Hodgkin lymphoma	Systemic lupus erythematosus
Chronic lymphocytic leukemia	Polyarteritis nodosa
Multiple myeloma	Systemic sclerosis
Chronic myeloid leukemia	Rheumatoid arthritis
Waldenström macroglobulinemia	Autoimmune thyroiditis
Castleman disease	Temporal arteritis
Myelodysplasia	Dermatomyositis-polymyositis
Thrombocytopenic thrombotic purpura	Henoch-Schönlein disease
Cold agglutinin disease	Sarcoidosis Pulmonary fibrosis Biliary cirrhosis Primary antiphospholipid syndrome Inflammatory bowel disease Endomyocardial fibrosis Pemphigus vulgaris

From Tedeschi A, Baratè C, Minola E, Morra E: Cryoglobulinemia. *Blood Rev* 2007 Jul;21(4):183–200.

- Laboratory studies
  - Serum evaluation: specimen must be obtained in warm tubes (37°C)
  - Types I and II precipitate within the first 24 hours
  - Type III cryoglobulins may require 7 days
  - RF is positive in types II and III
  - Serum cryoglobulin values usually do not correlate with clinical severity and prognosis of the disease
  - Complement levels
    - Low complement levels are frequently observed in patients with cryoglobulinemia related to autoimmune disorders
    - Type II HCV-related cryoglobulinemia presents with low levels of C4 and normal C3
- Treatment
  - Treatment of the underlying disorder
  - Nonsteroidal anti-inflammatory drugs (NSAIDs)
  - Immunosuppressives: corticosteroid therapy and/or cyclophosphamide or azathioprine, interferon-α (IFN-α), and ribavirin for HCV-associated disease
  - Plasmapheresis with other immunosuppressive treatment: in patients with severe manifestations of MC
  - Rituximab: B-cell lymphoproliferative disorders and in autoimmune diseases

Cryofibrinogenemia

- Cryofibrinogen
  - Precipitants of protein complexes made up of fibronectin, fibrinogen, and fibrin
  - Found in the plasma but not in the serum of some individuals
  - Reversibly precipitates in cooled plasma at 4°C and dissolves at 37°C
- Classification
  - Primary (essential)
  - Secondary and associated with
    - Carcinomas, infections, collagen-vascular diseases, thromboembolic diseases, cryoglobulins
- Clinical findings
  - Often clinically asymptomatic
  - Thrombotic vasculopathy characterized by ischemia, purpura, livedo reticularis, ecchymosis, ulcers, necrosis and gangrene, purpura (77%)
  - Histology: fibrin thrombi within superficial dermal vessels
- Treatment
  - Usually unresponsive to treatment; may respond to fibrinolytic therapy

Seronegative Spondyloarthropathies

- Chronic inflammatory diseases of the joints associated with the *HLA-B27* gene
- Characterised by shared rheumatic features including enthesitis, sacroiliitis, peripheral arthritis
- Also with associated extra-articular lesions notably psoriasis (Ps), uveitis, and inflammatory bowel disease
- Diseases
  - Ankylosing spondylitis/juvenile ankylosing spondylitis
  - Spondyloarthropathy of inflammatory bowel disease (IBD)
  - Psoriatic arthritis (PsA)
  - Reactive arthritis (ReA)/Reiter syndrome (RS)
  - Undifferentiated spondyloarthropathy
- Ankylosing spondylitis
  - Systemic rheumatic disorder of indeterminant etiology (but with a strong genetic predisposition), and sacroiliac (SI) joint inflammation (sacroiliitis)
  - HLA-B27: present in 95% of patients
- ReA
  - Previously called Reiter syndrome
  - Aseptic inflammatory arthritis, triggered by infection at a distant site in genetically susceptible people
    - Mainly affects patients 20 to 40 years old
    - Male to female ratio: 3:1
  - Human leukocyte antigen HLA-B27 (class 1 major histocompatibility complex gene)
    - Affects 45 to 90% of patients
    - Associated with more severe and prolonged disease, a higher prevalence of back pain, and are more likely to have mucocutaneous disease
    - HLA-B27 binds unique peptides of microbial or self-origin and presents them to CD8 positive T cells causing specific immune responses
    - Usually follows gastrointestinal or genitourinary infections (Table 22-5)
    - Sporadic cases of sexually acquired reactive arthritis (SARA) are usually due to infection with *Chlamydia trachomatis*
  - Clinical findings
    - Acute episode of arthritis, resolves spontaneously in 3 to 12 months
    - ACR definition: episode of peripheral arthritis of more than 1 month duration occurring in association with urethritis or cervicitis
      - ▲ Musculoskeletal manifestations
        - △ Arthritis (95% of patients): acute, asymmetric, knees, ankles, feet
        - △ Spondylitis: low back pain radiating to buttocks or thighs
        - △ Enthesitis: periarticular inflammation, can lead to "sausage digits"
      - ▲ Mucocutaneous involvement
        - △ *Keratoderma blennorrhagicum* (5–10% of patients): pustular psoriasis-like lesions on palms/soles, associated nail dystrophy
        - △ *Circinate balanitis/vulvitis*: painless gyrate white plaques eventually cover the entire surface of the glans penis
          - Painless shiny patches of the palate, tongue, and mucosa of the cheeks and lips

TABLE 22-5 Conditions to Which Arthritis May Be Reactive

	Probable	Possible
Respiratory infections		*Chlamydia pneumoniae* *Chlamydia psittaci* *Streptococcus pyogenes*
Genitourinary infections	*Chlamydia trachomatis*	*Mycoplasma fermentans* *Mycoplasma genitalium* *Neisseria gonorrhoeae* *Ureaplasma urealyticum*
Gastrointestinal infections	*Campylobacter jejuni* *Salmonella enteritidis* *Salmonella typhimurium* *Shigella flexneri* *Yersina enterocolitica* *Yersinia pseudotuberculosis*	*Brucella abortus* *Clostridium difficile* *Cryptosporidium* *Entamoeba histolytica* *Escherichia coli* *Giardia lamblia*

- Psoriasiform dermatitis of elbows/knees/scalp
- Pyoderma gangrenosum may also occur

▲ Ocular involvement: bilateral conjunctivitis (occurs in 30% of patients); also anterior uveitis

▲ Genitourinary involvement: urethritis or cervicitis: typically urethritis precedes conjunctivitis and arthritis; dysuria

▲ Gastrointestinal involvement: enteric acquired ReA usually presents 4 weeks after infection

▲ Renal involvement: immunoglobulin A (IgA) nephropathy

- Laboratory studies
  - Elevated ESR and CRP
  - Synovial fluid: leukocytosis; Gram stain/culture negative
  - Throat, stool, or urogenital tract cultures
  - Full blood count: neutrophilic leukocytosis, thrombocytosis, anemia of chronic disease
  - Synovial biopsy: polymorphous infiltrate indistinguishable from other chronic rheumatic diseases
  - Electrocardiogram: often normal but may show variable degrees of heart block
- Treatment
  - Usually self-limited course, with resolution of symptoms by 3 to 12 months; 50% may have recurrent arthritis
  - Empiric treatment for *Chlamydia*
  - NSAIDs
  - Sulfasalazine, methotrexate, TNF-α inhibitors

Psoriatic Arthritis (PsA)

- Found in 5 to 20% of patients with Ps that precedes the onset of PsA in 60 to 80% of patients
- CASPAR (classification criteria for psoriatic arthritis) criteria for the classification of PsA (Table 22-6): specificity of 98.7% and sensitivity of 91.4%
- Clinical findings
  - *Asymmetric oligoarthritis*: 50% of male patients
    - Involvement of hands and feet; DIPs, PIPs, spares MCPs
    - Leads to "sausage digits"
  - *Symmetric polyarthritis*: most common pattern in women
    - RA-like pattern of hands, feet, ankles
    - Unlike RA, may involve the DIP, RF negative
  - *DIP joint*: "classic," but uncommonly exclusively involved

TABLE 22-6 The CASPAR (Classification Criteria for Psoriatic Arthritis) Criteria

Requires the presence of inflammatory articular disease: joint, spine, or entheseal Also presence of 3 points from the following 5 categories: 1. Evidence of current psoriasis, a personal history of psoriasis, or a family history of psoriasis (first- or second-degree relative) 2. Typical psoriatic nail dystrophy: onycholysis, pitting, and hyperkeratosis 3. A negative test result for the presence of rheumatoid factor by any method except latex test 4. Either current dactylitis (swelling of an entire digit) or a history of dactylitis 5. Radiographic evidence of juxtaarticular new bone formation

- *Arthritis mutilans*: least common variant
  - Severe, rapidly progressive joint inflammation that results in digital shortening due to "telescoping" of digits and osteolysis (pencil in cup deformity on x-ray)
- *Spondylitis and sacroiliitis*: axial arthritis, knees also involved, may have peripheral joint involvement, HLA-B27 positive
- *Psoriatic-onychopachydermoperiostitis (POPP)*
  - Psoriatic nail lesions
  - Soft tissue thickening above the terminal phalanx and radiologic involvement of the phalanx with periosteal reaction

- Laboratory studies
  - Elevated ESR and CRP
  - Leukocytosis of synovial fluid
  - Radiologic findings: x-ray—pencil-in-cup deformity, fluffy periosteal bone formation
- Treatment
  - NSAIDs
  - MTX, sulfasalazine, and cyclosporine
  - TNF-α inhibitors: infliximab, etanercept, and adalimumab

Scleredema (Scleredema Adultorum of Buschke, Scleredema Diabeticorum)

- Benign self-limited cutaneous mucinosis with irreversible glycosylation of collagen that is collagenase resistant
- Pathogenesis: unknown, hypotheses implicating immune mechanisms, direct action of bacterial toxin, and effects of adrenal steroids released in response to infection
- Approximately 29% cases seen in children
- Type I: infection-association
  - Middle-aged women, preceding febrile illness, streptococcal, (tonsillitis, pharyngitis, and pyoderma), influenza, scarlet fever, measles, and mumps. Sudden-onset hardening of the cervicofacial region, with extension to the upper trunk and proximal extremities
  - Self-limited in several months
- Type II: monoclonal gammopathy-associated
  - Also associated with hyperparathyroidism, multiple myeloma, malignant insulinoma, rheumatoid arthritis, and Sjögren syndrome
  - Middle-aged women, no preceding illness
  - Similar course to type I
- Type III: diabetes and obesity associated
  - Middle-aged obese men
  - Slow-onset, persistent, erythema and induration of the posterior neck and back, peau d'orange
- Systemic findings
  - Serositis with possible pleural, pericardial, and peritoneal effusions
  - Dysarthria, dysphagia
  - Myositis
  - Parotitis
  - Ocular abnormalities: trophic corneal disturbances
  - Cardiac involvement: Wolff-Parkinson-White syndrome
- Histology: thickened dermis with deposition of mucin between thickened collagen bundles
- Treatment
  - Physical therapy
  - No known effective treatment

QUIZ

Questions

1. The most specific antinuclear pattern for SLE is:

   A. Rim
   B. Speckled
   C. Homogenous
   D. Nucleolar

2. Systemic lupus erythematosus is associated with:

   A. HLA-DR4
   B. HLA-DR2
   C. HLA-DQ4
   D. HLA-DQ2

3. Which statement is TRUE about acute cutaneous lupus erythematosus?

   A. ACLE occurs in 80 to 90% of patients with SLE.
   B. ACLE tends to spare the nasolabial folds.
   C. ACLE often flares with systemic disease.
   D. Alopecia is common in patients with ACLE.
   E. ACLE is the most photosensitive subtype of cutaneous lupus erythematosus.
   F. B, C, and D are true.
   G. B, C, D, and E are true.
   H. All are true.

4. Which of the following is NOT an ACR criterion of SLE?

   A. Complement deficiency
   B. Arthritis
   C. IgM antiphospholipid antibody positivity
   D. Oral ulcers
   E. Positive Smith
   F. Hemolytic anemia
   G. A and C are not
   H. A, C, and E are not
   I. All of the above are criteria

5. Which medication would NOT cause the following clinical scenarios?

   A. Hydrochlorothiazide and a patient with SCLE, photosensitivity, arthritis, and a positive ANA in a speckled pattern
   B. Griseofulvin and a patient with SCLE, photosensitivity, and a positive ANA in a speckled pattern

C. Phenytoin and a patient with a malar rash, photosensitivity, arthritis, pleurisy, and a positive ANA in a nucleolar pattern
D. Griseofulvin and a patient with a positive ANA in a homogenous pattern, arthritis, oral ulcers, hemolytic anemia, and pleurisy
E. Hydroxyurea and violaceous erythema over the knuckles, elbows, and knees, and a negative ANA

6. Which of the following is TRUE?

A. The risk of malignancy in adults with dermatomyositis is 35 to 40%.
B. Adults with dermatomyositis should have yearly malignancy screening for 2 years following their dermatomyositis diagnosis.
C. The heliotrope eruption is the most common and characteristic cutaneous features of dermatomyositis.
D. A patient with dermatomyositis with violaceous erythema on the elbows has Gottron sign.
E. Lipodystrophy, calcinosis cutis, and vasculopathic ulcers may occur in juvenile dermatomyositis.
F. D and E are true.
G. C, D, and E are true.

7. Scleroderma-like disorders can be seen in all of the following EXCEPT:

A. Stiff skin syndrome
B. Argyria
C. Crowe-Fukase syndrome
D. Vitamin K exposure
E. Paclitaxel

8. Which of the following statements about Shulman syndrome is FALSE?

A. Most cases have now been found to be associated with exposure to adulterated rapeseed oil.
B. Fascial involvement leads to contractures and the "groove sign."
C. It is characterized by increased expression of genes for TGF-β in fibroblasts.
D. It is usually steroid-responsive.
E. Approximately 75% of cases have associated hypergammaglobulinemia.
F. Approximately 10% of patients can progress to aplastic anemia.

9. Which of the following is NOT associated with the listed type of cryoglobulinemia?

A. Rheumatoid factor positivity and type I cryoglobulinemia
B. Peripheral sensory polyneuropathy and type II cryoglobulinemia
C. Monoclonal IgG and type I cryoglobulinemia
D. Type I cryoglobulinemia and acrocyanosis
E. Cryoglobulinemic glomerulonephritis and type II cryoglobulins

10. Which of the following is NOT a feature of reactive arthritis?

A. Gyrate white plaques on the penis
B. Shiny patches on the palate
C. Anterior uveitis
D. Trachyonychia
E. IgA nephropathy

Answers

1. A. Although a homogenous pattern is also highly specific for SLE and is the most common pattern in SLE, rim is the most specific. Both are associated with anti-DNA antibodies and antibodies to histone.
2. B. SLE is associated with HLA-DR2 and -DR3.
3. F. Localized ACLE (malar rash) occurs in only 20 to 60% of patients with SLE, spares the nasolabial folds (unlike dermatomyositis), often flares with systemic disease, and is often associated with alopecia (telogen effluvium–like). Although it is quite photosensitive, it is less so than SCLE.
4. A. Complement deficiency is the only item that is not an ACR criterion of SLE.
5. C. Phenytoin can cause drug-induced SLE, but cutaneous manifestations are usually not present, and the ANA pattern is rim or homogenous, corresponding with antihistone antibodies. Hydrochlorothiazide is a common cause of drug-induced SCLE, and can be associated with mild systemic symptoms and a positive Ro or La antibody. Griseofulvin can cause both drug-induced SLE (associated with antihistone antibodies and usually without cutaneous involvement) and drug-induced SCLE (associated with anti-Ro/La Abs). Hydroxyurea is associated with cutaneous findings consistent with dermatomyositis, with no associated evidence of muscle weakness, and usually with a negative ANA.
6. F. It is true that patients with violaceous erythema of the elbows, knees, or dorsal joints of the digits have Gottron sign and that lipodystrophy, calcinosis cutis, and vasculopathic ulcers are possible complications of JDM. The risk of malignancy in adults with DM is in fact 20 to 25%, and the risk remains elevated for at least 3 to 5 years, so that malignancy surveillance should be done annually for that period of time (perhaps longer). The most common lesion in DM is in fact the Gottron papule, not the heliotrope eruption.
7. B. A scleroderma-like disorder is not seen with argyria. Acrogeria, which sounds like argyria, is a premature aging syndrome that can be associated with scleroderma-like changes. Crowe-Fukase syndrome is another name for POEMS syndrome.

8. A. Toxic oil syndrome, which can present similarly to eosinophilic fasciitis, is associated with adulterated rapeseed oil exposure. However, it is a very small subset of patients with the clinical presentation. The other items are true.
9. A. Rheumatoid factor positivity is seen in types II and III cryoglobulinemia. The remaining associations are correct.
10. D. Trachyonychia is not commonly seen in patients with reactive arthritis (previously known as Reiter syndrome).

REFERENCES

Aggarwal K, Jain VK, Dayal S: Lupus erythematosus profundus. *Indian J Dermatol Venereol Leprol* 2002;68(6): 352–353.

András C, Ponyi A, Constantin T, et al. Dermatomyositis and polymyositis associated with malignancy: a 21-year retrospective study. *J Rheumatol* 2008;35(3):438–444.

Antic M, Lautenschlager S, Itin PH: Eosinophilic fasciitis 30 years after - what do we really know? Report of 11 patients and review of the literature. *Dermatology* 2006;23(2):93–101.

Baker WF Jr, Bick RL: The clinical spectrum of antiphospholipid syndrome. *Hematol Oncol Clin North Am* 2008;22(1):33–52, v-vi.

Belizna CC, Tron F, Joly P, Godin M, Hamidou M, Lévesque H: Outcome of essential cryofibrinogenaemia in a series of 61 patients. *Rheumatology (Oxford)* 2008;47(2):205–207.

Bernard P, Bonnetblanc JM: Dermatomyositis and malignancy. *J Invest Dermatol* 1993;100:128S–132S.

Bingham A, Mamyrova G, Rother KI, et al. Predictors of acquired lipodystrophy in juvenile-onset dermatomyositis and a gradient of severity. *Medicine (Baltimore)* 2008;87(2):70–86.

Bolognia JL, Jorizzo JL, Rapini RP, eds. *Dermatology*, 2nd Ed. Mosby: Elsevier; 2008.

Cepeda EJ, Reveille JD: Autoantibodies in systemic sclerosis and fibrosing syndromes: clinical indications and relevance. *Curr Opin Rheumatol* 2004;16(6):723–732.

Chung L, Lin J, Furst DE, Fiorentino D: Systemic and localized scleroderma. *Clin Dermatol* 2006;24(5):374–392.

Clements PJ, Furst DE, eds. *Systemic Sclerosis*. Baltimore: Williams & Wilkins; 1996.

Elyan M, Khan MA: Diagnosing ankylosing spondylitis. *J Rheumatol Suppl.* 2006;78:12–23.

Fernandez-Madrid F, Mattioli M: Antinuclear antibodies (ANA): immunologic and clinical significance. *Semin Arthritis Rheum* 1976;6:83.

Ferri C, Zignego AL, Pileri SA: Cryoglobulins. *J Clin Pathol* 2002;55:4–13.

Foti R, Leonardi R, Rondinone R: Scleroderma-like disorders. *Autoimmun Rev* 2008;7(4):331–339. Epub 2008 Jan 11.

Fritzler MJ: Antinuclear antibodies in the investigation of rheumatic disease. *Bull Rheum Dis* 1987;35:127–136.

Goldsmith LA et al. *Fitzpatrick's Dermatology in General Medicine*, 8th Ed. New York: McGraw-Hill; 2012.

Hamdulay SS, Glynne SJ, Keat A: When is arthritis reactive? *Postgrad Med J* 2006;82(969):446–453.

Hoffman, Robert W. DO; Greidinger, Eric L.: Mixed connective tissue disease. *Curr Opin Rheumatol* 2000;12(5):386–390.

Iorizzo LJ 3rd, Jorizzo JL: The treatment and prognosis of dermatomyositis: an updated review. *J Am Acad Dermatol.* 2008;59(1):99–112.

Kessel A, Toubi E, Rozenbaum M, Zisman D, Sabo E, Rosner I: Sjögren's syndrome in the community: can serology replace salivary gland biopsy? *Rheumatol Int* 2006;26(4):337–339. Epub 2005 Feb 10.

Klippel JH, Dieppe PA, eds. *Rheumatology*, 2nd Ed. London: Mosby; 1998.

Klippel JH, ed. *Primer on the Rheumatic Diseases*, 12th Ed. Atlanta: Arthritis Foundation; 2001.

McKee PH: *Pathology of the Skin: With Clinical Correlations*. London: Mosby-Wolfe; 1996.

Ortega-Loayza AG, Merritt BG, Groben PA, Morrell DS: Eosinophilic fasciitis in a female child. *J Am Acad Dermatol* 2008;58(5 Suppl 1): S72–S74.

Parmar RC, Bavdekar SB, Bansal S, Doraiswamy A, Khambadkone S: Scleredema adultorum. *J Postgrad Med* 2000;46(2):91–93.

Peterson LS, Nelson AM, Su WP: Classification of morphea (localized scleroderma). *Mayo Clin Proc* 1995;70:1068–1076.

Petrone D, Condemi JJ, Fife R, Gluck O, Cohen S, Dalgin P: A double-blind, randomized, placebo-controlled study of cevimeline in Sjögren's syndrome patients with xerostomia and keratoconjunctivitis sicca. *Arthritis Rheum* 2002;46(3):748–754.

Raffel GD, Gravallese EM, Schwab P, Joseph JT, Cannistra SA: Diagnostic dilemmas in oncology: case 2. Dermatomyositis and ovarian cancer. *J Clin Oncol* 2001;19(23):4341–4343.

Sigurgeirsson B, Lindelöf B, Edhag O, Allander E: Risk of cancer in patients with dermatomyositis or polymyositis: a population-based study. *N Engl J Med* 1992;326:363–367.

Sontheimer RD, Provost TT: *Cutaneous Manifestations of Rheumatic Diseases*, 2nd Ed. Philadelphia: Lippincott Williams and Wilkins; 2004.

Sparsa A, Liozon E, Herrmann F, et al. Routine vs extensive malignancy search for adult dermatomyositis and polymyositis: a study of 40 patients. *Arch Dermatol* 2002;138(7):885–890.

Provost T, Greenberg A, Falanga V: Localized cutaneous sclerosis. In R. Sontheimer, Provost T, eds. *Cutaneous manifestations of rheumatic diseases*. Philadelphia: Lippincott Williams & Wilkins: 2004;125–134.

Tan EM: Antinuclear antibodies: diagnostic markers for autoimmune diseases and probes for cell biology. *Adv Immunol* 1989;44:93.

Taylor W, Gladman D, Helliwell P: Classification criteria for psoriatic arthritis: development of new criteria from a large international study. *Arthritis Rheum* 2006;54(8):2665–2673.

Tedeschi A, Baratè C, Minola E, Morra E: Cryoglobulinemia. *Blood Rev* 2007;21(4):183–200.

Venables PJ: Mixed connective tissue disease. *Lupus* 2006;15(3): 132–137.

Wallace DJ, Hahn BH, eds. *Dubois' Lupus Erythematosus*, 5th Ed. Baltimore: Williams & Wilkins; 1997.

Zulian F: Systemic sclerosis and localized scleroderma in childhood. *Rheum Dis Clin North Am* 2008;34(1):239–255; ix.

Zulian F, Martini G: Childhood systemic sclerosis. *Curr Opin Rheumatol* 2007;19(6):592–597.

Zulian F, Woo P, Athreya BH, et al. The Pediatric Rheumatology European Society/American College of Rheumatology/European League against Rheumatism provisional classification criteria for juvenile systemic sclerosis. *Arthritis Rheum* 2007;57:203–212.

CHAPTER 23

METABOLIC DISEASES

JASON H. MILLER
ASRA ALI
NEIL FARNSWORTH

PORPHYRIAS

- Metabolic disorders of heme synthesis; may be hereditary or acquired
- Photosensitivity due to exposure of ultraviolet (UV) radiation in the Soret band (400–410 nm)

Classification of Porphyrias: Erythropoietic and Hepatic Forms (Based on the Primary Site of Expression of the Enzymatic Defect)

- Nonacute porphyrias: porphyria cutanea tarda (PCT), erythropoietic porphyria (EPP), congenital erythropoietic porphyria (CEP), and hepatoerythropoietic porphyria (HEP); most common cutaneous manifestation is photosensitivity
- Acute porphyrias: acute intermittent porphyria (AIP), variegate porphyria (VP), hereditary coproporphyria (HCP), and δ-aminolevulinic acid (ALA) dehydratase deficiency porphyria (plumboporphyria)
- Heme biosynthesis
  - Major sites of heme synthesis are bone marrow (85%) and in the liver
  - Initial reaction takes place in the mitochondrion within the cell
  - Condensation of 1-glycine and 1-succinylCoA by ALA synthase: this is the rate-limiting reaction of heme biosynthesis
  - Mitochondrial ALA is transported to the cytosol
  - ALA dehydratase (also called *porphobilinogen synthase*) dimerizes 2 molecules of ALA to produce porphobilinogen
  - Uroporphyrinogen I synthase, also called *porphobilinogen deaminase* or *PBG deaminase*, causes condensation of 4 molecules of porphobilinogen to produce intermediate hydroxymethylbilane
  - Hydroxymethylbilane undergoes enzymatic conversion to uroporphyrinogen III by uroporphyrinogen synthase plus a protein known as *uroporphyrinogen III cosynthase*
  - In the cytosol, the acetate substituents of uroporphyrinogen (normal uroporphyrinogen III or abnormal uroporphyrinogen I) are decarboxylated by uroporphyrinogen decarboxylase (UROD)
  - The resulting coproporphyrinogen III intermediate is transported to the interior of the mitochondrion, where, after decarboxylation, protoporphyrinogen IX results
  - In the mitochondrion, protoporphyrinogen IX is converted to protoporphyrin IX by protoporphyrinogen IX oxidase
  - Final reaction in heme synthesis takes place in the mitochondrion by ferrochelatase

ERYTHROPOIETIC PORPHYRIAS

Congenital Erythropoietic Porphyria (CEP)

GUNTHER DISEASE

- Autosomal recessive with complete absence of uroporphyrinogen III synthase (UROS) gene activity; affects uroporphyrinogen III synthase and the production of uroporphyrinogen III
- Results in massive accumulation and excretion of uroporphyrin I and coproporphyrin I
- Clinical findings (appear soon after birth)
  - *Cutaneous*: severe photosensitivity with burning, edema, bullae, mutilating scars, loss of brows/lashes, hypertrichosis, hyperpigmentation/hypopigmentation
  - *Ocular*: photophobia, kerato conjunctivitis, ectropion, symblepharon, loss of vision
  - *Other*: gallstones possible, cartilaginous breakdown, red/brown urine, erythrodontia (seen with Wood's lamp), splenomegaly, hemolytic anemia

- Laboratory findings
  - *Urine*: uroporphyrin I, coproporphyrin I
  - *Stool*: coproporphyrin I
  - *Blood*: plasma-uroporphyrin I, coprophorphyrin I; red blood cell (RBC): uroporphyrin I, coproporphyrin, and some protoporphyrin
- Other diagnostic tests: urine fluoresces reddish pink
- Treatment: strict photoprotection, splenectomy, blood transfusions, activated charcoal, hydroxyruea, oral ascorbic acid, and α-tocopherol

Erythropoietic Protoporphyria (EPP)

- Autosomal dominant, *FECH* gene mutation results in partial ferrochelatase deficiency
- Clinical findings
  - *Cutaneous* (photosensitivity): painful erythematous, edematous plaques after exposure to UV light that may heal with scarring, skin lichenification, waxy, leathery pseudovesicles, and nail changes
  - Hepatic: porphyrin gallstones (early age), liver disease (10% of patients): jaundice, cirrhosis
- Laboratory findings
  - *Urine*: normal (protoporphyrin IX is not water soluble)
  - *Stool*: protoporphyrin
  - *Blood* (RBC/plasma): protoporphyrin
- Treatment: photoprotection, β-carotene (60–300 mg/d), RBC transfusions, cholestyramine, activated charcoal
- Prognosis: normal life span if liver spared

CHRONIC HEPATIC PORPHYRIA

Porphyria Cutanea Tarda (PCT) (Fig. 23-1)

- Most common of the porphyrias
- Autosomal dominant
- UROD deficiency in the liver
- Three types: type 1: decreased hepatic UROD activity, but normal erythrocyte UROD activity (sporadic fashion); type II: decreased UROD activity in red cells and in the liver (occurs in multiples in a family); type III: decreased hepatic UROD activity and normal erythrocyte activity (occurs in multiples in a family)
- Clinical findings
  - *Cutaneous*: chronic bullae, vesicles and erosions on sun-exposed skin, bullae and vesicles rupture easily, hypertrichosis, milia, and sclerodermoid changes
  - *Hepatic*: associated with hepatitis C, hepatocellular carcinoma, increased liver iron stores with or without hemochromatosis. 40% of PCT patients of northern European descent carry a high Fe (HFE) gene with 1 of 2 mutations (C282Y or H63D)
  - *Other*: HIV (human immunodeficiency virus) infection, dermatomyositis

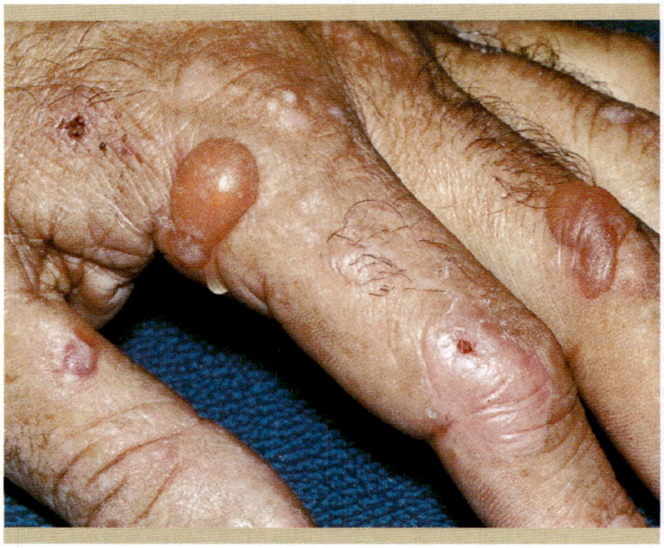

FIGURE 23-1 Porphyria cutanea tarda. (*Reproduced with permission from Goldsmith LA et al. Fitzpatrick's Dermatology in General Medicine, 8th Ed. New York: McGraw-Hill; 2012.*)

- Laboratory findings
  - *Urine*: uroporpyhrin I–III > coproporphyrin; coral-pink fluorescence of urine under Wood's lamp
  - *Stool*: isocoproporphyrins, coproporphyrin > uroporphyrin, tetracarboxyl porphyrins, protoporphyrin
  - *Blood*: RBC normal; plasma: increased uroporphyrin, serum iron increased
  - *Liver biopsy*: hepatocellular damage with fatty infiltration and hemosiderosis
- Treatment: photoprotection, phlebotomy (until serum transferrin saturation and serum ferritin levels are normalized, or hemoglobin level falls to 10 g/dL), antimalarials (hydroxychloroquine or chloroquine); recombinant erythropoietin for end-stage renal disease patients, avoidance of alcohol, estrogen, and iron supplements, interferon and ribavirin for hepatitis C

Hepatoerythropoietic Porphyria (HEP)

- Autosomal recessive
- Homozygous or compound heterozygous deficiency of UROD deficiency. In this case the deficiency exists in both the liver and the RBCs, as opposed to the liver—only in acquired UROD deficiency (PCT)
- Clinical findings
  - Resembles CEP, severe photophotosensitivity with burning, erythema, vesicles, bullae, mutilating scar formation, hypertrichosis, sclerodermoid skin changes
  - Other: hemolytic anemia, splenomegaly, dark urine at birth
- Laboratory findings
  - *Urine*: uroporphyrin I–III, isocoproporphyrin

  - *Stool*: uroporphyrin, coproporphyrin, isocoproporphyrin
  - *Blood*: RBC: protoporphyrin; plasma: uroporphyrin
- Treatment: photoprotection, red cell transfusion, hydroxyurea
- Prognosis: normal life span

ACUTE HEPATIC PORPHYRIAS

Acute Intermittent Porphyria (AIP)

- Autosomal dominant
- Mutation of porphobilinogen deaminase (PBGD) gene leading to deficient activity of the enzyme
- Attacks may be precipitated by drugs (barbiturates, sulphonamides), hormones, fever, smoking, infections, surgery, stress, or starvation
  - Clinical findings
  - No skin findings
  - Neuropathy, palsy, seizures, confusion, coma, abdominal pain, risk of hepatic carcinoma, hyponatremia common during acute attacks, due to inappropriate release of antidiuretic hormone
- Laboratory findings
  - Erythrocyte PBGD activity: reduced in type I and type III AIP patients; type II AIP patients show normal PBGD activity in erythrocytes, but have reduced PBGD activity in nonerythroid cells
  - *Urine*: latent: ALA and PBG; acute: ALA, PBG, uroporphyrin, and coproporphyrin
  - *Stool*: normal
  - *Blood*: normal
- Treatment: avoid precipitators, IV glucose loading and hematin infusions during attacks; supportive care
- Prognosis: acute attacks may be life threatening and leave residual neurologic deficits

Variegate Porphyria (VP)

- Most common in South Africans
- Autosomal dominant
- Protoporphyrinogen oxidase (PPO) deficiency
- Mixed porphyria: can present with neurological manifestations, cutaneous photosensitivity, or both
- Clinical findings
  - Skin lesions similar to PCT: fragility of skin, vesicles, bullae, erosions, milia, hyperpigmentation, hypertrichosis, and photosensitivity
  - Symptoms similar to AIP: abdominal pain, tachycardia, vomiting, constipation, hypertension, neuropathy, back pain, confusion, bulbar paralysis, psychiatric symptoms, fever, urinary frequency, dysuria, and hyponatremia
  - Attacks may be precipitated by alcohol, hormones, and drugs (dapsone, anticonvulsants, barbiturates, sulfonamides, griseofulvin)
- Laboratory findings
  - *Urine*: ALA, PBG, uroporphyrin elevated during attacks; coproporphyrin > protoporphyrin (acute and asymptomatic periods: helps distinguish from PCT, where uroporphyrins are always elevated)
  - *Stool*: protoporphyrin and coproporphyrin elevated
  - *Blood*: presence of plasma porphyrin (fluoresces at 626 nm)
  - *Biliary porphyrins*: increased risk of gallstones in VP, consist mainly of protoporphyrin
- Treatment: avoid precipitators, photoprotection, and intravenous/oral glucose. Treat acute attacks similar to AIP

Hereditary Coproporphyria (HCP)

- Autosomal dominant
- Coproporphyrinogen oxidase (CPO) deficiency
- Exacerbated by: barbiturates, endogenous or exogenous steroid hormones
- Clinical findings
  - Similar to AIP and VP, with gastrointestinal (GI) and neurologic attacks
  - *Cutaneous*: photosensitive bullae (30% of patients), hypertrichosis
  - Other: hemolytic anemia beginning in childhood, increased risk of hepatocellular carcinoma
- Laboratory findings
  - *Urine*: coproporphyrin III; ALA, PBG, and uroporphyrin also increased during attacks
  - *Stool*: coproporphyrin III
  - *Blood*: normal
- Treatment: avoid precipitators, photoprotection
  - Treat acute attacks as with AIP

δ-ALA Dehydratase Porphyria (ADP)

- Autosomal recessive
- ALA-D mutation → ALA dehydratase deficiency
- Clinical findings: no skin lesions. Symptoms similar to AIP
- Laboratory findings
  - *Urine*: ALA, coproporphyrin, uroporphyrin
  - *Stool*: coproporphyrin, protoporphyrin
  - *Blood*: protoporphyrin
  - Treatment: avoid offending agents such as alcohol and stress, intravenous infusion of glucose

SPHINGOLIPIDOSES (LIPID STORAGE DISORDERS)

- Diseases caused by defects in genes encoding proteins involved in the lysosomal degradation of sphingolipids
- Leads to lysosomal accumulation of the enzyme-specific sphingolipid substrate

- Diseases are named according to the identity of the storage material
- Mode of inheritance is autosomal recessive except for Fabry disease (X-linked recessive)

Fabry Disease (Angiokeratoma Corporis Diffusum)

- X-linked recessive
- Xq22, defective lysosomal α-galactosidase A
- Results in accumulation and deposition of glycosphingolipids (globotriaosylceramide, ceramide trihexoside) in plasma and lysosomes of vascular endothelial and smooth muscle cells
- Clinical findings (presents in adolescence)
  - *Ocular*: corneal and lenticular opacities
  - *Vascular*: ischemia, coronary artery disease, cerebrovascular accident (CVA), peripheral neuropathy
  - *Cutaneous*: angiokeratomas of lower trunk, thighs, oral/ocular mucosa (Fig. 23-2)
  - *Other* (renal failure, Maltese crosses in urine): lipid inclusions with characteristic birefringence, painful crises of the hands/feet (acroparesthesias), sensorineural deafness, hypohidrosis
- Treatment: Fabrazyme (agalsidase beta): enzyme replacement therapy arrests progression of disorder, dialysis, symptomatic pain management, phenytoin, and carbamazepine for paresthesias

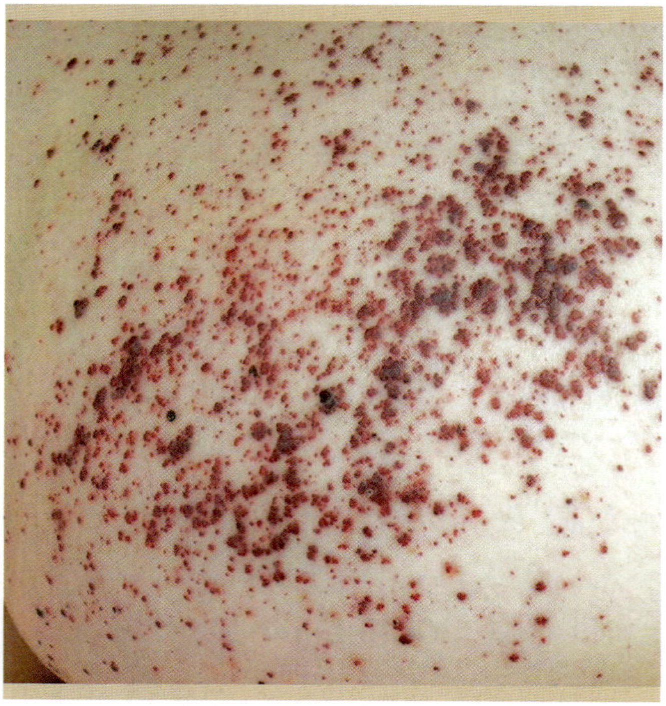

FIGURE 23-2 Angiokeratomas. (*Reproduced with permission from Wolff et al. Fitzpatrick's Dermatology in General Medicine, 7th Ed. New York: McGraw-Hill; 2008.*)

- Prognosis: death by fifth decade from myocardial infarction, CVA, and renal failure

Gaucher Disease

- Most common form of sphingolipidoses. Most common in patients of Ashkenazi Jewish descent
- Autosomal recessive
- Decreased β-glucocerebrosidase activity with resulting accumulation of glucocerebroside in histiocytes (Gaucher cells)
- Clinical findings
  - *Type I* (adult): attenuated form; diffuse hyperpigmetation, petechiae, ecchymoses, bone pain, fractures, aseptic necrosis of femoral head, hepatosplenomegaly, lymphadenopathy, pingueculae (limbal deposits on the eyes), and pancytopenia
  - *Type II* (infantile): acute form; central nervous system (CNS) involved with hypertonicity, neck rigidity, laryngeal spasm, dysphagia, hepatosplenomegaly, aspiration pneumonia, subset with severe congenital ichythosis and collodion membrane
  - *Type III*: (juvenile) subacute form; intermediate variant of types I and II
- Laboratory studies
  - Gaucher cell in the reticuloendothelial system: macrophages are enlarged with cytoplasmic inclusions
  - Elevated glucosylceramide, angiotensin-converting enzyme, ferritin, and acid phosphatase in plasma
  - X-ray: Erlenmeyer flask deformity of the distal femur
- Treatment
  - *Type I:* imiglucerase (Cerezyme), a recombinant-derived analogue of β-glucocerebrosidase; bone marrow transplant, splenectomy
  - *Type II*: supportive care, antibiotics (enzyme replacement is unable to cross blood-brain barrier); death at 1 to 2 years owing to aspiration
  - *Type III*: bone marrow or stem cell transplants

Niemann-Pick Disease (NPD)

- Autosomal recessive
- High incidence in patients of Ashkenazi Jewish descent
- Types A and B due to mutation in the sphingomyelin phosphodiesterase 1 (SMPD1) gene → acid sphingomyelinase (ASM) deficiency with sphingomyelin accumulation (foam cells)
- Type C is due to NPC-1 or NPC-2 gene deficiency
- Secondary drug-induced degradation of ASM → lysosomal storage of sphingomyelin (caused by tricyclic antidepressants)
- Clinical findings
  - Type A (most common): xanthomas, psychomotor deterioration, hepatosplenomegaly, failure to thrive, lymphadenopathy, blindness, and cherry red spots in fovea, deafness, pneumonia

- Type B: CNS spared, pulmonary infiltration, hepatosplenomegaly
- Type C: developmental delay, psychomotor deterioration, hepatosplenomegaly; cholesterol esterification defect (normal sphingomyelinase)
- Laboratory studies: Niemann-Pick cells: lipid-laden foam cells
- Prognosis
- *Type A*: death by 2 to 3 years with failure to thrive, pneumonia
- *Type B*: death in adolescence or adulthood; treatment with bone marrow transplant
- *Type C*: death in adolescence

Fucosidosis

- Autosomal recessive
- *FUCA 1* gene on chromosome 1p34 results in α-L-fucosidase deficiency: abnormal accumulations of glycosphingolipids, glycolipids, and glycoproteins (fucose-containing compounds)
- Clinical findings
    - Type I: neurologic changes, cardiomegaly, severe mental retardation, respiratory tract infections, hyperhidrosis, dysostosis multiplex, elevated sweat chloride, seizures
    - Type II: late infantile onset, short stature, coarse facies, mental retardation, hypertonia; sweat chloride normal, angiokeratomas (similar distribution to Fabry disease), longer survival than type I
- Treatment: laser therapy for angiokeratomas

Farber (Acid Ceramidase Deficiency, Lipogranulomatosis)

- Autosomal recessive
- *ASAH* gene → deficiency of lysosomal acid ceramidase and storage of ceramide in the lysosomes
- Clinical findings
- Subcutaneous nodules (lipogranulomas), painful and progressive joint deformations, periarticular swelling, mild macular degeneration of the eyes, pulmonary failure, progressive hoarseness, mental retardation
- Treatment: bone marrow transplantation, which improves the peripheral, but not the neurological manifestations

Mucopolysaccharidoses (MPS) (Lysosomal Storage Diseases)

- Inherited deficiency of enzymes that are involved in the degradation of glycosaminoglycans (GAGs); also referred to as *acid mucopolysaccharides* (Table 23-1)
- Dermatan sulfate, heparan sulfate, keratan sulfate (KS), and chondroitin sulfate are the main GAGs in tissues composed of sulfated sugar and uronic acid residues (except for KS)
- Diseases are autosomal recessive, except for MPS type II (Hunter), which is X-linked recessive
- Mucopolysaccharide staining
    - *Acid*: hematoxylin and eosin, Giemsa, colloidal iron mucicarmine, Alcian blue, pH 2.5, methyl and toluidine blue
    - *Neutral*: periodic acid–Schiff (PAS), gomori methenamine silver
    - *Sulfated*: aldehyde fuchsin, Alcian blue, pH 0.5

Hurler Syndrome (MPS-IH, Gargoylism)

- Autosomal recessive
- Defect in α-L-iduronidase → accumulation of dermatan and heparan sulfate
- Clinical findings
    - Coarse facies with macrocephaly, hypertelorism, hirsutism, valvular disease, umbilical hernias, upper respiratory infections, corneal opacities, short stature, dysostosis multiplex
- Scheie MPS-IS mild form of the MPS-IH, onset at 5 or 6 years, aortic valve disease, joint stiffness, claw hands, deformed feet, genu valgum, deafness, corneal clouding, normal intelligence, and life span
- Scheie and Hurler compound syndromes (MPS-IH/S): clinically intermediate between types IH and IS, healthy at birth; onset of symptoms at 3 to 8 years, corneal clouding, joint stiffness, dysostosis multiplex, and heart disease
- Course: deaths caused by upper airway obstruction and pulmonary complications
- Treatment: bone marrow transplantation for Hurler syndrome (not helpful for Hunter); laronidase: increases catabolism of GAGs; corrective surgery for joint contractures; corneal transplants; and valve replacement

Hunter Syndrome (MPS II)

- X-linked recessive
- Defect of iduronate 2-sulfatase → accumulation of heparan and dermatan sulfate
- Clinical findings
    - Type A: severe form, clinical features similar to MPS-IH
    - *Cutaneous*: ivory papules distributed symmetrically between the angles of the scapulae and posterior axillary lines; marker for the disease, hypertrichosis may result in synophrys
    - *Ocular*: atypical retinitis pigmentosa
- Type B: mild form, clinical features similar to MPS-IS, airway obstruction secondary to accumulation of mucopolysaccharide in the trachea and bronchi, deafness
- Treatment: symptomatic care; enzyme replacement

Sanfilippo Syndrome (MPS Type III)

- Heparan-*N*-sulfatase deficiency → accumulation of heparan sulfate
- Clinical: regression of psychomotor development, hyperactivity, autistic features, behavioral disorder

TABLE 23-1 Mucopolysaccharidoses (MPS)

Number	Syndrome Name	Enzyme Deficiency	Glycosaminoglycan Stored
MPS I (severe)	Hurler	α-L-iduronidase	Dermatan sulfate, heparan sulfate
MPS I (attenuated)	Scheie	α-L-iduronidase	Dermatan sulfate, heparan sulfate
MPS I (attenuated)	Hurler-Scheie	α-L-iduronidase	Dermatan sulfate, heparan sulfate
MPS II (severe)	Hunter (severe)	Iduronate sulfatase	Dermatan sulfate, heparan sulfate
MPS II (attenuated)	Hunter (mild)	Iduronate sulfatase	Dermatan sulfate, heparan sulfate
MPS IIIA	Sanfilippo A	Heparan *N*-sulfatase	Heparan sulfate
MPS IIIB	Sanfilippo B	α-*N*-acetyl-glucosaminidase	Heparan sulfate
MPS IIIC	Sanfilippo C	Acetyl CoA: α-glucosaminide acetyltransferase	Heparan sulfate
MPS IIID	Sanfilippo D	*N*-acetylglucosamine sulfatase	Heparan sulfate
MPS IVA	Morquio, type A	Galactose-6-sulfatase	Keratan sulfate, chondroitin 6-sulfate
MPS IVB	Morquio, type B	β-Galactosidase	Keratan sulfate
MPS VI	Maroteaux-Lamy	*N*-acetylgalactosamine 4-sulfatase (arylsulfatase B)	Dermatan sulfate
MPS VII	Sly	β-Glucuronidase	Dermatan sulfate, heparin sulfate, chondroitin 4-, 6 sulfates
MPS IX		Hyaluronidase	Hyaluronan

Morquio Syndrome (MPS Types IVA and IVB)

- Type A: *N*-acetylgalactosamine-sulfatase deficiency → accumulation of KS and chondroitin-6-sulfate
- Type B: β-Galactosidase deficiency → accumulation of chondroitin-6-sulfate
- Clinical findings: kyphoscoliosis, pectus carinatum, subluxation of the hips, aortic valvular disease, odontoid hyperplasia

Maroteaux-Lamy Syndrome (MPS Type VI)

- Arylsulfatase B (*N*-acetyl glucosamine-4-sulfatase) with accumulation of dermatan sulfate
- Clinical: first signs usually appear in the first 2 years of life, psychomotor retardation, clinically resembles Hurler syndrome
- Treatment: galsulfase enzyme replacement

Sly Syndrome (MPS Type VII)

- β-Glucuronidase deficiency
- Clinical findings: facial deformities: hypertelorism, prominent maxilla, depressed bridge of the nose; hydrops fetalis in neonatal form, hepatosplenomegaly

DISORDERS OF AMINO ACID METABOLISM

Alkaptonuria/Ochronosis

- Autosomal recessive
- Chromosome 3q, deficient homogentisic acid oxidase (HGA)
- Intermediate product of phenylalanine and tyrosine breakdown; excessive amounts of HGA are excreted in the urine and turn into a brown pigment on exposure to air causing the urine to appear dark
- Ochronosis is the connective tissue manifestation of alkaptonuria: in the body, polymerized HGA accumulates in connective tissues, such as the skin and cartilage resulting in pigmentation and degeneration
- HGA inhibits enzymes that are needed for the cross-linking of collagen fibers, which can result in degeneration of cartilage resulting in arthralgias
- *Exogenous ochronosis*: caused by medications such as quinacrine, carbolic acid, hydroquinone, phenol, resorcinol, picric acid, and antimalarials; metabolism of these medications results in an HGA polymer-like substance that differs from the polymer found in alkaptonuria

- Clinical findings
  - *Cutaneous*: macular blue-gray pigmentation on face, sclera, pinna, nasal ala, papules, milia, and nodules
  - *Skeletal*: narrowing of the joint spaces and disc calcifications, large joint arthropathy
  - *Other*: cardiac valve calcification, stenosis, coronary artery calcification, renal stones, black cerumen and sweat, dark urine at pH >7
  - *Exogenous ochronosis*: no joint involvement
- Diagnosis: urinary homogentisic acid level; darkening of urine with NaOH
  - *Histology*: ochronotic (yellow-brown) pigment in dermis, "yellow bananas," and within macrophages, homogenization and swelling of collagen bundles
  - Magnetic resonance imaging (MRI): thickened tendons, asymptomatic tears
  - Echocardiogram and computed tomography (CT): coronary artery calcifications and cardiac valve defects
  - Ultrasound and x-ray: renal stones
- Treatment (pigment changes persist): analgesics, physical therapy, supplemental vitamin C, nitisinone (inhibits homogentisic acid production)

Phenylketonuria (PKU)

- Autosomal recessive; chromosome arm 12q
- Deficiency of phenylalanine hydroxylase, cofactor required for hydroxylation of tyrosine (a precursor of dopamine) and hydroxylation of tryptophan (a precursor of serotonin)
- Clinical findings (presents at birth)
  - Toxic CNS effects: mental retardation, seizures, hyperreflexia, microcephaly, brain calcification, cataracts
  - *Cutaneous*: generalized hypopigmentation, blond hair, blue eyes; due to tyrosine deficiency, eczema, sclerodermoid skin (spares hands and feet), photosensitivity
  - Urine and sweat has "mousy" odor (due to phenylacetic acid)
- Diagnosis: check for serum elevation of phenylalanine, neonatal screening, and elevated urinary phenylpyruvic acid level
- Treatment: begin low-phenylalanine diet early to prevent CNS and skin changes; supplemental tyrosine, supplemental tetrahydobiopterin
- Course: normal life span if treated early

Homocystinuria

- Autosomal recessive
- Cystathionine β-synthetase deficiency, results in defect of methionine metabolism, and accumulation of homocystine
- Competitive inhibitor of tyrosinase
- Clinical findings (presents in early childhood)
  - *Cutaneous*: malar flush, livedo reticularis, pale and pink skin; due to tyrosine deficiency, buccal skin shows red macules, hyperhidrosis, xerosis, acrocyanosis, and leg ulcers
  - Occular: ectopia lentis with downward displacement, glaucoma
  - Vascular: cerebrovascular occlusions, deep venous thrombosis
  - *Other*: mental retardation, seizures, marfanoid habitus
- Treatment: low methionine, high-cystine diet, pyridoxine (300–600 mg/d), folic acid, betaine, and cyanocobalamin
- Course: death in third to fourth decade from vascular events

Richner-Hanhart Syndrome (Tyrosinemia II)

- Autosomal recessive
- Hepatic tyrosine aminotransferase (TAT) deficiency
- Tyrosinemia types I and III do not have skin involvement
- Clinical findings
  - *Ocular*: herpetiform corneal ulcers, photophobia, corneal clouding with central opacities, neovascularization, blindness
  - *Cutaneous*: focal or diffuse yellowish palmoplantar keratoderma, lesions associated with hyperhidrosis, erosions, bullae, hyperkeratotic plaques on elbows, knees in older patients
  - *Other*: mental retardation, seizures, self-mutilation
- Diagnosis: plasma amino acid and urine organic acid levels of tyrosine are elevated; urinary tyrosine metabolite levels are elevated
- Treatment: topical therapy, oral retinoids, low-phenylalanine/tyrosine diet can prevent skin and eye manifestations

DEPOSITION DISORDERS

Lipoid Proteinosis (Urbach-Wiethe Disease, Hyalinosis Cutis et Mucosae)

- Autosomal recessive
- Defect in extracellular matrix protein 1 (encoded by the *ECM1* gene); *ECM1* is known to inhibit bone mineralization, contribute to epidermal differentiation, and stimulate angiogenesis
- Accumulation of eosinophilic material composed of mucopolysaccharides, hyaluronic acid, neutral fat, lipids, and cholesterol
- Clinical findings
  - *Cutaneous*: patchy areas of alopecia may develop where hyaline deposits are present, early bullae formation on the face and distal extremities that heal with ice-pick scarring, infiltrated nodules on elbows, knees, and hands, skin becomes waxy, thickened, and yellow, beaded papules along the eyelid margins (moniliform blepharosis) (Fig. 23-3)
  - *Oral cavity*: cobblestone appearance to mucosa due to infiltrative papules on mucous membranes, large "wooden" tongue, parotiditis, dental anomalies

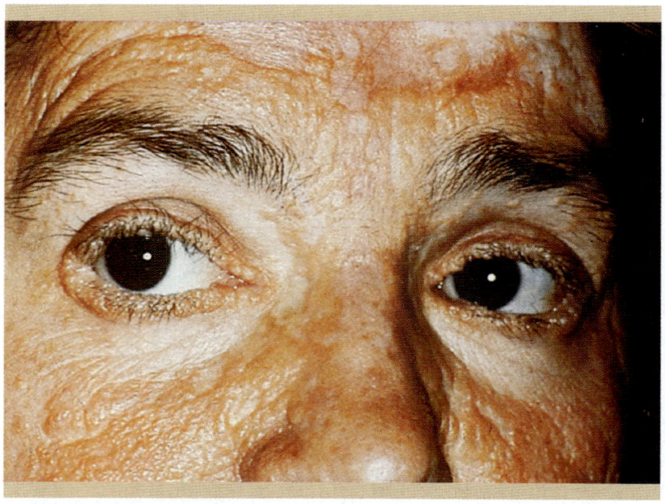

FIGURE 23-3 Lipoid proteinosis. (*Used with permission from O. Braun-Falco, Munich. Reproduced from Goldsmith LA et al. Fitzpatrick's Dermatology in General Medicine, 8th Ed. New York: McGraw-Hill; 2012.*)

  - *Neurologic*: psychiatric symptoms due to calcification of the termporal lobes
  - *Earliest sign*: hoarse cry due to vocal cord infiltration and possible airway compromise
- Diagnosis (CT or x-ray): hippocampal "bean-shaped" calcifications
- *Histology*: deposition of amorphous eosinophilic material at the dermal-epidermal junction, perivascularly and along adnexal epithelia. Hyaline material, PAS (+) and diastase resistant found perpendicular to the basement membrane. Arranged in "onion skin" layers around blood vessels; cytoplasmic vacuoles in dermal fibroblasts
- Treatment: oral dimethylsulfoxide, retinoids may be helpful, CO_2 laser for skin lesions, vocal cord lesions, and eyelid papules

Wilson Disease (Hepatolenticular Degeneration)

- Autosomal recessive
- Defect of *ATP7B* gene: copper-transporting adenosine triphosphatase (ATPase) in the liver
- Excessive absorption of copper from the small intestine
- Decreased excretion of copper by the liver; decreased serum ceruloplasmin and increased copper in the liver
- Diagnostic criteria: 7 criteria, including (1) presence of Kayser-Fleischer (KF) rings; (2) typical neurological symptoms; (3) decreased serum ceruloplasmin concentration; (4) Coombs negative hemolytic anemia; (5) elevated urinary copper excretion; (6) high liver copper value in the absence of cholestasis; and (7) mutational findings
- Clinical findings (seen in childhood to adulthood)
  - Copper accumulates in liver, brain, and cornea
  - *Hepatic*: hepatomegaly, cirrhosis
  - *Ocular* (KF ring): deposition of copper in Descemet membrane of cornea
  - *Cutaneous*: pretibial hyperpigmentation, blue lunulae, jaundice, varices, spider angiomas, and palmar erythema
  - *Other*: dysarthria, ataxia, dementia
- Diagnosis: low serum ceruloplasmin (copper carrier) levels, total serum copper levels are low and serum free-copper levels are elevated
- Treatment: D-penicillamine (risk of EPS), copper chelators, liver transplant, decreased copper intake. Symptoms reverse (except CNS) with early treatment

Hemochromatosis

- Autosomal recessive
- Mutations in the *HFE* gene; chromosome 6 (H63D and C282Y are the most common mutations)
- Hereditary hemochromatosis (HH) comprises a group of inherited disorders of iron metabolism that can result in progressive iron overload, morbidity, and mortality
- Increased iron absorption with solid-organ iron deposition
- Clinical findings (present in fifth decade)
  - *Cutaneous*: diffuse gray hyperpigmentation, sparse hair, koilonychia
  - *Hepatic*: hepatomegaly, cirrhosis, fibrosis, hepatocellular carcinoma
  - *Cardiac*: cardiac failure, arrhythmias
  - *Other*: diabetes, hypogonadism, polyarthritis
- Diagnosis: fasting serum transferrin saturation and ferritin levels elevated, serum iron levels increased, liver biopsy (fibrosis, cirrhosis)
- Treatment: serial phlebotomy, deferoxamine, supportive care of diabetes, arrhythmias
- Course: premature death owing to hepatic failure, hepatocellular carcinoma, heart disease

Amyloidosis

- Insoluble protein (misfolded plasma protein) fibrils accumulate extracellularly
- Up to 24 different proteins have been recognized; all share a common core structure that consists of a cross-β core and polypeptide chains (Table 23-2)
- Diagnosis: typing of systemic amyloidoses with refined immunohistochemical analysis and genetic testing
  - Systemic amyloidosis: histologic demonstration of amyloidosis within an organ; in AL amyloidosis fine needle aspiration of abdominal fat can substitute for histological demonstration of amyloidosis
- Histology: eosinophilic, amorphous, fissured masses of amyloid in dermis and subcutaneous tissue, extravasated RBCs, no lymph, intradermal bullae around blood vessels; amyloid rings (amyloid around individual fat cells)

TABLE 23-2 Classification of Amyloidoses

Amyloid Protein	Precursor	Systemic (S) or Localized (L)	Syndrome or Involved Tissue
AL	Immunoglobulin light chain	S, L	Primary Myeloma-associated
AH	Immunoglobulin heavy chain	S, L	Primary Myeloma-associated Familial
ATTR	Transthyretin	S	Senile systemic
Aβ_2M	β_2-Microglobulin	S	Hemodialysis
AA	(Apo)serum AA	S	Secondary, reactive
AApoA-I	Apolipoprotein A-I	S	Familial
AApoA-II	Apolipoprotein A-II	S	Familial
AGel	Gelsolin	S	Familial
ALys	Lysozyme	S	Familial
AFib	Fibrinogen α-chain	S	Familial
ACys	Cystatin C	S	Familial
ABri	ABriPP	L	Familial dementia
ADan	ADanPP	L	Familial dementia
Aβ	Aβ protein precursor (AβPP)	L	Alzheimer disease, aging
APrP	Prion protein	L	Spongioform encephalopathies
ACal	(Pro)calcitonin	L	C-cell thyroid tumors
AIAPP	Islet amyloid polypeptide	L	Islets of Langerhans Insulinomas
AANF	Atrial natriuretic factor	L	Cardiac atria
APro	Prolactin	L	Aging pituitary Prolactinomas
AIns	Insulin	L	Iatrogenic
AMed	Lactadherin	L	Senile aortic, media
AKer	Kerato-epithelin	L	Cornea; familial
A(tbn)	To be named	L	Pindborg tumors
ALac	Lactoferrin	L	Cornea; familial

- Stains
  - *Congo red* (brick red, apple-green birefringence)
  - *Cystal violet* (metachromasia [red])
  - *Methyl violet* (metachromasia)
  - *PAS + and diastase-resistant*
  - *Indirect immunofluoresence*: differentiates AA/AL
  - *Bone marrow*: 10% plasma cells (40% of patients)
  - *Bence-Jones protein*: monoclonal Ig light chain 90% in serum or urine
- *Immunoelectrophoresis*: monoclonal protein
- *Electron microscopy*: regular fibrillar structure
- X-ray diffraction: β-pleated sheet structure

Systemic Amyloidosis

- Fibril protein and related diseases, A amyloidosis protein (AA)
  - Formed by N-terminal proteolytic fragments of the acute-phase reactant serum amyloid A (SAA), a polymorphic apolipoprotein of high-density lipoproteins (HDL)
  - SAA is an acute-phase protein that increases secondary to chronic inflammatory stimuli (i.e., inflammatory arthritis, leprosy, osteomyelitis, tuberculosis, familial Mediterranean fever, Muckle Wells syndrome, Hodgkin disease, renal cell carcinoma)
- Clinical findings
  - *Cutaneous*: no skin findings
  - *Renal*: proteinuria, nephrotic syndrome, and progressive development of renal insufficiency
  - *Gastrointestinal*: constipation, diarrhea, and malabsorption
- Treatment: colchicine (to prevent AA amyloidosis in familial Mediterranean fever), treat primary inflammatory condition

AMYLOID LIGHT CHAIN (AL)

- Primary systemic ← formed by the N-terminal fragment of a monoclonal immunoglobulin light chain (usually λ subtype), comprising the variable region and a portion of the constant region, produced by a bone marrow plasma cell clone
- Clinical findings (almost any organ can be involved; multiple organ dysfunction is common)
  - *Renal*: nephrotic syndrome with peripheral edema
  - *Cardiac*: restrictive cardiomyopathy, arrhythmias
  - *Neurological*: neuropathies, carpal tunnel (17%)
  - *Mucocutaneous*: petechiae, soft tissues enlargement, papules, plaques, macroglossia, ecchymoses, pinch purpura (post-traumatic hemorrhage around orbits, umbilicus, axillae, perianal) (Fig. 23-4)
  - *Hepatic*: hepatosplenomegaly
  - *Gastrointestinal*: bleeding, weight loss

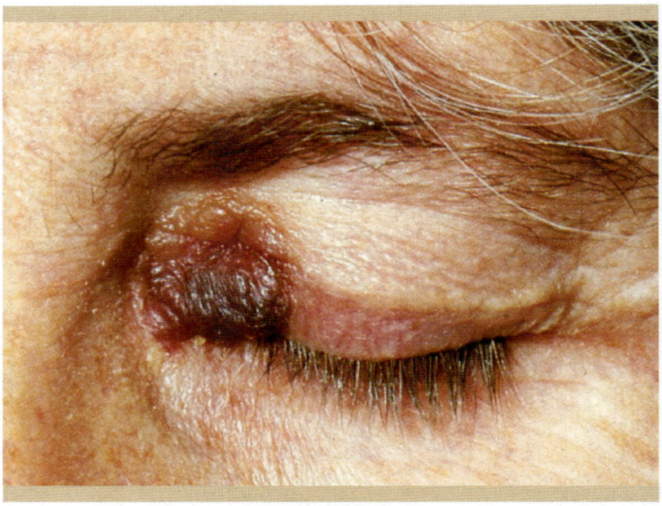

FIGURE 23-4 Amyloidosis of the eyelid. *(Reproduced with permission from Wolff et al. Fitzpatrick's Dermatology in General Medicine, 7th Ed. New York: McGraw-Hill; 2008.)*

HEREDITARY AMYLOIDOSIS

- Autosomal dominant, heterogenous group of diseases associated with mutations in apoliporoteins A1 and A2, fibrinogen A α chain, Gelsolin, lysozyme, cystatin C
- Clinical findings depend on the variant protein: deposits primarily in the peripheral nerves, heart, GI tract, and vitreous of eyes
- Familial amyloidotic polyneuropathy (FAP) types I/II
  - Mutation in transthyretin (TTR, transport protein synthesized in the liver and choroid plexus, transports thyroxine and retinol)
  - Most common type; treatment is liver transplantation
- FAP type III: mutation in apolipoprotein A1 mutation (lipid metabolism regulator)
- FAP type IV: mutation in Gelsolin (regulator of actin fiber organization). This form has cutis laxa
- Clinical findings: peripheral neuropathy, xerosis, seborrheic dermatitis, trauma or burn lesions, neuropathic ulcers, onychomycosis

DIALYSIS-RELATED AMYLOIDOSIS (DRA)

- β-2 Microglobulin protein accumulates in the serum
- Clinical findings: carpal tunnel syndrome, arthropathies, spondyloarthropathies, bone cysts, visceral amyloid deposition (heart, GI tract: macroglossia, bowel infarction and perforation; lungs)

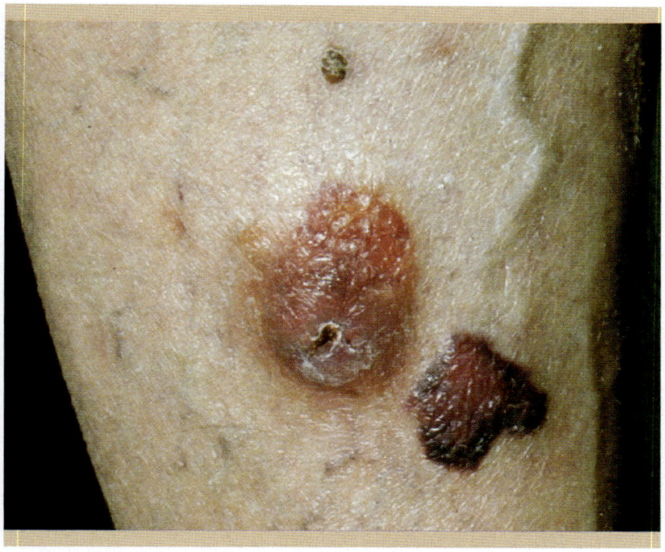

FIGURE 23-5 Nodular amyloidosis. (*Reproduced with permission from Freedberg IM et al. Fitzpatrick's Dermatology in General Medicine, 6th Ed. New York: McGraw-Hill; 2003.*)

Localized Cutaneous AL Amyloid (Nodular amyloidosis)

- Local production of fibril precursors derived from N-terminal cleavage fragments of monoclonal immunoglobulin light chains
- Deposition of AL protein; localized to the skin
- One or several nodules on legs/face (Fig. 23-5)
- Histology: atrophic epidermis, masses of amyloid dermis, subcutaneous fat, appears as "cracks in mud," lymphocytoplasmic infiltrate, Russell bodies: round hyaline, eosinophilic bodies inside/outside of plasma cells (with Ig), foreign-body giant cells
- Treatment: surgical excision, CO_2 laser
- Course: may develop systemic amyloidosis

MACULAR AND LICHEN AMYLOIDOSIS

- Due to altered keratin; amyloid deposits bind to antikeratin antibodies
- Usually idiopathic or friction related; also associated with connective tissue diseases (i.e., systemic lupus erythematosus [SLE])

Macular Amyloidosis

- Affects the upper back ← may result from constant scratching
- Clinical findings: pruritic brown-gray, reticulated, rippled, macules/patches mainly on upper back, notalgia paresthetica, some postinflammatory hyperpigmentation
- Diagnosis: *direct immunoflouresence*: IgM, C3, Ig, light chains
  - *Histology*: amyloid deposits in papillary dermis, globular, colloid deposition in dermis; do not involve blood vessels or adnexal structures

Lichen Amyloidosis

- Clinical findings: closely set, discrete brown-red papules, pruritic; commonly on the legs. Can be seen in multiple endocrine neoplasia type 2A (Sipple syndrome)
- Diagnosis: histology similar to macular amyloidosis but with irregular acanthosis
- Treatment: topical steroids, intralesional steroids, dimethyl sulfoxide (DMSO), calcineurin inhibitors, psoralen and ultraviolet A therapy, dermabrasion, acitretin

SENILE AMYLOIDOSIS

- Associated with Alzheimer disease, due to β amyloid = major fibril protein, amyloid precursor protein (APP)
- Senile/neuritic plaques: neurofibrillary tangles, vascular lesions, no skin lesions

XANTHOMAS

- Accumulations of lipid-laden macrophages; arise due to lipoprotein disorders
- Lipoproteins: lipids transported in plasma as complexes with specific apoproteins
- Lipoproteins: may be classified according to their buoyant density
  - *Chylomicrons*: dense collections of triglycerides (TG) that enter the circulation from the GI lymphatics and contain apolipoproteins C2 and E3/4 on their shell. In the peripheral tissues, these are hydrolyzed by lipoprotein lipase (LPL) into free fatty acids (FFA) and chylomicron remnants. Apo E3/4 then allows the remnants to be taken up by the liver via the LDL receptor. Hepatic lipase (HL) then hydrolyzes some TG to cholesterol, creating...
  - *Very low-density lipoproteins* (VLDLs): produced by the liver from chylomicron remnants, these lipoproteins contain less TG and more cholesterol, and have a tweaked Apo E and a new apolipoprotein, B-100, to facilitate their eventual return trip. VLDLs still carry Apo C2, allowing peripheral LPL to hydrolyze more TG, producing...
  - *Intermediate-density lipoproteins* (IDLs): now that LPL has worked on our particle a second time, the particle can return to the liver via Apo E and Apo B-100 binding to the and the LDL receptor. HL further hydrolyzes TG to cholesterol, forming...

- *Low-density lipoproteins* (LDLs): deliver cholesterol to the body for cell membranes, steroidogenesis, bile, and myelination. LDL can deliver unneeded cholesterol back to the liver via Apo B-100 and Apo E binding once again to the LDL receptor
- *High-density lipoproteins* (HDLs): take up unneeded free cholesterol from peripheral tissue and tack them onto IDL and LDL on their way back to the liver

PHENOTYPIC CLASSIFICATION OF HYPERLIPIDEMIAS (TABLE 23-3)

- Frederickson type I hyperlipidemia (familial chylomicronemia syndrome, autosomal recessive)
- Mutations in either LPL or apolipoprotein C2 (Apo C2) → impaired hydrolysis of chylomicrons into free fatty acids and remnants
  - Clinical findings
    - Eruptive xanthomas located over the buttocks, shoulders, and extensor surfaces, pancreatitis and lipemia retinalis
  - Laboratory: elevated TG, low LDL and HDL
  - Treatment: diet modification
- Frederickson type II hyperlipidemia (familial hypercholesterolemia, autosomal dominant)
- Genetic deficiency of the hepatic LDL receptor or of apolipoprotein B-100 (which along with Apo E binds to LDL receptor) → increased LDL in the serum
  - Clinical findings
    - Tendinous, tuberous, subperiosteal xanthomas, and xanthomatous plaques, as well as xanthelasmas
    - Treatment: high doses of statins, liver transplantation
- Frederickson type III hyperlipidemia (familial dysbetalipoproteinemia, broad-β disease)
- Accumulation of remnant lipoproteins (chylomicron remnants and VLDL remnants) due to a defective isoform of Apo E, named Apo E2 → poor hepatic uptake of chylomicron remnants, IDL, and LDL, leaving their plasma levels high
  - Clinical findings
    - Tuberous xanthomata, planar xanthomas, affecting the palms (xanthoma striatum palmare are fairly specific for this disorder)
  - Laboratory studies: cholesterol, TG increased; cholesterol to triglyceride ratio raised in VLDL
  - Treatment: fibric acids, nicotinic acid, statin
- Multifactorial hyperlipidemias
- Frederickson type IV hyperlipidemia (familial hypertriglyceridemia)
  - Liver overproduces VLDL and LDL
  - Xanthomas rare
  - Treatment: low fat diet, fibric acid
- Frederickson type V hyperlipidemia
  - Combined elevations in levels of chylomicrons and VLDL due to an unknown cause
  - Clinical findings
    - Eruptive xanthomas, pancreatitis
  - Treatment: low fat diet, fibric acids, weight reduction

Types of Cutaneous Xanthomas

- Xanthelasma palpebrarum (Fig. 23-6)
  - Most common of the xanthomas

TABLE 23-3 Frederickson Classification of Xanthoma

Frederickson Classification (Type)	Condition	Type of Xanthoma
I	Familial chylomicronemia	Eruptive xanthoma
IIa	Familial hypercholesterolemia Heterozygous Homozygous	Tendon, tuberous, plane (xanthelasma and intertriginous) 15% with xanthoma by second decade Xanthomata by age 6 years
IIb	Familial combined hypercholesterolemia	Palmar, tuberous, tuberoeruptive, xanthelasma
III	Familial dysbetalipoproteinemia	Palmar, tuberous, tuberoeruptive xanthoma, xanthelasma
IV	Familial hypertriglyceridemia	Rare eruptive xanthomas
V	Mixed hyperlipidemia	Eruptive xanthomas

Reprinted with permission from Wolff K et al. *Fitzpatrick's Dermatology in General Medicine*, 7th Ed. New York: McGraw-Hill; 2008

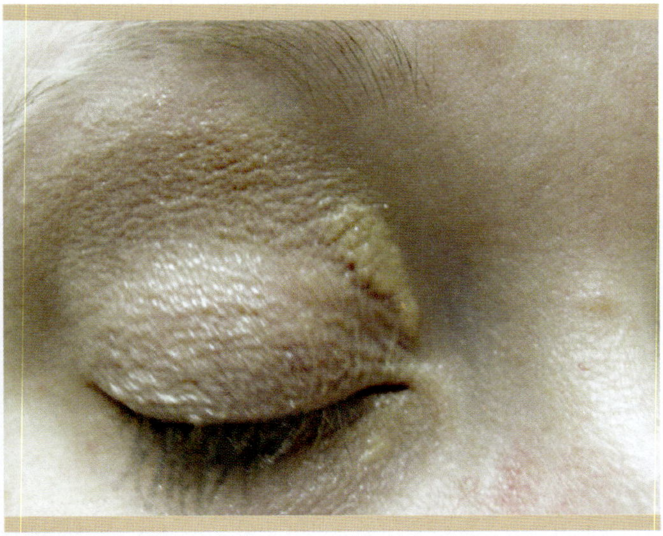

FIGURE 23-6 Xanthelasma palpebrarum. (*Used with permission from Dr. Asra Ali.*)

- Fifty-five percent of the patients may have hyperlipidemia
- Clinical: symmetric soft, velvety, yellow, flat, polygonal papules around the eyelids
- Treatment: trichloroacetic acid, surgical excision, cryotherapy, ablative laser treatment
- Tuberous xanthomas (Fig. 23-7)
  - Firm, painless, red-yellow nodules; can coalesce to form multilobulated tumors

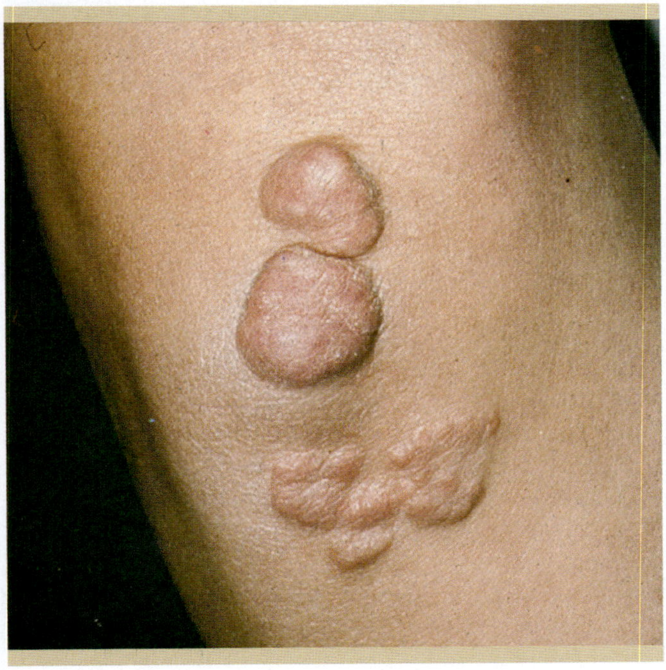

FIGURE 23-7 Tuberous xanthoma. (*Reproduced with permission from Goldsmith LA et al. Fitzpatrick's Dermatology in General Medicine, 8th Ed. New York: McGraw-Hill; 2012.*)

  - Develop in pressure areas, such as the extensor surfaces of the knees, the elbows, and the buttocks
- Tendinous xanthomas
  - Subcutaneous nodules related to the tendons or the ligaments
  - Most common locations are the extensor tendons of the hands, the feet, and the Achilles tendons
  - Often related to trauma
- Eruptive xanthomas
  - Crops of small, red-yellow papules on an erythematous base, pruritus is common
  - Most commonly arise over the buttocks, the shoulders, and the extensor surfaces of the extremities. May koebnerize
  - Types I, IV, and V hyperlipidemia, poorly controlled diabetics, hypothyroidism, oral retinoid therapy
  - May resolve spontaneously over weeks
- Planar xanthomas
  - Yellow macules, soft papules, commonly on palmar creases (xanthoma striatum palmare, common for type III hypercholesterolemia), eyelids (xanthelasma palpebrarum, 50% of patients normolipemic)
  - Generalized plane xanthomas: cover large areas of the face, neck, thorax, and flexures
  - May be associated with monoclonal gammopathy
- Xanthoma disseminatum
  - Occur in normolipemic patients
  - Red-yellow papules and nodules with a predilection for the flexures
  - Mucosa of the upper part of the aerodigestive tract is involved
  - Usually resolves spontaneously
- Verruciform xanthoma
  - Occurs in normolipemic patients (benign reactive condition)
  - Oral cavity of adults as a single papillomatous yellow lesion
  - Histology: vacuolated macrophages filled with lipid (foamy macrophages); lipids dissolved and removed from the tissue during histologic processing; multinucleated histiocytes (Touton giant cells)
- Treatment: local excision, topical trichloroacetic acid, electrodesiccation, laser therapy
- Prognosis: recurrences can occur

DIABETES-ASSOCIATED DISEASES

Acanthosis Nigricans

- Marker of insulin resistance
- Excessive amounts of circulating insulin bind with insulin-like growth factor (IGF-1) receptors on keratinocytes and dermal fibroblasts; increased proliferation of keratinocytes and fibroblasts

- Activation of tyrosine kinase receptors expressed on basal cells of the epidermis, → antiapoptotic and mitogenic effects on keratinocytes
- Associated conditions
    - Obesity: most common type; patients have higher fasting plasma insulin levels compared to control subjects
    - Syndromic
        - Type A syndrome: reduced number or dysfunction of insulin receptors, related to obesity
    - Hyperandrogenemia, insulin resistance, and acanthosis nigricans (HAIR-AN) syndrome
    - Polycystic ovaries or signs of virilization (hirsutism, clitoromegaly), high risk of developing diabetes
        - Type B syndrome: due to antibodies directed against the insulin receptor: uncontrolled diabetes mellitus, ovarian hyperandrogenism, or an autoimmune disease (SLE)
    - Examples of other associated syndromes and diseases: Cushing syndrome, connective tissue diseases (lupus erythematosus, scleroderma, dermatomyositis), hypothyroidism
    - Genetic benign (autosomal dominant): may develop at birth or during childhood; progresses until puberty, then stabilizes or regresses
    - Drug-induced: nicotinic acid, systemic corticosteroids, oral contraceptives
    - Malignant: most commonly adenocarcinoma of GI tract
- Clinical findings
    - Symmetric, hyperpigmented, velvety plaques with accentuation of skin markings (Fig. 23-8); develop in flexures, such as axillae, groin, and posterior neck
    - Tripe palms: thickening of the palms with accentuation of the ridges and furrows; thought to exist as a form of palmar acanthosis nigricans. Associated with acanthosis nigricans (75%), and with cancer (usually lung)
- Diagnosis
    - Laboratory findings: for patients with syndromic AN-glucose tolerance test; total testosterone, dehydroepiandrosterone sulfate (DHEA-S), gonadotropic concentrations, cortisol levels
    - Histology: hyperkeratosis, papillomatosis, and slight irregular acanthosis with minimal or no hyperpigmentation; the dermal papillae project upward as finger-like projections
- Treatment: correct the underlying disease, topical tretinoin, vitamin D3 analogs

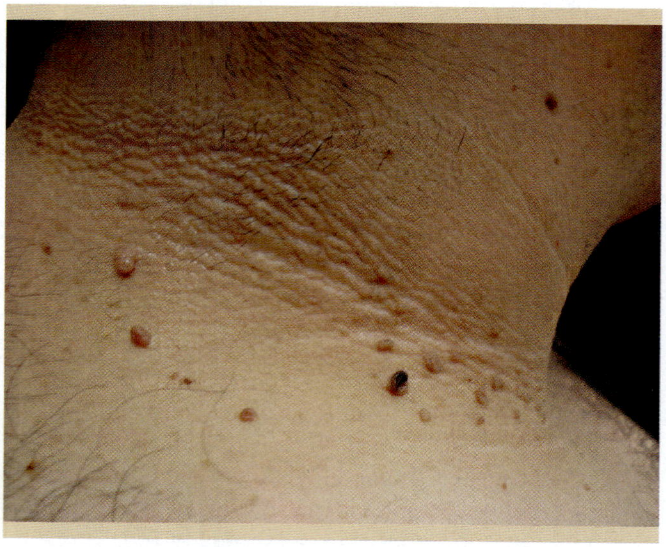

FIGURE 23-8 Acanthosis nigricans. (*Used with permission from Dr. Asra Ali.*)

Necrobiosis Lipoidica (Diabeticorum), NLD (Fig. 23-9)

- Degenerative disease of collagen in the dermis and subcutaneous fat
- Diabetics account for 14 to 65% of all cases; it occurs in 0.03% of diabetics
- Clinical findings
    - Well-circumscribed, symmetric, oval, or irregularly shaped indurated plaques with central atrophy, yellow pigmentation, and telangiectatic vessels on pretibial areas, periphery of lesions have red-brown or violaceous pigmentation

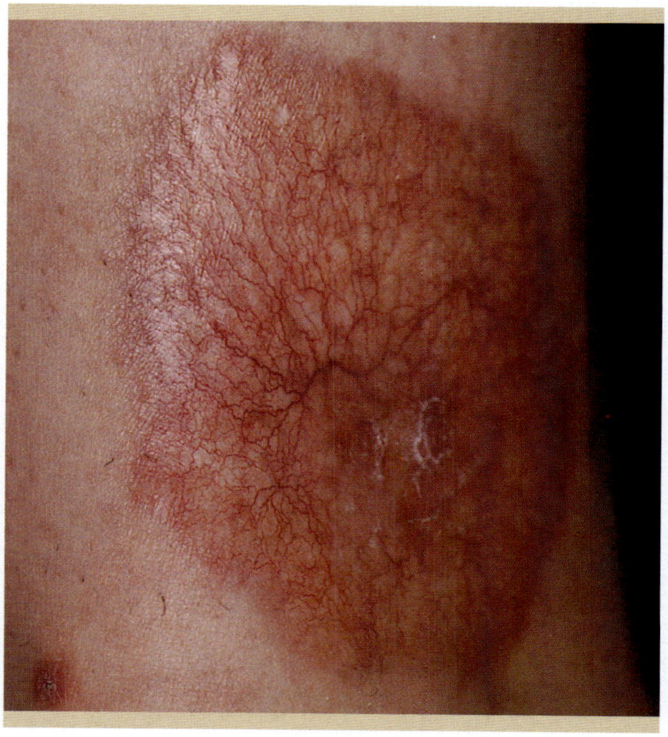

FIGURE 23-9 Necrobiosis lipoidica diabeticorum. (*Reproduced with permission from Goldsmith LA et al. Fitzpatrick's Dermatology in General Medicine, 8th Ed. New York: McGraw-Hill; 2012.*)

    - Koebner phenomenon present; decreased pinprick sensation
    - Lesions are typically multiple and bilateral and may ulcerate
- Diagnosis
    - Histology: neutrophilic vasculitis; granulomas are arranged in a tier-like fashion and are admixed with areas of collagen degeneration, thickening of the blood vessel walls; immune complex vasculitis
    - Direct immunofluorescence: may have immunoglobulin M, immunoglobulin A, C3, and fibrinogen in the blood vessels
    - Serum: increased fibronectin, factor VIII-related antigen, α_2-macroglobulin
- Treatment: topical and intralesional steroids, antiplatelet aggregation therapy with aspirin and dipyridamole; niacinamide, excision, and grafting
- Prognosis: progression of lesion does not correlate with glycemic level; course is indolent, spontaneous remission in less than 20% of patients

Diabetic Dermopathy

- Most common cutaneous finding in diabetes. More common in men
- Clinical findings
    - Round to oval atrophic hyperpigmented lesions on the pretibial ares of the lower extremities; sites of trauma
- Histology: edema of the papillary dermis, thickened superficial blood vessels, extravasation of erythrocytes, mild lymphocytic infiltrate
    - Course: resolves spontaneously

Bullosis Diabeticorum

- Confined to the extremities; occurs spontaneously; noninflammatory, 3 types:
    - Sterile with fluid: heals without scarring; histology shows intraepidermal cleavage without acantholysis
    - Hemorrhagic: heals with scarring, histology shows cleavage below the dermal-epidermal junction, destruction of anchoring fibrils
    - Multiple nonscarring bullae: sun-exposed areas, histology: cleavage at lamina lucida
    - Prognosis: runs a benign course

Diabetic Ulcers

- Ischemic ulcers, and/or neuropathic ulcers in patients with diminished sensation, especially on areas of pressure sites; present with a keratotic rim

Acquired Perforating Dermatosis

- Seen in patients with kidney failure associated with diabetes
- Kyrle disease (acquired perforating dermatosis): papules with a keratotic plug due to elimination of collagen and elastin, seen on the extensor surfaces of the lower extremities; histology shows hyperkeratosis surrounding a plug of degenerated material

GLUCAGONOMA SYNDROME

- Caused by glucagon-secreting tumors of the α cells of the pancreas, slow growing
- Associated with: hyperglucagonemia, diabetes mellitus, hypoaminoacidemia, cheilosis, normochromic, normocytic anemia, venous thrombosis, neuropsychiatric features
- Mucocutaneous findings: necrolytic migratory erythema (NME), predilection for the perineum, buttocks, groin, lower abdomen, and lower extremities; annular erythematous patches with blisters that erode atrophic glossitis, cheilosis, dystrophic nails, and buccal mucosal inflammation
- Prognosis: 50% of tumors are metastatic at the time of diagnosis

Carotenemia

- Associated with ingestion of yellow and green vegetables
- Slow conversion of β-carotene (provitamin A) to vitamin A in the small intestine
- Accelerated by thyroxine and hyperthyroidism
- Clinical findings: caratenoderma: yellow/orange color of skin, greatest concentration is in areas with increased sweating (nasolabial folds, forehead); lipophilic: may take months before color of skin returns to normal, sclerae and mucous membranes are spared (unlike in jaundice)
- Diagnosis: carotene excreted in the stool, skin, and urine

THYROID DERMOPATHY

- Associated with Graves disease (0.5–4%)
- Stimulatory autoantibodies directed at the thyrotropin receptor are the cause of hyperthyroidism
- Clinical findings
    - Graves disease is characterized by goiter, increased perspiration, heat intolerance, tachycardia, and exophthalmos
    - Cutaneous: warm and moist skin, with smooth texture; thin scalp hair, nails are thin, soft and friable with possible onycholysis with an upward curvature (Plummer nail); hyperpigmentation of the skin (diffuse or local)
    - Pretibial myxedema (PTM) (Fig. 23-10): due to deposition of hyaluronic acid in the dermis and subcutis; lateral or anterior aspect of the legs with pink to purple-brown bilateral, firm, nonpitting, asymmetric plaques or nodules, peau d'orange texture. IgG antibodies directed at the thyroid-stimulating hormone receptor (TSHR-Ab) are present in 80% of patients, elephantiasic form presents with verruciform plaques

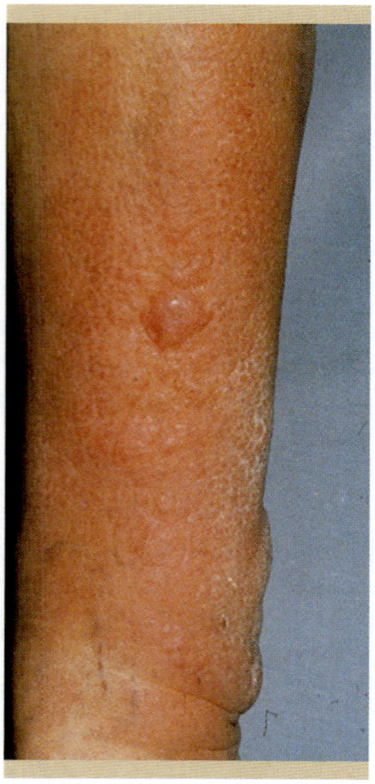

FIGURE 23-10 Thyroid dermopathy. Pretibial myxedema. (*Reproduced with permission from Wolff et al. Fitzpatrick's Dermatology in General Medicine, 7th Ed. New York: McGraw-Hill; 2008.*)

- Diagnosis
  - Histology: hyperkeratosis, mucin (GAGs) in the reticular dermis, and a Grenz zone of relatively normal papillary dermis; stains blue with Alcian blue, at a pH of 2.5, and colloidal iron stains; metachromasia with toluidine blue stain
  - Laboratory tests: serum thyroid function tests, thyroid-stimulating immunoglobulins
- Treatment: pretibial myxedema: topical or intralesional corticosteroids; plasmapheresis; octreotide

OSTEOMA CUTIS

- Presence of bone within the skin in the absence of a preexisting or associated lesion, such as
- Fibrodysplasia ossificans progressiva: AD; R206H substitution leading to ACVR1 mutation in bone morphogenic protein type 1 receptor leads to elevated bone morphogenic proteine-4 (BMP-4) levels in tissue, endochondral bone formation, early mortality
- Albright hereditary osteodystrophy: inactivating GNAS1 mutation (encodes α subunit of stimulatory G protein regulating adenylate cyclase, which may normally decrease bone formation), complex inheritance pseudohypoparathyroidism and pseudopseudohypoparathyroidism, short stature, round face, defective teeth, mental retardation, brachydactyly (short fourth metacarpals and metatarsals), tetany in patients with hypocalcemia, osteomas of the soft tissue and skin (intramembranous), miliary osteomas of the face, following acne, neurotic excoriation; milia-like ossification of syringomas in Down syndrome, progressive osseous heteroplasia (POH), intramembranous ossification, asymptomatic papules/nodules; "rice-grain" texture
- Plate-like osteoma cutis: a limited form of POH
- Secondary types: cutaneous ossification can also occur by metaplastic reaction to inflammatory, traumatic, and neoplastic processes
- Diagnosis
  - Laboratory findings: serum calcium and parathy-roid hormone (PTH) for hypoparathyroidism and pseudohypoparathyroidism (Albright)
  - Excisional biopsy
- Treatment: excision or laser resurfacing; tretinoin for miliary osteomas

NEPHROGENIC SYSTEMIC FIBROSIS (Nephrogenic Fibrosing Dermopathy)

- An acquired fibrosing disorder in patients with acute or chronic renal insufficiency, often after receiving Gadolinium dye for MRI
- Clinical findings
  - Symmetric, indurated plaques with brawny hyperpigmentation; may also present with distinct papules and subcutaneous nodules, extremities more commonly affected than trunk; face usually spared (distinguishing NFD from scleromyxedema, as does the lack of associated gammopathy), joint contractures with pain may be present; yellow plaques in sclera; fibrosis of heart, lungs, and skeletal muscle
- Diagnosis
  - Histology: thickened collagen bundles with surrounding clefts, mucin deposition, and proliferation of fibroblasts and elastic fibers; ± Gadolinium on tissue spectroscopy
  - Occasional CD34-positive and procollagen I positive dendritic fibroblasts ("circulating fibrocyte")
- Prognosis: course is progressive
- Treatment: there is no single treatment that has been shown to be effective

POLYCYSTIC OVARIAN SYNDROME

- Occurs in the presence of androgen excess with chronic anovulation without specific underlying disease of the adrenal or pituitary glands
- Other causes: congenital adrenal hyperplasia (CAH), ovarian and adrenal tumors, drugs (anabolic steroids, progestens, danazol)

- Diagnostic criteria requires the presence of 2 of the following 3 criteria:
  - Oligoovulation (<8 menses per 12-month period) and/or anovulation
  - Clinical hyperandrogenism and/or biochemical signs of hyperandrogenism
  - Polycystic ovaries (≥12 follicles in each ovary measuring 2–9 mm in diameter and/or increased ovarian volume [>10 mL]) by ultrasonography
- Cutaneous findings: acne vulgaris, seborrhea, androgenic alopecia, hirsutism, acanthosis nigricans; patients with virilization (secondary to severe hyperandrogenism): clitoromegaly, deepening of voice, increased muscle mass
- Other: secondary amenorrhea, infertility, menstrual alterations, obesity, insulin resistance with metabolic syndrome, risk of atherosclerosis
- Diagnosis
  - Laboratory: serum total testosterone, DHEA-S and prolactin; if total testosterone is greater than 200 ng/dL an ovarian tumor is suspected; if DHEA-S is over 8,000 ng/mL (normal is <4,000 ng/mL for women) an adrenal tumor is suspected; 17-hydroxyprogesterone to evaluate for late-onset CAH (abnormal is >3 ng/mL), deficient follicle stimulating hormone (FSH), increased luteinizing hormone (LH), evaluation of glucose intolerance
  - *Imaging*: transvaginal ultrasound for evaluation of ovarian tumor, CT scan of adrenal glands to exclude and adrenal mass
- Treatment: oral contraceptives, antiandrogens (i.e., spironolactone), metformin, oral contraceptive pills

HYPOPARATHYROIDISM/ PSEUDOHYPOPAR ATHYROIDISM

- Hypoparathyroidism can result from surgery, infiltrative disorders, autoimmune conditions, or may be idiopathic
- Pseudohypoparathyroidism is a heritable disorder of target organ unresponsiveness to parathyroid hormone
- Cutaneous findings: xerosis, hyperkeratosis, brittle nails, transverse ridging, coarse and sparse hair, eczematous dermatitis, Albright hereditary osteodystrophy (short neck, brachydactyly, subcutaneous ossifications)

CUSHING SYNDROME

- Results from chronic glucocorticoid excess, caused mainly by pituitary hypersecretion of adrenocorticotropic hormone (ACTH) or by nonpituitary tumors, adrenal hypersecretion of hyperinsulinism or exogenous administration of corticosteroids
- Clinical findings: progressive central (centripetal) obesity, fat deposition in the cheeks resulting in moon facies
  - *Cutaneous*: atrophic skin, loss of subcutaneous tissue, easy bruising, striae densae (violaceous > 1 cm) commonly seen on upper arms, shoulders, axillae, breasts, hips, buttocks, and upper thighs; hyperpigmentation may be generalized, most evident in areas exposed to light; vellus hair on forehead and cheeks; if androgen excess is present then hirsutism, oily facial skin, and acneiform rashes may occur
- Diagnosis: 24-hour urinary free cortisol (UFC), serum ACTH to define the source (low: adrenal; normal to high: pituitary; very high: ectopic)
- Treatment: dependent on the cause. Surgery for pituitary, adrenal, or ectopic tumors with possible radiation or chemotherapy; medications that inhibit steroid synthesis

ADDISON DISEASE

- Chronic primary adrenal insufficiency; most commonly an autoimmune adrenalitis, but can be due to infection, hemorrhage, neoplasia
- Clinical findings
  - Cutaneous: generalized hyperpigmentation due to increased melanin content in the skin, due to the melanocyte-stimulating activity of high plasma ACTH concentration; nails with longitudinal pigmented bands
- Diagnosis: cosyntropin (synthetic ACTH) stimulation test with serum cotisol measurements; plasma ACTH, hyponatremia, hyperkalemia, hyperchloremic metabolic acidosis; CT of adrenal glands
- Treatment: replace glucocoricoids

ACROMEGALY

- Due to excessive secretion of growth hormone (GH); usually due to a pituitary adenoma
- Clinical findings
  - Cutaneous: soft-tissue overgrowth, enlarged jaw (macrognathia), swollen hands and feet, thickened skin with a doughy feel, coarse facial features with accentuation of facial folds; thick eyelids, enlarged lips, thick and hard nails, hyperhidrosis (50%)
- Diagnosis: serum IGF-1, GH dependent; serum GH after a glucose load; MRI of pituitary gland
- Treatment: surgical resection of the pituitary tumor, somatostatin analogues

QUIZ

Questions

1. A 5-year-old child has a history of erythema, swelling, and crying within minutes of sun exposure, as well as red teeth and urine. A mutation in which enzyme could account for this disorder?
   A. Porphobilinogen deaminase
   B. Uroporphyrinogen decarboxylase
   C. Coproporphyrinogen oxidase
   D. Protoporphyrinogen oxidase
   E. Ferrochelatase

2. A patient presents with numerous itchy, reddish-yellow papules over his buttocks and dorsal arms. What condition would not be a potential cause?
   A. Apolipoprotein C2 mutation
   B. Diabetes
   C. Oral retinoid therapy
   D. Hyperthyroidism
   E. Lipoprotein lipase mutation

3. Which is the most common cutaneous manifestation of diabetes?
   A. Scar-like macule above the ankle
   B. Yellow, indurated plaque with a red rim on the shin
   C. Painless ulcer on the plantar metacarpophalangeal (MP) joint
   D. Blister on the dorsal foot
   E. Dark, velvety thickening of the axilla

4. In which of the following genes does mutation not characteristically lead to neuropsychiatric disturbances?
   A. Copper transporter P-type ATPase 7B
   B. Porphobilinogen deaminase
   C. Homogentisic acid oxidase
   D. Phenylalanine hydroxylase
   E. Cystathionine β-synthetase

5. Corneal changes are seen in all but which of the following conditions?
   A. α-L-iduronidase defect
   B. Sphingomyelinase deficiency
   C. α-Galactosidase deficiency
   D. Tyrosine aminotransferase deficiency
   E. ATPase 7B defect

6. A patient has scarring, hyperpigmentation, and milia on his dorsal hands, as well as facial hypertrichosis. Urinary coproporphyrins and uroporphyrins are equally elevated. What would be the most effective treatment for this patient?
   A. Antimalarials once to twice weekly
   B. Weekly phlebotomy
   C. Narrowband UVB phototherapy
   D. Interferon and ribavirin
   E. Glucose

7. A patient presents with patchy alopecia, ice-pick scarring on the face, moniliform blepharosis, cobblestone appearance of the oral mucosa, and a thickened, stiff tongue. Which of the following is also likely to be a finding?
   A. Antibodies to extracellular matrix protein-1
   B. Hyaline deposits encircling vessels
   C. Calcifications along the falx cerebri
   D. Cirrhosis
   E. Nephrotic syndrome

8. A patient has yellow papules along the palmar creases. Which condition does the patient probably have?
   A. Lipoprotein lipase deficiency
   B. Apolipoprotein E2 isoform
   C. Apolipoprotein C2 mutation
   D. Apolipoprotein B100 mutation
   E. LDL receptor defect

9. A short patient with brachydactyly, mild mental impairment, a round face, and a mutation in a stimulatory G-protein for cyclic adenosine monophosphate production would most likely have which finding?
   A. Progressive enchondral bone formation
   B. Precocious puberty
   C. Photosensitivity
   D. Firm dermal nodules and papules
   E. High serum calcium

10. A patient presents with a brownish-grey reticulated patch on the left upper back. Which is the most likely associated finding?
    A. λ Light chain deposition in the papillary dermis
    B. α Amyloid deposition in the papillary dermis
    C. Carpal tunnel syndrome
    D. Pheochromocytoma
    E. Notalgia paresthetica

Answers

1. B. While heterozygous mutation in uroporphyrinogen decarboxylase can lead to porphyria cutanea tarda, homozygosity causes hepatoerythropoietic porphyria, which can present with the features described. These features are also seen in congenital erythropoietic porphyria, (Gunther disease); however, uroporphyrinogen III synthase was not an answer choice.

2. D. Eruptive xanthomas come from elevated serum TG and have been associated with types I, IV, and V familial hypercholesterolemia, diabetes, oral retinoid therapy, and hypothyroidism. Hyperthyroidism is associated with warm, moist skin, thin hair and nails, and pretibial myxedema.
3. A. Diabetic dermopathy is the most common cutaneous sign of diabetes, occurring in up to half of patients as small, atrophic, reddish-brown macules, commonly on the lower extremities.
4. C. Alkaptonuria is characterized by dark urine (if pH >7), kidney stones, and arthritis, but not neuropsychiatric disturbance, unlike Wilson disease (ATP7A), AIP (homogentisic acid oxidase), PKU (phenylalanine hydroxylase), and homocystinuria (cystathione β-synthetase). Treatment for alkaptonuria is supplemental vitamin C.
5. B. Sphingomyelinase deficiency causes Niemann-Pick disease, which characteristically has a cherry-red spot on the fovea of the retina. Hurler (α-L-iduronidase), Fabry (α-galactosidase), and Richner-Hanhart (tyrosine aminotransferase) can all have corneal opacities, while Wilson disease (ATP7A) develops a characteristic Kayser-Fleischer ring of copper deposition in the corneal limbus.
6. E. Variegate porphyria and PCT may have similar cutaneous findings, with variegate porphyria more likely to have acute abdominal findings. The equal urine uroporphyrins and coproporphyrins show this case to be VP, as PCT would have a urine uro/copro ratio of at least 3:1. VP patients also have a characteristic plasma fluorescence at 626 nm during symptomatic periods. All of the answer choices are reported treatments for PCT (including narrowband UVB), except for glucose, which can be helpful when given orally or IV to patients with VP.
7. B. Lipoid proteinosis, also known as hyalinosis cutis et mucosae, will have globular or laminated hyaline deposits in the papillary dermis and around vessels. It is a deposition disease caused by a mutation in *ECM1* (not antibodies, as can be seen in some cases of lichen sclerosus et atrophicus). Sickle or bean-shaped calcifications are often seen around the sella turcica of the temporal lobes (not the falx cerebri as in Gorlin basal cell carcinoma syndrome). Cirrhosis is a potential complication of hemochromatosis, an iron deposition disorder. Nephrotic syndrome can be seen in systemic amyloidosis.
8. B. Xanthoma striatum palmare are characteristic of type III hyperlipidemia (broad-β disease, familial dysbetalipoproteinemia) caused by a defective Apo E isoform. LPL deficiency and Apo C2 mutations cause type I (familial chylomicronemia) and LDL receptor defects and Apo B100 mutations cause type II (familial hypercholesterolemia).
9. D. Albright hereditary osteodystrophy is characterized by intramembranous bone formation in the dermis, shortened fourth metacarpals with dimpling of the dorsal hand, and decreased calcium levels secondary to PTH hormone resistance (pseudohypoparathyroidism) which can lead to tetany. McCune-Albright syndrome is a completely separate entity, also resulting from a GNAS1 mutation (this one an activating mutation) characterized by precocious puberty, coast of Maine café-au-lait macules, and polyostotic fibrous dysplasia.
10. E. Macular amyloidosis is a keratin-derived deposition most commonly found on the upper back, and is commonly associated with notalgia paresthetica. Nodular amyloidosis comes from deposition of AL (light chain) amyloid by a localized plasma cell clonality. Carpal tunnel syndrome can be seen in primary systemic (AL), secondary systemic (AA), or hemodialysis-related (Ab2m) amyloidosis. Lichen amyloidosus is also keratin-derived but is most commonly found on the legs and can be associated with multiple endocrine Neoplasia 2a syndrome.

REFERENCES

Ayonrinde OT, Milward EA, Chua AC, Trinder D, Olynyk JK: Clinical perspectives on hereditary hemochromatosis. *Crit Rev Clin Lab Sci* 2008;45(5):451–484.

Azziz R: PCOS: a diagnostic challenge. *Reprod Biomed Online* 2004;8(6):644–648.

Bharati A, Higgins C, Ellis I, Wraith J: Fucosidosis: a therapeutic challenge. *Pediatr Dermatol* 2007;24(4):442–443.

Bolognia JL et al. *Dermatology*, 2nd Ed. London: Mosby-Elsevier; 2008.

Callen JP et al. *Dermatological Signs of Internal Disease*, 4th Ed. Philadelphia: Saunders-Elsevier; 2009.

Chemmanur AT, Bonkovsky HL: Hepatic porphyrias: diagnosis and management. *Clin Liver Dis* 2004;8(4):807–838.

Cowper SE et al. Nephrogenic fibrosing dermopathy. *Am J Dermatopathol* 2001;23:383–393.

Goldsmith LA et al. *Fitzpatrick's Dermatology in General Medicine*, 8th Ed. New York: McGraw-Hill; 2012.

Hanley WB: Adult phenylketonuria. *Am J Med* 2004;117(8):590–595.

Hermanns-Lê T, Scheen A, Piérard GE: Acanthosis nigricans associated with insulin resistance: pathophysiology and management. *Am J Clin Dermatol* 2004;5(3):199–203.

Jabbour SA: Cutaneous manifestations of endocrine disorders: a guide for dermatologists. *Am J Clin Dermatol* 2003;4(5):315–331.

Jensen TG: Strategies for long-term gene expression in the skin to treat metabolic disorders. *Expert Opin Biol Ther* 2004;4(5):677–682.

Keller JM, Macaulay W, Nercessian OA, Jaffe IA: New developments in ochronosis: review of the literature. *Rheumatol Int* 2005;25(2):81–85.

Kolter T, Sandhoff K: Sphingolipid metabolism diseases. *Biochim Biophys Acta* 2006;1758(12):2057–2079.

Lee AT, Zane LT: Dermatologic manifestations of polycystic ovary syndrome. *Am J Clin Dermatol* 2007;8(4):201–219.

Levin CY, Maibach H: Exogenous ochronosis. An update on clinical features, causative agents and treatment options. *Am J Clin Dermatol* 2001;2(4):213–217.

Lubics A, Schneider I, Sebök B, Havass Z: Extensive bluish gray skin pigmentation and severe arthropathy. *Arch Dermatol* 2000;136:547–552.

CHAPTER 24

DERMATOLOGIC MEDICATIONS

KARA E. WALTON
CHRISTOPHER T. BURNETT

SYSTEMIC MEDICATIONS

Androgenetic Alopecia Treatment

Finasteride

- Mechanism of action: inhibits type II 5α-reductase, which converts testosterone to dihydrotestosterone (DHT)
- Adverse effects: decreased libido, erectile dysfunction, decreased volume of ejaculate, teratogenicity (causes GU defects in male offspring)
- Pregnancy category X

Minoxidil

- Mechanism of action
  - Increases duration of anagen growth phase, gradually enlarges miniaturized hairs
  - Opens ATP-sensitive potassium channels; release of adenosine stimulates VEGF, a proposed promoter of hair growth
  - Stimulates prostaglandin production
- Adverse effects: irritant and allergic contact dermatitis (topical), hypertrichosis; may exacerbate angina pectoris (oral); caution in pulmonary hypertension, congestive heart failure, coronary artery disease, and significant renal failure (oral)
- Pregnancy category C

Spironolactone

- Mechanism of action: aldosterone antagonist, weak antiandrogen activity by blocking androgen receptor and inhibiting androgen biosynthesis; may be converted by progesterone 17-hydroxylase to active metabolites that decrease testosterone and DHT production
- Clinical use: dermatologic uses are off label and include acne vulgaris, androgenetic alopecia, hirsutism, hidradenitis suppurativa
- Adverse effects: menstrual irregularities, hyperkalemia, hyponatremia, potential teratogenicity as an antiandrogen (feminization of male fetus), gynecomastia
- Contraindications: renal insufficiency, hyperkalemia, pregnancy, abnormal uterine bleeding, family or personal history of estrogen-dependent malignancy
- Drug interactions: increased potential of hyperkalemia with angiotensin-converting enzyme inhibitors, thiazide diuretics, potassium supplements
- Increased levels of digoxin if taken with spironolactone
- Pregnancy category X

Antibiotics

Aminoglycosides

- Gentamicin, tobramycin, and amikacin
- Mechanism of action
  - Bind to 30S subunit of bacterial ribosomes to inhibit protein synthesis
- Active against aerobic gram-negative organisms
- Adverse effects: ototoxicity, nephrotoxicity, neuromuscular blockade, injection site necrosis
- Pregnancy category D

Beta-Lactam Antibiotics

- Include penicillins and cephalosporins
- Active against many gram-positive, gram-negative, and anaerobic organisms

Cephalosporins

- Mechanism of action: inhibit bacterial cell wall synthesis through inhibition of penicillin-binding proteins
- Treat soft tissue infections caused by *Streptococci*, methicillin-sensitive *Staphylococcus aureus*, some gram-negative bacilli
- Adverse effects: hypersensitivity, gastrointestinal (GI) upset, dizziness, Stevens-Johnson syndrome (SJS), toxic

epidermal necrolysis (TEN), *Clostridium difficile* colitis, serum sickness–like reaction (Cefaclor), acute generalized exanthematous pustulosis (AGEP), thrombocytopenia, neutropenia, eosinophilia; cross-reactivity with penicillins: 5 to 20%
- Drug interactions
  - Probenecid: increases levels of B-lactam medications
  - Allopurinol: increases hypersensitivity reaction of ampicillin
- Pregnancy category B

Penicillins

- Mechanism of action
  - Inhibit bacterial cell wall synthesis; lead to activation of autolytic enzymes that kill the bacteria
  - Active against gram-positive organisms and spirochetes
- Penicillinase-resistant penicillins include dicloxacillin, nafcillin, and oxacillin
- Beta-lactamase inhibitors: ampicillin-sulbactam, amoxicillin-clavulanic acid; used in the treatment of bite wounds; active against oral anaerobes, streptococci, anaerobes, and staphylococci
- Adverse effects: hypersensitivity reactions (mild morbilliform to anaphylaxis), hemolytic anemia, nephritis, TEN, erythema nodosum, cutis laxa, AGEP
- Ampicillin causes a morbilliform eruption when given to patients with infectious mononucleosis and when coadministered with allopurinol
- Pregnancy category B

Chloramphenicol

- Mechanism of action
  - Binds to 50S subunit of bacterial ribosomes and inhibits peptidyl transferase
- Used to treat *Salmonella, Haemophilus*, and pneumococcal and meningococcal meningitis in penicillin-sensitive patients; treats verruga peruana
- Adverse effects: gray baby syndrome, GI disturbances, anemia
- Pregnancy category C

Clindamycin

- Mechanism of action
  - Inhibits 50S bacterial ribosomal subunit to inhibit protein synthesis
- Active against gram-positive organisms (*S. aureus*, streptococci) and anaerobes (*Propionibacterium acnes*), aerobic and anaerobic streptococci (except enterococci)
- Adverse effects: photosensitivity, diarrhea, pseudomembranous colitis (owing to overgrowth of *C. difficile*), hepatic dysfunction, morbilliform rash, neuromuscular blockade, erythema multiforme, urticaria, anaphylaxis
- Pregnancy category B

Fluoroquinolones

- Ciprofloxacin, ofloxacin, gatifloxacin, levofloxacin, moxifloxacin, sparfloxacin, grepafloxicin, norfloxacin, enoxacin
- Mechanism of action
  - Inhibit bacterial DNA gyrase (bacterial topoisomerase 11)
- Active against gram-positive organisms (*S. aureus*, streptococci, except ciprofloxacin and ofloxacin) and gram-negative organisms (mycobacteria, *Neisseria gonorrhoeae*)
- Adverse effects: photosensitivity, flushing, hyperhidrosis, affect cartilage formation in children (contraindicated younger than 18 years), tendonitis and tendon rupture
- Drug interactions: absorption is decreased when administered with calcium-, magnesium-, or aluminum-containing antacids
  - Increased serum levels of warfarin
- Pregnancy category C

Macrolides: Erythromycin, Azithromycin, and Clarithromycin

- Mechanism of action
  - Bind to 50S bacterial ribosomal subunit to inhibit protein synthesis
- Active against gram-positive organisms (most streptococci and *S. aureus*)
- Adverse effects: GI distress, eosinophilia, oral mucosal lesions, xerosis; estolate formulation may cause cholestatic hepatitis (caution in liver disease)
- Drug interactions: certain macrolides inhibit hepatic cytochrome P450, thus decreasing metabolic clearance of certain drugs including phenytoin, theophylline, warfarin, digoxin, cyclosporine, carbamazepine, benzodiazepines, corticosteroids, omeprazole
  - Digoxin: elevated levels due to gut flora changes
  - Fluconazole: may increase clarithromycin levels
- Pregnancy category B for erythromycin and azithromycin; all others category C

Metronidazole

- Mechanism of action
  - Forms toxic metabolites in bacteria that inhibit nucleic acid synthesis
- Active against anaerobes, protozoa
- Adverse effects: glossitis, stomatitis, disulfiram-like reactions with ethanol, mucosal xerosis, vestibular dysfunction
- Pregnancy category B

Rifampin

- Mechanism of action
  - Inhibition of DNA-dependent RNA polymerase
- Activity: staphylococci, *Neisseria meningitidis*, *N. gonorrhoeae*, *Haemophilus influenzae*, *Mycobacterium tuberculosis*, and atypical mycobacteria, only drug bactericidal to *Mycobacterium leprae*; poor gram-negative coverage

- Rapid resistance, therefore, used synergistically with another agent
- Drug interactions (decreased effect): oral contraceptives, warfarin, corticosteroids, antiarrhythmics, phenytoin, phenobarbital, theophylline, β-blockers, fluoroquinolones, cyclosporine, dapsone, oral hypoglycemics
- Adverse effects: orange discoloration of urine and tears (permanent staining of soft contact lenses), bullous dermatoses, urticaria, mucositis

Sulfonamides (Trimethoprim-Sulfamethoxazole)

- Mechanism of action
  - Interfere with folic acid synthesis by inhibiting synthesis of dihydrofolate reductase (trimethoprim) and dihydropteroate synthase (sulfonamides)
- Active against gram-positive (*S. aureus*) and gram-negative organisms, *Chlamydia, Nocardia, Streptococcus pyogenes, Streptococcus viridans, Enterobacteriaceae, H. influenzae*
- Adverse effects: TEN, SJS; high doses may cause bone marrow depression (if signs occur, give leucovorin); caution in folate deficiency; hemolysis may occur in individuals with G6PD deficiency
- Drug interactions: increased warfarin effects; avoid in patients on methotrexate which also affects folic acid metabolism
- Pregnancy category C; contraindicated in third trimester due to risk of kernicterus

Tetracyclines: Tetracycline, Doxycycline, and Minocycline

- Mechanism of action
  - Bind to 30s subunit of bacterial ribosome, interfering with protein synthesis
- Active against *Mycoplasma pneumoniae, Chlamydia, Rickettsia, P. acnes* and *Vibrio* spp., *Borrelia burgdorferi, Mycobacterium marinum*
- Adverse effects: photosensitivity, GI disturbances, esophageal ulceration, enamel dysplasia (brown discoloration of gingival third) and delayed bone growth in children (younger than 9 years), photo-onycholysis, postacne osteoma cutis, psoriasis exacerbation, vertigo, pseudotumor cerebri, Fanconi anemia and uremia in renal disease patients
- Tetracycline: common cause of fixed drug eruption
- Minocycline: autoimmune hepatitis, systemic lupus erythematosus, blue-gray hyperpigmentation of nails, skin, scars, and sclerae, gray discoloration of mid-portion of permanent teeth, higher incidence of neurologic side effects
- Doxycycline and demeclocycline are the most phototoxic
- Reduce dose in renal impairment; doxycycline is the tetracycline of choice to use in renal failure patients
- Drug interactions: increased levels of warfarin, digoxin, lithium, insulin; increased risk of pseudotumor cerebri with isotretinoin, decreased absorption of tetracycline due to antacids, other cations (iron, zinc, bismuth, salts), cimetidine, and sodium bicarbonate
- Pregnancy category D

Antifungal Agents

Allylamines

- Butenafine, naftifine, terbinafine
- Mechanism of action: inhibits first step of ergosterol synthesis by blocking the activity of squalene epoxidase; fungicidal
- Adverse effects: GI upset, hepatocellular injury, dysgeusia (metallic taste), reversible agranulocytosis, lupus erythematosus, headache
- Pregnancy category B

Azoles

- Class members
  - *Imidazoles*: ketoconazole, clotrimazole, miconazole
  - *Triazoles*: fluconazole, itraconazole, voriconazole, posaconazole
- Mechanism of action: inhibit fungal lanosterol 14-α-demethylase blocking conversion of lanosterol to ergosterol; fungistatic
- Adverse effects
  - Neurologic: paresthesias in hands/feet (fluconazole), peripheral neuropathy (itraconazole)
  - GI: hepatitis (greatest risk with ketoconazole)
  - Cardiac: congestive heart failure (itraconazole)
  - Endocrine effects: gynecomastia, infertility, menstrual irregularities (ketoconazole); hypertriglyceridemia (itraconazole)
  - Cutaneous: development of squamous cell carcinoma (SCC), phototoxicity (voriconazole)
  - Visual disturbances: 30% with voriconazole; altered/enhanced visual perception, blurred vision, color vision change, and/or photophobia; reversible
- Drug interactions
  - Itraconazole and ketoconazole inhibit CYP3A4
  - Fluconazole inhibits CYP2C9; can increase INR when given with warfarin
- Pregnancy category C

Glucan Synthesis Inhibitors/Echinocandins: Caspofungin

- IV administration
- Mechanism of action: inhibits glucan synthesis (essential polysaccharide of the fungal cell wall)
- Activity: primarily *Candida, Aspergillus*
- Pregnancy category C

Griseofulvin

- Mechanism of action: interferes with microtubule function, causing metaphase arrest

- Activity: fungistatic for dermatophytes, not yeast
- Adverse effects: GI disturbance, headaches, hypersensitivity, photosensitivity, paresthesias, hepatotoxicity, amenorrhea, exacerbation of acute intermittent porphyria (contraindicated in patients with porphyria), lupus erythematosus
- Drug interactions: induces CYP450; decreases warfarin and oral contraceptive concentrations
- Pregnancy category C

Polyenes: Amphotericin B

- Mechanism of action: binds to ergosterol and forms amphotericin B–associated membrane pores, altering the fungal membrane permeability
- Adverse effects: hepatitis, infusion reactions, anemia, fever, flushing/generalized erythema, nephrotoxicity, hypotension
- Resistance: develops when binding of the drug to ergosterol is impaired or when ergosterol concentration in the membrane is decreased
- Pregnancy category B

Antihistamines

- Mast cells express high-affinity immunoglobulin E receptor (FCεRI) that can be cross-linked by an antigen, triggering release of histamine and other mediators
- H_1 and H_2 subclasses of histamine receptors are expressed in human skin; H_1 receptors are also found in the brain, smooth muscle cells, endothelial cells, adrenal medulla, and heart
- Inverse agonists at tissue receptor sites; binding is reversible
- Affect smooth muscle contraction, stimulation of nitric oxide formation, endothelial cell contraction, and increase vascular permeability
- Central nervous system effects are due to blockade of central muscarinic receptors
- *First-generation H_1 blockers*
- Lipophilic; sedating by crossing blood–brain barrier
  - Five classes
    - *Piperidine*: i.e., cyproheptadine, antiseratonin effects, preferred for cold urticaria and other physical urticarias, pregnancy category B
    - *Alkylamine*: i.e., chlorpheniramine, pregnancy category B (considered one of safest antihistamines in pregnancy)
    - *Ethanolamine*: i.e., diphenhydramine, also inhibits acetylcholine activity and may cause sedation, urinary retention, may exacerbate angle closure glaucoma, pregnancy category B
    - *Piperazine*: i.e., hydroxyzine, may exacerbate porphyria, may cause alterations in T waves on EKG, drowsiness, pregnancy category C
    - *Phenothiazine*: i.e., promethazine, pregnancy category C
- *Second-generation H_1 blockers*
  - Less lipid soluble and longer half-lives, allowing for less frequent dosing and less sedation compared to first-generation H_1 blockers
  - Cetirizine: metabolite of hydroxyzine; most sedating of second-generation H_1 blockers; minimal anticholinergic effects at high doses, pregnancy category B
- Others
  - Fexofenadine, desloratadine (pregnancy category C)
  - Loratadine, levocetirazine (pregnancy category B)
- Drug interactions
  - Increased antihistamine levels with CYP3A4 inhibitors: macrolide antibiotics, azole antifungals, protease inhibitors, SSRIs
  - Increased toxicity: CNS depressants, MAO inhibitors
- *H_2 blockers*
  - Cimetidine: antiandrogen (may cause gynecomastia, impotence) and immunomodulating effects; reduces hepatic oxidation of dapsone to hydroxylamine, limiting methemoglobin formation
- *Doxepin*
  - Tricyclic antidepressant with H_1- and H_2-antihistamine activity
  - Side effects: sedation, anticholinergic effects, prolonged QT interval, withdrawal syndrome (nausea, vomiting, diarrhea, headache, sleep disturbance, dizziness, akathisia)

Antimalarial agents

Hydroxychloroquine/Chloroquine/Quinacrine

- Mechanism of action
  - Not fully understood; impairs chemotaxis of inflammatory cells; may inhibit antigen-antibody complex formation and release of interleukin-2 (IL-2) from CD4+ T cells; decreases lysosomal size
- Adverse effects
  - *Ocular toxicity*: reversible premaculopathy (retinal pigment deposition without visual change) and corneal deposits (results in halos); irreversible true retinopathy ("bulls eye" pigment deposition, central scotoma); risk is greatest with chloroquine, no risk with quinicrine
  - *Hemolytic anemia* in patients with G6PD deficiency
  - *Mucocutaneous effects*: blue/gray hyperpigmentation (shins, face, palate) and transverse bands in nail beds due to hemosiderin and melanin; quinacrine → yellow skin pigmentation; chloroquine → progressive bleaching of hair roots
  - *Worsening of psoriasis*: mainly chloroquine
  - *Gastrointestinal*: nausea and vomiting
  - *Neuromuscular*: headache, psychosis, muscular weakness
- Eye studies: screening examination at baseline to rule out baseline maculopathy; annual screening to begin after 5 years on medication unless risk factors (elderly patients, high dose, or renal problems) or signs of toxicity

- Interactions with other medications
  - Cimetidine may increase serum levels of chloroquine; digoxin and cyclosporine levels may be elevated
- Pregnancy category C

Antimetabolic and Cytotoxic Agents

- Antimetabolites: mimic natural molecules and are most active while DNA is being synthesized in the S phase, i.e., proliferating target cell
- Side effects are most prominent in cells with an innately high proliferative index (e.g., bone marrow)
- Alkylating agents are cell-cycle nonspecific; affect proliferating populations of cells and cells that are not actively synthesizing DNA; greater propensity for mutagenicity

AZATHIOPRINE

- Mechanism of action
  - Azathioprine absorbed and converted into 6-mercaptopurine (6-MP) which is converted into 6-thioguanine via hypoxanthine-guanine phosphoribosyltransferase (HGPRT)
  - 6-Thioguanine (active metabolite), a purine analog, inhibits DNA/RNA synthesis and repair
  - Xanthine oxidase (XO) and thiopurine methyltransferase (TPMT) catabolize 6-MP into inactive metabolites
- Adverse effects
  - Malignancy: lymphoproliferative (especially patients with RA), SCC of skin
  - Gastrointestinal: GI distress (usually first 10 days), hepatitis, pancreatitis
  - Hypersensitivity syndrome (1–4 weeks after starting medication)
  - Myelosuppression: increased risk in patients with TPMT deficiency
  - Patients with Lesch-Nyhan syndrome lack HGPRT and are resistant to the cytotoxic effects of the drug
- Drug interactions
  - Allopurinol inhibits xanthine oxidase, causing increased toxicity
  - ACE inhibitors and folate antagonists can increase myelosuppression
  - Warfarin levels may be decreased
  - Check TPMT levels prior to initiating drug
- Pregnancy category D

CHLORAMBUCIL

- Mechanism of action: alkylating agent derived from nitrogen mustard, cell-cycle nonspecific, forms DNA cross-linkages
- Adverse effects
  - *Carcinogenic*: AML, lymphoma, SCC
  - *Hematologic*: leukopenia (common, dose-limiting), bone marrow suppression
  - *Mucocutaneous*: oral ulcers, alopecia, urticaria
  - *Others*: infertility (azoospermia, amenorrhea), generalized tonic-clonic seizures (especially in children with nephrotic syndrome or adults with seizure history)
- Pregnancy category D

CYCLOPHOSPHAMIDE

- Mechanism of action: alkylating agent derived from nitrogen mustard, cell-cycle nonspecific; forms DNA cross-linkages; suppresses B cells more than T cells (CD8 > CD4)
- Adverse effects
  - *Carcinogenic*: transitional cell bladder carcinoma, leukemia, non-Hodgkin lymphoma, SCC
  - *Hematologic*: thrombocytopenia, anemia, leukopenia, bone marrow suppression
  - *Gastrointestinal*: GI upset (dose-related)
  - *Genitourinary*: hemorrhagic cystitis, azoospermia
  - *Mucocutaneous*: acral erythema, anagen effluvium, diffuse hyperpigmentation, pigmented bands on teeth
- Acrolein metabolite of cyclophosphamide causes bladder toxicity; mesna (sodium 2-mercaptoethanesulfonate) binds to acrolein to reduce toxicity; screens for microscopic hematuria
- Pregnancy category D

HYDROXYUREA

- Mechanism of action: S phase specific; inhibits ribonucleotide reductase, a rate limiting step in DNA synthesis
- Adverse effects
  - *Hematologic*: megaloblastosis (all patients), anemia, acute leukemia (rare)
  - *Renal*: elevated BUN and creatinine
  - *Hepatic*: elevated transaminases, transient hepatitis
  - *Cutaneous*: leg ulcers, dermatomyositis-like eruptions, acral erythema, diffuse hyperpigmentation, radiation recall, poikiloderma
  - *Other*: flu-like symptoms
- Pregnancy category D

METHOTREXATE

- Mechanism of action
- S phase antimetabolite; competitively and irreversibly inhibits dihydrofolate reductase to prevent conversion of dihydrofolate to tetrahydrofolate, a cofactor in thymidylate and purine synthesis
- Adverse effects: GI upset, renal failure, hepatotoxicity, abortifacient, pancytopenia (first 4–6 weeks), acute pneumonitis, pulmonary fibrosis, nephrotoxicity, phototoxicity, acral erythema, radiation recall, lymphoma, ulcerative stomatitis
- Folic acid supplementation can decrease risk of pancytopenia and GI side effects
- Leucovorin (folinic acid) given for acute methotrexate-induced myelosuppresion

- Current guidelines on role of liver biopsy divide patients into 2 groups
  - High-risk (obesity, diabetes, overconsumption of alcohol, hepatitis): consider delayed biopsy after 2 to 6 months to establish efficacy and tolerability, then q 1.5 g
  - Low-risk: consider biopsy if persistently elevated liver function tests (LFTs); after 3.5- to 4-g cumulative dosage, consider biopsy, switch to other agent, or discontinue therapy
- Increased risk of hematologic toxicity with renal disease and concomitant use of NSAIDs, sulfonamides (especially TMP/SMX), salicylates, chloramphenicol, phenothiazine, phenytoin, tetracyclines (increase MTX levels by displacement of plasma proteins)
- Pregnancy category X

Mycophenolate Mofetil (MMF) and Mycophenolic Acid (MPA)

- Mechanism of action
  - MMF is hydrolyzed to MPA (active metabolite) after absorption
  - MPA noncompetitively inhibits inosine monophosphate dehydrogenase (IMPDH) and suppresses de novo purine synthesis in cells lacking salvage pathway (T and B lymphocytes)
- Adverse effects: GI effects (dose-dependent and most common), sterile pyuria, dysuria, urinary frequency, carcinogenicity (mostly in transplant patients), increased risk for infection (e.g., herpes zoster)
- Drug interactions
  - MMF can increase levels of phenytoin, acyclovir, ganciclovir, and theophylline
  - Antacids and iron decrease absorption
  - Cyclosporine and cholestyramine can decrease MPA levels
- Pregnancy category D

Antimycobacterial Agents

Clofazimine

- Red, fat-soluble, crystalline dye
- Mechanism of action: inhibits mycobacterial growth by binding preferentially to mycobacterial DNA
- Adverse effects: skin discoloration (diffuse red to red-brown vs.violet-brown to bluish discoloration); secretions discolored (red urine); ichthyosis; splenic infarction (rare), bowel obstruction, and GI bleeding; crystalline deposits of clofazimine in tissues, including intestinal mucosa, spleen, liver, and mesenteric lymph nodes
- Pregnancy category C

Ethambutol

- Mechanism of action: inhibits metabolite synthesis in susceptible bacteria, resulting in impaired cellular metabolism and cell death; bacteriostatic
- Useful for organisms resistant to streptomycin and isoniazid (no cross-resistance)
- Adverse effects: dose-dependent visual disturbances, neurotoxicity, hyperhidrosis, gout
- Pregnancy category C

Isoniazid

- Mechanism of action: disrupts mycobacterial cell walls, inhibits mycolic acid synthesis; bacteriostatic at most concentrations
- Elimination through acetylation; fast and slow acetylation of patient affects elimination half-life: fast = 70 minutes, slow = 180 minutes
- Adverse effects: neurotoxic, hepatotoxic, hemolysis in G6PD deficiency, lupus erythematosus, acneiform eruption, onycholysis, pellagra-like eruption, photosensitivity, pyridoxine (B_6) deficiency with high doses
- Pyridoxine supplementation can decrease risk of peripheral neuritis
- Pregnancy category C

Pyrazinamide (PZA)

- Mechanism of action: unknown
- Bacteriostatic or bactericidal against *M. tuberculosis* depending on concentration of drug attained at site of infection
- Adverse effects: photosensitivity, myalgias, hyperuricemia, GI irritation, red-brown change in skin color, alopecia, flushing, hepatic injury (most common and serious side effect); gout can be precipitated by inhibition of excretion of urate
- Pregnancy category C

Rifampin

- Macrocyclic antibiotic derived from *Streptomyces mediterranei*
- Rifabutin: semisynthetic rifampin; more effective in treating atypical mycobacteria
- Mechanism of action: bactericidal; inhibits DNA-dependent RNA polymerase, interfering with bacterial RNA synthesis
- Activity: *M. tuberculosis*, many gram-negative organisms, many chlamydiae
- Adverse effects: orange-red discoloration of skin, urine, tears; glossodynia; increased risk of deep venous thrombosis; antidrug antibodies; IgE-mediated anaphylaxis; thrombocytopenia (reversible)
- Drug interactions: potent inducer of multiple CYP enzymes
- Pregnancy category C

Streptomycin

- Mechanism of action: bactericidal antibiotic; interferes with normal protein synthesis

- Added as a fourth drug for *M. tuberculosis* treatment
- Adverse effects: renal tubular damage, vestibular damage, and ototoxicity; caution with myasthenia gravis, hypocalcemia, and conditions that depress neuromuscular transmission
- Pregnancy category D

Antiretroviral Agents

Fusion Inhibitors: Enfuvirtide

- Mechanism of action: binds to proteins on viral envelope and inhibits conformational change needed for fusion between viral envelope and CD4 cells
- Adverse effects: injection site reactions

Nonnucleoside Reverse Transcriptase Inhibitors

- Nevirapine, delavirdine, efavirenz
- Mechanism of action: bind directly to HIV-1 reverse transcriptase and noncompetitively inhibit DNA synthesis
- Adverse effects: morbilliform rash is common (within first 3–6 weeks), SJS, TEN, DRESS (SJS most common with nevirapine)

Nucleoside Reverse Transcriptase Inhibitors

- Mechanism of action: pyrimadine analogues; act as chain terminators
- Zidovudine (AZT, ZDV)
  - Resistance: due to mutations in the reverse transcriptase gene
  - Adverse effects: myelosuppression, blue-brown pigmentation of nails and mucosa, cutaneous hyperpigmentation, acral/periarticular reticulate erythema, eyelash hypertrichosis
- Didanosine (ddI)
  - Adverse effects: peripheral neuropathy and potentially fatal pancreatitis, optic neuritis
- Lamivudine (3TC), stavudine (d4T), and zalcitabine (ddC)
  - Adverse effects: paronychia, lipodystrophy, oral/esophageal ulcers, peripheral neuropathy, pancreatitis
- Abacavir (ABC)
  - Adverse effects: potentially fatal hypersensitivity reaction, Sweet syndrome
- Emtricitabine (FTC)
  - Adverse effects: palmoplantar hyperpigmentation, rare lactic acidosis with hepatic steatosis

Nucleotide Analogues: Tenofovir

- Mechanism of action: inhibits reverse transcriptase
- Adverse effects: peripheral wasting, facial wasting, breast enlargement, and cushingoid appearance; GI upset

Protease Inhibitors (PIs)

- Saquinavir, indinavir, nelfinavir, amprenavir, fosamprenavir, ritonavir, atazanavir, lopinavir, tipranivir, darunavir
- Mechanism of action: inhibit HIV protease activity, blocking Gag and Gag-Pol cleavage required for assembly of progeny virions
- Adverse effects abnormal fat deposits such as "buffalo hump" (indinavir), severe diarrhea (nelfinavir), hepatotoxicity, lipodystrophy, osteopenia, insulin resistance, severe lipid abnormalities, periungual pyogenic granulomas (indinavir)

Antiviral Agents

Acyclovir

- Mechanism of action
  - Inhibits DNA synthesis by inhibiting viral DNA polymerase; initial phosphorylation of acyclovir to acyclovir monophosphate is catalyzed by virus-induced thymidine kinase
- Activity: herpes simplex virus (HSV), varicella-zoster virus (VZV), Epstein-Barr virus (EBV); used to treat recurrent erythema multiforme secondary to HSV infection
- Adverse effects: reversible crystalluria-induced nephrotoxicity with IV infusion, seizures
- Resistant HSV: *thymidine kinase negative* (*tk* –) or *tk* mutant and hence does not phosphorylate and activate acyclovir; has an altered DNA polymerase that is not as greatly inhibited by the phosphorylated drug
- Pregnancy category B

Cidofovir

- Mechanism of action: nucleoside analog of deoxycytidine monophosphate
  - Converted by host cell enzymes to cidofovir diphosphate, which competitively inhibits viral DNA polymerase
  - Cidofovir is independent of thymidine kinase activation
- Adverse effects: renal toxicity (renal tubular damage), granulocytopenia may occur; with topical application, local irritation, pain
- Pregnancy category C

Famciclovir

- Mechanism of action
  - Prodrug of the antiviral agent penciclovir; converted to active form via deacetylation and oxidation
  - Action similar to acyclovir
- Activity: HSV, VZV
- Pregnancy category B

Foscarnet

- Mechanism of action: noncompetitively inhibits viral DNA polymerase by binding directly to the pyrophosphate-binding site
  - Does not require phosphorylation for antiviral activity

- Activity: acyclovir-resistant HSV infections in AIDS patients and cytomegalovirus (CMV) retinitis in immunocompromised patients
- Adverse effects: nephrotoxicity, electrolyte imbalances, genital and oral ulcerations
- Pregnancy category C

Ganciclovir

- Mechanism of action: nucleoside analogue that competes with deoxyguanosine for incorporation into viral DNA; hydroxymethylated derivative of acyclovir
    - Initially phosphorylated by virus-encoded kinases
    - Ganciclovir triphosphate competitively inhibits herpes virus DNA polymerase and also inhibits elongation of the nascent DNA chain
- HSV and VZV with thymidine kinase deficiency or with viral DNA polymerase mutations may be resistant to ganciclovir
- Activity: more active than acyclovir against CMV, especially CMV retinitis in immunocompromised patients
- Adverse effects: mucositis, hepatic dysfunction, seizures, granulocytopenia, and thrombocytopenia; may not be totally reversible after cessation
- Pregnancy category C

Interferons: Interferon-Alpha-2B

- Mechanism of action
    - Protein product manufactured by recombinant DNA technology
    - Induces differential gene transcription; inhibits viral replication; antiviral and immunomodulatory effects by suppressing cell proliferation; direct antiproliferative effects against malignant cells and modulation of host immune response
- Adverse effects: flu-like symptoms, GI upset, leukopenia, hepatitis, cardiovascular arrhythmias, eyelash hypertrichosis, spastic diplegia, rhabdomyolysis
- Pregnancy category C

Valacyclovir

- Mechanism of action
    - Valacyclovir (a prodrug) is the L-valine ester of acyclovir and exerts its action after being transformed into acyclovir during its first pass through the intestine and liver
- Bioavailability is 3 to 5 times greater than acyclovir
- At least as effective as acyclovir in shortening duration of pain from postherpetic neuralgia in herpes zoster patients
- Activity against HSV, VZV, and CMV
- Adverse effects: Thrombotic thrombocytopenic purpura/HUS syndrome in immunosuppressed patients (transplant, HIV) taking high doses, seizures
- Pregnancy category B

Valganciclovir

- Acts as a prodrug for ganciclovir; converted to active drug by intestinal and hepatic esterases
- Adverse effects: similar to parent compound
- Activity: CMV retinitis in patients with AIDS
- Pregnancy category C

Glucocorticosteroids

- Pharmacology
    - Cortisol-binding globulin (CBG, transcortin) binds 90 to 95% of plasma cortisol; the free fraction is the active form; CBG is increased by pregnancy, estrogen treatment, and hyperthyroidism; CBG is decreased by hypothyroidism, liver and renal disease, obesity
    - *Short acting*: cortisone and hydrocortisone; **mineralcorticoid potency** > **glucocorticoid** potency, with cortisone having the lowest glucocorticoid potency
    - *Intermediate acting*: prednisone, prednisolone, methylprednisolone, and triamcinolone; **glucocorticoid potency > mineralcorticoid potency**
    - *Long acting*: dexamethasone and betamethasone; glucocorticoid only
- Mechanism of action
    - Bind to cytosolic receptor, translocate to nucleus, and then bind to glucocorticoid response elements (GRE) on DNA
    - Corticosteroids (CS) reduce production of transcription factors AP-1 and NF-κB (nuclear factor-κB) resulting in decreased synthesis of proinflammatory molecules
    - CS-induced apoptosis in lymphocytes and eosinophils
    - *Glucocorticoid effects*: gluconeogenesis, protein catabolism, peripheral insulin resistance, lipolysis, fat redistribution
    - *Mineralocorticoid effects*: increased sodium retention → hypertension and congestive heart failure in susceptible patients, hypokalemia, decreased plasma adrenocorticotropic hormone (ACTH), decreased fibroblasts production of collagen
    - *GI effects*: peptic ulcer disease, fatty liver changes, esophageal reflux, nausea, and vomiting
    - *Skeletal effects*: osteoporosis, osteonecrosis
    - *Ocular effects*: posterior subcapsular cataracts
    - *Pulmonary effects*: increase surfactant production in fetal lungs
    - *Psychiatric effects*: euphoria, psychosis
    - *Cutaneous effects*: telogen effluvium, hirsutism, acne, increased infection risk, poor wound healing, purpura, cushingoid changes
    - *Other effects*: myopathy, pancreatitis, adrenal suppression
- Adverse effects may be reduced by alternate day dosing **EXCEPT** for risk of **osteoporosis, osteonecrosis, and cataracts**
- Interval between doses decreases chance of hypothalamic-pituitary-adrenal (HPA) axis suppression compared to actual dose of steroids

- Single dose in the AM decreases HPA axis suppression vs. split dosing
- Pregnancy category C

Immunobiologicals

- TNF inhibitors
  - CHF and family history of demyelinating disease or multiple sclerosis are relative contraindications; infections and known hypersensitivity are absolute; avoid live vaccines
  - Check PPD at baseline; start therapy for latent TB infection prior to initiation
  - Black box warning for serious infections and lymphoma/other malignancies

Adalimumab

- Fully human IgG1 monoclonal antibody to TNF-α only
- Mechanism of action: blocks TNF-α interaction with the p55 and p75 transmembrane TNF receptor
- Adverse effects: injection site reactions, infection, positive antinuclear antibody (ANA), demyelinating disorders, lymphoma, exacerbation of or new-onset CHF
- Pregnancy category B

Etanercept

- Fully human receptor fusion protein that comprises a dimer of the p-75 external domain of tumor necrosis factor-α (TNF-α) receptor linked to the Fc portion of human IgG1
- Mechanism of action: competitively binds to soluble and membrane-bound TNF-α and to TNF-β
- Adverse effects: injection site reaction, reactivation of latent tuberculosis, multiple sclerosis and CNS demyelinating disorders, positive ANA (11%), drug-induced lupus, exacerbation of or new-onset congestive heart failure (CHF), lymphoma, infection
- Pregnancy category B

Infliximab

- Mouse-human chimeric IgG1 monoclonal antibody specific for TNF-α
- Mechanism of action: binds to TNF-α and inhibits its binding to soluble and transmembrane TNF-α receptors
- Adverse effects: infusion reactions, risk of serious infections, reactivation of tuberculosis and Hepatitis B, positive ANA, serum sickness, hepatotoxicity, rare pancytopenia, lymphoma, CNS demyelinating disorders, exacerbation of or new-onset CHF
- Antidrug antibodies to the chimeric portion can form and reduce efficacy; methotrexate can decrease antibody formation and prolong efficacy
- Pregnancy category B

Alefacept

- Fully human dimeric fusion protein of leukocyte function antigen-3 (LFA-3) linked to the Fc portion of human IgG1; drug is no longer available as manufacture was voluntarily discontinued
- Mechanism of action: blocks the interaction of LFA-3 on antigen-presenting cells with CD2 on T cells (mostly memory CD45RO+ cells)
- Also links CD2 with CD16 (FcγIII receptor) on natural killer cells triggering apoptosis of selected memory T cells expressing high levels of CD2 on the surface
- Adverse effects: lymphopenia with low CD4+ counts (greatest at 6–8 weeks), malignancy (most commonly skin cancer), infection, hypersensitivity reactions, injection site reactions, increased LFTs, antidrug antibodies
- Monitoring: CD4+ T-lymphocyte counts should be monitored weekly during the 12-week dosing period; dose should be held if CD4+ T-lymphocyte counts fall below 250 cells/μL; medication should be discontinued if counts remain below 250 cells/μL for 1 month
- Pregnancy category B

Anakinra

- Mechanism of action: recombinant, nonglycosylated form of the human IL-1 receptor; blocks biologic activity of IL-1 in inflammatory and immunological responses
- Indicated for the treatment of rheumatoid arthritis; used to treat periodic fever syndromes (e.g., Schnitzler syndrome)
- Adverse reactions: neutropenia, serious infection (especially with TNF-α inhibitors), lymphoma, injection site reaction, headache, nausea, diarrhea, abdominal pain
- Pregnancy category B

Denileukin Diftitox

- Mechanism of action
  - Fusion protein of recombinant diphtheria toxin and the receptor-binding domain of human IL-2
  - Drug binds to high-affinity IL-2 receptors (cluster of differentiation 25 [CD25]), inhibits protein synthesis by translocation of the active portion of diphtheria toxin into the cytosol
- Approximately 50% of patients with mycosis fungoides or Sézary syndrome have malignant cells that express CD25; malignant cells may be tested for CD25 expression to see if this medication would be helpful
- Adverse effects: hypersensitivity/vascular leak syndrome (hypotension, edema, pleural effusions, weight gain), infusion reactions, hypoalbuminemia (occurs after 1–2 weeks), infection, visual changes (loss of visual acuity and color vision)
- Pregnancy category C

Efalizumab

- Humanized IgG1 monoclonal antibody against human CD11a subunit of LFA-1
- Mechanism of action: blocks the interaction of LFA-1 on T cells with intercellular adhesion molecule-1 (ICAM-1) on antigen-presenting cells
- No longer available due to possible risk of progressive multifocal leukoencephalopathy (PML)

Ipilimumab

- Mechanism of action: fully human monoclonal antibody that blocks cytotoxic T lymphocyte–associated antigen 4 (CTLA-4) on T lymphocytes; augments T-cell activation and proliferation
- Indicated for the treatment of unresectable or metastatic malignant melanoma
- Adverse reactions: fatigue, diarrhea, pruritus, colitis; may cause severe immune-mediated reactions due to T-cell activation including enterocolitis, hepatitis, SJS/TEN, neuropathy, endocrinopathies
- Pregnancy category C

Omalizumab

- Recombinant humanized monoclonal antibody against the high-affinity IgE receptor (FcεRI)
- Mechanism of action: reduces levels of free IgE and the high-affinity receptor for the Fc region of IgE (FcεRI), both of which are essential in mast-cell and basophil activation
- Clinical uses: FDA approved as add-on therapy for moderate-to-severe persistent allergic asthma; off-label use in chronic urticaria not controlled by antihistamines
- Adverse effects: anaphylaxis, injection site reaction, arthralgia, fever, fracture, fatigue thrombocytopenia, headache, infection, possible increased risk of malignancy
- Pregnancy category B

Rituximab

- Chimeric monoclonal antibody against CD20 on surface of mature B cells
- Mechanism of action: binds to CD20 on surface of mature B cells causing apoptosis
- Adverse effects: potentially fatal infusion reactions (hypoxia, pulmonary infiltrates, acute respiratory distress, myocardial infarction, ventricular fibrillation, cardiogenic shock), 80% after first infusion; acute renal failure; SJS/TEN; reactivation of hepatitis B
- Pregnancy category C

Thalidomide

- Mechanism of action: TNF-α and IL-12 suppressors, antiangiogenic; downregulates adhesion molecules
- Drug of choice for erythema nodosum leprosum
- Adverse effects: sedation, constipation, peripheral neuropathy (sensory), leukopenia, bradycardia, rash and fever (mainly in HIV patients), severe birth defects (malformations of extremities, microphthalmia, neural tube defects, cardiac and renal malfomations, esophageal fistulas, duodenal atresia, vaginal obstruction)
- Antagonized by thalidomides: acetylcholine, histamine, prostaglandins, serotonin
- Pregnancy category X

Trametinib

- Mechanism of action: specific inhibitor of MEK1 and MEK2; blocks MAP kinase pathway downstream of BRAF
- FDA approved for stages III and IV melanoma with BRAF V600E or V600K mutations
- May decrease incidence of development of cutaneous SCCs and KAs when used in combination with BRAF inhibitors
- Adverse effects: papulopustular skin rashes, diarrhea, peripheral edema, fatigue, decreased ejection fraction, central serous retinopathy
- Pregnancy category X

Ustekinumab

- Fully human monoclonal antibody targeting p40 subunit of interleukin-12 (IL-12) and interleukin-23 (IL-23); inhibits Th17 pathway
- 45- or 90-mg subcutaneous injection at weeks 0, 4, and then every 12 weeks
- Adverse effects: infection (individuals genetically deficient in IL-12/IL-23 susceptible to mycobacteria and salmonella); rare malignancy and reversible posterior leukoencephalopathy
- Pregnancy category B

Vemurafenib and Dabrafenib

- Mechanism of action: inhibit BRAF V600E protein kinase, leading to inhibition of tumor cell proliferation
- FDA approved for the treatment of patients with unresectable or metastatic melanoma with BRAF V600E mutation
- Adverse side effects: arthralgia, rash, photosensitivity, fatigue, alopecia, skin papillomas, transient elevations in liver enzymes, SJS/TEN, QT prolongation, cutaneous SSCs and keratoacanthomas, uveitis, new primary malignant melanoma
- Drug interactions: moderate CYP1A2 inhibitor, weak CYP2D6 inhibitor and CYP3A4 inducer; may increase warfarin levels; avoid use with strong CYP3A4 inhibitors (e.g., azole antifungals, clarithromycin, indinavir) and inducers (e.g., phenytoin, carbamazepine, phenobarbital, rifampin); avoid use with other medications that may prolong QT interval (e.g., cisapride, pimozide, amiodarone)
- Pregnancy category D

Vismodegib

- Mechanism of action: blocks Hedgehog signaling by binding to *smoothened* and inhibiting activation of downstream Hedgehog target genes

- FDA approved for the treatment of metastatic BCC or in patients with locally advanced BCC that has recurred after surgery or who are not candidates for surgery and are not candidates for radiation
- Adverse effects: dysguesia, alopecia, muscle spasms, fatigue, nausea, amenorrhea, decreased appetite, weight loss, hyponatremia, azotemia, hypokalemia, teratogenicity
- Drug interactions: potentiated by P-gp inhibitors (e.g., clarithromycin, erythromycin, azithromycin); antagonized by drugs that affect gastric pH (e.g., proton pump inhibitors, antacids, H_2-blockers)
- Pregnancy category D

Immunosuppressive Agents

Cyclosporine

- Mechanism of action
  - Binds to an immunophilin called *cyclophylin A* (CyPA) and inhibits calcineurin
  - Calcineurin regulates the transcription factor NFAT (nuclear factor of activated T cells) by dephosphorylating the cytoplasmic component (NFATc); NFATc translocates into the nucleus, where it binds NFATn
  - NFATn regulates cytokine-encoding genes, including interleukin-2 (IL-2) and interferon-γ (IFN-γ); impaired IL-2 leads to decreased activated CD4 and CD8 cells
- Adverse effects: hypertension, hyperkalemia, hyperuricemia, hypomagnesemia, hyperlipidemia, renal toxicity, hypertrichosis, gingival hyperplasia, neurotoxicity (headache, tremor, paresthesias), lymphoma (especially in transplant patients), increased incidence of skin cancer, osteoporosis, acne
- Discontinue or reduce dose if creatinine rises 25 to 30% above baseline
- Drug interactions: any medication that induces, inhibits, or competes for CYP3A4 (see Table 24-1); cyclosporine can increase risk of rhabdomyolysis when used with statins
- Pregnancy category C

Parasiticidals

Ivermectin

- Mechanism of action: blocks glutamate-gated chloride ion channels resulting in paralysis of the parasite
- Used to treat onchocerciasis, strongyloidiasis, Norwegian scabies
- Pregnancy category C

Thiabendazole

- Mechanism of action: inhibits helminth-specific enzyme fumarate reductase
- Used to treat cutaneous larva migrans and larva currens
- Adverse events: nausea, vomiting, diarrhea
- Pregnancy category C

Retinoids

- Hormones that possess vitamin A activity (natural and synthetic forms)
- Mechanism of action
  - Retinoic acid transported to nucleus by cytosolic retinoic acid–binding protein (CRABP) where it binds RAR or RXR receptors and acts as transcription factor for genes containing retinoic acid response element (RARE)
  - Two main families of intracellular receptors
    - *Retinoic acid receptor* (RAR; bound and activated by all-*trans* retinoic acid)
    - *Retinoid X receptor* (RXR; 9-*cis* retinoic acid is the proposed ligand)
    - Each family has 3 receptor subtypes: α, β, and γ; γ is the primary receptor subtype in the skin while β is absent
    - Each retinoid possesses unique receptor-binding profiles (Table 24-2)
  - Function in the regulation of cellular proliferation and the modulation of immune function and cytokine function
  - Enhance keratinocyte differentiation by increasing filaggrin production, keratohyaline granules, and Odland body secretion of lipids; downregulate keratins 6 and 16
  - Reduce size of sebaceous glands and decrease differentiation to mature sebocytes (isotretinoin)
  - Inhibit ornithine decarboxylase
- Side effects
  - *Mucocutaneous*: cheilitis, xerosis, pruritus, epistaxis, paronychia, periungual pyogenic granulomas, telogen effluvium, "sticky skin," photosensitivity
  - *Ophthalmologic*: blepharoconjunctivitis, blurred vision, abnormal night vision
  - *Teratogenicity*: retinoic acid embryopathy, central nervous system abnormalities (hydrocephalus, microcephaly), external ear abnormalities (anotia, small or absent external auditory canals), cardiovascular abnormalities (septal wall and aortic defects), facial dysmorphia, eye abnormalities (microphthalmia), thymus gland aplasia, and bone abnormalities
  - *Musculoskeletal*: diffuse idiopathic skeletal hyperostosis (DISH), premature epiphyseal closure, and possible osteoporosis; myalgias (may have increased CPK), arthralgias
  - *Neurologic*: headache, fatigue, lethargy, pseudotumor cerebri (increased with concomitant tetracyclines)
  - *Psychologic*: anxiety and depression
  - *Lipids*: increase in plasma lipids (dose-dependent), especially triglycerides
  - *Gastrointestinal*: elevated LFTs, most commonly the transaminases, occurs between 2 and 8 weeks; nausea, diarrhea, abdominal pain
  - *Endocrine*: central hypothyroidism (bexarotene)
  - *Hematologic*: reversible leukopenia (especially bexarotene)
- Pregnancy category X (see Table 24-2 for pregnancy recommendations after therapy)

TABLE 24-1 Examples of CYP3A4 Subfamily Substrates, Inducers, and Inhibitors*

CYP3A4 Substrates	CYP3A4 Inducers	CYP3A4 Inhibitors
Alprazolam	Carbamazepine	Cimetidine
Atorvastatin	Cortisol	Clarithromycin
Buspirone	Dexamethasone	Diltiazem
Busulfan	Griseofulvin	Erythromycin
Cyclosporine	Nevirapine	Nelfinavir
Digoxin	Omeprazole	Fluconazole (high dose)
Didanosine	Pantoprazole	Fluoxetine
Docetaxel	Phenobarbital	Fluvoxamine
Dofetilide	Phenylbutazone	Gestodene
Erythromycin	Phenytoin	Grapefruit
Felodipine	Prednisone	Indinavir
Fluconazole	Primidone	Itraconazole
Glyburide	Rifabutin	Ketoconazole
Indinavir	Rifampicin	Miconazole
Itraconazole	Rifampin	Mibefradil
Ketoconazole	Troglitazone	Nefazodone
Loratadine		Nifedipine
Lovastatin (statins)		Omeprazole
Metformin		Propoxyphene
Miconazole		Ritonavir
Midazolam		Saquinavir
Nifedipine		Verapamil
Pimozide		
Prednisone		
Quinidine		
Rifampin		
Ritonavir		
Saquinavir		
Sildenafil		
Simvastatin (statins)		
Tacrolimus		
Triazolam		
Verapamil		
Vincristine		
Warfarin		

*This is not a complete list, and readers should refer to the manufacturer's individual package insert for current information.
From Freedberg IM et al. *Fitzpatrick's Dermatology in General Medicine*, 6th Ed. New York: McGraw-Hill; 2003, p. 2445.

Sulfones and Sulfonamides

- Sulfonamides inhibit the enzyme dihydropteroate synthestase and are used extensively as antimicrobials
- Sulfonamides (antimicrobial agents) and sulfones (anti-inflammatory agents) differ in chemical structures and uses

DAPSONE

- Sulfone derivative
- Mechanism of action = inhibition of neutrophil myeloperoxidase and impairment of neutrophil chemotaxis
- Metabolism: **a**cetylation (by *N*-acetyltransferase) and *N*-hydroxylation by P450 occur in the liver; the metabolic products are responsible for the hematologic side effects
- Dose-dependent adverse effects
    - *Hemolytic anemia*: glucose-6 phosphate dehydrogenase (G6PD)-deficient patients are more susceptible
    - *Methemoglobinemia*: related to *N*-hydroxy metabolites; treat with methylene blue (not effective in G6PD-deficient patients); vitamin E and cimetidine shown to reduce methemoglobin formation

TABLE 24-2 Key Characteristics of Retinoids

Drug	Generation	Half-Life	Receptor Specificity	
			RAR	RXR
Tretinoin (all-trans-RA)	First	40–60 min†	α,β,γ	—
Isotretinoin (13-cis-RA)	First	20 h*	—	—
9-cis-retinoic acid (alitretinoin)	Second	—	α,β,γ	α,β,γ
Etretinate	Second	160 d**	—	—
Acitretin	Second	50 h**	—	—
Bexarotene	Third	9 h	—	α,β,γ
Adapalene	Third	—	β,γ>α	—
Tazarotene	Third	16 h	β>γ>α	—

† For systemic formulation.
*Avoid pregnancy for 1 month after therapy.
**Avoid pregnancy for 3 years after therapy due to conversion to etretinate by alcohol consumption.

- Dose-independent adverse effects
  - *Hypersensitivity syndrome*: hepatitis, fever, generalized cutaneous eruption
  - *Hematologic*: agranulocytosis (occurs within first 12 weeks)
  - *Hepatic*: hepatitis, cholestatic jaundice, hypoalbuminemia
  - *Neurologic*: peripheral neuropathy (predominantly motor), usually reversible; psychosis; higher risk in long-term use
  - *Cutaneous*: drug rash, including TEN
  - *Gastrointestinal*: GI upset, anorexia
- Interactions with other medications
  - May inhibit anti-inflammatory effects of clofazimine
  - Probenecid and folic acid antagonists (e.g., methotrexate) increase dapsone toxicity
  - Trimethoprim/sulfamethoxazole taken with dapsone may increase toxicity of both drugs
  - Rifampin, para-amino benzoic acid, and activated charcoal may decrease absorption
- Contraindications: documented hypersensitivity, known G6PD deficiency or methemoglobin reductase deficiency
- Pregnancy category C

Sulfasalazine

- Mechanism of action: unknown; inhibits neutrophil chemotaxis
- Adverse effects: GI upset, fatigue, headache, drug eruption, and photosensitivity; slow acetylators are prone to toxicity, agranulocytosis (within first 3 months of therapy)
- Pregnancy category B

Miscellaneous

Agalsidase Beta

- Mechanism of action: decreases globotriasosylceramide (GL-3) deposition in capillary endothelium of the kidney
- Indicated for treatment of Fabry disease
- Adverse effects: anaphylaxis or severe allergic reaction in 1% of patients, infusion reactions
- Pregnancy category B

Auranofin

- Mechanism of action: gold is taken up by macrophages, which in turn inhibit phagocytosis and lysosomal membrane stabilization
- Alters immunoglobulins, decreasing prostaglandin synthesis and lysosomal enzyme activity
- Adverse effects: lichen planus–like eruptions, pityriasis rosea–like eruptions, nitroid reaction after injection (flushing, hypotension, dizziness), pulmonary infiltrates, stomatitis, cheilitis, dysgeusia, thrombocytopenia, granulocytopenia, aplastic anemia
- Pregnancy category C

Cinacalcet

- Class II calcimimetic; targets calcium-sensing receptor of parathyroid gland chief cells

- Mechanism of action: induces conformation change in calcium receptor, increasing sensitivity to circulating calcium; lowers PTH levels and improves calcium-phosphorus homeostasis in hemodialysis patients
- Has shown to be useful in treatment of calciphylaxis
- Adverse effects: nausea, vomiting, hypocalcemia, seizures
- Pregnancy category C

Colchicine

- Mechanism of action: binds to tubulin dimers in neutrophils and inhibits microtubule assembly needed in metaphase; antimitotic
- Adverse effects: dose-dependent GI symptoms of cramping and watery diarrhea common; overdose can cause renal failure, hepatic failure, permanent hair loss, bone marrow suppression, numbness or tingling in hands and feet, disseminated intravascular coagulopathy, decreased sperm count
- Pregnancy category C (parenteral D)

Flutamide

- Mechanism of action: nonsteroidal antiandrogen; converted to 2-OH-flutamide, which competitively inhibits DHT binding
- Combined with oral contraceptive pills to treat hirsutism
- Adverse effects: hepatotoxicity with potentially fulminant liver failure, thrombocytopenia, leucopenia, photosensitivity
- Pregnancy category D

Intravenous Immunoglobulin (IVIg)

- Immunoglobulins are extracted from purified human plasma pool
- Proposed mechanism of action: blockade of Fc receptors, prevents complement-mediated effects, reduces circulating pathogens and antibodies, alters cytokine/cytokine antagonist ratios, anti-Fas receptor antibodies block Fas ligand/Fas receptor binding and inhibit apoptosis (likely important in treatment of TEN)
- Adverse effects: increased Cr and BUN, infusion reaction (within 1 hour; headache, flushing, chills, myalgia, wheezing, tachycardia, low back pain, nausea, and/or hypotension), anaphylactic reactions in patients with IgA deficiency having anti-IgA antibodies, acute renal failure, thromboembolic events
- Pregnancy category C

Penicillamine

- Mechanism of action: metal chelator used to treat arsenic poisoning; historical usage for scleroderma
- Adverse mucocutaneous effects: elastosis perforans serpiginosa, bullous diseases (pemphigus, pemphigoid), drug-induced lupus, pseudoxanthoma elasticum, cutis laxa, anetoderma, and lichen planus
- Pregnancy category D

Potassium Iodide

- Mechanism of action: unknown; may inhibit granuloma formation and suppress delayed-type hypersensitivity reactions by releasing heparin from mast cells
- Used to treat sporotrichosis, erythema nodosum
- Adverse effects: hypothyroidism from Wolff-Chaikoff effect (excess iodide blocks organic iodide binding in thyroid hormone synthesis); iododerma, acneiform, and vascular eruptions; may cause flare of dermatitis herpetiformis
- Pregnancy category D

Sodium Thiosulfate

- Mechanism of action: chelates calcium in the form of calcium thiosulfate salts, which are much more soluble; results in dissolution and inhibition of precipitation of calcium deposits
- Useful in treatment of calciphylaxis
- Adverse effects: metabolic acidosis, transient mild rhinorrhea, sinus congestion, nausea, vomiting, hypomagnesaemia, decreased zinc levels
- Pregnancy category C

Stanozolol and Danazol

- Synthetic derivatives of testosterone, attenuated androgens alkylated in the 17-α position; marked anabolic properties
- Mechanism of action: increase concentrations of several plasma glycoproteins synthesized in the liver, including inhibitor of the first component of complement; potent fibrinolytic properties
- Used to prevent angioedema attacks in hereditary angioedema; fibrinolytic activity useful in treatment of cryofibrinogenemia, lipodermatosclerosis, and livedoid vasculopathy
- Adverse effects: mild hirsutism, alopecia, acne, and menstrual irregularities in females; hypertension and CHF due to sodium retention; increased risk of myopathy with statins; microscopic hematuria and hemorrhagic cystitis
- Pregnancy category X

Phototherapy

- Ultraviolet B (UVB) 290 to 320 nm, narrow band UVB 311 to 313 nm, excimer laser 308 nm
- Mechanism of action: reduces DNA synthesis, induced expression of tumor suppressor gene p53; induces release of prostaglandins and cytokines, e.g., IL-6 and IL-1; alters antigen-presenting function of Langerhans cells
- Minimal erythema dose (MED): defined as lowest dose that causes a minimally perceptible erythema at 24 hours after irradiation; may be used as a reference value for dosimetry
- Adverse effects: erythema, xerosis, photoaging, carcinogenesis
- Goeckerman regimen: coal tar followed by UVB exposure

- Ingram method: anthralin application following a tar bath and UVB treatment
- Psoralen and ultraviolet A (wavelengths 320–400 nm) photochemotherapy (PUVA)
  - Uses the photosensitizing drug 8-methoxypsoralen (8-MOP) in combination with ultraviolet A (UVA) irradiation
  - Mechanism of action: interferes with DNA synthesis by inhibiting mitosis and binding covalently to pyrimidine bases in DNA when photoactivated by UVA; decreases cellular proliferation; induces apoptosis of cutaneous lymphocytes leading to a localized immunosuppression
  - Adverse effects of PUVA therapy: nausea, pruritus, and burning; carcinogenic, with risk being cumulative dose-dependent (SCC > BCC); photosensitivity (minimize exposure to outdoor or bright indoor light for 24 hours after each dose); PUVA lentigines; photo-onycholyis
  - Contraindications: diseases associated with photosensitivity
  - Pregnancy category C
- Extracorporeal photochemotherapy (photopheresis)
  - Oral administration of 8-MOP followed by passage of blood through photopheresis machine which harvests mononuclear cells; red cell fraction returned to patient; mononuclear cell fraction exposed to UVA and then reinfused into patient
  - Mechanism of action: exact mechanism unknown; proposed to stimulate CD8+ T cell–mediated antitumor responses; apoptotic tumor cells taken up by antigen-presenting cells leading to antitumor immunity; induces immunoregulatory cytokine shifts
  - FDA approved for CTCL; also has been used in graft-versus-host disease, atopic dermatitis, systemic sclerosis, pemphigus and systemic lupus erythematosus
  - Adverse effects: nausea, hypotension, vasovagal reflex during volume shifts; contraindicated in severe cardiac disease
- Photodynamic therapy
  - FDA approved for treatment of nonhypertrophic actinic keratoses; used off-label to treat BCC, photoaging, acne, and Bowen disease
  - Mechanism of action
    - Topical application of aminolevulinic acid (ALA) on skin leads to the accumulation of the endogenous photosensitizer protoporphyrin IX (PpIX) in epidermal cells
    - Rapidly proliferating skin cells convert more ALA to PpIX than do less rapidly proliferating normal epidermal cells
    - Subsequent illumination of the lesion with noncoherent blue light (417 nm) 3 to 6 hours after ALA application causes ALA to be enzymatically converted into the active endogenous photosensitizer PpIX
  - Results in apoptosis of malignant cells; may also modify cytokine expression and induce immune-specific responses
  - Methyl 5-aminolevulinate also can be used instead of ALA with red light (635 nm); other light sources are between 400 and 800 nm (visible spectrum) and include pulsed dye laser and intense pulsed light
  - Adverse effects: burning and pruritus; erythema and mild edema of the treated area; generalized cutaneous photosensitivity, photophobia, and/or ocular discomfort, dyspigmentation
  - Pregnancy category C

TOPICAL TREATMENTS

Acne Preparations

Azelaic Acid

- Mechanism of action: reduces production of keratin and inhibits growth of *P. acnes*, antityrosinase activity
- Used to treat acne and rosacea; some benefit in PIH, melasma
- Adverse effects: may produce hypopigmentation, skin irritation
- Pregnancy category B

Benzoyl Peroxide

- Mechanism of action: broad spectrum bactericidal agent with oxidizing activity
- Activity against: *P. acnes, S. capitis , Staphylococcus epidermidis, Staphylococcus hominis, P. avidum, P. granulosum, and Pityrosporum ovale*
  - No reported resistance; can suppress antibiotic-resistant bacteria
- Antibacterial effect greater than comedolytic effects
- Adverse effects: skin irritation and drying; contact allergy (1%); bleaching of hair, fabrics
- Pregnancy category C

Retinoids (see Topical Retinoids)

Salicylic Acid

- Keratolytic
- Adverse effects: erythema and peeling
- Systemic toxicity (occurs when blood concentrations exceed 35 mg/dL): nausea, vomiting, confusion, dizziness, delirium, psychosis, stupor, coma, death, respiratory alkalosis, metabolic acidosis, hypoglycemia, tinnitus, and hyperventilation

Sulfur

- Comedolytic, keratolytic, mild antibacterial
- Adverse effects: odor, application site reaction
- Combination sulfur–sodium sulfacetamide commonly used to treat acne and rosacea

Antiperspirants

Aluminum Salts

- Mechanism of action: reversibly inhibits eccrine gland secretion by obstructing eccrine pores and inducing transient secretory cell atrophy
- Aluminum chloride 10 to 30% in distilled water or 60% alcohol
- Adverse effects: irritant dermatitis
- Pregnancy category C

Botulinum Toxin

- See Chapter 26

Bleaching Agents

Hydroquinone

- Inhibits tyrosinase (causes oxidation of tyrosine to 3-, 4-dihydroxyphenylamine)
- Adverse event: exogenous ochronosis
- Pregnancy category C

Topical Anesthetics (See Chapter 25)

Topical Antibiotics

- See the Systemic Medications section on systemic therapy for mechanisms of other antibiotics

Dapsone

- Sulfone derivative with anti-inflammatory properties
- Mechanism of action: see systemic section above
- Indicated for acne
- Adverse events: oiliness, peeling, dryness, erythema, no cross-reactivity with sulfonamides (antimicrobial agents)
- Pregnancy category C

Mupirocin

- Produced by fermentation of *Pseudomonas fluorescens*
- Effective against *Staph* , including MRSA and *Strep*
- Mechanism of action: inhibits bacterial isoleucyl-tRNA synthetase and blocks bacterial RNA synthesis
- Pregnancy category B

Retapamulin

- Belongs to the pleuromutilin class
- Mechanism of action: inhibits the initiation of protein synthesis at the level of bacterial 50S ribosome; bacteriostatic
- Used for impetigo caused by *S. aureus* or *S. pyogenes*
- Pregnancy category B

Silver Sulfadiazine

- Gram-positive and gram-negative coverage (including *MRSA* and *Pseudomonas*)
- Mechanism of action: inhibiting DNA replication and modification of the cell membrane
- Adverse effects: early leukopenia (in postburn patients); brown-gray hyperpigmentation of skin due to systemic absorption (argyria); caution in sulfa-allergic patients

Topical Antifungals

Azoles, Allylamines, and Polyenes: See Antifungal Agents Section

Ciclopirox

- Mechanism of action: chelation of polyvalent metal cations (e.g., Fe^{3+} and Al^{3+}); inhibits metal-dependent enzymes responsible for the degradation of peroxides within microbial cells
- Activity against dermatophytes, yeasts, and saprophytes
- Adverse effects: contact dermatitis and pruritus
- Pregnancy category B

Selenium Sulfide

- Mechanism of action: increases fungal shedding by decreasing comeocyte production; sporocidal
- Adverse effects: skin irritation, hair loss
- Pregnancy category C

Zinc Pyrithione

- Mechanism of action: inhibitor of membrane transport in fungi
- Adverse effects: allergic contact dermatitis

Topical Antivirals

Acyclovir and Penciclovir

- Mechanism of action and side effects: See Antiviral Agents section

Bleomycin

- Cytodestructive agent; used as intralesional agent for verruca vulgaris, keratoacanthomas
- Mechanism of action: exact mechanism of action against HPV unclear; inhibits DNA by binding to DNA, leading to single-strand scission and altering DNA metabolism
- Adverse effects: local pain and burning at injection site, erythema, swelling, scarring, Raynaud phenomenon, nail dystrophy, flagellate hyperpigmentation

Cantharidin

- Vesiculating agent derived from the "blister beetle" *Lytta vesicatoria*
- Mechanism of action: interferes with mitochondria leading to epidermal cell death, acantholysis, and vesiculation; no direct antiviral effect
- Adverse effects: pain, dyspigmentation, blistering

Imiquimod

- Imidazoquinoline amine

- Mechanism of action
  - Induction of cytokines (IFN-α, IL-12, IFN-γ, TNF-α) after binding toll-like receptor (TLR) 7 leading to stimulation of cell-mediated immunity
- Adverse effects: local skin irritation (burning, stinging), erythema
- Pregnancy category C

Podophyllin and Podofilox

- Extracts from May apple plant
- FDA approved for treatment of condyloma acuminata
- Mechanism of action: antimitotic agent; reversibly bind to protein tubulin and arrest cells in metaphase; active ingredient is podophyllotoxin
- Podophyllin: pregnancy category X; podofilox: pregnancy category C

Topical Chemotherapy Agents

5-Fluorouracil

- Mechanism of action: cell-cycle specific pyrimidine antagonist; inhibits thymidylate synthetase, leading to inhibition of DNA synthesis and cell death
- Adverse effects: local pain, pruritus, hyper/hypopigmentation, irritation, inflammation, and burning at the site of application; allergic contact dermatitis (rare)
- Pregnancy category D

Nitrogen Mustard

- Mechanism of action: cytotoxic to cancer cells via DNA alkylation
- Adverse effects: delayed hypersensitivity (35–60%), more common with aqueous forms, can be overcome with use of topical steroids or desensitization; possible association with increased risk of nonmelanoma skin cancers; dyspigmentation
- Pregnancy category D

Topical Immunosuppressives

Topical Calcineurin Inhibitors

- Tacrolimus and pimecrolimus
- Macrolide derived from *Streptomyces tsukubaensis*
- Mechanism of action: similar to cyclosporine
  - Bind to FK-506 binding protein (receptor within cytoplasm) and the drug-protein complex inhibits ability of calcineurin (a calcium-dependent phosphatase enzyme) to dephosphorylate NFAT
  - NFAT cannot translocate to the nucleus and activate transcription of proinflammatory cytokines (e.g., IL-2, IL-3, IL-4, IL-5, IL-10, GM-CSF, and TNF-α)
  - Reduction in T-cell activation
  - Tacrolimus shown to reduce *S. aureus* colonization in lesional skin in patients with atopic dermatitis
- Adverse effects: minimally absorbed into the blood (caution in patients with significantly compromised epidermal barrier); application site stinging (usually transient), alcohol intolerance with tacrolimus (facial flushing, redness, heat intolerance); black box warning for increased risk of lymphoma (based on animal studies and few case reports)
- Pregnancy category C

Topical Corticosteroids

- Mechanism of action: similar to systemic corticosteroids
- Efficacy of an individual topical corticosteroid (TCS) is related to its potency
- Pharmacokinetics: clinical potency depends on 3 factors: structure, vehicle, and type of skin to which it is applied
  - Removing, replacing, or masking the hydroxyl group lipophilicity, solubility, percutaneous absorption, glucocorticoid receptor (GCR)–binding activity
  - Halogenation: augments glucocorticoid and mineralocorticoid activity
  - Fluorination or chlorination: enhances potency
  - Propylene glycol enhances percutaneous absorption
  - Occlusive vehicles enhance absorption by increasing hydration of stratum corneum (ointment more potent than cream or lotion)
  - Skin penetration enhanced by inflamed or diseased skin, increased hydration of stratum corneum, relative humidity and temperature, and inversely proportional to stratum corneum thickness
- Adverse effects: local: acne, tachyphylaxis, skin atrophy (striae, telangiectasia, and purpura), glaucoma/cataracts, delayed wound healing, allergic contact dermatitis (Table 24-3); systemic: may suppress HPA axis (rare); growth impairment due to premature epiphyseal closure
- Risk factors for adverse effects: young age, liver disease, renal disease, amount of topical steroid applied, potency of topical steroid, use of occlusion, location of topical application (face, neck, axilla, groin, upper inner thighs)

Topical Retinoids

- Mechanism of action: see systemic section for details; all normalize follicular epithelial differentiation and keratinization leading to decreased microcomedo formation
- Retinoid receptor specificity: see Table 24-2
- Systemic absorption higher on dermatitic skin; 1 to 2% of tretinoin absorbed in normal skin, 5% of tazarotene absorbed in normal skin (15% in psoriatic skin)
- *Tretinoin (all-trans retinoic acid)*
  - May decrease TLR-2 (important in pathogenesis of inflammatory acne)
  - Adverse effects: irritation, erythema, scaling, xerosis, photosensitivity
  - Pregnancy category C
- *Adapalene*
  - Retinoid properties from a synthetic naphtholic acid derivative
  - Pregnancy category C

TABLE 24-3 Allergenicity and Cross-reactivity of Corticosteroids

Structural Class	Representative Agents in Class	Patch-Screening Agent	Cross-reactivity
Group A	Hydrocortisone Methylprednisolone Prednisolone	Tixocortal-21-pivalate	Class D2
Group B	Triamcinolone Desonide Budesonide Fluocinonide	Budesonide	Class D2
Group C	Betamethasone Dexamethasone Desoximetasone	—	Least allergenic group
Group D1	Betamethasone dipropionate Betamethasone valerate Clobetasol Fluticasone Mometasone	Clobetasol-17-propionate	No significant cross-reactions
Group D2	Prednicarbate Hydrocortisone	Hydrocortisone-17-butyrate	Class A and budesonide

- *Tazarotene*
    - Prodrug is hydrolyzed rapidly in tissues to the active metabolite tazarotenic acid
    - Pregnancy category X
- *Alitretinoin (9-cis-retinoic* acid): used for Kaposi sarcoma
    - Pregnancy category D
- *Bexarotene*: used in stages IA and IB persistent or refractory CTCL
    - Pregnancy category X

Sunscreens

- Chemical blockers
    - Aromatic compounds conjugated with a carbonyl group
    - Absorb UV and produce excitation to higher energy state; energy is converted to lower-energy wavelength upon return to ground state

Ultraviolet A Filters

- *Oxybenzone (benzophenone)*
    - Absorbs well in UVA II wavelengths; primarily UVB absorbers, 270 to 350nm
    - Most common cause of sunscreen allergy
- *Menthyl anthranilate*
    - Absorbs mainly in the near UVA portion, 260 to 380nm, weak UVB
- Avobenzone (Parsol 1789), 320 to 400 nm; photolabile—must be photostabilized by combination with octocrylene and other compounds; the only available filter providing protecting in the long UVA range
- Dioxybenzone, 250 to 390nm
- *Ecamsule*

Ultraviolet B Filters

- *Aminobenzoic acid and derivatives*
    - Padimate O (PABA esters): most potent UVB absorber
    - High incidence of hypersensitivity
    - Cross-sensitivity with PABA: artificial sweeteners (e.g., saccharin, sodium cyclamate); ester-type anesthetics, Azo dyes (e.g., aniline, paraphenylenediamine), sulfonamide antibiotics, sulfonamide-based oral hypoglycemics, or thiazide diuretics
- *Cinnamates (Parsol MCX)*
    - Octyl methoxycinnamate (second most potent UVB absorber compared with padimate O)
    - Cross-sensitivity to balsam of Peru
    - Frequent cause of allergic reactions
- *Phenylbenzimidazole sulfonic acid*
    - Selective UVB filter; water soluble
- *Salicylates*
    - Octyl salicylate: used to augment the UVB protection in a sunscreen; weak UVB absorber on its own, 280 to 320 nm
- Weak UVB absorbers
    - *Octocrylene*
    - May be used in combination with other UV absorbers to achieve higher SPF

Physical Blockers

- Broad spectrum; reflect sunlight; low incidence of contact sensitivity
- *Titanium dioxide*
- *Zinc oxide*
  - Better UVA1 protection than titanium dioxide

Others

Anthralin

- Mechanism of action
  - Naturally occurring saturated dicarboxylic acid possessing antibacterial, comedolytic, and anti-inflammatory activities
  - Inhibits monocyte proinflammatory activity and induces extracellular generation of free radicals; anti-Langerhans cell effect
- Adverse effects: irritation, staining of clothing, hair, skin, and nails
- Pregnancy category C

Calcipotriene (Calcipotriol)

- Synthetic analog of calcitriol
- Mechanism of action
  - Inhibits proliferation of keratinocytes in culture; modulates epidermal differentiation
  - Promotes formation of cornified envelope by increasing involucrin and transglutaminase
  - Inhibits IL-2 and IL-6 production; blocks transcription of IFN-γ and GM-CSF
  - Inhibits cytotoxic T-cell and NK cell activity
- Degraded when combined with hydrocortisone valerate, ammonium lactate, or salicylic acid
- Adverse effects: hypercalcemia (usually in doses > 100 g per week), irritation, photosensitivity, allergic contact dermatitis (uncommon)
- Pregnancy category C

Castellani Paint

- Compounded solution of resorcinol (8 g), acetone (4 mL), magenta (0.4 g), phenol (4.0 g), boric acid (0.8 g), industrial methylated spirit 90% (8.5 mL), and water (100 mL)
- Fungicidal and bactericidal
- Adverse effects: magenta can stain clothing and skin; may be toxic in children because of phenol content; irritation
- Pregnancy category C

Eflornithine HCl

- Mechanism of action: inhibits enzyme ornithine decarboxylase (ODC)
  - Metabolic activity in the hair follicle decreases, and hairs grow in more slowly
- Adverse effect: mild skin irritation
- Pregnancy category C

Ingenol Mebutate

- Mechanism of action: macrocyclic diterpene ester from sap of *Euphorbia peplus* plant; suspected to induce rapid and direct cell death and immune responses mediated by protein kinase C delta, including neutrophil-mediated oxidative burst
- Indicated for field-directed topical therapy for actinic keratoses for 2 to 3 consecutive days
- Adverse effects: local skin reactions, pruritus, pain, local infection, periorbital edema, nasopharyngitis, headache
- Pregnancy category C

Brimonidine

- Mechanism of action: α_2-adrenergic receptor agonist; causes vasoconstriction
- 0.33% topical gel FDA approved for treatment of persistent facial erythema in adults with rosacea
- Adverse effects: erythema, flushing, skin burning sensation, contact dermatitis
- Pregnancy Category B

Timolol Maleate

- Mechanism of action: nonselective β-adrenergic receptor inhibitor approved in 1978 for the treatment of glaucoma
- 0.5% topical gel used for off-label use for small, nonulcerated infantile hemangiomas on nonmucosal surfaces
- Adverse effects: apnea, bradycardia, asthma, dizziness, and dissociated behavior have been seen with ophthalmic use
- Pregnancy category C

PHARMACOGENETICS

- Recent studies suggest an association between HLA alleles and susceptibility to drug hypersensitivity reactions
- HLA-B*1502: Carbamazepine-induced SJS/TEN in Han Chinese in Taiwan and Hong Kong, Thais, and Indians
- HLA-B*1502: Phenytoin-induced SJS in Han Chinese in Taiwan and Thais
- HLA-B*5801: Allopurinol-induced SJS/TEN and DIHS/DRESS in Han Chinese in Taiwan, Thais, Japanese, and Europeans
- HLA-A*0206: SJS/TEN with severe ocular complications in Japanese
- HLA-A*3101: Carbamazepine-induced SJS/TEN and DRESS in Japanese and Europeans
- HLA-B*5701: Abacavir-induced hypersensitivity in Europeans
- HLA-B*3505: Nevirapine-induced hypersensitivity in Thais
- HLA-DRB1*0101: Nevirapine-induced hypersensitivity in Europeans

TABLE 24-4 Cutaneous Side Effects of Systemic Medications

Side Effect	Associated Medications
Acanthosis nigricans	Nicotinic acid/niacin, OCPs, dilantin, estrogens, steroids
Acneiform eruptions	Phenytoin, isoniazid, iodides, phenobarbital, lithium, ethionamide, steroids, EGFR inhibitors
Acute generalized exanthematous pustulosis	β-lactam antibiotics, macrolide antibiotics, calcium channel blockers, antimalarials, terbinafine, imatinib
Aplasia cutis congenita	Methimazole
Blue-gray hyperpigmentation	Amiodarone, antimalarials, anticonvulsants, minocycline, imipramine, OCPs, clofazamine
Blue lunulae	5-FU, AZT
Bullous pemphigoid	Furosemide, penicillamine, captopril, gold, PCN, sulfonamides, PUVA, enalopril, NSAIDs, β-blockers
Cutis laxa	Penicillin, penicillamine
Dental abnormalities	Tetracyclines (gray discoloration)
Dermatomyositis	Hydroxyurea, penicillimine
Drug hypersensitivity syndrome/ DRESS	Carbamazepine, lamotrigine, phenobarbital, phenytoin, indinavir, nevirapine, sulfonamides, minocycline, allopurinol
EPS	Penicillamine
Erythema nodosum	OCPs, antibiotics (sulfonamides, tetracycline, PCN), 13-*cis* retinoic acid, gold, opiates, halogens
Fixed drug eruptions	NSAIDs, sulfonamides, pseudoephedrine (nonpigmented), phenopthaleine laxatives, tetracycline, barbiturates, carbamazepine
Gingival hyperplasia	Calcium channel blockers, cyclosporine, dilantin
Hypertrichosis	Cyclosporine, diazoxide, danazol, minoxidil, spironolactone, psoralen, phenytoin
Ichthyosis	Nicotinic acid
Leg ulcers	Hydroxyurea
Lichenoid eruptions	Lasix, penicillamine, gold, thiazides, chlorpropamide, antimalarials, methyldopa, phenylthiazides, β-blockers
Linear IgA	Vancomycin, β-lactam antibiotics, NSAIDS, ACE inhibitors (captopril), lithium, phenytoin
Livedo reticularis	Quinidine (photodistributed), amantadine
Melanonychia	AZT, cyclophosphamide, bleomycin, 5-FU, doxorubicin
Pellagra-like eruption	Isoniazid, azathioprine, 5-FU
Pemphigus vulgaris	Penicillamine, thiols (captopril)
Penile ulcers	Foscarnet
Photoallergic drug eruption	Griseofulvin, NSAIDs, phenothiazines, quinidine, sulfa drugs, thiazide diuretics

(Continued)

TABLE 24-4 Cutaneous Side Effects of Systemic Medications (Continued)

Side Effect	Associated Medications
Photo-onycholysis	Tetracycline, 8-MOP
Phototoxic drug eruption	Amiodarone, flouroquinolone, NSAIDS, phenothiazines (chlorpromazine), tetracyclines, psoralens, voriconazole
Pityriasis rosea–like eruptions	Barbiturates/bismuth, omeprazole, β-blockers, captopril, clonidine, griseofulvin, isotretinoin, metronidazole, penicillin
Porphyria cutanea tarda	Griseofulvin, rifampin, antimalarials, alcohol, busulfan, benzenes, hormones, iron, phenols, sulfonylurea
Pseudolymphoma	Anticonvulsants (phenytoin, phenobarbital), antihypertensives (β-blockers, ACE inhibitors, calcium channel blockers), tricyclic antidepressants, allopurinol
Pseudoporphyria	Tetracycline, isotretinoin, NSAIDs, griseofulvin, lasix, sulfonamides, hemodialysis for chronic renal failure
PXE	Penicillamine
Psoriasis	G-CSF, INH, interferon, NSAIDs, steroid withdrawal, lithium, ACE inhibitors, antimalarials, β-blockers, penicillamine
Pyogenic granulomas	Retinoids (isotretinoin), antiretrovirals (indinavir), estrogen
Serum sickness–like reaction	Cefaclor, ciprofloxacin, minocycline, PCN, sulfonamides, itraconazole, anticonvulsants, bupropion, fluoxetine, rituximab
SCLE	HCTZ, calcium channel blockers, terbinafine, sulfonylureas, griseofulvin, naproxen, gold, taxanes, azathioprine
SLE	Procainamide, hydralazine, dilantin, chlorpromazine, isoniazid, minocycline, penicillamine (induces native dsDNA), β-blockers
Sweet syndrome	G-CSF, all-trans retinoic acid, tetracyclines, TMP/SMZ, celecoxib, furosemide, norfloxacin
Toxic epidermal necrolysis/SJS	Sulfonamides, allopurinol, NSAIDs, anticonvulsants (phenytoin, phenobarbital, carbamazepine), pentamidine
Trichomegaly	Interferon, bimatoprost, EGFR inhibitors
Urticaria	Aspirin, NSAIDs, antibiotics (penicillin, cephalosporins, sulfonamides), contrast dye, ACE inhibitors (captopril)
Vasculitis	Penicillins, sulfonamides, cephalosporins, thiazides, furosemide, NSAIDs

*This is not a complete list but is intended to represent the agents most frequently associated with a given side effect.

PREGNANCY CATEGORIES

- All drugs are classified into the following categories:
  - A. Controlled studies show no risk
    - Adequate, well-controlled studies in pregnant women have failed to demonstrate risk to fetus
  - B. No evidence of risk in humans
    - Either animal findings show risk but human findings do not, or if no adequate human studies have been done, animal findings are negative
  - C. Risk cannot be ruled out
    - Human studies are lacking, and the animal studies are either positive for fetal risk or lacking; however, potential benefits may justify the potential risk

TABLE 24-5 Cutaneous Side Effects of Chemotherapeutic Agents

Side Effect	Associated Medications
Acral erythema/Hand-foot syndrome	Cytarabine, bleomycin, doxorubicin, etoposide, 5-FU, hydroxyurea, mercaptopurine, methotrexate, capecitabine, docetaxel, thiotepa, sorafenib, sunitinib, cyclophosphamide
Eccrine squamous syringometaplasia	Cytarabine, cyclophosphamide, busulfan, carmustine, taxanes, imatinib
Eruptive KAs, SCCs	Sorafenib, vemurafenib
Facial edema	Sunitinib, imatinib
Flagellate hyperpigmentation	Bleomycin
Hair/eyelash curling	EGFR inhibitors
Hair depigmentation	Sunitinib
Hair repigmentation	Imatinib
Hyperpigmentation under bandages	Carmustine, thiotepa
Hypopigmentation	Imatinib
Inflammed Aks	Capecitabine, sorafenib, 5-FU
Mycosis fungoides–like eruption	Sorafenib
Nail hyperpigmentation	Imatinib, idarubicin, taxanes
Neutrophilic eccrine hidradenitis	Cytarabine, bleomycin, G-CSF, anthracyclines, cyclophosphamide, cisplatin, topotecan, sunitinib
Ocular toxicity	Imatinib
Palmoplantar keratoderma	Tegafur
Papulopustular/follicular eruption	EGFR inhibitors (erlotinib, gefitinib, cetuximab)
Pityriasis rosea–like eruption	Imatinib
Pseudoscleroderma	Docetaxel, gemcitabine
Radiation recall	Taxanes, anthracyclines (doxorubicin), gemcitabine, capecitabine, actinomycin D, methotrexate, hydroxyurea
Raynaud	Bleomycin, vincristine
SCLE	Docetaxel, paclitaxel
Serpiginous pigmentation over veins	5-flourouracil
Subungal hemorrhage/paronychia/pyogenic granulomas	Paclitaxel, docetaxel, sorafenib, sunitinib, EGFR inhibitors
Trichomegaly	EGFR inhibitors
Yellow skin discoloration	Sunitinib

- D. Positive evidence for risk
  - Investigational or postmarketing data show risk to fetus; potential benefits may outweigh the potential risk
- X. Contraindicated in pregnancy
  - Studies in animals or humans or investigational or postmarketing reports have shown fetal risk that clearly overweighs any possible benefit to the patient

DRUG SIDE EFFECTS

Cutaneous Side Effects of Systemic Medications (Table 24-4)

Cutaneous Side Effects of Chemotherapeutic Agents (Table 24-5)

QUIZ

Questions

1. A 65-year-old Caucasian man is started on azathioprine for the treatment of bullous pemphigoid. Upon review of his laboratory work at his 2-month follow-up appointment, you note a WBC of 3000/mm^3 and a hemoglobin of 9 g/dL. He tells you he was recently started on a new medication by his primary care physician for joint pain. Which of the following medications was most likely started?

   A. Naproxen
   B. Colchicine
   C. Acetaminophen
   D. Allopurinol
   E. Prednisone

2. A 75-year-old African-American man presents for evaluation of a bilateral lower extremity rash. His rash is most consistent with stasis dermatitis and you start treatment with triamcinolone 0.1% ointment. At his follow-up appointment in 6 weeks, his condition is significantly worse and you are concerned about allergic contact dermatitis. Which of the following should be used to screen for allergy to triamcinolone?

   A. Budesonide
   B. Tixocortol-21-pivalate
   C. Hydrocortisone-17-butyrate
   D. Clobetasol-17-propionate
   E. Desoximetasone

3. You start a patient on dapsone for dermatitis herpetiformis. Which of the following drugs, when given concomitantly, may reduce the risk of methemoglobin formation?

   A. Ranitidine
   B. Vitamin C
   C. Cimetidine
   D. Zinc
   E. Folic acid

4. A 55-year-old Asian man from Taiwan presents with fever, conjunctival and penile erosions, as well as tender, erythematous, purpuric macules coalescing into patches on the torso. His history reveals that he suffered a CVA several months ago that was complicated by late-onset seizures and was started on phenytoin 2 weeks ago. Which of the following HLA types may have increased his risk for this adverse drug effect?

   A. HLA-A*0206
   B. HLA-B*5701
   C. HLA-B*3505
   D. HLA-B*5801
   E. HLA-B*1502

5. Match the biologic to its mechanism of action.

   A. Alefacept
   B. Etanercept
   C. Anakinra
   D. Ustekinumab
   E. Rituximab

   i. IL-1 receptor antagonist
   ii. Blocks interaction of LFA-3 on APC with CD2 on T cells
   iii. Binds to CD 20 on surface of mature B cells
   iv. Binds the p40 subunit on IL-12 and IL-23
   v. TNF-α inhibitor

6. Match the following chemotherapeutic agent to its appropriate cutaneous side effect.

   A. Sorafenib
   B. Thiotepa
   C. Cytarabine
   D. Methotrexate
   E. Bleomycin

   i. Flagellate hyperpigmentation
   ii. Neutrophilic eccrine hidradenitis
   iii. Eruptive KAs/SCCs
   iv. Hyperpigmentation under bandages
   v. Radiation recall

7. Which of the following represents the mechanism of action of vismodegib in the treatment of locally advanced basal cell carcinoma?

   A. Binds and inactivates *patched* resulting in constitutive activation of Gli and downstream Hedgehog target genes
   B. Binds and activates *smoothened* resulting in constitutive activation of Gli and downstream Hedgehog target genes
   C. Anti-Fas receptor antibodies block Fas ligand/Fas receptor binding and inhibit apoptosis
   D. Binds and inhibits *smoothened* to inhibit activation of downstream Hedgehog target genes
   E. Anti-Fas receptor antibodies simulate Fas ligand/Fas receptor binding and induce apoptosis

8. Match the antiviral medication with its side effect.

A. Zidovudine (AZT)	i. Reversible obstructive neuropathy
B. Foscarnet	ii. Exacerbation of psoriasis
C. Indinavir	iii. Penile ulcers
D. Interferon	iv. Hyperpigmented nail streaks
E. Acyclovir	v. Lipodystrophy

9. Which of the following is the likely mechanism of action for the beneficial effects of IVIg in the treatment of TEN?
   A. Suppression of antibody production by IgG binding via Fc fragment to cell surface receptors on B cells
   B. Anti-Fas receptor antibodies inhibit Fas ligand/Fas receptor binding and thereby inhibit apoptosis
   C. Inhibition of T-cell activation by downregulation of costimulatory molecules
   D. Binds to and inhibits pathogenic antibodies
   E. Binds to high-affinity IL-2 receptors to inhibit protein synthesis

10. A 39-year-old man who is status postrenal transplant develops painful grouped vesicles and crusted erosions on the right forehead, right upper eyelid, and nose that do not cross midline. He is started on treatment and develops abrupt onset of fever, thrombocytopenia, petechiae, and altered mental status. Which of the following medications was he most likely being treated with?
    A. Acyclovir
    B. Foscarnet
    C. Prednisone
    D. IVIg
    E. Valacyclovir

Answers

1. D. Allopurinol. Increased risk of bone marrow suppression may occur with concomitant use of azathioprine and allopurinol. Allopurinol inhibits xanthine oxidase, thus shunting more 6-MP to the HGPRT pathway. This creates an excess of toxic purine analogs and results in increased risk for myelosuppression. If azathioprine is to be given to patients taking allopurinol, the dose must be markedly reduced.
2. A. Budesonide. The patch test screening agent for suspected contact allergy to triamcinolone, a member of structural Class B, is budesonide. Tixocortol-21-pivalate is used to test for contact allergy to Class A corticosteroids, such as hydrocortisone acetate. Hydrocortisone-17-butyrate is the agent used to screen for allergy to Class D2 corticosteroids, such as hydrocortisone valerate. Clobetasol-17-propionate is used to test for contact allergy to Class D1 corticosteroids, which include betamethasone.
3. C. Cimetidine. Both cimetidine and vitamin E have been shown to reduce the risk of methemoglobin formation in patients taking dapsone by reducing the hepatic oxidation of dapsone to hydroxylamine.
4. E. HLA-B*1502. Individuals of Han Chinese descent possessing the HLA-B*1502 allele are shown to have an increased risk of developing SJS secondary to phenytoin. This HLA type is also associated with carbamazepine-induced SJS/TEN in Han Chinese, Thais, and Indians. HLA-A*0206 is associated with SJS/TEN with severe ocular complications in Japanese patients. HLA-B*5701 is associated with abacavir-induced hypersensitivity in Europeans. HLA-B*3505 is seen in association with nevirapine-induced hypersensitivity in Thais. HLA-B*5801 is seen with allopurinol-induced SJS/TEN and DIHS/DRESS in Han Chinese in Taiwan, Thais, Japanese, and Europeans.
5. A. ii; B. v; C. i; D. iv; E. iii. Alefacept is a human LFA-3/IgG fusion protein that inhibits the interaction of LFA-3 on antigen-presenting cells with CD2 on activated T cells. Etanercept is a human dimeric fusion protein of the TNF-α receptor and the Fc portion of human IgG1 which binds to and inhibits TNF-α. Anakinra is an IL-1 receptor antagonist which is used in the treatment of periodic fever syndromes and rheumatoid arthritis. Ustekinumab is a human monoclonal antibody that binds the p40 subunit of IL-12 and IL-23. Rituximab binds to CD20 on the surface of mature B cells.
6. A. iii; B. iv; C. ii; D. v; E. i. Sorafenib is associated with eruptive keratoacanthomas and squamous cell carcinomas. Thiotepa is reported to cause hyperpigmentation under bandages and other occluded areas such as the axillae. Cytarabine is frequently associated with neutrophilic eccrine hidradenitis. Methotrexate may cause radiation recall in which drug administration is associated with the reappearance of previous sunburn or previously irradiated area becomes inflamed. Bleomycin is associated with the development of flagellate hyperpigmentation.
7. D. Vismodegib acts in the treatment of locally advanced basal cell carcinoma by binding and inactivating *smoothened* which inhibits the activation of Gli and downstream Hedgehog signaling targets. Most basal cell carcinomas have abnormal Hedgehog signaling.
8. A. iv; B. iii; C. v; D. ii; E. i. Zidovudine may cause hyperpigmentation of the nails, oral mucosa, and skin. Penile erosions/ulcerations may occur in patients taking foscarnet. Protease inhibitors are associated with the development of lipodystrophy or abnormal fat deposits. Interferon may cause a flare of psoriasis. Acyclovir, when given intravenously, may cause a reversible obstructive neuropathy due to crystal deposition.
9. B. Fas ligand–mediated apoptosis is one of the proposed mechanisms in the development of TEN. It is thought that

IVIg is effective in the treatment of TEN due to the action of anti-Fas receptor antibodies that inhibit Fas ligand/Fas receptor binding and thereby inhibit apoptosis.

10. E. Use of valacyclovir at high doses in transplant patients is associated with severe, sometimes fatal, cases of thrombotic thrombocytopenic purpura/hemolytic uremic syndrome.

REFERENCES

Agero AL et al. Dermatologic side effects associated with the epidermal growth factor receptor inhibitors. *J Am Acad Dermatol* 2006;55(4):657-670.

Aihara M: Phamacogenetics of cutaneous adverse drug reactions. *J Dermatol* 2011;38:246-254.

Aoki M et al. New pharmacogenetic test for detecting an *HLA-A*31-01* allele using the InvaderPlus assay. *Pharmacogenet Genomics* 2012;22:441-446.

Balagula Y et al. The emergence of supportive oncodermatology: the study of dermatologic adverse events to cancer therapies. *J Am Acad Dermatol* 2010;65(3):624-635.

Bolognia JL, Jorizzo JJ, Rapini RP, eds: *Dermatology*, 2nd Ed. Edinburgh: Mosby; 2008.

Chan H et al. RCT of timolol maleate gel for superficial infantile hemangiomas in 5- to 24-week-olds. *Pediatr* 2013;131(6):e1739-e1747.

Chapman PB et al. Improved survival with vemurafenib in melanoma with BRAF V600E mutation. *N Engl J Med* 2011;364(26):2507-2516.

Dissemond J et al. Leg ulcer in a patient associated with hydroxyurea therapy. *Int J Dermatol* 2006;45:158-160.

Fowler J et al. Efficacy and safety of once-daily topical brimonidine tartrate gel 0.5% for the treatment of moderate to severe facial erythema of rosacea: results of two randomized, double-blind, and vehicle-controlled pivotal studies. *J Drugs Dermatol* 2013;12(6):650-656.

Heidary N et al. Chemotherapeutic agents and the skin: an update. *J Am Acad Dermatol* 2008;58(4):547-570.

Hodi FS et al. Improved survival with ipilimumab in patients with metastatic melanoma. *N Engl J Med* 2010;363(8):711-723.

Hu JC et al. Cutaneous side effects of epidermal growth factor receptor inhibitors: clinical presentation, pathogenesis, and management. *J Am Acad Dermatol* 2007;56(2):318-326.

Huang V et al. Dermatologic manifestations of cytotoxic therapy. *Dermatol Ther* 2011;24:401-410.

Johnson DB et al. Update on the targeted therapy of melanoma. *Curr Treat Options Oncol* 2013;14:280-292.

Kalb RE et al. Methotrexate and psoriasis: 2009 national psoriasis foundation consensus conference. *J Am Acad Dermatol* 2009;60(5):824-837.

Lebwohl M: Ingenol mebutate gel for actinic keratosis. *N Engl J Med* 2012;366:1010-1019.

Litt JZ, ed. *Drug Eruption Reference Manual 2002.* New York: The Parthenon Publishing Group, Inc.; 2002.

LoRusso PM et al. Phase I trial of Hedgehog pathway inhibitor vismodegib (GDC-0449) in patients with refractory, locally advanced or metastatic solid tumors. *Clin Cancer Res* 2011;17:2502-2511.

Marmor MF: Revised recommendations on screening for chloroquine and hydroxylchloroqine retinopathy. *Ophthalmology* 2011;188:415-422.

Maurer M et al. Omalizumab for the treatment of chronic idiopathic or spontaneous urticaria. *N Eng J Med* 2013;368(10):924-935.

Paul LJ et al. Paclitaxel-associated subungal pyogenic granuloma: report in a patient with breast cancer receiving paclitaxel and review drug-induced pyogenic granulomas adjacent to and beneath the nail. *J Drugs Dermatol* 2012;11(2):262-268.

Phillips EJ et al. Drug hypersensitivity: pharmacogenetics and clinical sydromes. *J Allergy Clin Immunol* 2011;127(3):S60-S66.

Thong BY et al. Epidemiology and risk factors for drug allergy. *Br J Clin Pharmacol* 2011;71(5):684-700.

Winnington P: What you should know about drugs in the pipeline. *Prac Dermatol* 2007;4(12):24-29.

Wolverton SE, ed. *Comprehensive Dermatologic Drug Therapy*, 2nd Ed. Philadelphia: W.B. Saunders; 2007.

CHAPTER 25

SURGERY AND ANATOMY

T. MINSUE CHEN
RUNGSIMA WANITPHAKDEEDECHA
TRI H. NGUYEN

ANATOMIC REVIEW OF ARTERIES AND VEINS AND LYMPHATICS

Arteries of the Head and Neck (Fig. 25-1, Table 25-1)

- Blood supply to the head and neck
- The internal carotid artery (ICA)
- External carotid artery (ECA) and their branches
- Intimate anastamoses between ICA and ECA in the region of the upper central face (nose, glabella, periorbital, and forehead)
- These connections are important clinically in that
  - Infections in this area may extend intracranially via ICA
  - Steroid injections in the periorbital skin may embolize to the retinal artery and cause blindness
- Named arteries give rise to unnamed branches and perforators that nourish overlying muscles, fascia, subcutaneous fat, and skin
  - *Septocutaneous arteries*: travel through septa to skin
  - *Musculocutaneous arteries*: perforate muscles to skin
  - *Subdermal plexus arteries*: at the junction of the subcutaneous fat and the deep reticular dermis
    - Arise from septocutaneous and musculocutaneous arteries
    - Main blood supply to the skin
    - Undermine at least below midfat to preserve the subdermal plexus as immediate subdermal undermining may compromise the subdermal plexus

Venous System of the Lower Extremities (Fig. 25-2, Table 25-2)

- Consists of the superficial (above muscular fascia) and deep (below muscular fascia) venous system
- The superficial and deep systems are connected via perforator veins
- Flow is unidirectional due to bicuspid valves in veins
  - Superficial veins drain into the deep veins via the perforators
  - Deep veins merge to form the common femoral vein
  - Venous valves permit only one-way flow (upward), when competent
  - Greatest density in the calf and progressively fewer valves in the thigh
- Calf muscles act as a muscular pump to propel venous blood upward
  - Venous blood is moved only during muscle contraction
  - Lying still or standing still does not drain the venous system

Lymphatics

Lymph Glands of the Head and Neck

- See Fig. 25-3

Lymph Glands of the Upper Extremity

- Divided into 2 sets: superficial and deep
  - Superficial lymph glands: few and of small size
  - Deep lymph glands: chiefly grouped in the axilla

Lymphatics of the Lower Extremity

- *Anterior tibial gland*: small and inconstant
- *Popliteal glands*: small in size and some six or seven in number; imbedded in the fat
- *Inguinal glands*: situated at the upper part of the femoral triangle

ANATOMIC REVIEW OF MUSCLES

See Tables 25-3 and 25-4.

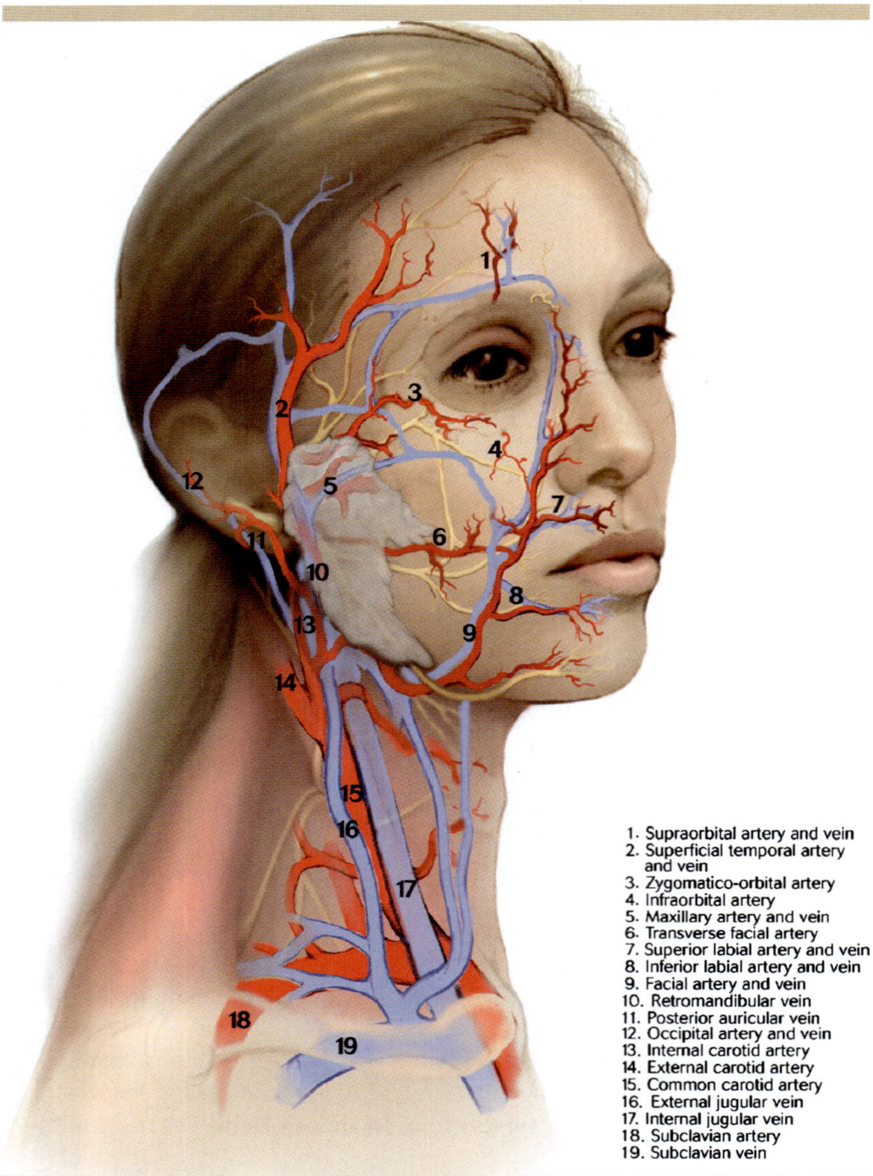

FIGURE 25-1 Arteries of the head and neck.

ANATOMIC REVIEW OF NERVES

Nerve Blocks: General Considerations

- Aspirate before injecting
  - Use a 30-gauge needle with a 60-degree beveled point
  - If pain/dysesthesia is elicited during insertion or injection, withdraw the needle slightly to avoid injuring the nerve itself
  - Do not inject the nerve directly; goal is to bathe the perineural space with local anesthetic
  - Wait at least 10 to 20 minutes for effective anesthesia
  - Most importantly: know your anatomy

Innervation of the Head and Neck (Tables 25-5, 25-6, and 25-7; Figs. 25-5 and 25-6)

- *Facial nerve (CN VII)*
  - Emerges from cranium through the stylomastoid foramen and runs in the deep body of the parotid in the lateral cheek/jaw
  - *Sensory* (minor role): sensation to the external auditory meatus along with auriculotemporal and vagus nerves
  - *Motor* (major function): 5 branches that innervate the muscles of facial expression are
    - Temporal
    - Zygomatic
    - Buccal

TABLE 25-1 Branches of the Carotid Artery

Internal Carotid Artery Branches	External Carotid Artery Branches
Supplies structures inside the skull, except for central facial arteries that nourish the periorbital skin, forehead, glabella, and nose: • Supraorbital • Supratrochlear • Infratrochlear • Dorsal nasal • External nasal arteries	• Superficial temporal • Maxillary – Anterior tympanic – Middle meningeal – Inferior alveolar – Accessory meningeal – Masseteric – Pterygoid – Deep temporal – Buccal – Sphenopalatine – Descending palatine – Infraorbital – Posterior superior alveolar – Middle superior alveolar – Pharyngeal – Anterior superior alveolar – Artery of the pterygoid canal • Posterior auricular • Occipital • Facial • Lingual • Ascending pharyngeal • Superior thyroid

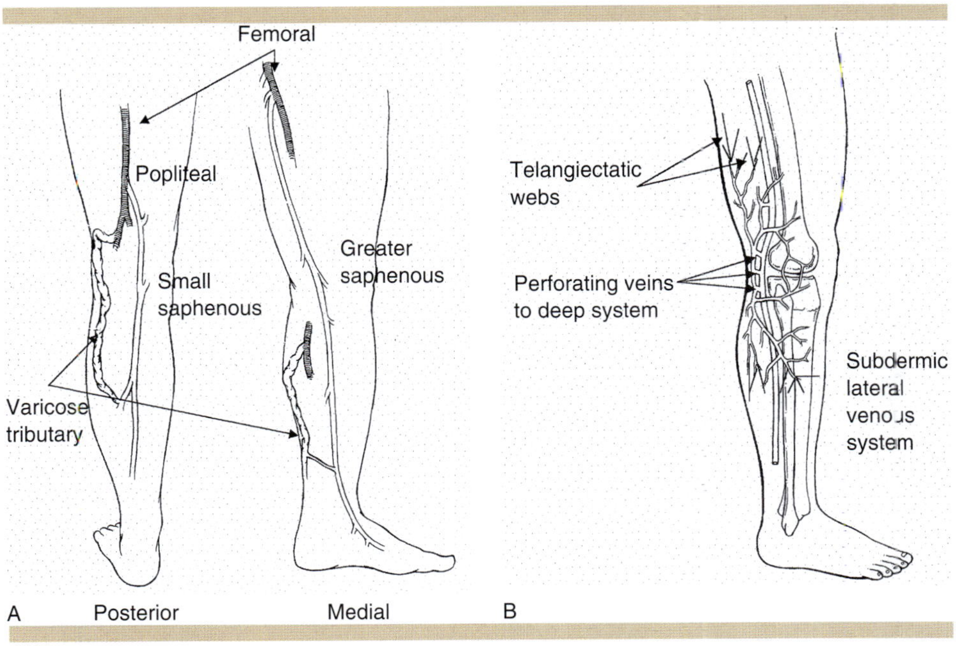

FIGURE 25-2 Venous system of lower extremities.

TABLE 25-2 Leg Veins

	Superficial Leg Veins	Deep Leg Veins
Location	Veins lie above the deep muscular fascia and drain into the deep venous system There are 3 major networks in the superficial venous system Great saphenous vein (GSV) • Originates from the dorsal arch veins of the foot, runs anterior to medial malleolus, up medial calf, knee, and inner thigh, and empties into the common femoral vein via the saphenofemoral junction (SFJ) • The longest superficial vein of the lower leg • Most common cause of superficial venous insufficiency Small saphenous vein (SSV) • Runs behind the lateral malleolus, up the posterior calf, and empties into the popliteal vein (where it empties may vary with individuals) within or near the popliteal fossa • Drains skin and superficial fascia of the lateral and posterior side of the foot and leg Lateral venous system (LVS) • Lateral venous system: series of veins on the lateral thigh that drain this area	Veins lie below the deep muscular fascia Tibial veins: anterior and posterior (aTV, pTV) • Drain into popliteal vein Popliteal vein (PV) • Drains into superficial femoral vein Femoral vein (FV) • Joins with deep femoral vein in thigh to form common femoral vein • This is a deep vein despite its name Deep femoral vein (DFV) Common femoral vein (CFV) • At the groin/upper thigh, this is the site of drainage for multiple veins: – GSV – Circumflex-iliac – External pudendal – Epigastric
Comment	• Anterolateral thigh vein: drains the lateral and anterior thigh; empties into the GSV; lateral segment is part of the lateral venous system • Venous thromboses in a superficial vein do not have to be treated with anticoagulation unless the thrombus is progressive or near the junction with a deep vein (proximal thrombus)	

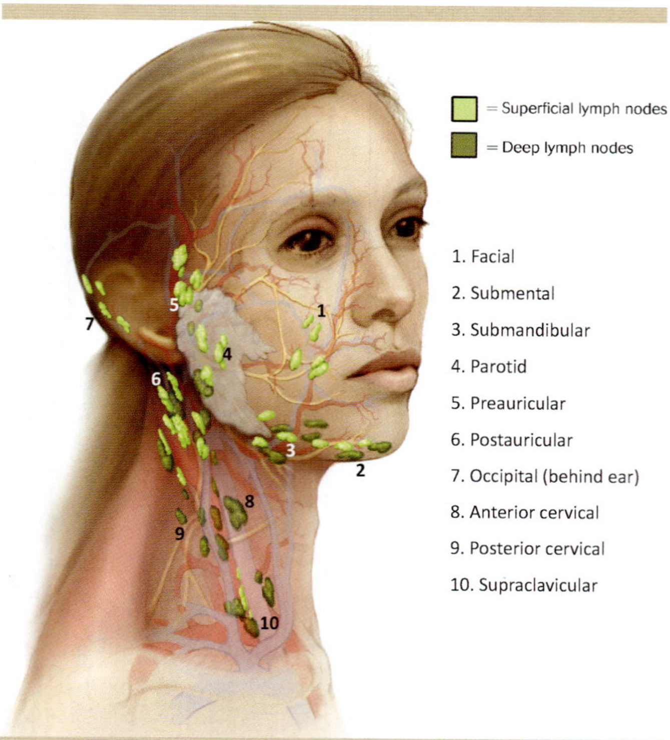

FIGURE 25-3 Lymph nodes of the head and neck.

TABLE 25-3 Embryology

Group	Muscles	Derived From	Comment
Muscles of mastication	Temporalis, masseter, medial pterygoid, lateral pterygoid	First branchial arch mesoderm	Trigeminal nerve (CNV)
Muscles of facial expression	See Fig. 25-4 and Table 25-4	Second branchial arch mesoderm	Facial nerve (CN VII)
Lower face muscles	Risorius, platysma, depressor anguli oris	Embryonic platysma	Tend to not have bony insertions or origins
Middle and upper face muscles	Muscles of the forehead, scalp, periorbital, upper mouth	Embryonic sphincter colli, profundus muscle	May have bony insertions

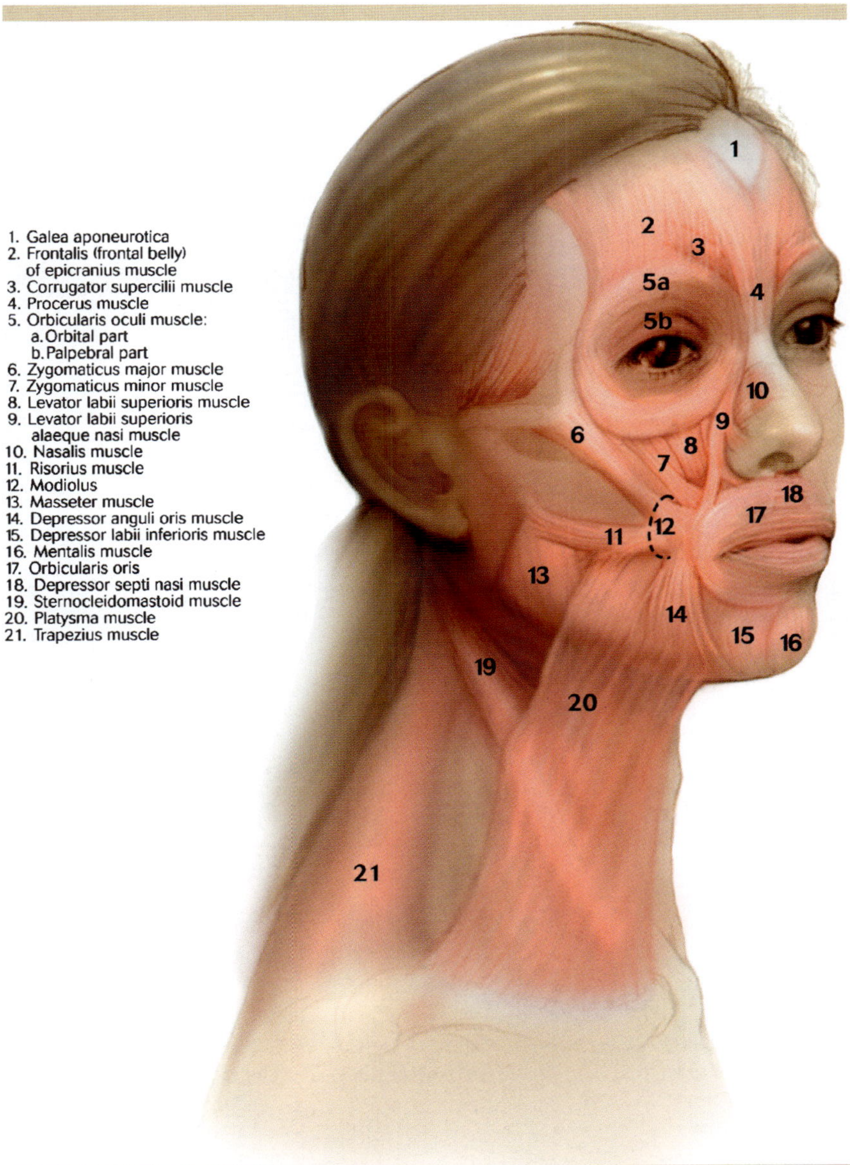

FIGURE 25-4 Muscles of facial expression.

TABLE 25-4 Muscles of Facial Expression With Innervations (Fig. 25-4)

Muscle	Action	Rhytids	Branch of Facial Nerve
Upper Face Muscles			
Scalp			
– Occipitalis	Moves scalp posteriorly		Postauricular
– Frontalis	Raises eyebrows Wrinkles forehead	Horizontal forehead lines	Temporal
Periorbital			
– Corrugator supercolli	Pulls eyebrows medially	Glabellar lines	Temporal
– Orbicularis oculi	Closes and squeezes eyelids shut	Crow's feet	Temporal Zygomatic
Nose			
– Procerus	Pulls skin over glabella inferiorly Wrinkles nose upward		Temporal Zygomatic
– Zygomaticus major and minor	Elevates corner of mouth		Zygomatic Buccal
– Nasalis	Dilates nares	Bunny lines	Buccal
– Depressor septi nasi	Pulls columella inferiorly		Buccal
Mouth-Lip Elevators			
– Levator labii superioris	Elevates upper lip		Buccal
– Levator labii superioris alaeque nasi	Lifts upper lip Dilates nares		Buccal
– Levator anguli oris	Elevates corner of mouth		Buccal
– Risorius	Pulls corner of mouth laterally		Buccal
Mouth-Lip Depressors			
– Buccinator	Flattens cheek Whistle, blow		Buccal
– Depressor anguli oris	Depresses corner of mouth (Marionette lines)		Buccal Marginal mandibular
– Depressor labii inferioris	Depresses lower lip		Marginal mandibular
– Mentalis	Protrudes lower lip	Mental crease	Marginal mandibular
– Orbicularis oris	Closes mouth Purses lips Pucker Protrudes lip	Vertical lip lines	Buccal Marginal mandibular
– Platysma	Pulls corner of mouth inferiorly Webs, tenses neck	Horizontal neck lines	Cervical

TABLE 25-5 Motor Nerves to the Face

Nerve	Innervates
Mandibular branch of trigeminal (CN V3)	Muscles of mastication
Facial nerve (CN VII)	Muscles of facial expression
Oculomotor (CN 3)	Levator palpebrae superioris (LPS)
Sympathetic innervation	Superior palpebral muscle of Müller (involuntary elevates upper eyelid in flight or fight situations)

    - Marginal mandibular
    - Cervical
- *Trigeminal nerve (CN V) (Table 25-6)*
- *Cervical plexus (Table 25-7)*
  - Facial nerve blocks
    - The most common facial nerve blocks target supraorbital (V_1), infraorbital (V_2), and mental (V_3) nerves which exit into the face through foramina of the same names
    - These 3 nerves line up vertically at the midpupillary line, which is 2.5 cm from the facial midline (Fig. 25-6)
    - Intracral approach to infraorbital and mental nerve is preferred to reduce patient discomfort, which is greater with transcutaneous injections
- Supraorbital nerve block
  - Supraorbital and supratrochlear nerves innervate the frontal part of scalp and forehead
  - Supraorbital foramen/notch may or may not be palpable. Use the midpupillary line as a guide to the supraorbital nerve
  - With patient in slight reverse Trendelenburg, stand behind the patient's head. This position will afford better access to the superior orbital rim and prevent the patient from seeing the needle approach
  - Raise a cutaneous wheal of anesthesia over the superior orbital rim in the midpupillary line. Insert the needle down to the rim until resistance is felt. Aspirate to ensure no blood return, and then inject 1 to 2 mL and massage the site to spread the anesthetic near the nerve
  - If no resistance is felt after inserting the needle 1 cm, then you are likely below the orbital rim or in the foramen itself. Withdraw the needle, and then insert it again, but redirect it to be above the rim

TABLE 25-6 Three Branches of the Trigeminal Nerve (CN V) (Provide Sensation to the Head) (Fig. 25-5)

CNV Branch	Ophthalmic Nerve (V_1 Sensory)	Maxillary Nerve (V_2 Sensory)	Mandibular Nerve (V_3 Sensory)
Location	Travels through superior orbital fissure (SOF) and passes through orbit Divides into 3 branches	Leaves the skull through the foramen rotundum Divides into 4 branches	Exits the cranium through the foramen ovale. Divides into 5 branches
Branches	Frontal nerve • Supraorbital nerve • Supratrochlear nerve Nasociliary nerve • Infratrochlear nerve • External nasal branch of anterior ethmoid Lacrimal nerve	Zygomaticotemporal Zygomaticofacial Infraorbital Nasopalatine • superior alveolar and palatine nerves (sensation to upper teeth, gingival, palate, nasal mucosa)	Buccal nerve Lingual nerve Mental nerve Inferior alveolar nerve Auriculotemporal nerve
Innervates	Forehead Scalp	Side of the nose Lower eyelid Upper lip	Mucous membranes of the mouth and cheek Anterior two-thirds of the tongue Lower teeth Skin of the lower jaw Side of the head and scalp Meninges of the anteriorand middle cranial fossae

TABLE 25-7 Cervical Plexus (3 Nerves) Supplies Sensation to the Neck (See Fig. 25-6)

Nerve	Innervation
Lesser occipital	Sensation to posterior neck, scalp, occiput, and upper posterior ear
Greater auricular	Sensation to earlobe and posterior auricle
Transverse cervical	Sensation to anterior neck

All exit in proximity at the posterior border of the sternocleidomastoid muscle in a region called Erb point (discussed in the section "Surgical Anatomy: Danger Zone").

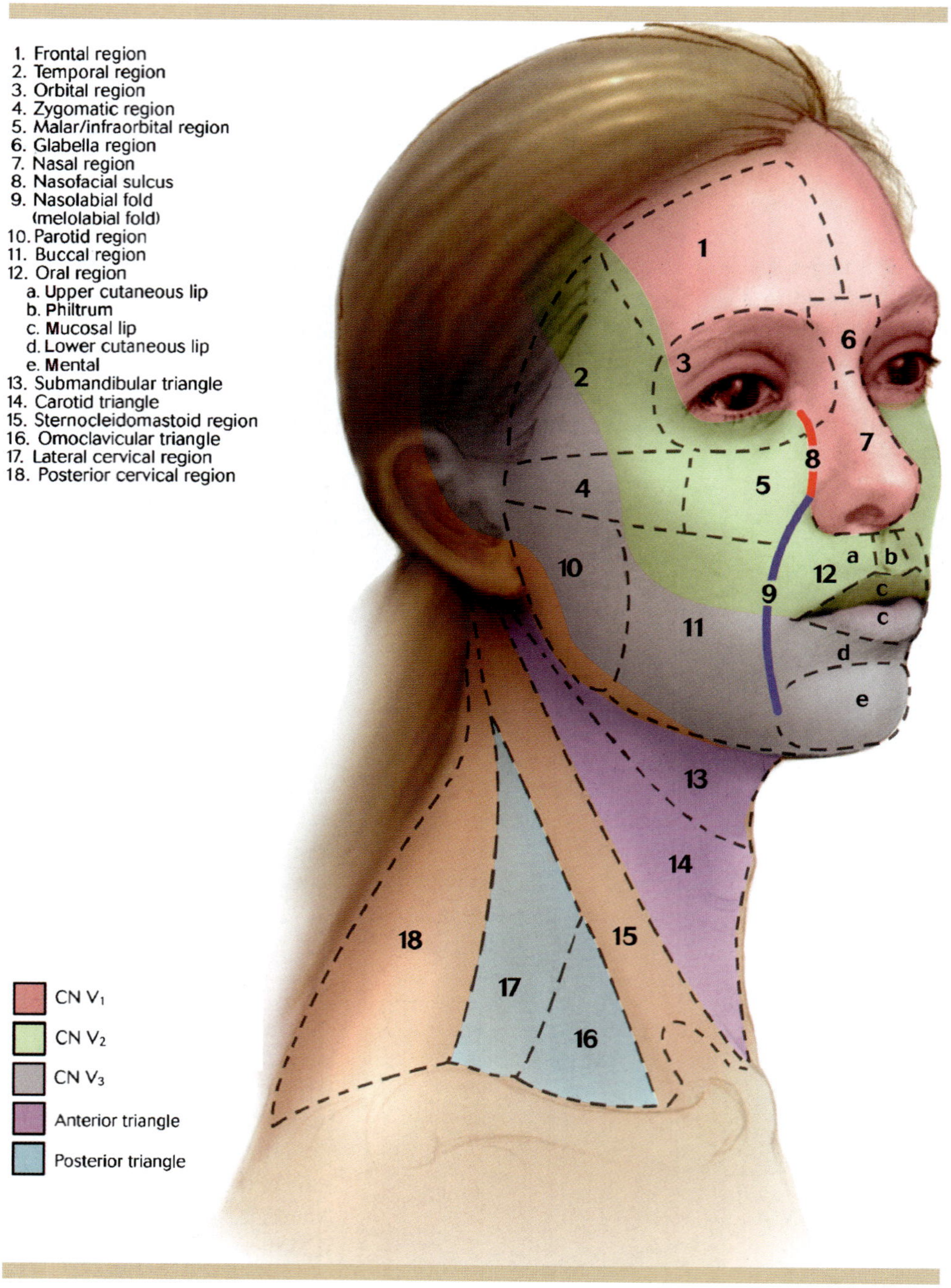

FIGURE 25-5 Facial subunits and sensory innervation.

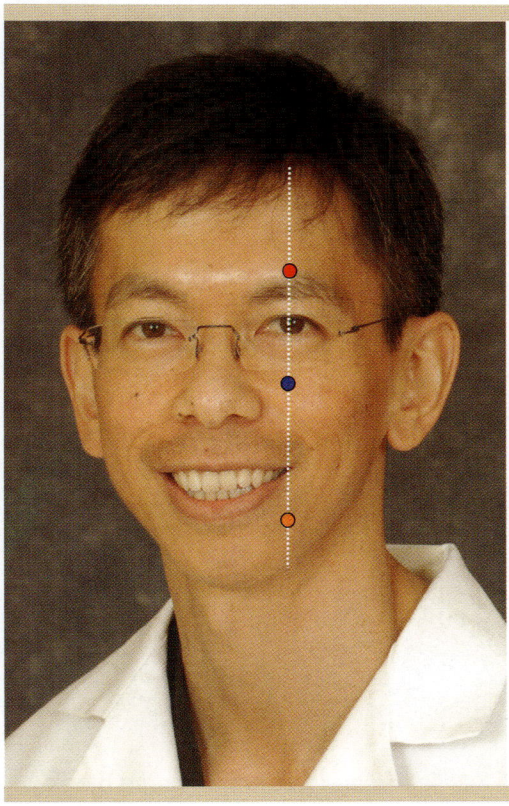

White line: midpupillary line.

Red dot: Supraorbital nerve block. Supraorbital notch at orbital rim and eyebrow.

Blue dot: Infraorbital nerve block. Infraorbital notch approximately 1 cm below infraorbital rim.

Orange dot: Mental nerve block. Mental nerve block approximately half way between corner of mouth and jawline.

FIGURE 25-6 Facial nerve blocks.

    - To extend the block medially or laterally, a bleb of anesthesia may be injected along the superior orbital rim medially and laterally from the supraorbital starting point
- Infraorbital nerve block (Fig. 25-7A)
    - Infraorbital nerve innervates the lower eyelid, medial aspect of the cheek, upper lip, and lateral portion of the nose
    - Intraoral (mucosal) approach is preferred
    - Use a 1-inch 30-gauge needle, and when possible, apply viscous lidocaine or EMLA cream to the gingival sulcus above the upper canines for 5 minutes prior to injection
    - Position yourself on the opposite side of the nerve to be blocked, and have the patient slightly turn his or her head toward you. For example, to block the right infraorbital nerve, stand at the patient's left side. This permits better access to the medially oriented foramen and causes less flexion of the injecting wrist
    - Place the third or fourth finger of the noninjecting hand over the infraorbital foramen (1 cm below the palpable infraorbital margin), and peel back the ipsilateral upper lip with the index finger and thumb of the same hand (use a gauze to lift up the lip to avoid slipping)
    - Inject a bleb of anesthesia at the gingival-labial sulcus above the apex of the canine fossa. Insert and aim the needle toward the foramen, or just below the overlying finger. Stop when resistance or bone is felt
    - Aspirate and confirm that no blood returns, and then inject 2 to 3 mL of local anesthetic. If you are in the proper location, then the finger overlying the infraorbital foramen should feel a bleb of anesthesia rise from underneath. Withdraw slightly, and inject another 1 to 2 mL laterally on each side of the infraorbital foramen. Massage the injected site
- Mental nerve block (Fig. 25-7B)
    - Mental nerve innervates the lower lip and chin
    - Intraoral (mucosal) approach is preferred
    - Use a 1-inch, 30-gauge needle, and when possible, apply viscous lidocaine or EMLA cream to the gingival-labial sulcus below the second bicuspid for 5 minutes prior to injection
    - Stand behind the patient's head with the patient body in reverse Trendelenburg. Mark the mental foramen position in the midpupillary line (rarely, the foramen may be palpable; the foramen is approximately midway between the oral commissure and the mandibular rim in the midpupillary line), and place the third or fourth finger of the noninjecting hand over this site. Peel the ipsilateral lower lip outward with the index finger and thumb of the same hand
    - Inject and raise a bleb of local anesthetic at the gingival-labial sulcus below the second bicuspid (second premolar). Insert and aim the needle toward the mental foramen, or below the overlying finger marking the site

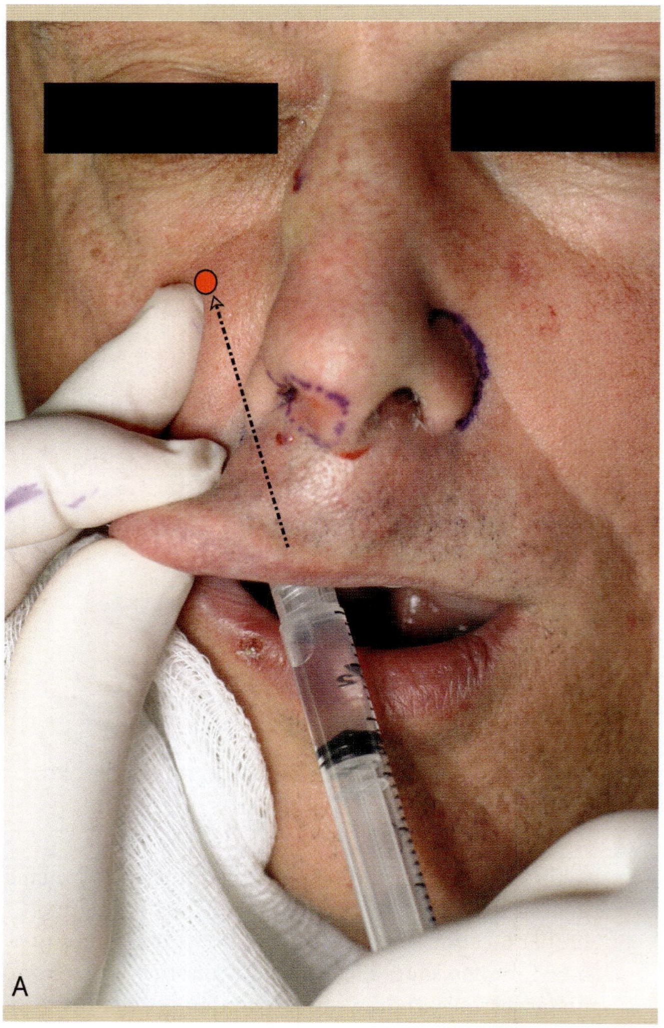

FIGURE 25-7A Technique for infraorbital nerve block. (A) Technique for infraorbital nerve block. Mucosal approach is less painful. Thumb and index finger everts lip outward. Middle or ring finger held over infraorbital foramen (red dot), which is approximately 1 cm below orbital rim. Injection is made at the gingivolabial sulcus at the superior canine, aiming upward under middle finger until needle abuts periosteum. Aspirate to avoid intravascular location, then inject slowly. If the needle is in the correct location, then a slow rise in swelling will be felt under the middle finger. Withdraw needle if patient feels shooting pain.

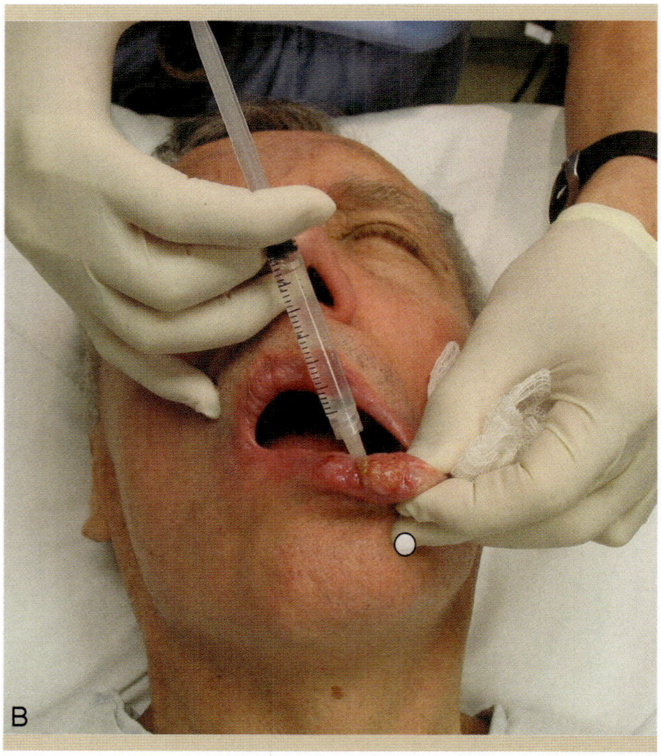

FIGURE 25-7B Technique for mental nerve block. (B) Technique for mental nerve block. Thumb and index finger everts lip outward. Middle finger held over mental foramen (white dot). Injection is made at the gingivolabial sulcus at the inferior canine, aiming downward under middle finger until needle abuts periosteum. Remaining steps similar to infraorbital nerve block.

- Aspirate and confirm that no blood returns, and then inject 2 to 3 mL of local anesthetic. If you are in the proper location, the finger overlying the mental foramen should feel a bleb of anesthesia rise from underneath. Withdraw slightly, and inject another 1 to 2 mL laterally on each side of the infraorbital foramen. Massage the injected site

- Regional anesthesia for the nose
  - Sensory innervation to the nose is via the infratrochlear (V_1: nasal root, middorsum, and sidewall), external nasal branch of the anterior ethmoid (V_1: distal nasal dorsum and tip), infraorbital (V_2: lower nasal sidewall and lateral ala), and branches of the nasopalatine (V_2: columella, nasal mucosa) nerves
- Regional anesthesia for the ear
  - For complete anesthesia of the external auricle (Fig. 25-8), 5 nerves must be targeted (great auricular, auriculotemporal, lesser occipital, facial, and vagus nerves). Four injection sites are required, and anesthesia is fanned peripherally in a ring-block fashion
- *Nerves of the hand and fingers (Fig. 25-9A and B, Table 25-8)*
  - Innervated by
    - Radial nerve
    - Ulnar nerve
    - Median nerve

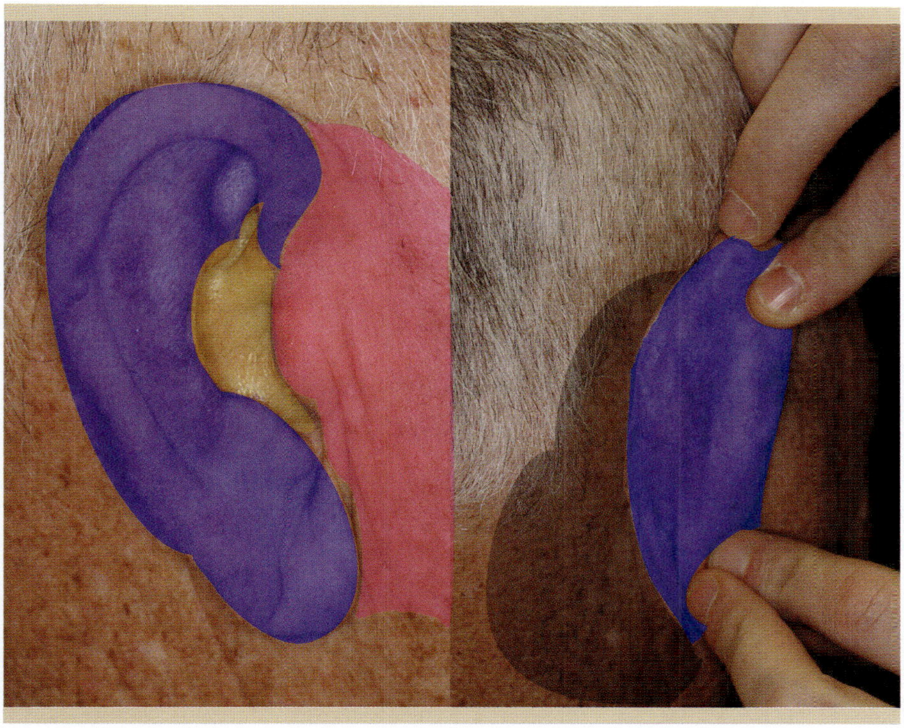

FIGURE 25-8 Sensory innervation of the ear.

- Hand blocks
  - Median nerve block (Fig. 25-10)
    - Median nerve innervates the skin of the palmar side of the thumb, the index and middle finger, half the ring finger, and the nail bed of these fingers. The lateral part of the palm is supplied by the palmar cutaneous branch of the median nerve
    - Nerve enters the hand between the flexor carpi radialis (radial side) and palmaris longus (ulnar side) tendons beneath the flexor retinaculum
    - Both tendons are identified by asking the patient to oppose the thumb and the fifth digit
    - Needle is angled at 45 degrees and enters between the tendons at the level of the proximal wrist crease
    - Inject 2 to 5 mL local anesthetic
    - If the patient has congenital absence of the palmaris longus muscle, the injection can be made on the medial aspect (toward the ulna) of the flexor carpi radialis tendon

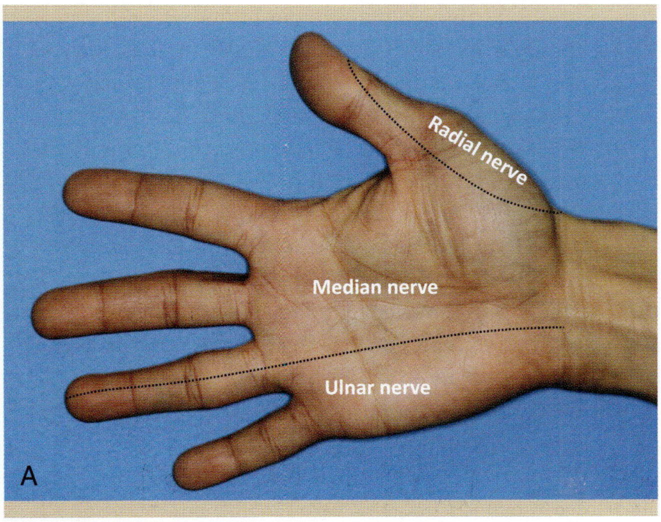

FIGURE 25-9A Innervation of the hand-palmar.

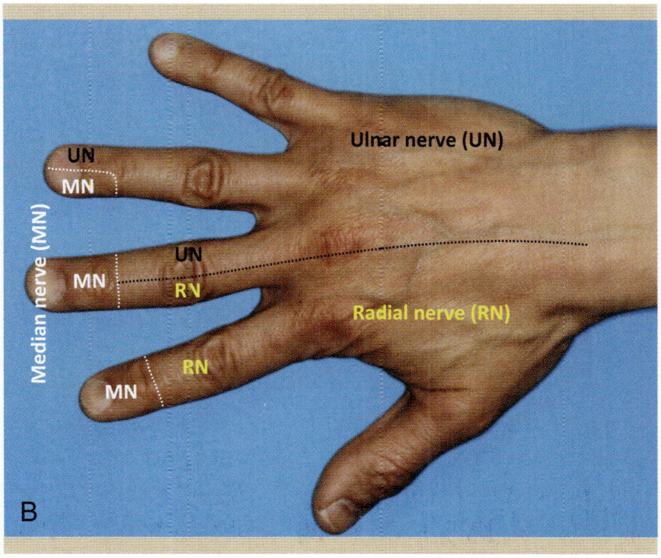

FIGURE 25-9B Innervation of the hand-dorsal.

TABLE 25-8 Innervation of the Hand and Fingers (Fig. 25-10)

	Radial	Ulnar	Median
Motor			
		Muscles of hypothenar eminence Ulnar 2 lumbricals 7 interossei Adductor pollicis muscle	Muscles of thenar eminence Radial 2 lumbrical muscles
Sensory			
Dorsum of hand	Skin of dorsum of thumb and 2½ digits as far as the distal interphalangeal joint	Ulnar 1½ digits and adjacent part of dorsum of hand	
Palm of hand		Ulnar nerve: sensory to skin of ulnar 1½ digits	Median nerve: sensory to skin of the palmar aspect of thumb and 2½ digits, including the skin on the dorsal aspect of the distal phalanges
Fingers	Dorsal digital nerves	Dorsal digital nerves Ventral digital nerves	Ventral digital nerves

- As the needle passes through the flexor retinaculum, a loss of resistance is felt, marking the point at which the injection should be made
- If paresthesias are elicited, the needle should be withdrawn slightly (i.e., approximately 2 mm) to avoid nerve damage or intraneural injection

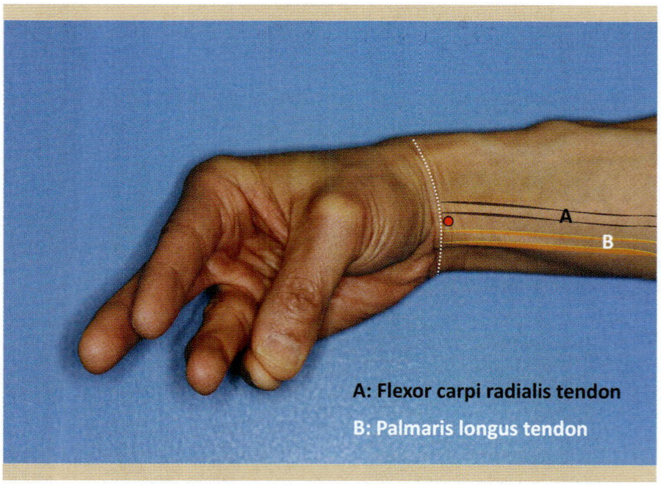

FIGURE 25-10 Technique for median nerve block of hand: to accentuate landmarks of the 2 tendons, have the patient oppose the thumb to touch the small finger while slightly flexing the wrist. Inject at the wrist crease (red dot) between the flexor carpi radialis (A) and the palmaris longus (B) tendons.

- Digital nerve block (Fig. 25-11)
  - On the dorsal surface of the fingers, the digital nerves are branches of the radial and ulnar nerves
  - On the ventral or palmar surface of the fingers, the digital nerves are branches of the median and ulnar nerves
  - The digital nerves that supply the toes are branches of the peroneal nerve on the dorsal surface, whereas the tibial nerve innervates the ventral or plantar surface of the toes
  - Avoid/circumferential injections, which may lead to digital ischemia
  - Limit injection volumes to 3 mL total
  - Epinephrine may be used cautiously in digital blocks (see discussion on epinephrine in section Local Anesthesia discussed later)
  - Block should be as far back as possible from the surgical site
  - Two nerves run on each side of the fingers and toes
  - These may be blocked with injections on each side of the digit
  - Needle is inserted perpendicular to the digit, midway between the palmar and dorsal surfaces of the digit, 1 to 2 cm distal to the web space
  - Once resistance or bone is felt, aspirate to ensure no blood return, then inject 0.5 mL
  - Withdraw the needle slightly, and redirect the needle to the dorsal surface, and inject 0.5 mL
  - Repeat 0.5 mL for the palmar surface

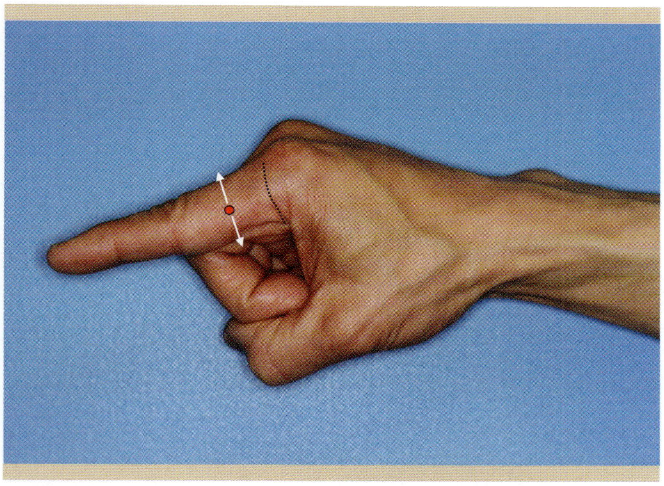

FIGURE 25-11 Digital block technique: The needle is inserted (red dot) perpendicular to the digit, midway between the palmar and dorsal surfaces of the digit and 1–2 cm distal to the webspace (black dotted line). Raise a bleb of local anesthesia and inject superior (dorsal) and inferior (palmar). Avoid circumferential ring block.

    - The side, palmar, and dorsal injections all may be done through 1 insertion point at the side of the finger by redirecting the needle
- Web space block (Fig. 25-12)
    - Provides digital nerve block
    - Needle is inserted from the dorsal aspect of the web space and advanced until the tip tents the palmar skin

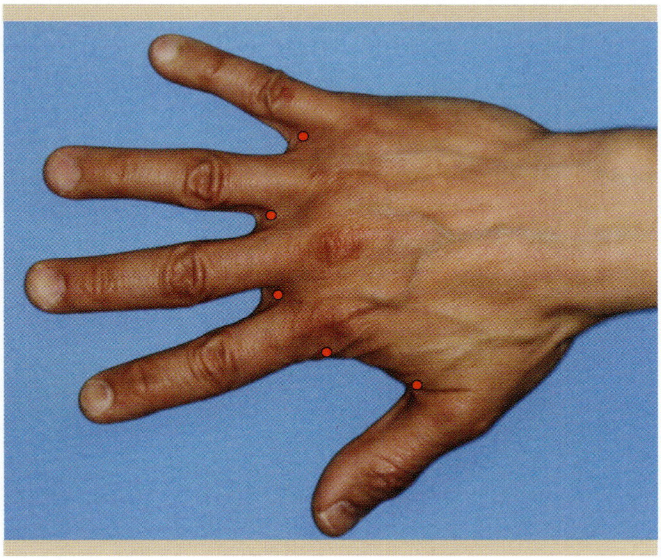

FIGURE 25-12 Web space block technique: The needle is inserted from the dorsal aspect of the web space (red dot) and advanced until the tip tents the palmar skin. The anesthetic is injected along the side of the digit as the needle is withdrawn.

    - Anesthetic is administered along the side of the digit as the needle is withdrawn
    - Epinephrine may be used with caution (see discussion on epinephrine aforementioned and in section Local Anesthesia)
- *Sensory nerves of the leg and ankle*
- Leg and ankle innervated by branches of the femoral nerve (Table 25-9)
    - Saphenous
    - Posterior tibial
    - Sural
    - Deep peroneal
    - Superficial peroneal
- Sensory innervation to the dorsum of the foot (3 nerves) (Fig. 25-13)
    - Dorsum, medial: saphenous nerve
    - Dorsum, lateral: superficial peroneal nerve
    - Between first and second toes: deep peroneal nerve
- *Sensory innervation of sole of the foot (2 nerves) (Fig. 25-13)*
    - Plantar surface (majority of): posterior tibial nerve
    - Lateral foot and fifth toe: sural nerve
- Nerve blocks for the foot
    - Dorsum of the foot nerve blocks: anterior ankle block
    - Superficial peroneal nerve block
        - Insert needle immediately above and anterior to the lateral malleolus
        - Inject 5 mL anesthetic subcutaneously between the anterior border of the tibia and the superior aspect of the lateral malleolus
    - Deep peroneal nerve block
        - Patient supine and the ankle in slight plantar flexion
        - Needle is inserted at the upper level of the malleoli between the tendons of the tibialis anterior and extensor hallucis longus
        - Tendons can be accentuated by dorsiflexing the ankle and the great toe against resistance
        - If the anterior tibial artery can be palpated, the needle should be inserted just lateral to the artery
        - Needle is advanced deep to the tendons just above the periosteum, and 5 mL of 1% lidocaine is injected after aspiration
    - Saphenous nerve block
        - Insert needle immediately above and anterior to the medial malleolus
        - Inject 3 to 4 mL anesthetic into the subcutaneous tissue around the great saphenous vein
- Sole of the foot nerve blocks: posterior ankle block
    - Sural nerve
        - Patient is positioned prone with the foot in slight dorsiflexion
        - Needle is inserted lateral to the Achilles tendon and 1 to 2 cm above the level of the distal tip of the lateral malleolus
        - Needle is redirected in a fan-shaped pattern from side to side as anesthetic is infiltrated

TABLE 25-9 Femoral Nerve Branches

Branch	Comment
Saphenous nerve	Largest cutaneous branch of femoral nerve Enters foot anterior to medial malleolus Provides sensory innervation to the medial aspect of the ankle and the medial-dorsal foot up to the first metatarsal bone
Sciatic nerve	Consists of the tibial nerve and common peroneal nerves
Tibial Nerve Divides Into → Posterior Tibial Nerve + Sural Nerve	
Posterior tibial nerve	Enters foot posterior to tibial artery at medial malleolus Gives rise to 2 nerves that supply most of the sensation to the sole of the foot Lateral plantar nerve: lateral sole of foot Medial plantar nerve: medial sole of foot
Sural nerve	Formed by branches of the common peroneal and tibial nerves Enters the foot posterior to lateral malleolus Sensation to lateral and posterior lower third of inferior leg Sensory to small portion of lateral margin of foot and lateral side of fifth toe
Common Peroneal Nerve Divides Into → Deep Peroneal Nerve + Superficial Peroneal Nerve	
Deep peroneal nerve	Underneath flexor retinaculum anteriorly Branch of the common peroneal nerve At level of the lateral malleolus, it is bounded medially by the tendon of the extensor hallucis longus and laterally by the anterior tibial artery Skin sensation between first and second toes
Superficial peroneal nerve	Above retinaculum Skin sensation of lateral dorsum of foot and toes except for the first interdigital space (deep peroneal nerve) and lateral aspect of the foot (sural nerve)

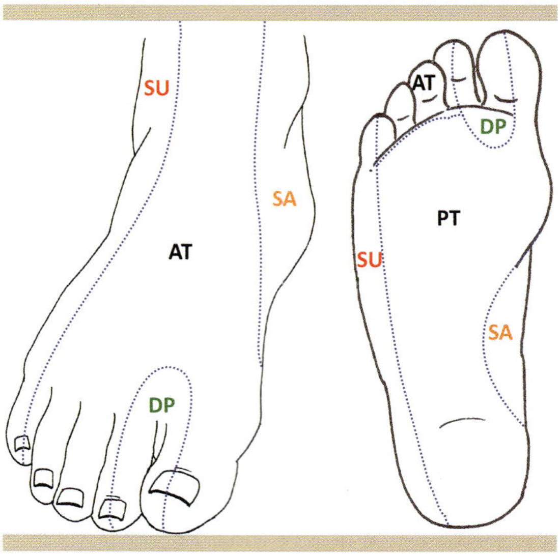

FIGURE 25-13 Innervation of the foot. AT, anterior tibial nerve; SU, sural nerve; SA, saphenous nerve; DP, deep peroneal nerve.

- Posterior tibial nerve
  - Patient is positioned prone with the foot in slight dorsiflexion. Feel for the posterior tibial artery pulsation (the nerve is just behind the artery)
  - Needle is inserted midway between the medial malleolus anteriorly and the Achilles tendon posteriorly. Raise a wheal at this site, and advance the needle toward the posterior tibial artery
  - Tibial nerve lies under the dense flexor retinaculum; advance the needle until a slight give is felt as the needle penetrates the retinaculum
  - Aspirate and confirm no blood return, and inject 5 mL of 1% lidocaine. Another 5 mL is injected as the needle is withdrawn

SURGICAL ANATOMY: DANGER ZONES

- The greatest danger is injury to a major motor nerve, especially at its proximal trunk, because permanent paralysis or weakeness may result, causing facial asymmetry and atrophy
- All motor nerves and major vessels lie below the superficial musculoaponeurotic system (SMAS) plane and muscle
  - Staying above the SMAS (when defined) or muscle (when the SMAS is ill defined) is always safe to avoid motor nerve injury
  - The SMAS-muscle plane, however, is thin or difficult to identify in 3 areas, which then are the 3 danger zones in the head and neck for motor nerve injury (Table 25-10)
- Facial layers (from most superficial to deepest) (Tables 25-11 and 25-12)
  - Epidermis (most superficial)
  - Dermis
  - Subcutaneous fat
  - SMAS
  - Muscle
  - Deep fat (variable)
  - Periosteum
  - Bone (deepest)
  - Other branches of the facial nerve: zygomatic, buccal
    - Rarely injured because they are well protected by a well-defined layer of SMAS and muscle
    - Injury to these nerves usually does not cause permanent injury because they have multiple rami and cross-innervate muscles
  - Nerves medial to a line connecting the lateral canthus to the oral commissure are usually well arborized, and permanent injury is rare medial to this line
- Undermining
  - Done to separate vertical and lateral fibrous/fascial attachments that restrict tissue mobility
  - Increases tissue mobility, decreases wound edge tension, and facilitates wound closure, thereby enhancing postoperative cosmesis
  - Undermining should always be above SMAS and muscle with few exceptions
  - Forehead: below the frontalis muscle, between the 2 superior temporal lines laterally
  - Nose: below the nasalis muscle
  - Disadvantages
    - Too deep: may injure vital structures (i.e., motor nerves or deep arteries)
    - Too superficial: may compromise tissue viability by thinning the vascular pedicle excessively

ANATOMIC REVIEW OF HEAD AND NECK

- SMAS (Fig. 25-15)
  - A fascial envelope that encircles the muscles of facial expression in a broad plane across the face via fibrous septa that extends and inserts into the dermis above
  - It also serves as a protective anatomic plane: all major motor and sensory nerve trunks and named vessels are deep (below) to the SMAS
  - With few exceptions, all motor nerves innervate their respective muscles on the muscle's underside. Therefore, staying above the SMAS and muscle will prevent motor nerve injury
  - Peripheral sensory nerves and vessels may perforate the SMAS and travel above it in a superficial plane, but the proximal roots are still sub-SMAS
  - The SMAS in the scalp and upper face and the SMAS of the lower face fuse at the zygoma
- Anatomic extensions of the SMAS include
  - Superficial fascia of the face and superficial temporalis fascia (also known as the temporal-parietal fascia)
  - Superficial fascia of the parotid
  - Platysma in the neck. (NOTE: Superficial fascia of the neck, however, is not SMAS. It is deep to the SMAS/platysma and represents the superficial leaflet of the deep cervical fascia)
  - Galea on the scalp and its forehead extension (below the frontalis muscle)
- The SMAS may be plicated and imbricated (done in face-lift surgery) to draw the facial skin tight, as well as, help to decrease wound tension during reconstruction
- Cosmetic units and subunits of the face
  - Figs. 25-16, 25-17, and 25-18 illustrate anatomy of the eyelid, nose, and ear, respectively

ELECTROSURGERY (TABLES 25-12 AND 25-13)

- Refers to the use of electric current in surgery to produce tissue destruction
- Tissue effects from electrosurgical energy are a function of waveform, power setting, electrode size and geometry,

TABLE 25-10 Danger Zones

Nerve	Danger Zone	Innervates	Injury
CNVII Temporal branch (Motor)	Temporal fossa Superior border: superior temporal line (line palpable from the frontal-temporal hairline to the lateral eyebrow) Inferior border: zygomatic arch Medial border: lateral orbital rim Posterior border: superficial temporal artery and temporal hairline Most vulnerable as it exits the superior parotid and crosses the zygomatic arch Next most vulnerable location: as it travels across the temporal fossa (temple) toward the lateral forehead. Nerve is protected medial to the superior temporal line because it now lies underneath the frontalis muscle	Frontalis	Drooping of affected eyebrow Flattening of the ipsilateral forehead
CNVII Marginal mandibular branch (Motor)	Nerve is relatively superficial as it enters the face where the anterior border of the masseter muscle and mandibular rim intersect (the facial artery also enters the face here) At this region, the marginal mandibular is superifical to the facial artery. The platysma above protects both the artery and the nerve. Nerve becomes even more superficial as it travels obliquely up toward the corner of the mouth. As long as one stays above the lip depressor muscles, however, the nerve will not be injured There is great variation, however, in where the nerve lies relative to the mandibular rim.	Lip depressors	Asymmetry of corners of mouth
CNXI Spinal accessory nerve (Motor)	Posterior cervical triangle at Erb's point (see Fig. 25-14): intersection of the following lines Draw a horizontal line connecting the mastoid to the mandibular angle At the midpoint of this line, a vertical line then is drawn inferiorly to intersect with the posterior border of the sternocleidomastoid muscle (SCM). The nerve is located within a 2- to 4-cm radius of this point. Several other nerves are at risk in this anatomic location: • Spinal accessory (motor) • Greater auricular (sensory) • Transverse cervical (sensory)	Trapezius muscle	Shoulder drooping Restricted shoulder elevation and abduction

activation time, surgical technique (orientation of electrode), and tissue impedance

- Definition of terms
    - *Electric current*: flow of electrons during a period of time, measured in amperes
    - *Circuit*: pathway for uninterrupted flow of electrons. Complete circuit must exist for electrical energy to flow
    - *Complete electrical circuit*: needs 3 basic system components, along with the patient—a power unit, an active electrode, and a dispersive or return electrode
    - *Active electrode*: i.e., handpiece
    - *Dispersive, return electrode*: i.e., grounding pad
    - *Resistance = impedance*: degree to which an object opposes electric current, measured in ohms

TABLE 25-11 SMAS Architecture[11]

SMAS Layer	Type 1: Distinct SMAS Layer	Type 2: Wispy or Membranous SMAS Layer
Characteristic	Meshwork of fibrous septa envelops lobules of fat cells	Meshwork of intermingled collagen and elastic fibers and muscle fibers
Region	Forehead, temple (Zone 1 in Fig. 25-15) Zygomatic, infraorbital region, and lateral part of the nasolabial fold (Zone 2 in Fig. 25-15)	Upper, lower lips (Zone 3 in Fig. 25-15) Medial part of the nasolabial fold (Zone 2 in Fig. 25-15)

- *Voltage*: force pushing current through the resistance, measured in volts
- *Direct current (DC):* electric current that flows in one direction (i.e., electrolysis and electrocautery)
- *Alternating current (AC):* electrons that alternate or regularly reverse direction
- *Frequency*: measure of the number of occurrences of a repeating event per unit time, measured in hertz
- *Hertz*: number of cycles of electric current flow (one direction and back) per second
- *Radiofrequency (RF):* an electric current occurring at high frequencies, usually more than 400,000 cycles per second (Hz)
- *Electrode*: a physical device; close to or in contact with the patient, through which electrosurgical energy is received or transmitted
- *AC electrical waveforms*: may be damped or undamped to produce tissue effects of coagulation, cutting, or fulguration (desiccation)
  - *Damped*: Waves produced are initially intense and strong and then diminish rapidly. The more rapidly the sine waves return to baseline, the more damped is the current. Damped current coagulates tissue, adding to hemostasis, but causes collateral tissue damage (i.e., electrofulguration, electrodesiccation, electrocoagulation, AKA coagulation)
  - *Undamped*: Waves produced are pure sine waves. Undamped current cuts tissue without hemostatic effect (i.e., electrosection, AKA cutting)
  - *Blended current*: combined characteristics of cutting and coagulation waveforms that result in cutting with moderate hemostasis
- *Monoterminal*: delivery of current using only 1 treatment electrode, without a dispersive electrode (i.e., electrofulguration, electrodesiccation with hyfrecator)
- *Biterminal*: delivery of current via 2 electrodes, 1 treatment electrode and 1 dispersive electrode (usually at a distance from the treatment end) (i.e., electrocoagulation, electrosection). May be unipolar or bipolar
- *Unipolar*: 1 treatment electrode and 1 dispersive electrode (usually a grounding pad at distant site)
- *Bipolar*: a forceps-like device contains both the treatment and the dispersive electrodes (dispersive pad is not required). Passage of current is restricted between these 2 tines, which results in substantially less tissue damage than in monopolar devices. Safest for patients with automatic implantable cardiac defibrillators (AICDs) or pacemakers

TABLE 25-12 Five Zones of SMAS

Zones of SMAS	Characteristics	Region	SMAS Architecture
Fronto-occipital	Galea together with frontalis and occipitalis muscles	Forehead	Type 1: distinct
Suprazygomatic	Musculoaponeurotic excursion covering the temporal aponeurosis, including the suprazygomatic periauricular muscles	Temporal and parotid	Type 1: distinct
Infrazygomatic	Musculoaponeurotic excursion covering the cheek	Cheek	Type 1: distinct
Perioral	Musculoaponeurotic excursion covering the paranasal and perioral area	Nose, perioral, upper and lower lips	Type 2: Wispy or membranous
Platysmal	Plastysma and its superficial fascia	Neck	Type 1: distinct

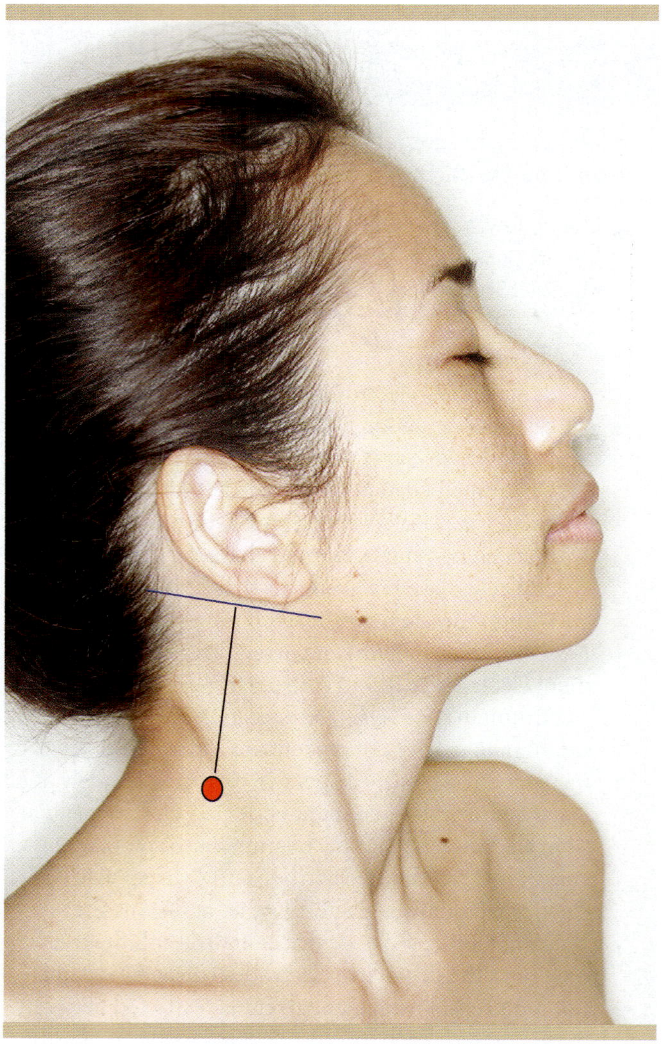

FIGURE 25-14 Erb point. Erb point, also known as "area nervosa" can be identified by drawing a line between the mastoid and jaw angle (blue line), and then drawing a line (black line) vertically down from the midpoint of the first line to the posterior border of the sternocleidomastoid muscle. Sensory nerves at risk in this region include the lesser occipital, great auricular, and transverse cervical nerves. Motor nerves at risk include the supraclavicular branches of the cervical plexus and the spinal accessory nerve.

- *Electrical surgery unit (ESU)*: generates the radiofrequency current in commercial electrosurgery machines
- *Ground-referenced ESU*: the current is referenced to a ground (i.e., the electric circuit is completed through a grounded object). If there is any interruption or high impedance in the normal return path, the current will seek an alternate path, possibly causing alternate-site burns
- *Radiofrequency (RF)–isolated units*: most monopolar ESUs are now this type. The isolation transformer inside the unit isolates the therapeutic current from the ground, and therefore the therapeutic current is only returned to the ESU and is not connected to the earth ground. This arrangement eliminates the flow of energy if there is no completed pathway to the ESU

- Complications of electrosurgery
  - ESU burn: occurs when the heat produced, over time, is not dissipated safely by the size or conductivity of the patient return electrode (i.e., poor grounding pad contact). Burn = heat × time/area
  - Interference with an implanted pacemaker
- Precautions in patients with an automatic implantable pacemaker and cardioverter/defibrillators (AICDs)
  - The risk of electrosurgery-induced arrhythmia is greater with an AICD than with a pacemaker
  - Electrosurgery current may mimic the electrical activity of the heart and stimulate the cardiac pacemaker/defibrillator, potentially causing an unnecessary shock (AICD) or an alteration of pacemaker function
  - Options for patients with pacemakers or AICDs
    - Electrocautery: safe; no electric current passes into the patient
    - Bipolar (biterminal) electrocoagulation: relatively safe in patients with pacemakers and AICDs because the current is restricted between the 2 forcep tips
    - Unipolar electrocoagulation (biterminal): may be used cautiously in patients with pacemakers and AICDs in the following circumstances
- Bursts of current are short (5 seconds or less)
- Lowest effective setting is used
- The dispersive pad/electrode is placed far away from the cardiac device such that the device is not in the path of the current flow
- The electrosurgery is not directly over the cardiac device
    - Magnet device: placed over a cardiac pacemaker to inhibit it during the procedure. Pacemaker then must be interrogated postoperatively to ensure function
    - AICD deactivation: requires rhythm monitoring and resuscitation abilities during the procedure

CRYOSURGERY (CRYOTHERAPY)

- Defined as the application of extreme cold to destroy abnormal or diseased tissue
- Mechanism of action can be divided into 3 phases: (1) heat transfer, (2) cell injury, and (3) inflammation (Tables 25-14 and 25-15)
- Cryosurgery is used to treat a number of diseases and disorders
  - *Benign lesions*: verruca, xanthelasma, seborrheic keratoses, milia, venous lake, hemangiomas, keloids,

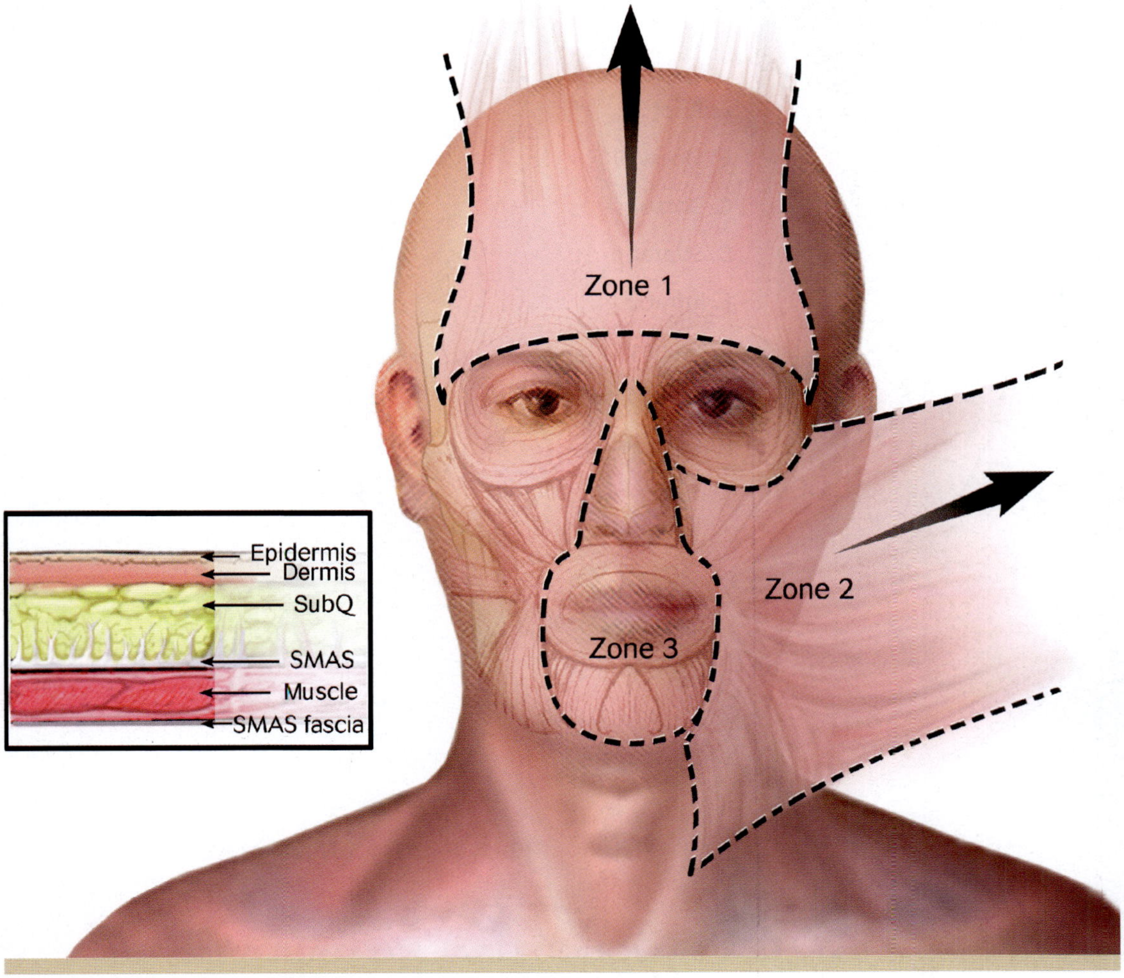

FIGURE 25-15 Superficial musculoaponeurotic system (SMAS).

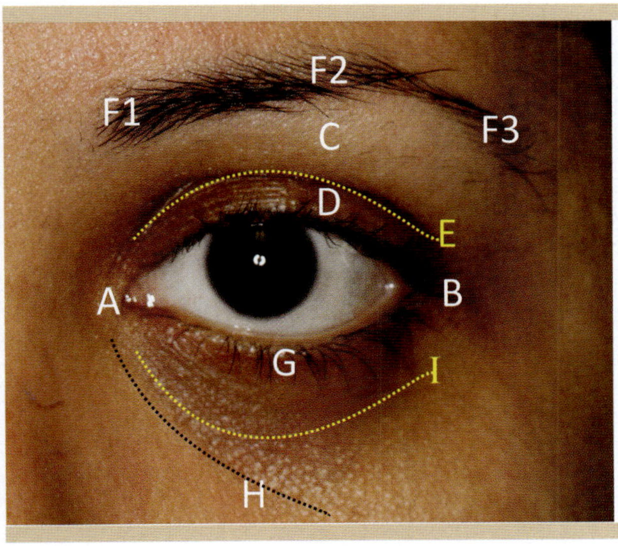

A. Medial canthus

B. Lateral canthus

C. Preseptal upper eyelid

D. Pretarsal upper eyelid

E. Superior palpebral sulcus

F. Eyebrow: F1-medial (head) F2-middle, F3- lateral (tail)

G. Lower eyelid

H. Nasojugal fold

I. Infraorbital crease

FIGURE 25-16 Eyelid anatomy

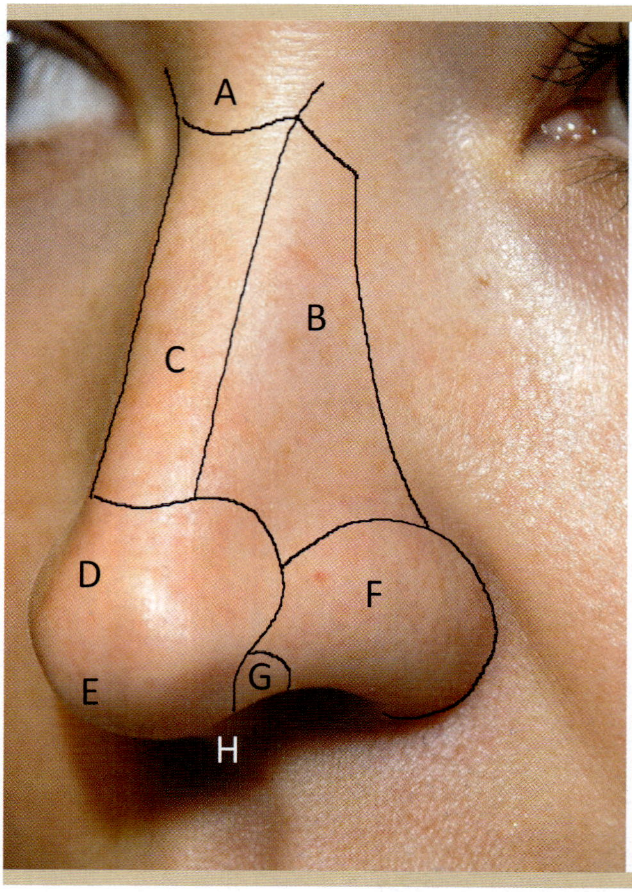

FIGURE 25-17 Nasal anatomy.

lentigines or other epidermal hyperpigmentation, granuloma annulare, prurigo nodularis, myxoid cysts, condyloma

- *Malignant lesions*: actinic keratosis, basal and squamous cell carcinomas, lentigo maligna, Kaposi sarcoma

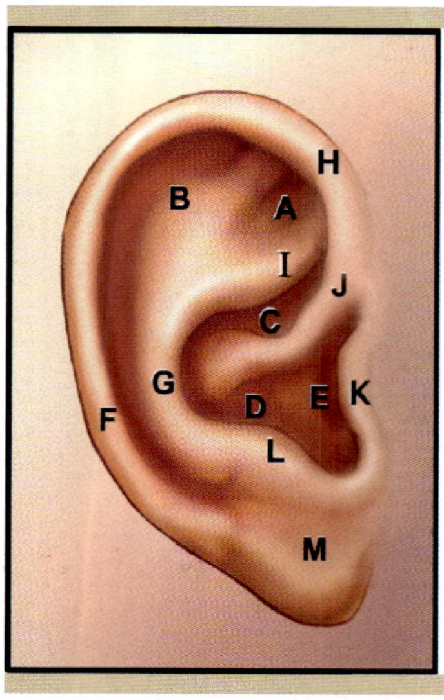

FIGURE 25-18 Ear anatomy.

WOUND HEALING (TABLES 25-16 TO 25-19)

- Wound healing is the restoration of tissue continuity after injury
- Original tissue is replaced with nonspecific connective tissue, which forms a functionally inferior scar
  - Forty eight hours: reepithelialization (sealing of wound)
  - Seven days: peak collagen formation
  - Three weeks: 20% of full wound tensile strength
  - Four months: 60% of full wound tensile strength (never exceeds 80% of full)
  - Six to twelve months: mature scar forms
- Macrophages are the most important cells for wound healing, releasing:
  - Transforming growth factors (TGFs)
  - Cytokines
  - Interleukin-1 (IL-1)
  - Tumor necrosis factor (TNF)
  - platelet-derived growth factor (PDGF)
- Neutropenic or lymphopenic patients do not have impaired wound healing, whereas macrophage-deficient (quantity or function) patients heal poorly

TABLE 25-13 Electrosurgery

Current	Electrosurgery	Mechanism of Action	Waveform	Spark Gap Outlet	Voltage	Amperage = Current/ Damage	Comments
DC	Electrolysis	• Galvanic electrolysis works by causing salt and water in the skin around the probe to be chemically altered to produce a small amount of sodium hydroxide, or lye. If enough is produced, it can damage the cells that cause hair growth.			Low	Low	Positive electrode = anode Negative electrode = cathode The chemical reaction is expressed like this: NaCl (salt) + H_2O (water) + direct current = NaOH (sodium hydroxide) + Cl (chlorine) + H (hydrogen)
DC	Electrocautery (heat)	• Heats electrodes • Rate at which heat is produced determines whether a waveform vaporizes tissue or creates a coagulum.			Low	High	• High heat: vaporization • Low heat: coagulum
AC	Electrodesiccation (coagulation of tissue)	• Damped waveform • Treatment electrode is in direct contact with tissue • No spark is generated	Intermittent	Markedly damped	High	Low/ moderate	Monoterminal

(*Continued*)

TABLE 25-13 Electrosurgery (Continued)

Current	Electrosurgery	Mechanism of Action	Waveform	Spark Gap Outlet	Voltage	Amperage = Current/ Damage	Comments
AC	Electrofulguration (coagulation of tissue)*	• AKA noncontact surface coagulation • Damped waveform • Intermittent short bursts of high voltage produce superficial coagulation and tissue char • Treatment electrode is not in contact with tissue • Electric current "sparks" from the electrode tip across the air gap onto the tissue. The electrode is close enough for sparks to bridge the air gap	Intermittent	Markedly damped	High	Low/ moderate	Monoterminal
AC	Electrocoagulation (coagulation)†	• Damped waveform that turns on and off several times per second	Intermittent	Moderately damped	Moderate	Moderate/ high	• Biterminal • Unipolar or bipolar • Excellent for hemostasis of small blood vessel diameter (< 2 mm) (> 2 mm may need suture ligation) • Some degree of collateral tissue damage with electrocoagulation
AC	Electrosection (cut)	• Undamped waveform concentrates energy in a small area for quick, clean cutting • Causes extreme heating and vaporizing of intracellular fluid that bursts cells	Continuous	Undamped	Low	High/high (vaporized)	• Biterminal • Bipolar

*Electrofulguration and electrodessication are identical in electrical properties, except that the former is noncontact, and the latter has contact with the treated tissue. Owing to direct tissue contact, charring depth may be slightly deeper in electrodesiccation than in electrofulguration

†Both electrodesiccation and electrofulguration cause superficial coagulation and have hemostatic effects. However, they are technically not electrocoagulation. Average power of coagulation current is less than that of a cutting current

TABLE 25-14 Cyrosurgery Mechanism of Action

	Heat Transfer	Cell Freeze	Cell Injury	Inflammation
Event	• Cryogen (heat sink) is applied to the skin • Heat is transferred from the skin to the cryogen • Cryogen evaporates as boiling point is reached	• Formation of ice crystals (−5 to −10°C) • Intracellular ice crystals: form with fast freeze; more destructive • Extracellular ice crystals: form with slow freeze; less tissue damage	• Occurs during cellular thaw	• Inflammation is the response to cell death and helps in local cell destruction
Comment	• Rate of heat transfer depends on the temperature difference between the skin and cryogen	• Greatest destruction seen with rapid freeze, slow thaw • Significant vascular stasis occurs during thaw, contributing to cellular death • May cause basement membrane separation and vesicle (blister) formation	• Cell sensitivity to cryogen damage - 4 to -7° C: Melanocytes (most delicate; reason for hypopigmentation with cryotherapy) - 20 to - 30°C: Keratinocytes - 30 to - 35°C: Dermal fibroblasts (most resistant) 50°C: Malignant tumors (core tissue temperature for optimal destruction) - 20 to - 25°C: Benign lesions	• Observed as erythema and edema

ANTISEPTICS

- Infection control
  - Minor procedures (i.e., biopsies): cleanse with isopropyl alcohol and use nonsterile gloves
  - More invasive procedures (i.e., excisions with layered closure, flaps, grafts): prepare skin with either povidone-iodine or chlorhexidine scrub, followed by placement of sterile towels or drapes around the field
  - Preoperative shaving of hair has been associated with an increase in wound infections. Hairs may be trimmed but not shaved
- Antiseptic (Table 25-20)
  - Agent that kills or inhibits the growth of microorganisms on the external surfaces of the body

TABLE 25-15 Commonly Used Cryogens and Their Temperatures

Cryogen	Boiling Point STP (°C)
Carbon dioxide (solid)	~ 78.5 (~ 109.3°F)
Nitrous oxide (liquid)	~ 89.5 (~ 129.1°F)
Liquid nitrogen	~ 195.8 (~ 320.4°F)

From Graham GF, George MN, Patel M: Cryosurgery, in Nouri K, Leal-Khouri S, eds. *Techniques in Dermatologic Surgery.* London: Mosby; 2003.

TABLE 25-16 Categories of Wound Healing

Category	First Intention	Second Intention
Wound	Seen in clean, well-perfused, incised surgical wounds and casual wounds inflicted by sharp-edged objects where there is minimum destruction of tissue	When the wound is large, when there has been significant loss or destruction of tissue such that the edges cannot be apposed
Healing	Primary subtype: edges of the wound are closely apposed shortly after injury, and healing occurs without complication Delayed primary subtype: If the wound edges are not reapproximated immediately, delayed primary wound healing transpires	See Table 25-17: Phases of Wound Healing Process

TABLE 25-17 Phases of Wound Healing Process

Phase	Hemostasis	Inflammation	Granulation Reepithelialization	Remodeling
Timing	• Immediate	• First 6–8 hours	• Days 5–7; can last up to 4 weeks in the clean and uncontaminated wound	• Begins after third week; can last for years
Comment	• Vasoconstriction • Coagulation with fibrin clot	• Monocytes also exude from the vessels and become macrophages once in tissue • Neutrophils flood the wound via TGF-β	• Fibroblasts have migrated into the wound, producing glycosaminoglycans (GAGs) and fibronectin • Formation of new vasculature (endothelial bud formation) • Reepithelialization via migration of cells from the periphery of the wound and adnexal structures	• Dynamic continuation of collagen synthesis and degradation • Highly vascular granulation tissue undergoes a process of devascularization as it matures into less vascular scar tissue

TABLE 25-18 Growth Factors in Wound Repair

	Growth Factor	Effect
EGF TGF-β	Epidermal growth factor Transforming growth factor β	Reepithelialization
KGF	Keratinocyte growth factor	Reepithelialization
HBEGF	Heparin-binding epidermal growth factor	Reepithelialization, fibroblast proliferation
PDGF	Platelet-derived growth factor	Fibroblast chemotaxis, proliferation, and contraction
IGF	Insulin-like growth factor	Fibroblast proliferation, extracellular matrix production
aFGF-1 bFGF-2	Acidic fibroblast growth factor Basic fibroblast growth factor	Fibroblast proliferation, angiogenesis
VEGF	Vascular endothelial growth factor	Angiogenesis
TGF-β	Transforming growth factor β	Fibroblast chemotaxis and contraction, extracellular matrix production, protease inhibitor production

TABLE 25-19 Macrophage Effects

Activity	Effect
Phagocytosis and killing of microorganisms	Wound decontamination
Phagocytosis of tissue debris	Wound debridement
Growth factor release	Formation of new tissue

Data from Bello Y, Falabella A, Eaglstein WH: Wound healing modalities, in Nouri K, Leal-Khouri S, eds. *Techniques in Dermatologic Surgery*. London: Mosby; 2003 and Lie J, Kirsner RS: Wound healing, in Robinson JK, Hanke WC, Sengelmann RD, et al., eds., *Surgery of the Skin: Procedural Dermatology*. London: Elsevier; 2005.

TABLE 25-20 Topical Antiseptics

	Alcohol	Chlorhexidine Gluconate	Iodine Iodophores	Hexachlorophene	Triclosan
Mode of action	Denaturation of proteins, DNA, RNA, lipids, etc.	Disruption of the microbial cell membrane with precipitation of cell contents	Iodine precipitates microorganism proteins by forming salts via direct halogenation (oxidation-substitution) Results from the combination of molecular iodine and polyvinylpyrrolidone	Disruption of the microbial cell membrane Chlorinated bisphenol antiseptic	Disruption of the microbial cell membrane Derived from phenol
Gram-positive bacteria	Excellent	Excellent	Excellent	Excellent	Good
Gram-negative bacteria	Excellent	Good	Good	Fair/Poor	Good (can use for *Pseudomonas*)
Mycobacterium tuberculosis	Good	Fair	Good	Fair	
Virus	Good	Good	Good	Fair	Unknown
Onset of action	Very rapid	Intermediate	Intermediate	Slow to intermediate	Intermediate
Residual activity	None	Excellent	Minimal	Excellent	Excellent
Toxicity/side effects	Volatile	Ototoxicity Keratitis	Absorbed through the skin; possible toxicity and irritation	Absorbed through intact skin Neurotoxic, especially in neonates	Under investigation
Precautions	Avoid open flame	Avoid contact with eyes, external auditory meatus	Molecular iodine can be very toxic for tissues; therefore, iodine is combined with a carrier, decreasing iodine availability	Avoid use on neonates, pregnant women	Avoid contact with eyes

- Unlike antibiotics that act selectively on a specific target, antiseptics have multiple targets and a broader spectrum of activity, which include bacteria, fungi, viruses, and protozoa

ANTIBIOTICS

- Antibiotics and surgical procedures
  - Risk of wound infection after skin surgery or surgical site infection (SSI) is small (1–2%) but may be higher depending on wound types (class I–IV wounds)
    - Class I: Clean (intact, noninflamed skin, no break in aseptic technique. SSI risk is low, < 2–4%)
    - Class II: Clean-contaminated (mucosal lips, oral, perineum, inguinal, axilla, or minor break in aseptic technique. SSI risk is higher, 4–10%)
    - Class III: contaminated (acute, nonpurulent, traumatic wounds, or major breaks in aseptic technique. SSI rate is 20–30%)
    - Class IV: dirty, infected wounds (inflamed, purulent, foreign body [i.e., ruptured cyst]. SSI risk is 30–40%).
  - Routine prophylactic antibiotics are usually indicated for
    - All Class III and IV wounds, immunosuppressed patients, smokers, diabetes, and those at risk for endocarditis or joint infections (Tables 25-21 and 25-22)
    - Anatomic sites at greater risk for infection: Some class II wounds are oral mucosa, ears, perineum, below the knee
  - If antibiotics are given, they must be in the bloodstream at time of surgery in order to be effective (i.e., 30–60 minutes before incision, but may depend on antibiotic half-life). The American Heart Association states that antibiotics may be given up to 2 hours after the procedure if it was not given preoperatively.
  - Open wounds almost never become infected, whereas closed wounds with hematomas or a large amount of necrotic tissue are at increased risk for infection
  - Prophylactic antiherpesvirus medications for susceptible patients undergoing lip surgery, including laser procedures
    - Regimens for procedures on infected skin, skin structure, or musculoskeletal tissue
    - Staphylococci and (β)-hemolytic streptococci are likely to cause infective endocarditis
    - Patients with the conditions listed in Table 25-21 below who undergo a surgical procedure that involves infected skin, skin structure, or musculoskeletal tissue, should receive prophylactic antibiotics

WOUND CLOSURE

- The wound closure algorithm (Fig. 25-19) is not all inclusive
  - The type of repair of a wound greatly depends on the defect location (i.e., a 1-cm defect on the nose demands greater consideration and complexity than the same sized wound on the cheek)
  - *Wound defect sizes*: Small (< 1 cm), medium (1–3 cm), large (> 3 cm)
  - *Location of a wound is critical*
    - Defects greater than 3 mm in depth will likely heal with a contour depression (unless in concave area),

TABLE 25-21 Cardiac and Prosthetic Joint Conditions Associated With the Highest Risk of Adverse Outcome for Which Antibiotic Prophylaxis Is Reasonable

Prostatic cardiac valve or prosthetic material used for cardiac valve repair
Previous infective endocarditis
Congestive heart disease (CHD)*
• Unrepaired cyanotic CHD, including palliative shunts and conduits
• Completely repaired congenital heart defect with prosthetic material or device, whether placed by surgery or by catheter intervention, during the first 6 months after the procedure†
• Repaired CHD with residual defects at the site or adjacent to the site of a prosthetic patch or prosthetic device (which inhibit endothelialization)
Cardiac transplantation recipients who develop cardiac valvulopathy
Joint replacement within first 2 years
History of prosthetic joint infection
Joint replacement in patients with hemophilia, diabetes Type 1, HIV, malignancy, malnutrition, and other immunosuppressed states.

*Except for the conditions listed above, antibiotic prophylaxis is no longer recommended for any other form of CHD.
† Prophylaxis is reasonable because endothelialization of prosthetic material occurs within 6 months after the procedure.

TABLE 25-22 Prophylactic Antibiotics Regimens

Situation	Agent	Dose (All Doses given 30-60 Minutes Preoperatively)	
		Adults	Children
Oral	Amoxicillin	2 g	50 mg/kg
Unable to take oral medication	Ampicillin Cefazolin or ceftriaxone	2 g IM or IV 1 g IM or IV	50 mg/kg IM or IV 50 mg/kg IM or IV
Allergic to penicillins or ampicillin—oral	Cephalexin* Clindamycin Azithromycin or clarihromycin	2 g 600 mg 500 mg	50 mg/kg 20 mg/kg 15 mg/kg
Allergic to penicillins or ampicillin and unable to take oral medication	Cefazolin or cetriaxone clindamycin	1 g IM or IV 600 mg IM or IV	50 mg/kg IM or IV 20 mg/kg IM or IV

IM, intramuscular; IV, intravenous.

Or other first- or second-generation oral cephalosporin in equivalent adult or pediatric dosage. Cephalosporins should not be used in an individual with a history of anaphylaxis, angioedema, or urticaria with penicillins or ampicilllin.

especially if overlying convex surfaces or sebaceous skin
  - Small, superficial defects in concave areas are ideal for second intention healing. Avoid second intention if bare bone, tendon, or neurovascular structures are exposed
  - Large defects will also heal well if superficial. However, anticipate significant wound contraction and its impact, if any, on free margins or function
- *Full thickness skin graft (FTSG):* consists of the epidermis and the whole thickness of the dermis, may be applied to any defect that is well vascularized
  - Superficial defects with FTSG will maintain contour
  - If deep defects are repaired with FTSG, contour depressions may result unless delayed (partial granulation to fill the depth) skin grafting is performed
- *Split thickness skin graft (STSG):* consists of the epidermis and part of the dermis, have less metabolic demand and survive better in poorly vascularized defects. However, significant graft contraction (with potential effect on free margins) is assured compared to FTSG
- *Composite grafts*: consists of epidermal keratinocytes seeded on a fibroblast-containing collagen matrix, work best for small deep wounds at free margins. Due to their bulk and high metabolic demand, composite grafts survive poorly if sized greater than 1.5 cm
- *Combination closures*: may involve flap + flap, flap + graft, or flap + second intention; should be considered in wounds involving multiple subunits

FLAPS (TABLE 25-23 AND FIGS. 25-20 TO 25-33)

- Transfer of tissue (donor site) with its attached vascular supply into a wound defect (recipient site) for closure
- Tissue may be directly connected to the defect or nearby but not contiguous
- Usually performed when a primary straight-line closure is not possible (owing to excess tension or potential anatomic/functional distortion)
- A secondary defect is always created
- May be categorized by the following characteristics
  - Location with respect to the surgical defect (i.e., local, regional, or distant)
  - Movement (i.e., advancement, rotation) (NOTE: In reality, flaps may have more than one movement)
  - Vascular supply (i.e., random pattern, axial, or microvascular)
  - Stage (i.e., single or multistage)
  - Configuration (i.e., note, rhomboid, bilobed, banner, etc.)
  - Eponym (i.e., Abbe, Rieger, Mustarde, etc.)
  - No single classification accounts for every design or definition variation
  - Eponyms should generally be avoided
  - Most flaps in cutaneous surgery are local (adjacent and contiguous skin) and regional (nearby but not directly adjacent)
  - Within this context, the most useful classification scheme is based on *movement* and *vascular supply*

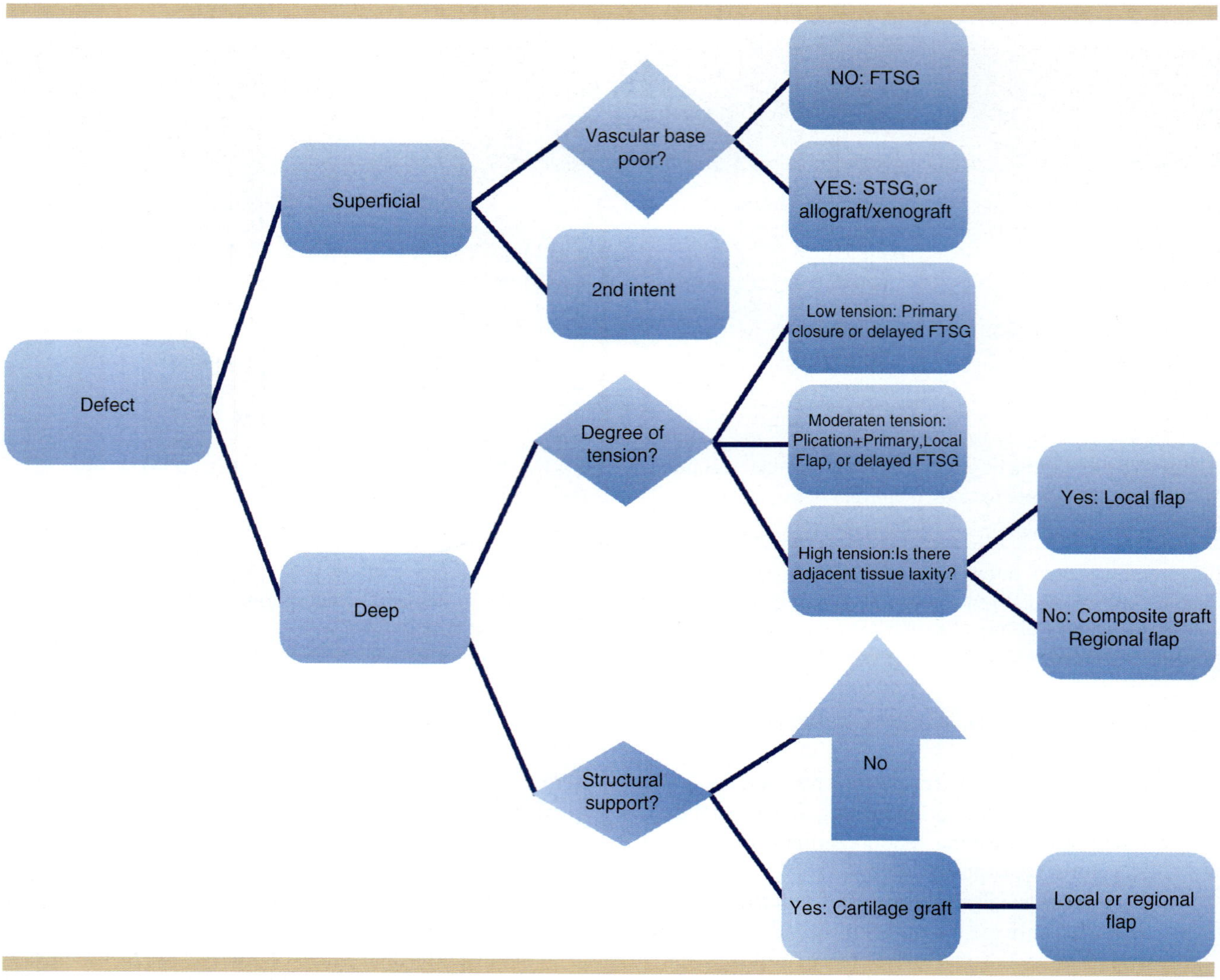

FIGURE 25-19 Wound closure algorithm.

- Definition of terms: general
  - *Tension vector*: the direction of pull or stress on a wound during its closure (Fig. 25-25)
  - *Primary defect*: the wound that requires closure (Fig. 25-25)
  - *Secondary defect*: the wound that results from closure of the primary defect (Fig. 25-25)
  - *Primary movement*: the motion (advancement, rotation, or transposition) and tension vectors required for closure of the primary defect. Rotation and transposition flaps have in common a pivoting or arclike motion, whereas advancement flaps have a sliding motion in straight lines (Fig. 25-25)
  - *Secondary movement*: the motion and tension vectors required to close the secondary defect (Fig. 25-25)
  - *Bürow triangle (dog-ear, standing cutaneous cone)*: redundant skin that is removed as wounds are closed
  - *Primary Bürow triangle*: The dog-ear directly connected to the primary defect that is removed during closure (Fig. 25-24)
  - *Secondary Bürow triangle*: the dog-ear directly connected to the secondary defect that is removed during closure (Fig. 25-24)
  - *Subunit*: a surface area demarcated by either natural or arbitrary lines that has unique textural, cosmetic, or functional characteristics (i.e., upper lip has 4 subunits, the left and right upper cutaneous lips, the philtrum, and the mucosal lip). In general, repairs within a subunit or incisions placed at junctions of subunits yield the best cosmetic results
  - *Local flap*: adjacent and contiguous
  - *Regional flap*: nearby but not directly adjacent
  - *Advancement flap*: a random-pattern flap where the primary flap movement is linear and provides the least

TABLE 25-23 Flap Types Based on Type of Movement

Flap Design	Advancement Flap (Linear Sliding Movement, Straight or Perpendicular Lines)	Rotation Flap (Curvilinear Pivoting Movement, Curved or Angulated Lines)
Examples	Unilateral designs 1. Bürow wedge advancement (Fig. 25-20) 2. Crescentic advancement (can be unilateral or bilateral (Fig. 25-21) 3. V–Y (V–Y flaps should no longer be referred to as island pedicle flaps) (Fig. 25-22) Bilateral designs 1. H-plasty 2. A–T bilateral advancement (Fig. 25-23) Interpolation flap subtypes with advancement movement 1. Retroauricular-staged flap (This is a staged flap that has a linear movement. However, it may also be classified as a transposition design because it crosses over intervening island of normal skin to reach the defect.)	Rotation (Fig. 25-24—lip, Fig. 25-25—scalp) 1. Dorsal nasal rotation (Rieger, hatchet) (Fig. 25-26) 2. Cervicofacial rotation (Fig. 25-27) 3. O to Z bilateral rotation (Fig. 25-28) 4. Innervated myocutaneous lip and cheek (Karapandzic) 5. O–T bilateral rotation 6. Comet flap Transposition subtype 1. Rhombic or Rhomboid (Limberg 60 degree, Dufourmental) 2. Webster 30 degree Note or Banner flap (Fig. 25-29) 3. Bilobe (Fig. 25-30) 4. Rhombic transposition with Z-plasty or Trilobe (Fig. 25-31) Interpolation flap subtypes with rotation movement 1. Paramedian forehead flap (Fig. 25-32) 2. Lip-switch (Abbe) flap 3. Cheek-to-nose (melolabial) interpolation (Fig. 25-33)
Movement	Linear	Pivotal (movement is in an arc)
Vascular supply	Random pattern	Random pattern or axial (paramedian forehead flap, lip-switch flap)
Flap:defect ratio	2–4:1	2-4:1 (flap:defect ratio may be greater with axial flap)
Tension	Tension is reduced and redistributed but is not redirected	Tension is reduced, redistributed, and redirected
Mobility	Recruits some adjacent tissue laxity laterally	Optimizes recruitment of lax donor tissue lateral and distant from the defect
Restraint	Lateral restraint	Pivotal restraint (Fig 25-24) Arises from inherent tissue stiffness at the flap's pivot point and prevents the flap's tip from reaching distal margin of the operative defect. Secondary movement expected at the primary defect.

mobility among the different flap types. Flap lines are straight and angles are often perpendicular at right angles

- *Rotation flap*: a random- or axial-pattern flap where the donor tissue pivots in a curved or arclike motion. Flap lines are often semicircular or curvilinear
- *Transposition flap*: a subset of either a rotation or advancement flap where the donor tissue is nearby but not directly adjacent to defect. The flap, therefore, must move across and over an intervening segment of normal skin to close the defect. Flap lines are often at acute angles (< 90 degrees)
- *Interpolation flap*: a subset of transposition flap that is usually indicated for larger defects and typically requires at least 2 separate stages of surgery (usually separated by 3 weeks between stages) (i.e., melolabial interpolation flap, paramedian forehead flap)

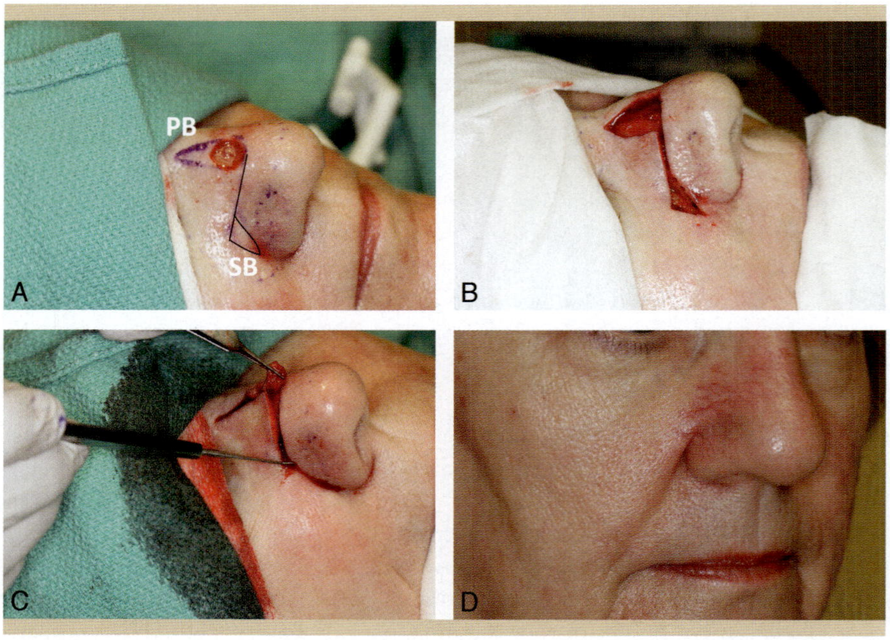

FIGURE 25-20 Bürow wedge advancement flap. (A) Standing cones (Bürow triangles) designed. PB- primary Bürow, SB—secondary Burow. (B) Cones excised. (C) Flap advanced to close defect. (D) Result at 4 months.

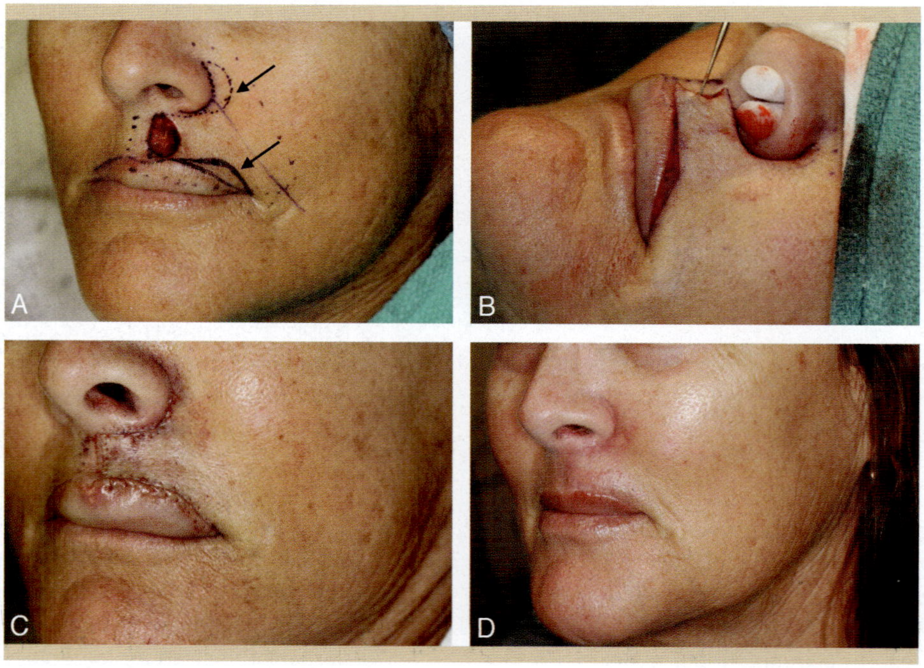

FIGURE 25-21 Crescentic advancement flap. (A) Standing cones excised as "crescents" (black arrows). (B) Flap advanced medially. (C) Flap sutured. (D) Result at 2 months.

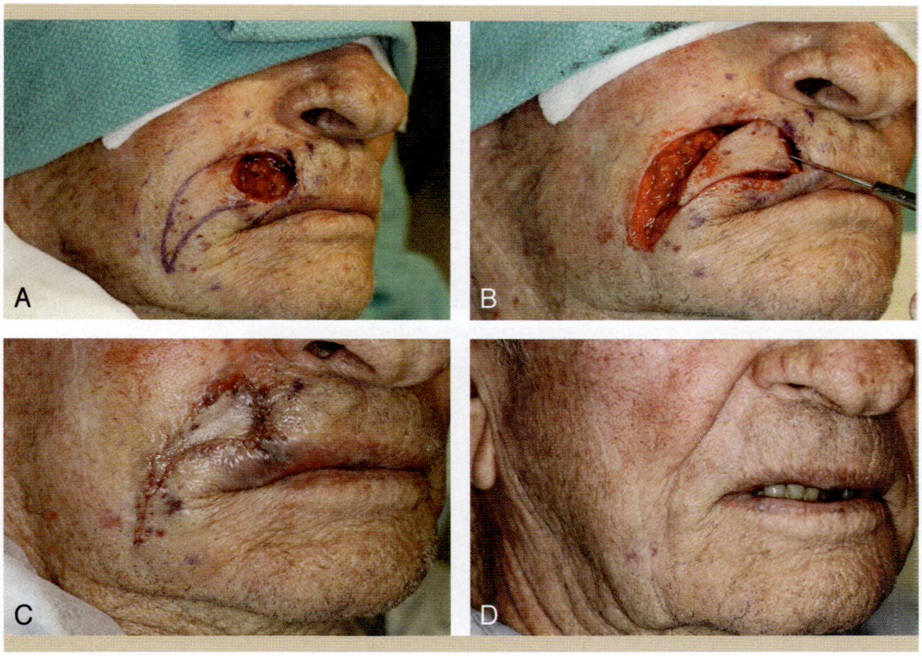

FIGURE 25-22 V-Y advancement flap. (A) Flap designed as "curved triangle." (B) Pedicle is myocutaneous and underneath the flap. (C) Flap sutured. (D) Result at 12 months.

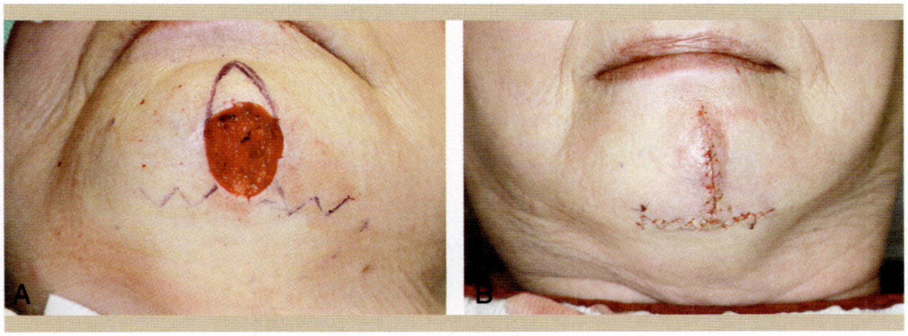

FIGURE 25-23 A-T bilateral advancement.

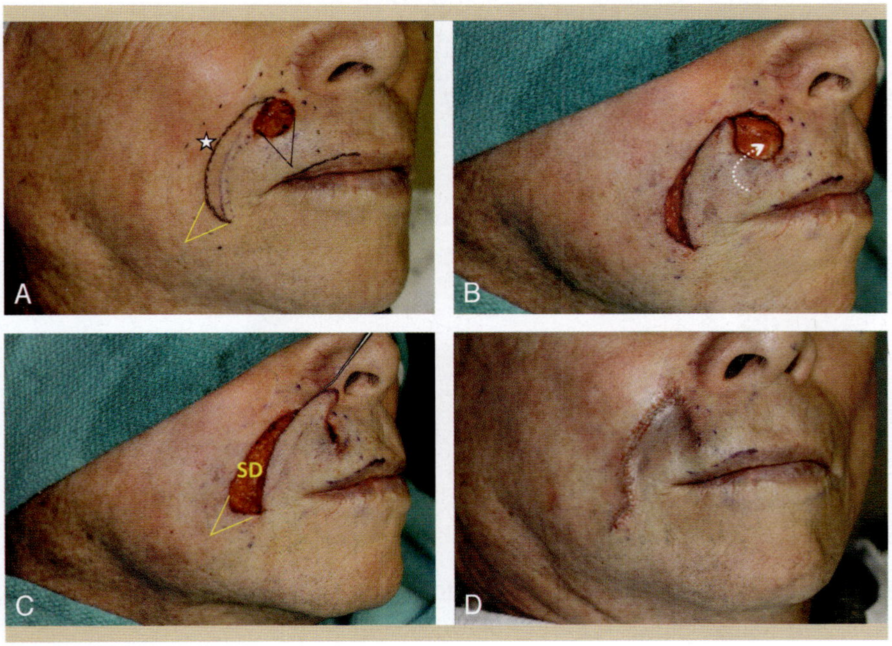

FIGURE 25-24 Rotation flap-lip. (A) Flap incision is curvilinear (star). Primary Bürow (black triangle) closes primary defect and secondary Bürow (yellow triangle) closes secondary defect. (B) Curved arrow-pivotal restraint, reduced with undermining. (C) Note secondary defect (SD) as flap rotates

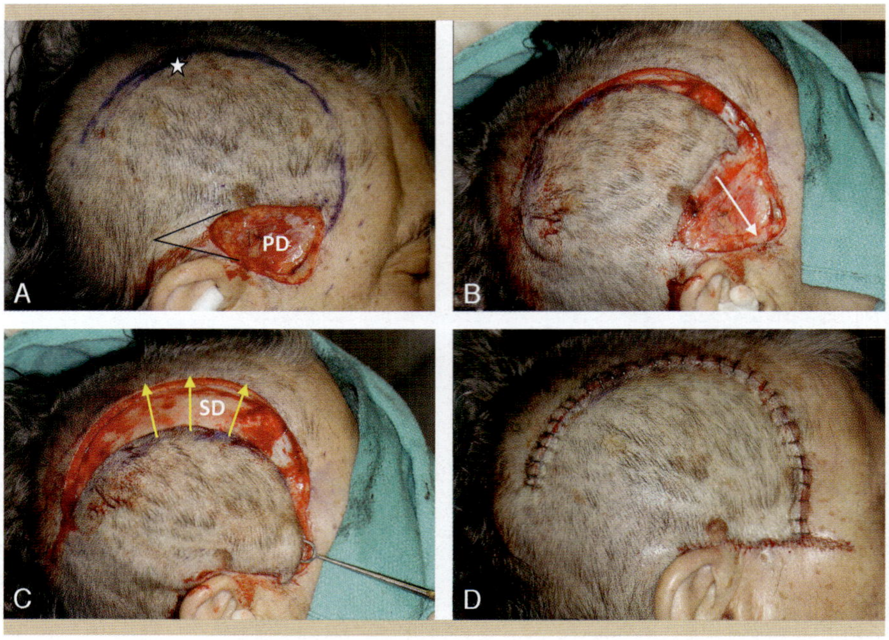

FIGURE 25-25 Rotation flap-scalp. (A) PD-primary defect. (B) White arrow—primary movement and tension vector. (C) Large secondary defect (SD) results when flap closes PD. Yellow arrow is secondary movement and tension vector to close donor site. (D) Flap sutured.

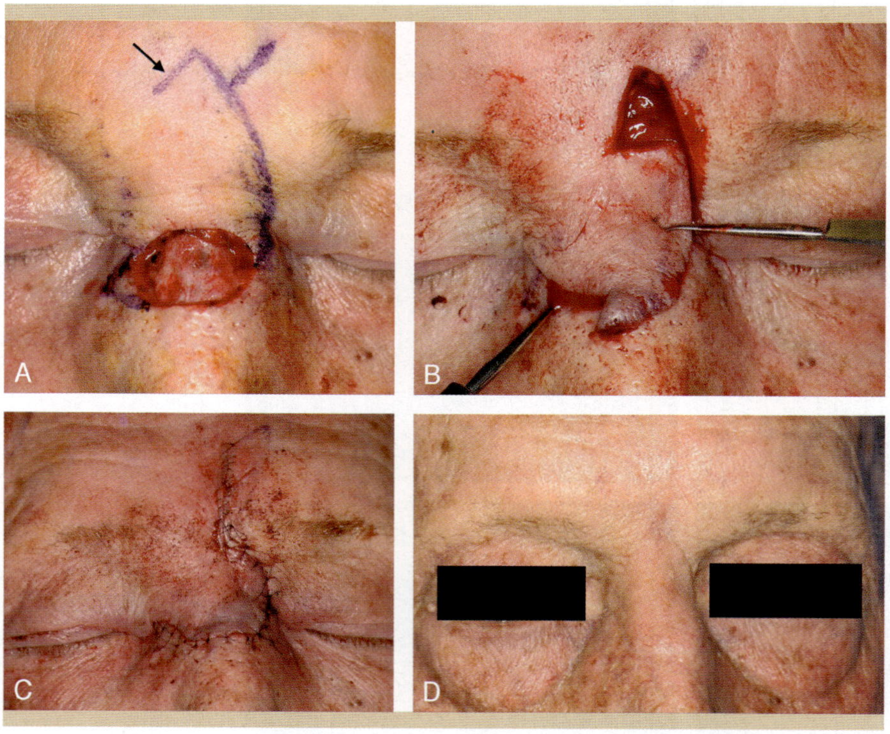

FIGURE 25-26 Dorsal nasal rotation flap (Rieger or hatchet flap). (A) Black arrow identifies backcut, a relaxing incision to facilitate flap rotation.

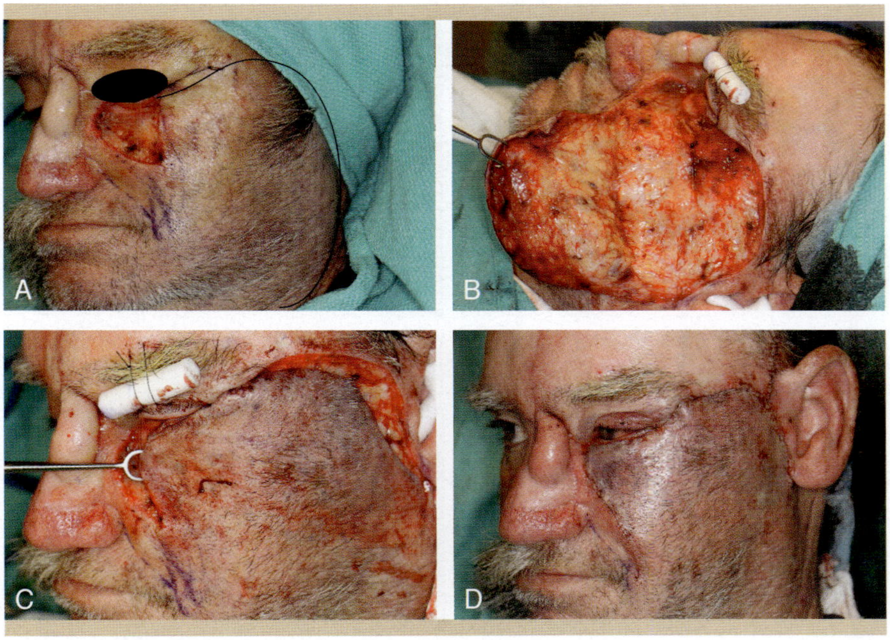

FIGURE 25-27 Cervicofacial rotation flap. A rotation flap that extends to the neck to recruit tissue laxity. Reserved for larger wounds.

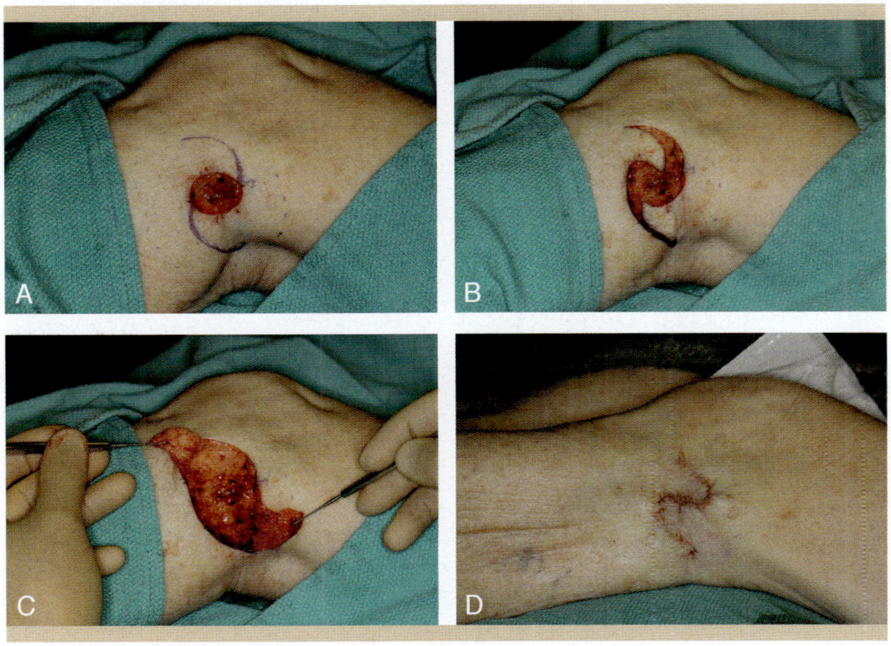

FIGURE 25-28 O-Z bilateral rotation flap.

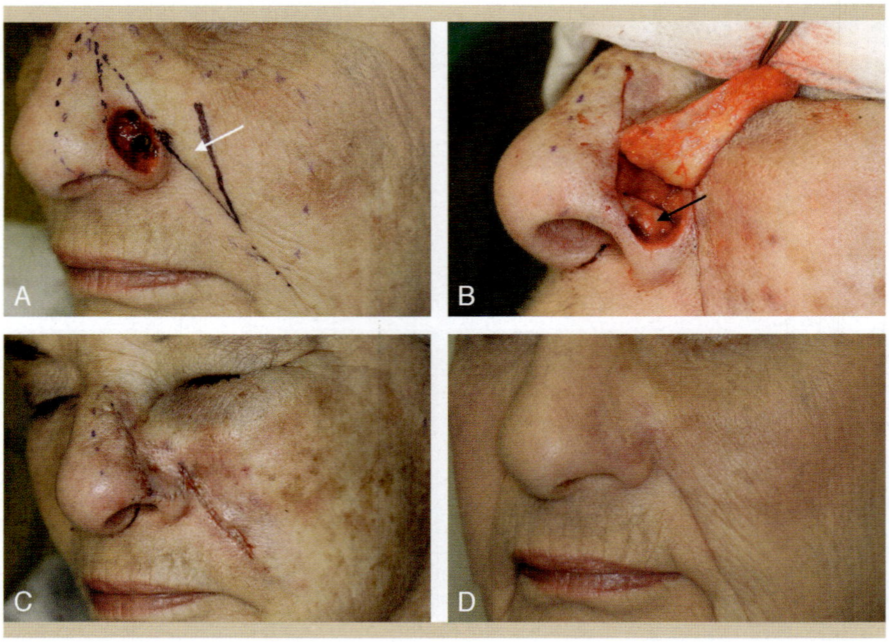

FIGURE 25-29 Note or Banner flap (single-stage melolabial transposition flap). (A) Flap recruited from cheek (white arrow) (B) Flap crosses over melolabial fold to cover alar defect (black arrow—cartilage graft at base of wound). (C) Flap sutured. (D) Result at 4 months

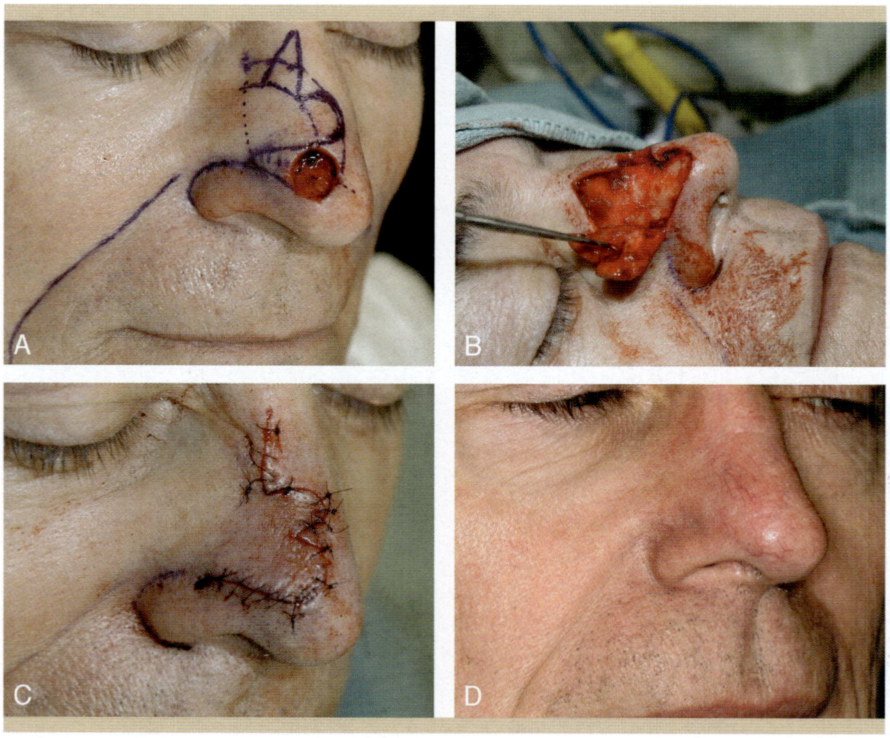

FIGURE 25-30 Bilobe transposition flap.

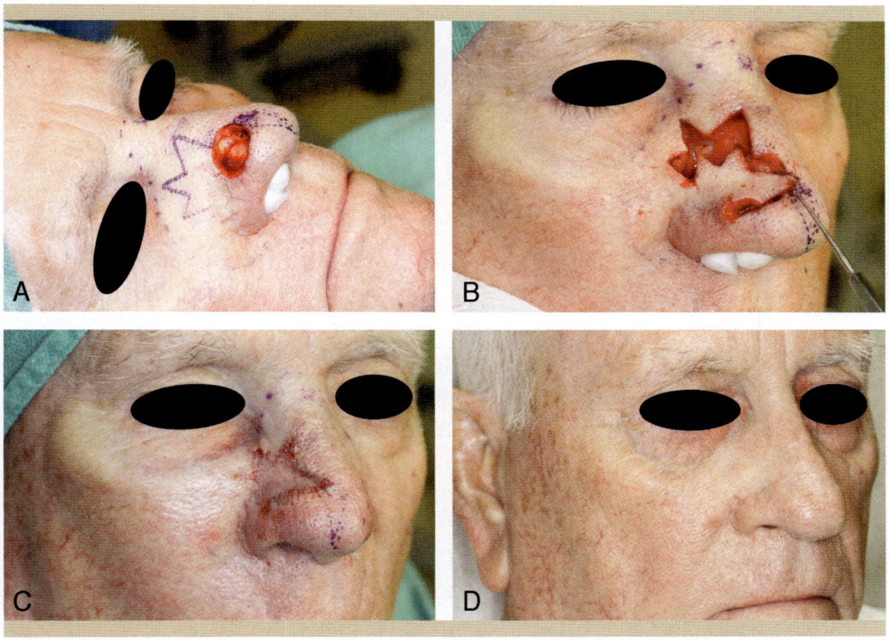

FIGURE 25-31 Transposition flap with Z-plasty (variant of trilobe transposition f ap)

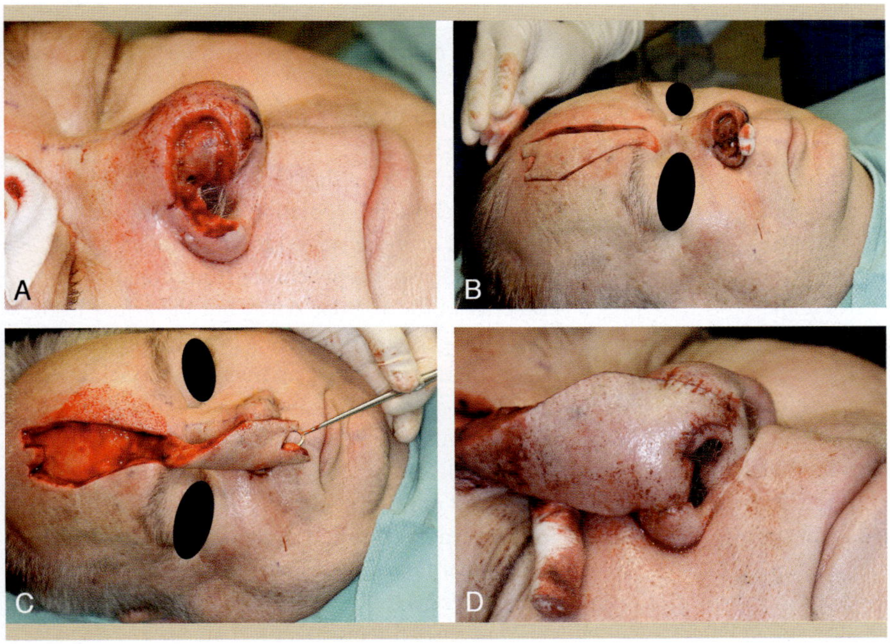

FIGURE 25-32A Paramedian forehead flap—Stage I: pedicle based on supratrochlear artery (B). Flap rotated down to cover nose (C & D). Flap inset for 3 weeks.

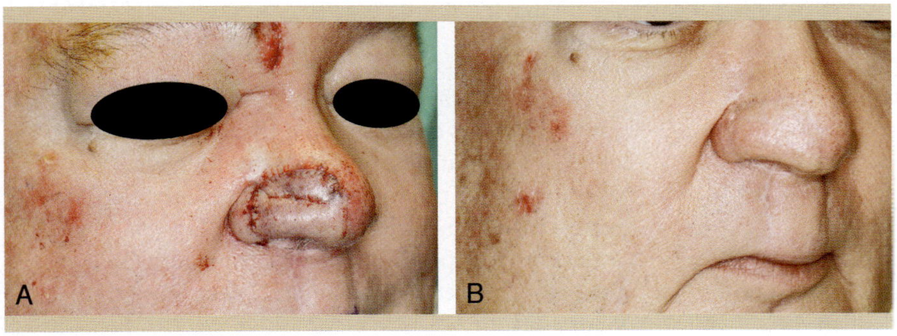

FIGURE 25-32B Paramedian Forehead flap—Stage II: (A) Pedicle divided in 3 weeks. (B) Result in 2 years.

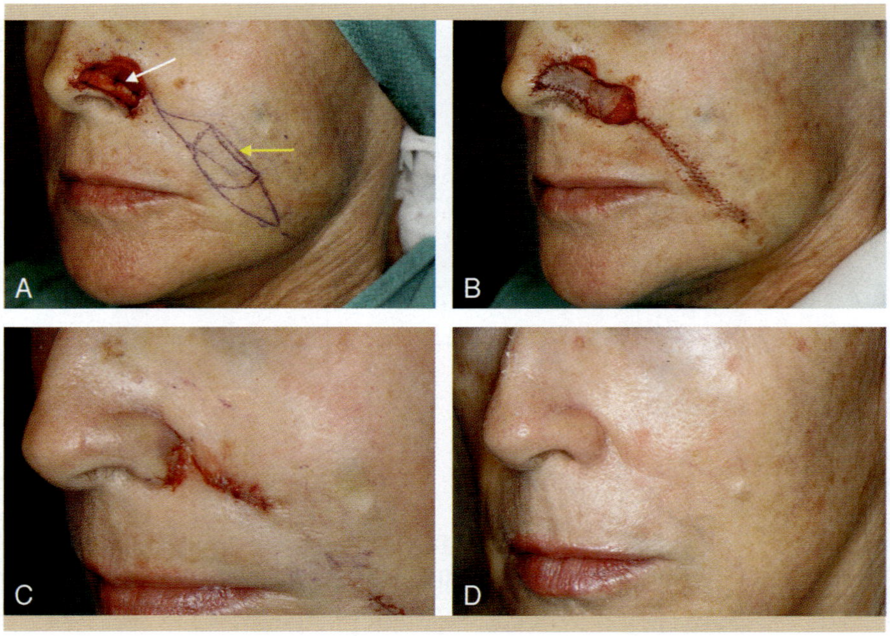

FIGURE 25-33 Cheek-to-nose interpolation flap (2-stage melolabial transposition flap). (A) Cartilage graft to support ala (white arrow). Flap recruited from medial cheek (yellow arrow). (B) Pedicle based on branches of angular artery but is random pattern (no named artery in flap). (C) Division of flap in stage 2.

- *V-Y advancement flaps:* a random-pattern flap where the flap is completely separated from the surrounding skin (literally an island) and subcutis except for an underlying subcutaneous pedicle. The term island pedicle flap (IPF) historically described V-Y advancement flaps. However, this term is archaic and should no longer be used for V-Y flaps performed in dermatologic surgery. The term IPF is now reserved for large, named axial artery flaps with substantial myocutaneous pedicles that are tunneled to their defects.
- *Backcut*: a relaxing incision on the far end of a rotation curve to release lateral flap restraints and facilitate movement (Fig. 25-26)
- *Z-plasty*: distinct form of transposition often used for scar revision. (Fig. 25-34) A Z-plasty will change both a scar's length (makes scar longer, more angulated, zigzag broken lines) and its direction or orientation (Table 25-24). The extent of scar lengthening and change in direction depends on the degree of transposition of the Z-plasty. Z-plasties may be designed as 15, 30, or 60 degrees of transposition. Scars that may benefit from Z-plasty revision include: 1) contracted or webbed scars, especially over joint spaces or concavities, 2) scars that are oriented incorrectly
  - Lengthening and breaking up of a scar into multiple zigzag lines.
- *Pedicle*: the vascular supply to a flap (blood vessels are contiguous with the flap)
- *Random-pattern flap*: flap that is nourished by unnamed vessels from underlying arterial perforators. Random flaps rely on a rich vascular plexus of subcutaneous tissue that directly connects with the flap
- *Axial-pattern flap*: flap that has a named vessel for its pedicle
  - Paramedian forehead flap (supratrochlear artery) (Fig. 25-32)
  - Cheek interpolation flap (angular artery) (Fig. 25-33). A cheek interpolation flap is a staged flap (requires 2 or more stages) but it is not an axial flap. Its vascular supply comes from non-named branches of the angular artery but the artery itself is not in the pedicle. Similarly, a postauricular staged flap is an interpolation flap but not an axial flap
- *Abbe (lip-switch) flap* (Fig. 25-35): The *Abbe flap* is most commonly harvested from the lower lip, to repair an upper lip defect (up to 50% loss). *Abbe* flaps repair midline or off of midline lip defects. Its pedicle is either the inferior (most common) or superior labial artery. *Abbe Estlander* flaps repair lip defects at the oral commissure. Whereas the *Abbe flap* is a 2-staged repair, the *Abbe Estlander* flap requires only 1 stage

GRAFTS (TABLES 25-25 AND 25-26)

- Autologous skin grafts
- Skin that is detached completely from its blood supply, removed from its donor site, and transplanted to a recipient site for wound closure in the same individual
- All grafts contract to some degree, but contraction is greatest with split-thickness skin grafts
- Graft survival depends on the establishment of new vasculature between the wound recipient site and the donor graft

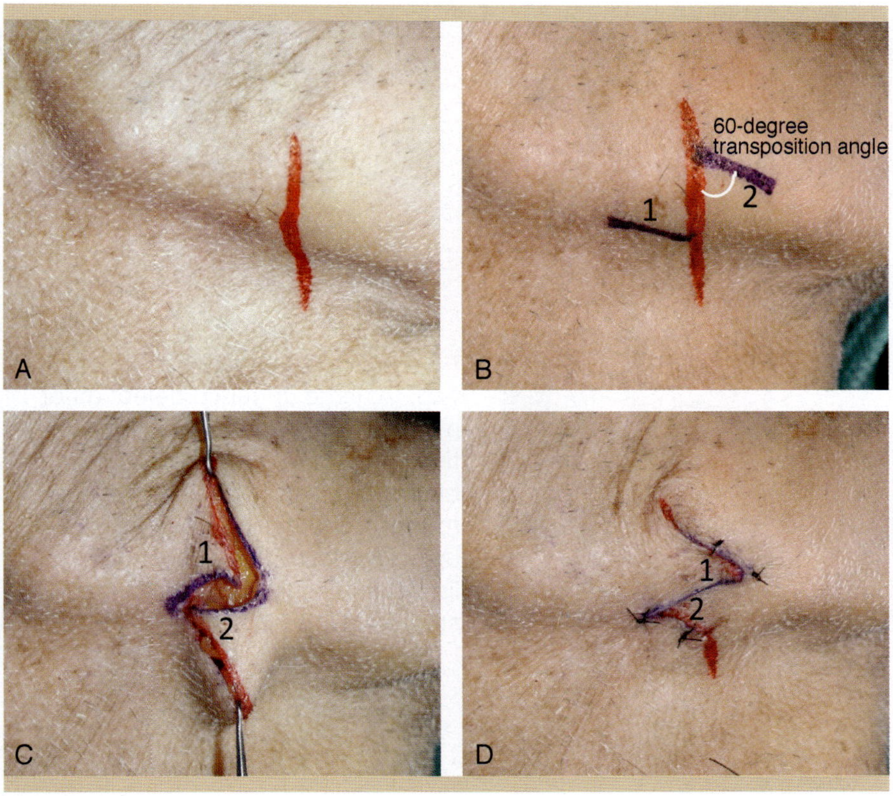

FIGURE 25-34 Z-plasty. A) Vertical scar across jawline. (B) 60-degree Z-plasty to change scar direction from vertical to horizontal. Design creates 2 flaps—1 and 2. (C) Flaps are transposed and exchange positions, with Flap 1 now above and flap 2 below. (D) Note lengthening of flap after Z-plasty and change of scar's direction.

LOCAL ANESTHESIA (TABLES 25-27 TO 25-29)

- Mechanism of action
  - Anesthetics block membrane Na+/K+ channels, thus preventing effective depolarization and nerve transmission
  - Unmyelinated C-type nerve fibers (slow conduction) conduct temperature and pain (blocked more easily)
  - Myelinated A-type fibers (fast conduction) carry pressure and motor fibers
- Side effects
  - Vasovagal reaction with hypotension and bradycardia (most frequent)
    - Place patient in Trendelenburg position to increase cerebral perfusion; supportive care; atropine for severe reactions
    - Bruising and edema, especially in periorbital area
    - Transient motor nerve paralysis
    - Prolonged paresthesia (nerve injury can occur in nerve blocks if needle traumatizes nerve)
  - Allergy to anesthetic
    - True allergy is rare (more common with esters than amides)
    - Allergic reactions are usually IgE-mediated type I reactions with urticaria, angioedema, or anaphylaxis with hypotension and tachycardia
  - Cocaine (ester group) is vasoconstricting; all other anesthetics are vasodilating
  - Longer-lasting anesthetics (> 2-hour duration) are more protein bound (bupivacaine, etidocaine)
- Lidocaine 1% with 1:100,000 epinephrine
  - Most common local anesthetic for skin surgery
  - Very acidic (low pH)
  - Addition of $NaHCO_3$ to lidocaine with epinephrine neutralizes solution, reducing burning on injection and facilitating anesthetic diffusion
  - Lidocaine toxicity
    - Maximum dose of lidocaine: 5 mg/kg of 1% lidocaine plain; 7 mg/kg of 1% lidocaine with 1:100,000 epinephrine

TABLE 25-24 Z-Plasties and Scar-Lengthening Properties (Fig 25-34)

Degree of Transposition	Extent of Scar Lengthening (%)
30°	25
45°	50
60°	75

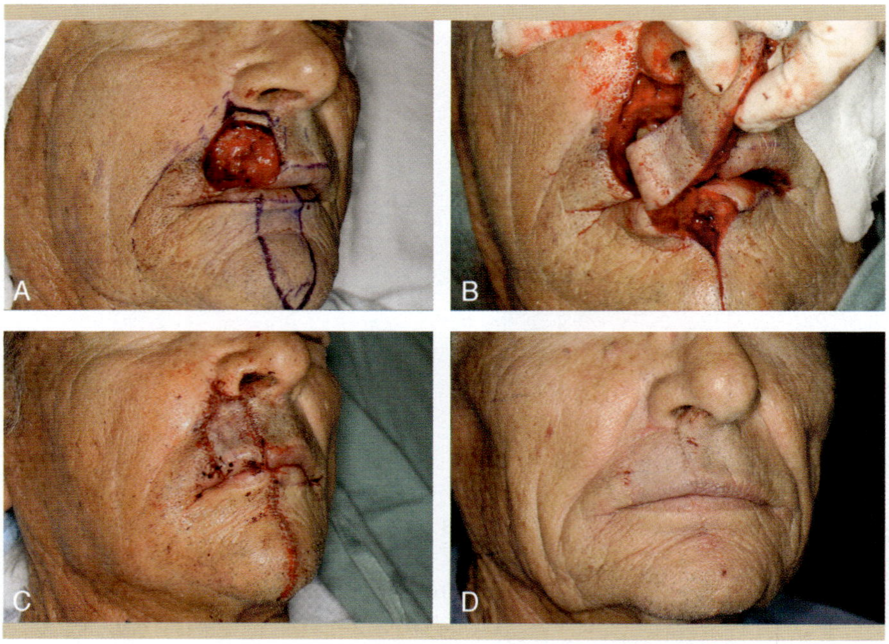

FIGURE 25-35 *Abbe* or lip-switch flap. (A) large upper lip defect off of midline. (B) Lower lip donates flap tissue (mucosa, muscle, dermis) based on inferior labial artery. Flap rotates from midline lower lip to repair upper lip defect. Residual upper lip defect tissue excised. (C) Flap sutured. (D) Result in 4 months.

TABLE 25-25 Graft Take

Phase	Timing	Comment
Plasma imbibition	First 48 hours	Imbibition means to take in or absorb fluid, causing swelling Ischemic and edematous phase of graft because no blood flow established Grafts survive the first 1–2 days by absorbing wound exudate and passive diffusion of nutrients Fibin also forms between the recipient bed and graft, promoting graft adhesion and reducing infection
Inosculation	Days 2–3	Initial establishment of vessels between the recipient bed and graft New vessels form from the recipient bed and migrate to anastamose with vasculature from the graft Fibrin mesh established during imbibition facilitates vessel migration
Capillary ingrowth, revascularization	Days 4–7	Additional vascular anastamoses occur between wound base and graft Blood flow evident by days 5 to 7
Keratinocyte activation	Day 4 to week 4	Epidermal activation and proliferation, greater in split-thickness skin grafts Lymphatic flow reestablished
Sensory innervation	Begins after 2–3 months	Starts at edge of graft and moves centrally

TABLE 25-26 Types of Autologous Skin Grafts

	Full-Thickness Skin Graft (FTSG)	Split-Thickness Skin Graft (STSG)	Composite Grafts
Definition	Entire epidermis and a dermis harvested Dermis may be of varying thickness depending on donor site	Epidermis and only partial-thickness dermis Thin (0.005–0.012 in) Intermediate (0.012–0.018 in) Thick (0.018–0.030 in)	Contains 2 different tissue layers (i.e., skin and cartilage)
Advantages	Minimal contraction during healing phase Potential for good match with recipient site if donor site properly selected Donor site is usually sutured or closed	Much thinner, requires less metabolic support, and survives better than FTSGs. Able to cover large wounds, line cavities, resurface mucosal deficits, exposed bone, close donor sites of flaps, and resurface muscle flaps.	Provides scaffolding (cartilage) as well as soft tissue covering (skin)
Disadvantages	Donor site morbidity FTSGs require more metabolic support (thicker) and do not survive as well as STSGs	Requires more equipment Significant graft contraction Cosmetically poor compared to FTSGs Discomfort and appearance of donor site (donor site heals by second intention; a rectangular discolored patch is typical postoperative appearance)	Most metabolically demanding of all graft types. Most composite grafts over 1 cm do not survive completely
Donor sites	Selected based on matching qualities for thickness, texture, pigmentation, actinic damage, and morbidity of donor harvesting (i.e., upper eyelid, nasolabial fold, pre- and postauricular regions, conchal bowl, and the supraclavicular fossa)	Harvested from any surface of the body (i.e., thigh, buttock, abdomen, scalp)	Donor site is usually crux of the helix to include skin and cartilage

  - Systemic lidocaine toxicity: starts with circumoral numbness and tingling; can progress to seizures and cardiovascular collapse with severe overdosage; toxic effects are exacerbated by acidosis and hypoxia
- Prilocaine toxicity
  - Metabolizes to ortho-toluidine, an oxiding agent capable of converting hemoglobin to methemoglobin, potentially causing methemoglogbinemia
  - Patients at risk of methemoglobinemia include
    - Patients younger than 1 year old
    - Patients with G-6-PD deficiency
    - Methemoglobinemia-inducing agents: dapsone, nitroglycerin, nitrofurantoin, antimalarials, sulfonamides, phenobarbitol, phenytoin, nitroprusside, acetaminophen
    - See EMLA below
- Bupivacaine toxicity
  - Risk of cardiac toxicity, with ventricular arrhythmias and cardiovascular collapse
- Epinephrine
  - Epinephrine prolongs duration of anesthesia by 100% to 150% and decreases the anesthetic's systemic toxicity by slowing absorption
  - Epinephrine is hemostatic in a dilution of up to 1:1,000,000
  - Epinephrine use in digital anesthesia (fingers/toes)

TABLE 25-27 Two Main Groups of Local Anesthetics: Esters and Amides—Groups Differentiated by Their Intermediate Chain

Anesthetic	Amide	Ester
Metabolized	• *N*-dealkylated and hydrolyzed by microsomal liver enzymes cytochrome P450 3A4	• Hydrolyzed by tissue pseudocholinesterases • Excreted by kidney
Caution	• Lidocaine is class B in pregnancy; avoid complex procedures in the first trimester; small volumes of lidocaine without epinephrine may be used for essential procedures • Possible drug interaction with medications that are metabolized via liver cytochrome P450 enzymes • End-stage liver disease (altered drug metabolism)	• Pseudocholinesterase deficiency • Severe renal compromise • Allergy to PABA compounds (esters cross-react with PABA): sulfonamides, sulfonylureas, thiazides, and paraphenylene diamine
Comment	• Amide anesthetics have 2 "i"s in the name	• Ester anesthetics only have 1 "i"

TABLE 25-28 Local Anesthetics

Generic Name	Trade Name	Primary Use	Relative Potency	Onset	Duration* Plan	Maximum Dose† Plan	Maximum Dose With Epinephrine†
Amides							
Bupivacaine Dibucaine Etidocaine Lidocaine	Marcaine Nupercaine Duranest Xylocaine	Infiltration Topical Infiltration Infiltr/ topical	8 6 2	2–10 min Rapid 3–5 min Rapid	30–10 h Short 3–10 h 1–2 h	175 mg 300 mg 300 mg	250 mg 400 mg 500 mg (3,850 mg dilute)
Mepivacaine	Carbocaine	Infiltration	2	3–20 min	2–3 h	300 mg	400 mg
Prilocaine	Citanest	Infiltration	2	Rapid	2–4 h	400 mg	600 mg
Prilocaine/ lidocaine	EMLA	Topical		30–120 min	Short		
Esters							
Benzocaine	Anbersol, etc.	Topical		Rapid	Short		
Chloroprocaine Cocaine Procaine	Nesacaine Novocaine	Infiltration Topical Infiltration	1 1	Rapid 2–10 min Slow	0.5–2 h 1–3 h 1–1.5 h	600 mg 200 mg 500 mg	600 mg
Proparacaine	Ophthaine	Topical	Rapid	Short			
Tetracaine	Pontocaine	Infiltration	8	Slow	2–3 h	20 mg	
Tetracaine	Cetacaine	Topical	Rapid	Short			

*Clinically, duration of anesthesia may be less than stated above, especially for head and neck; addition of epinephrine prolongs anesthesia by factor of 2.

†Maximum doses are for a 70-kg person.

TABLE 25-29 Lidocaine Toxicity

Organ System	Signs	Treatment
Central nervous system		
Early (1–5 mcg/ml)	Tinnitus, circumoral pallor, metallic taste in mouth, lightheadedness, talkativeness, nausea, emesis, diplopia	Recognition, observation, hold lidocaine
Middle (8–12 mcg/ml)	Nystagmus, slurred speech, hallucinations, muscle twitching, facial, hand tremors, seizures	Diazepam, airway maintenance
Late (20–25 mcg/ml)	Apnea, coma	Respiratory support
Cardiovascular system	Myocardial depression, bradycardia, atrioventricular blockade, ventricular arrythmias, vasodilation, hypotension	Oxygen, vasopressors, cardiopulmonary resuscitation
Allergy	Pruritus, urticaria, angioedema, nausea, wheezing, anaphylaxis	Antihistamines; epinephrine 0.3 mL 1:1000 SQ, oxygen, airway
Psychogenic	Pallor, diaphoresis, hyperventilation, lightheadedness, nausea, syncope	Trendelenburg position, cool compresses, observation

    - Safe to use in digital blocks and local anesthesia as long as these guidelines are followed
    - Epinephrine dilution of 1:200,000 or greater
    - Volumes injected are minimal (digital block should not exceed 3 mL—1.5 mL max per side)
    - Circumferential injection (ring block) is avoided
    - Patients with vascular compromise are avoided (smokers, diabetes, peripheral vascular disease, Raynaud phenomenon)
  - Contraindications
    - Absolute: uncontrolled hyperthyroidism and pheochromocytoma
    - Relative contraindications: hypertension, blood pressure instability, severe cardiovascular disease, pregnancy, and narrow-angle glaucoma, β-blockers, phenothiazines, monoamine oxidase inhibitors, and tricyclic antidepressants
    - Epinephrine may be used by diluting it to 1:500,000; use sparingly
  - Side effects
    - Self-limited palpitations, anxiety, fear, diaphoresis, headache, tremor, weakness, and tachycardia
    - Serious side effects: arrhythmias, ventricular tachycardia, ventricular fibrillation, cardiac arrest, and cerebral hemorrhage
- Topical anesthetics
  - Conjunctiva anesthetized with: proparacaine or tetracaine eyedrops
  - Superficial mucous membrane anesthesia: Surfacaine, Topicale, Dyclone, Anbesol, viscous lidocaine, and lidocaine jelly
  - Intranasal mucosa: 4 to 10% cocaine solution is effective, and hemostatic
  - EMLA (eutectic mixture of local anesthetics) cream contains 2.5% lidocaine and 2.5% prilocaine; applied under occlusion 1 to 2 hours preoperatively depending on location
    - Should be applied to intact skin only and in patients older than 1 year of age
    - Application to denuded skin or to large surface areas may result in substantial prilocaine absorption and risk of systemic methemoglobinemia
  - Approximately 30 to 40% lidocaine in acid-mantle cream may also be applied under occlusion 1 to 2 hours before a procedure
  - ELA-Max (4% lidocaine) liposomal delivery; thus no occlusion necessary; no chance of methemoglobinemia as with EMLA. Available over the counter; comes in 5- and 30-g tubes
  - Iontophoresis of lidocaine also can achieve superficial skin anesthesia
- Tumescent anesthesia (TA)
  - TA is the use of dilute lidocaine (i.e., 0.05–0.1%) and epinephrine (i.e., 1:1,000,000) for local anesthesia
  - Large volumes of TA may be infiltrated subcutaneously to achieve complete anesthesia and effective hemostasis
  - TA pharmacology applies only to dilute lidocaine and epinephrine; it cannot be extrapolated to other anesthetics (i.e., bupivacaine cannot be substituted for lidocaine)
  - Originally developed for liposuction

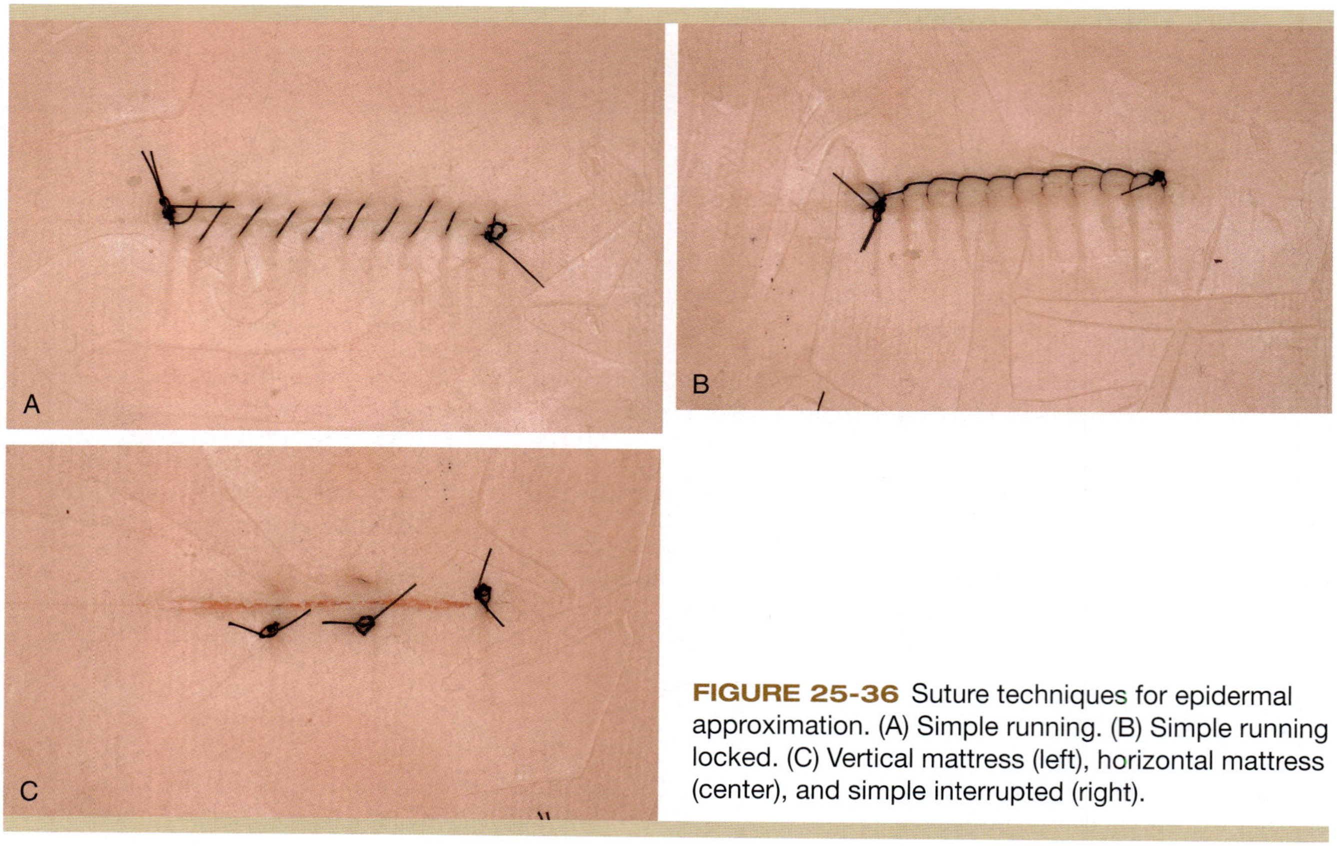

FIGURE 25-36 Suture techniques for epidermal approximation. (A) Simple running. (B) Simple running locked. (C) Vertical mattress (left), horizontal mattress (center), and simple interrupted (right).

TABLE 25-30 Suture Materials

Material (Trade Name)	Type	Memory	Tissue Reactivity	Tensile Strength Half-Life
Nonabsorbable				
Cotton	Twisted	Low	Very high	—
Nylon (Ethilon, Demalon)	Monofilament	High	Low	—
Nylon (Nurolon, Surgilon)	Braided	Low	Low	—
Polybutester (Novafil)	Monofilament	High	Low	—
Polyester, uncoated (Mersilene)	Braided	Low	Low	—
Polyester, coated (EthiGoodd)	Braided	Low	Low	—
Polypropylene (Prolene, Surgilene)	Monofilament	Very high	Very low	—
Silk	Braided/twisted	Very low	High	—
Stainless steel	Monofilament/braided/twisted	Very high	Very low	—
Absorbable				
Gut, fast absorbing/mild chromic	Twisted	Very high	High	2 d
Gut	Twisted	Very high	High	4 d
Gut, chromic	Twisted	Very high	High	1 wk
Polyglactin 910 (Vicryl)	Braided	Very low	Low	2 wks
Polyglycolic acid (Dexon)	Braided	Very low	Low	2 wks
Poliglecaprone 25 (Monocryl)	Monofilament	Low	Very low	1 wk
Polyglyconate (Maxon)	Monofilament	Low	Very low	1 mo
Polydioxanone (PDS)	Monofilament	High	Very low	1 mo

From Weitzul S, Taylor RS: Suturing techniques and other closure materials, in Robinson JK, Hanke WC, Sengelmann RD, et al., eds., *Surgery of the Skin: Procedural Dermatology*. London: Elsevier; 2005.

TABLE 25-31 Epidermal Suture Applications

Suture Technique	Comments
Simple running (Figure 25-36)	Fast epidermal closure May not approximate skin as precisely as simple interrupted May unravel if one segment is severed
Simple interrupted (Figure 25-36)	Time consuming Best for correcting minor differences in overlapping edge Most accurate for skin approximation
Vertical mattress (Figure 25-36)	Suture line perpendicular to wound edge Time consuming Best suture for additional wound edge eversion May strangulate wound edge if tied too tightly
Horizontal mattress (Figure 25-36)	Suture line parallel to wound edge Time consuming Moderate wound edge eversion Helpful in hemostasis for nonspecific wound edge oozing
Running subcuticular	Entire suture is buried in the superficial dermis except for an entry and exit point on either ends of the wound edge Time consuming Beneficial for closure that requires epidermal support > 1 wk; running subcuticular suture may be left in place > 1 wk and removed later without railroad tracks on skin

Note: All epidermal sutures will leave cross-marks of railroad-track lines on skin if not removed within 1 week.

- Other uses: face-lift surgery, reconstruction, ambulatory phlebectomy, ablative laser resurfacing, hair transplantation, endovenous radiofrequency ablation
- Advantages of TA
- Increases maximum safe dose of lidocaine to 55 mg/kg
- Dilute epinephrine achieves pronounced vasoconstriction of subdermal vessels, thereby limiting systemic absorption while achieving excellent hemostasis
  - Some procedures (liposuction, phlebectomy, endovenous ablation) cannot be done safely in an outpatient setting without TA
- Disadvantages of TA
  - Requires equipment and understanding of tumescent pharmacology
  - Swelling of subcutaneous space is typical but may be prolonged in the lower extremities
- Alternatives to esters and amides for local anesthesia
  - Diphenhydramine hydrochloride (Benadryl) 12.5 mg/mL
  - Normal saline injected intradermally (transient brief anesthesia)
  - Cryoanesthesia with ice or cryogen (i.e., fluoroethyl or frigiderm) for superficial procedures (i.e., dermabrasion)

SUTURE REVIEW (TABLES 25-30 AND 25-31)

- Suture characteristics (Fig. 25-33)
  - *Tensile strength*: measure of a material or tissue's ability to resist deformation and breakage
  - *Knot strength*: force required for a knot to slip
  - *Configuration*
    - Monofilament (less risk of infection)
    - Braided multifilament (easier to handle and tie)
  - *Elasticity*: degree suture stretches and returns to original length
  - *Memory or suture stiffness*: inherent capability of suture to return to or maintain its original gross shape
  - *Plasticity*: measure of the ability to deform without breaking and to maintain a new form after relief of the deforming force
  - *Pliability*: ease of handling of suture material; ability to adjust knot tension and to secure knots (related to suture material, filament type, and diameter)

QUIZ

Questions

1. Where do the internal carotid and external carotid arteries *not* anastamose?

   A. Perinasal
   B. Glabella
   C. Mentum
   D. Periorbital

2. Put the following items in order from least to most sensitive to cryogen exposure:
   1. Melanocytes
   2. Keratinocytes
   3. Fibroblasts

   A. 1, 2, 3
   B. 1, 3, 2
   C. 2, 1, 3
   D. 2, 3, 1
   E. 3, 2, 1
   F. 3, 1, 2

3. Matching:

Patient	Wound Healing
1. Neutropenic	A. Not impaired
2. Lymphopenic	B. Impaired
3. Macrophage deficient	

4. Matching:

Term	Definition
1. Sterilization	A. Destruction of ALL infectious agents from an environment. This includes algae, bacteria, fungi, protozoa, viruses dormant endospores and poorly characterised agents such as viroids and the agents that are associated with spongiform encephalopathies
2. Disinfection	B. Refers to the removal of some microbes from an environment that may cause disease
3. Antisepsis	C. Less harsh in their action than are disinfectants

5. Matching:

Antibiotic prophylaxis	Indication
1. Keflex	A. Cutaneous defect
2. Amoxicillin	B. Mucosal defect
3. Clindamycin	C. Cutaneous defect, penicillin allergic
4. Azithromycin	D. Mucosal defect, penicillin allergic

6. How much will a scar lengthen with a 60-degree Z-plasty transposition?

   A. 10%
   B. 25%
   C. 50%
   D. 55%
   E. 75%

7. Which of the following in *not* a risk factor for a patient developing methhemoglobinemia while using topical EMLA?

   A. Patient younger than 1 year old
   B. Patient with G-6-PD deficiency
   C. Patient with sickle cell anemia
   D. Patient taking dapsone
   E. Patient taking phenobarbitol

8. When does inosculation occur after skin graft placement?

   A. First 48 hours
   B. Days 2 to 3
   C. Days 4 to 7
   D. Day 4 to week 4
   E. After 2 to 3 months

9. How is procaine metabolized?

   A. Pseudocholinesterase
   B. Microsomal liver enzymes
   C. Monoamine oxidase
   D. Peroxidase
   E. Glutathione S-transferase

10. Which nonabsorbable suture has more tissue reactivity?

   A. Polypropylene
   B. Silk
   C. Polyglactin 910
   D. Gut

11. Which absorbable suture has less tissue reactivity?
    A. Polypropylene
    B. Silk
    C. Polyglactin 910
    D. Gut

12. Which of these interpolation flaps is not an axial flap?
    A. Paramedian forehead flap
    B. Cheek-to-nose staged flap
    C. Lip-switch flap
    D. *Abbe flap*

13. Which of these patients do not require prophylactic antibiotics preoperatively to prevent endocarditis?
    A. Adult male with prominent mitral valve regurgitation
    B. Woman with aortic valve prosthesis
    C. Student with cardiac transplantation and mitral valve regurgitation
    D. Man with history of infective endocarditis

Answers

1. C. Mentum. Blood supply to the head and neck is via the internal carotid artery (ICA) and external carotid artery (ECA) and their branches. Intimate anastamoses between ICA and ECA occur in the region of the upper central face (nose, glabella, periorbital, and forehead). These connections are important clinically in that: (1) infections in this area may extend intracranially via ICA; (2) steroid injections in the periorbital skin may embolize to the retinal artery and cause blindness.
2. E. 3, 2, 1 (fibroblast, keratinocyte, melanocyte). Different cells and tissues demonstrate a range of temperature sensitivity. Melanocytes are more sensitive than keratinocytes, and with cold injury, dyspigmentation should be discussed as an adverse outcome when treating dark skinned individuals. Fibroblasts and other stromal structures are less sensitive to cold, which may contribute to the lack of scarring after superficial cold injury and/or cryosurgery.
3. 1, A; 2, A; 3, B. The inflammatory response is an important component after wounding of the skin. Macrophages are the most important cells for wound healing, releasing numerous growth factors and cytokines. Neutropenic or lymphopenic patients do not have impaired wound healing, whereas macrophage-deficient (quantity or function) patients heal poorly.
4. 1, A; 2, B; 3, C. Infection control is extremely important to prevent infection. Techniques used to destroy all infectious agents from an environment are called sterilization. In contrast, disinfection and antisepsis are terms that should be used to reduce microbe burden, with disinfection utilizing harsher agents that, in general, would not be used on human tissue (i.e., undiluted bleach).
5. 1, A; 2, B; 3, C,D; 4, C,D. Although the risk of wound infection after skin surgery is small (1–2%), routine prophylactic antibiotics are usually indicated for: 1) certain patient populations—immunosuppressed, debilitated patients, and those with reduced blood flow to the surgical site (i.e., peripheral vascular disease, diabetes mellitus); 2) anatomic sites at greater risk for infection—ears, perineum, legs, and feet. Prophylactic antiobiotic regimen depends on the endogenous flora of the operative site, as well as, patient specific issues (i.e., penicillin allergic).
6. E. 75%. The Z-plasty is a form of transposition flap that is often used for scar revision for scar length and changing scar orientation. It alters the change (redirection) of tension vectors of the original wound/scar, in addition to lengthening and breaking up of a scar into multiple zigzag lines. The extent of scar lengthening depends on the degree of transposition of the Z-plasty.
7. C. Sickle cell anemia. EMLA (eutectic mixture of local anesthetics) cream contains 2.5% lidocaine and 2.5% prilocaine. Prilocaine is metabolized to ortho-toluidine, an oxiding agent capable of converting hemoglobin to methemoglobin, potentially causing methemoglogbinemia. Patients at risk of methemoglobinemia include patients younger than 1 year old, patients with G-6-PD deficiency, and patients taking methemoglobinemia-inducing agents (dapsone, nitroglycerin, nitrofurantoin, antimalarials, sulfonamides, phenobarbitol, phenytoin, nitroprusside, and acetaminophen).
8. B. Day 2 to 3. A skin graft is any skin that is detached completely from its blood supply, removed from its donor site, and transplanted to a recipient site for wound closure in the same individual. Graft survival depends on the establishment of new vasculature between the wound recipient site and the donor graft through the following phases: imbibition, inosculation, capillary ingrowth and neovascularization, keratinocyte activation, and finally, sensory innervation.
9. A. Pseudocholinesterase. Several major enzymes and pathways are involved in drug metabolism. Amide anesthetics are *N*-dealkylated and hydrolyzed by microsomal liver enzymes cytochrome P450 3A4. Ester anesthetics are hydrolyzed by tissue pseudocholinesterases and excreted by kidney. Procaine is an ester anesthetic.
10. B. Silk. Suture characteristics include tensile strength, knot strength, configuration, elasticity, memory or suture stiffness, plasticity, and pliability. Suture reactivity is another characteristic defined as the amount of inflammatory response that is elicited, which is dependent on the material from which it is made. Synthetic sutures are made from synthetic collagen derived from polymers and are broken down by hydrolysis as opposed to enzymatic degradation in natural sutures, causing less tissue reaction. In contrast, natural sutures are made

from natural materials such as collagen derived from the gastrointestinal tract of animals, woven cotton, raw silk, linen, or steel. Of the answer choices listed, polypropylene and silk are nonabsorbable suture made from synthetic and natural materials, respectively.

11. C. Polyglactin. Suture characteristics include tensile strength, knot strength, configuration, elasticity, memory or suture stiffness, plasticity, and pliability. Suture reactivity is another characteristic defined as the amount of inflammatory response that is elicited, which is dependent on the material from which it is made. Synthetic sutures are made from synthetic collagen derived from polymers and are broken down by hydrolysis as opposed to enzymatic degradation in natural sutures, causing less tissue reaction. In contrast, natural sutures are made from natural materials such as collagen derived from the gastrointestinal tract of animals, woven cotton, raw silk, linen, or steel. Of the answer choices listed, polyglactin 910 and gut suture are absorbable suture made from synthetic and natural materials, respectively.
12. Answer B. The cheek-to-nose staged flap is NOT an axial flap. It receives vascular supply from branches of the angular artery but the angular artery itself is not in the pedicle. The paramedian forehead flap's pedicle is the supratrochlear artery, the lip-switch and the Abbe Estlander flaps' pedicles are from either the inferior labial artery or superior labial artery.
    A. Paramedian forehead flap
    B. Cheek–to-nose staged flap
    C. Lip-switch flap
    D. *Abbe Estlander flap*
13. Answer A. Mitral valve regurgitation was once an indication for prophylactic antibiotics to prevent endocarditis. Without other risk factors, mitral regurgitation no longer requires preoperative prophylactic antibiotics.

REFERENCES

Baker S, Swanson N: *Local Flaps in Facial Reconstruction*. London: Mosby; 1995.

Bello Y, Falabella A, Eaglstein WH: Wound healing modalities, in Nouri K, Leal-Khouri S, eds. *Techniques in Dermatologic Surgery*. London: Mosby; 2003.

Castro-Ron G, Pasquali P: Cryosurgery, in Robinson JK, Hanke WC, Sengelmann RD, et al, eds. *Surgery of the Skin: Procedural Dermatology*. London: Elsevier; 2005.

Graham GF, George MN, Patel M: Cryosurgery, in Nouri K, Leal-Khouri S, eds. *Techniques in Dermatologic Surgery*. London: Mosby; 2003.

Hurst EA, Grekin RC, Neuhaus IM: Infectious complications and antibiotic use in dermatologic surgery. *Semin Cutan Med Surg* 2007;26(3):47-53.

Larrabee WF, Makielski KH, Henderson JL: *Surgical Anatomy of the Face*, 2nd Ed. Baltimore: Lippincott Williams & Wilkins; 2004.

Lie J, Kirsner RS: Wound healing, in Robinson JK, Hanke WC, Sengelmann RD, et al, eds. *Surgery of the Skin: Procedural Dermatology*. London: Elsevier; 2005.

Nguyen TH: Topical and local anesthesia, in Narins RS, ed. *Cosmetic Surgery*. New York: Marcel Dekker; 2001:411-441.

Nouri K, Trent J, Lodha R: Aseptic techniques, in Nouri K, Leal-Khouri S, eds. *Techniques in Dermatologic Surgery*. London: Mosby; 2003.

Putz R, Pabst R: Sobotta *Atlas of Human Anatomy*, vol. 1, 13th Ed. Baltimore: Lippincott Williams & Wilkins; 2001.

Robinson JK, Anderson R Jr.: Skin structure and anatomy, in Robinson JK, Hanke WC, Sengelmann RD, et al, eds. *Surgery of the Skin: Procedural Dermatology*. London: Elsevier; 2005.

Rohrer, TE, Cook JL, Nguyen TH, Mellete JR: *Flaps and Grafts in Dermatologic Surgery*. Philadelphia: Saunders Elsevier; 2007.

Rossie AM, Mariwalla K: Prophylactic and empiric use of antibiotics in dermatologic surgery: a review of the literature and practical considerations. *Dermatol Surg* 2012;38:1898-1921.

Soon SL, Washington CV: Electrosurgery, electrocoagulation, electrofulguration, electrodessication, electrosection, electrocautery, in Robinson JK, Hanke WC, Sengelmann RD, et al, eds. *Surgery of the Skin: Procedural Dermatology*. London: Elsevier; 2005.

Soriano TT, Lask GP, Dinehart SM: Anesthesia and analgesia, in Robinson JK, Hanke WC, Sengelmann RD, et al, eds. *Surgery of the Skin: Procedural Dermatology*. London: Elsevier; 2005.

Weiss RA, Feied CF, Weiss MA: *Vein Diagnosis & Treatment: A Comprehensive Approach*. New York: McGraw-Hill; 2001.

Weitzul S, Taylor RS: Suturing techniques and other closure materials, in Robinson JK, Hanke WC, Sengelmann RD, et al, eds. *Surgery of the Skin: Procedural Dermatology*. London: Elsevier; 2005.

CHAPTER 26

COSMETIC DERMATOLOGY

MELISSA A. BOGLE

SKIN AGING

- Intrinsic aging: natural or chronologic aging, influenced by genetics
  - Begins in the mid-20s, but signs may not be visible for decades
  - Collagen production and cell turnover slows
  - Loss of subcutaneous fat and bone loss contribute to volume issues
- Extrinsic aging: caused by environmental factors
  - Largest contributors are ultraviolet (UV) radiation (photoaging) and smoking
  - Facial expressions, sleeping positions, nutrition, and airborne particles (pollution) are additive factors
  - Solar elastosis or dermatoheliosis: term applied to the chronic inflammatory changes and degradation of elastin and collagen

OXIDATIVE STRESS (FREE RADICAL THEORY OF AGING)

- Reactive oxygen species (ROS) derived from the environment and oxidative cell metabolism damage cellular components and lead to aging
  - Mitochondria are the main endogenous source of ROS
- ROS activate signal transduction pathways including mitogen-activated protein kinases, c-jun N-terminal kinase (JNK), and extracellular signal related kinases, which upregulate the nuclear transcription factor activator protein 1 (AP-1)
- AP-1 activates matrix metalloproteinase (MMP) genes for MMP-1 (collagenase), MMP-3 (stromolysin), and MMP-9 (gelatinase)
- MMPs degrade collagen types I and III
- AP-1 inhibits transforming growth factor B (TGF-B), a profibrotic cytokine, and downregulates type II TGF-B receptors so cells cannot respond to TGF-B and less type I procollagen is produced
- Antioxidants such as vitamins A, C, and E, ubiquinone and glutathione may help to minimize ROS-induced damage
- All-trans-retinoic acid (tretinoin) acts like an antioxidant to inhibit the accumulation of c-jun protein, thereby preventing the formation of AP-1 and the upregulation of MMPs
- Tretinoin also induces TGF-B to enhance production of procollagen types I and III

Ultraviolet Radiation

- UVA: 320 to 400 nm; largest contributor to *A*ging due to deeper penetration depth and ability to generate ROS
  - UVA1: 340 to 400 nm (longest wavelength and deepest penetration of all ultraviolet light)
  - UVA2: 320 to 340 nm
- UVB: 290 to 320 nm; *B*urning rays; absorbed by the epidermis, mainly causing damage to keratinocytes in the form of pyrimidine dimers
  - Narrowband UVB: 311 to 312 nm
  - UVC: 100 to 290 nm; has negligible effect on skin as nearly all is blocked by the atmosphere
- UVA rays make up 95% of UV radiation reaching the Earth's surface; however UVB rays are more intense
- Both contribute to skin cancer, photoaging (wrinkles, discoloration, telangiectasias), and ocular changes (cataracts, pterygium)
- UV radiation downregulates gene expression in types I and III procollagen in dermal fibroblasts
- UV radiation activates transcription factor nuclear factor κB (NF-κB), resulting in transcription of proinflammatory cytokines such as IL-1β, tumor necrosis factor α, IL-6, and IL-8. Proinflammatory cytokines bind receptors on the cell surface to further activate AP-1 and NF-κB, escalating the photoaging response
- Activation of MMP-1 and NF-κB are iron dependent mechanisms, so iron chelators such as kojic acid may be included in topical antiaging preparations

Telomeres and Aging

- Telomeres form the ends of human chromosomes; defend the ends of chromosomes from instability
- Comprised of repeats of the DNA base sequence (TTAGGGG) (T = thymine, G = guanine, A = adenosine)
- DNA polymerase (the enzyme that synthesizes new DNA) cannot act on the end DNA bases during replication, so telomeres are shortened with each cell replication cycle
- When telomeres become too short, the cell will no longer divide; leads to apoptosis and premature cell cycle arrest
- Telomeres in keratinocytes and fibroblasts have a slower rate of loss of approximately 25 base pairs per year (vs. 100 or more base pairs in the body in general), suggesting telomere loss is not as predominant a factor in skin aging as ultraviolet radiation and oxidative stress
- UV radiation enhances telomere disruption; TT (dithymidine) residues are particularly targeted and concentrated in the telomere region of the chromosome

HORMONAL INFLUENCES ON AGING SKIN

- Decreased levels of sex hormones (estrogen, progesterone, and testosterone) are the primary influences
- Contributes to
  - Reduction of skin lipids and dryness
  - Wrinkling, epidermal atrophy, and collagen breakdown
  - Loss of skin elasticity
  - Changes in hair growth: increased facial hair in women, thinning of hair on the scalp, extremities, and public region
  - Loss of vascular tone: increase in varicose veins, enlargement of dorsal hand veins
- Estrogens act on the skin via 2 estrogen receptors ER-α and ER-β
  - Keratinocytes express ER-α
  - Fibroblasts express both ER-α and ER-β
- Estrogen/progesterone replacement therapy during early menopause may help to ameliorate changes associated with intrinsic aging

Fitzpatrick Scale

- Classification of the response of different types of skin to UV light
- Measures several components: genetic disposition, reaction to sun exposure, and tanning ability (Table 26-1)

STRUCTURAL CHANGES IN THE AGING FACE

- Bone resorption and remodeling, fat atrophy/hypertrophy, and muscular changes all play an interrelated role
- The skeleton framework is continually remodeled in a process of resorption and differential growth; overall trend is toward a decrease in volume
- Subtle changes over time alter the shape of the face and the way the overlying soft tissues fit
  - The frontal bone moves anteriorly and inferiorly
  - The maxilla moves posteriorly and superiorly
  - The mandible loses both length and height, with a blunting of the posterior angle
  - The eye socket enlarges
  - Loss of projection and support in the brow and nose
- The face has multiple distinct fat compartments (Fig. 26-1). Some hypertrophy over time (jowls, submentum), most are prone to atrophy (Fig. 26-2)
  - Restoration of volume loss and ptosis in the midface region play a large role in rejuvenation
  - Goal is to balance facial proportions (ideal is the "upside down egg" or "inverted triangle" shape
- Repeated movements of the muscles of facial contraction lead to shortening of the muscle and an increase in resting tone
  - Contributes to rhytides in the glabella, forehead, periocular region, lateral nasal sidewall, neck/upper chest, and perioral region

TABLE 26-1 Fitzpatrick Skin Types

Skin Type	I	II	III	IV	V	VI
Clinical appearance	Very white, very fair skin	White, fair skin	Beige skin, most common Caucasian skin type	Beige with an olive to brown tint	Dark brown	Black
Reaction to sun exposure	Always burns	Usually burns	Sometimes burns	Rarely burns	Very rarely	Never burns
Tanning ability	Never tans	Tans with difficulty	Gradually tans to light to medium brown	Tans with ease to a moderate brown	Tans very easily	Always tans, deeply pigmented

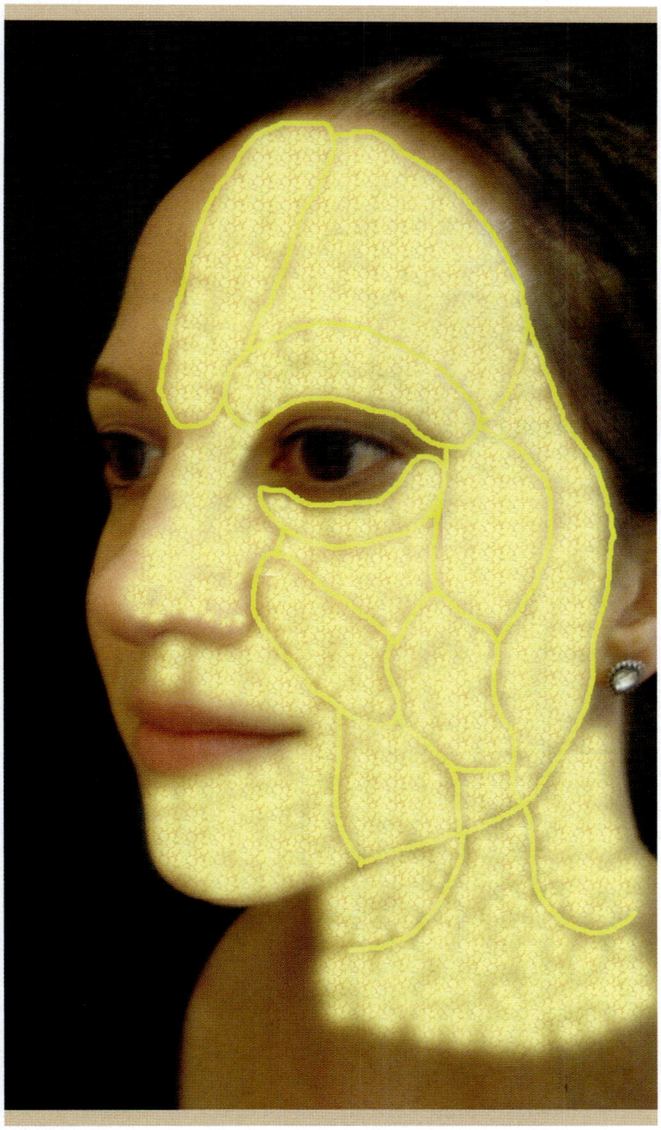

FIGURE 26-1 The subcutaneous fat of the face is partitioned into multiple, distinct anatomical compartments. How these compartments change with time plays a significant role in facial aging. (*Used with permission from Melissa A. Bogle, MD, The Laser and Cosmetic Surgery Center of Houston.*)

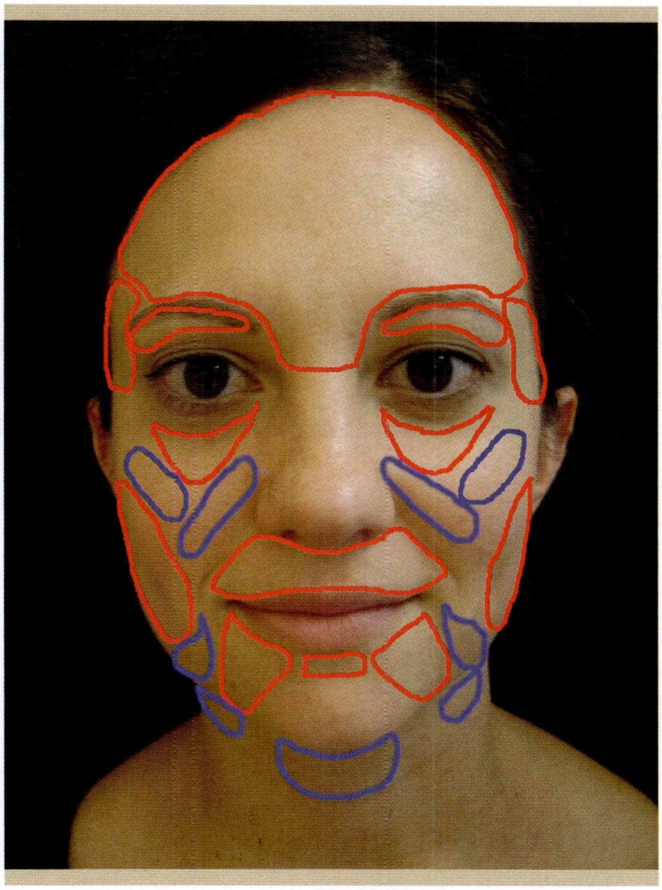

FIGURE 26-2 Certain parts of the aging face are prone to fat atrophy (red), particularly the upper face/temples, lateral face, periorbital region, upper cheeks and chin. Other areas are prone to weight-dependent hypertrophy (blue), such as the lower cheeks, jowls, submental and submandibular regions. (*Used with permission from Melissa A. Bogle, MD, The Laser and Cosmetic Surgery Center of Houston.*)

  - Shortened muscles may also displace underlying fat compartments
  - Compensatory increases in muscular tone may be a response to skin laxity (forehead)

ELECTROMAGNETIC RADIATION

- Electromagnetic radiation (EMR): energy comprised of photons that moves through space as a wave, organized along an electromagnetic spectrum (Fig. 26-3)
- LASER (light amplification by stimulated emission of radiation)
  - Atoms have a positively charged nucleus and negatively charged electrons which orbit around the nucleus
  - The electrons closest to the nucleus are in the ground state and have the lowest energy. If energy is placed into the system, electrons can be jumped to the excited state, which is furthest away from the nucleus
  - Electrons in the excited state inherently want to go back to the ground state. To do this, they have to give off energy in the form of light called a photon
  - When photons are emitted from an electron going from the excited state back to the ground state, they can crash into another excited system, causing a duplication of 2 photons coming out of that system

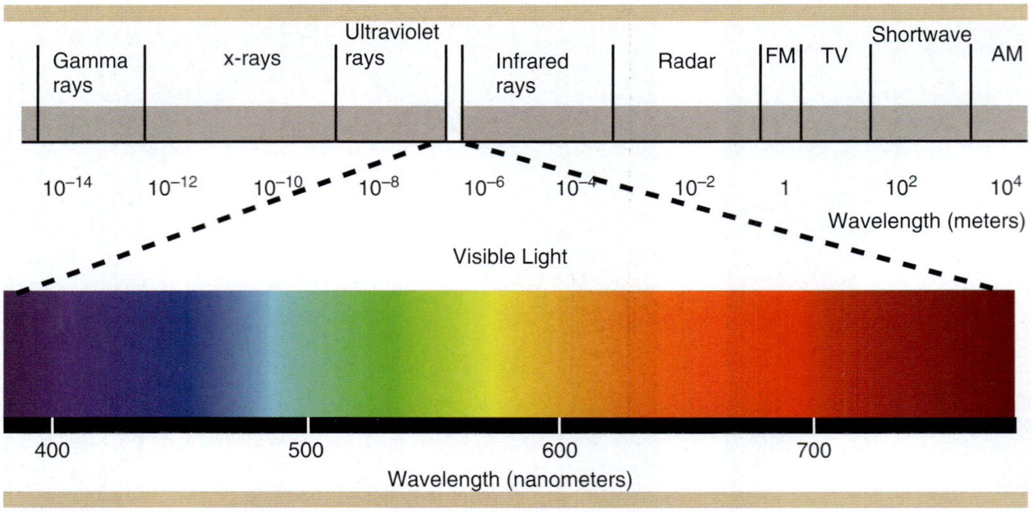

FIGURE 26-3 Electromagnetic spectrum.

- These 2 photons will propagate to 4 and then 8 and so on in an amplification of a mass amount of light, all of the same wavelength
- Photons display both particle-like and wave-like behavior

Characteristics of Lasers (Table 26-2)

- Monochromaticity: single, discrete wavelength; active medium determines the emission wavelength, which is restricted to a very narrowband
- Coherency: laser light is in a single direction so that the wavelengths are running in parallel to one another; this is different from incoherent light (light from a light bulb), which emits light in different directions
- Collimation: light in parallel fashion to achieve its propagation across long distances without light divergence (constant diameter beam)
- Intensity: amplification process allows the emission of high-energy level laser

Skin Optics

- Reflection: waves encounter a surface or other boundary that does not absorb the energy of the radiation and bounces the waves away from the surface
- Absorption: energy is deposited in a chromophore
- Transmission: direction of photon path is unchanged
- Scattering: energy is redirected elsewhere in the skin; longer wavelengths typically penetrate deeper due to less scatter; however, this is not true for ablative lasers
  - Tyndall effect: short (blue) wavelengths are scattered more than long (red) wavelengths
- Depth of penetration depends on absorption and scattering
  - Amount of scattering of laser energy is inversely proportional to the wavelength of incident light
  - In general depth of penetration increases with wavelength
  - Classically, the 1064 nm Nd:YAG laser penetrates the deepest into the skin
  - For wavelengths greater than this, depth of penetration is typically limited due to absorption by water in the upper dermis; the exception to this is with some fractional resurfacing lasers where the depth of penetration is largely dependent upon energy

Laser-Tissue Interactions

- Photothermal reaction: light energy transformed and dissipated as heat; most lasers
- Photomechanical/photoacoustic reaction: rapid absorption of a laser pulse resulting in a rapid temperature change along with sudden tissue vaporization, shock wave, or pressure wave formation (the pulse occurs so fast, a shock wave is created)
  - Q-switched lasers
  - Ideal for "popping" thin growths off the surface such as pigmented seborrheic keratosis (Fig. 26-4)
- Photoablative reaction: tissue is heated so quickly and thoroughly, tissue is ablated
  - Ablative resurfacing lasers (carbon dioxide, erbium:YAG)
- Photochemical reaction: reaction of an endogenous or exogenous photosensitizer with UV or visible light (i.e., light energy starts a chemical reaction)
  - Photodynamic therapy (PDT): photosensitizer is administered to the patient by one of several routes (topical, oral, intravenous) and allowed to be taken up by the target cells; the photosensitizer is then activated with a specific wavelength of light
  - Common photosensitizers: topically applied aminolevulinic acid (ALA) and methylaminolevulinate (MAL)

TABLE 26-2 Laser Characteristics

LASER Characteristic	Symbol	Unit of Measurement	Notes
Wavelength	λ	Nanometer (nm)	
Spot size	d (diameter) s (square)	Centimeter (cm)	Larger spot sizes penetrate deeper
Pulse duration	T (exposure time)	Seconds (s)	Must be shorter than the thermal relaxation time to effectively heat the target For blood vessels: pulse duration close to thermal relaxation time improves results; there is an increasing risk of purpura with decreasing pulse duration
Energy	E (energy or work)	Joules (J)	Suitable for measuring energy in a single pulse of a pulsed laser
Fluence	Φ Energy density or Energy per square centimeter of treatment area	J/cm^2	Fluence is dependent on spot size. 10 J/cm^2 with a 12 mm spot is *not* equivalent 10 J/cm^2 with an 18 mm spot. The larger spot size would have a greater energy delivered. Increasing the fluence can increase the depth of penetration into to tissue Fluence is generally the most important parameter in efficacy
Power	P (power) Energy delivery per unit time	Watts (W) = J/s	Applicable to continuous wave lasers. Power is the rate at which the energy is expended
Irradiance *(not to be confused with intensity)*	Power delivered per unit area (radiative flux)	W/cm^2	Applicable to continuous wave lasers Intensity refers to the brightness of a light source

- ALA-PDT: classically associated with blue light activation; major absorption peak for ALA is seen in the blue light range (410–420 nm)
- MAL-PDT: classically associated with red light activation; red light has a deeper penetration than blue light and MAL is thought to penetrate deeper due to its lipophilic nature
- Other activating sources such as pulsed dye lasers and intense pulsed light (IPL) have also been used with success

Selective Photothermolysis

- Controlled destruction of a targeted lesion while sparing significant thermal damage to surrounding normal tissue
- Different chromophores in the skin absorb different wavelengths of light (Fig. 26-5)
  - Hemoglobin
  - Water
  - Melanin
  - Exogenous pigment (tattoo ink)
  - Fat
- Pulse duration or exposure time should be shorter than the thermal relaxation time of the target (defined as the time required for the targeted site to cool to one-half its peak temperature); this allows the intended target to be heated before the heat has time to dissipate to surrounding structures
- Small targets cool faster than larger ones, so small targets like melanosomes or tattoo particles do best with very short pulses (nanosecond range vs. millisecond range)
- Summary: targets in the skin (blood, water, pigment) can be selectively treated when the right wavelength is used; the target has to be treated fast, before it has a chance to cool

Lasing Media

- Wavelength is determined by the lasing medium, which can be solid crystal, gas, liquid dye, or semiconductor (Fig. 26-6)
- Solid-state lasers: Ruby, alexandrite, or neodymium: yttrium-aluminum garnet (Nd:Yag) lasers

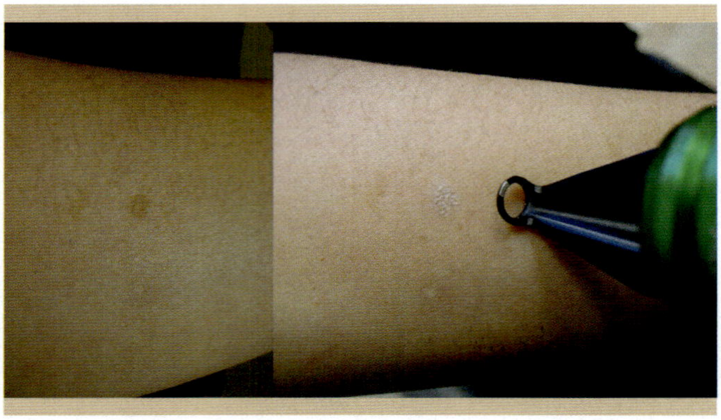

FIGURE 26-4 "Stuck on" growths such as macular seborrheic keratoses can be treated with Q-switched lasers by taking advantage of the photomechanical/photoacoustic effect and "popping" them off the surface. Treatment is less successful with devices that have a pure photothermal reaction. (*Used with permission from Melissa A. Bogle, MD, The Laser and Cosmetic Surgery Center of Houston.*)

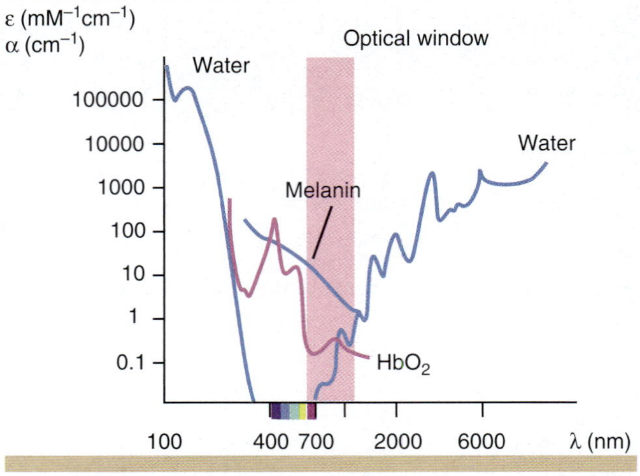

FIGURE 26-5 Absorption spectra of cutaneous chromophores.

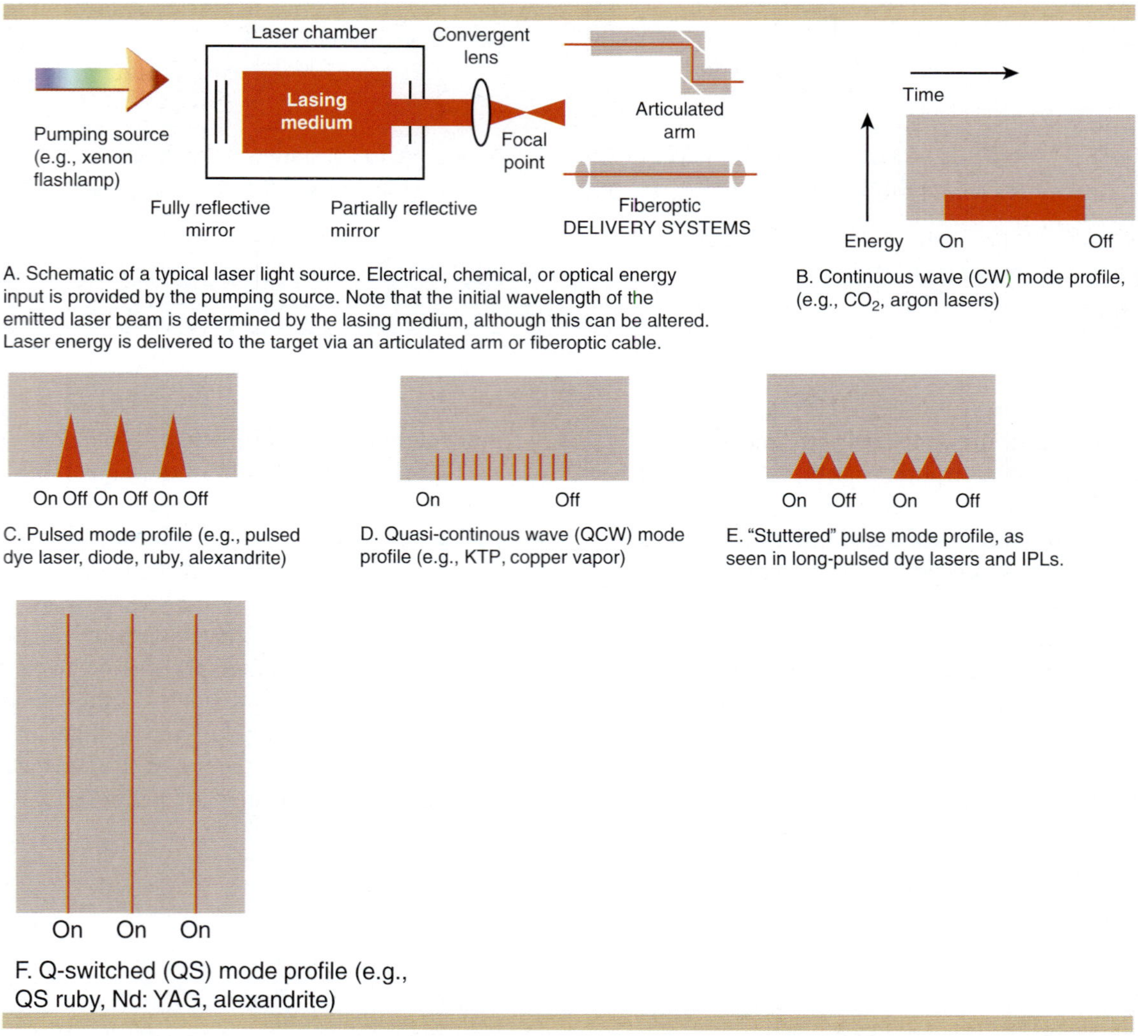

FIGURE 26-6 Laser beam types (Reprinted with permission from Wolff K et al. Fitzpatrick's Dermatology in General Medicine, 7th Ed. New York: McGraw-Hill; 2008.)

- Gas lasers: carbon dioxide (CO_2), excimer lasers
- Liquid medium lasers: pulsed dye laser
- Semiconductor lasers: diode lasers

LASER MODES OF OPERATION

- Continuous wave (CW): power output is essentially continuous over time
- Quasicontinuous wave (QCW): continuous wave mechanically shuttered to deliver pulses of light
- Pulsed lasers: power output takes the form of pulses of light at some duration and repetition rate; reduces the amount of thermal damage that occurs adjacent to the target area
- Q-switched lasers: allows buildup of high energy in the laser cavity before discharge in short pulses with an extremely high peak power

TYPES OF LASERS AND THEIR APPLICATIONS

- The various types of lasers used in cutaneous applications are described in Table 26-3
- Laser treatment for tattoo pigments is described in Table 26-4

Nonlaser Light and Energy Sources

- IPL
  - Noncoherent light within 500 to 1200 nm
  - Cutoff filters are used to eliminate shorter wavelengths
  - Single-, double-, or triple-pulse sequences; pulse durations of 2 to 25 ms and delays between pulses ranging from 10 to 500 ms
- Light-emitting diodes (LEDs)
  - Low-intensity light photons of the proper parameters interact with subcellular chromophores to activate cells to induce or inhibit activity in a nonthermal, nonablative fashion
  - Emit light in a pulsed or continuous fashion and in either a single color (red, yellow, blue) or multiple colors of light to maximize the therapeutic approach
- Narrowband light
  - Emit noncoherent light; restricted wavelength range of ±20 nm; pulse signal to stimulate mitochondria in fibroblasts
- Radio-frequency devices
  - Used primarily for skin tightening and endovenous closure
  - Heat is generated due to the natural resistance of tissue to the movement of electrons within a radio-frequency field as governed by Ohm law
  - Tissue resistance, called impedance, generates heat relative to the amount of current and time by converting electrical current to thermal energy
  - Energy is dispersed to three-dimensional volumes of tissue at controlled depths
  - The configuration of electrodes in a radio-frequency device can be monopolar or bipolar
- Ultrasound devices
  - High-intensity focused ultrasound (HIFU) used primarily for skin tightening
  - When an intense ultrasound field vibrates tissue, friction is created between molecules, causing them to absorb mechanical energy and leading to secondary generation of heat

Laser Safety

- The vast majority of laser accidents involve eye injuries
  - The retina is particularly affected by the wavelengths 400 to 1400 nm (pulsed dye, diode, alexandrite, ruby, or Nd:YAG lasers) due to its high density of vascular and melanocytic targets
  - The cornea is more vulnerable to lasers that target water (Erbium:YAG, carbon dioxide, nonablative infrared lasers)
- Hazards of plume: viral particles are aerosolized in smoke plume exhaust; use smoke evacuator with clean filters and tubing and particle masks if appropriate (particularly important for laser hair removal, ablative resurfacing and laser treatment of warts)
- Reflection hazard: collimated beams can be reflected back by high gloss instruments; this is not as much of an issue with focused hand pieces as the laser beam spreads out and becomes less powerful with distance
- Fire prevention
  - Wet drapes or cloths should be used intraoperatively with ablative lasers
  - Exposed hair-bearing areas should be kept moist with ablative lasers
  - Alcohol-based skin preps should be thoroughly dried before use of the laser
  - Care should be taken with tanks of compressed gas (liquid nitrogen, oxygen)

Topical Anesthetic Compounds

- Can be applied under occlusion for 30 to 90 minutes before treatment
- EMLA cream: lidocaine 2.5% and prilocaine 2.5%
  - Prilocaine component has risk of methemoglobinemia
- LMX: 4 or 5% lidocaine
- Life-threatening side effects can occur with application over large body surface areas or with excessive exposure to abraded or torn skin due to high plasma concentrations; occlusion may enhance absorption

Possible Laser Side Effects and/or Expected Healing Course

- Expected healing course: erythema, edema, purpura are transient and expected, depending on the procedure

TABLE 26-3 Types of Lasers

Laser	Wavelength (nm)	Color	Chromophore	Output
Excimer	308	Ultraviolet	Protein	QCW
Narrowband blue light	407–420	Violet/blue	Endogenous porphyrins	CW
Argon	488/514	Blue	Vascular and pigmented lesions	CW
Pulsed dye (PDL)	510	Yellow	Pigmented lesions, vascular lesions	Pulsed
Copper vapor	511/578	Yellow/green	Pigmented lesions, vascular lesions	CW
Krypton	530/568	Yellow/green	Pigmented lesions, vascular lesions	CW
Potassium-titanyl-phosphate (KTP), Frequency-doubled Nd:YAG	532	Green	Pigmented lesions, red tattoos	QS
Argon-pumped tunable dye	577/585	Yellow	Vascular lesions	CW
Pulsed dye laser (PDL)	585–595	Yellow	Vascular lesions, hypertrophic/keloid scars, striae, verrucae, nonablative dermal remodeling	Pulsed
Ruby, normal mode	694	Red	Hair removal	Pulsed
QS ruby	694	Red	Pigmented lesions, blue/black/green/tattoos	QS
Alexandrite, normal mode	755	Red	Hair removal, leg veins	Pulsed
QS alexandrite	755	Red	Pigmented lesions, blue/black/green tattoos	QS
Diode	800–810	Red	Hair removal, leg veins	Pulsed
Qs Nd:YAG	1,064	Infrared	Pigmented lesions, blue/black tattoos	QS
Nd:YAG, normal mode	1,064	Infrared	Hair removal, leg veins, nonablative dermal remodeling	Pulsed
Nd:YAG, normal mode	1,320	Infrared	Water: nonablative dermal remodeling	Pulsed
Diode	1,450	Infrared	Water: nonablative dermal remodeling	Pulsed
Thulium	1,927	Infrared	Water: dermal remodeling	Pulsed
Erbium:Yttrium Scandium Gallium Garnet (YSGG)	2,790	Infrared	Water: ablative resurfacing	CW
Erbium:YAG	2,940	Infrared	Water: ablative resurfacing	CW or Pulsed
Erbium:Glass	1,540	Infrared	Water: nonablative dermal remodeling	Pulsed
Erbium:Glass	1,550	Infrared	Water, dermal remodeling	Pulsed
CO_2	10,600	Infrared	Water (vaporization and coagulation): actinic cheilitis, verrucae, rhinophyma Ablative resurfacing, epidermal/dermal lesions	CW or Pulsed

Note: CW, continuous-wave; Nd, neodymium; QCW, quasicontinuous wave; QS, quality-switched; YAG, yttrium-aluminum-garnet.

TABLE 26-4 Laser Treatment of Tattoo Pigment

Laser Type	Wavelength	Tattoo Pigment Color
QS Nd:YAG, frequency-doubled	532 nm	Red, orange, yellow
QS ruby	694 nm	Blue, black Occasionally green and brown
QS alexandrite	755 nm	Blue, black, and green
QS Nd:YAG	1,064 nm	Blue, black

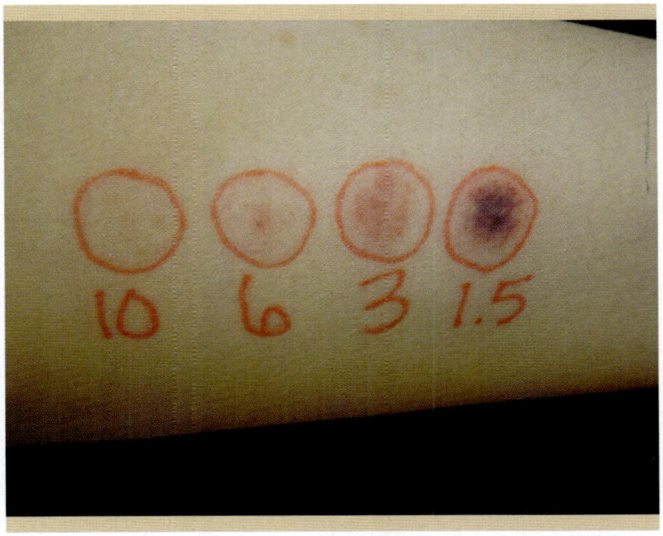

FIGURE 26-7 Forearm skin treated with the pulsed dye laser at 10 J/cm^2 at decreasing pulse durations (left to right: 10, 6, 3, 1.5 ms). Purpura formation increases with shorter pulse durations. (*Used with permission from Melissa A. Bogle, MD, The Laser and Cosmetic Surgery Center of Houston.*)

- Side effects
  - Hyperpigmentation or hypopigmentation, erythema, pain, scar, incomplete removal of target
  - Laser tattoo or pigmented lesion removal: purpura, crusting expected; hypopigmentation or scarring may occur
  - Laser treatment of vessels: purpura; vesiculation, crusting
    - Incidence of purpura particularly high with the pulsed dye laser used at shorter pulse durations (Fig. 26-7)
  - Laser hair removal: erythema common and expected; edema, purpura, vesiculation, crusting
  - Ablative laser skin resurfacing
    - Short term: edema and exudation expected; risk of infection (*Herpes simplex virus*, *Candida*, or bacterial)
    - Medium term: acne/milia, pruritus, hyperpigmenation, dermatitis
    - Permanent: hypopigmentation, scar, ectropion
  - Nonablative resurfacing: edema, vesiculation, crusting

Skin Cooling

- Allows use of higher fluences (most important parameter in efficacy) while protecting the epidermis and reducing collateral thermal damage
- Increases treatment options for darker skin types
- Decreases pain
- Timing:
  - Precooling: heating by laser pulse is instantaneous; cooling is slow, so cooling needs a head start
  - Parallel cooling: important to avoid overheating with long pulse durations
  - Postcooling: prevents retrograde heating from damaging the skin surface
- Types of cooling
  - Cryogen spray: good spatial confinement of cooling to epidermis and upper dermis, high heat transfer coefficient (efficient), potential for cryoinjury under certain conditions
  - Surface contact (sapphire window or copper plate): precooling, parallel cooling, and postcooling, can compress skin (good for hair, bad for vessels)
  - Forced air convection: no beam interference, poor special confinement of cooling; low heat transfer coefficient, but heat extraction can be significant at longer application times; excellent analgesia
  - Iced/chilled rollers: best for postcooling; can use as precooling when needed

Chemical Peels

- Depth of peels
  - Superficial: necrosis of all or part of the epidermis
  - Medium: necrosis extends to the papillary dermis
  - Deep: wounding extends to the upper or mid reticular dermis
- Indications: actinic keratoses, superficial scarring, hyperpigmentation and melasma, acne, photoaging, keratosis pilaris, epidermal growths
- Chemical peel strengths
  - Depends on the amount of free acid present
    - Free acid availability (pKa) = pH at which half is in acid form
    - Lower pKa = more free acid available

- Affected by
  - Percentage of acid
  - Type of vehicle used
  - Buffering
  - pKa of acid preparation
  - Contact time
  - How much solution is applied
  - Aggressive application technique (rubbing, etc.)
  - Number of passes
  - Aggressive defatting
  - Peeling agent (Table 26-5)
- Defatting: acetone or rubbing alcohol; essential for optimal penetration as most peeling agents are not lipid soluble
- Frost formation: whitish tint of skin due to keratin agglutination; depth of trichloracetic acid peels can be correlated with intensity of frost (Fig. 26-8)
  - No frost: stratum corneum
  - Patchy light frost: superficial epidermis
  - Uniform white frost with some pink showing through: full thickness epidermis
- Peels such as salicylic acid can have a "pseudofrost" formation due to precipitation of crystals in the peel solution (Fig. 26-9); this is not a measure of the depth of the peel
- Microdermabrasion may be performed prepeel to enhance penetration and allow a more even coverage
- Complications of chemical peels
  - Hyperpigmentation or hypopigmentation
  - Scarring
  - Infection
  - Prolonged erythema
  - Acne
  - Milia
  - Arrhythmias (need electrocardiogram and pulse oximeter monitoring with phenol peels)

MICRODERMABRASION

- Produces a superficial ablation, primarily in the stratum corneum or upper epidermis
- Indicated for superficial skin conditions, early photoaging, superficial scarring; requires a series of treatments for best results
- Contraindications: active infection, cold sores, inflammatory skin conditions
- Crystals may cause corneal abrasion—use eye protection

DERMABRASION

- Manual abrasion, wound healing by second intention allows reepithelialization to occur from the underlying adnexal structures
- Highly operator-dependent process and depends on coarseness of the dermabrading tip (fraise) or sanding paper, number of brush strokes, pressure exerted, and tissue contact time
- Indicated for scarring, actinic keratosis, photoaging or deep rhytides, tattoos
- Contraindications: isotretinoin use within 6 to 12 months, history of hypertrophic scarring, active infection
- Side effects: scarring, hyperpigmentation, milia, infection, permanent hypopigmentation

BOTULINUM TOXIN (BoNT OR BTX)

- Botulinum toxin acts by binding presynaptically to high-affinity sites on cholinergic nerve terminals and decreasing the release of acetylcholine, causing a neuromuscular blockade (Fig. 26-10)
- Requires 24 to 72 hours to start to take effect; full effect by 2 weeks
- Lasts approximately 3 to 5 months
- Effects wear off through proximal axonal sprouting and reinnervation by formation of a new neuromuscular junction
- Seven toxin serotypes (A–G) bind to different sites on the motor nerve terminal and within the motor neuron
  - Botulinum toxin type A and type B are commercially available; A is the most potent
- Each toxin serotype is composed of 3 domains: binding, translocation, and enzymatic
  - Serotypes A and E cleave synaptosomal-associated protein (SNAP-25), a presynaptic membrane protein required for fusion of neurotransmitter vesicles
  - Serotypes B, D, F, and G cleave a vesicle-associated membrane protein (VAMP), also known as synaptobrevin
  - Serotype C acts by cleaving syntaxin, a target membrane protein
- The BoNT molecule is synthesized as a single chain and then cleaved to form a dichain molecule with a disulfide bridge
  - The 50-kD light chain acts as a zinc (Zn^{2+}) endopeptidase similar to tetanus toxin; it blocks acetylcholine-containing vesicles from fusing with the N-terminal membrane of the motor neuron (SNARE complex)
  - Zinc supplementation may enhance the effect and duration of BoTX injections
  - The 100-kD heavy chain provides cholinergic specificity, is responsible for binding of the toxin to presynaptic receptors, and promotes light chain translocation across the endosomal membrane
  - SNARE (synaptosomal-associated protein receptor) proteins are presynaptic proteins involved in exocytosis of acetylcholine

TABLE 26-5 Peeling Agents

Chemical Agent	Characteristics
Alpha-hydroxy acid (AHA)	Glycolic, lactic, citric, and malic acids Dependent on the contact time with the skin Carboxylic acids normally found in many foods Thins the stratum corneum, although the epidermis thickens May increase photosensitivity
- Glycolic acid	Derived from sugar cane Concentrations range from 20–70% Decreases corneocyte cohesion by promoting exfoliation of the outer layers of the stratum corneum Neutralize with sodium bicarbonate Dispersal of melanin pigmentation and a return to a more normal rete pattern
- Lactic acid (LA)	Derived from sour milk Acts as a humectant (causes the skin to hold onto water), keratolytic
Beta-hydroxy acid (BHA) -Salicylic acid	Derived from willow bark, wintergreen leaves, or sweet birch Concentrations of 20 or 30% (OTC preparations contain only 2%) Exhibits anti-inflammatory capabilities, producing less irritation Lipophilic, good for acne and oily skin Penetrates the follicular sebaceous material (anticomedogenic effect) Does not need to be neutralized, visible "frost" is not a true frost, but rather precipitation of salicylic acid crystals No need to time the peel: after 2 minutes, there is very little absorption of the active agent Contraindicated in pregnancy, breast-feeding, and aspirin allergies Adverse effect: salicylism (nausea, disorientation, and tinnitus)
Jessner solution	14% salicylic acid, 14% lactic acid, 14% resorcinol in alcohol Keratolytic effects
Carbon dioxide (CO_2)	Boiling point: 78°C Physical peeling method Solid block of CO_2 ice dipped in an acetone-alcohol mixture Applied to the skin for 5–15 seconds
Resorcinol	1,3-Dihydroxybenzene Concentrations of 20–50%
Trichloroacetic acid	Can be used for superficial, medium, and less often deep peels No need to neutralize No systemic toxicity Causes coagulation of proteins in the skin (results in frost)
Baker Gordon phenol	Phenol 88%, 2 mL distilled water, 8 drops Septisol, and 3 drops croton oil Septisol (triclosan) causes deeper penetration of phenol and a deeper peel Croton oil (especially the toxic fraction solubilized in phenol) causes a deeper peel Exfoliation to middle reticular dermis New zone of collagen forms Occluded method uses zinc oxide tape or other artificial barrier product to prevent evaporation of the phenol from the skin, thus enabling the solution to penetrate deeper *Litton formula*: replaces Septisol (triclosan) with glycerin *Beeson McCollough formula*: uses aggressive defatting and heavier application of Baker Gordon solution Risk of permanent hypopigmentation

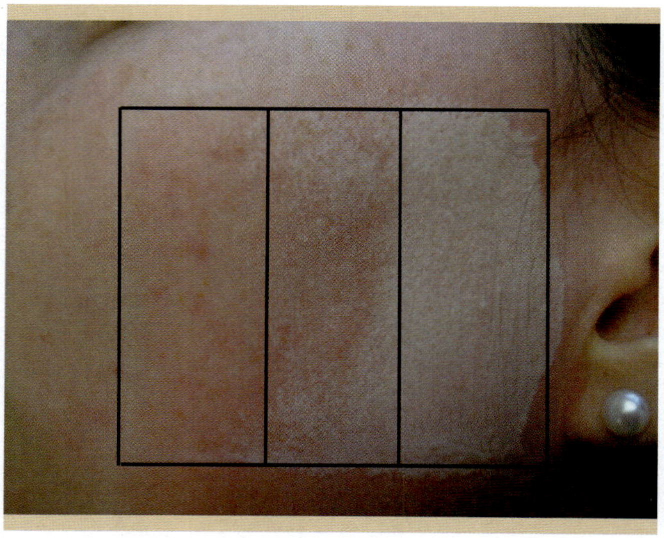

FIGURE 26-8 Depth of trichloracetic acid peels can be correlated with intensity of frost formation. The left segment has no frost formation with a 5% TCA peel indicating penetration only of the stratum corneum. The middle segment has patchy light frost formation with a 15% TCA peel indicating penetration of the superficial epidermis. The right segment has a uniform white frost with some pink showing through with heavy application of a 30% TCA peel indicating full thickness penetration through the epidermis and into the upper dermis. (*Used with permission from Melissa A. Bogle, MD, The Laser and Cosmetic Surgery Center of Houston.*)

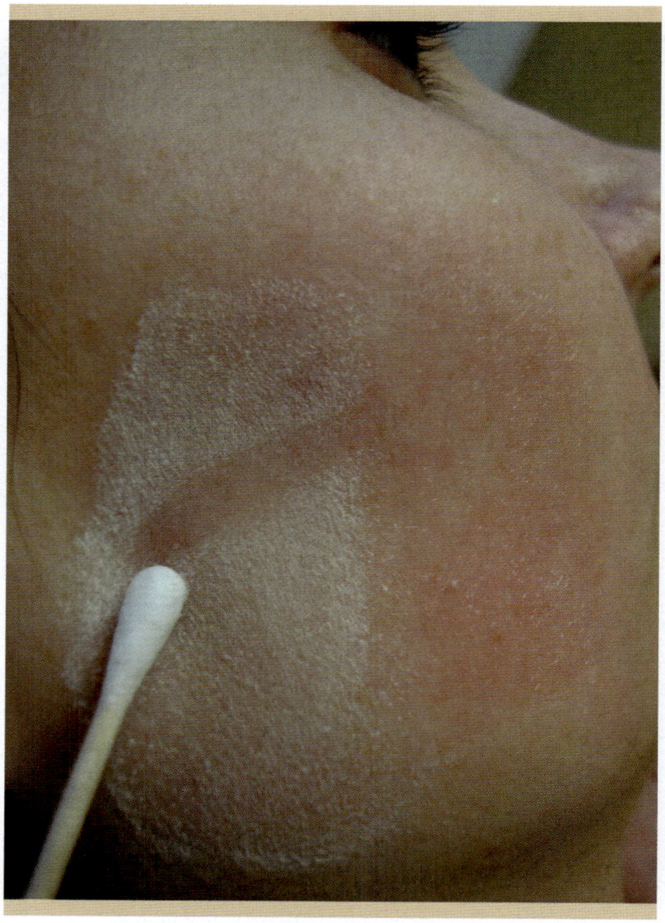

FIGURE 26-9 Pseudofrost formation due to precipitation of crystals with a 30% salicylic acid peel. The crystals can be easily wiped off the skin, which is not the case with a true frost. (*Used with permission from Melissa A. Bogle, MD, The Laser and Cosmetic Surgery Center of Houston.*)

- The potency of BoNT-A is measured in mouse units (MU); 1 MU = the amount of toxin that kills 50% of a group of 20-g Swiss-Webster mice within 3 days of intraperitoneal injection (LD50)
  - Units between BoNT-A brand preparations are not equivalent
- Commercially available preparations in the United States
  - Onabotulinumtoxin A (Botox [BoTX], Botox Cosmetic)
    - Botox: Cervical dystonia, severe primary axillary hyperhidrosis, strabismus, blepharospasm, chronic migraine, upper limb spasticity, neurogenic detrusor overactivity in the bladder
    - Botox Cosmetic: Moderate-to-severe glabellar lines
  - Abobotulinumtoxin A (Dysport): cervical dystonia, moderate-to-severe glabellar lines
  - Incobotulinumtoxin A (Xeomin): cervical dystonia, blepharospasm
  - Rimabotulinumtoxin B (Myobloc): cervical dystonia
- Antibodies to Botox
  - Antibodies may rarely develop to the binding site on the heavy chain of the BTX molecule
  - Prevents BTX binding to its receptor and thereby cripples the actions of the BTX
  - Increased risk of antibody formation at doses of more than 300 units at a time
  - Myobloc binding domain distinct from Botox (i.e., antibodies that neutralize BoTX A would not neutralize BoTX B, and vice versa)
- Common uses for BoTX on the face and neck
  - Glabellar furrows: procerus, corrugator, and depressor supercilii muscles (Fig. 26-11)
  - Horizontal forehead rhytides: frontalis muscle (Fig. 26-12)
  - Crow's feet: orbicularis oculi (Fig. 26-13)
  - Bunny lines on the nose: levator labii aleque nasi, transversalis nasalis (see Fig. 26-13)
  - Gummy smile: levator labii superioris, levator labii superioris alaeque nasi, and zygomaticus minor (Fig. 26-14)

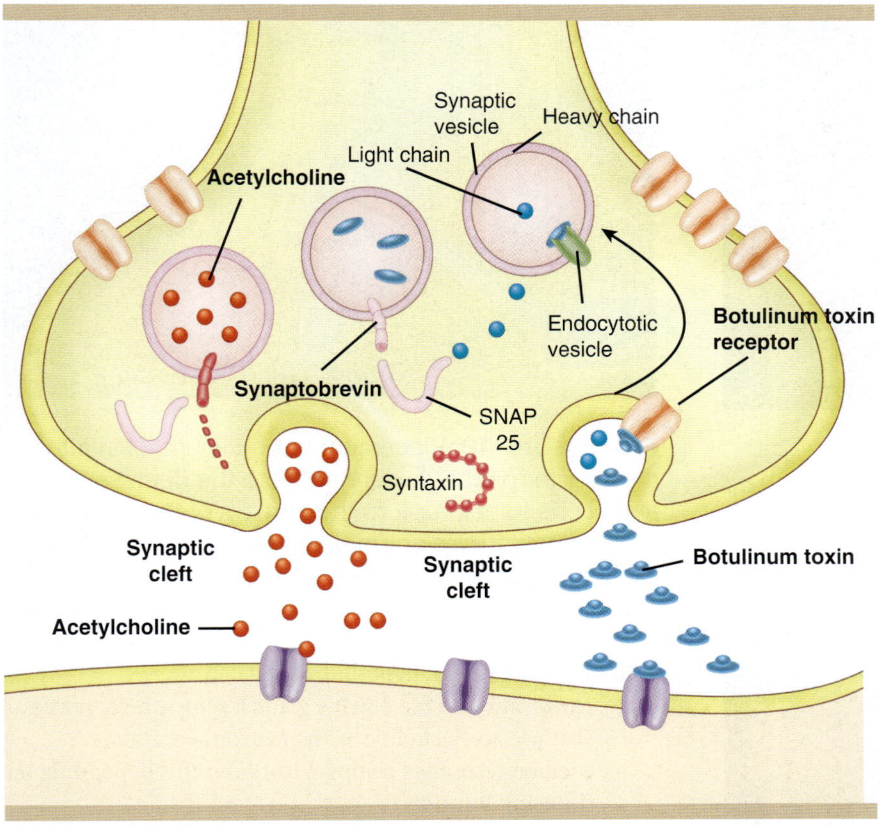

FIGURE 26-10 Botulinum toxin mechanism of action. (*Reprinted with permission from Baumann L: Cosmetic Dermatology: Principles and Practice, 2nd Ed., New York: McGraw-Hill; 2009.*)

- Lip lines: orbicularis oris (Fig. 26-15)
- Downturned mouth: depressor anguli oris (Fig. 26-16)
- Pebbly chin texture: mentalis muscle (see Fig. 26-16)
- Neck: platysma muscle (Fig. 26-17)
- Complications
  - Eyelid ptosis may develop when BTX affects the levator palpebrae superioris muscle, which normally elevates the eyelid
  - May persist for 2 to 4 weeks
  - Risk is minimized by the correct injection volume and site of injection
    - Stay 1 cm above the orbital ridge
    - Have the patient stay vertical for 4 hours
    - Avoid manipulating injection site
  - Apraclonidine 0.5% eye drops (Iopidine) 1 to 3 drops three times a day to the affected side

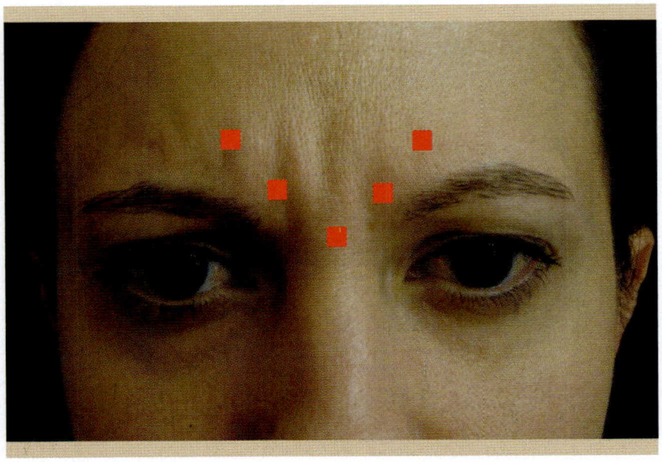

FIGURE 26-11 Placement of botulinum toxin into the glabellar complex. (*Used with permission from Melissa A. Bogle, MD, The Laser and Cosmetic Surgery Center of Houston.*)

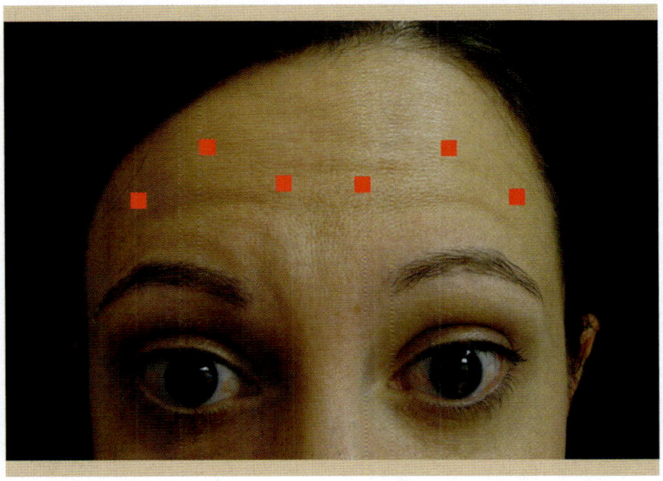

FIGURE 26-12 Placement of botulinum toxin into the frontalis muscle. (*Used with permission from Melissa A. Bogle, MD, The Laser and Cosmetic Surgery Center of Houston.*)

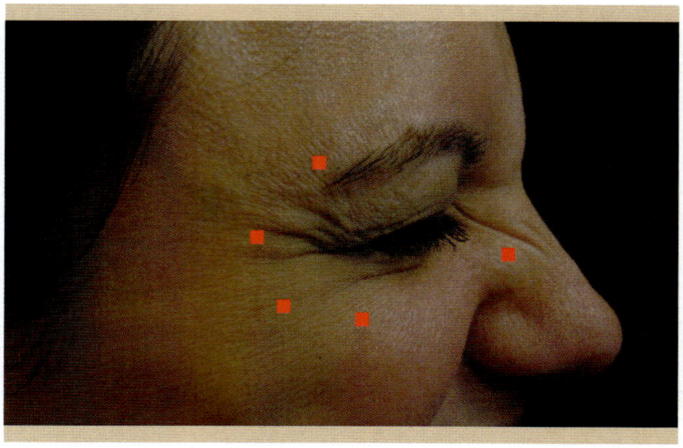

FIGURE 26-13 Placement of botulinum toxin into the crow's feet and bunny lines. (*Used with permission from Melissa A. Bogle, MD, The Laser and Cosmetic Surgery Center of Houston.*)

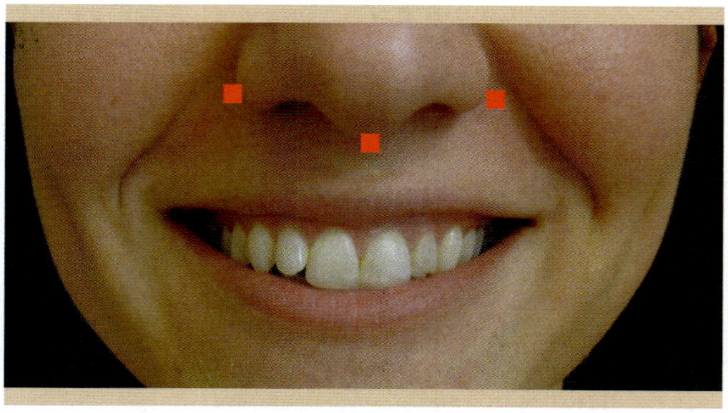

FIGURE 26-14 Placement of botulinum toxin for treatment of a gummy smile. (*Used with permission from Melissa A. Bogle, MD, The Laser and Cosmetic Surgery Center of Houston.*)

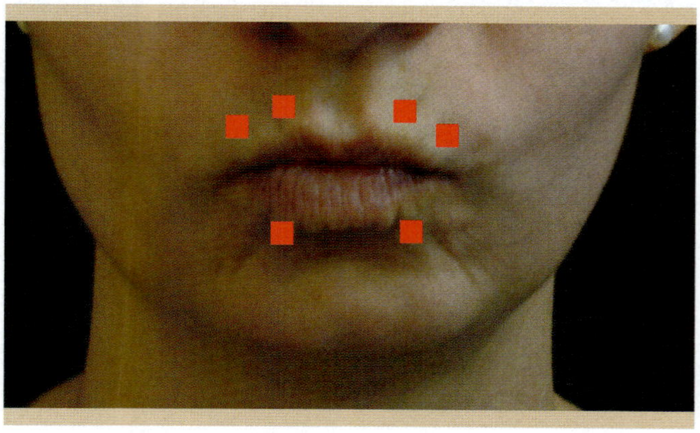

FIGURE 26-15 Placement of botulinum toxin for the treatment of perioral rhytides. (*Used with permission from Melissa A. Bogle, MD, The Laser and Cosmetic Surgery Center of Houston.*)

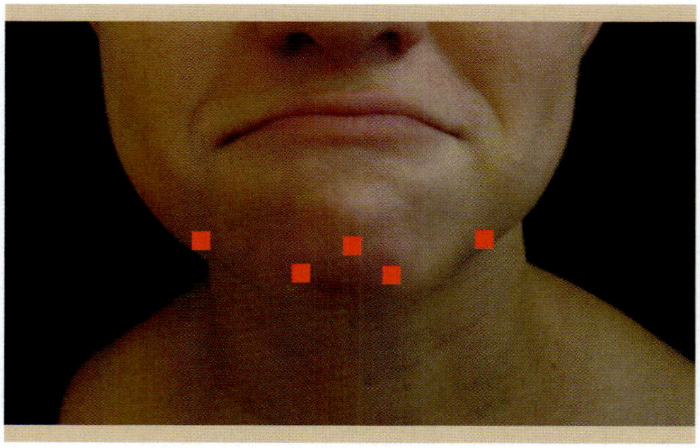

FIGURE 26-16 Placement of botulinum toxin into the chin for pebbly texture and into the depressor anguli oris to help upturn the corners of the mouth. (*Used with permission from Melissa A. Bogle, MD, The Laser and Cosmetic Surgery Center of Houston.*)

- BoTX treatment of hyperhidrosis
  - Innervation of the eccrine glands: sympathetic nerves that use acetylcholine as the neurotransmitter
  - Median responses lasting 6 to 19 months depending on dose and location
  - Extent of hyperhidrosis: evaluated by performing an iodine starch test of axillae, palms, or soles (Fig. 26-18)
- Contraindications to use of BoTX
  - History of a neuromuscular disease (Eaton-Lambert syndrome, amyotrophic lateral sclerosis, or myasthenia gravis)
  - Known history of sensitivity to BoTX or human albumin
  - Aminoglycosides can interfere with neuromuscular transmission
  - Pregnancy or lactation

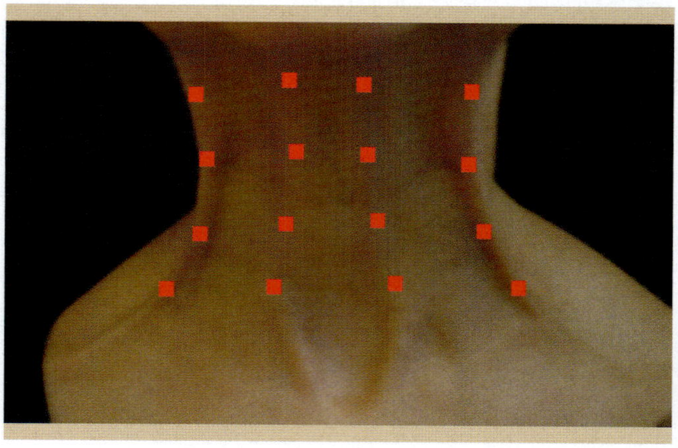

FIGURE 26-17 Placement of botulinum toxin into the platysma muscle for reduction of neck banding. (*Used with permission from Melissa A. Bogle, MD, The Laser and Cosmetic Surgery Center of Houston.*)

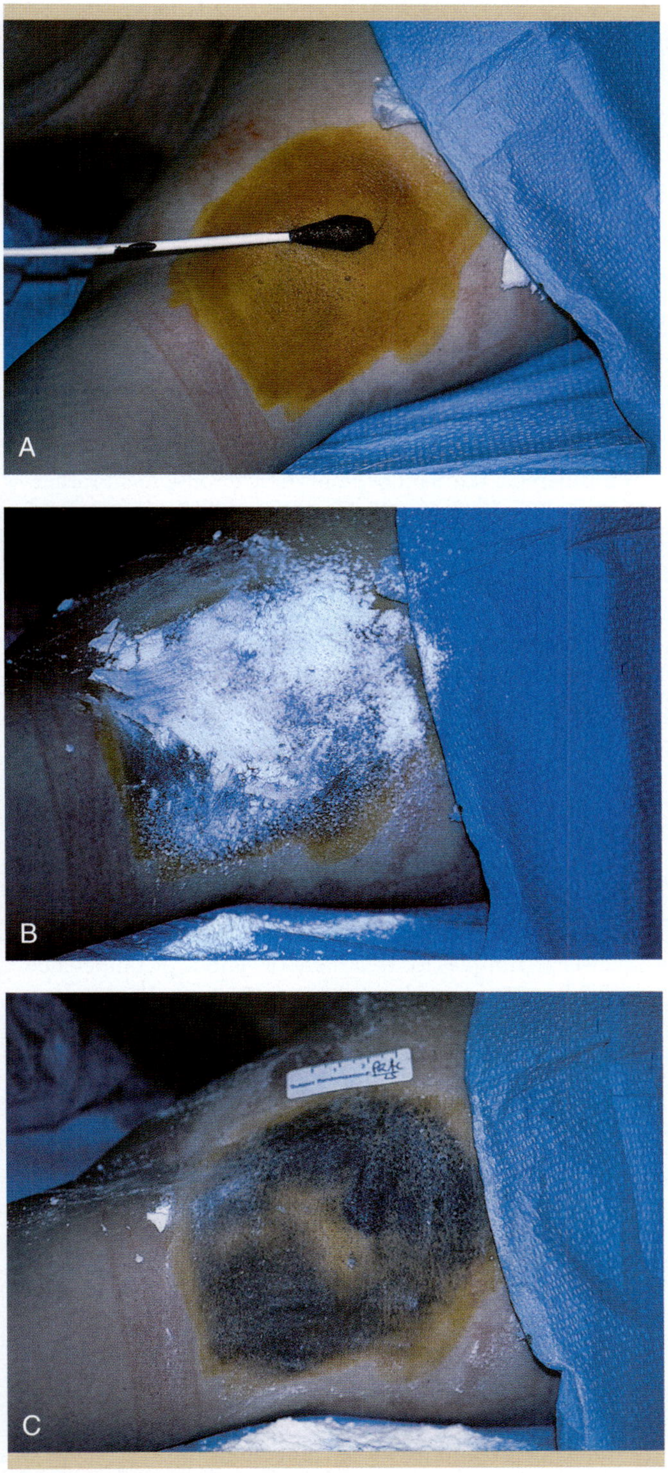

FIGURE 26-18 Iodine starch test for evaluation of hyperhidrosis. (A) An iodine solution is applied to the affected area. (B) Potato starch is then sprinkled over the area. (C) The starch turns black in reaction to sweat, clearly delineating affected areas.

SOFT-TISSUE AUGMENTATION/ INJECTABLE FILLERS

- Collagen fillers
  - Bovine (cow) collagen: Zyderm I and II, Zyplast: skin allergy test required (~3% risk of allergy in general population)
  - Porcine (pig) collagen: Evolence; no skin allergy testing required
  - Human collagen: Cosmoderm, Cosmoplast
  - Postfiller necrosis was first reported after collagen injections into the glabella, but any filler may cause necrosis and it may also occur in any area; necrosis can result from direct intravascular injection or vascular compression due to edema or excessive filler
- Hyaluronic acid
  - Naturally occurring polysaccharide that is ubiquitous in the extracellular matrix of all animal tissues; the most commonly used filler agent worldwide
  - Nonanimal stabilized hyaluronic dermal filler (NASHA): Restylane, Perlane, Juvederm Ultra, Juvederm Ultra Plus, Prevelle Silk; produced by fermentation in bacterial cultures of equine streptococci
  - Animal-derived hyaluronic dermal filler: Hylaform (derived from avian source [rooster combs])
  - When injected too superficially, a bluish Tyndall effect can be seen, which represents visible hyaluronic acid seen through the translucent epidermis
  - Product can be dissolved with the injection of commercially available hyaluronidase
  - Results generally last 6 to 12 months
- Radiesse
  - Calcium hydroxyapatite in a cellulose carrier gel
  - The cellulose gel degrades over several months, leaving behind calcium hydroxyapatite microspheres to stimulate reactive collagen formation
  - Several injection sessions may be required, results can last up to 2 years
- Sculptra
  - Freeze dried poly-L-lactic acid powder, reconstituted in sterile water; pure stimulatory filler
  - Poly-L-lactic acid is also used to make dissolvable sutures
  - Poly-L-lactic acid particles stimulate reactive collagen formation
  - Multiple treatments over several months are required, results can last up to 2 years
- Artefill
  - Polymethylmethacrylate (PMMA) beads suspended in bovine collagen
  - Pretreatment skin allergy test is required due to the bovine collagen carrier (pretest contains only bovine collagen, no PMMA)

    - Collagen degrades, leaving behind PMMA beads which stimulate a local inflammatory response and resulting fibrous connective tissue
    - The only US FDA approved permanent filler
- Autologous fat
    - Fat is harvested from the patient's own stores and injected via 18 gauge needle or microcannula
    - Fat is a large molecule, subcutaneous filling substance best for deep volumetric enhancement and large atrophic defects that include skin and fat
    - About 20 to 30% of injected fat generally grafts and survives, results last months to years, multiple injection sessions recommended for best results
    - Fat is source of human stem cells; may play an additional role in rejuvenation of tissue area after injection
    - Longevity is highly variable (1–5 years or longer)
- Autologous cell therapy
    - LaViv (Azficel-T), formerly Isologen
    - Autologous cultured human fibroblasts
    - Multiple punch biopsies are taken from behind the ear and sent to the company, where the skin's fibroblast cells are isolated and grown into a concentrated broth
    - Therapy consists of a series of injection sessions using the fibroblast broth with the goal of increasing the number of fibroblasts at the injection site so that body will produce collagen there
    - Best for injection directly into a wrinkle or scar, results more subtle when used as a true dermal filler; results last 1 year or longer
- Silicon-1000
    - Approved by the US FDA for certain ophthalmologic applications; use as a permanent cosmetic filler is strictly off-label
    - Microdroplet technique; fibrosis around silicone droplets localizes the material and provide "bulk"
    - In the hands of a trained practitioner, its use can yield excellent cosmetic results; in untrained hands or with nonmedical grade silicone, results can be disastrous with chronic inflammatory reaction and granulomatous response

FILLER INJECTION TECHNIQUES

- Serial puncture: multiple small aliquots of filler along the length of the defect
- Linear threading or tunneling: the needle pierces the skin once and is advanced parallel to the defect
- Fanning: the needle insertion site remains the same with multiple threading injections extended across the defect in a "fan" shape
- Cross-hatching: layered linear injections perpendicular to one another in a defect or anatomical segment
- Depot: bolus of filler injected in the subcutaneous tissue or above the bone

Leg Veins

- The lower extremity has both a superficial and a deep venous system, connected by communication vessels called perforating veins
    - The deep venous system includes the femoral, popliteal, anterior tibial, posterior tibial, peroneal veins, and others
    - The superficial system highly variable and includes the great and short saphenous veins and other unnamed veins
    - The great and short saphenous veins may connect by intersaphenous veins, such as the Giacomini vein
- Clusters of veins and telangiectasias on the lateral thigh are from the lateral subdermic plexus of Albanese and considered a remnant of embryonic development rather than a sign of venous insufficiency
- Any concern about underlying saphenous vessel insufficiency should warrant an investigation of the lower extremities by duplex ultrasonography
    - The presence of clusters of telangiectatic veins on the medial or lateral ankles is commonly the result of incompetence in the great saphenous vein (medial) or small saphenous vein (lateral)
    - Telangiectatic veins along the medial thigh or knee areas should generate suspicion of incompetence in the great saphenous vein
- Traditionally, ligation of the saphenous vein at its deep vein junction and removal of the abnormal saphenous vein segments has been used to treat venous incompetence
- Newer techniques for treatment of venous incompetence include endovenous laser ablation (ELA) and radiofrequency ablation (RFA); used to safely ablate the great and small saphenous veins, the anterior and posterior accessory great saphenous vein, the superficial accessory saphenous vein, and the anterior and posterior circumflex veins of the thigh
- Common sclerosants include the following:
    - Detergents: disrupt the cellular membrane of the vein via denaturation; may be mixed with air to create a foamed solution to enhance contact with the vessel wall of larger vessels
        - Sodium tetradecyl sulfate (Sotradecol)
        - Polidocanol (Asclera)
        - Sodium morrhuate (Scleromate)
        - Ethanolamine Oleate (Ethamolin)
    - Osmotic agents: damage the cell by shifting the water balance through cellular gradient (osmotic) dehydration and cell membrane denaturation
        - Hypertonic sodium chloride solution
        - Sodium chloride solution with dextrose (Sclerodex)
    - Chemical irritants: damage the cell wall by direct caustic destruction of the vascular endothelium
        - Chromated glycerin (Sclermo)
        - Polyiodinated iodine (Variglobin, Sclerodine)

QUIZ

Questions

1. Which of the following wavelengths is most appropriate for ablative laser skin resurfacing?

   A. 532 nm
   B. 595 nm
   C. 755 nm
   D. 1,064 nm
   E. 2,940 nm

2. Which of the following chemical peel agents is most likely to cause cardiac arrhythmias?

   A. Trichloracetic acid
   B. Salicylic acid
   C. Jessner's solution
   D. Phenol
   E. Glycolic acid

3. Which of the following wavelengths penetrates most deeply into the skin?

   A. 532 nm
   B. 595 nm
   C. 755 nm
   D. 1,064 nm
   E. 10,600 nm

4. Endovascular venous ablation techniques using laser or radio frequency can be most safely applied to which of the following veins?

   A. Peroneal vein
   B. Femoral vein
   C. Anterior tibial vein
   D. Great saphenous vein
   E. Popliteal vein

5. Uniform white frost with pink showing through correlates with what depth of injury after a trichloroacetic acid peel?

   A. Stratum corneum
   B. Superficial epidermis
   C. Full thickness epidermis
   D. Papillary dermis
   E. Reticular dermis

6. What neurotransmitter is blocked by botulinum toxin?

   A. Epinephrine
   B. Dopamine
   C. Norepinephrine
   D. Gamma aminobutyric acid
   E. Acetylcholine

7. What does Botox cleave?

   A. Synaptosomal-associated protein
   B. Vesicle-associated protein
   C. Syntaxin
   D. Cholinergic receptor
   E. Acetylcholine

8. Neutralization of which of the following chemical peels is important to prevent excess penetration?

   A. Trichloracetic acid
   B. Jessner's solution
   C. Phenol
   D. Glycolic acid
   E. Salicylic acid

9. Which of the following lasers operates in the red portion of the electromagnetic spectrum?

   A. Alexandrite
   B. Pulsed dye
   C. Carbon dioxide
   D. Nd:YAG
   E. Potassium titanyl-phosphate (KTP)

10. Treatment with which of the following lasers most commonly results in purpura?

    A. Alexandrite
    B. Pulsed dye
    C. Carbon dioxide
    D. Nd:YAG
    E. Er:YAG

11. Local skin necrosis following the use of soft-tissue filler for the correction of dermal rhytides occurs most frequently at which of the following sites?

    A. Glabella
    B. Cheeks
    C. Nasolabial folds
    D. Lips
    E. Temples

Answers

1. E. Traditional ablative laser skin resurfacing is most commonly accomplished with the 2,940 nm Erbium:YAG and 10,600 nm carbon dioxide lasers.
2. D. Cardiac arrhythmias are a potential complication in phenol face peeling. All patients who undergo phenol peels should have cardiac monitoring and careful attention to their fluid status and hydration. Cardiac arrhythmias typically develop during phenol peels when the peeling solution is applied too rapidly resulting in systemic accumulation of excess phenol. To help avoid this problem, individual facial segments (cheeks, forehead, perioral, periorbital, and nose should be

treated with at least a 15 minute time delay between them.

3. D. In general, depth of penetration increases with wavelength, however this is not true for traditional ablative lasers such as the 10,600 nm carbon dioxide laser. The longer infrared laser wavelengths are absorbed efficiently by water in the superficial dermis such that penetration is limited.
4. D. Endovenous laser ablation (ELA) and radio-frequency ablation (RFA) have replaced stripping and ligation as the technique of choice for elimination of saphenous vein reflux. The other veins listed all fall within the deep venous system of the lower extremity.
5. C. After defatting the skin, chemical peeling agents are applied to the skin. Skin keratin begins to agglutinate. Depth of peel can be correlated with the intensity of the frost: no frost (stratum corneum), irregular light frost (superficial epidermis), and uniform white frost with pink showing through (full thickness epidermis).
6. E. Neurotransmitters are chemicals used to signal between a neuron and another cell. They are present in the presynaptic element, bind to postsynaptic receptors, and must be in sufficient quantity to affect the postsynaptic cell. Botulinum toxin blocks neurotransmitter release at peripheral cholinergic nerve terminals. Epinephrine, dopamine, norepinephrine, gamma aminobutyric acid, melatonin, serotonin and glutamic acid are other neurotransmitters.
7. A. Seven botulinum toxin serotypes (A–G) bind to different sites on the motor nerve terminal and within the motor neuron. Botox is botulinum toxin type A, and Myobloc is botulinum toxin type B. Synaptosomal-associated protein (SNAP-25) is cleaved by serotypes A and E. Vesicle-associated membrane protein (VAMP, synaptobrevin) is cleaved by serotypes B, D, F, and G. Syntaxin 1 is cleaved by serotype C1. Cleavage of these proteins prevents exocytosis of acetylcholine into the synapse between the motor neuron and the skeletal muscle cell.
8. D. Glycolic acid peeling agents do not induce enough coagulation of skin proteins and therefore cannot neutralize themselves. They must be neutralized using copious amounts of water or a weak buffer agent such as sodium bicarbonate.
9. A. The alexandrite laser emits red light at a wavelength of 755 nm. The pulsed dye laser emits yellow light at 585 to 595 nm. The KTP laser emits green light at 532 nm. Neither the Nd:YAG nor carbon dioxide lasers emit light in the visible spectrum.
10. B. The pulsed dye laser is frequently associated with purpura formation, particularly when used at shorter pulse durations.
11. A. Local skin necrosis most commonly occurs after injection of dermal fillers in the glabella, but may occur in any location. Necrosis is thought to occur either by direct injection of filler into a vessel that supplies the area or from compression of vessels in the area by edema or the bulk of excessive filler.

REFERENCES

Battie C, Verschoore M: Cutaneous solar exposure and clinical aspects of photodamage. *Indian J Dermatol Venereol Leprol* 2012;78:S9.

Bogle MA, Dover JS: Tissue tightening technologies. *Dermatol Clin* 2009;27:491.

Carruthers J, Carruthers A: Botulinum toxin (botox) chemodenervation for facial rejuvenation *Facial Plast Surg Clin North Am* 2001 May;9(2):197–204,Vii.

Dudelzak J, Goldberg DJ. Laser safety. *Curr Probl Dermatol* 2011;42:35.

Ezzat WH, Keller GS: The use of poly-L-lactic acid filler in facial aesthetics. *Facial Plast Surg* 2011;27:503.

Fitzgerald R, Graivier MH, Kane M, et al. Update on facial aging. *Aesthet Surg J* 2010;30:11S.

Holliday R: Telomeres and telomerase: the commitment theory of cellular aging revisited. *Sci Prog* 2012;95:199.

Kim JE, Sykes JM: Hyaluronic acid fillers: history and overview. *Facial Plast Surg* 2011;27:523.

Lee Y, Baron ED: Photodynamic therapy: current evidence and applications in dermatology. *Semin Cutan Med Surg* 2011;30:199

Matarasso SL, Glogai RG: Chemical face peels. *Dermatol Clin* 1991;9:131.

Murina AT, Kerisit KG, Boh, EE: Mechanisms of skin aging. *J Cosmet Dermatol* 2012;25:399.

Pessa JE, Rohrich RJ: Discussion: Aging changes of the midfacial fat compartments: a computed tomographic study. *Plast Reconstr Surg* 2012;129:274.

Phillips TJ, Demircay Z, Sahu M: Hormonal effects on skin aging. *Clin Geriatr Med* 2001;17:661.

Rubin MG: Trichloroacetic acid peels, in *Manual of Chemical Peels*: Superficial and Medium Depth. Philadelphia: J.B. Lippincott Company; 1995, p. 110–129.

Tansavatdi K, Mangat DS: Calcium hydroxyapatite fillers. *Facial Plast Surg* 2011;27:510.

Weiss RA, McDaniel DH, Geronemus RG, Weiss MA: Clinical trial of a novel non-thermal LED array for reversal of photoaging: clinical, histologic, and surface profilometric results. *Lasers Surg Med* 2005;36:85

Zouboulis CC, Makrantonaki E: Hormonal therapy of intrinsic aging. *Rejuvenation Res* 2012;15:302.

CHAPTER 27

IMMUNOLOGY REVIEW

KURT Q. LU
ROBERTO A. NOVOA

THE IMMUNE RESPONSE (FIG. 27-1)

- The human body can respond to antigen via innate and/or adaptive immunity
- Innate immunity (nonspecific, nonclonal, no anamnestic characteristics)
  - Characteristics
    - Immediate first-line defense against pathogens composed of 3 major components
      - ▲ Nonspecific physical and chemical barriers
      - ▲ Recruitment and activation of leukocytes
      - ▲ Release and/or activation of extracellular humoral mediators (i.e., cytokines, complement)
    - Exists prior to exposure to a given microbe or antigen (requires no previous exposure) and is rapidly available on pathogen encounter (minutes)
  - Key components
    - Physical and chemical barriers to pathogen invasion
      - ▲ Skin, mucous membranes, cilia, and secretions (mucous and sweat) cover body surfaces and prevent microorganisms and other potentially injurious agents from entering the tissues beneath
        - △ Mucus traps, dissolves, and sweeps away foreign substances
        - △ Sweat contains lactic acid and other substances that maintain the surface of the epidermis at an acidic pH, thereby decreasing colonization by bacteria and other organisms
        - △ Chemical barrier antimicrobial substances include enzymes that can directly injure or kill microbial pathogens

Complement

Alternate pathway of complement can be spontaneously activated by microbial surfaces in the absence of specific antibodies

Antimicrobial Peptides

- Produced by keratinocytes; include cathelicidins and β-defensins
  - Defensins (α or β) and cathelicidins have multiple receptor-mediated effects on the immune cells
  - Defensins are secreted by resident epithelial cells or by transient leukocytes that coat and destabilize the cell membrane of pathogens
  - Beta-Defensins interact with chemokine receptor 6 (CCR6) which results in attraction of dendritic cells and memory T cells
  - Defensins may facilitate microbial antigen delivery to dendritic cells
  - Cathelicidins are secreted by neutrophils, keratinocytes, epithelial cells, mast cells, and monocytes-macrophages

Pattern Recognition Receptors (PRRs)

- Phagocytic cell PRRs recognize highly conserved pathogen amino acid sequences and result in a variety of signals
  - Examples of PRRs:
    - *Toll-like receptors* (TLRs): mediate innate immune response in host defenses; expressed in peripheral blood leukocytes (monocytes, B cells, T cells, granulocytes, and dendritic cells). Modulate inflammatory responses via cytokine release. Activation of TLRs can lead to tissue injury (e.g., TLR2 activation by *Propionibacterium acnes* induces inflammatory responses in acne which result in tissue injury, but TLR2 activation by

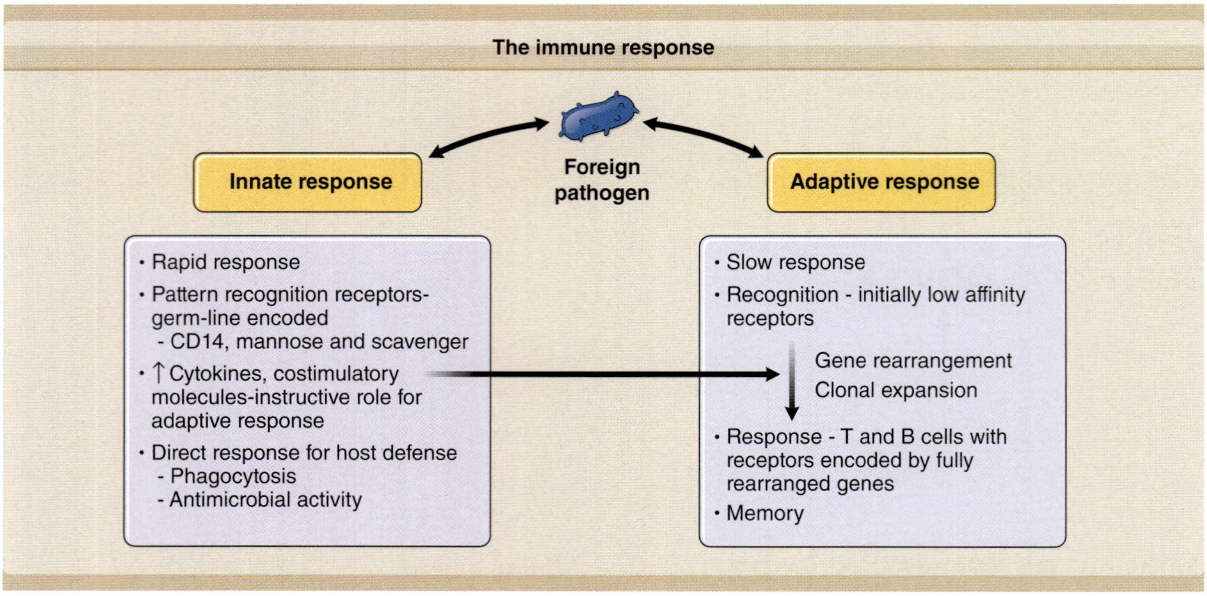

FIGURE 27-1 The immune response. (*Reprinted with permission from Goldsmith LA et al.* Fitzpatrick's Dermatology in General Medicine*, 8th Ed. New York: McGraw-Hill; 2012.*)

Staphylococcus epidermidis may also induce β-defensins that protect against infection by pathogenic bacteria.
  - Innate transmembrane receptors that recognize different types of pathogen-associated molecular patterns (PAMPs), which are molecular patterns unique to pathogens
  - Ligands include lipopolysaccharide, peptidoglycan, CpG DNA
  - Humans have at least 10 different TLRs
  - TLRs identify the nature of the pathogen and result in NFκB activation, which results in appropriate cytokine and chemokine expression, along with increased expression of additional immune system receptors
  - Triggering receptors expressed on myeloid cells (TREM): amplify innate immune responses

CELLS OF THE INNATE IMMUNE SYSTEM

- Phagocytes
  - Integral to the innate immune response and are composed of macrophages and polymorphonuclear cells; activity is sometimes regulated by TLR's and complement receptors
  - Phagocytes can also be activated by cells of the adaptive immune system: CD4+ cells can activate macrophages to produce TNF-α, IL-1, IL-12, interferon-γ, and nitric oxide
  - Phagocytic cells (macrophage, neutrophils) recognize pathogens via cell-surface PRRs
  - Macrophage mannose receptor: only on macrophages, recognizes certain sugar molecules found on bacteria and some viruses (HIV), direct phagocytic receptor (transmembrane bound)
  - Endocytosed pathogens are taken up and processed, with antigenic proteins binding in the major histocompatibility complex (MHC) II cleft and then moving to the cell surface, where they can be presented to circulating CD4+ cells.
  - A CD4 cell that recognizes the MHC II molecule will activate the macrophage, binding its CD40L to the macrophage's CD40 receptor and secreting interferon-γ, which will activate the macrophage.
  - Scavenger receptors: recognize anionic polymers and also acetylated low-density lipoproteins, involved in the removal of old red blood cells and pathogens
- Natural killer (NK) cells
  - Large granular lymphocytes: approximately 2% of the circulating lymphocytes. Kill pathogens within infected cells through perforin/granzyme- or Fas/FasL-dependent mechanisms or indirectly through cytokine secretion activated by IFN-γ, IFN-β, and macrophage-derived cytokines (TNF-α, IL-12)
  - Reside in blood, spleen, lung, and liver, gastrointestinal (GI) tract, and uterine epithelium
  - Main function is to search for and eradicate virally infected cells and neoplastic cells through both antibody-independent and antibody-dependent pathways
  - Respond early to microbial assault and interact with other cells of the innate immune system; able to nonspecifically kill target cells without prior sensitization

- While they express neither a T-cell receptor nor a B-cell receptor, NK cells demonstrate specificity in their ability to recognize targets
- NK cells recognize killer inhibitory receptors on MHC class I molecules which results in a negative signal to the NK cell. The NK cell recognizes the cell as self and does not kill the cell
- Express distinct surface molecules
  - CD16 is a receptor for the Fc portion of Ig (used in antibody-dependent cellular cytotoxicity)
  - CD56 is a neural adhesion molecule that can bind to CD56 on other cells
- Activated by IL-2, IL-7, IL-12, and IL-18
  - NK cells express the β chain of the IL-2 receptor; therefore, resting NK cells can respond directly to IL-2
  - Capable of producing cytokines following activation, such as IFN-γ and TNF-α, which can affect the proliferation and differentiation of other cell types
- Mechanisms of cytotoxicity
  - NK cells lyse targets through calcium-dependent release of preformed granules that contain perforin and granulysin
- Perforin, like complement, intercalates into the target cell membrane, forming pores
- Granulysin is a cationic protein that can induce apoptosis by initiating DNA fragmentation; may potentiate the activity of perforin in the lysis of target cells
  - Receptor-induced apoptosis
    - ▲ Activated NK cells will induce apoptosis or lysis of target cells expressing certain receptors such as FAS and TRAIL ligands death receptor-4 and death receptor-5
    - ▲ NK cells are also capable of killing specifically when they are provided with an antibody (antibody-dependent cellular cytotoxicity [ADCC]); ADCC occurs via binding of the antibody to the Fcγ receptor (CD16) located on the NK cell, leading to apoptosis of the target cell
    - ▲ NK cell cytotoxic activity can be regulated by interaction with MHC-I on the target cell via the killer cell inhibitory receptor (KIR)
    - ▲ Dendritic cells are stimulated to move from the periphery to the lymph node by TNF-α, where they mature from phagocytes into nonphagocytic efficient antigen-presenting cells
- Eosinophils
  - Develop and mature from CD34+ hematopoietic progenitor cells and are released into the circulation as mature cells
  - Bilobed nucleus
  - IL-5 (released by Th_2 cells) increases the production of mast cells in the bone marrow
  - Possess chemokine receptors that, when bound, activate, degranulate, and coordinate chemotaxis
  - Membrane bound core containing secondary granules which contain basic proteins
  - *Four basic proteins*: major basic protein (MBP), eosinophil cationic protein (ECP), eosinophil peroxidase (EPO), eosinophil-derived neurotoxin (EDN)
  - *Primary granules*: lack a core and have variable sizes; contain Charcot-Leyden crystal protein (galectin-10)
  - Cyclooxygenase and 5- and 15-lipoxygenase which are required to synthesize prostaglandins and leukotrienes
  - *Activation of eosinophils*: various mediators activate eosinophils: cytokines (TNF-α, GM-CSF, IL-3, and IL-5), complement components (C3a and C5a), lipid mediators (LTC4 and PAF [platelet-activating factor]), chemokines and IgA and IgG Fc receptors. CC chemokine subfamily (CCL5, CCL7, CCL11, CCL14, and CCL240) bind to the chemokine receptor CCR3
  - Eosinophil activating cytokines IL-3, IL-5, and GM-CSF enhance cell survival, eosinophil maturation, chemotactic responses, and leukotriene production
  - *Types of eosinophil activation*: expression of P selectin on endothelial surface, induction by nonspecific activators such as IL-1 and TNF- α, induction by IL-4 and IL-13
  - After cytokine and chemokine activation, the high affinity IgE receptors (FceRI) are expressed along with an increase in complement receptors
  - Degranulation releases major basic protein, which causes degranulation of mast cells and basophils
- Basophils
  - Growth factors include IL3, IL-5, and GM-CSF
  - TGF-β IL-3 suppresses eosinophil differentiation and promotes basophil differentiation
  - Eotaxins attract and degranulate (release histamine and IL-4)
  - Pathogens coated with fragments of the complement protein C3 bind strongly to B cells
- Keratinocytes
  - Can activate an immune and/or inflammatory response through secretion of cytokines, arachadonic acid metabolites, complement components, and antimicrobial peptides
  - Following appropriate stimuli, the following cytokine response may occur:
    - Initiation of inflammation: IL-1, TNF- α, IL-6
    - Modulation of langerhan cells: IL-1, GM-CSF, TNF-α, IL-10, IL-15
      - ▲ T-cell activation: IL-15, IL-18
      - ▲ T-cell inhibition: IL-10, TGF-β
      - ▲ Th_1 response: IL-12, IL-18, Th_2 response: thymic stromal lymphopoietin or Th_{17}: IL-23

- Bridging innate immunity to adaptive immunity
  - Macrophages and dendritic cells present antigens to T cells
  - Interaction of PAMPs and TLRs on the surface of dendritic cells triggers secretion of innate immune cytokines (INF-α, INF-β, IL-12, TNF-α) and chemokines, which may affect both T and B cells

ADAPTIVE IMMUNITY

- An antigen-specific immune response resulting in the activation of humoral and cell-mediated immunity, mediated by specific antibodies
- T-lymphocytes and B-lymphocytes differentiate from a common lymphoid stem cell in the bone marrow
- B-lymphocytes (B cells): antibody-producing cells
  - Represent 5 to 10% of the lymphocytes found in the blood
  - Express cell membrane immunoglobulin (Ig): majority expresses both IgM and IgD
  - A small minority of B cells expresses surface IgG or IgA
  - Possess a variety of receptors on their surface (complement receptors, class I and II MHC molecule receptors)
  - Analogous to T cells, B cells have specific antigen receptors, which are immunoglobulins (Ig)
  - On activation and cross-linking of surface Ig by specific antigen, B cells undergo proliferation and differentiation to produce plasma cells
  - Plasma cells are nondividing, specialized cells whose only function is to secrete Ig
  - Immunoglobulins (Igs) (Fig. 27-2)
    - Proteins with exquisite specificity for antigen achieved by a mechanism of genetic recombination unique to Ig and T-cell receptor genes
    - The antigen-binding site consists of a highly variable sequence created by the juxtaposition of 2 constituent polypeptides: heavy (H) chain and 1 of 2 alternative light (L) chains, κ, or λ
    - These polypeptides can be divided into 2 segments: antigen-binding amino-terminal *variable domain* and 1 or more carboxy-terminal *constant (nonvariable)* domains that are generally responsible for biologic functions and activities of the molecules
    - Ig antigen receptor
      - ▲ A virtually limitless array of antigen-specific receptors is possible
      - ▲ The great variability is accomplished by recombination of genomic segments that encode the variable portions of Ig
      - ▲ The products of these rearranged genes provide the B cell with its own unique receptor

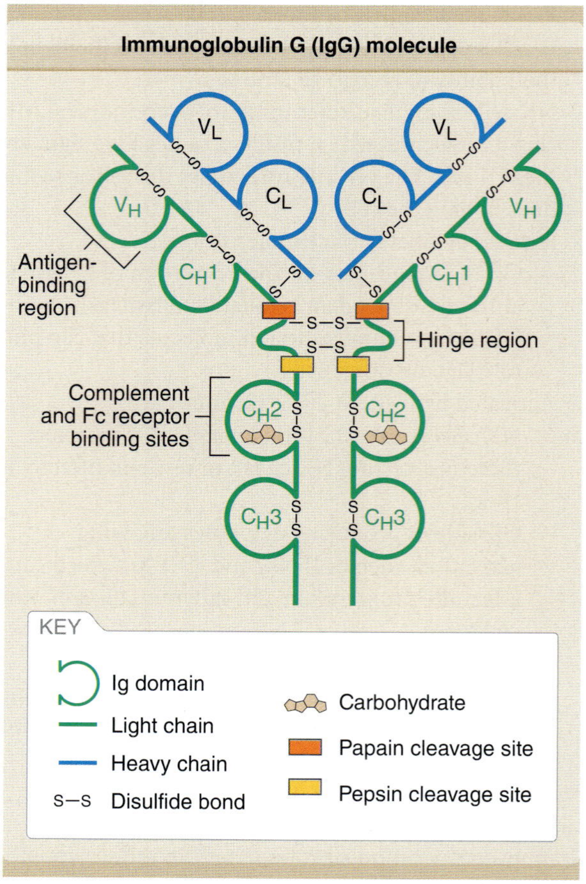

FIGURE 27-2 Immunoglobulin (Ig) molecule. (*Reprinted with permission from Goldsmith LA et al.* Fitzpatrick's Dermatology in General Medicine, *8th Ed. New York: McGraw-Hill, 2012.*)

      - ▲ The mature receptor consists of the products of 2 or 3 such rearranged segments
        - △ V (variable) and J (joining) for IgL (light) chains
        - △ V, D (diversity), and J for IgH (heavy) chains
      - ▲ DNA rearrangement
        - △ Controlled by recombinases
        - △ Sequential and carefully regulated process
        - △ Leads to translation of 1 receptor of unique specificity for any given B-lymphocyte
        - △ Unique specificity is achieved through a process termed *allelic exclusion* (only 1 member of a pair of allelic genes potentially contributing to an Ig is rearranged at a time)
      - ▲ Somatic hypermutation
        - △ A feature of the V-region construction that is unique to B cells
        - △ As antigen is introduced into the germinal centers of lymphoid follicles through

dendritic cells, mature B cells remain genetically responsive to the antigenic environment
    - △ Higher-affinity B cells are preferentially activated at exposure to the antigen and proliferate
    - △ These higher-affinity B cells outcompete other B cells. As a result, the average affinity of antibodies produced during the course of an immune response increases (termed *affinity maturation*)
- Secretion of Ig molecules
    - ▲ The cell-surface antigen receptors can be secreted in large quantities as antibody molecules
    - ▲ The effector functions of antibodies can be carried out in solution or at the surface of other cells
    - ▲ Secretion is accomplished by alternative splicing of Ig transcripts to include or exclude a transmembrane segment of the Ig heavy chains
- Ig classes (isotypes) (Table 27-1)
    - ▲ Five major classes in order of abundance: IgG, IgM, IgA, IgD, and IgE
    - ▲ Determined by the sequence of the constant region of its heavy chain (Ch)
    - ▲ Isotype or class switching: B cell can change the class of antibody molecule that it synthesizes by using different Ch genes without changing its unique antibody specificity
    - ▲ IgG1 through IgG4 are 4 subclasses of IgG, and these are determined largely by differences in the constant region of the heavy chains.
        - △ IgG1 is the most common subclass
        - △ IgG4 is the rarest subclass, and does not appear to activate complement or bind well to the Fc receptor. It may be implicated in variety of autoimmune diseases, ranging from pemphigus and pemphigoid to fibrosing diseases with high levels of IgG4, such as Reidel thyroiditis, retroperitoneal fibrosis, and autoimmune pancreatitis.

- T lymphocytes
    - T-cell development: progenitor cells exit the bone marrow and undergo further maturation and selection in the thymus; they express antigen receptors needed for self/nonself discrimination (Fig. 27-3)
        - In the thymus: T cells rearrange their specific T-cell antigen receptors (TCRs) and then express CD3 along with the TCRs on their surface
        - The TCR for antigen is a heterodimeric membrane molecule expressed exclusively by T-lymphocytes
        - T-cell subpopulations are based on surface expression of CD4 and CD8, as well as by their function in the immune response
        - Skin contains twice as many T cells as are circulating in the blood
    - *Helper T cells* (Th cells): express CD4 surface molecules and recognize antigen bound to class II MHC molecules
    - Play a central role in the initiation and regulation of immune responses through the secretion of cytokines and activation of macrophages
    - Important effectors of cell-mediated immunity
    - Essential contributors to the generation of chronic inflammatory responses
    - Cytotoxic activity either through the elaboration of cytotoxic cytokines (i.e., lymphotoxin, tumor necrosis

TABLE 27-1 Classes of Immunoglobulin

Characteristic	IgG	IgA	IgM	IgD	IgE
Heavy chain	γ	α	μ	σ	ε
Light chain	κ, λ	κ, λ	κ, λ	κ, λ	κ, λ
J chain	–	+	+	+	–
Molecular weight	150,000	160,0002–400,000	900,000	180,000	190,000
Serum half-life (days)	23	6	5	3	2
Serum concentration	1,200	140–400	20–50	4	0.02
Complement fixation	+	±	+	–	–
Placental transfer	+	–	–	–	–

Used with permission from Freedberg IM et al.: Fitzpatrick's Dermatology in General Medicine, *5th Eed. New York: McGraw-Hill;, 1999, p. 380.*

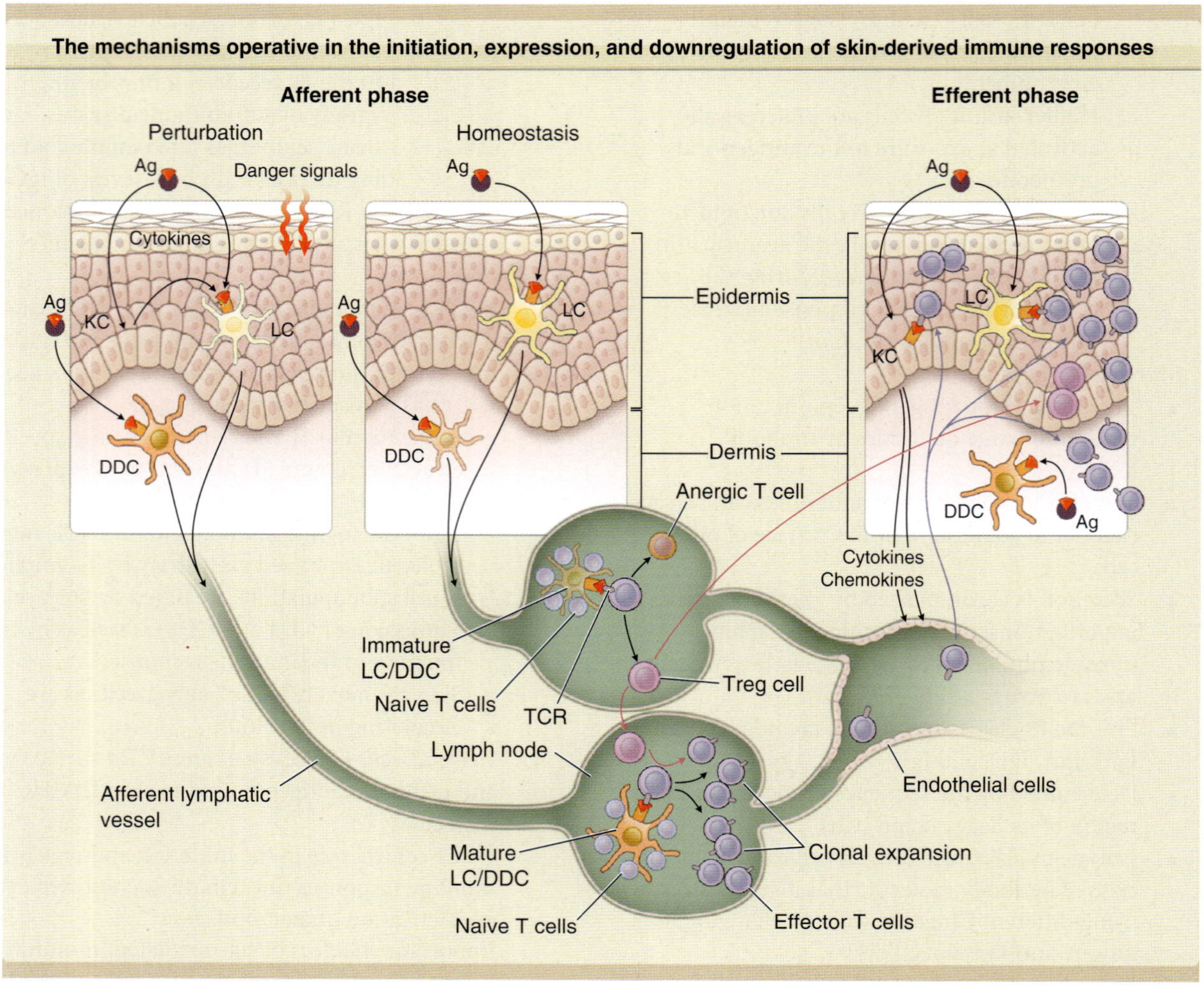

FIGURE 27-3 T-cell development. (*Reprinted with permission from Goldsmith LA et al.* Fitzpatrick's Dermatology in General Medicine, *8th Ed. New York: McGraw-Hill; 2012.*)

factor (TNF)-α) or directly through interaction with antigen bound to MHC class II molecules

- Function depends on the cytokine profile produced, and falls into 1 of several categories
- Naïve CD4+ cells differentiate into immature effector T cells (T_H0). depending on activation signals and the cytokine milieu in the microenvironment, T_H0 can differentiate into several different classes of cells: (1) T_H1 (2) T_H2, (3) T_H17, (4) regulatory T cells, (5) natural killer T cells (see section "Cells of Innate Immune System" discussed earlier)
  (1) T_H1 cells: produce primarily IFN-γ, IL-2, and TNF-α; important in cell-mediated immunity to intracellular pathogens. Excess activation may be linked to significant inflammation and tissue destruction. The ulcers generated by cutaneous and mucosal leishmaniasis are examples of pronounced T_H1 responses (see Fig. 27-3)
  (2) T_H2 cells: produce predominantly IL-4, IL-5, IL-6, IL-10, IL-13, and IL-15; they predominate in immediate or allergic type I hypersensitivity
  (3) T_H17 cells: produced directly from naïve CD4+ cells exposed to a particular cytokine milieu, including TGF-β, IL-6, IL-21, and IL-23
    - ▲ These cells have been described in the past 10 years and are important in protecting against extracellular pathogens and some viral infections
    - ▲ T_H17 cells appear to play a role in the recruitment and activation of neutrophils
    - ▲ The cells can produce IL-17A, IL-17F, IL-21, IL-22, and IL-23
    - ▲ IL-23 activates IL-23 receptors on Th_{17} cells through RORγt, helping to maintain the Th_{17} response
      - △ Ustekinumab, a new antibody used in psoriasis, targets the p40 subunit of IL-12 and IL-23, with its function in large part due to downregulation of the Th_{17} pathway
    - ▲ Many of these cytokines function by inducing transcription of signal transducer and activator of transcription 3 (STAT3)

- ▲ Genetic defects in STAT3, result in autosomal dominant hyper IgE syndrome (previously known as Job syndrome)
  - △ Recurrent "cold" abscesses, without adequate inflammatory response
    - *Staphylococcus*
    - *Candida*
  - △ Pulmonary infections resulting in pneumatoceles
  - △ Retained deciduous teeth
  - △ Facial dysmorphism
  - △ Dermatitis, often present at birth
- ▲ DOCK8 (belonging to a guanine nucleotide exchange factor family) deficiency causes a phenotypically similar clinical picture, with elevated IgE levels, recurrent infections, atopic dermatitis, with a few key differences
  - △ Widespread, persistent viral infections (HSV, HPV, molluscum)
  - △ No dysmorphism or retained deciduous teeth
  - △ Autosomal recessive
  - △ Severe asthma, allergies, anaphylactic reactions
- ▲ T_H17 cells appear to play an important role in a variety of autoimmune diseases, ranging from psoriasis to rheumatoid arthritis to multiple sclerosis

(4) Regulatory T cells: (Treg cells)

- ▲ Function as suppressors or downregulators of immune responses
- ▲ Molecular basis of this activity is being defined. Several classes of regulatory T cells have been described
- ▲ These cells express CD4 and CD25 (IL-2 receptor). Naturally occurring circulating CD4+/CD25^{hi} cells are the best characterized population
  - △ The CD4+/CD25hi regulatory T cells have been found to express *FOXP3*, a gene encoding a transcription factor important in the regulation of regulatory T cells
  - △ Mutation in *FOXP3* in humans leads to a rare disease with regulatory cell dysfunction called IPEX (immune dysregulation polyendocrinopathy enteropathy X-linked)
  - △ Mechanism of suppression is via direct contact with target cells

- Other regulatory T-cell populations have been described and have been generated in vitro including
  - Th_3 cells which are CD4+. Mechanism of suppression is via production of IL-TGF-β
  - Tr1 cells which are CD4+/CD25low
  - CD8+ cells have also been described. Mechanism of suppression is via production of IL-10 and TGF-β
  - CD28−/CD8+ regulatory T cells. Mechanism of suppression is thought to be via direct cell contact and also via induction of regulatory receptors on other cells
  - Thought to involve the production of nonspecific inhibitory cytokines
  - Currently some investigations examining the role of low-dose IL-2 in conditions such as graft-versus-host disease, based on a mechanism of selective activation of $CD25_{high}$ T reg cells
- *Cytotoxic T cells* (Tc cells): cytotoxic effectors that can target infected or damaged host cells
- Cytotoxic CD8+ T cells can further differentiate into Tc1 or Tc2 cells
  - Express CD8 surface molecules and recognize antigen bound to class I MHC molecules
  - Capable of direct killing of target cells expressing an appropriate viral peptide bound to a self-MHC class I molecule
  - Highly specific process that requires direct apposition of Tc cell and target cell membrane
  - Following killing, Tc cell is capable of detaching from target and seeking another target cell
  - Destruction of target cells requires the insertion of perforins from the Tc cell into the target cell membrane that results in fragmentation of target cell nuclear DNA (apoptotic)

Cell-Mediated and Humoral Immune Response

- Antibodies, dissolved in blood, lymph, and other body fluids, bind the antigen and trigger a response to the antigen (i.e., release cytokines)
- T-cell response
  - Viruses and intracellular parasite antigens are processed into peptides within antigen-presenting cells (APCs) and are bound to the heavy chain of an MHC class I and presented to a CD8+ (cytotoxic) T cell
  - If a specific antigen encounters its specific T-cell receptor, IL-2 is released, and T-cell activation, along with expansion of the antigen-specific cytotoxic T-cell (Tc) line, follows
  - If an antigen-specific Tc cell encounters a cell expressing its specific antigen, the activation signal that ensues results in exocytosis of granzymes (granules containing enzymes), perforins, cytolysins, lymphotoxins, and serine esterases, which kill the APC
- Extracellular antigens
  - Taken up by APCs by pinocytosis and then processed into peptides
  - Peptides are presented in the context of an MHC class II molecule to a CD4+ T cell
- After activation, CD4 and CD8 cells may differentiate toward T_H1 or T_H2 cytokine profiles depending on cytokine milieu
  - *T_H1 cell activation*

- Goal: macrophage activation and increased cell-mediated immunity
- T_H1 cytokine profile: IL-2, IFN-γ, TNF-α, and IL-12
  - ▲ IL-2: T- and B-cell activation
  - ▲ IFN-γ: activator of macrophages and NK cells
  - ▲ TNF-α: activates macrophages and stimulates the acute-phase response along with IL-1
  - ▲ IL-12 activates CD8+ (Tc) cell proliferation
  - ▲ Antigen binding to receptors results in release lytic agents (perforins, cytolysins, lymphotoxins)
- *T_H2 cell activation*
  - Goal: B-cell activation
  - IL-2 production by Th_1 cells induces the CD4+ Th_2 cells to transform, differentiate, and divide
  - Th_2 cytokine profile: IL-4, IL-5, IL-10, and IL-13
    - ▲ IL-4: promotes the synthesis of antibodies by stimulating B-cell differentiation
    - ▲ Downregulates IFN-γ; therefore, can suppress cell-mediated immunity
    - ▲ Can cause production of IgE
    - ▲ IL-5: helps with B-cell differentiation
    - ▲ Facilitates IgA synthesis
    - ▲ Stimulates growth of eosinophils
    - ▲ IL-4, IL-10, and IL-13 can inhibit Th_1 cell release of IFN-γ and IL-2; thus capable of suppressing cell-mediated immunity
    - ▲ ADCC reactions
    - ▲ Target cell is linked to the T cell by an antibody bridge
    - ▲ Fab portion of the antibody binds to a specific membrane antigen on the target cell
    - ▲ Fc portion of the antibody binds to the Fc receptor on the T cell
- B-cell response
  - Like T cells, B cells contain membrane bound IgM antibody specific for the antigen epitope
  - Primary immune response: initial encounter
    - Antigen bound to the APC receptor along with cytokines IL-2 and IL-4 (stimuli for T cells) triggers the antigen-specific B cell to differentiate and divide
    - IgM is secreted initially, and subsequent gene arrangements result in a switch to IgG, IgA, and IgE
    - B memory cells of all classes are generated and migrated to various lymphoid tissues, where they have extended survival
    - Plasma cell: B cell that secretes antibodies
  - Secondary immune response: subsequent exposure to the same antigen
    - Activation of antigen-specific B cell results in more efficient antibody synthesis and faster isotype switching from IgM to IgG
    - A greater amount of IgG with higher affinity for the antigen during subsequent encounters
    - Predominance of IgA secretion in mucosal tissues

Myeloid Progenitor Cell

- Dendritic cells express costimulatory molecules and cytokines in response to pathogen antigens
  - Proteoglycans first recognized by PRRs
  - Then costimulatory molecules and cytokines are upregulated via toll-like receptor-2

Langerhans Cells and Other Dendritic Cells

- Bone marrow derived leukocytes that can migrate and present antigen
- *Langerhans cells* (LCs) are found in all stratified squamous epithelia
- The following molecules are expressed by LCs
  - Langerin (CD207): calcium dependent lectin; helps identify LC cells, CD1a, MHC class II antigens: HLA-DR, HLA-DP, HLA-DQ; and CD39
  - Birbeck granules: pentilaminar cytoplasmic structures that appear as a tennis racket shape with electron microscopy
  - LCs are activated under inflammatory conditions. LCs express chemokine receptors CCR2 and CCR6 (their ligands are secreted by endothelial cells and keratinocytes)
- *Dendritic leukocytes* (DCs) are found in the dermis
  - Express the following molecules: CD1b and CD1c and factor XIIIa, MHC class II molecules DEC205/CD205
- DCs enter the skin secondary to CCR2-dependent cell migration; other dendritic cells also migrate to the skin (plasmacytoid DCs and inflammatory dendritic epidermal cells)
- Dendritic cells: stimulate antigen-specific responses in naïve, resting T cells. (T cells are not able to recognize soluble protein antigen)
- CD1-dependent antigen presentation: CD1 family expressed by LCs and DCs
- Antigens presented to T cells bound to MCH class II molecules are recognized by CD4 cells, while antigens bound to MCH class I are recognized by CD8+ cells
- Second signals: MHC-peptide complexes provide the first signal to T cells, but this first signal is insufficient for the full activation of naïve T cells, costimulatory molecules deliver second signals which are induced by surface receptors triggered by ligands secreted by other somatic cells or by microbial products
- Examples of costimulatory molecules and their ligands
  - ICAM-1 binds to LFA-1 and LFA-3 (ligand of T cell expressed CD2), CD24/CD24L, CD40/CD40L, CD70/CD70L, receptor activator of nuclear factor KB (RANK)/RANKL
  - B7-CD28 is a prototypical costimulatory molecule, with B7 expressed on the APC and CD28 on the T cell (see Fig. 27-3)
  - CTLA-4 (CD152) is a receptor on T cells that can inhibit CD28 and block the costimulatory response.

It binds to B7 and competes with CD28, but also triggers downstream inhibition of T-cell activation
- CTLA-4 is often upregulated 48 hours after T-cell activation and serves to downregulate the T cell's responsiveness
- Abatacept and belatacept are fusion proteins of CTLA-4 and IgG that bind to B7 and prevent costimulation and immune activation. They are meant to block CD28-B7 binding and downregulate a hyperactive immune response
  - Abatacept is currently approved for rheumatoid arthritis
  - belatacept is currently in trials for organ transplant graft survival extension
- Ipilimumab is an antibody to CTLA-4 that prevents downregulation of the immune response
  - It increases the likelihood of costimulation and helps prevent the immune tolerance that some cancers create
  - It is FDA approved for use in metastatic melanoma, but causes side effects such as autoimmune diarrhea, hypophysisitis, and vitiligo
- The programmed death-1 (PD-1) receptor and PD-1 ligand (PD-1L) are another set of interacting cell surface proteins that have important biological implications
  - PD-1 belongs to the family of CD28 and CTLA-4 molecules, but is expressed on activated T cells, macrophages, and B cells
  - PD-1L is expressed on inflamed tissues and can bind to PD-1, downregulating the immune response. This has several important contexts
    - Chronic viral infections (HCV, HIV) often result in chronic inflammation and PD-1 activation, downregulating the immune response and leading to T cell dysfunction and "exhaustion"
    - Cancer cells can express high levels of PD-1, helping to shut down the immune response. Novel anti-PD-1 and anti-PD-1L antibodies are showing promise for immunologic treatment of advanced malignancies

CYTOKINES

- Polypeptides serve as intercellular messengers in order to mediate immune responses
  - Autocrine in nature: affect the cell that releases the cytokine
  - Paracrine in nature: affect the adjacent cells
  - Endocrine in nature: affect distant cells
- Produced by inflammatory cells (lymphocytes, monocytes) as well as resident cells in the skin (keratinocytes, Langerhans cells, and endothelial cells)
- Variable effects: see Table 27-2 on specific cytokines, their actions, and major sources of the cytokines
- Involved in innate immunity (occurs without the activation of B or T cells) or adaptive immunity (depends on a B or T cell reacting to a specific antigen)
- Primary cytokines: can initiate all events required to bring about leukocyte infiltration in tissues (i.e., IL-1 and TNF), can be viewed as part of the innate immune system
- Secondary cytokines: induced after stimulation by IL-1 and/or TNF family molecules Th_{17}: IL-17
- Jak/STAT pathway: common cell surface to nucleus pathway used by the majority of cytokines. Jaks (Janus family kinases) are upregulated after stimulation of cytokine receptors (such as IFN-γ), Jak kinases phosphorylate STATs (signal transducers and activators of transcription) through Src homology 2 (SH2) domains; STATs translocate to the nucleus and stimulate transcription of specific genes (see Fig. 27-3)
- Jaks play an important role in the signal transduction of inflammatory cytokines involved in the T_H1 and T_H17 pathways
- Patients with germline Jak3 inactivating mutations have severe combined immune deficiency with no T cells, no NK cells, and present but nonfunctioning B cells. Jak3 appears to be preferentially expressed in hematopoietic cells.
- Activating somatic Jak2 mutations (particularly V617F) have been found in essential thrombocythemia, polycythemia vera, and myelofibrosis
- Oral Jak2 inhibitors have been developed for these diseases, but because of their role in inhibiting cytokine-related signal transduction, they are finding applications in inflammatory diseases
- Ruloxitinib is a Jak2 inhibitor with some potential promise in psoriasis, and tofacitinib is a Jak1 and Jak3 inhibitor that has efficacy in rheumatoid arthritis and possibly in other autoimmune disease as well
- The IL-1 family shares a common signaling domain with the TLRs: Toll/L-1 receptor (TIR) domain. When activated by TIR domain-containing proteins (i.e., MyD88), TIR will activate IL-1R-associated kinase (IRAK) and ultimately activation of nuclear factor κB (NFκB), IL-1 accessory protein (RAcP), and TNF receptor-associated factor (TRAF)
- NFκB
- TNF-α can trigger apoptosis and/or nuclear factor KB activation
- Medications that target cytokines include receptor fusion proteins (etanercept), monoclonal antibodies (infliximab and adalimumab), and receptor antagonists

CHEMOKINES

- Class of cytokines that express both chemoattractant and cytokinetic properties
  - Leukocytes can respond to a panel of different chemokines
  - Neutrophils are recruited first, while monocytes and immature dendritic cells are recruited later

TABLE 27-2 Cytokines of Particular Importance for Cutaneous Biology

Cytokine	Major Sources	Responsive Cells	Features of Interest	Clinical Relevance
IL-1α	Epithelial cells	Infiltrating leukocytes	Activate from stored in keratinocytes	IL-1Ra used to treat rheumatoid arthritis
IL-1β	Myeloid cells	Infiltrating leukocytes	Caspase 1 cleavage required for activation	IL-1Ra used to treat rheumatoid arthritis
IL-2	Activated T cells	Activated T cells, Treg cells	Autocrine facto for activated T cells	IL-2 fusion toxin targets CTCL
IL-4	Activated Th_2 cells, NKT cells	Lymphocytes, endothelial cells, keratinocytes	Causes B-cell class switching and Th_2 differentiation	—
IL-5	Activated Th_2 cells, mast cells	B cells, eosinophils	Regulates eosinophil response to parasites	Anti-IL-5 depletes eosinophils
IL-6	Activated myeloid cells, fibroblasts, endothelial cells	B cells, myeloid cells, hepatocytes	Triggers acute-phase response, promotes immunoglobulin synthesis	—
IL-10	T cells, NK cells	Myeloid and lymphoid cells	Inhibits innate and acquired immune response	—
IL-12	Activated APCs	Th_1 cells	Promotes Th_1 differentiation, share p40 subunit with IL-23	Anti-p40 inhibits Crohn disease and psoriasis
IL-13	Activated Th_2 cells	Monocytes, keratinocytes, endothelial cells	Mediates tissue response to parasites	—
IL-17	Activated Th_{17} cells	Multiple cell types	Mediates autoimmune diseases	Potential drug target in autoimmune disease
IL-23	Activated dendritic cells	Memory T cells, Th_{17} cells	Directs Th_{17} differentiation, mediates autoimmune disease	Anti-p40 inhibits Crohn disease and psoriasis
TNF-α	Activated myeloid, lymphoid, and epithelial cells	Infiltrating leukocytes	Mediated inflammation	Anti-TNF-α effective in psoriasis
IFN-α and IFN-β	Plasmacytoid dendritic cells	Most cell types	Major part of antiviral response	Elicited by topical imiquimod
IFN-γ	Activated Th_1 cells, CD8 T cells, NK cells, dendritic cells	Macrophages, dendritic cells, naive T cells	Macrophage activation, specific isotype switching	IFN-γ used to treat chronic granulomatous disease

APC, = antigen-presenting cell; CTCL, = cutaneous T-cell lymphoma; IFN, = interferon; IL =, interleukin; NK =, natural killer; NKT, = natural killer T cell; Th =, T helper; TMF =, tumor necrosis facto; Treg =, T regulatory.

- Structures contain a 4-cysteine motif with a disulfide bond between cysteines 1,3 and 2,4 along with an N-terminus critical for receptor recognition and activation
- Four subfamilies, based on the position of the first 2 of 4 conserved cysteines (α, β, γ, and κ)
- Multiple cell types can produce the same chemokine, and a cell can produce many different chemokines in response to a single stimulus
- Chemokine receptors
  - Members of the large family of G protein–coupled receptors possessing 7 transmembrane-spanning domains
  - One receptor is capable of binding to various chemokines
  - Binding of the ligand to the chemokine receptor induces conformational changes in the receptor and leads to activation of G proteins
  - The G protein causes exchange of GDP for GTP and begins a chain of events resulting in intracellular signaling responses
- Biologic effects of chemokines
  - Influence leukocyte trafficking at all stages of maturation
  - Regulate cells trafficking within primary and secondary lymphoid organs (i.e., from bone marrow to the spleen, lymph node, or thymus)
  - Control the type of inflammatory infiltrate at a site of inflammation
  - Regulate the expression and activity of adhesion molecules on the leukocyte surface to increase the adhesion of leukocytes to activated endothelium
  - Recruitment and activation of neutrophils and mononuclear cells to sites of inflammation
  - Regulate proliferation of subsets of mature stem cells and immature progenitor cells
- Secretion of chemokines
  - Released by endothelial cells, leukocytes, and tissue cells at the sites of inflammation
  - Locally retained on cell surface proteoglycans, establishing a chemokine chemical gradient that begins at the endothelium surface and increases as the cell approaches the focus of inflammation
  - Thought to be upregulated in inflammatory foci and certain inflammatory diseases (i.e., glomerulonephritis, rheumatoid arthritis, ulcerative colitis, and Crohn disease)

EICOSANOIDS

- Large, complex family of immunomodulatory and vasoactive compounds derived from arachadonic acid (AA) generated by mast cells, basophils, eosinophils, and mononuclear leukocytes
- General
  - Peroxidation of AA by phospholipases generates prostaglandins (via the cyclooxygenase [COX] pathway) or thromboxanes and leukotrienes (via the lipooxygenase [LO] pathway)
    - Play a key role in inflammatory and anaphylactoid responses
- Arachadonic acid
  - Polyunsaturated fatty acid with 20 carbon atoms and 4 double bonds
  - Resides in cell membrane lipids
  - Derived from dietary sources or synthesized by desaturation and elongation of linoleic acid
- Cyclooxygenase (COX) pathway
  - Key enzyme in the pathway, cyclooxygenase (COX), has 2 different isoforms
    - COX-1: constitutively expressed in cells and associated with cellular homeostasis
    - COX-2: requires specific induction, upregulated in inflammatory conditions, and associated with synthesis of proinflammatory prostaglandins
    - COX-1 and COX-2 are inhibited by nonsteroidal anti-inflammatory drugs
    - COX-2 inhibitors were specific for COX-2 and had fewer GI side effects, but several drugs were linked with increased risk of death and cardiovascular events
  - Derivatives of the cyclooxygenase pathway
    - Prostaglandins (PGs)
      - ▲ *PGD2*
        - △ Released by activated mast cells
        - △ Generated very rapidly after IgE-dependent activation
        - △ Enhances venular permeability
        - △ Promotes leukocyte adherence to vascular endothelial cells
        - △ Coronary and pulmonary vasoconstrictor
        - △ Peripheral vasodilator
        - △ Potent inhibitor of platelet aggregation
        - △ Chemokinetic for neutrophils and in conjunction with LTD4 can induce the accumulation of neutrophils in the skin
        - △ Important hypotensive effects, particularly in mastocytosis, suggesting that it is probably an important contributor to the anaphylactic response
        - △ Metabolite of PGD2 is elevated in patients with systemic mastocytosis
      - ▲ *PGE2*
        - △ Proinflammatory effects
        - △ Released in response to infection with ameba (specifically *Entamoeba histolytica*) and parasites
        - △ Released by endothelial cells following trauma, leading to tissue inflammation

      - △ Plays an important role in the secondary immunosuppression following surgical stress
      - △ Synthesized by the synovial lining in rheumatoid arthritis
    - ▲ *PGI2 and PGE2*
      - △ Potent vasodilators
      - △ Enhance capillary permeability and edema formation
- Derivatives of lipoxygenase (LO) pathway
  - *Thromboxanes/thromboxane A2*
    - Promotes platelet aggregation, bronchoconstriction, and vasoconstriction
    - Contributes to the pulmonary hypertension and acute tubular necrosis that occurs in shock
    - Predominately found in platelets and monocytes
    - Aspirin inhibits thromboxane in platelets
  - *Leukotrienes*
    - Mediate wheal and flare reactions, edema formation, and bronchial constriction
    - Combined with histamine can result in hypotension
    - One of the major inflammatory mediators involved in asthma pathogenesis
    - Enhances airway hyperresponsiveness and smooth muscle hypertrophy
    - Causes mucus hypersecretion and mucosal edema
    - Induces influx of eosinophils into the airway tissue key players in anaphylactic reactions and IgE-mediated syndromes
    - Mediators of the vascular sequelae of anaphylaxis as well as of shock states resulting from sepsis or tissue injury
    - Leukotriene receptor antagonist montelukast can be used in asthma
    - LTB4
    - Predominantly formed and released by neutrophils
    - Neutrophil chemoattractant
    - LTC4
    - Derived from activated mast cells, basophils, and eosinophils
    - Potent vasodilator

COMPLEMENT

- General
  - Group of plasma and cell membrane proteins that play a role in inflammation, tissue injury, hemostasis, and immune response to antigens
  - Some of the proteins exist as precursor (inactive) enzymes that are cleaved by proteolysis; products then act as a catalyst for the next step in the cascade
  - The central step of the complement pathway is the generation of C3b cleavage by C3 convertases and subsequent assembly of C5b-9, the membrane attack complex (MAC)
- Main functions
  - Lysis of cells
  - Generate inflammatory mediators and chemotactic fragments
  - Opsonization for enhanced phagocytosis
- Three pathways for complement activation
- Classical pathway
  - Activated primarily by antibody-antigen complexes
  - Also activated by oligosaccarides, porins from gram-negative bacteria, ligand-bound C-reactive protein
  - The starting point of the classical pathway is C1
  - Steps of classical pathway (Fig. 27-4)
    - ▲ Aggregation of IgG or IgM activates C1
    - ▲ C1 is a calcium-dependent complex of 3 subunits: C1q, C1r, and C1s
    - ▲ Activated C1 then cleaves C4 to C4a and C4b
    - ▲ C4a is a weak anaphylatoxin
    - ▲ C4b binds C2 in the presence of Mg^{2+}
    - ▲ C1 cleaves the attached C2 into C2b and C2a
    - ▲ C2b is released, cleaved by plasmin, and has kinin-like activity
    - ▲ C2a stays bound to C4 to form C4b2a—the classical pathway C3 convertase that generates C3
  - Alternative pathway
    - Activation usually occurs independent of antibody
    - May be activated by bacterial surfaces, virus-infected cells, certain viruses, abnormal erythrocytes, and lymphoblastoid cell lines
    - The starting point of the alternative pathway is C3b
    - Steps of the alternative pathway (Fig. 27-5)
      - ▲ Starts with internal hydrolysis of C3 on interaction with water to form C3 (H_2O)
      - ▲ C3 (H_2O) then binds factor B and magnesium
      - ▲ Factor D then cleaves the bound factor B into Ba and Bb
      - ▲ Ba is released
      - ▲ Bb stays bound to C3 (H_2O) to form C3 (H_2O), which is the initial C3 convertase of the alternative pathway that cleaves C3
      - ▲ C3 is cleaved to C3a and C3b
      - ▲ C3a is released and becomes a potent anaphylatoxin
      - ▲ C3b binds factor B in the presence of magnesium, and factor B is cleaved by factor D into Bb and Ba
      - ▲ Ba is released
      - ▲ Bb stays bound to form C3bBb, the C3 convertase of the alternative pathway
  - Lectin pathway
    - C4 activation can be achieved without antibody and C1 participation
    - Pathway is initiated by 3 proteins: a mannan-binding lectin (MBL) (mannan-binding protein [MBP]),

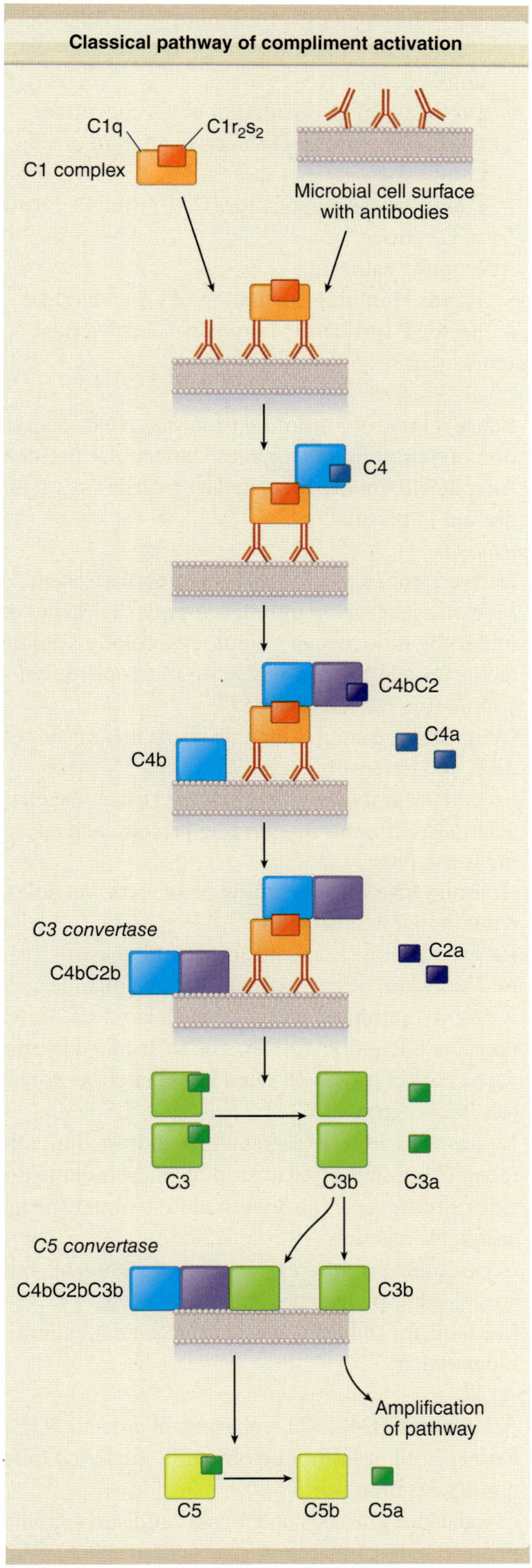

FIGURE 27-4 Classical pathway of complement activation. (*Reprinted with permission from Goldsmith LA et al.* Fitzpatrick's Dermatology in General Medicine, *8th Ed. New York: McGraw-Hill; 2012.*)

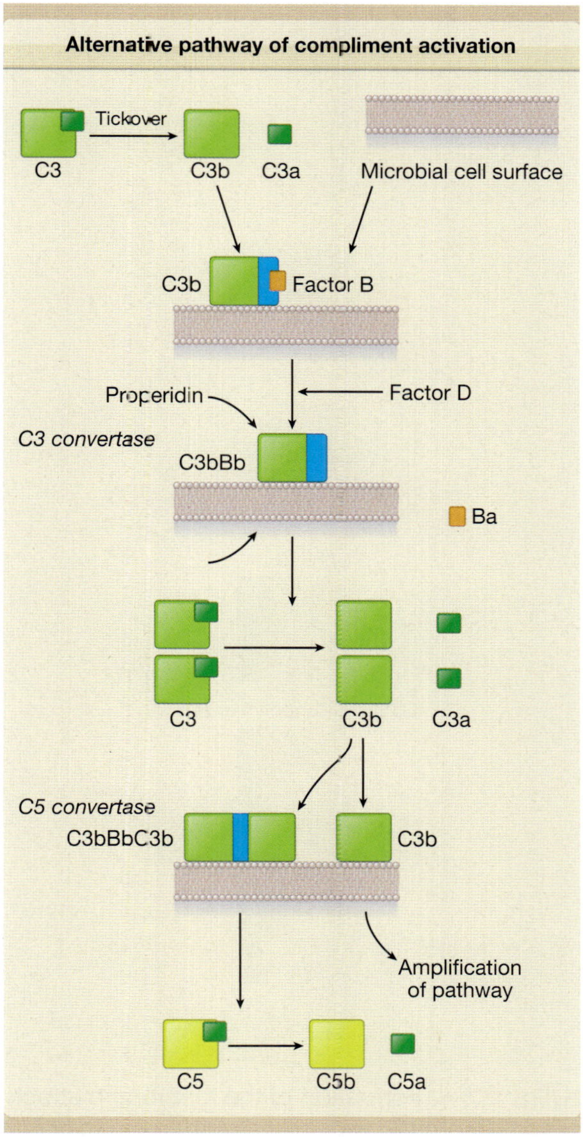

FIGURE 27-5 Alternate pathway of complement activation. (*Reprinted with permission from Goldsmith LA et al.* Fitzpatrick's Dermatology in General Medicine, *8th Ed. New York: McGraw-Hill; 2012.*)

which interacts with 2 mannan-binding lectin–associated serine proteases (MASP and MADSP2), analogous to C1r and C1s
  - This interaction generates a complex analogous to C1qrs and leads to antibody-independent activation of the classical pathway
- Common portion of pathway/membrane attack complex (Fig. 27-6)
  - At this point, the classical, alternative, and lectin pathways all have generated C3b using their respective C3 convertases, C4b2a, and C3bBb
  - The 2 convertases assist in the cleavage of C3 to C3a (an anaphylatoxin) and C3b

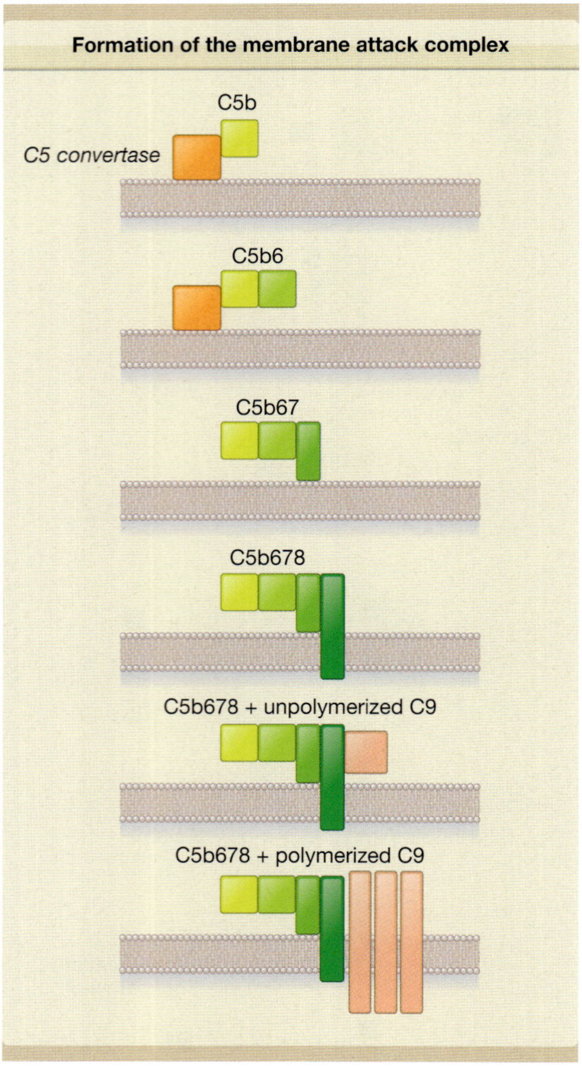

FIGURE 27-6 Formation of the membrane attack complex. (*Reprinted with permission from Goldsmith LA et al.* Fitzpatrick's Dermatology in General Medicine, *8th Ed. New York: McGraw-Hill; 2012.*)

- C3b binds to the next protein, C5
- C5 is also cleaved by the C3 convertases into C5a and C5b
- C5a is released and becomes the most potent anaphylatoxin
- C5b becomes the point of assembly for MAC (membrane attack complex)
- C5b associates with target cell membrane and C6
- C5b6 then associates with the assembly of C7, C8, and C9
- C5b6789 is the MAC that forms transmembrane channels (holes) in the cell membrane that allows an influx of water and ions to cause cell swelling and lysis

- Points of regulation
  - Classical pathway
    - C1 is inhibited by C1 inhibitor (C1 INH)
    - C1 esterase inhibitor (C1 INH) deficiency causes angioedema
    - Factor I inhibits formation of C3 convertase
    - C4-binding protein inhibits formation of C3 convertase
    - Decay accelerating factor (DAF) inhibits formation of C3 convertase
  - Alternative pathway
    - Factor H inhibits formation of C3 convertase
    - Factor P (properdin) protects C3 convertase
- Anaphylatoxins
  - C3a, C5a, C4a
  - Cause release of histamine from mast cells, degranulation of basophils, and increase in vascular permeability
  - Anaphylatoxins are regulated by a carboxipeptidase present in plasma
- *Neutrophils*
  - Derived from a pluripotent hematopoietic stem cell
  - Myeloblasts develop into neutrophils, the stages are under the influence of granulocyte colony-stimulating factor (G-CSF) and granulocyte-macrophage colony stimulating factor (GM-CSF)
  - Cytoplasmic granules include lysozyme, myeloperoxidase, and defensins
  - Secondary granules include lactoferrin, collagenase, gelatinase, vitamin B_{12}-binding protein, and complement receptor 3
  - Granules fuse with incoming phagocytic vacuoles that contain ingested bacteria
  - IL-8 is a potent chemoattractant and neutrophil activator, other chemoattractants include *N*-fromlymethionyl-leucyl-phenylalanine, C5a, leukotriene B4, and PAF. IL-8 is often secreted by macrophages but can be secreted by other cells expressing toll-like receptors
  - Neutrophils adhere to sites along endothelium after recognizing sites of activation (e.g., chemokine expression) and traverse the endothelium to enter the tissue and fight infection
  - Neutrophils produce cytokines that stimulate and attract other phagocytes and lymphocytes
  - Mechanisms of killing may be oxygen dependent or independent
- *Mast cell*
  - Arise from CD34+, KIT+ pluripotent progenitor stem cell
  - Primary cell in immunoglobulin E–mediated inflammatory reactions
  - Cytoplasmic granule content, size, and susceptibility to pharmacologic treatments vary with location of the cells
  - All mast cells contain tryptase, histamine, proteoglycans (heparin and chondroitin sulfate E)
  - Types of mast cells
    - TC mast cells (MCTC): contain tryptase and chymase, located in submucosal tissue

  - T mast cells (MCT): contain tryptase and lack chymase; increased in allergic and parasitic diseases, decreased in GI mucosa in patients with HIV
  - Chymase only mast cells: located in skin, lymph nodes, intestinal submucosa
- Mast cell activation and mediators: see Table 27-3
- Preformed secretory mediators are released in response to aggregation of the high-affinity IgE receptor
- Histamine and tryptase are relased after activation of mast cells
- Histamine receptors: H_1 on epithelial cells, vascular and perivascular cells; H_2 on epithelial cells of the GI tract, H_3 are found in the brain and GI tract and may be associated with headache; H_4 expressed on bone marrow cells, eosinophils, and mast cells

EXAMPLES OF IMMUNE-MEDIATED DERMATOLOGIC DISEASES

Hypersensitivity Reactions: Resulting From Humoral Immunity or Cell-Mediated Immunity

- *Type I reactions*: anaphylaxis reactions (IgE-mediated)
  - Immediate hypersensitivity reactions: symptoms begin within 30 minutes of the exposure
  - Clinical classification of Type I reactions
    - *Local*: allergic rhinitis, allergic asthma, contact urticaria (stinging nettles)
    - *Systemic: anaphylaxis*: a hypersensitive response in genetically susceptible individuals to small amounts of antigen to which they have been sensititized previously

TABLE 27-3 Selected Mast Cell Mediators

Mediators	Biologic Effects	Possible Consequences
Pre-formed		
Histamine	Vasodilation, increased vascular permeability, gastric hypersecretion, brochoconstriction	Hypotension, flushing, urticaria, abdominal pain; (peptic, colic) diarrhea, malabsorption
Heparin	Anticoagulant, inhibition of platelet aggregation	Prolonged bleeding time
Tryptase	Endothelial cell activation, fibrinogen cleavage, mitogenic for smooth muscles cells	Osteoporosis/osteopenia, disruption of cascade systems (clotting, etc.)
Chymase	Converts angiotensin I to II, lipoprotein degradation	Hypertension
Newly Synthesized		
Leukotrienes	Increase vascular permeability, brochoconstriction, vasoconstriction	Bronchospasm, hypotension
Prostaglandins	Vasodilation, bronchoconstriction	Flushing, urticaria
Cytokines		
Stem cell factor	Growth and survival of mast cells, chemotaxis of KIT^{+}cells	Mast cell hyperplasia, focal aggregates
Tumor necrosis factor-α	Activation of vascular endothelial cells, cachexia, fatigue	Weight loss, fatigue
Transforming growth factor-β	Enhanced production of connective tissue components	Fibrosis
IL-5	Eosinophil growth factor	Eosinophilia
IL-6	Growth and survival of mast cells	Fever, bone pain, osteoporosis/osteopenia
IL-16	Lymphocyte accumulation	Focal aggregates

Hypertension IL = interleukin.

- Early signs and symptoms include angioedema, dyspnea, vomiting, and abdominal cramping. Late signs include tachycardia, conjunctival edema, hypotension, and upper airway edema leading to potential respiratory arrest. Generalized vasodilation and increased vascular permeability can lead to hypotension, shock, and ultimately death
- Common triggers of anaphylaxis are foods (peanuts, eggs, shellfish), drugs (aspirin, radiocontrast media, penicillin, and other β-lactam antibiotics), *Hymenoptera* venom, and pollens
- Mechanism
  - Sensitization to a particular antigen occurs after an initial exposure by injection, ingestion, inhalation, or insect sting
  - IgE antibody is produced, which then binds to its receptor on the surface of mast cells and basophils
  - After reintroduction of antigen to the sensitized host, the antigen binds to several cell-bound IgE antibody molecules, resulting in cross-link and signal transduction
  - Mast cells degranulate and release histamine, leukotriene, serotonin, and bradykinin, resulting in vasodilation, increased vascular permeability, contraction of smooth muscle in brochi, and increased secretions
  - Primary mediators include TNF-α, IL-1, IL-6, prostaglandins, leukotrienes, and histamine
  - Treatment: epinephrine, diphenhydramine, aminophylline, and corticosteroids

- *Type II reactions*: cell surface antigen-antibody cytotoxicity reactions (antibody-mediated)
  - Antibody is directed against an antigen that may be intrinsic (innately part of the host tissues) or extrinsic (absorbed onto host tissue surfaces during exposure)
  - IgG and IgM antibodies bound to these antigens form in situ complexes that activate the classical pathway of complement and generate mediators of acute inflammation at the site
  - ADCC: NK cells destroy antibody-coated target cells via perforins and serine proteases, which results in pore formation and cell lysis
  - In some cases, formation of the antigen-antibody complexes does not lead to activation of the complement system but still can lead to cell injury
  - In other cases, such as Graves disease, antibodies do not injure the cell, but bind to receptors and lead to receptor activation and downstream effects.
  - Examples of Type II reactions: transfusion reactions, reactions to certain drugs (penicillin, quinidine, methyldopa), myasthenia gravis, and autoimmune hemolytic anemia or thrombocytopenia
- *Type III reactions*: antigen-antibody complex reactions
  - Circulating antibodies bind to antigen and form complexes that, in the presence of excess antigen, escape phagocytosis and deposit on the surface of blood vessels or tissues
  - Antigen-antibody complexes activate complement and release C5a that acts as a potent neutrophil chemotactic factor and anaphylatoxin; clotting factors are also activated
  - Neutrophils are attracted to the area of complex deposition and release lysosomal enzymes, causing tissue destruction
  - Examples of antigen-antibody complex reactions
    - *Arthus reaction*: local Type III reaction usually seen when antigen is injected into the skin
      - ▲ An IgG antibody directed against the antigen forms immune complexes that bind Fc receptors on leukocytes and mast cells
      - ▲ The immune complexes also activate complement and release of chemotactic factors (C3a, C5a), leading to neutrophil infiltration and activation
    - *Serum sickness*: allergic vasculitis characterized by joint pain, fever, pruritic rash, and lymphadenopathy that leads to a complement-mediated systemic immune complex reaction
      - ▲ Occurs by the injection of foreign serum or its products into the blood
      - ▲ Antibody-antigen complexes activate the complement cascade and also trigger ligation of the FcγRIII mast cell receptor, resulting in histamine release
      - ▲ Associated medications include sulfonamides, penicillin, cephalosporins, phenytoin, thiourea, lamotrigine, and streptokinase
- *Type IV reactions*: delayed-type hypersensitivity (DTH) reactions
  - Consequence of cell-mediated immunity (antigen-specific T cells): appears in 24 to 48 hours. Patients become sensitized through the creation of memory T cells, and subsequent exposures lead to more robust responses
  - Three clinical examples of Type IV reactions
    - *Delayed-type hypersensitivity:* Tuberculin skin test (purified protein derivative)
    - *Contact hypersensitivity*: antigen in the form of haptens from a topical exposure (i.e., Rhus dermatitis, nickel)
    - *Gluten-sensitive enteropathy*: antigen introduced parenterally
    - *Diabetes mellitus Type 1*

Vitiligo

- Clinical: depigmented patches of skin in various distributions on the body
- Etiology: loss of melanocytes from the epidermis
- Considered by most to be an autoimmune phenomenon

- Both melanocyte autoantibodies and T cells are involved in the pathogenesis
- CD4+/CD8+ ratio is reversed, with predominant CD8+ T cells suggesting a role of CD8+ mediated cytotoxicity to melanocytes in disease etiology
- Associated with other autoimmune diseases as well as organ-specific autoantibodies: diabetes mellitus, pernicious anemia, systemic lupus erythematosus, thyroid disease (Graves disease)
- Treatment: steroids, immune modulators: calcineurin inhibitors, phototherapy, punch grafts

Psoriasis

- Clinical: a systemic inflammatory disorder that manifests as sharply dermarcated red plaques with silvery white scales on the extensor surfaces and scalp
- Types
  - *Plaque psoriasis*: raised lesions most common on the extensor surfaces of the knees, elbows, scalp, and trunk (Fig. 27-7)
  - *Guttate psoriasis*: drop-like lesions; may follow streptococcal pharyngitis
  - *Inverse psoriasis*: flexural surfaces, intertriginous areas
  - *Pustular psoriasis*: diffuse erythema with pustular eruption, can occur with fever, tachycardia, and systemic inflammation in rare cases leading to adult respiratory distress syndrome (ARDS)
  - *Nail psoriasis*: nail pitting, oil spots, and onycholysis
  - *Scalp psoriasis*: erythema and silvery scale
  - *Erythrodermic psoriasis*: widespread inflammation and exfoliation; exacerbation of unstable plaque psoriasis
  - *Inflammatory progressive arthritis*: approximately 10 to 30% of patients; asymmetric destructive oligoarthritis occurs in as many as 70% of patients with psoriatic arthritis
- Pathogenesis
  - T cells and macrophages can be detected in newly forming lesions

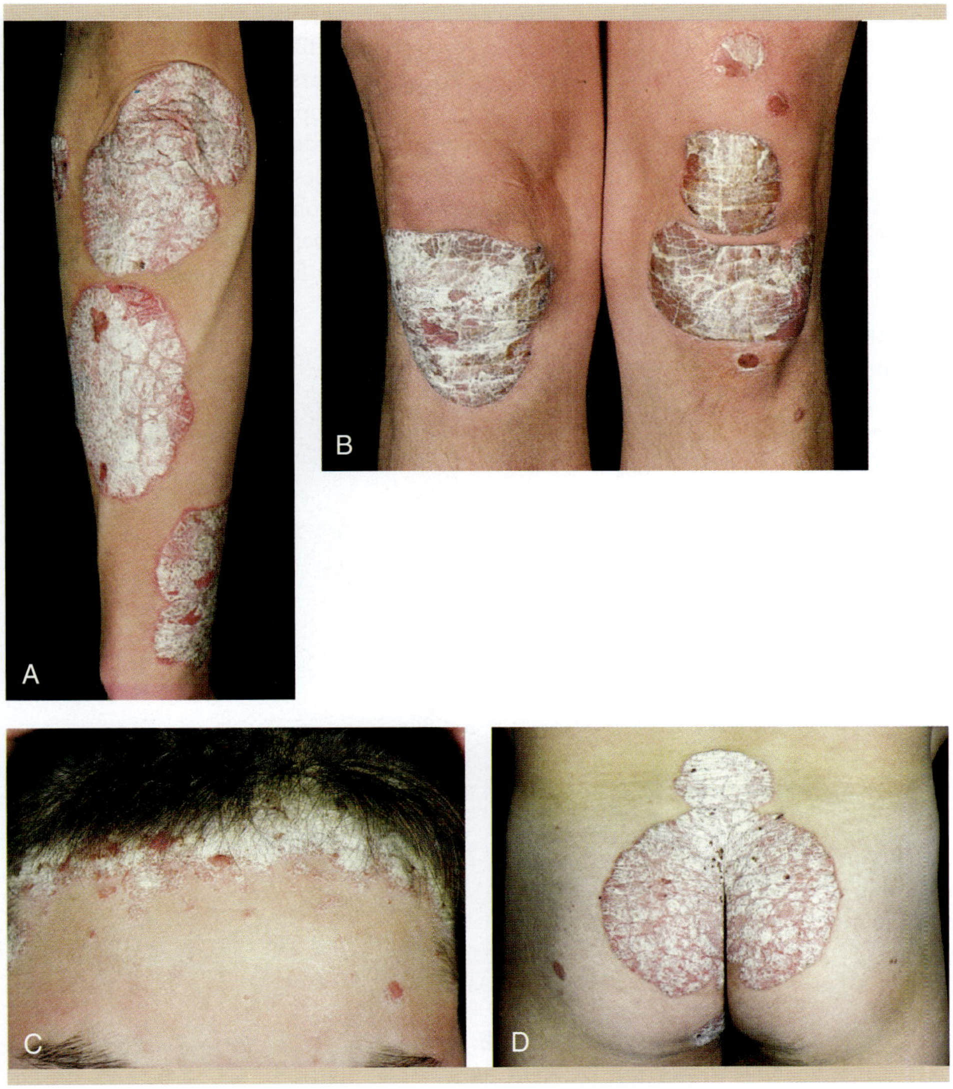

FIGURE 27-7 Psoriasis. (*Reprinted with permission from Wolff K et al.* Fitzpatrick's Dermatology in General Medicine, *7th Ed. New York: McGraw-Hill; 2008.*)

- Activated memory T-lymphocytes release proinflammatory cytokines, which results in proliferation of keratinocytes and leukocyte recruitment
- CD4 + and CD8 + T cells are both present in the dermal and epidermal infiltrate, respectively
- Th_1 cytokines (IL-2, IFN-γ, IL-6, IL-12, and TNF-α) are produced by the T cells, keratinocytes, and antigen-presenting cells
- IL-23 is overproduced by dendritic cells and possibly keratinocytes in psoriatic lesions. It stimulates Th_{17} cells to produce cytokines that stimulate keratinocytes proliferation
- Th_{17} family of cytokines include IL-17A, IL-17F, IL-21, IL-22, and TNF-α
- Elevated TNF-α levels lead to increased production of proinflammatory cytokines by T cells and macrophages

- Treatment: targets T cells or their cytokines
- Skin-directed therapies: topical corticosteroids; topical calcipotriene; coal tar; topical tazarotene; ultraviolet A (UVA) light; psoralen plus UVA light (PUVA); UVB light; Goeckerman regimen (coal tar followed by UVB exposure); Ingram method, (anthralin cream is applied to the skin after a tar bath and UVB treatment)
- Systemic therapies
  - Oral retinoids
  - Immunosuppressive medications: methotrexate; cyclosporine
  - Biologic agents: alefacept, efalizumab (discontinued due to progressive multifocal leukoencephalopathy)
    - TNF inhibitors: infliximab; etanercept, adalimumab
    - IL-12/23 (p40 subunit) inhibitor: ustekinumab
    - IL-17 inhibitors: currently in clinical trials, with anti-IL-17 and anti-IL-17 receptor antibodies showing promise as possible therapies
    - Patients should avoid oral steroids owing to rebound effect

Alopecia Areata (AA)

- Clinical: an autoimmune nonscarring alopecia; usually localized; however, more severe forms may affect the entire scalp (alopecia totalis) or body (alopecia universalis)
- Pathogenesis
  - Associated with certain HLA alleles (HLA-DR4, -DR6, -B12, -B18, -B13, and -B27)
  - CLA+ CD4 and CD8 T lymphocytes are thought to be involved in the pathogenesis
  - Associated autoimmune diseases: diabetes mellitus, systemic lupus erythematosus, Graves, and vitiligo
- Treatment: intralesional corticosteroids, induction of allergic contact dermatitis using sensitizers

Sarcoid

- Clinical: a multisystemic disorder of unknown etiology. Clinical manifestations include cutaneous lesions in 25% of patients. Manifestations are categorized as specific or nonspecific based on the histologic presence or absence of noncaseating epithelioid granulomas, respectively; systemic involvement is seen in 70% of cutaneously involved patients
- The skin disease does not correlate with prognosis or extent of visceral involvement (except in erythema nodosum which is a self-limiting condition)
  - Nonspecific lesions seen in sarcoidosis (biopsy does not show granulomas)
    - *Erythema nodosum (EN)*: most common nonspecific lesion; tender, erythematous nodules most commonly on legs; associated with a better prognosis
    - May be self-limited and asymptomatic; better prognosis
  - Specific lesions (biopsy shows granulomatous inflammation)
    - *Lupus pernio* (Fig. 27-8): violaceous patches and plaques most commonly on the nose; more common in women and associated with pulmonary involvement; resolution with scarring is possible; marker for aggressive disease; progresses over many months. The cheeks, ears, digits, and toes may be similarly affected. Complications include ulceration and involvement of underlying structures
    - Papules/plaques/nodules
    - Head and neck more common for papules
    - Legs: plaques; *angiolupoid sarcoid* (plaques with telangectasias); marker for pulmonary fibrosis

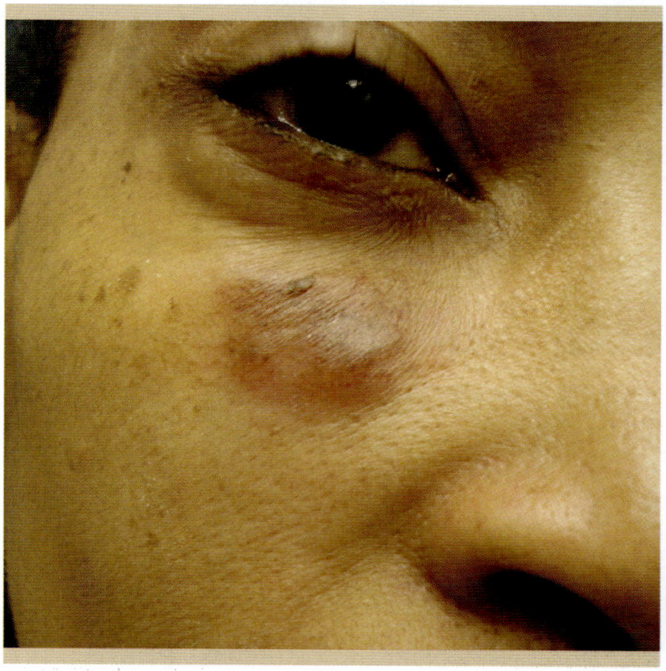

FIGURE 27-8 Lupus pernio. (*Used with permission from Dr. Asra Ali.*)

- *Subcutaneous nodules (Darier-Roussy)*: firm, painless, subcutaneous nodules that represent sarcoidosis; this subset is higly associated with systemic disease
  - Scar sarcoidosis (i.e., vaccination site, tattoos)
- Unique variants: ulcerative (legs), ichthyosiform lesions, scarring/nonscarring alopecia

- Syndromes
  - *Lofgren syndrome*: hilar adenopathy, EN, fever, migrating polyathritis, and acute iritis
  - *Heerfordts-Waldenstrom syndrome (uveoparotid fever)*: parotid gland enlargement, fever, cranial nerve palsy, anterior uveitis
- Systemic disease manifestations
  - Pulmonary
    - Interstitial lung disease may be subclinical
    - Symptoms: dyspnea, dry cough
    - Fifty percent clear spontaneously
  - *Lymphadenopathy*: hilar, cervical, axillary, inguinal
  - *Ophthalmic*: anterior uveitis
  - *Cardiac*: occurs in approximately 2% of patients. Can be asymptomatic. Can cause conduction abnormalities, dilated cardiomyopathy, acute myocarditis, and sudden cardiac death
  - *Gastrointestinal*: hematemesis, 10% with granulomas
  - *Neurologic*: CN VII palsy
  - *Endocrine*: overproduction of 1 to 25 dihydroxy vitamin D by granulomas leading to hypercalcemia, sometimes severe, with altered mental status, nephrolithiasis, and nephrotoxicity
  - *Muscle*: biopsy: granulomas, no symptoms
  - *Bone*: If hands involved, check for bone cysts; joint pain in 25 to 40%
- Diagnosis
  - Histology
    - Naked (absent to sparse inflammation at periphery), noncaseating granulomas, Schaumann bodies (round, laminated, calcified body), asteroid bodies (star-shaped eosinophilic structure)
    - Must exclude infection, foreign-body reaction (zirconium, beryllium, silica, etc.), other inflammatory disorders (granulomatous rosacea, cutaneous Crohn, etc.), and neoplastic disorders (granulomatous MF and sarcoidal response to underlying lymphoma)
      - ▲ Tuberculoid leprosy will be paucibacillary, but it can be differentiated from sarcoid by the perineural distribution of granulomas
  - Chest x-ray
    - Stage I: hilar adenopathy
    - Stage II: hilar adenopathy with infiltrates
    - Stage III: pulmonary infiltrates with adenopathy
    - Stage IV: end-stage fibrosis
  - *Kveim-Siltzbach test*: injection of sarcoidal spleen extract into a patient with suspected sarcoid results in typical granulomatous reaction 4 to 6 weeks later; false-positive results are possible
  - Laboratory studies
    - Angiotensin converting enzyme (ACE) levels may be elevated in two-thirds of patients; used for predicting disease progression with serial measurements. Lysozyme can be elevated as well
    - Increased erythrocyte sedimentation rate (ESR) in two-thirds of patients
    - Lymphopenia with a reduced CD4:CD8 ratio
    - 24-hour urine
    - Serum Ca^{2+}: elevated
- Treatment
  - Corticosteroids
  - Antimalarials (hydroxychloroquine [Plaquenil] and chloroquine [Aralen])
  - Antimetabolites: methotrexate, chlorambucil, imuran
  - Tetracycline antibiotics
  - Retinoids
  - Thalidomide
  - Biologics that target T cells or TNF may be useful. Caution should be exercised with etanercept, as there are reports of etanercept-induced sarcoidosis and possible flares of disease

Urticaria/Angioedema

- Edema formation in specific layers of the skin
- Clinical
  - *Urticaria* involves only the superficial portion of the dermis, presents as well-circumscribed wheals with erythematous, raised, serpiginous borders and blanched centers; may coalesce to become giant wheals; usually pruritic
    - Can involve any area of the body from the scalp to the soles of the feet
    - Appears in crops, with old lesions fading within 24 hours as new ones appear
  - *Angioedema* presents as well-demarcated, localized edema involving the deeper layers of the skin, including the subcutaneous tissue
    - Angioedema often occurs in the periorbital region involving the lips
    - Although self-limited in duration, angioedema involvement of the upper respiratory tract may be life threatening owing to laryngeal obstruction
  - Recurrent episodes of urticaria and/or angioedema of less than 6 weeks' duration are considered acute; more than 6 weeks' duration are designated as chronic
- Pathology: dermal edema characterizes urticaria, sometimes with perivascular infiltrates of neutrophils and eosinophils; edema of both the dermis and subcutaneous tissue characterizes angioedema; collagen bundles are widely separated, venules are often dilated

- Classification based on etiology
  - *Ig-E dependent*: due to specific antigen sensitivity (pollens, foods, drugs, fungi, molds, *Hymenoptera* venom, helminthes)
    - Mechanism
      - ▲ A sensitized individual possesses IgE antibodies against a specific antigen
      - ▲ IgE antibodies are attached to the surfaces of mast cells
      - ▲ When rechallenged with the same antigen, the result is release of biologically active products from the mast cells, the most important being histamine
    - *Physical urticaria*: numerous types
    - *Dermographism*: linear wheals following minor pressure or scratching of the skin
    - *Solar urticaria*: characteristically occurs within minutes of sun exposure
    - *Cold urticaria*: precipitated by exposure to the cold, and, therefore, exposed areas usually are affected
      - ▲ In some cases, the disease is associated with abnormal circulating proteins, more commonly cryoglobulins and less commonly cryofibrinogens and cold agglutinins
      - ▲ Additional systemic symptoms include wheezing and syncope, thus explaining the need for these patients to avoid swimming in cold water
  - *Cholinergic urticaria*: precipitated by heat, exercise, or emotion; characterized by small wheals with relatively large flares; occasionally associated with wheezing
- Complement-mediated
  - Hereditary/acquired angioedema
    - Caused by C1 inhibitor (C1 INH) deficiency: hereditary angioedema (HAE)-low levels of the plasma protein C1 INH
    - Acquired angioedema (AAE) caused by consumption of C1 INH
    - C1 INH inhibits klikerein and factor Xia; therefore, kinin forming pathway is augmented when C1 INH is missing
    - *Hereditary angioedema (HAE)*: type 1 (85%), autosomal dominant; suppressed C1 INH levels due to abnormal secretion or intracellular degradation; type 2 (15%), autosomal dominant, leads to synthesis of dysfunctional C1 INH, therefore, levels may be normal or elevated
    - HAE: normal c1q, depressed C4 levels
    - Occurs without accompanying urticaria
    - Trauma often precipitates attacks
    - Results in massive local swelling and occasionally fatal laryngeal edema
    - *Aquired angioedema*: may be associated with B-cell lymphoma or connective tissue disease with consumption of C1 INH; may also be associated with autoimmune disorders with circulating IgG antibody to C1 INH
      - ▲ Aquired angioedema has depressed C1q levels and depressed C4 levels
    - Bradykinin is the mediator of the swelling in both hereditary and acquired angioedema
    - Angiotensin-converting enzyme inhibitors can cause angioedema: swelling also caused by increased bradykinin (due to a decreased degradation)
  - Infections
    - Acute urticaria may be associated with upper respiratory tract infections due to viruses; hepatitis B virus has also been associated with urticaria
  - Abnormalities of arachidonic acid metabolism
    - Urticaria/angioedema may occur in reponse to aspirin
- Nonimmunologic
  - *Direct mast cell–releasing agents*: opiates, antibiotics, curare, D-tubocurarine[Ed.11], radiocontrast media
  - *Agents that alter arachidonic acid metabolism*: aspirin and other NSAIDs, azo dyes, benzoates
    - Blocks the production of prostaglandins from arachidonic acid
    - The pathway is then shifted to the production of other metabolites, including leukotrienes
    - Leukotriene release ultimately results in release of vasoactive substances (histamine) that alter vascular permeability and produce dermal edema (urticaria)
- Idiopathic
  - *Chronic idiopathic urticaria*
    - Autoantibodies to the high-infinity IgE receptor or to IgE itself have been identified in these patients
    - Autoantibodies possess histamine-releasing activity
    - Wheals and itching daily for at least 6 weeks
      - ▲ Hashimoto thyroidetis and Grave disease are associated with CIU
      - ▲ Laboratory: thyroid function, antithyroid peraxide, and thyroglobulin antibody titers

Urticarial Vasculitis (Immune Complex–Mediated)

- Sometimes a reflection of an underlying systemic illness such as lupus erythematosus, Sjögren syndrome, hereditary complement deficiency, serum sickness, or infections such as hepatitis B or C infection
- Individual erythematous wheals last longer than 24 hours and usually develop central petechiae that can be observed even after the urticarial phase has resolved
- On biopsy, there is a leukocytoclastic vasculitis of the small blood vessels
- Laboratory findings: patients should have CH50, C3, C4, and C1q levels checked, along with an ANA panel and both HBV and HCV serologies
- Treatment

- Any suspected medication should be discontinued
- Avoidance of precipitating factors may be helpful for some of the physical urticarias, such as solar and cold urticaria
- Symptomatic therapy usually includes H_1 antihistamines given on a regular rather than an intermittent, as-needed basis
- The tricyclic antidepressant doxepin (Sinequan) is also effective and has been shown to have both H_1 and H_2 antihistamine activity

Graft-Versus-Host Disease (GVHD)

- Occurs when immunologically competent cells are introduced into an immunoincompetent host
- Most commonly seen in hematopoietic cell transplantation (HCT), both allogeneic (between 2 individuals) and autologous (from the same individual)
- Solid-organ transplants, blood transfusions, and maternal-fetal transfusions also have been reported to cause GVHD
- The skin often is the earliest organ affected
- GVHD remains a primary cause of morbidity and mortality after HCT
- Classifications: arbitrarily defined based on days from transplant
  - Acute GVHD
    - Occurs within the first 100 days of a transplant
    - Consists of a triad of dermatitis, enteritis, and hepatitis
    - Usually begins as scattered erythematous macules and papules that may evolve into a generalized erythroderma or bullous eruption
    - Mediated by T_H1 cells
    - Graded in 5 steps (0–IV)
      - ▲ Grade 0: no clinical evidence of disease
      - ▲ Grade I: rash on less than 50% of skin and no gut or liver involvement
      - ▲ Grade II: rash covering more than 50% of skin, bilirubin 2 to 3 mg/dL, diarrhea 10 to 15 mL/kg per day, or persistent nausea
      - ▲ Grade III or IV: generalized erythroderma with bulla formation, bilirubin greater than 3 mg/dL, or diarrhea more than 16 mL/kg per day
  - Chronic GVHD
    - Develops after 100 days
    - Consists of an autoimmune syndrome directed toward multiple organs
    - May occur as a late phase of acute GVHD or as a distinct entity
    - The skin is the primary organ involved and may be characterized as localized or generalized with lichen planus–like or sclerodermoid lesions commonly encountered
    - Mediated by T_H2 cells
- Pathophysiology
  - Three components are required for the development of GVHD
    - The graft must contain immunologically competent cells
    - The host must appear foreign to the graft
    - The host must be incapable of reacting sufficiently against the graft
  - Disease is caused by recognition of epithelial target tissues as foreign by the immunocompetent cells and subsequent induction of an inflammatory response and eventual apoptotic death of the target tissue (regardless of whether the immunoreactive T cells are derived from a nonidentical donor or from the recipient)
  - While T cells may orchestrate the initial inflammatory response, many cell types (e.g., CD4+, CD8+ T-cell subsets, and natural killer cells) are found at sites of epithelial injury
- Histology
  - Acute: epidermal basal vacuolization, followed by epidermal basal cell apoptotic death with lymphoid infiltration; satellite cell necrosis (direct apposition of a lymphocyte to a necrotic keratinocyte)
  - Chronic: basal cell degeneration and necrosis, epidermal atrophy, and dermal fibrosis; lichenoid changes with mononuclear infiltrates, epithelial cell necrosis
- Treatment
  - Immunosuppression is the mainstay of therapy: limiting the graft-versus-host tissue response while maintaining the graft-versus-tumor effect is crucial
  - T-cell depletion with Campath 1H or thymoglobulin during transplant is useful
  - Prophylaxis with cyclosporine, mycophenolate mofetil, and tacrolimus is common; however, exacerbations of GVHD frequently require prednisone
  - Newer biologicals (CTLA-4-Ig, infliximab, etanercept, and anti-CD25 agents such as daclizumab) appear interesting and may prove useful
  - Immune modulation with photopheresis or phototherapy also has been helpful

Atopic Eczema (Atopic Dermatitis)

- Clinical: pruritic poorly demarcated, erythematous scaly patches, small vesicles, excoriations, crusting, lichenification and impetiginization that have a predilection for the skin flexures (neck, antecubital fossa, and popliteal fossa) in children and extensors in adults
- Chronic scratching and rubbing can lead to hyperpigmentation and lichenification; periorbital fold (Denny Morgan sign) may be present
- Pathogenesis: believed to be multifactorial
  - Allergens (house dust mites, pollen, animal dander), outdoor pollution, climate, diet, and prenatal or early-life factors such as infections

- Patients appear to have a genetic predisposition that can then be exacerbated by these numerous factors
- Atopic skin has decreased human β-defensin 3 predisposing patients to frequent skin infections
- Patients appear to have elevated levels of T_H2 cytokines, and increased levels of IgE production
- Recent studies show a potential role for the T_H17 pathway, with increased circulating T_H17 cells in atopic patients, and increased T_H17 cells in acute eczematous lesions. A decreased number of T_H17 cells in chronic lesions argues for a dynamic role for the T_H17 pathway

- Histology: edema within the epidermis (spongiosis) and infiltration with lymphocytes and macrophages in the superficial dermis
- Diagnosis
  - Made by the typical morphology and distribution of the lesions
  - Family and personal history of atopy (asthma, allergic rhinitis, or atopic dermatitis) also can help with the diagnosis
- Prognosis: there is currently no cure; however, various interventions exist to control symptoms
  - Can be expected to clear in 60 to 70% of children by their early teens, although relapses may occur
- Treatment
  - Includes emollients, oral antihistamines, topical corticosteroid ointments, topical tacrolimus, topical pimecrolimus
  - More severe cases sometimes use UVB phototherapy or PUVA
  - Occasionally, a short course of systemic steroids is necessary to bring the disease under control
  - Steroid wet wraps and baths are helpful in treating acute atopic dermatis
  - Avoidance of environmental factors that enhance itching is important
  - Moisturizers reduce dry skin and itching
  - Topical and/or oral antibiotics, bleach baths for bacterial superinfection
  - Given elevated levels of IgE in atopic patients, anti-IgE therapy with omalizumab has been attempted, with a small randomized clinical trial showing few clinical benefits. Patients required increased amounts of allergen to experience type I hypersensitivity reactions, but experienced few other benefits
  - Nevertheless, there are reports of refractory disease responding to omalizumab, and other studies showing improvements in patients with both atopic dermatitis and eczema
- Omalizumab: Anti-IgE therapy in allergy. Kopp MV. Curr Allergy Asthma Rep. 2011 apr;11(2):101-6. Review.

Seborrheic Dermatitis

Take a look at 2 recent papers in 2011 on seborrheic dermatitis

1. Kerr K, Darcy T, Henry J, et al. A description of epidermal changes associated with symptomatic resolution of dandruff: Biomarkers of scalp health. *Intl J Derm* 2011;50:102-113.
2. Kerr K, Schwartz J, Filloon T, et al. Scalp stratum corneum histamine levels: Novel sampling method reveals correlation to itch resolution in dandruff/seborrheic dermatitis. *Acta Derm Venereol* 2011;91:404-408.

- A common problem affecting 3 to 5% of the healthy population
- Waxing and waning course that parallels the increased sebaceous gland activity occurring in infancy and after puberty
- Clinical: erythematous patches and plaques with indistinct margins and yellowish, greasy-appearing scales affecting sebaceous hairy regions of the body (scalp, eyebrows, nasolabial creases, ears, chest, intertriginous areas, axilla, groin, buttocks, and inframammary folds); variable amount of pruritus
  - Refractory or more widespread disease may be associated with underlying HIV infection (approximately one-third of patients with AIDS and AIDS-related complex) or neurologic disorder (i.e., Parkinson disease)
- Pathogenesis
  - Thought to be an inflammatory reaction to the resident skin yeast, *Malassezia*
  - *Malassezia* is a lipophilic yeast that is normally found on the seborrheic regions of the skin. May be due to the lipolytic activity of *Malassezia* freeing free fatty acids that have a proinflammatory effect
  - Epidermis becomes hyperproliferative and parakeratotic, with neutrophil migration and a breakdown in the barrier function of the skin. Elevated levels of IL-1 and IL-8 correlate with disease activity
- Diagnosis: usually made on clinical grounds alone
- Treatment
  - Antiseborrheic shampoos containing zinc pyrithione, selenium sulfide, or ketoconazole are the mainstay of treatment
  - Topical steroids
  - Topical antifungals

Other Systemic Inflammatory Diseases

- Familial Mediterranean fever
  - Autosomal recessive
  - MEFV gene; chromosome 16, mutation in the gene *pyrin* (*Marenostrin*)
  - Clinical findings: self-limited attacks of fever accompanied by peritonitis, pleurisy, and arthritis, erysipelas-like eruption on lower legs, urticaria, Henoch-Schönlein purpura
  - Treatment: colchicine, anti-TNF

- Muckle-Wells
  - Autosomal dominant
  - CIAS1, encoding cryopyrin, a component of the inflammasome. This defect results in high levels of IL-1β
  - Clinical findings: urticaria, fever, paresthesias, limb pain, deafness, renal, abdominal pain, polyarthralgia, conjunctivitis, systemic amyloidosis (25%)
  - Treatment: IL-1 receptor antagonist
- Other autoinflammatory disorders

QUIZ

Questions

1. CTLA-4 binds to ____, and serves to ____T-cell activation. _____binds to and inhibits CTLA-4.

   A. B7, inhibit, Abatacept
   B. CD28, stimulate, Etanercept
   C. B7, stimulate, Ipilimumab
   D. PD-1, inhibit, Adalimumab
   E. B7, inhibit, Ipilimumab

2. A patient presents with recurrent MRSA abscesses, thrush, and chronic lung infections. Physical examination reveals facial dysmorphism and retained deciduous teeth. The most likely mutation is in_____.

   A. FoxP3
   B. IL-23
   C. STAT3
   D. LFA-3
   E. NFAT

3. A patient presents with recurrent MRSA abscesses, thrush, and chronic lung infections. Laboratory examination reveals extremely elevated levels of IgE. Hyper IgE syndrome in DOCK8 deficiency can be distinguished from that occurring in STAT3 deficiency by:

   A. Facial dysmorphism in cases of DOCK8 deficiency
   B. Increased incidence of severe asthma and food allergies in STAT3 deficiency
   C. Staphylococcal infections in STAT3 deficiency
   D. Pneumatoceles in DOCK8 deficiency
   E. Viral infections in DOCK8 deficiency

4. A 6-month-old boy presents to the emergency department with fever and tachypnea, and is found to be in diabetic ketoacidosis. He has a history of intractable watery diarrhea and a gradually worsening eczematous dermatitis. His older brother had many of the same conditions, along with hypothyroidism, and died in early childhood. This likely represents a defect in _____, a key signaling molecule in _____

   A. STAT3, T_H17 cells
   B. RAG1, T cells,
   C. STAT3, B cells
   D. FoxP3, Treg cells
   E. WASP, macrophages

5. All of the following are considered type II immune reactions, except:

   A. Graft-versus-host disease
   B. Graves disease
   C. Myasthenia gravis
   D. Pernicious anemia
   E. Autoimmune hemolytic anemia

6. A 30-year-old man presents with recurring fevers, urticaria, deafness, joint pains, foamy urine, and peripheral neuropathy. His mother died of renal failure. This autosomal dominant disease of the inflammasome is caused by a defect in ____, resulting in high levels of _____ that can be treated by a targeted antibody.

   A. CIAS1, IL-1β
   B. MEFV, IL-6
   C. WASP, IL-17
   D. CIAS1, TNF-α
   E. NEMO, IL-8

7. PD-1 belongs to the family of _____ molecules and is increased in the presence of which of the following:

   A. B7, chronic viral infections
   B. B7, malignant cells
   C. CD45, basophils
   D. CD 28, malignant cells
   E. CD40, chronic viral infections

8. IL-8 is a potent chemoattractant for:

   A. Eosinophils
   B. Macrophages
   C. Neutrophils
   D. Langerhans cells
   E. B cells

9. Germline Jak3 mutations have been found in _____, while somatic Jak2 mutations have been found in _____.

   A. Common variable immune deficiency, acute lymphoblastic leukemia
   B. Severe combined immune deficiency, polycythemia vera
   C. Severe combined immune deficiency, psoriasis
   D. Chronic granulomatous disease, psoriasis
   E. Common variable immune deficiency, polycythemia vera

10. In the classical pathway, C4 is cleaved by ______. C4 level is an important laboratory test to order in ________.

    A. C3, atopic dermatitis
    B. C5, urticarial vasculitis
    C. C1, atopic dermatitis
    D. C1INH, angioedema
    E. C1, urticarial vasculitis

11. All of the following are manifestations of sarcoidosis, except:

    A. Hypocalcemia
    B. Arthritis
    C. Sudden cardiac death
    D. Interstitial lung disease
    E. Ichthyosis

Answers

1. E. CTLA-4 is a regulatory molecule expressed on T-cells that binds to B7 on antigen-presenting cells and downregulates T-cell activation. Ipilimumab is a monoclonal antibody that inhibits CTLA-4, inhibiting the inhibitor and increasing T-cell activation. Ipilimumab has been shown to have modest survival benefits in metastatic melanoma.

2. C. Hyper IgE syndrome is characterized by patients with recurrent MRSA abscesses, thrush, and chronic lung infections leading to bronchiectasis and pneumatoceles. Hyper IgE syndrome can be caused by both STAT3 mutations and DOCK8 mutations, but patients with STAT3 mutations tend to have "coarse," dysmorphic facies and retained deciduous teeth, while patients with DOCK8 mutations tend to have viral infections and severe food allergies.

3. E. Hyper IgE syndrome is characterized by patients with recurrent MRSA abscesses, thrush, and chronic lung infections leading to bronchiectasis and pneumatoceles. Hyper IgE syndrome can be caused by both STAT3 mutations and DOCK8 mutations, but patients with STAT3 mutations tend to have "coarse," dysmorphic facies and retained deciduous teeth, while patients with DOCK8 mutations tend to have viral infections and severe food allergies.

4. D. The patient likely has IPEX (immune dysregulation, polyendocrinopathy, enteropathy, X-linked) syndrome, characterized by early onset of Type 1 diabetes, chronic diarrhea, and an eczematous dermatitis that often proves refractory to common treatments and can continue to erythroderma. The disease is often rapidly progressive, with diverse described manifestations, including sepsis, hypogammaglobulinemia, and arthritis, and often results in death within the first years of life. These patients have defects in FoxP3 and have dysfunctional Treg cells which may switch to an inflammatory T_H17 phenotype.

5. A. A type II immune reaction is characterized by the interaction between an antibody and an antigen, with consequent downstream effects. Graves disease is caused by the binding of anti-TSH antibodies to the TSH receptor, with consequent hyperstimulation of the thyroid, leading to gland enlargement and hyperthyroidism. Myasthenia gravis is caused by antibodies to the acetylcholine receptor at the postsynaptic neuromuscular junction, with consequent neuromuscular weakness. Pernicious anemia can be caused by autoantibodies to either parietal cells or to intrinsic factor itself, both resulting in decreased levels of intrinsic factor and vitamin B_{12} deficiency. Autoimmune hemolytic anemia is caused by antibodies that result in erythrocyte destruction and hemolysis. While antibodies may be involved in the pathogenesis of graft-versus-host disease, most manifestations of the disease are caused by T-lymphocytes from the graft targeting host tissues, with prominent manifestations in the skin, the gut, and the liver.

6. A. Muckle-Wells is an autoinflammatory periodic fever syndrome. It can be inherited in an autosomal dominant fashion, with a CIAS1 mutation causing increased levels of cryopyrin, leading to elevated levels of IL-1β. Targeted treatment can be achieved with anakinra, an antibody against IL-1.

7. D. PD-1 is a costimulatory molecule in the CD28 family and is expressed on chronically activated T lymphocytes, B lymphocytes, and macrophages. It binds to the PD-L1 and PD-L2 ligands and downregulates the immune response, particularly in effector T cells. Malignant cells express large amounts of PD-L1, and this may suppress the host immune response.

8. C. IL-8 is often secreted by macrophages and acts as a powerful chemokine for neutrophils.

9. B. Germline Jak3 mutations are seen in some types of severe combined immune deficiency, with loss of T cells, NK cells, and present but nonfunctioning B cells. Somatic Jak2 mutations have been found in polycythemia vera and essential thrombocytosis. Jak inhibitors developed to treat these medications may have efficacy against psoriasis and other inflammatory skin diseases.

10. E. In the classical complement pathway, C4 is cleaved by C1 into C4a and C4b; C4a is a weak anaphylotoxin, while C4b binds to C2a and can trigger the complement cascade. C4 is consumed and low in

hypocomplementemic states such as lupus erythematosus and urticarial vasculitis. Low C4 in urticarial vasculitis raises the concern for systemic vasculitis and renal disease.

11. A. Sarcoidosis is characterized by the formation of granulomas in a variety of different tissues. These granulomas express high levels of 1α hydroxylase, resulting in high levels of the active form of vitamin D and hypercalcemia. All the other choices are possible manifestations of sarcoidosis.

REFERENCES

Asadullag K, Sterry W: Analysis of cytokine expression in dermatology. *Arch Dermatol* 2002;138(9).

Assmann T, Ruzicka T: New immunosuppressive drugs in dermatology (mycophenolate mofetil, tacrolimus): unapproved uses, dosages, or indications. *Clin Dermatol* 2002;20:505–514.

Athman R, Philpott D: Innate immunity via toll-like receptors and Nod proteins. *Curr Opin Microbiol* 2004;7(1):25–32.

Blauvelt A: T-Helper 17 cells in psoriatic plaques and additional genetic links between IL-23 and psoriasis. *J Invest Dermatol* 2008;128:1064–1067.

Brahmer JR, Tykodi SS, Chow LQ, et al. Safety and activity of anti-PD-L1 antibody in patients with advanced cancer. *N Engl J Med* Jun 28 2012;366(26):2455–2465.

Craze M, Young M: Integrating biologic therapies in to a dermatology practice: practical and economic considerations. *J Am Acad Dermatol* 2003;49:S139–S142.

Day CL, Kaufmann DE, Kiepiela P, et al. PD-1 expression on HIV-specific T cells is associated with T-cell exhaustion and disease progression. *Nature* Sep 21 2006;443(7109):350–354. Epub 2006 Aug 20.

Dempsey PW, Vaidya SA, Cheng G: The art of war: innate and adaptive immune responses. *Cell Mol Life Sci* 2003;60(12):2604, 2621.

Gilhar A, Landau M, Assy B, Shalaginov R, Serafimovich S, Kalish RS: Mediation of alopecia areata by cooperartion between CD4+ and CD8+ T lymphocytes: transfer to human scalp explants on Prkdc (scid) mice. *Arch Dermatol* 2002;138(7):916–922.

Greaves MW: The immunopharmacology of skin inflammation: the future is already here! *Br J Dermatol* 2000;143(1):47–52.

Holland SM, DeLeo FR, Elloumi HZ et al. STAT3 mutations in the hyper-IgE syndrome. *N Engl J Med* Oct 18 2007;357(16):1608–1619.

Janeway CA Jr, Medzhitov R: Innate immune recognition. *Annu Rev Immunol* 2002;20:197–216.

Koga C, Kabashima K, Shiraishi N, Kobayashi M, Tokura Y: Possible pathogenic role of Th17 cells for atopic dermatitis. *J Invest Dermatol* 2008;128:2625–2630.

Lai Y, Cogen AL, Radek KA, et al. Activation of TLR2 by a small molecule produced by Staphylococcus epidermidis increases antimicrobial defense against bacterial skin infections. *J Invest Dermatol* Sep 2010;130(9):2211–2221.

Heil PM, Maurer D, Klein B, Hultsch T, Stingl G: Omalizumab therapy in atopic dermatitis: depletion of IgE does not improve the clinical course - a randomized, placebo-controlled and double blind pilot study. *J Dtsch Dermatol Ges* Dec 2010;8(12):990–998.

Lan RT, Ansari AA, Lian ZX, Gershwin ME: Regulatory T cells: development, function and role in autoimmunity. *Autoimmun Rev* 2005;4(6):351–363.

Mackel SE, Jordan RE: Leukocytoclasitc vasculitis. A cutaneous expression of immune complex disease. *Arch Dermatol* 1982; 118(5):296–301.

Nomura I, et al. Cytokine milieu of atopic dermatitis, as compared to Psoriasis, skin prevents induction of innate immune response genes. *J Immunol* 2003;171:3262–3269.

Sakaguchi S, Yamaguchi T, Nomura T, Ono M: Regulatory T cells and 2013 Mar 27;93(2):131-7. doi: 10.2340/00015555-1382.

Schwartz JR, Messenger AG, Tosti A, et al. A comprehensive pathophysiology of dandruff and seborrheic dermatitis–towards a more precise definition of scalp health. *Acta Derm Venereol* Mar 27 2013;93(2):131–137. doi: 10.2340/00015555–1382.

Stanley MA: Imiquimod and the imidazoquinolones: mechanism of action and therapeutic potential. *Clin Exp Dermatol* 2002;27(7):571–577.

Stone JH, Zen Y, Deshpande V: IgG4-related disease. *N Engl J Med* Feb 9 2012;366(6):539–551.

Topalian SL, Hodi FS, Brahmer JR, et al. Safety, activity, and immune correlates of anti-PD-1 antibody in cancer. *N Engl J Med* Jun 28 2012;366(26):2443–2454.

Victor FC, Gottlieb AB, Menter A: Changing paradigms in dermatology: tumor necrosis factor alpha blockade in psoriasis and psoriatic arthritis. *Clin Dermatol* 2003:21(5):392–397.

Williams JDL, Griffiths CEM: Cytokine blocking agents in dermatology. *Clin Exp Dermatol* 2002;27(7):585.

CHAPTER 28

BASIC SCIENCES

BASSEL H. MAHMOUD
CHRISTOPHER T. BURNETT

INTRODUCTION

- Skin is the largest organ in the body. It weighs over 5 kg in a 70-kg individual and contains a variety of complex adnexal structures, including hair, nails, glands, and specialized sensory structures
- The anatomic structures of the skin are similar in most regions of the body
- Specialized regions of skin have modified forms of these structures, such as the palms, soles, genitalia, and scalp
- Human skin consists of a stratified, cellular epidermis, and an underlying dermis of connective tissue. Beneath the dermis is a layer of subcutaneous fat

EPIDERMIS AND DERMIS

Epidermis

- The epidermis contains 3 major resident populations of cells: keratinocytes, melanocytes, and Langerhans cells
- Approximately 0.4 to 1.5 mm thick and consisting mostly of keratinocytes (Fig. 28-1)
- Epidermis is formed by division of cells in the basal layer which give rise to the spinous layer
- Under basal conditions, differentiated keratinocytes require approximately 2 weeks to reach the stratum corneum (SC) and an additional 2 weeks to be shed from the SC
- Keratinocytes have the capacity to increase rates of proliferation and maturation to levels far greater than this, when stimulated to do so by injury, inflammation, or disease
- Divided into 4 main layers with characteristic cell shape, specialized intracellular structures, types of keratin, accessory cells, and proteins (Table 28-1): SC, stratum granulosum, stratum spinosum, stratum basale
- *Stratum disjunction*: outer SC cells are more prone to desquamation
- *Stratum compactum*: cells of the lower SC; thicker cells and more densely packed, organized parallel arrays of keratin filaments, more fragile cornified envelope
- Stratum lucidum is an additional layer present between the strata granulosum and corneum in palmoplantar skin. It appears as an electron-lucent zone and contains nucleated cells
- Differentiation from basal cell to corneocyte involves the loss of the nucleus and extrusion of cellular contents except for keratin filaments and filaggrin matrix
- The most obvious function of epidermis lies in the SC, a semipermeable surface which serve as a physiologic barrier

SPECIALIZED CELLS

- *Merkel cell*
  - Type I mechanoreceptor (slow-adapting, low threshold)
  - Located amongst basal keratinocytes and are mainly found in hairy skin, tactile areas of glabrous skin, taste buds, the anal canal, labial epithelium, and eccrine sweat glands
  - Thought to be derived from ectoderm/neural crest but recent studies have demonstrated that mammalian Merkel cells are derived from an epidermal rather than neural crest lineage
  - Scattered throughout the epidermis of vertebrates and constitute 0.2 to 5% of epidermal cells
  - Contain granules with neurotransmitter-like substances; nonspecific enolase present
  - Members of the amine precursor uptake and decarboxylation (APUD) system
  - They are identified by the presence of cytoplasmic dense core granules, cytokeratin 20, and neuropeptides
  - Keratins found in merkel cells: K20 is specific; also contain K18, K8, K19
  - Sun-exposed skin may contain twice as many Merkel cells as nonsun-exposed skin

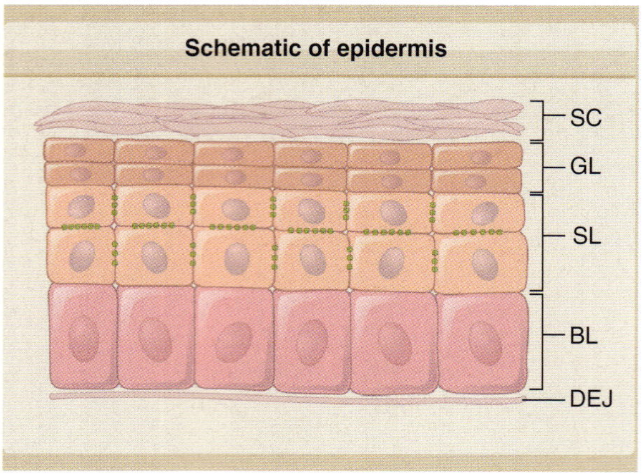

FIGURE 28-1 Epidermis. (*Reprinted with permission from Goldsmith LA et al. Fitzpatrick's Dermatology in General Medicine, 8th Ed. New York: McGraw-Hill; 2012.*)

TABLE 28-1 Layers of the Skin and Characteristics

	Cell Shape	Types of Cells	Types of Keratin	Additional Structures	Associated Proteins
Stratum corneum Stratum disjunctum (outer stratum corneum cells)	Flattened polyhedral-shaped horny cells with loss of nucleus	Keratinocytes		Cornified cell envelope	Loricrin Profilaggrin Filaggrin Involucrin
Stratum compactum (cells of the lower stratum corneum)					Cornifin Trichohyalin TGM 1/2/3 Envolplakin SPR 1/2
Stratum granulosum	Diamond shaped with characteristic dense basophilic granules		K2 K11	Basophilic keratohyaline granules	Profilaggrin Loricrin
Stratum spinosum	Polyhedral with round nucleus; "spiny appearance"	Keratinocytes Langerhans cell Transient amplifying cells	K1 K10 K9	Lamellar granules Desmosomes Gap junctions	Desmoglein II/III Desmocollin I
Stratum germinativum	Columnar with round nucleus	Keratinocytes stem cells (10%) Transient amplifying cells (50%) Postmitotic differentiated cells (40%) Melanocytes Merkel cell Langerhans cell	K5 K14 K19		BPAG 1

- Circulating autoantibodies against Merkel cells have been described in pemphigus and graft-versus-host disease. Merkel cells are absent in vitiligo lesions, in keeping with an autoimmune destruction or neural involvement
- *Melanocytes*
  - Pigment-producing cells located in the skin, inner ear, choroid, and iris of the eye
  - Neural crest–derived dendritic cell; forms along the dorsal neural tube. They can also arise from Schwann cell precursors located along nerves in the skin
  - Mainly confined to basal layer
  - Extend above and below basal layer but do not form junctions with keratinocytes
  - Contains 2 types of the pigment melanin
    - Eumelanin (brown and black coloration)
    - Pheomelanin (red or yellow coloration)
  - Melanocytes are functional at birth, but newborn skin is not fully pigmented and subsequently darkens over the first few months of life
  - By the time of birth, dermal melanocytes have disappeared with the exception of certain anatomic sites (e.g., presacral, head/neck, and dorsal hands), which correspond to common locations for dermal melanocytoses and blue nevi
  - Melanocyte function, development, and differentiation are under the control of the paired box (PAX3) and the microphthalmia-associated transcription factor (MITF) genes. (Mutations in PAX3 and MITF result in Waardenburg syndrome.)
  - Melanocytes migrate dorsoventrally in the eighth week of fetal development
  - Melanin synthesis begins in the head region in the third month of fetal development
  - Melanin is also found in the retina, uvea, cochlea/vestibular apparatus, and leptomeninges; therefore, diseases of skin pigmentation also may have abnormalities in these areas
  - In all races, density of melanocytes is a consistent ratio of about 1 melanocyte for every 10 keratinocytes
  - Melanocytes reside in the basal layer and send dendrites containing melanosomes (containing the pigment melanin) into contact with keratinocytes
  - Melanocytes do not form desmosomes with adjacent keratinocytes; they may form contact via E-cadherin adhesion molecules
  - Melanocytes do not form hemidesmosomes with the basement membrane
- *Melanosomes*
  - Melanosomes are secretory organelles developed from specialized exocrine cells of neural crest origin
  - *Epidermal melanin unit*: each melanocyte secretes melanosomes into several keratinocytes (approximately 36)
  - Differences in skin pigmentation are due to differences in size and distribution of melanosomes
    - Dark skin = larger and single melanosomes
    - Light skin = smaller and grouped melanosomes
  - Four stages of melanosome development
    - Stage I—premelanosome
      - ▲ Round in shape
      - ▲ No melanin
    - Stage II—melanosome
      - ▲ Eumelanosomes with oval, lamellar structure
      - ▲ Pheomelanosomes with round, irregular structure
      - ▲ Start of melanin deposition
      - ▲ High tyrosinase activity
    - Stage III—melanosome
      - ▲ Partially melanized
      - ▲ Decrease in tyrosinase activity
      - ▲ Acid phosphatase present
    - Stage IV—melanosome
      - ▲ Complete melanization
      - ▲ Very little tyrosinase activity
      - ▲ Acid phosphatase present
      - ▲ Pathway of melanin formation
  - Melanosome structure is formed within melanocytes
  - Tyrosinase enzyme necessary for melanin formation is formed from Golgi apparatus of melanocyte
  - Tyrosinase is transported to melanosome and begins melanin formation
  - Melanosome is transferred to keratinocyte
  - Melanosome is degraded during ascent to cornified layer
  - Melanin is ultimately removed with loss of SC
- *Melanin*
  - Pigment that absorbs UV and visible light over a wide range of wavelengths without a distinct peak of absorption
  - Able to absorb free radicals
  - Tyrosinase is the main enzyme for melanin formation and catalyzes the first step: hydroxylation of tyrosine to dopa
  - Tyrosinase is copper dependent
  - Tyrosine → dopa → dopaquinone: both these steps are catalyzed by tyrosinase
  - The type of melanin produced depends on presence of other factors
    - Eumelanin—brown-black pigment
      - ▲ Formed if divalent cations are present with dopaquinone
      - ▲ Found in dark, oval melanosomes
    - Pheomelanin—yellow-red pigment
      - ▲ Formed if cysteine (or glutathione) is present with dopaquinone
      - ▲ Found in round, lamellar melanosomes

- Control of melanin production
  - Pigmentation is either constitutive (level of pigment determined genetically) or facultative (inducible by UV exposure, "tan")
  - Stimulated by melanocyte-stimulating hormone (MSH), which is derived from the larger precursor proopiomelanocortin (POMC); POMC is also the precursor for adrenocorticotropic hormone (ACTH); this explains the hyperpigmentation of Addison disease
  - Stimulated by estrogens and progesterones
- Melanocytic protein associated conditions: (see Chapter 9, Pigmentary Disorders)
- *Langerhans cell*
  - Dendritic, bone marrow–derived (mesoderm) antigen-presenting cell (APC)
  - Density in fetal skin remains low early in gestation and increases to adult levels during the third trimester
  - Langerhans cells, in combination with macrophages and dermal dendrocytes, represent the skin's mononuclear phagocyte system. They are capable of phagocytosis, antigen processing, antigen presentation, and interactions with lymphocytes
  - Have characteristics distinct from other dendritic cells in that they are more likely to induce Th2 responses than the Th1 responses that are usually necessary for cellular immune responses against pathogens
  - Involved in T-cell responses (i.e., contact hypersensitivity and graft-versus-host disease)
  - Process antigen and present it to T cells in the presence of major histocompatability complex (MHC) class II
  - Produces interleukin 1 (IL-1) to promote lymphocyte chemotaxis and activation
  - Under pathological stimulation, adjacent Langerhans cells may exchange antigens between cells
  - Can be distinguished by their characteristic dendritic morphology; expression of CD45, HLA-DR, and CD1c; and high levels of ATPase activity. Langerin expression precedes CD1a acquisition
  - Contains distinctive racket-shaped Birbeck granules that are formed when an antigen is internalized by endocytosis
  - Ultraviolet B (UVB) decreases number and antigen-presenting ability of Langerhans cell
  - Can be infected with HIV

Specialized Structures

- *Desmosomes*
  - Desmosomes are multiprotein complexes that function as cell-cell adhesion structures in epidermal cells
  - They also provide attachment sites for the keratin intermediate filament cytoskeleton of keratinocytes
  - Tissues that are exposed to a significant amount of mechanical stress, are often affected by desmosomal defects
  - Prominent in the stratum spinosum
  - Anchoring junctions that connect adjacent keratinocytes (Fig. 28-2)
  - Keratin filaments extend from desmosome to desmosome to form keratin cytoskeleton
  - Desmosomes also function as signaling centers, for example, by controlling the cytoplasmic pool of signaling molecules
  - Structure consists of a desmosomal plaque on the interior of the cell membrane, transmembrane glycoproteins, and a central plate that crosses the intercellular space between 2 keratinocytes
  - Plaque contains polypeptides
    - Desmoplakins 1 and 2—mediate attachment of keratins to plaque
    - Desmocalmin—important for calcium regulation
    - Band 6 protein
    - Plakoglobin—mediates attachment of keratins to plaque
    - Desmoyokin—associated with cell membrane

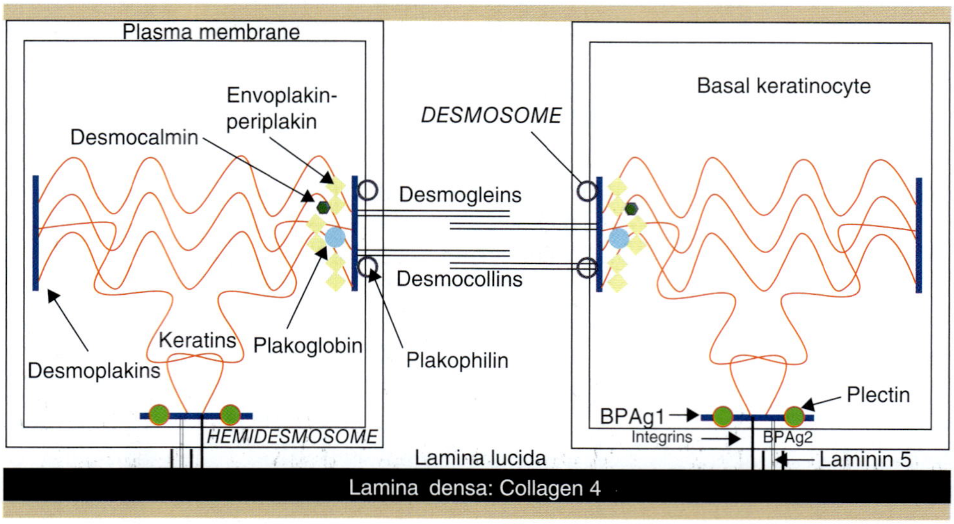

FIGURE 28-2 Desmosomes. *(Modified with permission from Freedberg IM et al. Fitzpatrick's Dermatology in General Medicine, 6th Ed. New York: McGraw-Hill, 2003; p. 93.)*

- *Adherens junctions*
  - Adherens junctions contribute to epithelial assembly, adhesion, barrier formation, cell motility and changes in cell shape
  - Cadherins (Ca^{2+} dependent cell-cell adhesion molecules) provide adhesion
  - Complex of cytoplasmic plaque proteins, catenins, also known as plakoglobin
  - Actin attaches to cadherins via α, β, and γ catenins
- *Tight junctions*
  - Seal the intercellular space, thus preventing the free diffusion of macromolecules
  - In the granular layer of the epidermis, they maintain the water barrier function of the epidermis
  - Composed of structural proteins called claudins
  - Mutation in claudin-1 has been linked to a rare ichthyosis
- *Gap junctions*
  - Gap junction communication is essential for cell synchronization, differentiation, cell growth and metabolic coordination of avascular organs, including epidermis
  - Made of connexins
    - Mutation in connexin-26 results in Vohwinkel syndrome and keratitis-ichthyosis-deafness syndrome (KID)
    - Mutation in connexin-30 results in Clouston syndrome
    - Mutation in connexin-30.3 and connexin-31 result in erythrokeratodermia variabilis
  - Apart from the connexins, vertebrates contain pannexins, however, no human abnormalities of pannexins have been reported
- *Lamellar granules (Odland bodies)*
  - First apparent in upper spinous layer, but primary site of action is the granular layer where they migrate towards the periphery of the cells as they enter the granular cell layer
  - 0.2 to 0.3 μm in diameter, membrane-bound secretory granules
  - Contain glycoproteins, glycolipids, phospholipids, free sterols, acid hydrolases, and glucosylceramides (precursors to ceramides that contribute to corneum lipid layer)
  - Discharge their contents of lipids and enzymes into the intercellular space, where the lipid is rearranged to lipid sheets
  - Create a hydrophobic barrier between the granular and cornified layers and play an important role in intercellular cohesion within the SC
- *Keratohyaline granules*
  - Located in the granular layer
  - Filaggrin (cleaved from profilaggrin) becomes the major protein of keratohyaline granules
  - In SC, the cells become flattened and the keratin filaments align into disulphide cross-linked macrofibres, under the influence of filaggrin, the protein component of the keratohyalin granule, responsible for keratin filament aggregation
  - Involved in formation of cornified cell envelope (CCE)
  - Rich in sulfur
  - Loss-of-function mutations in the filaggrin gene is the cause of the genetic disorder ichthyosis vulgaris and a risk factor for the development of atopic dermatitis, atopic asthma, and systemic allergies
- *CCE*
  - An extremely durable protein-lipid polymer
  - Assembled on the interior of the keratinocyte
  - Eventually resides on the exterior of the corneocyte
  - Provides a mechanical and chemical barrier
  - CCE is 7 to 15 nm thick
  - Impermeability of this layer is achieved by the action of calcium-dependent transglutaminases (TGs) that bind (cross-link) loricrin, keratin, desmosomal proteins, involucrin, elafin, and other proteins to the cell membrane, creating a proteinaceous and insoluble shield
  - Epsilon-gamma-glutamyl-lysine-isopeptide cross-links make the CCE insoluble
  - Mutations in TG1 underlie some cases of lamellar ichthyosis or nonbullous congenital ichthyosiform erythroderma; mutations in TG5 result in autosomal recessive skin peeling syndrome

Specialized Proteins

- Profilaggrin/filaggrin (*fil*ament *aggr*egate prote*in)*
  - Profilaggrin is a protein made up of 10 to 12 tandem repeat units of filaggrin
  - Profilaggrin is converted to monomers of filaggrin in a stepwise conversion by 3 proteases and dephosphorylation
  - Filaggrin is thought to provide a protein matrix for keratin filament aggregation in corneocytes
- *Loricrin*
  - A protein composing 70% of the CCE
  - Hydrophobic, cysteine-rich protein
  - Gene is located on chromosome 1q21 as part of the epidermal differentiation complex
  - Encoded along with other proteins required for the terminal differentiation of epidermis
  - Loricrin is localized to the desmosome in association with desmoglein
- *Involucrin*
  - Glutamine-rich, acidic protein
  - Resistant to denaturing and unchanged by retinoic acids
  - Early marker of keratin differentiation
  - Serves as a scaffold for other proteins to bind during keratinization

Dermis

- The dermis provides structural and nutritional support. It is composed of a mucopolysaccharide gel held together by a collagen- and elastin-containing fibrous matrix

- The origin of the dermis varies depending on the body site
- Vascular structures, accompanied by nerves and mast cells, course through the dermis to provide nutrition, recirculating cells, and cutaneous sensation
- Collagen is major protein composed of fibroblasts. Mainly type I in adult skin and type III in fetal skin
- Two regions
  - Papillary dermis
    - Superficial
    - Small collagen bundles
    - Fine meshwork of microfibrils (fibrillin) organized into elaunin and oxytalan fibers
  - Reticular dermis
    - Below papillary dermis
    - Large collagen bundles
    - Mature, branching elastic fibers
- Main components of dermis
  - Ground substance (mucopolysaccharides)
  - Subpapillary vascular plexus
  - Deeper vascular plexus that envelops hair follicles and eccrine sweat glands
  - Fibroblasts, macrophages, and mast cells
  - Afferent nerves (stain for S-100)
    - Unmyelinated nerve fibers (C-type fibers)
      - ▲ Detect temperature, pain, and itch
      - ▲ Located in papillary dermis and possibly basal layer
      - ▲ Encapsulated nerve endings detect touch and pressure
    - Meissner corpuscles
      - ▲ Located in dermal papillae
      - ▲ Detect light pressure
      - ▲ More prevalent in palms and soles
      - ▲ "Pine cone" appearance
    - Vater-Pacini corpuscles
      - ▲ Located in deep dermis of palms, dorsum of hands, and soles; also skin of nipples and anogenital region
      - ▲ Detect deep pressure and vibration
      - ▲ "Pearl onion" appearance in cross section
    - Mucocutaneous end organs (Krause end bulbs)
      - ▲ Located in papillary dermis
      - ▲ Found in skin at mucocutaneous junction (vermilion border of lips, glans penis, clitoris)

DERMAL-EPIDERMAL JUNCTION (DEJ)

- The boundary between epidermis and dermis consists of a specialized aggregation of attachment molecules, known as the basement membrane zone (BMZ)
- Mediates adhesion between the basal keratinocytes and the dermis and provides resistance against shearing forces on the skin
- Thickness of 0.5 to 1.0 mm
- Visualized with periodic acid–Schiff (PAS) staining
- The major biochemical components of the BMZ are type IV collagen and a number of collagenous glycoproteins, including laminin 332
- *Function*
  - Main function of BMZ is as supportive structure to anchor the epidermis to the dermis: anchoring occurs through the cytoskeleton in keratinocytes that bind to laminin 332 in the lamina lucida, which, in turn, binds to type VII collagen in lamina densa
  - Other basement membranes functions include: tissue repair; matrices for cell migration; influence differentiation, morphogenesis, and apoptosis of epithelial cell layers; and permeability barriers for cells and macromolecules
- Hemidesmosome (anchoring complex) (Fig. 28-3)
  - Attaches basal cells of epidermis to the basement membrane (link keratin cytoskeleton to laminin 332 in the lamina lucida)
  - Structurally different from desmosomes
  - Consists of a cytoplasmic portion (attachment plaque), transmembrane portion bullous pemphigoid (BP) antigen 2 (180 kD) and integrin, and an extracellular portion (anchoring filaments and subbasal dense plate)
  - Cytoplasmic attachment plaque
    - Consists of BP antigen 1 (230 kD) and plectin (HD-1)
    - Keratin filaments (K5, 14) attach to plaque
    - Desmocalmin and desmoplakin bind keratin to plaque
    - Intracellular portion of BP antigen 2 (180 kD) (BPAG2) and collagen XVII are also present
  - Transmembrane portion
    - Consists of BP antigen 180 (BPAG2)—type II transmembrane configuration
    - Contains $\alpha 6\beta 4$ integrin, which likely interacts with laminin 5 to form anchoring filaments
  - Subbasal dense plate and anchoring filaments
    - Located below the hemidesmosome in the lamina lucida
    - Integrins and BPAG2 cross the membrane and attach to plate
    - Anchoring filaments then extend from the subbasal plate into the lamina densa, providing a point of deeper attachment
- Three zones of basement membrane zone
  - *Lamina lucida*
    - Named for appearance on electron microscopy (EM) as electron lucen
    - 8 nm wide
    - Weakest of layers—able to split with heat or salt

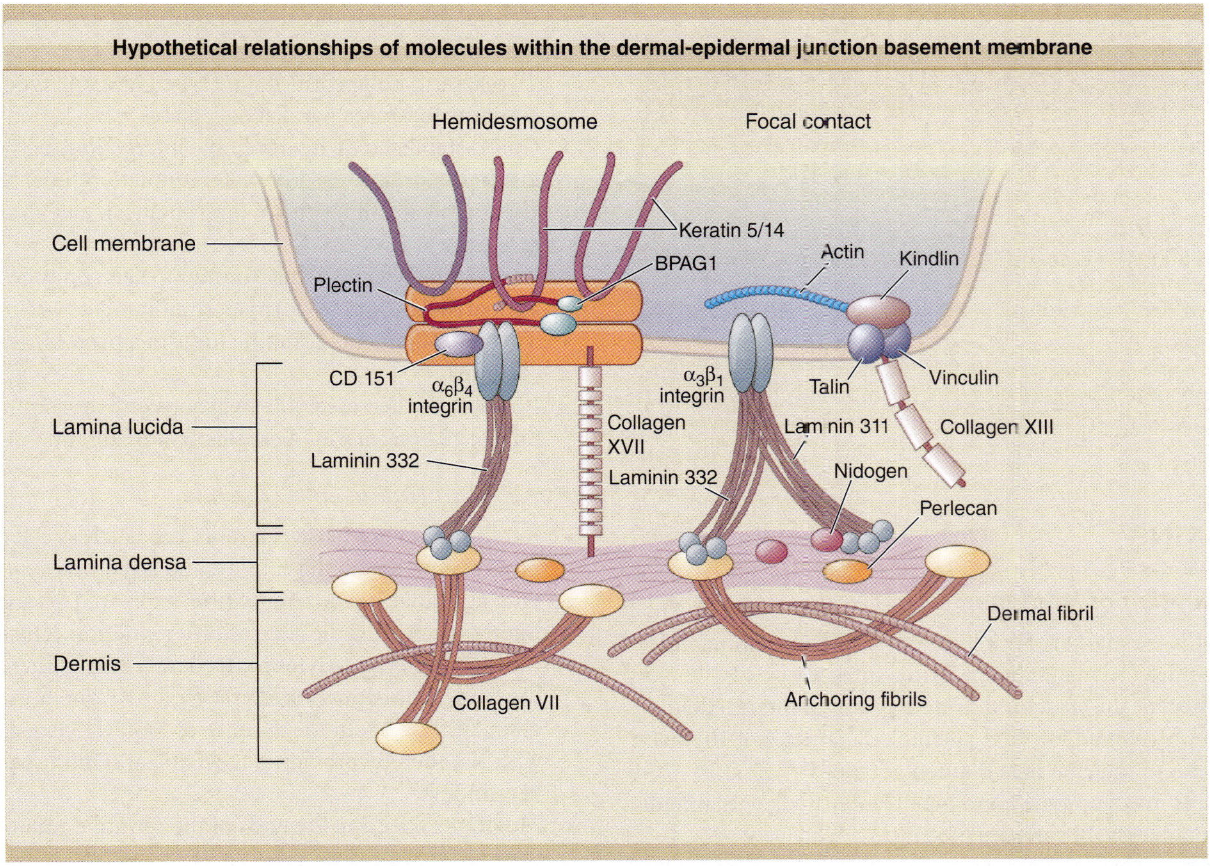

FIGURE 28-3 Hemidesmosome. (*Reprinted with permission from Goldsmith LA et al. Fitzpatrick's Dermatology in General Medicine, 8th Ed. New York: McGraw-Hill; 2012, p. 582.*)

- Composed of laminin 1, nidogen (entactin), and fibronectin
- Anchoring filaments cross lamina lucida
  - ▲ Filaments contain laminin-332 (composed of one α3, β3, and γ2 chain), formerly known as laminin 5 (aka. epiligrin, kalinin, and nicein)
  - ▲ One side connects to attachement plaque of plasma membrane; the other side connects to the subbasal dense plate

- *Lamina densa*
  - Major components of the lamina densa include type IV collagen, laminin, and heparan sulfate proteoglycan (PG)
  - Composed of type IV collagen (unique to dermal-epidermal junction)
  - Also contains entactin (nidogen): binds laminin, collagen IV, perlecan, and fibulins (calcium-binding extracellular matrix proteins)
    - ▲ Fibulins function is to support the structural network of different basement membranes by joining other supramolecular structures, elastic fibers, and aggregates
    - ▲ Fibulin-4 and fibulin-5 are involved in the pathogenesis of recessive and dominant forms of cutis laxa
  - Contains heparan sulfate PG, which is negatively charged owing to disulfide bridges and renders the dermal-epidermal junction impermeable to negatively charged substances
- *Sublamina densa*
  - Contains network of anchoring fibrils composed of type VII collagen
  - Anchoring fibrils originate in lamina densa, dip down into the dermis, and attach to an anchoring plaque or loop back to reinsert into the lamina densa
  - Fibrils appear as "wheatstacks" on EM
  - Contains interstitial collagen fibers of types I, III, V, and VI
  - Contains microfibils composed of fibrillin: 2 types of microfibrils
    - ▲ Elaunins—horizontal
    - ▲ Oxytalins—perpendicular to elaunins
  - Contains microthread-like fibers of the glycoprotein linkin

TABLE 28-2 Classification of Keratins

Type I	Type II
Acidic (pK 4.5–5.5)	Basic or neutral (pK 5.5–7.5)
Smaller in size (40–56.5 kDa)	Larger in size (52–67 kDa)
Keratins K9–K20 Ha1 to Ha4, Hax	Keratins K1–K8 Hb1 to Hb4, Hbx
Chromosome 17q12-21	Chromosome 12q11-13

KERATINS

Classification of Keratins

- Keratins are markers for keratinocyte differentiation and are required to maintain epidermal integrity
- Members of the structural protein group of intermediate filaments (named for their assembled diameter of 10 nm)
- Six types of intermediate filaments (types I–VI)
- Keratins make up type I and type II intermediate filaments
- Approximately 40 varieties of keratin
- Spontaneously form pairs consisting of a type I and a type II; an acidic and a basic protein, respectively (Table 28-2)

Structure of Keratins

- Polypeptides consisting of a central rod domain of approximately 310 amino acids (Fig. 28-4)
- Central domain is composed of 4 highly conserved α-helical regions (designated 1A, 2A, 1B, and 2B)
- Regions are connected by 3 nonhelical linking sequences thought to provide flexibility (designated L1, L12, and L2)
- Central domain is flanked by an amino head and carboxy tail
- Two keratin polypeptides (one type I and one type II) combine to form a parallel coiled coil
- Coil is stabilized by hydrophobic interactions between the 2 strands; structure is now a keratin heterodimer
- Keratin heterodimers form long chains in a head-to-tail sequence
- Two chains of keratin heterodimers then combine in antiparellel fashion to form a protofilament (2–3 nm)
- Two protofilaments combine to form a protofibril (4.5 nm)
- Protofibrils then assemble in groups of 3 or 4 strands to form a 10-nm intermediate filament of keratin

Keratins in Health and Disease

- Keratin influence basic cell functions, such as cell cycle progression, metabolic activity, and apoptosis
- During epidermal differentiation, expressed keratins are highly specific for the state of differentiation. The mitotically active keratinocytes in the basal compartment of the epidermis express the keratin pair K5 and K14, less abundantly, K15. In the absence of K14, K15 can assemble with K5, thereby providing mechanical stability to the keratinocyte
- Mutations affecting the ends of the central domain prove the most deleterious (Table 28-3)

ADHESION MOLECULES

- Adhesion molecules contribute to
  - Cell-to-cell adhesion
  - Interaction between cells
  - Cell signaling
  - Inflammation

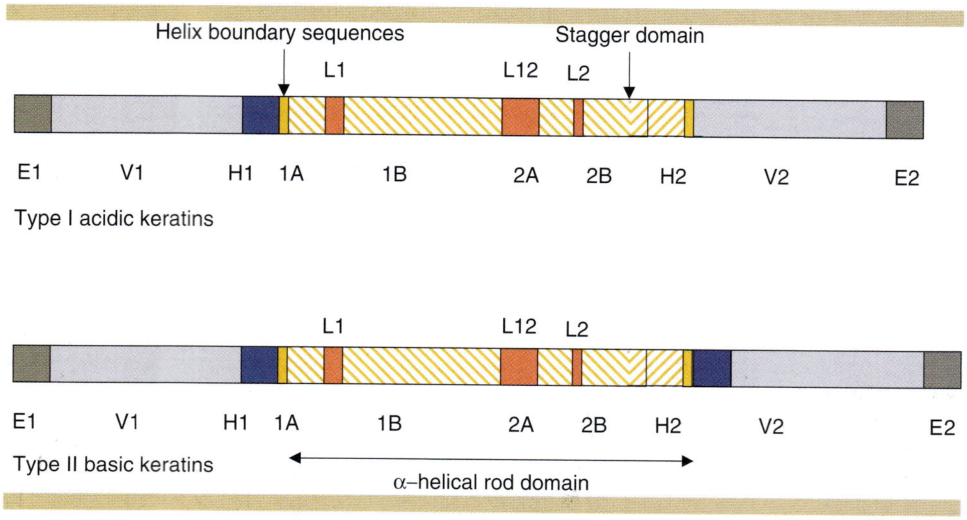

FIGURE 28-4 Keratin polypeptides. *(Reprinted with permission from Freedberg IM et al. Fitzpatrick's Dermatology in General Medicine, 6th Ed. New York: McGraw-Hill, 2003, p. 96.)*

TABLE 28-3 Keratin Expression Patterns and Keratin-Associated Diseases

Type II	Type I	Physiologic Location of Expression	Hereditary Diseases
1	10	Suprabasal keratinocytes	Bullous congenital ichthyosiform erythroderma
1	9	Palmoplantar suprabasilar keratinocytes	Epidermolytic PPK Diffuse nonepidermolytic PPK Epidermolytic PPK with polycyclic psoriasiform plaques
2e	10	Upper spinous and granular layer	Ichthyosis bullosa of Siemens
3	12	Cornea	Meesmann corneal dystrophy
4	13	Mucosal epithelium	White sponge nevus
5	14	Basal keratinocytes	Epidermolysis bullosa simplex
6a	16	Outer root sheath, hyperproliferative keratinocytes, palmoplantar keratinocytes	Pachyonychia congenita type I, focal nonepidermolytic PPK
6b	17	Nail bed, epidermal appendages	Pachyonychia congenita type II Steatocystoma multiplex
8	18	Simple epithelium	Cryptogenic cirrhosis
	19	Embryonic	
Hb, 1, 3, 5, 6	Ha 1, 2, 3a, 3b, 4–8	Hair follicle	Monilethrix (Hb1 and 6)

Reprinted with permission from Freedberg IM et al. *Fitzpatrick's Dermatology in General Medicine*, 6th Ed. New York: McGraw-Hill; 2003, p. 91.

- Migration of cells
- Wound healing
- Embryogenesis

- Families of adhesion molecules
  - Cadherins
    - Calcium-dependent cell-cell adhesion molecules
    - Main adhesion molecule in early embryogenesis
    - Structure: single-pass transmembrane glycoprotein
    - Bind to catenins (link cytoskeleton to adherens junction)
    - Two types
      - ▲ Classic cadherins—found at adherens junctions and interact with cytoplasmic anchoring structures
        - △ E cadherin: found on all epithelium; chromosome 16q
        - △ N cadherin: found on nerve, muscle, epithelium
        - △ P cadherin: found on placenta and basal epithelium
      - ▲ Desmosomal cadherins—found in desmosomes; associate with keratin filaments via plakoglobin and desmoplakin
        - △ Desmoglein—membrane bound; pemphigus vulgaris—autoimmunity against desmoglein 3; pemphigus foliaceous—autoimmunity against desmoglein 1
        - △ Desmocollins—membrane bound
        - △ Plakoglobin—cytoplasmic
        - △ Desmoplakin—cytoplasmic: only molecule known to be present in both desmosomes and adherens junctions
  - Integrins—integrate intracellular cytoskeleton with extracellular matrix
    - Large family of transmembrane molecules composed of 2 noncovalently bound polypeptide subunits (α, β)
    - Most integrins recognize and bind peptide sequence of arginine-glycine-aspartic acid (commonly found on matrix proteins like collagen)

- Subfamily depends on β subunit
- β1—binds cells to extracellular matrix: this subfamily is also known as VLA (very late activation) 1–6
- β2—binds leukocytes to endothelium or other inflammatory cells
  - ▲ Three members: leukocyte function antigen-1 (LFA-1), macrophage activation antigen 1 (Mac 1), and P150, 95
  - ▲ Abnormality leads to leukocyte adhesion problems and chronic infection/abscess
- β3—interaction between platelets and neutrophils at sites of inflammation or vascular damage: contains 2 members: platelet glycoprotein IIb/IIIa and vitronectin receptor
- β4—$\alpha 6\beta_4$ is the most notable of this subfamily
  - ▲ Localized to hemidesmosomes of basement membrane
  - ▲ Binds to laminin 5 in anchoring filaments
  - ▲ Plays an important role in junctional epidermolysis bullosa
- Summary of integrins (Table 28-4)

• Selectins
  - Family of proteins that function in cell-cell adhesion; mediate recruitment of inflammatory cells
  - Three classes
    - ▲ L-selectin (leukocyte): expressed on leukocytes
    - ▲ P-selectin (platelet)
      - △ Stored preformed in Weibel-Palade bodies (WPBs) of endothelium; released rapidly to membrane in response to stimulation and then can be reinternalized
      - △ Also found on α-granules of platelets and megakaryocytes
    - ▲ E-selectin (endothelial): produced on endothelial cells in response to IL-1 and tumor necrosis factor (TNF)

• Immunoglobulin supergene family
  - Extensive group of cell surface-binding proteins that contain one or more Ig/Ig-like domain (disulfide-bridged loops)
  - *Cellular adhesion molecule* (CAM)
  - Primary function is antigen recognition and cell-cell adhesion
  - Can be inducible or constitutively expressed on endothelium
  - Members
    - ▲ Intercellular adhesion molecule 1 (ICAM 1) CD54
      - △ Expressed constitutively on endothelial cells, certain epithelial cells, and antigen presenting cells
      - △ Can be induced for surface expression on other cells by cytokines (αIFN)
      - △ ICAM 1 allows inflammatory cells to attach and infiltrate lesions in skin (e.g., psoriasis)
      - △ Ligand is LFA-1
      - △ Interaction of LFA-1 and ICAM allows T cells to come into close contact with an APC, which is a key step in activating a T-lymphocyte
      - △ ICAM 1 is the receptor for rhinovirus on respiratory epithelium
    - ▲ Intercellular adhesion molecule 2 (ICAM 2)
      - △ Constitutively expressed
      - △ A second ligand for LFA-1
    - ▲ Leukocyte function antigen 3 (LFA-3) CD58
      - △ Expressed on APCs and forms a ligand with CD2 receptor on T-cell surface
      - △ This is a secondary signal in the activation of T cells
      - △ Important target for current psoriasis therapies
    - ▲ Vascular cell adhesion molecule 1 (VCAM 1)
      - △ Expressed on endothelial cells on activation
      - △ Expression induced by IL-1 and TNF-α
      - △ Directly involved in endothelium-lymphocyte interactions
      - △ Mediates recruitment of lymphocytes into areas of inflammation

EXTRACELLULAR MATRIX OF CONNECTIVE TISSUE

Four major classes of extracellular matrix components:

(a) Collagen fibers, which provide tensile strength to allow skin to serve as a protective organ against external trauma
(b) Elastic structures, which provide elasticity and resilience to normal human skin
(c) Noncollagenous glycoproteins, such as fibrillins, fibulins, and integrins, which often serve as organizers of the matrix and facilitate cell-matrix interactions
(d) PG/glycosaminoglycan (GAG), which provide hydration to the skin

COLLAGEN

- Major extracellular matrix component in the dermis
- Produced by ribosomes within fibroblasts
- Provide tensile strength to the skin to serve as a protective organ against external trauma
- Represents 70 to 80% of dry weight of the dermis
- Basic collagen structure is 3 α chains combined in a triple-helix formation with cross-linking hydrogen bonds
- Twenty nine distinct collagens have been identified in vertebrate tissues, and are referred to by Roman numeral

TABLE 28-4 Summary of Integrins

Integrin	Alternate Name	Expressed on	Matrix Ligand	Endothelial Ligand
β1 Subfamily				
α1β1	VLA-1	T cells	Collagen I, IV Laminin	
α2β1	VLA-2	T cells	Collagen I, IV Laminin	
α3β1	VLA-3	T cells	Collagen Laminin 1, 5 Fibronectin Epiligrin	
α4β1	VLA-4	T cells	Fibronectin	VCAM-1
α5β1	VLA-5	T cells	Fibronectin	
α6β1	VLA-6	T cells	Laminin	
β2 Subfamily				
α1β2	LFA-1	Neutrophils Monocytes		ICAM-1 ICAM-2
αmβ2	Mac-1	Neutrophils Monocytes	C3bi Fibronectin	ICAM-1
αxβ2	P150, 95	Neutrophils Monocytes	C3b Fibronectin	
β3 Subfamily				
Platelet Glycoprotein Iib/IIIa		Platelets	Fibrinogen Fibronectin von Willebrand factor Vitronectin	
Vitronectin Receptor		Vitronectin Fibrinogen vWF		
β4 Subfamily				
α6β4		Keratinocytes (basal)	Laminin 1, 5	

designation (I–XXIX) in the order of their discovery, many of them being present in the skin

- Typical sequence of collagen: GLY-X-Y (Fig. 28-5)
  - GLY = glycine, always the third residue, 33% of amino acids in collagen
  - X = frequently proline
  - Y = frequently hydroxyproline or hydroxylysine
- Genetically distinct collagens can be divided into different classes
  - Types I, II, III, V, and IX align into large fibrils and are designated as fibril-forming collagens
  - Type IV is arranged in an interlacing network within the basement membranes
  - Type VI is a distinct microfibril-forming collagen

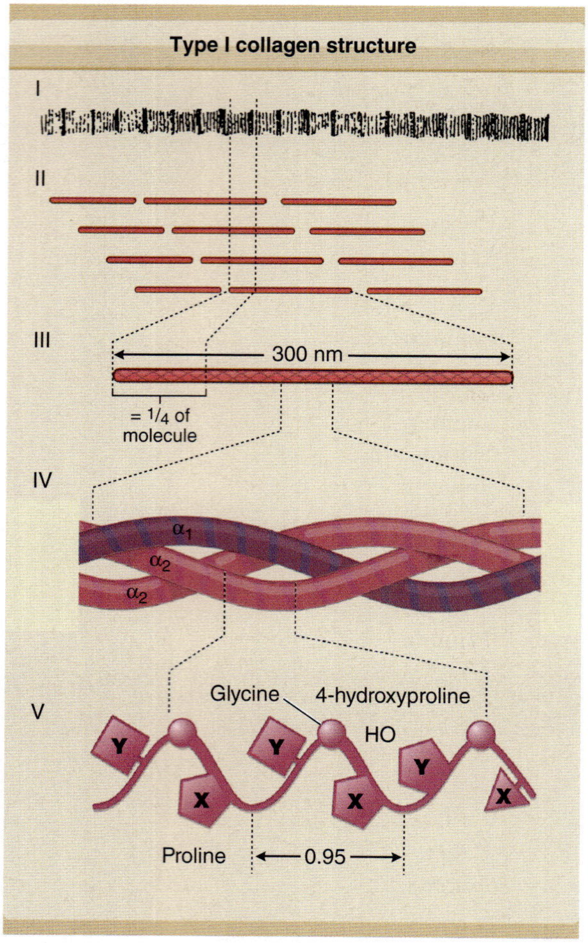

FIGURE 28-5 Typical sequence of collagen. *(Redrawn from Uitto J et al. Collagens structure, function, and pathology. In: Progress in Diseases of the Skin, vol. 1, edited by R. Fleischmajer. New York: Grune & Stratton, 1981, p. 103.)*

- Type VII collagen forms anchoring fibrils
- FACIT collagens (fibril-associated collagens with interrupted triple helices) include types IX, XII, XIV, XIX, XX, and XXI
- Collagen biosynthesis (Fig. 28-6)
  - Pretranslational
    - Occurs in the nucleus
    - Transcription of genes for procollagen
    - messenger ribonucleic acid (mRNA) is formed
  - Cotranslational
    - mRNA is transferred to ribosomes of rich endoplasmic reticulum (RER)
    - Preprocollagen is formed and contains a signal peptide that indicates that the peptide is to be excreted from the cell
    - During passage through the RER the following occurs:
      - ▲ Hydrolytic cleavage of signal peptide
      - ▲ Hydroxylation of proline and lysine residues by prolyl hydroxylase or lysyl hydroxylase (deficient in type VI Ehlers-Danlos syndrome); hydroxylation requires oxygen, vitamin C, ferrous iron, α-ketoglutarate
      - ▲ Glycosylation of hydroxylysine residues and asparagine with N-linked oligosaccharides
  - Postranslational
    - While in the RER, 3 procollagens are aligned and form disulfide bonds between chains to stabilize the structure; this occurs first on the amino end and then on the carboxy end
    - Three procollagens form a triple helix (carboxy-to-amino end)
    - Procollagen is transferred from the RER to the Golgi complex and is secreted continuously from the cell into the extracellular space
    - Once excreted, neutral calcium-dependent proteinases cleave the extra peptide extensions on the end of the procollagen to form tropocollagen
    - Tropocollagen then combines to form collagen fibrils, which are stabilized by cross-links
    - Cross-linking is catalyzed by lysyl oxidase, which uses copper as a required cofactor (enzyme is defective in type IX Ehlers-Danlos syndrome)
    - Fibrils combine to create a collagen fiber
- Factors that affect collagen production
  - Ascorbic acid—stimulates
  - Transforming growth factor β (TGF-β)—stimulates
  - IL-1—inhibits by stimulating PGE2
  - Glucocorticoids—inhibit collagen gene transcription
  - Retinoic acid—increases collagen synthesis
  - Interferon-γ (INF-γ)—potent inhibitor of collagen gene transcription
  - TNF-α—inhibits gene transcription
  - D-penicillamine—interferes with collagen cross-linking
  - Minoxidil—inhibits expression of lysyl hydroxylase
  - Distribution of types of collagens (Table 28-5)
  - Heritable connective tissue diseases (Table 28-6)

ELASTIC TISSUE

- Provides resilience and elasticity to the skin, to allow skin to return to normal shape after being deformed or stretched, they can be stretched by 100% or more and still return to their original form
- Composed of elastic fibers and is a relatively minor component in normal sun-protected adult skin, being less than 2 to 4% of the total dry weight of the dermis
- Elastic fibers are visualized with special stains: Verhoeff-van Gieson, Orcein, or Resorcin-Fuchsin
- Elastic fibers are made of protein filaments embedded in an amorphous matrix of mostly elastin; this elastin core is surrounded by microfibrils that contain fibrillin

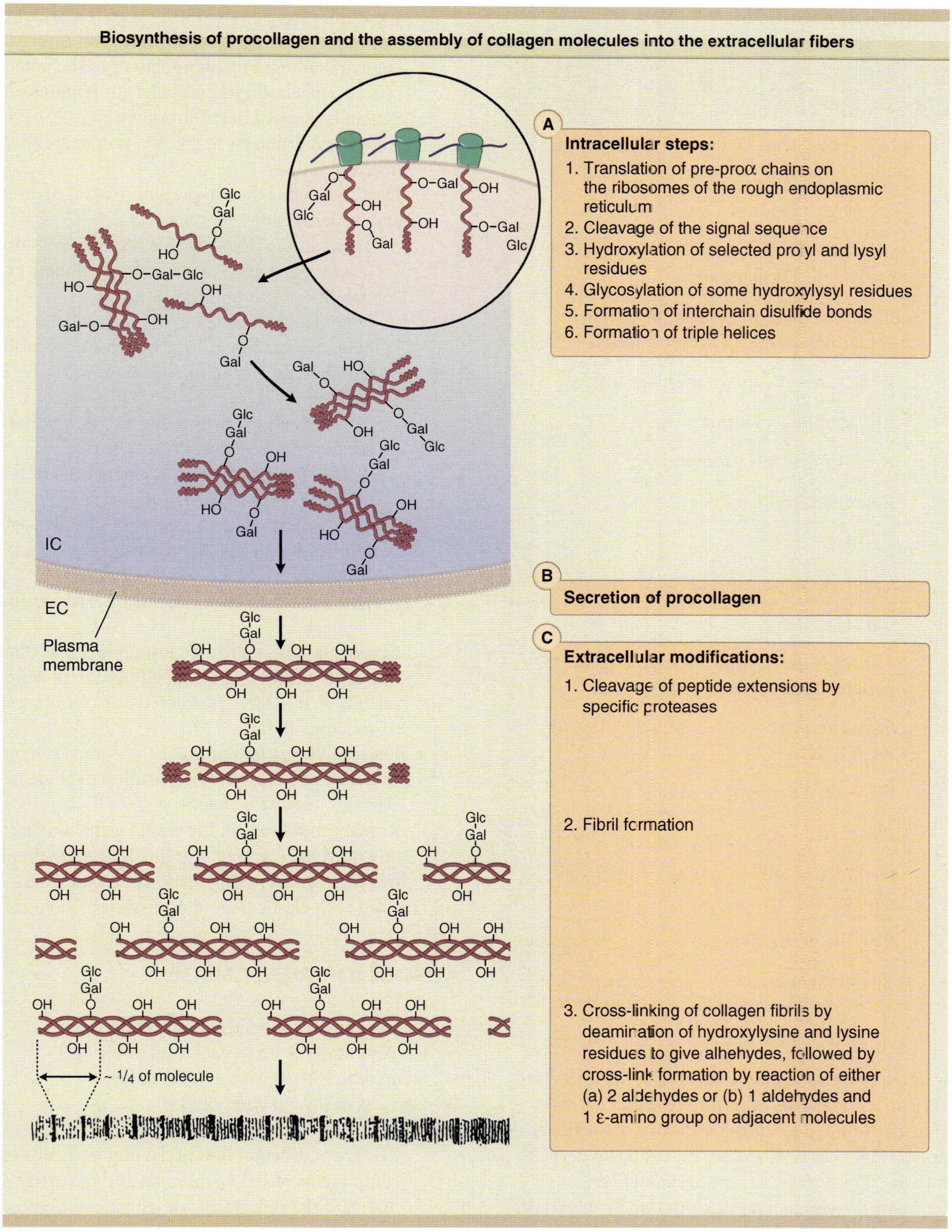

FIGURE 28-6 Collagen biosynthesis. (*Reprinted with permission from Goldsmith LA et al. Fitzpatrick's Dermatology in General Medicine, 8th Ed. New York: McGraw-Hill; 2012.*)

TABLE 28-5 Distribution of Types of Collagens

Collagen	Distribution
I	Skin, bone, tendon, dentin (80% of total adult collagen)
II	Cartilage, vitreous
III	Blood vessels, gut, fetal skin (predominant cartilage), chorioamnion
IV	Basement membrane (lamina densa), epidermal appendages, blood vessels
V	Wide spread except in hyaline cartilage
VI	Aortic intima, placenta
VII	Anchoring fibrils, amnion
VIII	Endothelial cells, cornea
IX	Cartilage
X	Cartilage (hypertrophic)
XI	Cartilage
XII	Cartilage, fibroblasts, FACIT collagen, perichondrium, periosteum, cornea
XIV	Cartilage, skin, tendons, muscle, placenta, FACIT collagen
XV	Placenta, basement membrane
XVI	Placenta
XVII	Hemidesmosomes (bullous pemphigoid antigen 2)
XVIII	Placenta, liver, kidney, basement membrane
XIX	Rhabdomyosarcoma, basement membrane

- In fully developed elastic fibers, ver 90% of the total content is elastin with relatively few microfibrillar components, mostly confined to the outer surface of the fibers
- Papillary dermis—elastic fibers are thin and run perpendicular to the skin surface; named *oxytalan fibers*
- Reticular dermis—elastic fibers are thick and run parallel to the skin surface; named *elaunin fibers,* which interconnect to provide a network structure
- Elastin
  - Synthesized as a precursor polypeptide, "tropoelastin," which consists of approximately 700 amino acids with a molecular mass of approximately 70 kDa
  - Secreted mainly by skin fibroblasts
  - Keratinocytes have also been suggested to express the elastin gene, but the level of expression is very low in comparison to dermal fibroblasts and the potential significance of elastin in the epidermis remains unclear
  - Elastin is mapped to chromosome 7
  - Composed primarily of glycine, alanine, valine, proline, and lysine
  - Elastin contains the unique amino acids of desmosine and isodesmosine
    - These amino acids provide sites for cross-linking (catalyzed by lysyl oxidase); cross-linking creates stability and insolubility
    - Desmosine is formed in the extracellular space by oxidative deamination of lysyl residues to allysine and then the fusion of 3 allysines with a lysyl residue
    - This is catalyzed by the enzyme lysyl oxidase, with copper and oxygen as cofactors
    - Anetoderma = loss and fragmentation of skin owing to decreased desmosine
- Expression of elastin is activated early in embryogenesis and continues at a steady rate until age 40, when it drops off precipitously
- Degradation of elastic fibers occurs by elastases (proteolytic enzymes)
  - Classic elastases—degrade insoluble elastic fibers at neutral or mildly alkaline pH; found in polymorphonuclear cells (PMNs); inhibited by α_1-antitrypsin, α_2-macroglobulin
  - Elastase-like metalloproteases—degrade soluble elastin, oxytalan, and elaunin fibers; cannot degrade insoluble elastases; requires calcium
  - Primary mutations in the elastin gene have been demonstrated in cutis laxa, a group of diseases that manifest with loss or fragmentation of elastic fibers
- Diseases with elastic fiber abnormalities (Table 28-7)

GROUND SUBSTANCE

- Component of connective tissue of dermis
- Consistency of a viscous solution or thin gel
- Stains with PAS or with toluidine blue
- Consists of several types of PGs
- PGs
  - PGs are of different functional importance as critical components of cell membranes and the extracellular matrix of the skin during development, homeostasis, and disease
  - Macromolecule with a core of protein and covalently attached GAGs
  - Abundance of hydroxyl, carboxyl, and sulfate groups make PGs hydrophilic and polyanionic; this creates an intensely hydrated molecule that can bind up to 1000 times of its own volume

TABLE 28-6 Heritable Connective Tissue Diseases With Cutaneous Involvement

Disease	Inheritance*	Mutated Genes	Affected Protein
Ehlers-Danlos syndrome	AD, AR	COL1A1, COL1A2, COL3A1, COL5A1, COL5A2	α chains of types I, III, and V collagens
	~	PLOD	Procollagen-lysine 2-oxoglutarate 5-dioxygenase (lysyl hydroxylase)
		ADAMTS-2	Procollagen N-peptidase
		TNX	Tenascin-X
		B4GALT-7	Xylosylprotein 4-β-galactosyltransferase
Osteogenesis imperfecta	AD, AR,	COL1A1, COL1A2	α1 and α2 chains of type I collagen
Cutis laxa	AD, AR, XR†	ELN MNK-1 (ATP7A)	Elastin ATP-dependent copper transporter
Homocystinuria	AR	CBS	Cystathionine β-synthase
Menkes syndrome	XR	MNK-1 (ATP7A)	ATP-dependent copper transporter
Focal dermal hypoplasia	XD	ND	
Tuberous sclerosis (shagreen patches)	AD	TSK-1 TSC 1 plus 2	Hamartin 1 Tuberen
Familial cutaneous collagenoma	AD	ND	
Epidermolysis bullosa VII and XVII collagens	AD, AR	COL7A1, COL17A1	α1 chains of types VII and XVII collagens

*AD, autosomal dominant; AR, autosomal recessive; XD, X-linked dominant; XR, X-linked recessive; ND, not determined.

†Most cases involve abnormalities in the elastic fibers, and in some cases, mutations in the elastin gene (ELN) have been disclosed. Occipital horn syndrome, a copper deficiency syndrome, allelic to the Menkes syndrome gene (MNK-1), was previously known as X-linked cutis laxa and also Ehlers-Danlos syndrome IX.

Reprinted with permission from Freedberg IM et al. *Fitzpatrick's Dermatology in General Medicine*, 6th Ed. New York: McGraw-Hill; 2003, p. 178.

  - This hydration affects volume and compressibility of the dermis
  - PGs also play a role in binding growth factors and acting as adhesion sites for other molecules
- GAGs—repeating units of disaccharides (Table 28-8)
- Skin conditions associated with GAG include
  - Mucopolysaccharidoses (Hunter, Hurler, Sanfilippo) result from defective lysosomal enzymes; the defect causes accumulation of GAGs in many tissues
  - Aging results in increases of dermatan sulfate and decreases in chondroitin-6-sulfate
  - In wound healing, hyaluronic acid increases shortly after injury and then decreases as chondroitin sulfate increases
  - Hyaluronic acid is a GAG produced without synthesis of a core protein; it is synthesized by a complex of enzymes at the plasma membrane, with subsequent extrusion into the extracellular space
  - Hyaluronic acid plays an important role in providing physicochemical properties to the skin, mediated by its hydrophilicity and viscosity in dilute solutions
  - During wound healing, the physicochemical properties of hyaluronanic acid may serve to expand the matrix and thus aid cell movement

ENDOTHELIAL CELLS

- The innermost component of the blood vessels is the endothelium, consisting of adjoining endothelial cells that surround the lumen

TABLE 28-7 Clinical Features, Histopathology, Inheritance, Associated Biochemical Findings, and Predisposing Clinical Conditions in Cutaneous Diseases With Elastic Fiber Abnormalities*

Disease	Inheritance†	Clinical Manifestations	Histopathology of Skin	Biochemical Findings‡ Related to Elastic Fibers and Predisposing Clinical Conditions
Pseudoxanthoma elasticum	AR, sporadic§	Yellowish papules coalescing into plaques Inelastic skin Cardiovascular and ocular abnormalities	Accumulation of pleomorphic and calcified elastic fibers in the mid-dermis	Deposition of calcium apatite crystals, excessive accumulation of glycosaminoglycans on elastic fibers; D-penicillamine treatment; mutations in the *ABCC6* gene
Buschke-Ollendorf syndrome	AD	Dermatofibrosis lenticularis disseminata and osteopoikilosi	Accumulation of interlacing elastic fibers in the dermis	Increased desmosine content in the skin
Cutis laxa	AR, AD, or NH	Loose, sagging, inelastic skin Pulmonary emphysema Tortuosity of aorta Urinary and gastrointestinal tract diverticuli	Fragmentation and loss of elastic fibers	Decreased desmosine content and reduced elastin mRNA levels; increased elastase activity in some cases; D-penicillamine treatment, inflammatory and urticarial skin lesions (e.g., drug reaction); mutations in the ELN or FBLN5 gene in limited cases
De Barsy syndrome	AR	Cutis laxa-like skin changes Mental retardation Dwarfism	Rudimentary, fragmented elastic fibers	Reduced elastin mRNA levels
Wrinkly skin syndrome	AR	Decreased elastic recoil of the skin Increased number of palmar and plantar creases	Decreased number and length of elastic fibers	
Mid-dermal elastolysis	NH	Fine wrinkling of the skin, primarily in exposed areas	Fragmentation and loss of elastin in the mid-dermis	Inflammatory; sun-exposure related
Anetoderma	NH	Localized areas of atrophic, sac-like lesions	Loss and fragmentation of elastic fibers in the dermis	Reduced desmosine content in the lesions; often secondary to inflammatory lesions
Elastosis perforans serpiginosa	NH	Hyperkeratotic papules, commonly on the face and neck	Accumulation and transepidermal elimination of elastic fibers	D-Penicillamine–induced abnormalities in elastin cross-linking

(Continued)

TABLE 28-7 Clinical Features, Histopathology, Inheritance, Associated Biochemical Findings, and Predisposing Clinical Conditions in Cutaneous Diseases With Elastic Fiber Abnormalities* (Continued)

Disease	Inheritance†	Clinical Manifestations	Histopathology of Skin	Biochemical Findings‡ Related to Elastic Fibers and Predisposing Clinical Conditions
Elastoderma	Unknown	Loose and sagging skin with loss of recoil	Accumulation of pleomorphic elastotic material without calcification in the mid- and lower dermis and the subcutaneous tissue	
Isolated elastomas	NH	Dermal papules or nodules	Accumulation of thick elastic fibers in the dermis	
Elastofibroma dorsi	NH	Deep subcutaneous tumor, usually on subscapular area	Accumulation of globular elastic structures encased in collagenous meshwork	Trauma on the lesional area
Actinic elastosis	NH	Thickening and furrowing of the skin	Accumulation of irregularly thickened elastic fibers in upper dermis	Chronic sun exposure
Marfan syndrome	AD	Skeletal, ocular, and cardiovascular abnormalities, hyperextensible skin; striae distensae	Fragmentation of the elastic structure in the aorta	Mutations in the *FBN1* gene Fibrillin 1 protein
Congenital contractural arachnodactyly	AD	Camptodactyly and joint contractures		Mutations in the *FBN2* gene Fibrillin 2 protein
Williams syndrome	AD	Supravalvular aortic stenosis; velvety skin; dysmorphic facies	Disruption of smooth muscle and matrix relationship affecting blood vessels	Allelic deletion of the ELN gene; contiguous gene deletion syndrome

*Most of these conditions represent a group of diseases with clinical, genetic, and biochemical heterogeneity.

†AD, autosomal dominant; AR, autosomal recessive; NH, not a heritable disease.

‡The biochemical abnormalities have been demonstrated in only a limited number of patients in each group, and it is not known whether the biochemical changes are the same in each patient with given disease.

§Rare cases with a distinct acquired form of pseudoxanthoma elasticum have been described.

Reprinted with permission from Freedberg IM et al. *Fitzpatrick's Dermatology in General Medicine*, 6th Ed. New York: McGraw-Hill; 2003, p. 187.

TABLE 28-8 Glycosaminoglycans

Glycosaminoglycan	Distribution and Collagen Interaction
Hyaluronic acid	Found in dermis, umbilical cord, synovial fluid, cartilage, vitreous. No interaction with collagen High levels associated with nonscarring wound healing (i.e., fetal)
Dermatan sulfate	Found in structures formed by collagen fibers; dermis, tendon, ligaments, heart valves, arteries, fibrous cartilage Interaction with type I collagen Decorin—small dermatan sulfate, found along surface of collagen fibrils and assist with lateral fibrils into fibers; low levels in hypertrophic scars
Chondroitin 4- to 6-sulfate	Hyaline and elastic cartilage, arterial medial layer, nucleus pulposus Interact with type II collagen
Heparan sulfate	Basement membrane, structures with reticular fibers: smooth muscle, liver, spleen nerves Interact with type III collagen

- At the ultrastructural level, endothelial cells possess many of the common cellular organelles, including the rough and smooth endoplasmic reticulum, mitochondria, and lysosomes, and micropinocytotic vesicles are also evident
- Flattened epithelial-like cells
- Thickness <10 μm
- Usually form a continuous monolayer with gap junctions between cells
- Endothelial cells rest on a basal lamina of laminin 1, collagens, fibronectin, nidogen (entactin), and heparan sulfate
- Endothelial cells have a polarized structure with differences between apical (lumen) aspect and basal surface
- They are the major source of angiotensin-converting enzyme as well as various cytokines and adhesion molecules
  - Integrin receptors for ground substance/matrix molecules on basal surface
  - Leukocyte receptors on apical (lumen) side
- Endothelial cells have a number of specialized structures
  - WPBs
    - Contain von Willebrand factor (vWF), P selectin, and CD63, factor XIII-related antigen, and GMP-140, a protein that was first described in platelet α-granules
      - ▲ P selectin (CD62P) mediates leukocyte adhesion
      - ▲ CD63 is a lysosomal membrane glycoprotein that interferes with neutrophil adhesion
    - vWF: amino acid protein; one specific domain binds to factor VIII, other domains perform other specific functions
  - Fenestrae
    - Sieve-plate structure of membrane
    - 175 nm in diameter
    - Unique to endothelial cells
    - Capillaries composed of endothelial cells with fenestrae are more permeable to water and small-molecular-weight solutes
    - Located in capillaries in lymph nodes, renal glomerulus, intestine, hepatic sinusoids, and bone marrow sinusoids
    - Negative charge of fenestrae prevents transfer of negatively charged plasma proteins
- Caveolae
  - "Little caves" or vesicles associated with the plasma membrane via the protein caveolin
  - Serve as storage compartments for growth factor receptors structural components
- Tight (occludens) junctions
  - Provide dual function of sealing off paracellular space and dividing the cell into distinct apical and basolateral segments
  - Appear as continuous interlocking belt-like strands that associate laterally with tight junctions of adjacent cell
  - Consist of transmembrane proteins occludin and claudins
  - Also associated with cytoplasmic proteins ZO-1, ZO-2, and ZO-3
- Adherens junctions
  - Composed of cadherin adhesion molecules
  - Presence of junctions regulates paracellular transport and adhesion of molecules to one another
  - Cadherins link adjacent cells via a cytoplasmic plaque structure connected to the cytoskeleton
  - The plaque is composed of transmembrane proteins cadherin 5 (CD144) and PECAM 1 (CD31)
  - Cadherin 5 is now renamed *vascular endothelial cadherin* (VE cadherin)

- The cadherins are attached to the actin cytoskeleton by catenins
- Gap junctions
  - Clusters of transmembrane channels formed by 6 connexin monomers
  - Connexin 37, 40, and 43
  - Allow direct exchange of ions and small molecules between endothelial cells
- Complexus adherentes
  - Endothelial cells have no desmosomes
  - However, the desmosomal protein desmoplakin is located to complexus adherentes and participates in a distinct type of cell contact separate from desmosomes

- Endothelial cells play a critical role in cutaneous inflammation
  - Endothelial cells produce a number of cytokines
    - IL-1
      - ▲ Responsible for upregulation of ICAM-1, VCAM-1, and E selectin
      - ▲ Induces platelet-activating factor, prostaglandins, and nitric oxide
      - ▲ Activates T cells, serves as chemoattractant for lymphocytes, and stimulates proliferation of B cells
    - IL-6: has few effects on normal endothelium but plays a critical role as a growth factor for Kaposi sarcoma neoplasms
    - IL-8: likely plays a role as a chemoattractant for inflammatory cells
    - G-CSF
    - M-CSF
    - GM-CSF
  - Endothelial cells express a variety of adhesion molecules that play a vital role in inflammation
    - ICAM-1 (binds LFA-1 on leukocytes)
    - ICAM-2 (binds LFA-1 on leukocytes)
    - E selectin (binds memory T cells, especially in chronic inflammation)
    - P selectin (binds Lewis X, which is important in initial binding of PMNs to endothelium)
    - VCAM-1 (binds $\alpha 4\beta 1$ integrin of leukocytes)
    - MHC I, II (bind CD8 and CD4 on T cells)
    - LFA-3 (binds CD2 on T cells)
    - CD44 (binds hyaluronic acid)

SWEAT GLANDS: ECCRINE AND APOCRINE

- Eccrine glands
  - Eccrine sweat glands begin to develop during the first trimester and are fully developed by the second trimester
  - Primary function of the eccrine unit is thermoregulation: cooling effects of evaporation of sweat on the skin surface
  - Highest density of eccrine glands is seen on the palms, soles, and axillae
  - Consists of 2 segments: secretory coil and a duct
  - Coil: composed of 3 distinct cell types: clear (secretory), dark (mucoid), and myoepithelial cells
  - Duct: outer ring of peripheral cells (basal) and an inner ring of luminal cells (cuticular); the coiled duct (proximal) is more active than the distal (straight) portion
  - Duct is referred to as the *acrosyringium* because it spirals through the epidermis and opens directly onto the skin surface
  - Eccrine sweat is produced via merocrine secretion in the coiled gland and is composed of water, sodium, potassium lactate, urea, ammonia, serine, ornithine, citrulline, aspartic acid, heavy metals, organic compounds, and proteolytic enzymes
  - Stimulation of eccrine sweat production is mediated predominantly through postganglionic C fiber production of acetylcholine
  - Ectodermal dysplasias are a large, heterogeneous group of genetic disorders that are characterized by developmental abnormalities in 2 or more major ectodermal appendages such as hair, teeth, nails, and sweat glands
  - Hypohidrotic ectodermal dysplasia is caused by mutations in genes encoding components of the ectodysplasin A (EDA) signaling pathway, which is critical for the initiation of sweat gland, hair follicle, and tooth morphogenesis
- Apocrine sweat gland
  - Derive their name from the way that their secretion appears, pinching off parts of the cytoplasm
  - Outgrowths of the superior portions of pilosebaceous units
  - Respond mainly to cholinergic stimuli
  - It consists of a coiled gland in the deep dermis or at the junction of the dermis and subcutaneous fat and a straight duct that traverses the dermis and empties into the isthmus (uppermost portion) of a hair follicle
  - Secretion is decapitation, a process where the apical portion of the secretory cell cytoplasm pinches off and enters the lumen of the gland
  - Apocrine glands secrete very small quantities of an oily fluid (sialomucin), which may be colored. This secretion is odorless on reaching the surface, and bacterial decomposition is responsible for the characteristic odor; trans-3-methyl-2-hexanoic acid, which is water soluble, is one of the substances which contributes to the odor
  - Specialized variants: the Moll glands seen on the eyelids, the cerumen (ear wax–producing) glands of the external auditory canal, and the milk-producing glands of the breasts
  - Fox-Fordyce disease
    - Chronic pruritic disease
    - Usually in women

  - Characterized by small follicular papular eruptions in apocrine areas
  - Caused by obstruction and rupture of intraepidermal apocrine ducts
- Apoeccrine sweat gland
  - Readily distinguished from classic eccrine and apocrine glands
  - Develop during puberty from eccrine-like precursor glands and are found in as many as 50% of the axillary glands in patients with hyperhidrosis
  - Long duct, opens onto skin surface (similar to eccrine glands)
  - Cholinergic and adrenergic, secretory rate is 10 times that of the eccrine glands because of its large glandular size
  - Thick segment of the duct is similar in morphology to apocrine glands
- Disorders of the eccrine glands and apocrine glands
  - Hyperhidrosis, or excessive eccrine sweat secretion
    - Localized hyperhidrosis of the palms and soles is often due to emotional stressors
  - Hypohidrosis: decreased eccrine sweating; anhidrosis: absent sweating seen in hereditary disorders such as the ectodermal dysplasias or in acquired conditions such as heat stroke or heat exhaustion
  - Miliaria crystallina: excessive heat and humidity causes duct obstruction within the SC, asymptomatic superficial vesicles, and no surrounding inflammation
  - Miliaria rubra (prickly heat): obstruction is found deeper in the epidermis; pruritic or tender red macules or papules that are often located on the thorax and neck
  - Miliaria profunda: duct obstruction at or below the dermal-epidermal junction; asymptomatic skin-colored papules
  - Apocrine miliaria: inflammation follows intraepidermal rupture of apocrine ducts
  - Hidradenitis suppurativa: intense inflammation owing to follicular obstruction
  - Syringomas: most common benign sweat gland tumor; skin-colored papules on lower eyelids of adults

MATRIX METALLOPROTEINASES

- Group of zinc-dependent enzymes (endopeptidases) that degrade varying components of the extracellular matrix in both normal and diseased tissue
- MMPs can be subdivided into several groups based upon substrate specificity, include collagenases, gelatinases the stomelysins, the matrilysins, metalloelasstases, enamelysins, and the membrane-type matrix metalloproteinases (MMPs) (Table 28-9)
- Synthesized as inactive proenzymes; limited proteolysis or treatment with an organomercurial compound sets up a chain of events causing conversion to the fully active form by complete removal of a propeptide (gelatinase A, MMP-2, can only be activated by the second mechanism)
- Cells secrete extracellular matrix (ECM) MMPs in a complex pattern of response to multiple growth factors and oncogenes
- Squamous cell carcinomas (SCCs) can secrete MMP-13 (collagenase-3), which preferentially cleaves type II collagen and gelatin, mediating their invasiveness
- UV irradiation releases cytokines from the epidermis and generates of reactive oxygen species, which induce inflammatory processes and stimulate expression and activation of matrix MMPs and serine proteinases such as elastase, which can degrade ECM networks. In particular, UVA1 most effectively stimulates MMPs and therefore can be used in the treatment of sclerotic skin conditions
- Tissue inhibitors of MMPs (TIMPs) are considered to be the major tissue inhibitors; these are secreted proteins that are tightly regulated during tissue remodeling and physiologic processes
- Inhibitors can modulate proteolysis once proenzymes have been activated
  - α_2-Macroglobulin, a nonspecific antiproteinase, accounts for more than 95% of the inhibitory activity

HAIR DEVELOPMENT

- Hair has very important psychological functions
- Both, loss of hair from the scalp and the growth of body or facial hair in excess of the culturally accepted norm is distressing
- Follicle formation is initiated by signals from the dermis to form focal thickenings, called placodes
- Hair cycling through anagen, catagen, and telogen continues throughout life, but become asynchronous after birth
- Most hairs become thicker and coarser leading to vellus and then adult-like terminal hairs on the scalp and in the eyebrows
- The hair follicle bulge, which is located deep to the sebaceous gland and adjacent to the arrector pili muscle attachment site, and harbor hair follicle stem cells
- Hair follicle bulge cells are multipotent and provide an important ectodermal reserve after severe wounds
- See Chapter 1: Hair Findings, for details

NAIL DEVELOPMENT

- The nail bed on the dorsal digit is the first skin structure to keratinize distally and then toward the proximal nail fold
- Preliminary nail is shed easily and replaced by the hard
- See Chapter 3: Nail Findings, for details

TABLE 28-9 Matrix Metalloproteinases

Enzyme	MMP Number	Alternate Name	Proenzyme Mol. Wt.	Known Matrix Substrates
Interstitial collagenase	MMP-1	Type 1 collagenase	52,000	Collagens I, II, III, VII, VIII, X, entactin, tenascin, aggrecan, denatured collagens, IL-1β, myelin basic protein, L selectin
Neutrophil collagenase	MMP-8		75,000	Collagens I, II, III, V, VII, VIII, X, gelatin, aggrecan, fibronectin
Collagenase-3	MMP-13		52,000	Collagens I, II, IV, IX, X, XIV, aggrecan
Gelatinase A	MMP-2	72-kDa type IV collagenase	72,000	Denatured collagens, collagens IV, V, VII, X, XI, XIV, collagen 1, species-dependent, elastin, fibronectin, laminin, aggrecan, myelin basic protein
Gelatinase B	MMP-9	92-kDa type IV collagenase	92,000	Denatured collagens, collagens IV, V, VII, X, XIV, elastin, entacin, aggrecan, fibronectin, osteonectin, IL-1β, plasminogen, myelin basic protein
Stromeylsin-1	MMP-3	Proteoglycanase	57,000	Proteoglycan core protein, laminin, fibronectin collagens I, IV, V, IX, X, XI, gelatin, elastin, tenascin, aggrecan, myelin basic protein, entactin, decorin, osteonectin
Stromelysin-2	MMP-10	Transin-2	55,000	Proteoglycan core protein, collagens III, IV, V, laminin, fibronectin, elastin, aggrecan
Stromelysin-3	MMP-11		61,000	α1 Proteinase inhibitor
Matrilsyin	MMP-7	PUMP matrilysin-1	28,000	Collagen IV, denatured collagens, laminin, fibronectin, elastin, aggrecan, tenascin, myelin basic protein
Matrilsyin-2	MMP-26	Endometase	28,000	Gelatin, α1 proteinase inhibitor
Membrane type matrix metalloproteinase-1	MMP-14	MT1-MMP	63,000	Progelatinase A, denatured collagen, fibronectin, laminin, vitronectin, entactin, proteoglycans
Membrane type matrix metalloproteinase-2	MMP-15	MT2-MMP	72,000	Progelatinase A
Membrane type matrix metalloproteinase-3	MMP-16	MT3-MMP	64,000	Progelatinase A
Membrane type matrix metalloproteinase-4	MMP-17	MT4-MMP	70,000	Unknown
Membrane type matrix metalloproteinase-5	MMP-24	MT5-MMP	73,000	Progelatinase A

(Continued)

TABLE 28-9 Matrix Metalloproteinases (Continued)

Enzyme	MMP Number	Alternate Name	Proenzyme Mol. Wt.	Known Matrix Substrates
Membrane type matrix metalloproteinase-6	MMP-25	MT6-MMP	63,000	Unknown
Metalloelastase	MMP-12		54,000	Elastin, collagen IV, vitronectin, plasminogen, laminin, entactin, fibrinogen, fibrin, fibronectin
Enamelysin	MMP-20		54,000	Amelogenin, aggrecan
MMP-19	MMP-19	RASI-1	57,000	Gelatin, aggrecan, fibronectin
MMP-21	MMP-21		Unknown	Unknown
MMP-22	MMP-22		Unknown	Unknown
MMP-23	MMP-23		44,000	Unknown
Epilysin	MMP-28		56,000	Unknown

Reprinted with permission from Freedberg IM et al. *Fitzpatrick's Dermatology in General Medicine*, 6th Ed. New York: McGraw-Hill; 2003, p. 201.

SKIN AS AN IMMUNOLOGIC ORGAN

- Both innate and adaptive, protects skin from infection
- Adaptive immunity depends on lymphocytes and antibodies that are specifically recruited to recognize foreign materials
- Failure of immunity leads to infection. Examples infectious skin diseases illustrate lost or defective immunity in some patients
- Faulty immunity leads to autoimmunity by failure in distinguishing "self" from infection
- Failure of immunity may lead to cancer as immune responses also protect against malignancy, especially cutaneous melanoma and SCC, which is a known complication of immunosuppression in solid organ transplant recipients

SKIN STEM CELLS

Stem cells are responsible for maintaining and repairing the tissue they reside in. The epidermis, dermis, appendages, and melanocytes are each maintained by different stem cell compartments. Stem cells undergo asymmetric division, generating one new stem cell and one daughter transit amplifying (TA) cell, which differentiates into lineage-specific cell types

Importance of microRNAs in skin morphogenesis and diseases

MicroRNAs (miRNAs) are small noncoding RNAs involved in posttranscriptional gene silencing. miRNAs regulate several developmental and physiological processes, including stem cell differentiation and the immune response. Recent findings report their involvement in hair follicle morphogenesis, in psoriasis, in autoimmune diseases affecting the skin, such as SLE and ITP, in wound healing, and in skin carcinogenesis. Researchers worldwide are interested in miRNAs as potential therapeutic targets (such as in the case of psoriasis) and potential diagnostic biomarkers (such as in case of SLE).

QUIZ

Questions

1. Renewal of the epidermis takes approximately:

    A. 13 to 14 days
    B. 1 to 14 days
    C. 14 to 26 days
    D. 26 to 28 days
    E. 28 to 32 days

2. Fibulin-2 is capable of binding

    A. Fibrinogen
    B. Versican
    C. Aggrecan
    D. All of the above
    E. None of the above

3. Stratum lucidum is a layer present between the granular and cornified layer found in:
   A. Palmoplantar skin
   B. Mucosa
   C. Nail
   D. Axillary skin
   E. Scalp skin

4. Seventy percent of the cornified cell envelope consists of:
   A. Profillagrin
   B. Loricrin
   C. Involucrin
   D. Filaggrin
   E. Keratin

5. Krause end bulbs or mucocutaneous end organs are found in:
   A. Mucocutaneous junction
   B. Hands and soles
   C. Nipples/areola
   D. Scalp skin
   E. Nail apparatus

6. Which is the only protein known to be present in both desmosomes and adherens junctions:
   A. Desmoplakin
   B. Integrin
   C. Desmocollins
   D. BP antigen 2 (180 kD)
   E. BP antigen 1 (230 kD)

7. The postganglionic neurotransmitter mediating eccrine sweat production is:
   A. Acetylcholine
   B. Epinephrine
   C. Dopamine
   D. Norepinephrine
   E. Serotonin

8. Matrix metalloproteinases can be upregulated during normal development and physiologic tissue repair. Under pathologic conditions, squamous cell carcinomas can secrete:
   A. Collagenase-1
   B. Stromelysin-3
   C. MMP-13
   D. Gelatinase-9
   E. Matrilsyin-2

9. Which type of collagen is found in cartilage?
   A. I
   B. III
   C. XI
   D. XV
   E. XVII

10. At what week of development do neural crest–derived melanocytes produce melanin?
    A. 8th week
    B. 10th week
    C. 12th week
    D. 16th week
    E. 18th week

11. Which keratin is most specific to Merkel cells?
    A. K8
    B. K18
    C. K1
    D. K20
    E. K10

12. Basal cell layer is associated with the following protein:
    A. BPAG1
    B. Desmoglein II
    C. Desmocollin I
    D. Loricrin
    E. Profilaggrin

13. Mutation in Gap junctions' proteins can result in:
    A. Ichthyosis vulgaris
    B. Lamellar ichthyosis
    C. Marfan syndrome
    D. Cutis laxa
    E. Erythrokeratodermia variabilis

14. The following stain is used to visualize BMZ:
    A. H & E
    B. PAS
    C. Sudan III
    D. Acid Orcein
    E. Melan A

15. Epidermolytic palmoplantar keratoderma (PPK) shows a defect in which types of keratins:
    A. Keratins 1 and 10
    B. Keratins 3 and 12
    C. Keratins 1 and 9
    D. Keratins 5 and 14
    E. Keratins 4 and 13

16. Weibel-Palade bodies are present within the following cells:
    A. Basal keratinocytes
    B. Langerhans cells
    C. Neutrophils
    D. Plasma cells
    E. Endothelial cells

17. Moll glands are specialized variants of:
    A. Eccrine glands
    B. Apocrine glands
    C. Sebaceous glands
    D. Parotid gland
    E. Thyroid gland

18. Anchoring fibrils are composed of the following type of collagen:
    A. X
    B. VII
    C. XVI
    D. II
    E. III

19. The rate-limiting enzyme in melanin synthesis is dependent on:
    A. Copper
    B. Gold
    C. Zinc
    D. Selenium
    E. Sulfur

20. The following factor stimulates collagen production:
    A. IL-1
    B. Glucocorticoids
    C. Ascorbic acid
    D. TNF-α
    E. INF-γ

Answers

1. D. It takes 13 to 14 days for maturation of keratinocytes from the basal layer to the corneum and another 13 to 14 days for shedding.
2. D. Fibulins are calcium-binding extracellular matrix proteins that do not form large aggregates but are capable of joining other supramolecular structures. Fibulin-2 is capable of binding fibrinogen, fibronectin, nidogen, PGs, aggrecan, and versican.
3. A. The layer appears as an electronlucent zone and contains nucleated cells.
4. B. Loricrin accounts for the majority of proteins in the cornified cell envelope. It is insoluble and is highly hydrophobic. It is cross-linked by transglutaminase-3 to form homodimers and heterodimers with other proteins to increase solubilization.
5. A. These structures are found at the vermillion border of the lips, glans penis, and clitoris.
6. A. Desmoplakin bind intermediate filaments at their carboxy-terminal site. In adherens junctions, the N-terminus of desmoplakin can bind plakoglobin and plakophilin and in desmosomes, it can bind plakoglobin, plakophilin, and desmocollin.
7. A. Eccrine glands are highest in density in the palms, soles, and axillae. They are principally mediated by cholinergic stimulation.
8. C. Invasive SCCs can secrete MMP-13 (collagenase-3) which preferentially cleaves type II collagen and gelatin.
9. C. Many types of collagens can be found in cartilage including collagen II, IX, X, XI, XII, and XIV.
10. C. At the 8th week of fetal development melanocytes develop from the neural crest cells. It is not until the 12th week that melanocytes begin synthesis of melanin beginning in the head region.
11. D. K20 is most specific to Merkel cells.
12. A. Basal cell layer is associated with BPAG I.
13. E. Mutation in Gap junctions' proteins, which are connexins can result in erythrokeratodermia variabilis.
14. B. PAS stain is used to visualize BMZ.
15. C. Epidermolytic PPK shows a defect in keratins 1 and 9, which are located in palmoplantar suprabasal keratinocytes.
16. E. Weibel-Palade bodies are present within endothelial cells.
17. B. Moll glands are specialized variants of apocrine glands.
18. B. Anchoring fibrils are composed of collagen type VII.
19. A. The rate-limiting enzyme in melanin synthesis is copper dependent.
20. C. The only factor that stimulates collagen production from the answers is ascorbic acid.

REFERENCES

Agren UM, Tammi M, Ryynänen M, Tammi R: Developmentally programmed expression of hyaluronan in human skin and its appendages. *J Invest Dermatol* 1997;109:219–224.

Alberts B et al. *Molecular Biology of the Cell*, 4th Ed. New York: Garland Science; 2002.

Amagai M: Adhesion molecules: I. Keratinocyte-keratinocyte interactions; cadherins and pemphigus. *J Invest Dermatol* 1995; 104:146–152.

Blume U, Ferracin J, Verschoore M, et al. Physiology of the vellus hair follicle: hair growth and sebum excretion. *Br J Dermatol* 1991;124:21–28.

Buac K, Pavan WJ: Stem cells of the melanocyte lineage. *Cancer Biomark* 2007;3:203–209.

Burgeson RE, Christiano AM: The dermal-epidermal junction. *Curr Opin Cell Biol* 1997;9:651–658.

Dai Y et al. Microarray analysis of microRNA expression in peripheral blood cells of systemic lupus erythematosus patients. *Lupus* 2007;16:939–946.

Ebling FJG: Apocrine glands in health and disease. *Int J Dermatol* 1989;28:508–511.

Franzke CW, Bruckner P, Bruckner-Tuderman L: Collagenous transmembrane proteins: recent insights into biology and pathology. *J Biol Chem* 2005;280:4005–4008.

Frienkel RK, Woodley D: *The Biology of the Skin*. New York: Parthenon; 2001.

Fuchs E, Weber K: Intermediate filaments: structure, dynamics, function, and disease. *Annu Rev Biochem* 1994;63:345–382.

Gaur A et al. Characterization of microRNA expression levels and their biological correlates in human cancer cell lines. *Cancer Res* 2007;67:2456–2468.

Goldsmith LA et al. *Fitzpatrick's Dermatology in General Medicine*, 8th Ed. New York: McGraw-Hill; 2012.

Hornyak TJ, Hayes DJ, Chiu LY, Ziff EB: Transcription factors in melanocyte development: distinct roles for pax-3 and Mitf. *Mech Dev* 2001 Mar;101(1-2):47–59.

Houben E, De Paepe K, Rogiers V: A keratinocyte's course of life. *Skin Pharmacol Physiol* 2007;20:122–132.

Jurisic G, Detmar M: Lymphatic endothelium in health and disease. *Cell Tissue Res* 2009;335:97–108.

Katz AM, Rosenthal D, Sauder DN: Cell adhesion molecules: structure, function, and implication in a variety of cutaneous and other pathologic conditions. *Int J Dermatol* 1991;30:130–161.

Kimayai-Asadi A, Kotcher LB, Jih MH: The molecular basis of hereditary palmoplantar keratodermas. *J Am Acad Dermatol* 2002;47(3):327–343.

Lai-Cheong JE, Arita K, McGrath JA: Genetic diseases of junctions. *J Invest Dermatol* 2007;127:2713–2725.

Midwood KS, Schwarzbauer JE: Elastic fibers: building bridges between cells and their matrix. *Curr Biol* 2002;12:R279.

Mohr RE, Takashima A: Epidermal Langerhans cell movement in situ: a model for understanding immunologic function in the skin. *Arch Dermatol* 2007;143:1438.

Moll I et al. Human Merkel cells—aspects of cell biology, distribution and functions. *Eur J Cell Biol* 2005;84:259–271.

Myllyharju J, Kivirikko KI: Collagens, modifying enzymes and their mutations in humans, flies and worms. *Trends Genet* 2004;20:33–43.

Nicosia RF, Madri JA: The microvascular extracellular matrix. Developmental changes during angiogenesis in the aortic ring-plasma clot model. *Am J Pathol* 1987;128:78–90.

Niessen CM: Tight/adherens junctions: basic structure and function. *J Invest Dermatol* 2007;127:2525–2532.

Paus R, Cotsarelis G: Mechanisms of disease: the biology of hair follicles. *N Engl J Med* 1999;341(7):491–497.

Roitt I, Brostoff J, Male D: *Immunology*, 6th Ed. St. Louis: Mosby; 2001.

Smack DP, Korge BP, James WD: Keratin and keratinization. *J Am Acad Dermatol* 1994;30(1):85–102.

Swerlick RA, Lawley TJ: Role of microvascular endothelial cells in inflammation. *J Invest Dermatol* 1993;100(1):111S–114S.

Timpl R, Sasaki T, Kostka G, Chu ML: Fibulins: a versatile family of extracellular matrix proteins. *Nat Rev Mol Cell Biol* 2003 Jun;4(6):479–489. Review.

Vestweber D: Molecular mechanisms that control endothelial cell contacts. *J Pathol* 2000;190:281–291.

Villone D, Fritsch A, Koch M: Supramolecular interactions in the dermoepidermal junction zone: Anchoring fibril-collagen VII tightly binds to banded collagen fibrils. *J Biol Chem* 2008;238:24506–24513.

Yaar M, Gilchrest BA: Human melanocyte growth and differentiation: a decade of new data. *J Invest Dermatol* 1991;97(4):611–617.

CHAPTER 29

BIOSTATISTICS

ALICE Z. CHUANG
STEPHANIE F. CHAN

RANDOM VARIABLE AND PROBABILITY

In a clinical study, 1 or more outcomes are observed or measured. Outcomes vary from subject to subject and may or may not be numerical values. For example, the outcome could be "success" or "failure" for a drug treatment or "number of bacteria" in a tissue culture. However, for a statistical analysis, we often want to represent outcomes as numbers.

A random variable is a function that associates a unique numerical value with every possible outcome of a study. There are 2 types of random variables—discrete and continuous.

- A discrete random variable has either a finite or a countable number of distinct values. Examples are as follows
  - The number of patients that visited a doctor's office in a day is countable, such as 0, 1, 2, etc
  - Of 10 participants in a pilot study, the number of study patients experiencing adverse effects after the treatment must be a finite number of distinct values, 0, 1, 2, ..., 10
- A discrete random variable has a probability distribution which provides the possible values of the random variable and their corresponding probabilities. Let P(x) denote the probability that the random variable X equals x. The properties of a probability distribution P(x) are
  - $0 \le P(x) \le 1$
  - The sum of P(x) for all possible X equals 1.
- A probability distribution can be expressed as a table, graph, or mathematical formula. Examples are as follows
  - Suppose a disease can be classified into 5 stages (0–4). The probabilities associated with its classification after a treatment can be expressed as a table (Table 29-1) or a graph (Fig. 29-1)
  - The binomial distribution is one of the most common discrete probability distributions in clinical studies. The binomial random variable is defined as the number of "successes" in *N* independent binary trials such that each trial has 2 possible outcomes, for example, "yes/no" or "success/failure." The probability of success, *p*, is the same on every trial
- A continuous random variable is one which can take on any value within an interval (or range) of values. It has infinite number of possible values. Continuous random variables are usually measurements such as height, weight, age, or temperature
- A continuous random variable is not defined at specific values. The probability of observing any single value is equal to 0, $P(X = x) = 0$, since the number of possible values is infinite. Instead, it is defined over a range of values, such as $P(X < 5)$ or $P(2 < X < 10)$ and is equal to the area under a continuous probability distribution curve. The curve, continuous probability distribution *f(x)*, must satisfy the following
  - *f(x)* has no negative values for all x
  - The total area under the curve is equal to 1

The most important family of continuous probability distributions is the normal (Gaussian) distribution. It has the following characteristics

- It is graphically categorized by a bell-shaped curve (Fig. 29-2)
- The most frequently occurring value is in the middle of the range, and other probabilities tail off symmetrically in both directions
- The mean and median are identical
- The probability that a measurement will fall within 1.96 standard deviations of the mean is 0.95

Many statistical tests rely on the assumption that analyzed data are derived from a population that has a normal (Gaussian) distribution. Regression, correlation, *t* tests, and analysis of variance all depend on a normal distribution assumption

DESCRIPTIVE STATISTICS

Descriptive statistics are used to describe the basic features of the data in a study. They provide simple summaries about the study variables such as central tendency, variability, skewness, kurtosis, and associations of variables

TABLE 29-1 Example of Probability Distribution

X = Disease classification	0	1	2	3	4	Sum
P(X = x)	0.40	0.25	0.20	0.10	0.05	1.00

Discrete Variable

The following statistics are often used to summarize discrete random variables and their probability distribution

- **Frequency**: The number of times the event occurred in a study
- **Probability** (P) = frequency/total number of trials: A number, between 0 and 1, that indicates how likely an event is to occur on the basis of the number of events per the number of trials.
- **Percentage** = $P \times 100\%$
- **Odds** = $P/(1-P)$: ratio of the probability of an event occurring (P) to the probability of the event not occurring ($1-P$)
- **Odds ratio (OR)**: the ratio of the odds of an event occurring in one group to the odds of it occurring in another group. These groups might be case and control, or any other 2 groups' classification. If the probabilities of the event in each of the groups are P_1 (first group) and P_2 (second group), then the odds ratio (OR) is

$$OR = \frac{P_1}{1-P_1} \times \frac{1-P_2}{P_2}$$

The odds ratio measures whether a certain *exposure* (case) is associated with a specific disease and is often used in a retrospective case-control study

- **Relative Risk (RR)**: ratio of the probability of event occurred in one group (P_1) to the probability of event occurred in the other group (P_2)

$$RR = \frac{P_1}{P_2}$$

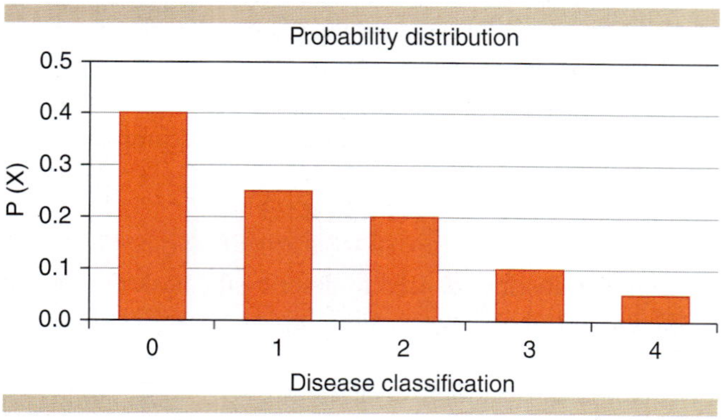

FIGURE 29-1 Illustration of probability distribution.

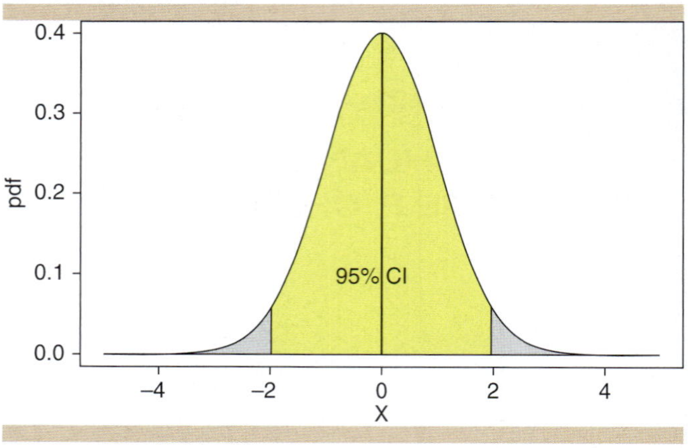

FIGURE 29-2 Normal distribution and 95% confidence interval.

These groups are often classified as exposed to certain condition (group 1) vs. nonexposed (group 2). RR is often used in prospective cohort studies (Table 29-2)

- If RR = 1: the probability that the event occurred (risk) in exposed individuals is same as the probability that the event occurred in nonexposed individuals
- If RR >1: the risk in exposed individuals is greater than the risk in nonexposed
- If RR <1: the risk in exposed individuals is less than the risk in nonexposed
- OR is closed to RR, if P_1 and P_2 approach to 0. It means the event is rare

TABLE 29-2 Calculating Probability, Odds, Odds Ratio, and Relative Risk

	Event Occurred	Event Did NOT Occur	Total
Group 1	A	B	A+B
Group 2	C	D	C+D

Note:
A, B, C, and D are frequencies
Probability of event occurred:
P_1 = A/(A+B) for group 1 and
P_2 = C/(C+D) for group 2
Odds = A/B for group 1 and C/D for group 2
OR = AD/BC
RR = [A/(A + B)]/[C/(C + D)]
Attributable risk = $P_1 - P_2$ = [A/(A + B)] − [C/(C + D)]

- **Disease Incidence**: the number of ***new*** disease cases in the population during a specific time divided by the number of individuals at risk of developing the disease during that specific time. It is used to determine the probability of developing a specific disease and to detect etiologic factors. A prospective cohort study, following a cohort over a given time interval, is often conducted to investigate disease incidence
- **Disease Prevalence**: the number of ***current*** disease cases at a *specific time* (a single time point or a specific period of time) divided by the number of individuals in the population at that specific time. It is frequently used to measure the amount of illness in the community and to determine health care needs of the community. The illness could be
- Old: persistence of an active disease contracted previously
- New: onset of an active disease

A cross-sectional survey is usually conducted to estimate the disease prevalence

Continuous Variable

The following statistics are often used to summarize continuous random variables and characteristics of their probability distribution curves:

- *Central Tendency* (Fig. 29-3)
  - Sample mean (Arithmetic average): sum of all the values divided by the number of observations. Outliers (extreme values) weigh heavily on the sample mean but it does provide a central value representative of the entire collection of numbers
  - Median: Middle value of a set of data; where 50% of the values are below this point, and 50% of the values are above it. It provides a central value that is not influenced by high and low extremes in the data
  - Mode: Represents the value occurring most frequently in a data set. A data set has no mode when all the values appear in the data with the same frequency. A data set has multiple modes when 2 or more values appear with the same frequency

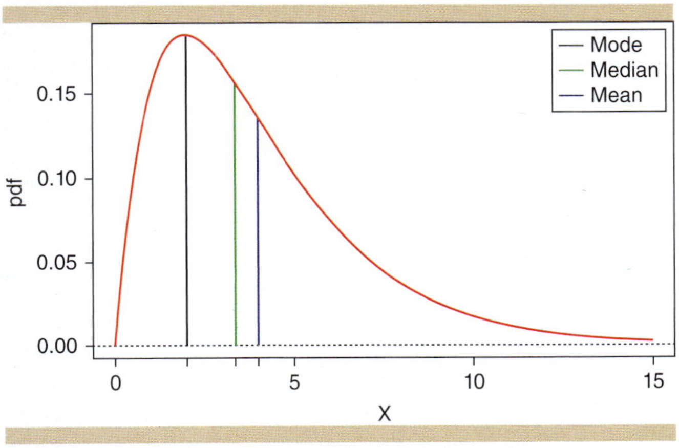

FIGURE 29-3 Illustration of measurements for central tendency.

- *Variability*

The following properties measure the spread or variability of a distribution

- Variance [$V(X)$ or σ^2]: the average value of the squared difference between measurements and their mean. Variance is small if many data points are close to their mean and is zero if all data points are equal. Variances are typically useful only when the measurements follow a normal or at least a symmetric distribution
- Standard deviation (SD or σ): the standard deviation, also called the root-mean-square deviation, is equal to the square root of the variance. It has the same measuring scale as the random variable. If the distribution of the random variable is normal (Gaussian), 68% of outcomes are within 1 SD; 95% of the outcomes are expected to be within 2 standard deviations of the mean (see Fig. 29-2); and 99.7% of outcomes are within 3 SDs.
- Standard error of mean (SEM) = $SD/\sqrt{N}$, where N is the sample size: the sample mean is a random variable which has a distribution with the same mean as the samples and a standard deviation equal to SEM. It has the following properties:
  - SEM falls as the sample size increases
  - SEM increases as standard deviation increases
- Standard deviation (SD) vs. standard error of mean (SEM): SD measures how widely ***measurements*** are scattered, and SEM evaluates the accuracy of estimation of mean by the sample mean
- Range = largest measurement−smallest measurement: the length of smallest interval that contains all the data
- *Skewness*

Positively skewed data are represented by a distribution that has a long right tail while negatively skewed data are represented by a distribution that has a long left tail (Fig. 29-4)

- *Kurtosis*

The kurtosis of a distribution is positive when the tails are narrow with a steep peak and negative when the data distribution curve has wide tails with a flat peak (Fig. 29-5)

- *Correlation coefficient*

The correlation coefficient (R) measures the ***linear*** relationship between 2 continuous random variables. The range of the coefficient is −1 to +1. Zero equals no association, +1 equals a perfect positive ***linear*** correlation (Fig. 29-6A, red), and −1 equals a perfect negative ***linear*** correlation (Fig. 29-6A, green). The strength of the relationship between 2 continuous variables is determined by how far the correlation coefficient is from zero (absolute value)

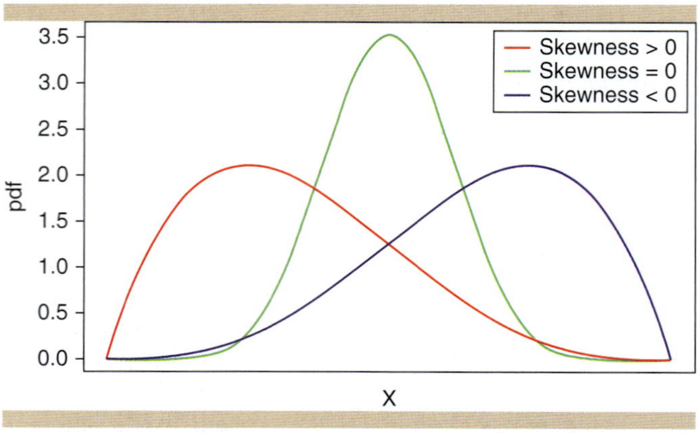

FIGURE 29-4 Illustration of skewness.

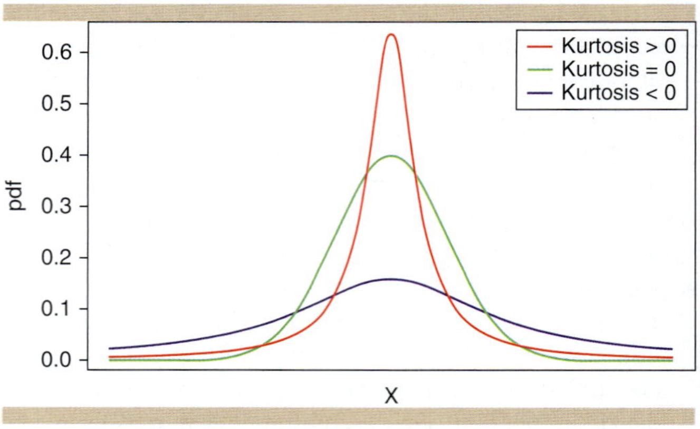

FIGURE 29-5 Illustration for kurtosis.

CONFIDENCE INTERVAL

The descriptive statistics described before uses a single value to describe the data. If we repeat the study several times, the descriptive statistics such as mean and/or standard deviation will vary. The confidence interval is the estimated range of values which is likely to include an unknown population parameter

- The probability that the confidence interval produced will contain the true parameter value is through the selection of a confidence level for an interval
- Common choices for the confidence level are 0.90, 0.95 (most commonly used), and 0.99
- If we repeat a study 1,000 times and construct a 95% confidence interval, there should be approximately 950 intervals containing the unknown parameter (Fig. 29-7)
- For example, a 95% confidence interval for population mean is

$$\text{Sample mean} \pm Z_{1-0.05/2}\ \text{SEM}$$

where $Z_{1-0.05/2}$ is 97.5 percentile of a normal distribution with mean 0 and SD = 1.

- Decreasing the level of confidence will decrease the Z value, resulting in a decrease in the length, b–a, of the corresponding interval
- Increasing the sample size will decrease SEM, which decreases the length of the confidence interval without reducing the level of confidence

HYPOTHESIS TESTING

A hypothesis test is an algorithm used to make statistical decisions by minimizing the risk of making wrong decisions using study data. It contains the following components

- Before data are collected, the following must be determined
  1. Random variable and its distribution (described earlier in the chapter)
  2. Null hypothesis and alternative hypothesis
  3. Test statistics
  4. Distribution of test statistics
  5. Significance level and rejection region
  6. Power and sample size

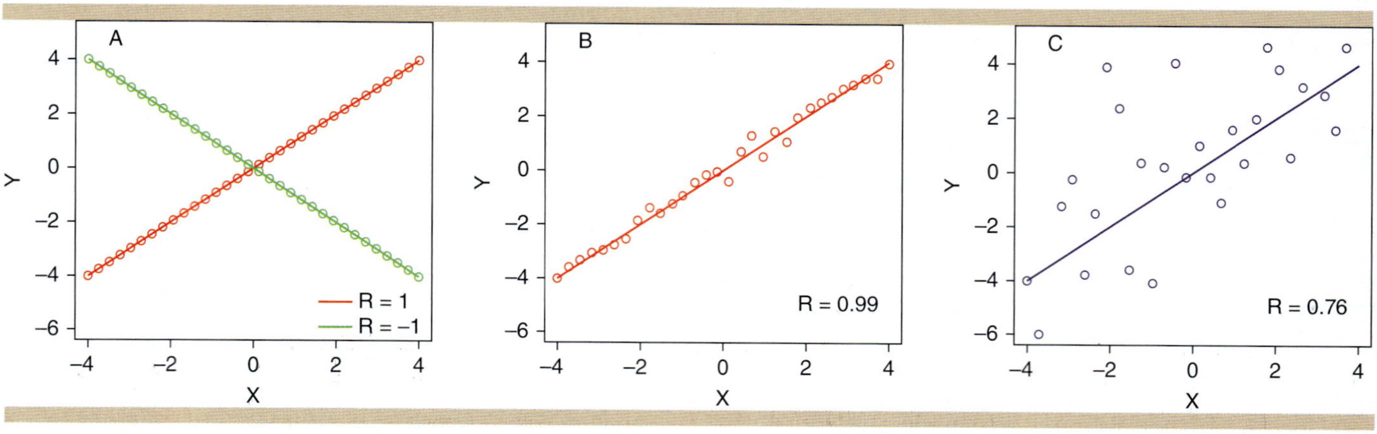

FIGURE 29-6 Examples of correlation coefficients.

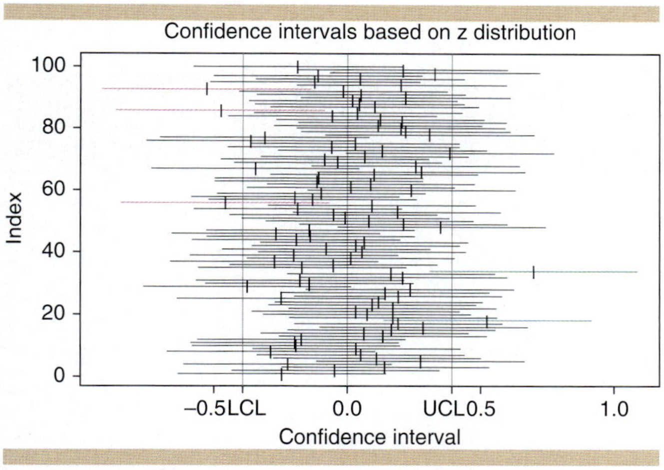

FIGURE 29-7 One hundred simulated confidence intervals based on 25 normal distributed samples. The confidence interval covers 95% of the means.

- After data are collected
  7. Calculate test statistics and *p*-value
  8. Determine if the test statistics are in the rejection region or if the *p*-value is smaller than significance level
  9. Conclusion: the null hypothesis is rejected, if *p*-value is less than the significance level or the test statistics fall in rejection region; otherwise, the null hypothesis is not rejected

However, since any test has a possibility of making wrong decisions, it is important to minimize the risks of making mistakes

Null Hypothesis (H_0) and Alternative Hypothesis (H_a)

A null hypothesis (H_0) is a hypothesis set up to be nullified or refuted in order to support an alternative hypothesis (H_a). When used, the null hypothesis is presumed true until statistical evidence, in the form of a hypothesis test, indicates otherwise

- The null hypothesis asserts that any observed difference in samples is due to chance or sampling error, while the alternative hypothesis asserts that there is a significant systematic association
- The null hypothesis assumes that a hypothesis may not be correct (i.e., no effect of a treatment) and attempts to gather evidence against that assumption (i.e., tries to reject H_0 and accept the alternative hypothesis)
- In general, there are 2 types of hypotheses
  - Two-tailed test, for example

$$\begin{cases} H_0 : \mu_1 = \mu_2 \\ H_a : \mu_1 \neq \mu_2 \end{cases}$$

  - One-tailed test, for example

$$\begin{cases} H_0 : \mu_1 \leq \mu_2 \\ H_a : \mu_1 > \mu_2 \end{cases} \quad \text{or} \quad \begin{cases} H_0 : \mu_1 \geq \mu_2 \\ H_a : \mu_1 < \mu_2 \end{cases}$$

- It should be noted that the equal sign is always in the H_0, and $\mu_1 - \mu_2$ is called effect size.

Test Statistics and Their Distributions

There are many test statistics in the literatures. The following 3 tests are frequently mentioned in clinical research.

t Test

The *t* test employs t statistics which follows a student t distribution and is commonly used in the following situations

- Test whether the mean is different from a constant (1 sample *t* test)
  - H_0: $\mu = C$
  - t statistics

$$t = \frac{sample\ mean - C}{SEM}$$

with degrees of freedom = $N - 1$ where N is the sample size

- Test whether 2 means are different (2 sample *t* tests)
  - H_0: $\mu_1 - \mu_2 = 0$
  - t statistics

$$t = \frac{Difference\ between\ 2\ sample\ means}{Standard\ error\ of\ the\ difference\ in\ sample\ means}$$

with degrees of freedom = $N_1 + N_2 - 2$ *where* N_1 *and* N_2 are sample sizes for each group

The larger the ratio, *t statistics*, the more likely it is to demonstrate a statistical difference from H_0.

F Test

The F test employs F statistics which follows an F distribution and is commonly used in the following situations

- Test whether 2 variances are equal
  - $H_0 : \frac{\sigma_1^2}{\sigma_2^2} = 1$
  - F statistics

$$F = \frac{Group\ 1\ sample\ variance}{Group\ 2\ sample\ variance}$$

with degrees of freedom, $df_1 = N_1 - 1$ and $df_2 = N_2 - 1$, where N_1 and N_2 are sample sizes for each group

- Test whether samples obtained from $K(>2)$ groups are actually from the same distribution
  - $H_0: \mu_1 = \mu_2 = \ldots = \mu_k$
  - F statistics

$$F = \frac{\textit{Sum of squared group means deviated from the grand mean} / (K-1)}{\textit{Sum of squared observations deviated from their group means} / (N-K)}$$

with degrees of freedom, $df_1 = K - 1$ and $df_2 = N - K$, where N is sample size and K is the number of groups

Chi-Square Test

The *chi-square* test employs the chi-square statistics which follows a chi-square distribution and is commonly used in the following situations

- Test for homogeneity: answers the proposition that several populations ($K > 1$) are homogeneous with respect to some characteristic, that is

$$H_0: P_1 = P_2 = P_2 = \ldots = P_k$$

- Test of independence: tests the null hypothesis, which states that 2 criteria of classification, when applied to a population of subjects, are independent
- For both situations, the test for homogeneity and the test for independence, the observed frequencies can be tabulated in an R × C contingency table (Table 29-3). Under the null hypothesis,
  - The expected frequency for cell (i, j) is

$$E_{ij} = \frac{n_{iT} \times n_{Tj}}{N}$$

  - The chi-square statistics is

$$\sum_{\textit{all } i \textit{ and } j} \frac{(n_{ij} - E_{ij})^2}{E_{ij}}$$

with degrees of freedom = (R − 1) × (C − 1) where R and C is number of rows and columns, respectively

- Goodness of fit: used to determine if differences exist between observed and expected frequencies from a distribution or a model. As in the example mentioned before, suppose a disease can be classified into 5 stages (0–4). The probabilities associated with its classification after a treatment can be expressed as in Table 29-1. A researcher treated 250 patients and observed the disease classification in their 1 year follow-up visits and tabulated the results in Table 29-4. The chi-square statistics is 18.89 with degrees of freedom, $df = 5 - 1 = 4$.

TABLE 29-3 Example of R × C contingency Table

	Column 1	Column 2	...	Column C	Total
Row 1	n_{11}	n_{12}		n_{1C}	n_{1T}
Row 2	n_{21}	n_{23}		n_{2C}	n_{2T}
...					
Row R	n_{R1}	n_{R2}		n_{RC}	n_{RT}
Total	n_{T1}	n_{T2}		n_{TC}	N

These 3 common test statistics, *t*, F, and chi-square tests, are based on the assumptions that samples are obtained from a known distribution. *t* test and Ftest assume that samples are from a normal distribution and that the sample variances are essentially equal among groups, while chi-square test assumes that samples are from a binomial (or multinomial) distribution or a known distribution, like the example in Table 29-4.

Nonparametric Tests

Nonparametric tests do not make any assumptions about the underlying distribution of the data; they are less powerful than parametric tests, meaning nonparametric tests are less likely than parametric tests to detect a difference if one exists.

Type I Error (α) and Significance Level

- In hypothesis testing, rejecting the null hypothesis when it is in fact true results in a false positive study (Fig. 29-8)

TABLE 29-4 Example of Chi-Square Test for Goodness of Fite

X = Disease classification	0	1	2	3	4	Sum
P(X = x)	0.40	0.25	0.20	0.10	0.05	1.0
Observed frequency	115	40	67	18	10	250
Expected frequency [250 x P(X = x)]	100.0	62.5	50.0	25.0	12.5	250
$\frac{(\textit{Observed} - \textit{Expected})^2}{\textit{Expected}}$	2.25	8.10	5.78	1.96	0.50	**18.89**

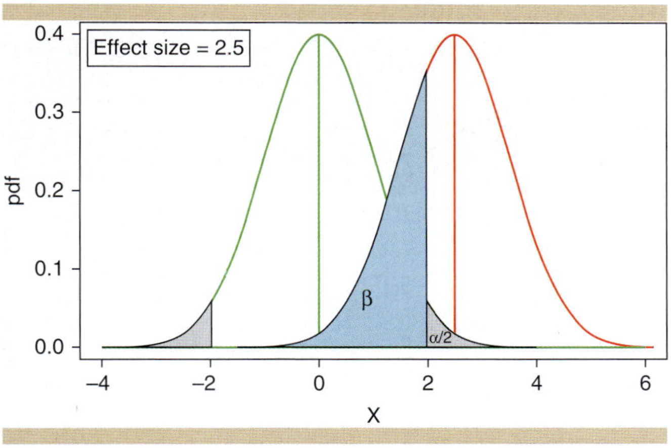

FIGURE 29-8 Illustration of type I and type II errors.

- For example, the testing result from observed data shows a difference where the true difference (unobservable) doesn't exist (Table 29-5)
- Probability of a type I error: P(type I error) = significance level = α
- The significance is usually set at 0.05

Type II Error (β)

- In hypothesis testing, failing to reject a false null hypothesis results in a false-negative study that rejects a true alternative hypothesis (see Fig. 29-8)
- For example, a study shows that no difference exists when in fact it does (Table 29-5)
- Probability of a type II error: P(type II error) = β
- Type I and type II errors are inversely related; for any set of data, the smaller the risk of one, the higher the risk of the other

Power

- The probability that the test will reject a *null hypothesis* when alternative hypothesis is true
- 1 − β = Power
- As the power increases, the chances of a type II error decreases
- Power is commonly set at 80 or 90%; maximum power a test can have is 1, the minimum is 0. The goal of a study is to have the power as close to 1 as possible
- The power of a study depends on α, β, effect size (small effect size decreases the power), sample size (a small sample size decreases the power of a study), and variance (large variance decreases power of a study)

To minimize the risks of making wrong decisions, we need to minimize both α and β. In general, we fix α and minimize β by increasing sample size, because we can control neither variance nor effect size

Rejection Region and *p*-Value

- The set of test statistics for which we should reject the null hypothesis is the rejection region (see Fig. 29-8, gray area)
- The rejection region depends on the probability distribution of the test statistics, the significance level, and the hypotheses (one- or two-tailed)
- The size of the rejection region is equal to α
- The *p*-value is the *probability* of obtaining a value of the test statistic *at least* as extreme as the one that was actually observed, given that the null hypothesis is true
- The lower the *p*-value, the lower the chance that the difference occurred by chance alone as opposed to the intervention being tested
- If the *p*-value is less than the significance level, it indicates that the test statistics falls in the rejection region

STATISTICAL METHODS FOR MULTIVARIATE ANALYSIS

When there is more than 1 variable in a study or the data may be raised from more than 2 populations, the principal idea of statistical analysis is still the same: describe the data and make a decision to reject or accept the research hypothesis. However, the statistical models used to describe the data are

TABLE 29-5 Understanding Hypothesis Testing*

Study Results	Reality	
	Treatments Are Not Different	Treatments Are Different
Treatments are *not* different	Correct decision (probability = 1 − α)	Type II error (probability = β)
Treatments *are* different	Type I error (probability = α)	Correct decision (probability = 1 − β = Power)

*Note: Only pertains to outcomes of a randomized controlled trial.

TABLE 29-6 Summary of Statistical Methods for Multivariate Analysis

Independent Variables	Outcome Variable: Discrete	Outcome Variable: Continuous	Outcome Variable: Survival
Discrete	Pearson chi-square Or Fisher exact test	*t* test (2 groups) ANOVA (2 or more)	Kaplan-Meier survival curve
Continuous	Logistic Regression	Regression	Cox Regression
Mixed	Logistic regression with indicator variables*	Regression with indicator variables	Cox regression with indicator variables*

*Dichotomized a discrete random variable into 0 and 1.

much more complicated (Table 29-6), but the following are common in multivariate analysis

- It is used to examine the relationship between a single outcome (or called dependent) variable and multiple predictor variables (risk factors, treatments, etc.)
- One can ascertain the relationship between a predictor variable and the outcome variable independently and account for the effects of other predictor variables

Two most frequently used methods are analysis of variance (ANOVA) and regression analysis

Analysis of Variance

- Used to determine whether means from several populations (>2) are same
- Does not allow you to compare which groups are more likely to differ from another
- Several post ad-hoc multiple comparison techniques are available to compare among groups

Regression Analysis

Regression analysis is a model relating multiple predictor variables (risk factors, treatments, etc.) to a single response or dependent variable

- Types of regression analysis: linear (most common), weighted, and logistic
- If the dependent variable is a continuous variable, then we model the dependent variable as a linear combination of independent variables
- If the dependent variable is dichotomies, the relation between dependent variables and independent variables is modeled by logistic regression model
- Many survival time data, that is, time from the treatment to disease recurrent, contains censoring observations, in which their survival times are not observable due to reaching the end of clinical trial, patient death, patient leaving the study early, etc. Thus, the linear regression cannot be applied to survival time data. If the dependent variable is survival time, the relation between survival time and the discrete independent variables is often modeled by a Kaplan-Meier survival curve. When there is at least 1 continuous variable, we use a proportional hazard regression model (called Cox regression model) to model the relation between survival time and the independent variables

Table 29-6 summarizes statistical methods for multivariate analysis based on type of outcome variables and type of independent variables

RELIABILITY OF MEASUREMENTS

Before data being collected, the researchers need to assess the reliability of measurements, just like we need to check the reliability of a ruler for measuring height, or scale for measuring weight, or skin test for detecting TB, or a questionnaire for detecting depression, etc. Again, to assess the reliability of measurement depends on whether the variable is continuous or discrete. For the discrete case, the assessments focus on specificity and sensitivity, while for a continuous measurement, the assessments focus on precision, accuracy, and validity

Discrete Variable

A diagnostic test (an instrument or a set of evaluation criteria) can result in the following outcomes (Table 29-7)

- *True positive*: the test is positive and the disease is present
- *False positive*: the test is positive and the disease is absent
- *True negative*: the test is negative and the disease is absent
- *False negative*: the test is negative and the disease is present

A good diagnostic test should have high true positive and true negative as well as low false positive and false negative.

TABLE 29-7 Understanding Diagnostic Test Performance

Diagnostic Test Results	Disease Status		Total
	Present	Absent	
Positive	A (True positive)	B (False positive)	A + B
Negative	C (False negative)	D (True negative)	C + D
Total	A + C	B + D	N

Sensitivity = A/(A + C)
Specificity = D/(B + D)
PPV = A/(A + B)
NPV = D/(C + D)

The following are the statistics for evaluating outcomes of a diagnostic test (see Table 29-7)

- *Sensitivity* = True positive/(true positive + false negative) = A/(A + C) is the ability of a screening test to identify correctly those who *have* the disease. It is used to assess the validity of a diagnostic test. A test with high sensitivity has few false-negative results and is *independent* of disease prevalence
- *Specificity* = True negative/(true negative + false positive) = D/(C + D) is the ability of a screening test to identify correctly those who *do not have* the disease. It is used to assess the validity of a diagnostic test. A test with high specificity has few false-positive results and is *independent* of disease prevalence
- *Positive Predictive Value (PPV)* = True positive/(true positive + false positive) = A/(A + B) is the probability that a patient has a disease when the test for the disease is positive. It is used to assess the reliability of a positive test. It is affected by 2 factors
  - Disease prevalence: higher disease prevalence results in a higher PPV
  - Specificity (only when disease is infrequent): higher specificity results in a higher PPV (with infrequent diseases)
- *Negative Predictive Value (NPV)* = True negative/(True negative + False negative) = D/(B + D) is the probability that the patient does *not have* disease when the result is negative. It is used to assess the reliability of a negative test. It is affected by 2 factors
  - Disease prevalence: lower disease prevalence results in a higher NPV
  - Sensitivity effect is minimized at a low prevalence and results in a more reliable negative test

Continuous Variable

An ideal measurement should be both accurate and precise which means all measurements are close to and tightly clustered around the known reference value or the gold standard (Fig. 29-9A)

Precision of a Measurement

- Reduced by random error
- Measures by repeatability (test-retest consistency) and reproducibility (inter-observer consistency)
- Commonly used statistics for measuring precision are
  - Measure random error by standard deviation
  - Measure test-retest consistency by Spearman-Brown coefficient
  - Measure inter-observer consistency by intraclass correlation (ICC) or Cohen Kappa

Accuracy of a Measurement

- Measured by the difference between the mean and the reference value. This difference is also known as the bias
- Reduced by systematic error
- In psychometrics, they need to develop a set of questions to measure some subjective outcomes. The accuracy is usually validated through the following
  - *Internal validity*: a study with no major methodological problems thus minimizing the error in correctly

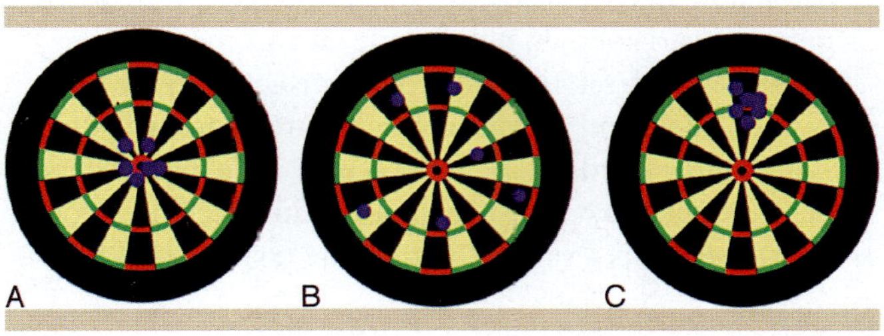

FIGURE 29-9 Illustration for accuracy and precision. (A) high accuracy and high precision; (B) low accuracy and low precision; and (C) low accuracy and low precision.

finding a causal relationship between the experimental treatment and the observed effect
- *Construct validity of cause*: support for the intended interpretation of the result. The observed effect is attributable to the specific experimental intervention and not other variables of effect
- *External validity*: relates to the generalizability of the study. Could the observed effect be produced in other settings, beyond the studied populations and at other times?
- *Statistical conclusion validity*: are the conclusions reached justifiable on statistical grounds? Does the effect generalize to the population from which the sample was drawn?

ISSUES IN STUDY DESIGN

Research Questions

The 5 characteristics of a good research question are feasible, interesting, novel, ethical, and relevant.

Trial Design

The classifications based on different characteristics of studies are

- Observational versus experimental
- Retrospective versus prospective
- Cross-sectional versus longitudinal

(See Types of Study section)

Outcome Variables

Outcome variables should be chosen on the basis of the appropriateness of the measure to the research question; the statistical characteristics of the measure; and the number of outcome variables necessary to answer the research question. In many research studies, primary and secondary outcome variables are chosen for study

- *Primary outcome variables* are the key variables in the study that will prove or disprove the null hypothesis or research question
- *Secondary outcome variables*, in addition to the primary outcome variables, do not directly answer the research question; however, they do provide insight into the intervention effect and provide areas for further investigation
- Both primary and secondary outcome variables are dependent variables in a statistical model. The outcome (dependent) variable is a variable that we are trying to predict

Predictor Variables (Risk Factors or Independent Variables)

- Variables that might influence outcome variables
- Might be variables that we can control, like a treatment, or variables that cannot be controlled, like an exposure
- Might also represent a demographic factor like age or gender
- Any variable that is used to make predictions of outcome variables is a predictor (or an independent) variable

Confounding Variables

A confounding variable is a variable that has correlation with both the *independent* (predictor) and *dependent* (outcome) variables

- Confounding is a major threat to the validity of inferences made about cause and effect (regression analysis)
- Confounding variables cannot be defined in terms of statistical notions alone; some causal assumptions are necessary

Research Error

There are 2 types of research errors

- Random error: handled with the use of statistical tests and methods
- Systematic error: uncontrolled error that may change the results and/or interpretation of research

Selection Bias

Selection bias is a nonrandom systematic error in the design or conduct of a study

- Types of selection bias
  - *Sampling bias*: results from failure to ensure that all members of the reference population have a known chance of being selected for inclusion in the sample
  - *Allocation bias*: results from systematic differences in the characteristics of those assigned to treatment vs. control groups in a controlled study
  - *Selection bias*: results when one of the following occurs: (1) self-selection of individuals to participate in a survey or experimental study; (2) selection of samples or studies by researchers to support a particular hypothesis
  - *Nonresponder bias*: results if the survey results differ substantially from those that would have been generated if the response rate was 100%
  - *Interviewer bias*: results from the personal prejudice of the individual conducting the interview

The following characteristics of studies can decrease bias: randomization (minimizes selection bias), blinding, matching, prospective studies (may decrease the chance of patient selection bias)

Randomization

- Best means of avoiding allocation bias
- Balances the groups for prognostic factors (i.e., disease severity)
- Eliminates overrepresentation of any one characteristic within the study group
- Should be concealed from the clinicians and researchers of the study to help eliminate conscious or unconscious bias

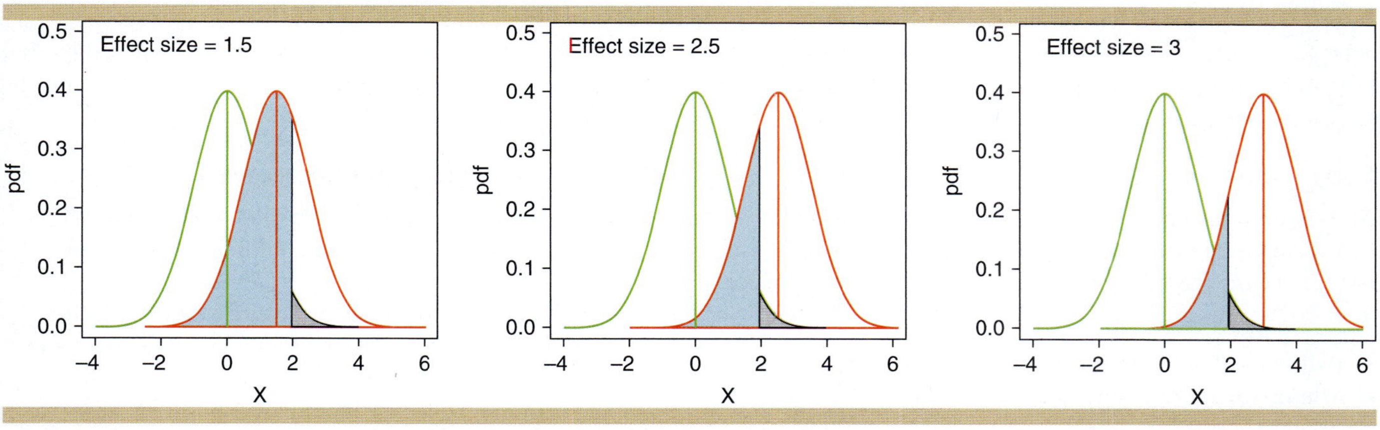

FIGURE 29-10 Relationship between effect size and power.

Blinding (Masking)

- People involved in the study do not know which treatments are given to which patients
- With double blinding, neither the patient nor the clinician knows which treatment is being administered
- Eliminates bias and preconceived notions as to how the treatments should be working

SAMPLE SIZE DETERMINATION

Specifications needed to determine the sample size in a randomized trial are as follows

- Whether the test should be one- or two-tailed
- Level of statistical significance (α): the lower the significance level, the greater the required sample size
- Level of power ($1 - \beta$): the higher the power specification, the greater the required sample size
- Effect size: the size of effect on the primary outcome variable to be detected
- Estimated SD

Relationship among significance level, power, effect size, SD, and sample size:

- When α increases, β decreases, thus power increases; while holding effect size, SD, and sample size constant
- When effect size increases, β decreases, thus power increases (Fig. 29-10); while holding α, SD, and sample size constant
- When SD increases, SEM = $SD/\sqrt{N}$ increases, β increases, thus power decreases (Fig. 29-11); while holding α, effect size, and sample size constant
- When sample size increases, SEM = $SD/\sqrt{N}$ decreases, β decreases, thus power increases; while holding α, effect size, and SD constant

Data Reliability

To obtain reliable data, we are required to have

- Reliable measurements (see Reliability of Measurements section), and
- A reliable data collection scheme

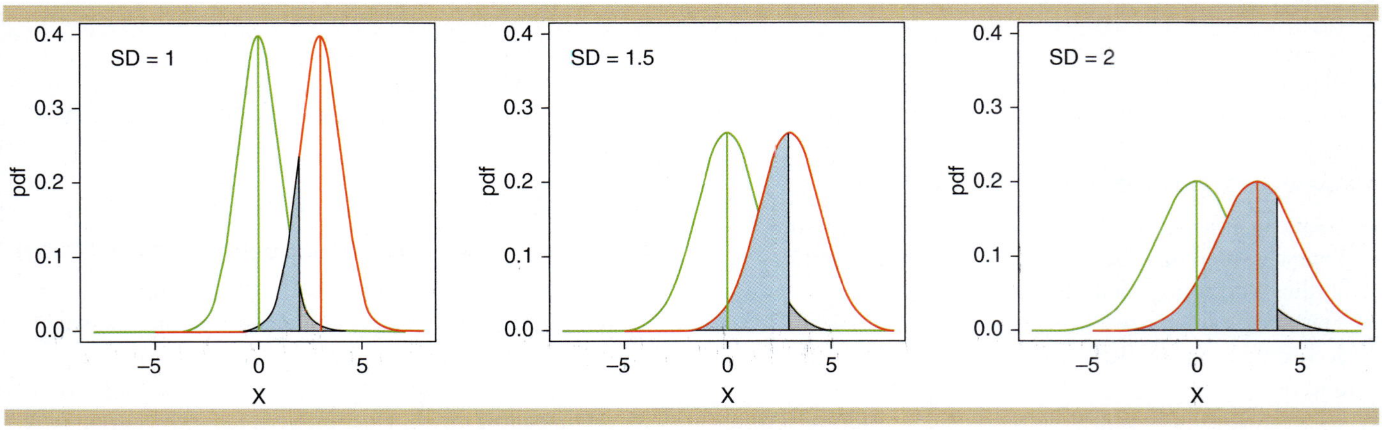

FIGURE 29-11 Relationship between SD and power.

"Gold Standard"

The *gold standard* provides objective criteria (e.g., laboratory test not requiring interpretation) or a current clinical standard (e.g., a venogram for deep venous thrombosis) for diagnosis

Intention to Treat Principle

All randomized subjects should be analyzed according to the treatment group to which they were assigned, even if they did not receive the intended treatment or received only a portion of it

- Reflects real-world nonadherence to treatment
- Minimizes nonresponder and transfer bias

TYPES OF STUDIES

Classification based on different characteristics of studies

- *Observational versus Experimental*
  - *Observational*: investigator does not intervene in any way, but merely observes outcomes (case series, case-control studies, cross-sectional surveys, and cohort studies)
  - *Experimental*: investigator intervenes in some way to effect the outcome
- *Retrospective versus Prospective*
  - *Retrospective:* the events of interest transpired before the onset of the study
  - *Prospective*: the direction of inquiry is forward from the cohort inception and that the events of interest transpire after the onset of the study
- *Cross-sectional versus Longitudinal*
  - *Cross-sectional studies* are used to survey one point in time
  - *Longitudinal studies* follow the same patients over multiple points in time

Retrospective Studies—Literature Review and Chart Review

Case Report

- A report on a single patient
- Reports of cases with no control groups with which to compare outcomes; they have no statistical validity

Meta-Analysis (Systematic Literature Review)

- Focus on a clinical topic and answer a specific question
- Extensive literature searches are conducted to identify studies with sound methodology
- The studies are reviewed, assessed, and summarized according to the predetermined criteria of the review question
- Uses statistical techniques to combine the results of several studies as if they were 1 large study

Case Series (Retrospective Study)

A case series is a noncomparative study looking at the effect of treatment of individual patients, presentation of interesting or unusual observations

Case-Control Study (Retrospective Study)

- A group of individuals with the *condition* (cases) and a group of people *without the condition* (controls) are identified
- The effect of an individual's exposure to various factors is evaluated in terms of the development of the outcome being studied
- Information is collected about past exposure to suspected etiological factors in the case and control individuals by looking at their records or by questioning
- Bias may arise in this type of study (bias occurs when there is a systematic difference between the true results and those that are observed in the study)
- Less reliable than randomized controlled trials and cohort studies because a statistical relationship does not mean that one factor necessarily caused the other
- Can only determine odds ratio (OR) of developing the condition

Cohort Study (Prospective or Retrospective Study)

- Groups of *exposed* and *nonexposed* individuals are followed to compare the incidence of disease (or rate of death from disease) in the 2 groups
- Can determine incidence (new cases) of disease and determine if a temporal relationship exists
- Types of cohort studies
  - Concurrent (concurrent prospective or longitudinal): original population is defined at the start of the study, and subjects are followed through time until the disease does or does not develop
  - Retrospective cohort (historical cohort, nonconcurrent prospective): exposed population is defined by historical records, and outcome is determined at the time the study begins
- Not as reliable as randomized controlled studies because the 2 groups may differ in ways other than the variable under study
- Longitudinal study
- RR is used to assess the effect of a risk factor in a cohort study

Prospective Studies—Clinical Trials

Randomized Controlled Studies (Prospective Study)

- Study the effect of a therapy or test on patients with randomization and with large enough sample size to avoid confounding and selection bias
- Include methodologies that reduce the potential for bias and that allow for comparison between intervention groups and control groups (no intervention)

- Evidence for questions of diagnosis is found in prospective trials that compare tests with a reference or "gold standard" test
- From the results, an estimate of the number of patients who would need to be treated (NNT) to prevent one adverse outcome is calculated by

NNT = 1/(Rate in untreated group − Rate in treated group)

- NNT helps to estimate the effect that might be expected to be observed by using the new treatment or preventive measure but is limited by not taking into account quality of life

Crossover Studies (Prospective Study)

- Similar to randomized controlled studies, however, each subject receives treatments being compared or both the treatment and control
- The order of the treatments is randomly assigned
- Used for patients who have a stable, usually chronic condition during both treatment periods
- Used for reducing the variation of outcome variable among subjects

Phases of Clinical Trials

- *Phase I*: studies to obtain preliminary information on dosage, absorption, metabolism, and the relationship between toxicity and the dose-schedule of treatment
- *Phase II*: studies to determine feasibility and estimate treatment activity and safety in diseases (or, e.g., tumor types) for which the treatment appears promising and generates hypotheses for later testing
- *Phase III*: comparative trial to determine the effectiveness and safety of a new treatment relative to standard therapy. These trials usually represent the most rigorous proof of treatment efficacy (pivotal trials) and are the last stage before product licensing
- *Phase IV*: postmarketing studies of licensed products

Cost-Identification Studies

Cost-identification studies evaluate the cost of providing treatments

Cost-Effectiveness Analysis

- Evaluates the costs and clinical outcome
- Results are reported as cost per clinical outcome

Cost-Benefit Analysis

- Evaluation of costs and benefits of a specific treatment
- Results are reported in monetary units

Cost-Utility Analysis

- Evaluation of cost and utility of a specific treatment
- Results are reported as cost per quality-adjusted life-year (QALY)

PRACTICE GUIDELINES

- Evidence-based developed statements to assist practitioners about appropriate health care for specific clinical circumstances
- Guidelines review and evaluate the evidence and then make explicit recommendations for practice

QUIZ

Questions

1. Your office has just purchased a new screening test for fungal infections. You decide to use the test along with the gold standard culture. Calculate the sensitivity and specificity of the test using the information below. What do these results mean to you?

Results of Screening Test	Fungal Infection	No Fungal Infection
Positive	25	1
Negative	2	100

2. You wish to find further information about this screening test. A trial is performed in a clinic population similar to the one that you treat and has produced the following results. Calculate the positive and negative predictive value of the test. What do these numbers tell you?

	Population		
Test Results	Fungal Infection	No Fungal Infection	Total
Positive	200	10	210
Negative	20	770	790
Total	220	780	1,000

3. Which of the following can be used to summarize the variability of a continuous outcome variable?

   A. Mean
   B. Median
   C. Standard deviation
   D. Standard error of mean

4. Which is true for a normal (Gaussian) distribution?
   A. The graph normally has 2 peaks
   B. When the data are distributed normally, the mean and median are very close and may be identical
   C. It only applies to cross-sectional trials
   D. The most frequently occurring value is on either end of the curve

5. A study which is done in a very specific population that is not generalizable to the population that you treat, would be said have low:
   A. Construct validity
   B. Internal validity
   C. External validity
   D. Statistical validity

6. The results of a randomized controlled trial using therapy to treat a severe skin malignancy showed a mortality rate of 18% in the untreated group and 5% in the treated group. Calculate the number needed to treat (NNT) to determine how many people would need to be treated in order to prevent one death.

7. When looking at the possible outcomes of a randomized controlled trial that compare 2 treatments, you generate a table based on your conclusions about treatment and what the true outcome is. Identify in the table, which would be a "correct decision," "type II error," and "type I error." (Hint: 2 of the boxes are a "correct decision.")

	Truth	
Your decision	Treatments are not different	Treatments are different
Treatments are not different		
Treatments are different		

8. The power of a test has the following qualities, EXCEPT:
   A. It is equal to (1 – the probability of making a type II error)
   B. It is the probability of correctly concluding that the treatments do in fact differ.
   C. It is the probability of making a type I error.
   D. It can be expressed as $1 - \beta$.

9. The dermatology consult records from a large university hospital from the year 1980, which were examined in 1999 to see if their recorded effects of a treatment was related to the development of lymphoma by 2002. This is an example of:
   A. A cross-sectional study
   B. A case-control study
   C. A concurrent cohort study
   D. A retrospective cohort study
   E. A randomized controlled trial

10. A study was conducted to assess the risk of stroke in relation to the use of an oral therapy that you wish to use for your patient. A standard questionnaire was administered to patients who were admitted with a stroke as well as to a control set of patients who were admitted for nonstroke-related problems to determine their use of this medication. They found that 10 of the 70 patients who had a stroke took the medication and that of 1,200 patients who did not have a stroke, 200 of those patients had a history of taking the medication. Calculate the odds ratio for these data.

11. What are characteristics of a phase 3 trial?
    A. These are small studies intended to provide preliminary information on dosage, metabolism, toxicity, and absorption.
    B. They involve fairly large comparative trials based on previous information from smaller trials to determine the effectiveness and safety of a new treatment relative to standard therapy.
    C. They only provide information on feasibility.
    D. They do not focus on generalizability to the population.

12. You just completed a randomized clinical trial comparing new treatment A with old treatment B. The result shows a 20% improvement with the new treatment, p-value = 0.058. What is the most appropriate interpretation of this result?
    A. Two treatments are comparable.
    B. Treatment A is definitely inferior to Treatment B.
    C. Treatment A is not statistically superior to Treatment B.
    D. Treatment A is definitely superior to Treatment B.

13. What is the reason that blinding (masking) the examiner is important in a clinical trial?
    A. It helps maintain objectivity in assessment of clinical events.
    B. It preserves type I error rate.
    C. It avoids treatment assignment bias.
    D. It balances for prognostic factors.

Answers

1. Sensitivity: (True positive/[True positive + False negative]) 25/[25 + 2] = 93%. Of all the people *with* the disease, the number that will have a *positive test.* Specificity: (True negative/[True negative + False positive]) 100/[100 + 1] = 99% Of all the people *without* the disease, the number that will have a *negative test.*

2. Positive predictive value: (True positive/[True positive + False positive]) 200/[200 + 10] = 95%. Of all the people with a *positive test*, the number that *will* have the disease.
   Negative predictive value: (True negative/[True negative + False negative]) 770/[770 + 20] = 97%. Of all the people with a *negative test*, the number that *will not* have the disease.
3. C. Standard deviation measures how widely measurements are scattered around the mean, while standard error of mean measures the accuracy of estimation of mean.
4. B. A normal distribution is a bell-shaped curve (1 peak) where approximately 68% of the results fall within 1 standard deviation and about 95% within 2 standard deviations. Since the mean is the average number and the median is the value that half the population falls below, these numbers can be very close when values follow a normal distribution.
5. C. One major objective of trials is to have the results apply to those outside of the study population. When a trial has low external validity, the therapy is found to be best for the population studied only. Internal validity takes into account whether the trial was done properly and had valid findings.
6. NNT = 1/[(Rate in untreated group) − (Rate in treated group)] = 1/(18 − 5%) = 1/0.13 = 8
7. Your decision that a treatment is not different when it really is not different is a correct answer. Similarly, concluding that the treatments are different when in reality they are different is also a correct answer. A type I error is committed when there is no difference between treatments but on the basis of the study, the investigators erroneously conclude that they are different. The probability of making this error is the *p*-value (or α). A type II error occurs when there really is a difference between therapies but on the basis of the study, it is erroneously concluded that there is no difference. The probability of making this error is β. Since the total of all probabilities are equal to 1, the probability that the investigators correctly decide on the basis of their study that the treatments are correctly different is $1 - \beta$ (or power).

	Truth	
Your decision	Treatments are not different	Treatments are different
Treatments are not different	Correct decision	Type II error
Treatments are different	Type I error	Correct decision

8. C. The power of a study tells the investigator how good the study is at correctly identifying a difference between the treatments being tested, if in reality they actually are different. In other words, how likely is the study NOT to miss a difference if one really exists? Thus all are true statements except for C. The probability of making a type I error is the *p*-value (or α).
9. D. A cohort design involves a study population that is followed for a long period of time to determine whether an outcome of interest has occurred, i.e., it begins with exposed and nonexposed subjects.
   In a concurrent cohort study (also known as prospective or longitudinal), the study follows the subjects through time until the point at which the outcome develops or not. This is problematic when studying something that takes a long time to develop. Using data from 1980, the observation time will be shortened. For this reason it is called a retrospective cohort (or a historical cohort or nonconcurrent prospective study). In the end, exposed and nonexposed groups will be compared. In a cross sectional study both exposure and disease outcome are determined at the same time for each subject. It looks only at one point in time. Case control studies start with those who have the disease outcome and compares them to those without. Randomized controlled trials involve 2 groups that are randomized to an intervention and followed for the outcome.
10. OR = ([A × D]/[B × C]) = (10 × 1000)/(200 × 60) = 0.83

	Cases With Stroke	Cases Without Stroke
History of medication	A = 10	B = 200
No history of medication	C = 60	D = 1,000

11. B. The U.S. Food and Drug Administration follows a standard protocol in testing new pharmaceutical agents. Phase 1 are small studies that evaluate the agent for toxins and pharmaceutical effects while Phase 2 are larger studies that look for efficacy and safety. Phase 3 are large randomized controlled trials that test for effectiveness and safety, which if successful would then be approved for marketing. Phase 4 studies are postmarketing surveillance studies that will continue the study for safety and effectiveness as it is used by the public.
12. C. Although there is a measurement difference between treatments (20%), the conventional type I error, 0.05, has been exceeded; therefore, you cannot conclude that A is superior to B. In addition, the reported *p*-value is very close to 0.05; you cannot conclude comparability of the treatment without more information.

13. A. Blinding (masking) in a clinical trial can reduce the likelihood of biased behavior on the part of investigators, patients, or other study personnel. For example, if an investigator knows the treatment assignment, he/she may look harder for certain drug effects.

REFERENCES

Alford L: On differences between explanatory and pragmatic clinical trials. *N Zealand J Physiother* 2006;35(1):12–16.

Altman DG, Bland JM: Standard deviations and standard errors. *BMJ* 2005;331(7521):903.

Altman DJ, Bland JM: Treatment allocation in controlled trials: why randomise? *BMJ* 1999;318:1209–1209.

Day SJ, Altman DJ: Blinding in clinical trials and other studies. *BMJ* 2000;321:504.

Easton V, McColl JH: STEPS Statistics Glossary v1.1, web version, 1997.

Egger M, Smith GD, Phillips AN: Meta-analysis: principles and procedures. *BMJ* 1997;315:1533–1537.

Glantz S: *Primer of Biostatistics*, 7th Ed. New York: McGraw-Hill; 2012.

Gordis L: *Epidemiology*, 3rd Ed. Philadelphia: Saunders; 2004.

Kocher MS, Zurakowski D: Clinical epidemiology and biostatistics: a primer for orthopaedic surgeons. *J Bone Joint Surg Am* 2004;86-A(3):607–620.

Lau FH, Chung KC: Survey research: a primer for hand surgery. *J Hand Surg Am* 2005;30(5):893.e1–893.e11.

Livingston EH: The mean and standard deviation: what does it all mean? *J Surg Res* 2004;119(2):117–123.

Morales AJ: Study design for the evaluation of treatment. *Semin Reprod Endocrinol* 1996;14(2):111–118. Review.

Overholser BR, Sowinski KM: Biostatistics primer: part 2. *Nutr Clin Pract* 2008;23(1):76–84.

Petrie A: Statistics in orthopaedic papers. *J Bone Joint Surg Br* 2006;88(9):1121–1136.

Pocock SJ: *Clinical Trials: A Practical Approach*. New York: John Wiley; 2004.

Rochon PA, Gurwitz JH, et al. Reader's guide to critical appraisal of cohort studies: 1. Role and design. *BMJ* 2005;330:895–897.

Schwartz D, Lellouch J: Explanatory and pragmatic attitudes in therapeutical trials. *J Chronic Dis* 1967;20(8):637–648.

Sibbald B, Roberts C: Understanding controlled trials Crossover trials. *BMJ* 1998;316:1719–1720.

CHAPTER 30

HISTOLOGIC STAINS AND SPECIAL STUDIES

HAFEEZ DIWAN
VICTOR G. PRIETO
RICHARD R. JAHAN-TIGH

HEMATOXYLIN AND EOSIN (H&E)

Used for elucidation of basic histologic features, prior to the use of special stains or immunohistochemical studies as needed; among other features, calcification and microorganisms such as fungi and bacteria may be detected by H&E and confirmed by additional studies

STAINS FOR CARBOHYDRATES

- Periodic-acid Schiff (PAS)
  - Stains glycogen red—diastase labile; therefore, diastase pretreatment will remove glycogen
  - Stains mucopolysaccharides red—diastase stable
  - Stains fungi red—diastase stable
  - Stains basement membrane red—diastase stable
- Colloidal iron
  - Stains mucin blue
- Alcian blue
  - Stains mucopolysaccharides blue
    - At pH 2.5: acid (carboxylated or sulfated mucopolysaccharides)
    - At pH 1.0: acid (sulfated mucopolysaccharides)
    - With hyaluronidase: only epithelial mucins will stain (connective tissue mucins will be digested and will not stain)
  - With PAS: acid mucopolysaccharides will stain blue and neutral polysaccharides will stain magenta; also, the yeast of *Cryptococcus* will stain red and the capsule will stain blue with this method
- Mucicarmine
  - Stains epithelial mucins red (also stains capsule of *Cryptococcus* red)

STAINS FOR PIGMENTS

- Fontana-Masson (Fig. 30-1)
  - Stains melanin and argentaffin granules black (nuclei will be red); useful for quantifying melanocytes (e.g., in vitiligo) and in cases of minocycline pigmentary alteration
  - Also stains *Cryptococcus and the phaeohyphomycotic organisms*
- Grimelius argyrophil stain
  - Argentaffin and argyrophil substances will stain black
- Tyrosinase (DOPA-oxidase)
  - Requires fresh tissue
  - Stains melanin-containing cells brownish-black (due to tyrosinase acting on DOPA, the substrate for this reaction)

STAINS FOR MINERALS

- Von-Kossa
  - Stains calcium salts black; useful for detecting calcification of vessel walls and elastic tissue (calcinosis cutis, pseudoxanthoma elasticum, calciphylaxis, elastosis, and elastofibroma)
- Alizarin red S
  - Stains calcium red
- Prussian blue stain (Fig. 30-2)
  - Stains iron blue (the Prussian blue reaction: tissue treated with dilute hydrochloric acid and potassium ferrocyanide) (Note: if it's granular and staining blue, it's likely an iron stain)

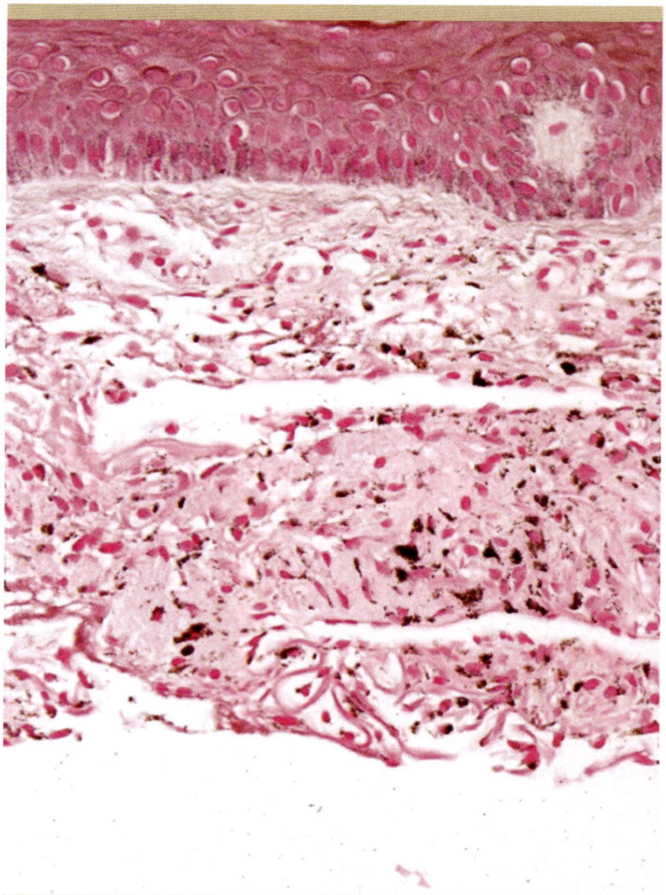

FIGURE 30-1 Fontana-Masson stains melanin black in this biopsy of minocycline pigmentation (200x) (also see Fig. 30-3).

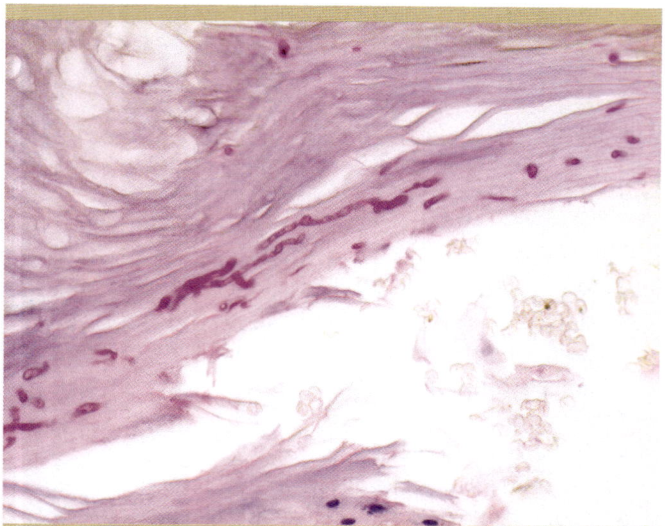

FIGURE 30-2 PAS stain showing dermatophytes in stratum corneum (200x).

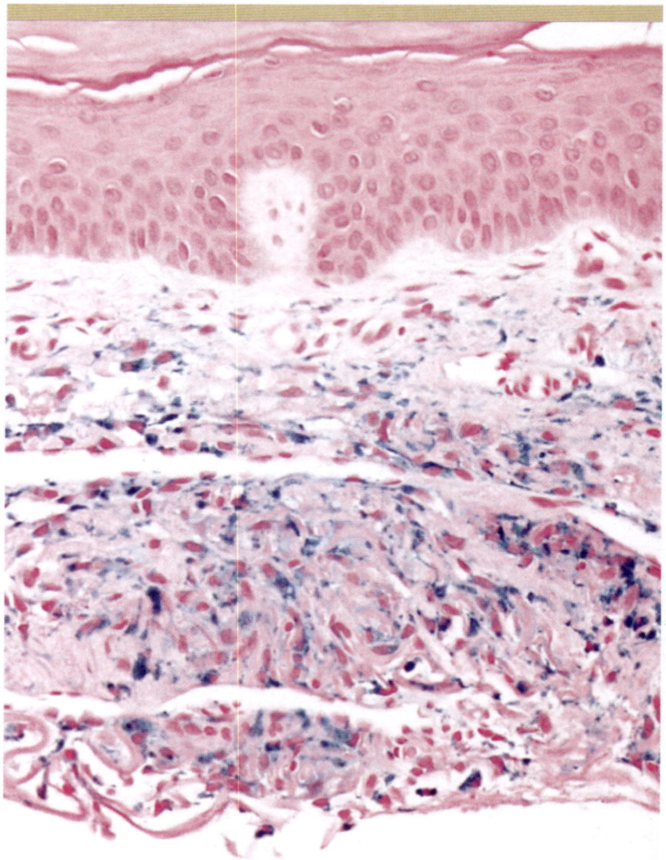

FIGURE 30-3 Prussian blue stains iron blue (200x). This is a case of minocycline pigmentation, which was also Fontana-Masson positive.

- Gomori methenamine silver (GMS) (Fig. 30-3)
  - Stains urates (e.g., gout) black. (Note: urates are lost if tissue is processed in formalin)
  - Tissue must be processed with alcohol to prevent loss of urates
  - Also see section "Stains for Microorganisms"

STAINS FOR CONNECTIVE TISSUE COMPONENTS

- Trichrome
  - Stains collagen blue or green and muscle red, depending on the type of reagents used
- Verhoeff-van Gieson
  - Stains elastic fibers black, collagen red, and muscle yellow (also red cells will stain yellow)
- Acid-Orcein
  - Stains elastic fibers brown. When combined with giemsa, stains amyloid "sky-blue"

- Gomori aldehyde fuchsin
  - Elastic fibers are stained purple

STAINS FOR AMYLOID

- Congo red
  - Stains amyloid pinkish-red; gives apple-green birefringence to amyloid (the most specific method for amyloid)
- Thioflavin T
  - Amyloid shows yellow fluorescence
- Crystal violet
  - Stains amyloid purple-violet
- Acid-Orcein Giemsa
  - Amyloid highlighted "sky blue"

STAINS FOR FAT

- Oil red O
  - Stains fat red; needs frozen/fresh tissue (once tissue is fixed and processed into paraffin blocks, this method does not work). This may be very helpful in seeing the fat globules in sebaceous carcinoma
- Osmium tetroxide
  - Paraffin-embedded tissue; stains fat black
- Sudan black B
  - Paraffin-embedded tissue; stains fat black

STAINS FOR MICROORGANISMS

- H&E
  - May demonstrate fungi, bacteria
- Gram
  - Stains gram-positive bacteria (also *Nocardia*) dark blue and gram-negative organisms red
- Giemsa
  - For *Leishmania* and granuloma inguinale
- GMS (see Fig. 30-3)
  - Stains fungi, *Pneumocystis jiroveci* (formerly *carinii*), and protothecosis black
  - Grocott methenamine silver is a modified Gomori and looks the same
- PAS
  - Stains fungi and protothecosis pink
- Fontana-Masson (see Fig. 30-1)
  - Stains *Cryptococcus* and the *phaeohyphomycoses*
- Warthin-Starry
  - Stains spirochetes black
- Ziehl-Neelson stain
  - Uses carbol fuchsin; stains mycobacteria red
    - usually too harsh for *Mycobacterium leprae* and Fite stain is preferred

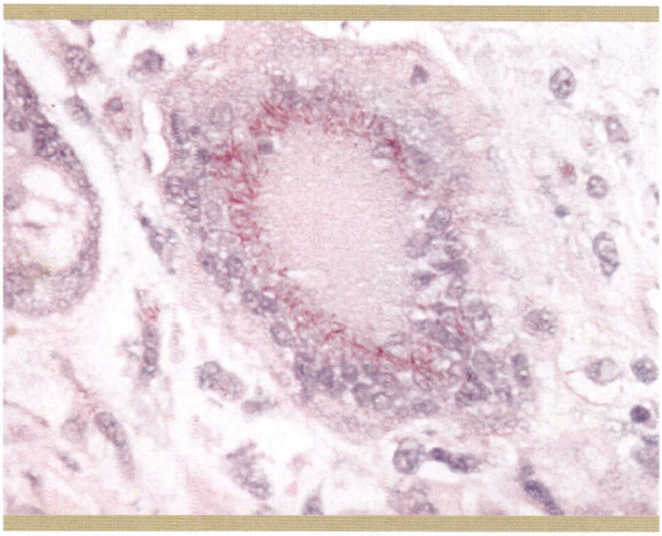

FIGURE 30-4 Fite stain showing atypical mycobacteria pink inside giant cells (400x). This case was thought to be erythema nodosum clinically.

- Fite stain (Fig. 30-4)
  - Modification of Ziehl-Neelson; stains *M. leprae* and *Nocardia*
  - It also detects atypical mycobacteria
- Dieterle stain
  - Stains spirochetes, bacillary angiomatosis, Donovan bodies black (uses silver nitrate)

STAINS FOR MAST CELLS

Giemsa and toluidine blue are metachromatic stains for mast cells; also chloroacetate esterase (Leder stain) (Table 30-1 is a summary of information on special stains used in dermatopathology)

IMMUNOHISTOCHEMICAL STUDIES

Uses primary antibodies (polyclonal or monoclonal) to a particular antigen, followed by secondary antibody complexed to an enzyme; subsequently, a chromagen is added, which is acted on by the enzyme, releasing a colored product that is evaluated histologically

STUDIES FOR EPITHELIA

- Cytokeratins (CK) are intermediate filaments found in epithelial cells, the following antibodies and cocktail antibodies are useful (Figs. 30-5 and 30-6):
- AE1/AE3—a cocktail antibody recognizing a broad spectrum of keratin; it labels most squamous cell carcinomas

TABLE 30-1 Special Stains Used in Dermatopathology

Color	What is Staining	Stain Name	Comment:
Black			
Black-Brown structures with **Yellow** background	Spirochetes, bacillary angiomatosis, Donovan bodies	Dieterle or Steiner	Basically looks like a Warthin-Starry
Black structures with **Yellow** background	Spirochetes, Donovan bodies, rhinoscleroma	Warthin-Starry	
Black structures with variable background color	Melanocyte tyrosinase	Dopa	
Black structures with light **Pink/Purple** background	Melanin	Fontana-Masson	Useful in vitiligo. Do not forget it stains some fungal organisms with melanin in their cell walls (e.g., cryptococcus, the phaeohyphomycoses, *Hortaea werneckii*)
Black structures with **Green** background	Fungal hyphae, spores, nocardia, actinomyces	Gomori methenamine silver (GMS)	Protothecosis "Soccer balls" (Morulae) will stain
Black structures with **Green** background	Fungal hyphae, spores, nocardia, actinomyces	Grocott	Looks identical to Gomori
Black structures with variable background	Reticulin fibers and melanin (both black)	Silver nitrate	
Black fibers with **Pink** background	Elastic fibers black, collagen pink	Verhoeff-van Gieson	Useful in perforating disorders, anetoderma, mid-dermal elastolysis, cutis laxa, scarring alopecias, collagenomas
Black structures with **Pink** background	Calcium, urates (gout) both black	Von-Kossa	Urates only stain if fixed in other than formalin (e.g., 95% ethanol). Urates on H&E look light brown
Black-Blue staining of globular deposits either within cells or in stroma	Intracellular or extracellular lipids stained bluish-black	Sudan black	Requires fresh tissue (i.e., not placed in formalin). Could be used in Mohs for sebaceous carcinoma or other tumor with sebaceous differentiation
Red/Pink			
Red granular structures with **orangish** background	Calcium	Alizarin red	
Pink/red granular within cells—background varies	Mast cell granules	Leder stain (naphthol chloroacetate esterase, a.k.a. specific esterase)	

(*Continued*)

TABLE 30-1 Special Stains Used in Dermatopathology (Continued)

Color	What is Staining	Stain Name	Comment:
Pinkish-red nodular material on lighter pink background	Amyloid	Congo red	Polarized light yields the "apple green" birefringence
Red bacterial forms on a **Blue** background	AFB (including *Mycobacterium leprae*), nocardia, actinomyces	Fite	
Red bacterial forms on a **Blue** background	AFB, actinomyces	Ziehl-Neelson	Stain may miss *M. leprae*
Red cords on **blue-green** background	Muscle/keratin stains red, collagen blue/green, nuclei red	Trichrome	
Red structures on **Yellow** background	Cryptococcus capsule red, pagets, and extramammary pagets stain red	Mucicarmine	
Red droplets within cells with variable background color	Intracellular or extracellular lipids stain red	Oil red O	Requires fresh tissue (i.e., not placed in formalin). Could be used in Mohs for sebaceous carcinoma or other tumor with sebaceous differentiation
Blue			
Bright **blue** stain on **pink/ purple** background(varies)	Mucopolysaccharides	Alcian blue	
Light **purple** epidermis, **pink** dermis with dark **brown** fibers	Amyloid stains "sky blue"	Acid Orcein-Giemsa	Unpolarized: looks somewhat like an H&E, but with brown elastin fibers staining in the dermis. Must polarize to see the "Sky Blue" amyloid
Blue granules on variable color background	Iron (hemosiderin)	Perls Prussian blue	
Bluish staining throughout dermis or around follicles with **pink** background	Mucopolysaccharides	Colloidal iron	Used in cutaneous lupus, follicular mucinosis, scleromyxedema
Red cords on **blue-green** background	Muscle/keratin stains red, collagen blue/green, nuclei red	Trichrome	
Purple			
Pink/Purple granules within cells on a light **blue** background	Mast cell granules purple, leishmaniasis	Giemsa	Heparin is what is being stained in the mast cell granule
Purple fibers in dermis with faint **blue** background	Elastin fibers purple	Gomori aldehyde fuchsin	

(Continued)

TABLE 30-1 Special Stains Used in Dermatopathology (Continued)

Color	What is Staining	Stain Name	Comment:
Purple granules within cells on a **bluish-purple** background	Mast cell granules purple	Toluidine blue	
Brown			
Brown fibers on **grayish-blue** background	Elastic fibers stain brown	Acid-Orcein	

(SCC), basal cell carcinomas (BCC), adnexal tumors, and Merkel cell carcinomas but it may not label spindle cell SCC

- CAM5.2—useful for eccrine tumors, Paget disease (PD), extramammary PD (EMPD), Merkel cell carcinoma, and will also label sebaceous carcinoma and a minority of BCC; SCC is mostly negative

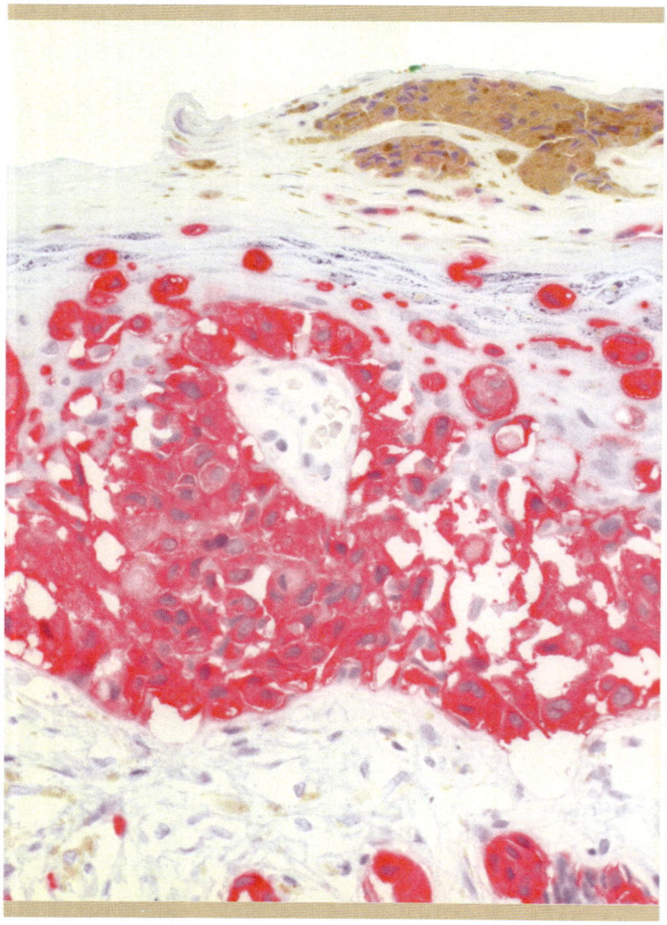

FIGURE 30-5 Melan-A positivity in a case of melanoma, showing pagetoid spread of atypical melanocytes (200x).

- CK5/6—useful for SCC, including spindle cell SCC; it has been shown to label the majority of primary cutaneous adnexal neoplasms and may be useful in distinguishing these from metastatic adenocarcinoma to the skin (fewer of these are reactive with anti-CK5/6)
- CK7—Very useful for demonstrating PD and EMPD; present in less than a quarter cases of Merkel cell carcinoma
- CK20—Merkel cell carcinoma will typically exhibit perinuclear dot-like positivity
- CEA (carcinoembryonic antigen)
  - Antibody to CEA, which is an oncofetal antigen, will demonstrate glandular differentiation (helpful in eccrine and apocrine adnexal neoplasms)

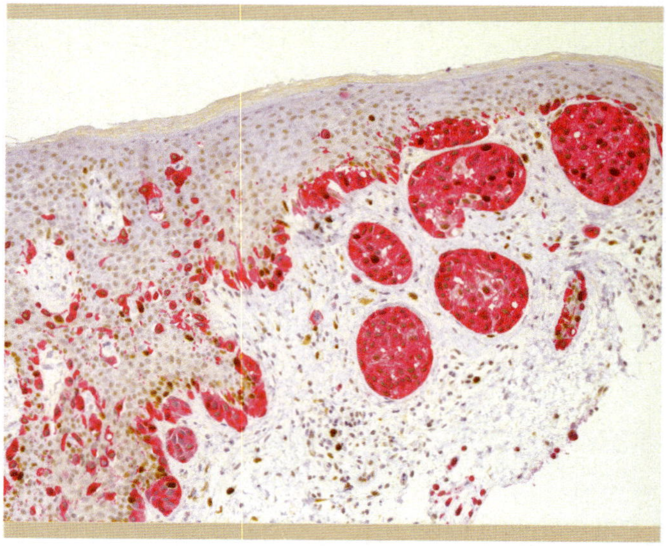

FIGURE 30-6 Pan-melanoma + Ki-67 double immunohistochemical stain in a case of melanoma (100x). The pan-melanoma component labels the cytoplasm of melanocytic cells pink/red. The brown Ki-67 component labels nuclei. Cells exhibiting both components are proliferative melanocytic cells.

- It will also be positive in the ducts of sebaceous carcinoma
- It is extremely useful to demonstrate EMPD but may not be as good for PD
- EMA (epithelial membrane antigen)
  - Positive in numerous tumors: EMPD, PD, adnexal neoplasms especially sebaceous neoplasms, perineuriomas, and focally positive in most SCC and in epithelioid sarcoma; also positive in plasma cells and some CD30 anaplastic large cell lymphomas
- GCDFP (gross cystic disease fluid protein)
  - Positive in PD, EMPD, and adnexal neoplasms; breast carcinomas are also labeled
- Adipophilin
  - Positive in sebaceous neoplasms, as it labels intracellular lipid microvesicles in a membranous pattern
- p63
  - Positive in SCC; also useful in distinguishing primary cutaneous adenocarcinoma (positive) from adenocarcinoma metastatic to the skin (expected to be negative)
- CD10
  - Positive in atypical fibroxanthoma (AFX); generally negative in SCC. Although sensitive for AFX, it has poor specificity
- D2-40
  - Antibody against podoplanin found on lymphatic endothelium. Positive in dermatofibroma, lymphangioma, Kaposi sarcoma

STUDIES FOR MESENCHYMAL TISSUE

- Actin antibodies (smooth muscle actin)
  - Useful in demonstrating leiomyoma/leiomyosarcoma, glomus tumors, and dermatofibroma
  - Cellular neurothekeoma will also exhibit positivity in 50% of cases
- Desmin
  - For leiomyoma/leiomyosarcoma, angiomyofibroblastoma
- CD34
  - Very useful for dermatofibrosarcoma protuberans (DFSP); it is positive in vascular tumors such as hemangioma, angiosarcoma, Kaposi sarcoma, and lymphangioma and is also positive in nearly half the cases of epithelioid sarcoma
- CD31
  - It is positive in vascular neoplasms: angiosarcoma, hemangioma, lymphangioma, Kaposi sarcoma; also positive in macrophages (which is a possible pitfall)

STUDIES FOR NEUROECTODERMAL LESIONS

- S-100
  - Not very specific but extremely sensitive for primary melanoma (including desmoplastic melanoma), metastatic melanoma, and nevi; also positive in a variety of other tumors such as breast carcinoma, Rosai-Dorfman disease, granular cell tumor, neurofibroma, schwannoma, myxoid neurothekeoma, chondroid syringoma, syringoma, and Langerhans cell histiocytosis
- S-100A6 is positive in cellular neurothekeomas and some melanocytic lesions
- MART-1 (melanoma antigen recognized by T cells): two main antibodies (M2 and A103)
  - Less sensitive and more specific than S-100 for melanocytic lesions; only a minority of cells in a proportion of desmoplastic melanoma label with this marker
- It is also positive in adrenocortical carcinoma and angiomyolipoma (among others), particularly the clone A103
- HMB45 and Ki-67
  - HMB45 is less sensitive and more specific than S-100 for melanocytic lesions; it reacts with gp100, a glycoprotein present in premelanosomes
  - Only a minority of cells in a proportion of desmoplastic melanoma label with this marker
  - This is a useful marker to demonstrate maturation in melanocytic lesions: that is, melanocytic cells in the dermis label at the top of benign melanocytic lesions but not at the bottom; in suspicious lesions, demonstration of maturation may be helpful in arguing against a diagnosis of melanoma
  - Ki-67 is an antigen present in all cells not in G_0 (resting) phase. The most common antibody is Mib-1
  - Regarding blue nevi versus spindle cell melanoma, the former are strongly, diffusely positive with HMB45; HMB45 is especially useful in this context when used together with Ki-67, a marker of proliferation
  - Melanocytic cells in the dermis that show maturation with HMB45 and show low proliferation (less than approximately 5% of cells reacting with Ki-67) are less likely to be melanoma
- Pan-melanoma + Ki-67
  - The pan-melanoma component stains melanocytes, and the Ki-67 antibody (Mib-1) is a surrogate marker for proliferation (see above). Therefore, a cell that shows cytoplasmic reactivity for pan-melanoma and nuclear staining for Ki-67 is a melanocytic cell that is proliferative. If numerous such cells (with both pan-melanoma and Ki-67 immunopositivity) are seen, then, taken together with the histologic features, the findings may point toward melanoma. The usefulness of this study derives from the fact that there are many K-67 positive cells such as lymphocytes, and by this method melanocytic cells that are Ki-67 positive are highlighted
- CK20 (see above)
- Synaptophysin and chromogranin
  - Both of these markers may be positive in Merkel cell carcinoma

- CD57
  - Labels a small proportion of cellular neurothekeoma and neurofibroma
- PGP9.5
  - It is positive in cellular neurothekeoma; it is not very specific, though, and is positive in many other tumors, including Merkel cell carcinoma and dermatofibroma
- NKI/C3
  - It is a macrophage marker positive in cellular neurothekeoma, but is not very specific
- MiTF
  - Nuclear stain that targets micropthalmia transcription factor expressed in melanocytes. Very sensitive and specific for melanoma, but not desmoplastic melanoma. Much cleaner staining pattern than MART-1, but can be positive in histiocytes
- SOX10
  - Nuclear transcription factor that is currently the most sensitive and specific marker for desmoplastic melanoma. Also highlights peripheral nerve and eccrine duct nuclei (Note: Remember MiTF and SOX10 from Waardenburg syndrome types II [deafness, no dystopia canthorum] and IV [Hirschsprung], respectively)

STUDIES FOR HEMATOPOEITIC LESIONS

- CD1a
  - Marker for Langerhans cells (and therefore useful in Langerhans cell histiocytosis)
- CD3
  - Marks T cells
- CD4
  - Marks T cells (T-helper cells), Langerhans cells, and macrophages; in mycosis fungoides, typically CD4 predominates over CD8
- CD5
  - Marks T cells; it is also positive in B cells in chronic lymphocytic leukemia (CLL) and mantle zone lymphoma. CLL lymphocytes would be expected to be CD5 and CD20 positive
- CD7
  - Marks T cells
  - It may be useful in MF in the following manner: it may not be present on epidermal lymphocytes that mark with CD4 and CD3, for example, suggesting loss of expression; however, inflammatory lesions may also exhibit this feature
- CD8
  - Marks T cells (T-cytotoxic/suppressor cells) (see CD4 above); hypopigmented mycosis fungoides more often shows CD8 predominance over CD4
- CD20 (Figs. 30-7 and 30-8)
  - Marks B cells; may be useful, along with CD3, kappa and lambda in showing that a lymphoid infiltrate in the skin is composed of heterogenous cells, and therefore likely to be reactive rather than neoplastic

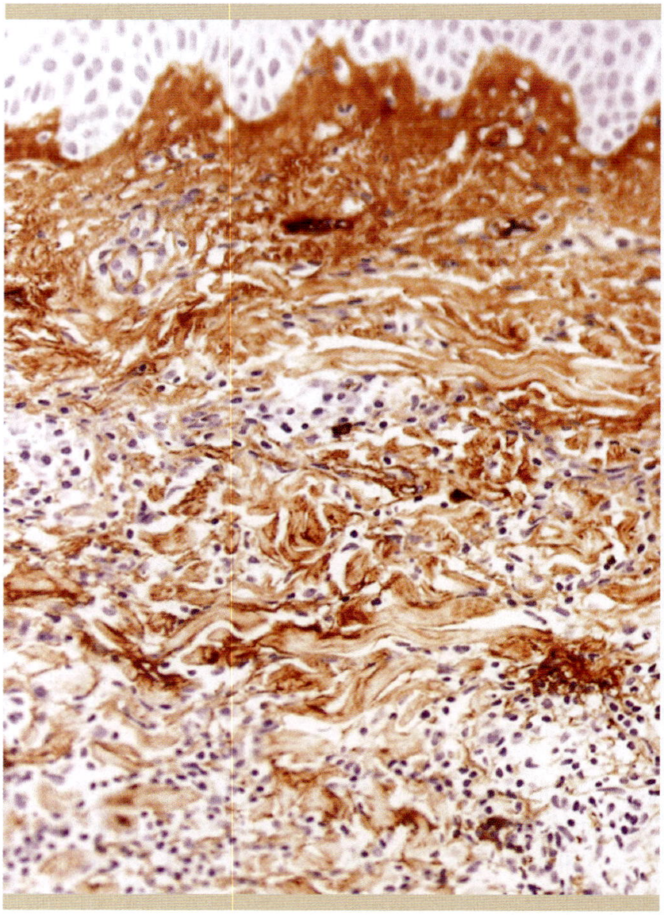

FIGURE 30-7 Kappa immunoreactivity in cutaneous marginal zone lymphoma (200x). The majority of the plasma cells were kappa positive and lambda negative.

- CD21
  - Marks B cells and follicular dendritic cells; positive in follicular dendritic cell sarcoma
- CD30
  - Marks activated T cells (among others)
  - It labels the majority of cells in anaplastic T-cell lymphoma (ALCL) (primary cutaneous ALCL shows less positivity for ALK-1 as compared to systemic ALCL; nevertheless, ALK-1 may be positive in a minority of primary cutaneous ALCL)
  - CD30 also labels large cells in lymphomatoid papulosis (types A and C; also, to a lesser extent, type B)
  - It is very rarely found in cutaneous B-cell lymphoma
- CD34
  - Helpful marker for leukemia cutis
- CD35
  - Marks follicular dendritic cells; positive in follicular dendritic cell sarcoma

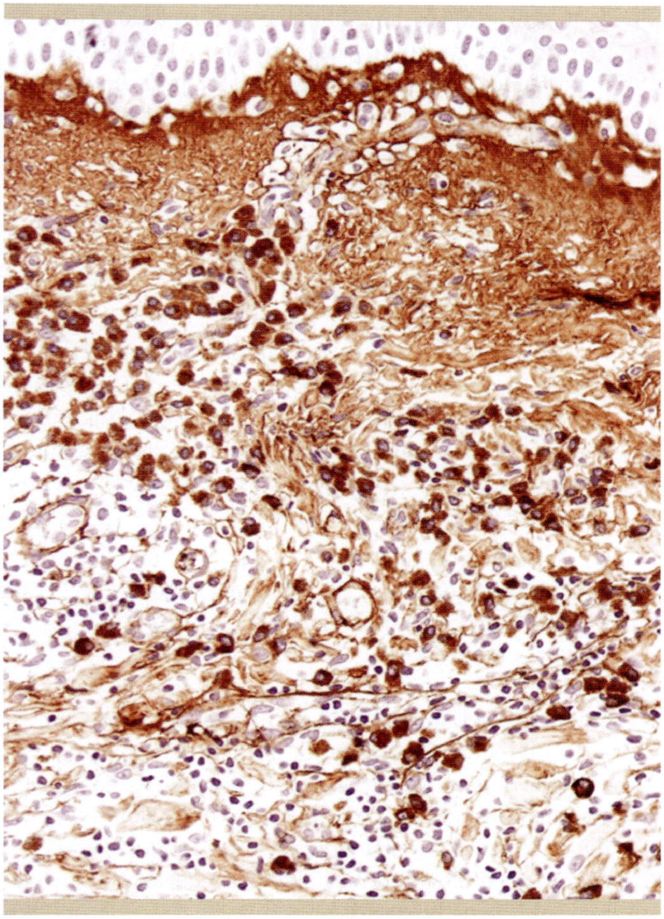

FIGURE 30-8 Lambda positive immnoreactivity. Only rare plasma cells are lambda positive in this case of marginal zone lymphoma (200x).

- CD45
  - Marks most hematopoeitic cells (ALCL may be negative)
- CD45RA
  - Labels naïve T cells
- CD45RO
  - Labels activated memory T cells
- CD56 (neuronal cell adhesion marker [NCAM])
  - Marker for NK cell lymphoma
  - Leukemic cells may be positive as well; also positive in neural neoplasms such as neurofibroma, myxoid neurothekeoma, and in desmoplastic melanoma
- CD57 (see above)
- Mast cell tryptase
  - Positive in mast cells
- CD117 (c-KIT)
  - A tyrosine kinase receptor for stem cell factor (SCF)
  - Labels mast cells, melanocytes; leukemic cells may also be positive for CD117
- CD207 (Langerin)
  - Positive in Langerhans cells (CD207/langerin is a component of Birbeck granules which are found in Langerhans cells)
- Myeloperoxidase (MPO)
  - Antibody to MPO may label leukemic cells; also labels neutrophils and monocytes (note that there is a histochemical stain for MPO as well, with similar usefulness)
- Kappa and lambda
  - Presence of light-chain restriction, that is, a plasmacytic infiltrate that is either kappa or lambda positive is seen in conditions such as myeloma and marginal zone lymphoma. Normally, a mixture of both with kappa predominance is expected
- Cytotoxic T-cell markers
  - These are granzyme B, TIA, and perforin. Lymphomas positive for these markers include subcutaneous T-cell lymphoma, primary cutaneous aggressive epidermotropic CD8-positive T-cell lymphoma, and cutaneous gamma/delta lymphoma
- β-F1
  - This is a marker for T-cell receptor (TCR) αβ, and is seen in subcutaneous panniculitic T-cell lymphoma (which would also be positive for CD8). In contrast cutaneous gamma/delta lymphoma is negative for β-F1 (and is negative for CD4 and CD8, but is positive for CD56)

STUDIES FOR INFECTIOUS DISEASES

The following is a list of useful antibodies:

- HHV-8: Kaposi sarcoma
- Spirochetal antibody: syphilis
- Herpes-simplex antibody: for demonstrating *Herpes simplex* virus
- Herpes-zoster (varicella-zoster) antibody: for demonstrating zoster

QUIZ

Questions

1. Biopsy of a lesion on the thigh of a 65-year-old man shows pagetoid cells in the epidermis. Immunohistochemical studies show these pagetoid cells to be positive for CK7 and CEA. Which of the following statements is untrue?

   A. The diagnosis is most likely extramammary Paget disease (EMPD)
   B. S-100 and Mart-1 stains are most likely to be positive
   C. Adipophilin is unlikely to be positive
   D. Another stain which might be helpful is Cam5.2

2. A biopsy shows large cells in sheets in the dermis. Immunohistochemical studies reveal that these are CD45, CD34, and myeloperoxidase (MPO) positive. The best diagnosis is:

   A. Leukemia cutis
   B. Cutaneous lymphoid hyperplasia
   C. Marginal zone lymphoma
   D. Chronic lymphocytic leukemia

3. Which of the following may be helpful in evaluating mucin?

   A. Antityrosinase antibody
   B. Antitryptase antibody
   C. Colloidal iron
   D. Fontana-Masson

4. A skin biopsy reveals "small blue cells." Immunohistochemical studies reveal the following profile: CK20—positive in a "dot-like" pattern; pan-cytokeratin—also positive, similar to CK20; TTF-1—negative. The diagnosis is:

   A. Merkel cell carcinoma
   B. B-cell lymphoma
   C. Poorly differentiated carcinoma
   D. Sebaceous carcinoma

5. You are suspecting a diagnosis of calciphylaxis. Which of the following stains may be helpful in evaluating a biopsy of the lesion?

   A. Prussian blue
   B. Von-Kossa
   C. Mucicarmine
   D. Alcian blue at pH 1.0

6. A 54-year-old patient presents with a 1.5 cm nodular lesion on his back. Biopsy shows a dense "top-heavy" lymphoid infiltrate with germinal centers. There are abundant plasma cells present. Immunohistochemical studies show the following: CD3—positive, sparing germinal centers; CD20—positive in germinal centers; kappa—positive; lambda—negative. The best diagnosis is:

   A. Marginal zone lymphoma
   B. Mantle cell lymphoma
   C. Secondary syphilis
   D. Lupus

7. Which of the following antibodies labels Langerhans cells?

   A. CD1a
   B. CD30
   C. CD8
   D. CD34

8. A 30-year-old African-American woman has hypopigmented patches on the trunk and elbows. You suspect hypopigmented mycosis fungoides and perform a biopsy. Which of the following combination of studies may be useful in this case?

   A. CD3, CD20, kappa, lambda
   B. CD45, CD30, CD34, CD117
   C. CD3, CD4, CD7, CD8
   D. CD1a, CD207, S-100, CD34

9. An upper eyelid lesion on frozen section reveals clear cells in the epidermis, with pagetoid spread. The histological differential diagnosis is melanoma in situ, sebaceous carcinoma and pagetoid squamous cell carcinoma in situ. An Oil red O stain is positive on a frozen section slide. The diagnosis is most likely:

   A. Melanoma in situ
   B. Pagetoid squamous cell carcinoma in situ
   C. Sebaceous carcinoma in situ
   D. None of the above

10. You biopsy a lesion of suspected Kaposi sarcoma, and write on the requisition form, "HIV patient, please rule out Kaposi". The pathologist reports a diagnosis of acroangiodermatitis. You call the pathologist to discuss the case, because you are pretty sure of your clinical diagnosis. Which of the following is a question that you may ask the pathologist?

    A. "Did you perform a Congo red stain?"
    B. "Did you perform a Leder stain?"
    C. "Did you do a CMV immuno study?"
    D. "Did you do an HHV-8 immuno study?"

Answers

1. B. In EMPD, CK7, CEA, and Cam5.2 should be positive. CK20 positivity is seen less frequently, but may be seen associated with underlying gastrointestinal malignancy. The CK7 and CEA immunopositivity indicates that this is EMPD. Therefore, S-100 and Mart-1 will be expected to be negative, since they would be positive in melanoma in situ. Adipophilin labels the lipid microvesicles in sebaceous cells, and therefore this too should be negative in this case.
2. A. Leukemic cells from acute myeloid leukemia may be positive for myeloperoxidase, CD34, CD117, and CD45 (leukocyte common antigen).
3. C. Colloidal iron stains mucin blue. Antibody to tyrosinase would be positive in melanocytic cells. Antitryptase antibody labels mast cells. Fontana-Masson stain is used for melanin.
4. A. Merkel cell carcinoma shows characteristic dot-like CK20 positivity, cytokeratin positivity, and is positive with Cam5.2 and CD56.

5. B. In order to demonstrate calcium (which may, on occasion, be difficult to find) a Von-Kossa stain would be helpful. Calcium salts are stained black.
6. A. Marginal zone lymphoma can be "top-heavy" infiltrate of lymphocytes in the dermis, with germinal centers and can therefore resemble cutaneous lymphoid hyperplasia. A clue to the diagnosis on H&E is the presence of plasma cells around the aggregates of lymphocytes. Immunohistochemical studies to show that the plasma cells are either kappa or lambda (known as "light chain restriction") are essential in arriving at the correct diagnosis.
7. A. Langerhans cells are CD1a, CD207, and S-100 positive. An important thing to remember is that S-100 positive intraepidermal cells are not always melanocytic cells—they may be Langerhans cells.
8. C. Hypopigmented mycosis fungoides is often CD8 positive and negative for CD4. Epidermotropic lymphocytic cells in the epidermis will therefore be expected to be CD8 and CD3 positive, and negative for CD4. CD7 immunoreactivity is often lost.
9. C. In cases of sebaceous carcinoma, a fat stain (such as an Oil red-O stain that gives fat a red-orange color) is very useful. It generally works in the frozen section setting, since the process of fixation leads to loss of fat.
10. D. In cases of Kaposi sarcoma, an HHV-8 immunohistochemical study would be expected to be positive. Severe stasis dermatitis (acroangiodermatitis) can histologically resemble Kaposi sarcoma, and so an HHV-8 study can be very useful in this setting.

REFERENCES

Carson FL, Hladik C: *Histotechnology. A Self-Instructional Text*, 3rd Ed. Chicago: ASCP Press; 2009.

Elder DE, Elenitsas R, Johnson BL Jr, Murphy GF, Xu X: *Lever's Histopathology of the Skin*, 10th Ed. Philadelphia: Lippincott Williams & Wilkins; 2008.

Smoller B: *Practical Immunopathology of the Skin*. Totowa, NJ: Humana Press; 2002.

Weedon D: *Weedon's Skin Pathology*, 3rd Ed. Churchill Livingstone: Elsevier; 2009.

CHAPTER 31

DERMOSCOPY

ROBERT H. JOHR

SYNONYMS

- Dermatoscopy
- Skin surface microscopy
- Epiluminescence microscopy (ELM)
- Digital dermoscopy/digital ELM
- Auflichtmikroscopie (German)
- Dermoscopia/dermatoscopia (Spanish)
- Dermoscopy and dermatoscopy are used interchangeably by experienced dermoscopists and in the literature

DEFINITION

- Dermoscopy is an in vivo, noninvasive technique in which oil or fluid (e.g., mineral oil, gels, alcohol, and water) is placed on the lesion
  - Fluid eliminates reflection of light from the surface of the skin allowing visualization of color and structure in the epidermis, dermoepidermal junction, and papillary dermis
  - The color and structure visualized cannot be seen with the naked eye or with typical magnification that clinicians use
  - Polarizing light and digital instrumentation do not require fluid
- When using polarized light dermoscopy
  - Light from a polarized light source penetrates the stratum corneum with less scatter
  - A second polarizer screens out scattered surface light resulting in the physician seeing primarily light from the deeper structures
  - This removes the need for contact with the skin and the need for immersion fluids, resulting in faster examination times
- There is noncontact and contact polarized dermoscopy
  - Gels can be used with contact polarized dermoscopy to enhance the appearance of vessels or eliminate the negative effects of dry skin
- There is contact nonpolarized dermoscopy
  - Some criteria can be better visualized with polarized dermoscopy such as small vessels, blue-white color, etc.
  - Some criteria can be better visualized with nonpolarized contact dermoscopy such as milia-like cysts seen in seborrheic keratosis and melanocytic lesions
  - Crystalline (a.k.a. shiny white structures) can only be seen with polarized dermoscopy
  - All the criteria needed to make a dermoscopic diagnosis can be made using any form of the technique

BENEFITS OF DERMOSCOPY

- Helps to differentiate melanocytic from nonmelanocytic skin lesions
- Helps to differentiate benign from malignant skin lesions
- With dermoscopy, the sensitivity to diagnose melanoma is 85% and better compared to 65 to 80% when the technique is not used
- Increases the diagnosis of early melanoma
  - Increases the diagnosis of amelanotic and hypomelanotic melanoma
- Increases the diagnosis of melanoma incognito (false negative melanoma)
- Increases the diagnosis of inflammatory lesions (i.e., lichen planus, psoriasis, seborrheic dermatitis)
- Increases the diagnosis of infestations (i.e., scabies, head and crab lice)
- Increases the diagnosis of hair shaft pathology (i.e., monilethrix, trichorrhexis invaginata)
- Helps to avoid unnecessary surgery
- Helps to plan surgery
- Helps to work better with a pathologist (asymmetrical high-risk criteria, dermoscopic–pathologic correlation)
- Patient reassurance
- Allows for follow-up of patients with multiple nevi digitally to find changes over time

DERMOSCOPIC DIGITAL MONITORING

- There are pigmented skin lesions that are not high risk enough to warrant immediate histopathologic diagnosis, yet not so banal that there is no concern at all
- There are melanomas that do not appear to be high risk clinically or with dermoscopy
- They are only diagnosed after monitoring for dermoscopic changes over time when comparing baseline with subsequent digital images
- Short-term monitoring is performed every 3 or 4 months
    - Any change over time could be a melanoma
- Long-term monitoring is done at 6-month to yearly intervals
    - Important changes include asymmetrical enlargement, the appearance of high-risk criteria, new colors, or regression
- Single or multiple suspicious pigmented skin lesions can be chosen for digital monitoring

THE 2-STEP ALGORITHM

- The analysis of a suspicious skin lesion is a 2-step process
    - Step one: determine if it is melanocytic or nonmelanocytic
    - Step two: if it has the criteria for a melanocytic lesion, the second step is to determine if it is low, intermediate, or high risk using the melanocytic algorithm of your choice
- Pattern analysis was the first melanocytic algorithm developed for this purpose and is most often used by experienced dermoscopists. Variations of pattern analysis have also been developed, including
    - The ABCD rule of dermatoscopy (Table 31-1)
    - Menzies method (11-point checklist) (Table 31-2)
    - The 7-point checklist (Table 31-3)
    - The 3-point checklist (Table 31-4)

Step One: Identification of Criteria

Look for the criteria associated with a melanocytic lesion. If one does not find them, the search is on for the criteria associated with seborrheic keratosis, basal cell carcinoma, dermatofibromas, vascular lesions, and others (Table 31-5)

- Not all of the possible criteria are needed to make a diagnosis
- When there is absence of criteria for a melanocytic lesion, seborrheic keratosis, basal cell carcinoma, dermatofibroma, or vascular lesion, you are now dealing with a melanocytic lesion by default
- The "default category" is the last criterion used to diagnose a melanocytic lesion (Fig. 31-1)

TABLE 31-1 ABCD Rule of Dermatoscopy: Identify Criteria and Assign Points to Determine Total Dermatoscopy Score (TDS)

Dermoscopic Criterion Definition Score Weight Factor
*A*symmetry: In 0, 1, or 2 perpendicular axes; assess contour, colors, and structures 0–2 *B*order: Abrupt ending of pigment pattern at periphery in 0–8 segments 0–8 *C*olor: Presence of up to 6 colors (white, red, light brown, dark brown, blue-gray, and black) 1–6 *D*ermoscopic structures: Presence of network, structureless (homogeneous) areas, branched streaks, dots, and globules 1–5 Formula for calculating TDS: (A score × 1.3) + (B score × 0.1) + (C score × 0.5) + (D score × 0.5) = TDS. Interpretation of total score: <4.75. Benign melanocytic lesion 4.75–5.45; suspect lesion (close follow-up or excision recommended); >5.45, lesion highly suspect for melanoma

CRITERIA DEFINED

- Melanocytic lesion
    - *Pigment network/network/reticulation*
        - On the trunk and extremities
        - Shades of black or brown

TABLE 31-2 Menzies Scoring Method: 11-Point Check List

Dermoscopic Criteria
1. Symmetry of pattern (negative feature)
2. Presence of single color (negative feature)
Positive Features
3. Blue-white veil (color)
4. Multiple brown dots
5. Pseudopods (streaks)
6. Radial streaming (streaks)
7. Scar-like depigmentation
8. Peripheral black dots/globules
9. Multiple (5 or 6) colors
10. Multiple blue/gray dots
11. Broadened network (irregular pigment network)

For melanoma to be diagnosed, both negative features must be absent and 1 or more of the 9 positive features must be present.

TABLE 31-3 7-Point Checklist

Dermoscopic Criteria	Scores
1. Irregular pigment network (**major criteria**)	2
2. Blue-whitish veil (color)	2
3. Polymorphous vascular pattern	2
4. Irregular streaks (**minor criteria**)	1
5. Irregular dots/globules	1
6. Irregular blotches	1
7. Regression	1

By simple addition of the individual scores a minimum total score of 3 is required for the diagnosis of melanoma, whereas a total score of less than 3 is indicated of nonmelanoma.

- Honeycomb-like, reticular, web-like line segments (elongated and hyperpigmented rete ridges) with hypopigmented holes (dermal papilla)

- *Pseudonetwork/Pseudopigment network*
  - Because the skin of the head and neck is thin and does not have well-developed rete ridges, one sees
    - ▲ Appendageal openings/adnexal structures (sebaceous glands, hair follicles)
    - ▲ Uniform, round white or yellowish structures
  - When they penetrate areas of diffuse pigmentation, reticular-like structures are formed that is referred to as the pseudonetwork
  - Gray pseudonetwork associated with benign (i.e., lichen planus–like keratosis) and malignant pathology (i.e., melanoma) can be seen on the face, nose, and ears
  - Monomorphous appendageal openings can often be seen on the skin of the face without any pigmentation
  - They should not be confused with the milia-like cysts seen in seborrheic keratosis
  - It is not always possible to make the differentiation

TABLE 31-4 3-Point Checklist to Diagnose High-Risk Lesions (Melanoma, Basal Cells)

1. Asymmetry of color and/or structure
2. Irregular pigment network
3. Blue and/or white color
2 out 3, 3 out 3 → Excise

The 3-point checklist is based on simplified pattern analysis and is intended to be used by nonexpert dermoscopists as a screening technique. Its aim is to diagnose melanocytic and nonmelanoctyic potentially malignant pathology.

TABLE 31-5 Criteria for Various Lesions

Criteria for a melanocytic lesion	Pigment network (trunk and extremities) Aggregated brown globules Homogeneous blue color (blue nevus) Parallel patterns on acral sites By default (when there is an absence of criteria for a melanocytic lesion, seborrheic keratosis, basal cell carcinoma, hemangioma, or dermatofibroma, the lesion should be considered melanocytic by default)
Criteria for a seborrheic keratosis	Milia-like cysts Pseudofollicular openings Fissures/furrows and ridges Fat fingers Hairpin vessels Sharp demarcation
Criteria for a basal cell carcinoma	Absence of of pigment network Arborizing blood vessels Pigmentation Ulceration Spoke-wheel structures
Criteria for a dermatofibroma	Central white patch Peripheral pigment network
Criterion for a vascular lesion	Vascular spaces called lacunae

  - Consequences could be misdiagnosing lentigo maligna for a seborrheic keratosis
  - This criterion can be seen with nonmelanocytic lesions (i.e., solar lentigo, lichen planus–like keratosis)
  - It is not diagnostic of a melanocytic lesion

- *Dots and Globules*
  - Roundish structures distinguished only by their relative sizes
  - Dots (0.1 mm) are smaller than globules (>0.1 mm)
  - Black, brown, gray, or red
    - ▲ When black, they can represent atypical melanocytes in the epidermis or transepidermal elimination of pigment
    - ▲ Regular brown dots and globules represent nests of melanocytes at the dermoepidermal junction
    - ▲ Irregular brown dots and globules represent nests of atypical melanocytes at the dermoepidermal junction

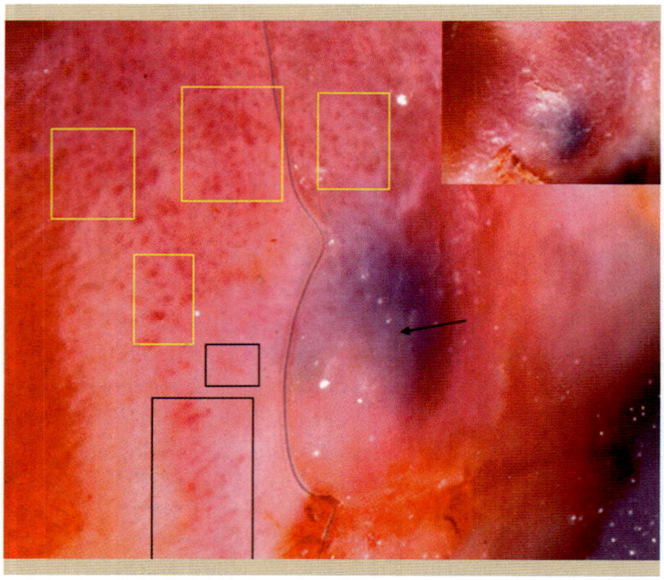

FIGURE 31-1 Amelanotic melanoma. This is a melanocytic lesion by default because there is an absence of criteria for a melanocytic lesion, seborrheic keratosis, basal cell carcinoma, dermatofibroma, or hemangioma. The blue-white color (arrow) is a clue that this might be a melanocytic lesion. There are pinpoint/dotted (yellow boxes) and irregular linear (black boxes) vessels plus a general milky red background color. Note: This interdigital melanoma was mistakingly treated as a tinea for 2 years.

  - ▲ Grayish dots ("peppering") represent free melanin and/or melanophages in the papillary dermis, which can be seen in regression or alone in benign pathology such as late stage lichen planus–like keratosis or posttraumatic
  - ▲ Reddish globules (milky red globules) can be seen in melanoma (neovascularization)
- – It is written and taught that aggregated brown globules identify a melanocytic lesion with no mention of the smaller dots. The reality is that both dots and globules define a melanocytic lesion (Fig. 31-2)

- *Homogeneous blue pigmentation*
  - – Structureless blue color in the absence of local criteria such as pigment network, dots or globules (Fig. 31-3)
  - – Different shades of homogeneous blue color usually represents a blue nevus
  - – The history is important because there is a differential diagnosis which could include
    - ▲ A lesion as banal as a radiation tattoo to one more ominous such as nodular or cutaneous metastatic melanoma
- *Parallel patterns/acral patterns/palms and soles*
  - – Fissures/furrows and ridges on the skin of the palms and soles (dermoglyphics)

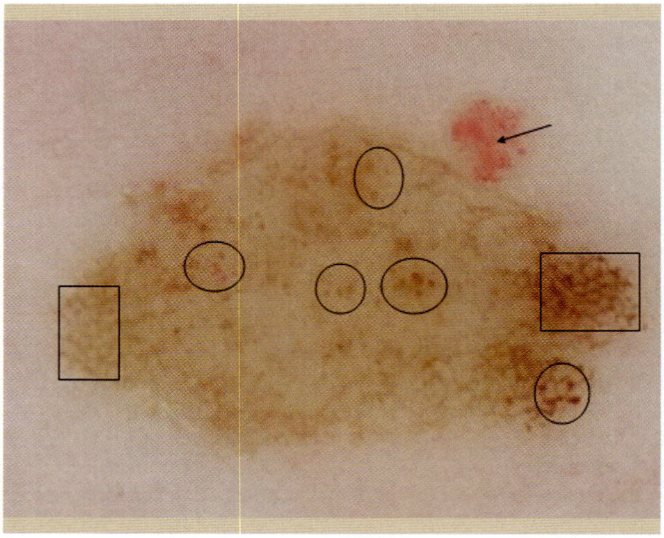

FIGURE 31-2 Acquired nevus. This is a melanoctic lesion because it has pigment network (black boxes) and aggregated brown globules (circles). There is a small hemangioma adjacent to the nevus (arrow).

  - – Can create parallel patterns
    - ▲ Parallel lines can also be seen on all nonglabrous skin/mucosal surfaces (i.e., lips, genitalia)
- *Parallel-furrow pattern (benign pattern)*
  - – Thin brown parallel lines in the furrows of the skin (crista superficialis limitans)
  - – Variations include 2 thin lines with or with out dots and globules (Fig. 31-4)
- *Lattice-like pattern (benign pattern)*
  - – Thin brown parallel lines in the furrows
  - – Thin brown parallel lines running perpendicular to the furrows forming a ladder-like picture (Fig. 31-5)

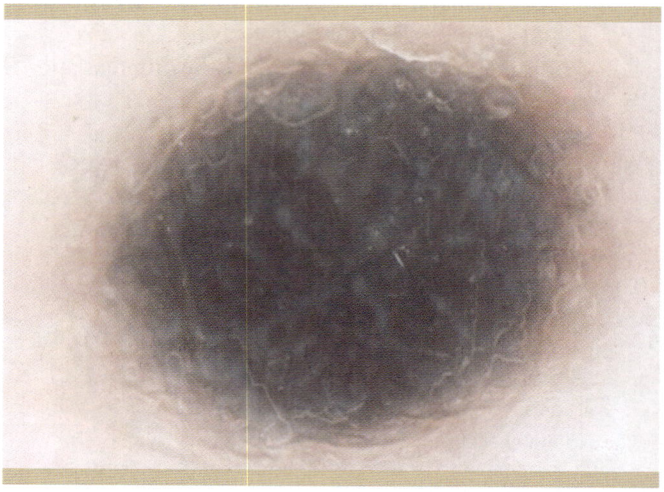

FIGURE 31-3 Blue nevus. The classic homogenous blue color of a blue nevus.

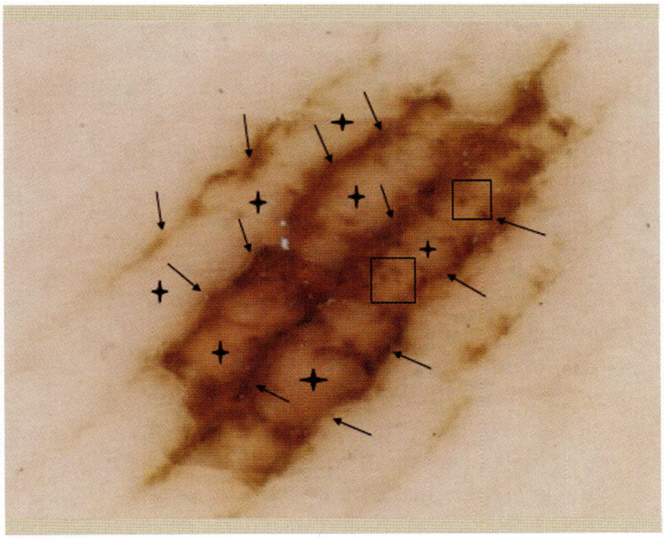

FIGURE 31-4 Acral nevus. This is a melanocytic lesion on acral skin with the benign parallel-furrow pattern. Pigmentation is in the thin furrows (arrows) with globules (boxes) in the ridges (stars).

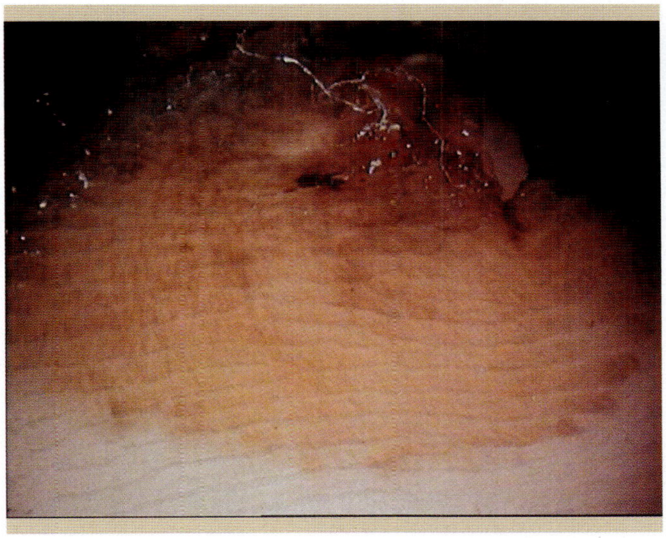

FIGURE 31-6 Acral melanoma. The parallel-ridge pattern diagnoses this acral melanoma with pigmentation in the thicker light brown ridges. The thin white lines are the furrows.

- *Fibrillar pattern (benign pattern)*
  - Fine brown lines
  - Run in an oblique (/////) direction
  - Pressure can change the lattice-like pattern into a fibrillar pattern
- *Globular pattern (benign)*
  - Brown globules without a parallel component
- *Reticular pattern (benign)*
  - A lesion with only pigment network
- *Homogeneous pattern (benign)*
  - Brown homogeneous color

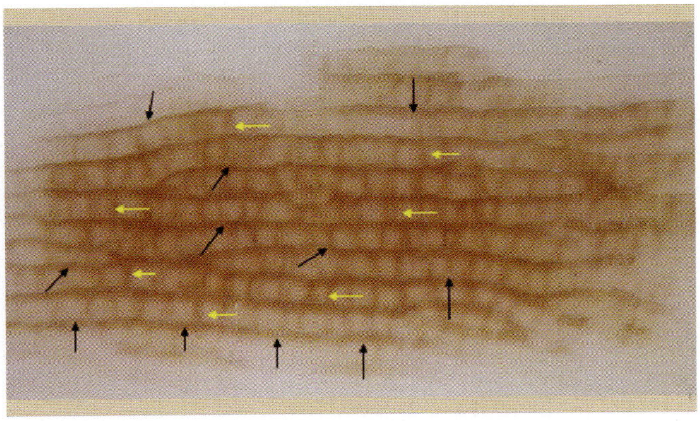

FIGURE 31-5 Acral nevus. Brown lines in the furrows (black arrows) and perpendicular to the furrows (yellow arrows) characterize the lattice-like pattern. Pressure on the foot can change this into the fibrillar pattern with fine oblique (/////) lines.

- *Parallel-ridge pattern (thin/early melanoma)*
  - Pigmentation is in the thicker ridges of the skin (crista profunda intermedia) (Fig. 31-6)
  - Sometimes there are monomorphous round white structures in the ridges that represent the acrosyringia of the sweat ducts "string of pearls"
  - The acrosyringia are always in the ridges
  - An important landmark when one has to determine if pigmentation is in the furrows or ridges. Benign (furrows) vs. malignant(ridges) pathology
  - Foci of the parallel-ridge pattern can be seen in more advanced acral melanomas with a multicomponent global pattern and melanoma-specific criteria (i.e., regression, irregular blotches, blue color, polymorphous vessels)
  - Parallel-ridge pattern created by blood (talon noir, black heel) (Fig. 31-7)
  - Parallel-ridge pattern in darker skinned races (Fig. 31-8)
  - Macules seen in the Peutz-Jeghers syndrome
  - This pattern is not 100% diagnostic of melanoma
- *Diffuse variegate pattern (melanoma)*
  - Irregular pigmented dark blotches
  - Black, brown, or gray
- *Multicomponent pattern (melanoma)*
  - Filled with regular and irregular criteria
  - Multiple colors plus areas with acral benign patterns (fibrillar, parallel-furrow)
- *Nonspecific pattern (melanoma)*
  - If one cannot determine any of the above benign or malignant patterns, this represents a "red flag" of concern

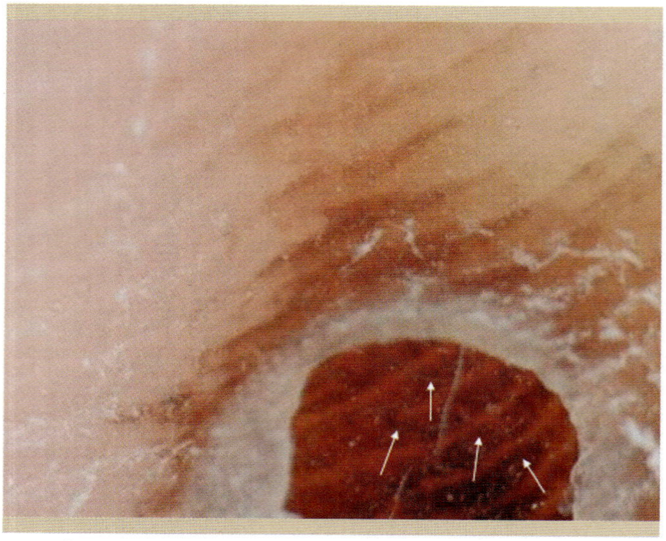

FIGURE 31-7 Acral hemorrhage. The parallel-ridge pattern created by blood (white arrows).

Pearls

- There can be exceptions to every dermoscopic rule
- The history and clinical appearance of a lesion are important and should not be ignored
- Negative "gut" feelings should not be ignored
- If an acral lesion is rapidly changing yet has a benign appearance, it still could be melanoma

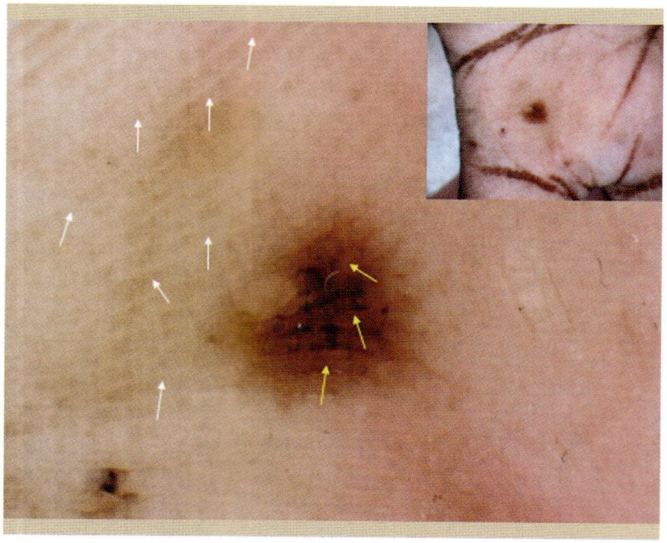

FIGURE 31-8 Acquired nevus. There is an increased incidence of acral melanoma in darker skinned races. This nevus on the palm of an African-American was without change and demonstrates the benign parallel-ridge pattern. Pigmentation is seen in the ridges of the nevus (yellow arrows) and in the ridges of the entire palm (white arrows).

- A supposedly benign acral pattern with irregularity of some components could be high risk
- The presence of blood at acral sites (palms, soles, nails) can be associated with melanoma
- Look carefully for other high-risk criteria when blood is seen
- If in doubt, cut it out!

- ***Seborrheic keratosis***
  - *Milia-like cysts*
    - Variously sized white or yellow structures
    - Small or large, single or multiple
    - They can appear opaque or bright-like "stars in the sky" (epidermal horn cysts)
  - *Pseudofollicular openings/comedo-like openings*
    - Sharply demarcated roundish structures
    - Pigmented or nonpigmented
    - Shapes can vary, not only within a single lesion, but from lesion to lesion in an individual patient
    - When pigmented, they can be brownish yellow or even dark brown and black (oxidized keratin-filled invaginations of the epidermis)
    - Pigmented pseudofollicular openings can be hard to differentiate from the pigmented dots and globules of a melanocytic lesion (see Fig. 31-9)
  - *Fissures and ridges*
    - Fissures (sulci) and ridges (gyri) seen in seborrheic keratosis can create several patterns

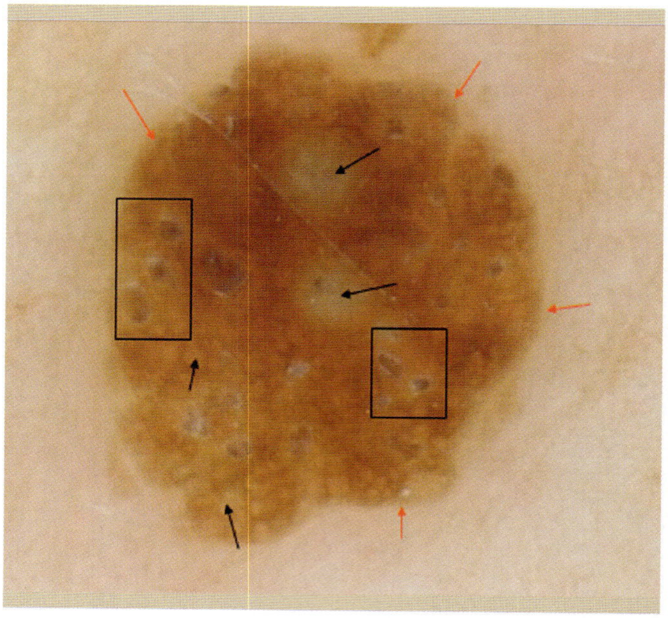

FIGURE 31-9 Seborrheic keratosis. Sharp borders (red arrows) milia-like cysts (black arrows) and pseudofollicular openings (boxes) characterize this seborrheic keratosis.

- Large irregularly shaped keratin-filled fissures are called crypts
  - ▲ Fissures and ridges can also be seen in papillomatous melanocytic lesions
  - ▲ Cerebriform or brain-like in which they resemble a saggital section through the cerebral cortex
  - ▲ Mountain-like with variously sized or uniformly roundish structures representing mountains (ridges) and fine pigmented lines representing valleys (fissures)
    - △ Possible to confuse the mountain and valley pattern with the globular or cobblestone pattern of a melanocytic lesion
  - ▲ Pigmented lines should not be confused with an irregular pigment network
  - ▲ Hypo- and hyperpigmented ridges can be digit-like (straight, kinked, circular, or branched) and are referred to as "fat fingers"
  - ▲ "Fat fingers" might be the only clue that a lesion could be a seborrheic keratosis
- All these patterns are commonly seen in this ubiquitous most commonly encountered benign skin lesion (Fig. 31-10)

• *Fingerprint pattern*
  - Brown fine/thin parallel line segments that resemble fingerprints
    - ▲ The lines can be arched, swirled, or look like branched fungal hyphae
    - ▲ The lines can fill the lesion or be broken up

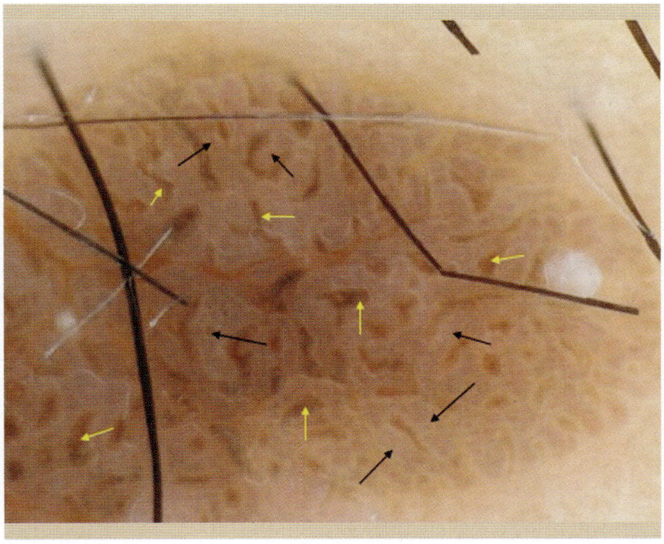

FIGURE 31-10 Seborrheic keratosis. A striking brain-like pattern created by pigmented fissures (yellow arrows) and light ridges (black arrows). Many of the ridges look like "fat fingers."

  - Differ from the pigment network where the line segments are honeycomb-like or reticular
    - ▲ Network-like structures/ pseudonetwork can be seen in seborrheic keratosis created by fissures and ridges not elongated and hyperpigmented rete ridges of the true pigment network
  - Fingerprint pattern can be seen in flat seborrheic keratosis or in solar lentigines
  - Some authors believe that solar lentigines are flat seborrheic keratosis (see below and Fig. 31-23)

• *Hairpin vessels*
  - Elongated vessels (capillary loops) resembling hairpins (Fig. 31-11)
  - May or may not be surrounded by hypopigmented halos
  - Light halo indicates a keratinizing tumor and may be found in keratoacanthomas
  - Irregular and thick hairpin vessels can be seen in melanoma

• *Moth-eaten borders*
  - Flat or slightly raised brown seborrheic keratoses and solar lentigines
  - Well-demarcated, concave borders that are felt to resemble a "moth-eaten" garment

• *Sharp demarcation*
  - The majority of seborrheic keratoses have sharp, well-demarcated borders
  - Not always indicative of melanoma in a pigmented lesion (Fig. 31-9)

• **Basal cell carcinoma**

• *Absence of a pigment network*

• *Arborizing vessels*
  - One of the most sensitive and specific vascular structures seen with dermoscopy

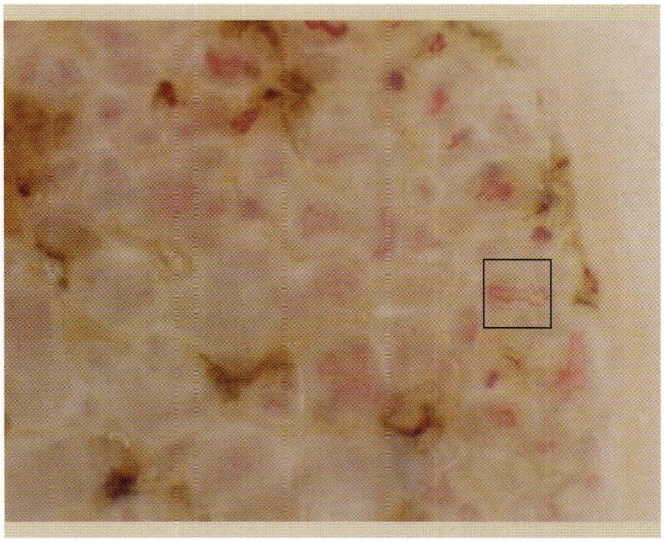

FIGURE 31-11 Seborrheic keratosis. An especially well-formed hairpin vessel in a seborrheic keratosis (black box).

- Not all basal cell carcinomas contain arborizing vessels
  - ▲ Red tree-like branching telangiectatic blood vessels
  - ▲ Can be thick or thin lines that are in focus because of their superficial location
- Out-of-focus arborizing vessels are a clue that the lesion might be a melanoma
  - ▲ Most often, there are different caliber vessels in a single lesion
- Can also be found in
  - ▲ Benign nevi
  - ▲ Sebaceous gland hyperplasia
  - ▲ Scars
  - ▲ On sun-damaged skin
  - ▲ Melanoma
  - ▲ Merkel cell carcinoma

• ***Pigmentation***
- Basal cell carcinoma may or may not contain pigment (pigmented nests or island of basal cell carcinoma in the dermis) that can range from
  - ▲ Fine dots to large leaf-like structures (bulbous extensions forming a leaf-like pattern)
  - ▲ Blue-gray ovoid nets
  - ▲ Multiple blue-gray dots and globules
  - ▲ Colors that can be seen
    - △ Black
    - △ Brown
    - △ Gray
    - △ Blue
    - △ Red
    - △ White
- Not necessary to try to determine if "leaf-like" structures ("maple leaf–like areas") are present because in reality this is a difficult task (Fig. 31-12)

• *Ulceration*
- Single or multiple areas where there is loss of epidermis with oozing blood or congealed blood and crusts (Fig. 31-13)
- Mutifocal ulceration is associated with superficial basal cell carcinomas
- There should be no recent history of trauma

• *Spoke-wheel structures*
  - ▲ Can be found in up to 10% of basal cell carcinomas
- Diagnostic of basal cell carcinoma
  - ▲ May or may not be associated with the other criteria used to make the diagnosis
- Well-defined pigmented radial projections meeting at a darker central globule/central axle/hub
- Complete or incomplete variations of this structure can be seen and one often has to use their imagination to make the identification
- Streak-like structures referred to as pseudostreaks represent incomplete spoke-wheel structures and could be confused with true steaks of a melanocytic lesion

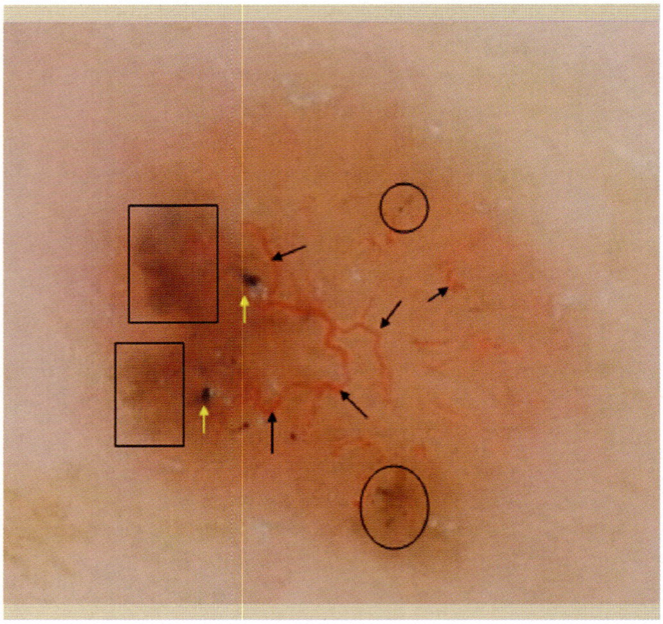

FIGURE 31-12 Basal cell carcinoma. This pigmented basal cell carcinoma has classic arborizing vessels (black arrows), gray blotches (boxes), blue globules (yellow arrows), and fine gray dots (circles). The 3 different presentations of pigmentation point out how variable this criterion can be.

- Finding spoke-wheel structures might be the only clue to the correct diagnosis

Pearl

At times, one cannot differentiate melanoma from basal cell carcinoma. If there is pigment network in any form, then it cannot be a basal cell carcinoma.

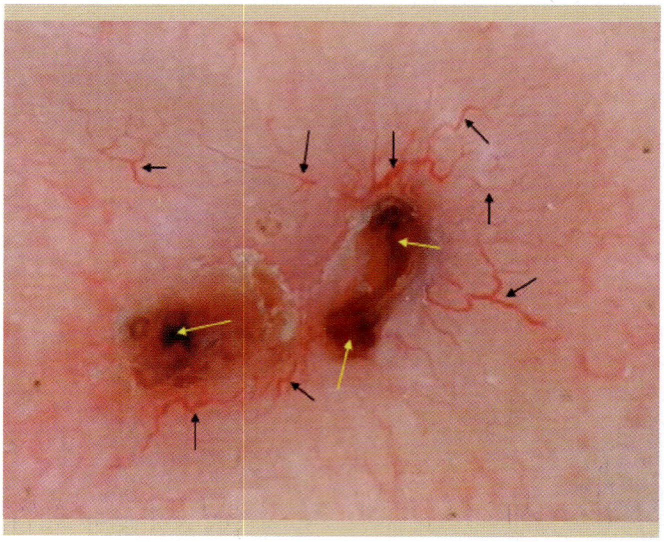

FIGURE 31-13 Basal cell carcinoma. Arborizing vessels (black arrows) and ulceration (yellow arrows) characterize this nonpigmented basal cell carcinoma.

- Dermatofibroma
  - *Central white patch*
    - Most typical presentation of this criterion is
      - ▲ Centrally located
      - ▲ Scar-like
      - ▲ Bony or milky white
      - ▲ Homogeneous area (scarring in this fibrohistiocytic tumor)
    - Several variations such as white network–like structures (negative pigment network, reticular depigmentation) which can also be seen in Spitz nevi and melanoma
    - Telangiectatic vessels (i.e., pinpoint vessels) with different shapes can also be found anywhere in the lesion
    - Not all dermatofibromas have a central white patch
    - The clinically firm feel should be used to help make the diagnosis
  - *Pigment network*
    - Dermatofibromas are one of the nonmelanocytic lesions that can have a pigment network; solar lentigines are another
      - ▲ In most cases, a fine peripheral pigment network with thin brown lines is seen
      - ▲ Ring-like structures which are a variation of a pigment network (Fig. 31-14)
      - ▲ Not all dermatofibromas have a pigment network
    - Atypical dermatofibromas with the following features are melanoma simulators that warrant a histopathologic diagnosis

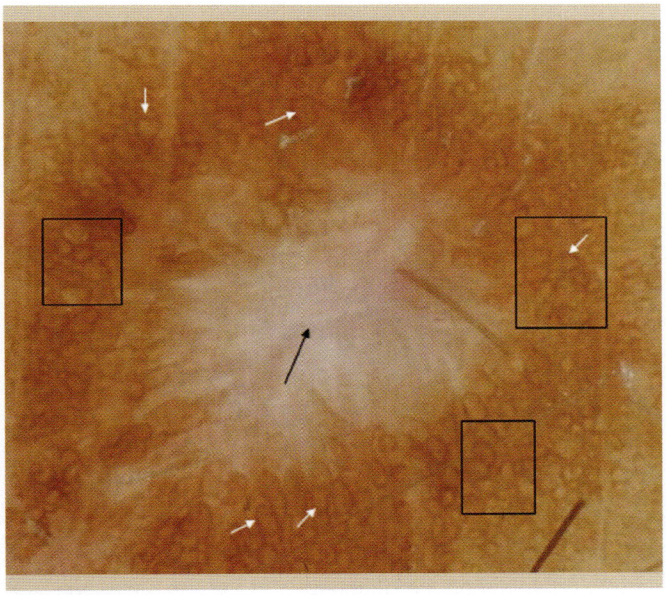

FIGURE 31-14 Dermatofibroma. A classic central white patch (black arrow) and pigment network (black boxes) characterize this dermatofibroma. In this instance, ring-like structures (white arrows) make up the pigment network.

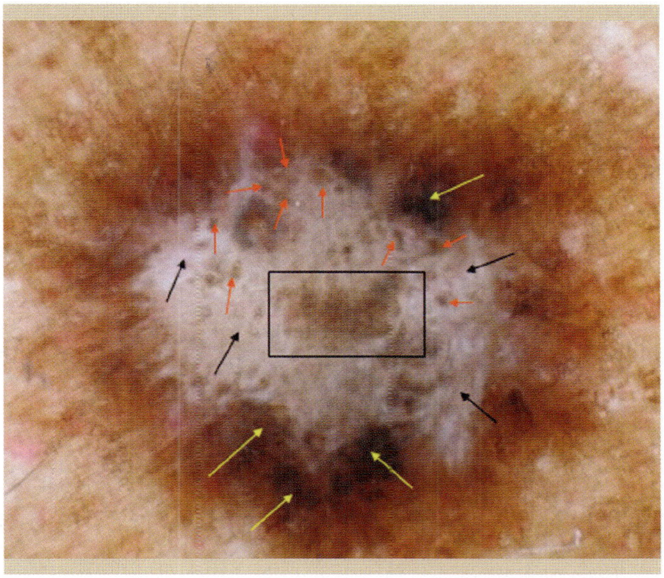

FIGURE 31-15 Atypical dermatofibroma. Regressive melanoma is in the dermoscopic differential diagnoses of this atypical dermatofibroma. There is asymmetry of color and structure, the multicomponent global pattern, irregular pigment network (box), irregular globules (red arrows) and irregular blotches (yellow arrows). This warrants a histopathologic diagnosis.

      - ▲ Irregular pigment network
      - ▲ Irregular dots/globules/ dark blotches
      - ▲ Pink color
      - ▲ Irregular regression–like white color
      - ▲ High-risk vascular structures/polymorphous vessels with different shapes (Fig. 31-15)
- Vascular lesions
  - ***Lacunae/lagoons/saccules***
    - Sharply demarcated bright red to bluish round or oval structures (dilated vascular spaces in the dermis) (Fig. 31-16)
      - ▲ Different colors can be seen in a single hemangioma
      - ▲ The deeper the vessels, the darker the color (dark blue)
      - ▲ Lacunae should not be mistaken for the milky red globules seen in pigmented and amelanotic melanoma which can have "out-of-focus" reddish globular-like structures
      - ▲ Black homogeneous structureless areas represent thrombosis
      - ▲ Significant scale or dryness (hyperkeratosis) can be seen in angiokeratomas
    - Patchy white color or blue-white veil (blue and/or white color) is commonly seen in hemangiomas
    - Linear white lines can fill the lesion and represent fibrous septae

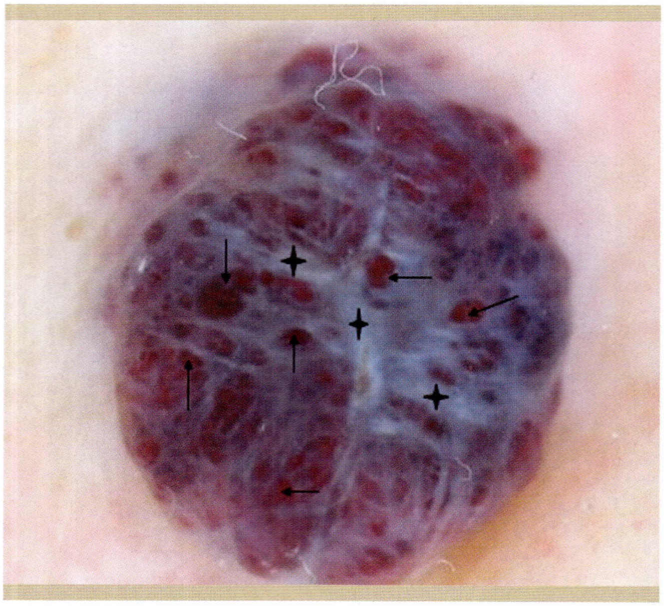

FIGURE 31-16 Hemangioma. Well-demarcated dark red lacunae (arrows) and blue-white color (stars) characterize this classic hemangioma. The linear blue-white color represents fibrous septae.

- Blue and/or white color or fibrous septae should not be mistaken for regression found in melanomas
- Cutaneous metastatic melanoma can be indistinguishable from a hemangioma
  - ▲ A history of a previous melanoma will help make the diagnosis (Fig. 31-17)

Pearl

- There is a significant learning curve with dermoscopy. It is essential to learn the definitions of the criteria and patterns and be able to recognize the classic examples because there are innumerable variations that one will see in daily practice. This is the weak link in the chain for those who attempt to master this tissue-sparing life-saving technique. One cannot learn dermoscopy by osmosis and one cannot see what one does not know.

STEP TWO: Analysis of a Melanocytic Lesion

Pattern Analysis Defined

Identify as many criteria in the lesion as possible and see if they fit into the known patterns associated with the variants of

- Melanocytic nevi
  - Congenital
  - Acquired
  - Recurrent
  - Halo
  - Combined
  - Blue
  - Dysplastic
  - Spitz
- Melanoma
  - In situ
  - Superficial spreading
  - Nodular
  - Hypo and amelanotic
  - Nail apparatus
  - Acral
- Even though pattern analysis is considered a melanocytic algorithm, the same principles are used to diagnose all the lesions that can be identified with the technique
  - Melanocytic
  - Nonmelanocytic
  - Benign
  - Malignant
  - Inflammatory

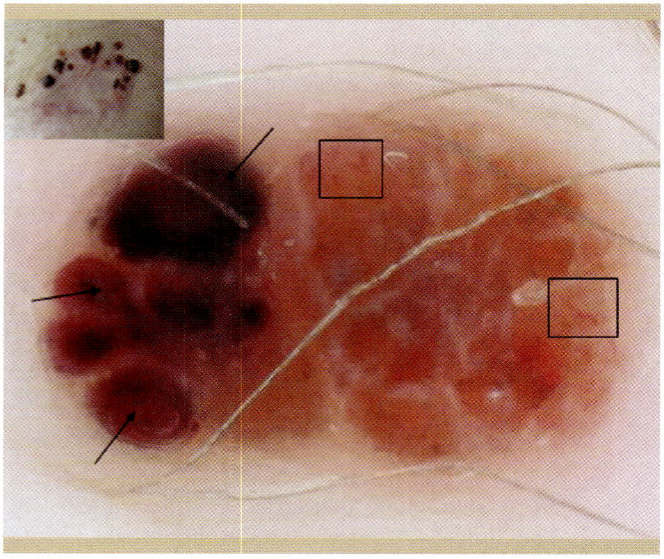

FIGURE 31-17 Cutaneous metastatic melanoma. This is one of many generalized cutaneous metastatic lesions in a 27-year-old white man with a history of a 7-mm melanoma on his back. There are well-demarcated lacunae-like areas (arrows) and irregular vessels (boxes). Milky red color fills most of the lesion. A collision tumor, hemangioma, and amelanotic melanoma are in the dermoscopic differential diagnosis.

Pearls

- Do not focus on 1 or 2 criteria and make a diagnosis before checking for all the criteria. You could be lead astray.
- Try to identify all of the criteria in a lesion.
- High-risk criteria that are present are not always easy to find. Beware!

Pattern Analysis Method

- *Step #1*
  - Determine symmetry or asymmetry of color and/or structure using the mirror image technique
    - Contour of the lesion is not important with this algorithm
    - The lesion is bisected by 2 lines that are placed 90 degrees to each other
    - The lines should attempt to create the most symmetry as possible and should be visualized with that point in mind
    - Is the color and/or the structure on the left half of the lesion a mirror image of the right half
  - Repeat the analysis for the upper and lower half of the lesion
  - Perfect symmetry of color and structure is not often found in nature, and inter-observer agreement is not good with this assessment even among experienced dermoscopists
  - Symmetry or asymmetry can also be determined along any axis through the center of the lesion
  - Significant asymmetry of color and/or structure is a very important clue that you might be dealing with high-risk pathology
  - Raise a "red flag" of concern and proceed with focused attention to what else you might find
- *Step #2*
  - Determine the global/overall pattern of the lesion. The predominant criteria seen throughout the lesion could be
    - Reticular
    - Globular
    - Cobblestone
    - Homogeneous
    - Parallel
    - Starburst
    - Multicomponent
    - Nonspecific
    - There can be combinations of criteria in a single lesion such as reticular and homogeneous or reticular and globular
    - The "reticular homogeneous pattern" or "reticular globular pattern"
- *Step #3*
  - Identify the local criteria in the lesion
    - Pigment network
    - Dots and globules
    - Streaks (also called pseudopods and radial streaming)
    - Blotches
    - Blue-white veil
    - Regression
    - Colors
    - Vascular structures
- *Step #4*
  - Determine if the criteria seen are:
    - Regular or irregular
    - Good or bad
    - Low, intermediate, or high risk
  - Melanoma-specific criteria are defined as criteria that can be seen in benign and malignant lesions but are more specific for high-risk pathology such as
    - Dysplastic nevi
    - Spitzoid lesions
    - Melanoma
  - All of the high-risk criteria can be seen in benign pathology and one should never tell a patient that they have melanoma 100%
  - Due to the different characteristics of the skin in these locations, the criteria are different on
    - Trunk and extremities
    - Face, nose, ears, neck
    - Palms, soles, and genital mucosa
  - Thinner skin on the head and neck vs. the trunk and extremities and thicker skin on the palms and soles with fissures and ridges
  - The criteria found on the head, neck, palms, soles, and genital mucosa are referred to as *site-specific criteria*

Global Patterns

- *Reticular*
  - Pigment network filling most of the lesion
- *Globular*
  - Dots and globules filling most of the lesion
- *Cobblestone*
  - Larger angulated globules resembling street cobblestones filling most of the lesion (Fig. 31-18)
- *Homogeneous*
  - Diffuse pigmentation in the absence of local criteria such as pigment network, dots, and globules
- *Starburst (Spitzoid)*
  - Streaks and/or dots and globules at the periphery of the lesion
- *Multicomponent*
  - Three or more different areas within a lesion
  - Each zone can be composed of a single criterion or multiple criteria
- *Nonspecific*
  - None of the above global patterns can be identified

Local Criteria

- *Regular pigment network*
  - Various shades of brown
  - Honeycomb-like (web-like, reticular) line segments
  - Uniform color, thickness, and holes
  - The lighter holes seen between the line segments represent the dermal papilla

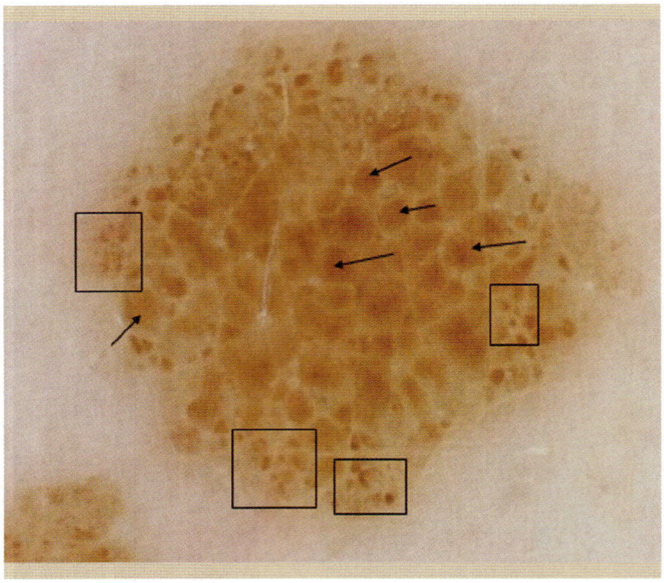

FIGURE 31-18 Acquired nevus. Small dots and globules (boxes) and larger angulated globules (arrows) characterize this benign nevus. The cobblestone global pattern. The mountain and valley pattern seen in seborrheic keratosis is in the dermoscopic differential diagnosis. A positive wobble sign in which the soft nevus moves from side to side with movement of instrumentation versus a stiff immoveable seborrheic keratosis helps to make the differentiation.

- *Irregular pigment network*
  - Black, brown, or gray
  - Line segments that are thickened, branched, and broken up (enlarged, irregular fused rete ridges)
  - There may be a diffuse distribution or foci of irregular pigment network
- *Regular dots and globules*
  - Brown roundish structures
    - Usually clustered
    - Dots (0.1 mm) are smaller than globules (>0.1 mm)
    - Size, shape, and color are similar with an even distribution in the lesion (nest of melanocytes at the dermoepidermal junction)
  - Dots and/or globules only found at the periphery can be seen in Spitz or actively changing nevi
  - Actively changing means if followed digitally the nevus will invariably enlarge within a short period of time
  - Peripheral dots and globules are usually seen in younger patients with benign pathology
  - Beware of this pattern in a newly acquired nevus in an adult
- *Irregular dots and globules*
  - Black, brown, gray, or red roundish structures
    - Different sizes and shades of color
    - Usually but not always asymmetrically located in the lesion
- *Regular streaks*
  - Black or brown linear projections of pigment can stand alone
  - Can be associated with a pigment network or dark regular blotch
  - At all points along the periphery of the lesion
  - Pseudopods and radial streaming are similar structures clinically and histopathologically (aggregates of tumor cells running parallel to the epidermis that can be seen in Spitz nevi or represent the radial growth phase of melanoma) that are difficult to differentiate from each another
  - To simplify the identification, the term "streaks" is now used by many but not all experienced dermoscopists to encompass all variations of this criterion
  - The shape of the linear projections does not determine if they are regular or irregular, rather their distribution at the periphery of the lesion
- *Irregular streaks*
  - Black or brown linear projections
  - Can stand alone or be associated with a pigment network or a dark blotch
  - Irregularly distributed at the periphery of a lesion
  - Some but not all points at the periphery, foci of streaks
- *Regular blotches*
  - Black, brown, or gray
  - Structureless (i.e., absence of network, dots or globules) areas of color
  - Bigger than dots and globules
  - Uniform shape and color symmetrically located in the lesion (aggregates of melanin in the epidermis and/or dermis)
- *Irregular blotches*
  - Black, brown, or gray structureless areas
  - Irregular in size and shape asymmetrically located in the lesion
- *Blue-white veil*
  - Irregular, structureless area of confluent blue color
  - Does not fill the entire lesion
  - Overlying whitish ground glass appearance
    - Orthokeratosis
    - Acanthosis
    - Hypergranulosis
  - Can also represent heavily pigmented tumor cells in the dermis
  - In lectures, publications, and books the use of the term blue-white veil is loosely used and quite often does not meet the definition of the criterion. Any blue and/or white color is often called the "veil"
- *Regression*
  - Bony or milky white scar-like depigmentation (fibrosis)
  - With or without gray or blue pepper-like granules "Peppering"
  - Gray color is much more commonly seen than blue in areas of regression

- Gray irregular blotches can be associated with peppering
- Peppering represents free melanin and/or melanophages in the dermis
- The white color should be lighter than the surrounding skin
- Regression by itself is an independently potentially high-risk criterion
- The more regression seen, the greater the chance the lesion is a melanoma

- ***Blue-white color***
  - It is not always possible to identify classic regression on blue-white veil
  - Blue and/or white color of any intensity, shape, or distribution
  - A "red flag" of concern should be raised
- ***Crystalline structures***
  - Also called shiny white streaks
  - White, shiny, linear structures
  - Only visible with polarized dermoscopy
  - Represents dermal fibrosis/fibroplasia
  - Seen in melanoctyic, nonmelanocytic, benign, malignant, and inflammatory pathology
  - Basal cell carcinoma, melanoma, Spitz nevi, dermatofibromas, lichen planus
  - If seen in a melanocytic lesion, it favors the diagnosis of melanoma
- ***Hypopigmentation***
  - Commonly seen featureless areas of light brown color in all types of melanocytic lesions both benign and malignant
  - Multifocal hypopigmentation is a common feature of dysplastic nevi
  - Asymmetrical irregular hypopigmentation seen at the periphery can be seen in melanoma
  - Inexperienced dermoscopists can have trouble differentiating hypopigmentation from the white color seen with true regression
  - An important clue to make the differentiation is that hypopigmentation does not have any gray color or peppering
- ***Colors seen with dermoscopy***
  - Eumelanin has a brown color
  - Its location in the skin will determine the colors one sees with dermoscopy (the Tyndall effect)
  - Black indicates melanin is superficially located in the epidermis (i.e., in the stratum corneum)
  - Black color in a nodular lesion usually represents invasive melanoma
  - Black is not always an ominous color but can be seen in benign pathology as well as in melanoma
  - Light and dark brown indicates pigment is at the dermoepidermal junction
  - Gray in the papillary dermis represents free melanin and melanophages ("peppering")

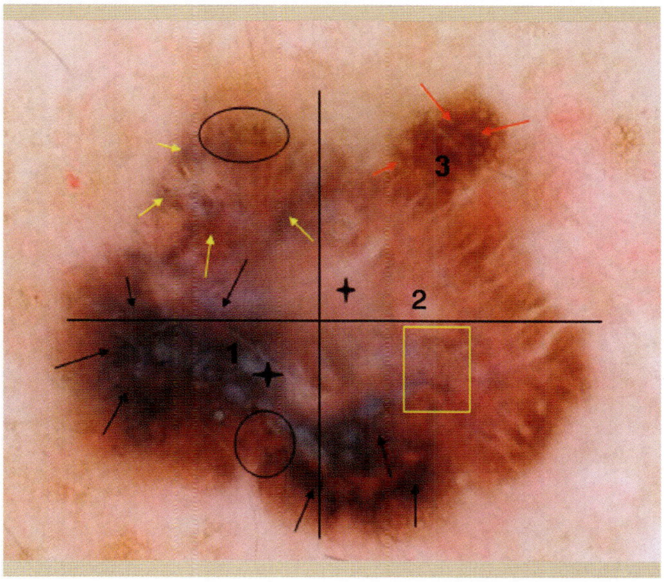

FIGURE 31-19 Melanoma. This is a melanocytic lesion because there is a pigment network (red arrows) and aggregated brown globules (circles). There is asymmetry of color and structure (+) plus the multicomponent global pattern (1, 2, 3). Local criteria includes irregular pigment network (red arrows), irregular dots and globules (circles), irregular dark blotches (black arrows), and blue-white color (stars). The classic blue-white veil is not seen. Peppering (yellow box) and gray blotches (yellow arrows) are part of the regression. More than 5 colors are seen including red.

  - As the pigment gets into the deeper dermis, it looks blue (the Tyndall effect)
  - Red and/or pink color can be created by inflammation or neovascularization
  - Sebaceous material and hyperkeratosis can look yellow
  - The more colors seen, the greater chance one is dealing with high-risk pathology (Figs. 31-19, 31-20, and 31-21)
- ***Polymorphous vascular pattern/polymorphous vessels***
  - Three or more different shapes of telangiectatic vessels
  - Telangiectatic vessels that can be seen in melanoma are nonspecific; they can also commonly be found in other lesions, including
    - Benign
    - Malignant
    - Inflammatory
  - When identified, they should raise a "red flag" of concern, including
    - Dotted/pinpoint (dots resembling the head of a pin)
    - Linear (regular and irregular)
    - Arborizing
    - Glomerular

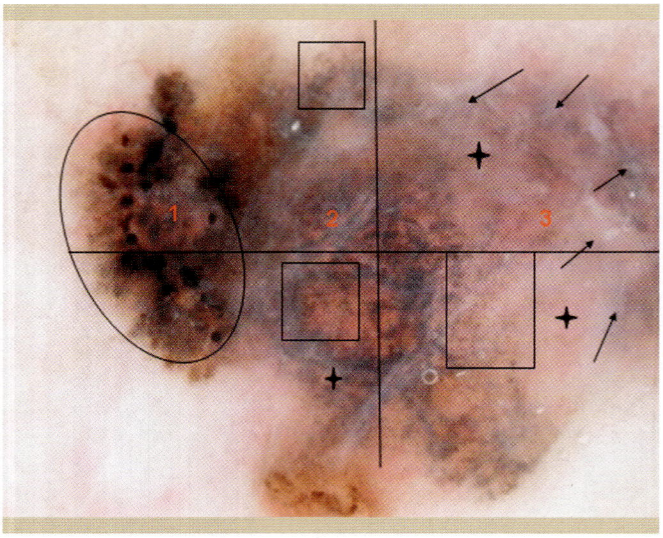

FIGURE 31-20 Melanoma. There is a melanocytic lesion because there are aggregated dark brown/black globules (circle). There is asymmetry of color and structure (+) plus the multicomponent global pattern (1, 2, 3). Local criteria includes irregular dots and globules (circle), blue-white color (stars), and peppering (boxes). The classic blue-white veil is not seen. More than 5 colors, including red, are another melanoma-specific criterion.

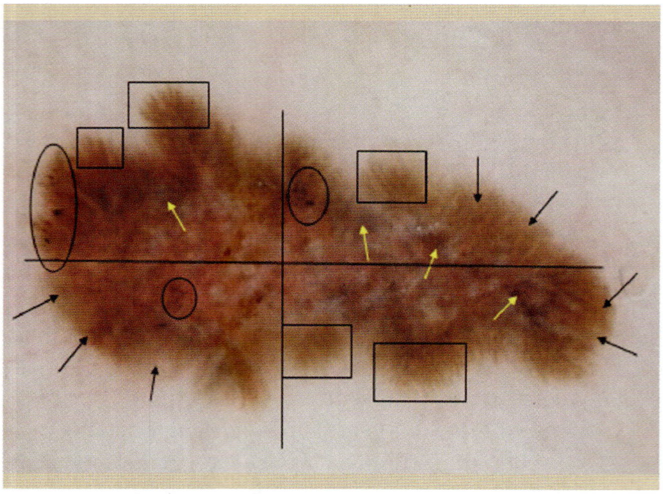

FIGURE 31-21 Melanoma. This is a melanocytic lesion because there are aggregated brown globules (circles). There is an irregular starburst (Spitzoid) global pattern with foci of streaks at the periphery (boxes). Local criteria includes; irregular dots and globules (circles), irregular streaks (boxes) and regression. The white and gray blotches (yellow arrows) make up the regression. The black arrows point out where there are no streaks. Five colors, including red, round off the melanoma specific-criteria.

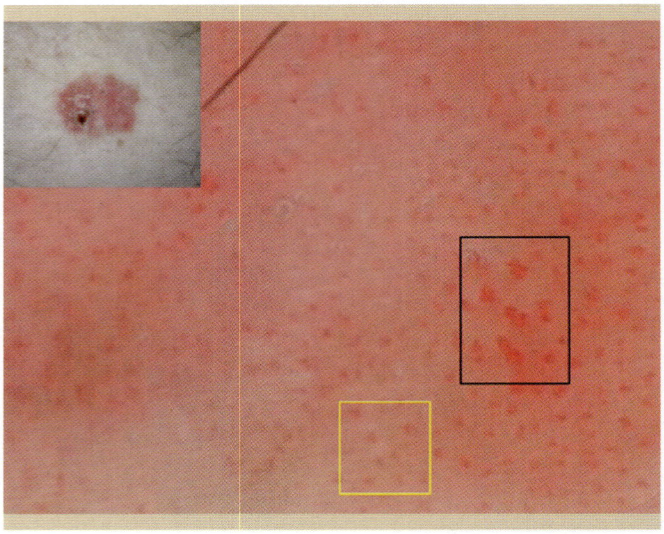

FIGURE 31-22 Bowen disease. Typical glomerular vessels (black box) and smaller dotted/pinpoint vessels (yellow box) help diagnose this nonspecific pink scaly patch. A psoriatic plaque could have the same clinical and dermoscopic picture.

    - Irregular torturous/corkscrew (irregular, thick, coiled)
    - Irregular hairpin (irregular and thick hairpin shaped)
    - Many shapes can be seen that have not been described
  - One must focus his/her attention to make out the shapes of these small vessels (Fig. 31-22)
- ***Milky red areas***
  - Localized or diffuse (seen in pigmented, hypo-, or amelanotic melanoma) pinkish white color
  - Milky-red/pink color can also be seen in benign pathology both melanocytic and non- melanocytic (i.e., nevi, acute lichen planus-like keratosis)
  - With or without reddish and or bluish out-of-focus/fuzzy globular structures (neovascularization)
  - Not to be confused with the in focus lacunae seen in hemangiomas
- ***Glomerular vessels***
  - Diffuse or clustered fine coiled vessels that can be seen in
    - Bowen disease (see Fig. 31-22)
    - Melanoma
    - Acute pink lichen planus–like keratosis
    - Stasis dermatitis
    - Psoriasis
  - Pinpoint and larger glomerular vessels represent a variation of the same criterion
- ***Asymmetrical pigmentation around follicular openings***
  - Seen only on the face, nose, and ears
  - Irregular brown color outlining parts of the round follicular openings
  - The color does not completely encircle the openings (early proliferation of atypical melanocytes)

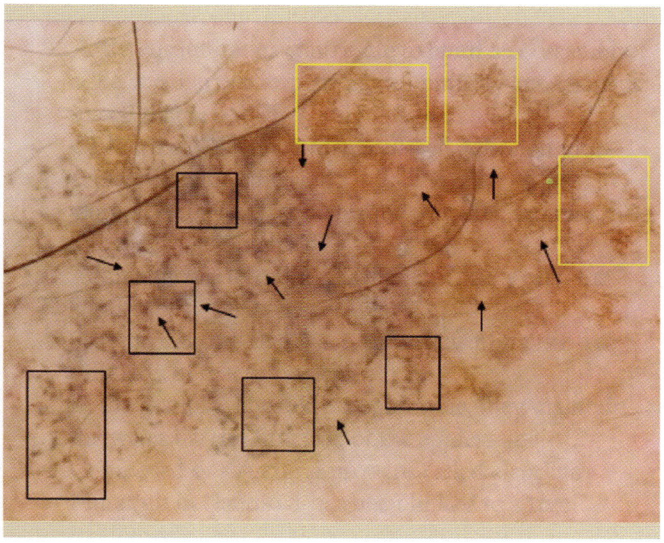

FIGURE 31-23 Lichen planus–like keratosis. Remnants of a fingerprint pattern (yellow boxes) with faint brown parallel lines of a solar lentigo are clues that this is not lentigo maligna. Gray annular-granular pattern (black boxes) around follicular openings (arrows) are are also seen. The gray dots represent melanophages and free melanin in the papillary dermis, not atypical melanocytes. A subset of lichen planus–like keratosis are thought to represent an immunologic event against flat seborrheic keratosis of solar lentigines.

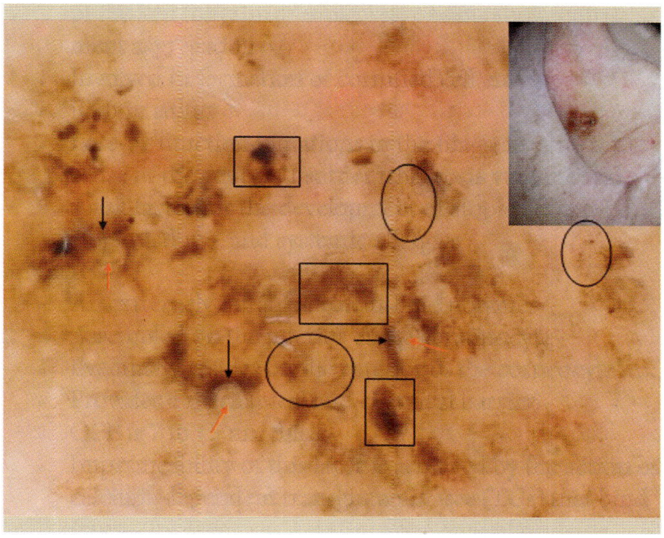

FIGURE 31-24 Lentigo maligna (ear lobe). This case demonstrates variations of the classic criteria. The lesion is suspicious clinically but has a differential diagnosis that includes a seborrheic keratosis. The dermoscopic criteria for a seborrheic keratosis are not present. There is asymmetry of color and structure, asymmetrical pigmentation (black arrows) around follicular openings (red arrows), annular-granular structures (circles), and irregular dark blotches (boxes). One should have a mental checklist of the melanoma-specific criteria for this site-specific area because they are not always easy to find and identify. "One cannot see what one does not know."

- ***Annular-granular pattern/structures***
  - Seen only on the face, nose, and ears
  - Brown or gray fine dots that surround follicular openings (melanophages and/or atypical melanocytes)
  - This criterion can be seen in
    - Lentigo maligna, lentigo maligna melanoma
    - Pigmented actinic keratosis
    - Posttraumatic
    - Late stage lichen planus–like keratosis (Figs. 31-23 and 31-24)
- ***Rhomboid structures***
  - Seen only on the face, nose, and ears
  - Rhomboid is a parallelogram with 2 pairs of parallel lines in which the opposite sides have equal length and there are obtuse angles
  - Black, brown, or gray thickening completely surrounding the follicular openings
  - In reality true rhomboids are not regularly formed
  - Any pigmented thickening around follicular openings is worrisome
- ***Circle within a circle***
  - Not well-studied criterion associated with melanoma on the face, nose, and ears
  - Central hair shaft (inner circle)
  - Outer ring of gray color (outer circle)
  - Gray color can represent atypical melanocytes and/or melanophages

Pearls

- A large patch of brown color typically seen on the face of older people cannot be excised to make a histopathologic diagnosis. Commonly, it can have dermoscopic features associated with solar lentigo, actinic keratosis, and melanoma. Use the area and/or areas with atypical features to make an incisional biopsy. For example, biopsy the foci with asymmetrical follicular pigmentation or circle within a circle.
- If you think a lesion is lentigo maligna yet the pathology report does not make the diagnosis, seek another histopathologic opinion or biopsy of another area of the lesion.
- There should always be a good clinico-dermoscopic-pathologic correlation

- ***Benign pigmented nail bands (melanonychia striata)***
  - Single or multiple nail involvement with brown longitudinal parallel lines
  - Uniform color, spacing, and thickness
  - Variable presence of a diffuse brown background
  - A single band in a lighter skinned person with these findings is still worrisome and could represent dysplastic histology or in situ melanoma
- ***Malignant pigmented nail bands (atypical melanonychia striata)***
  - Loss of parallelism(broken up line segments) with brown, black, or gray parallel lines that demonstrate different shades of color, irregular spacing, and thickness (Fig. 31-25)

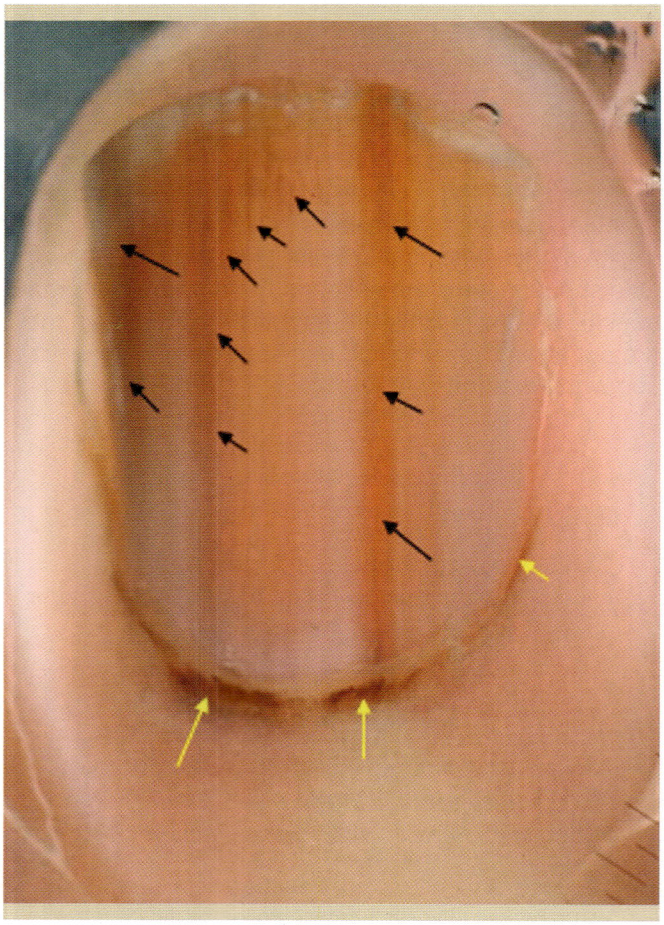

FIGURE 31-25 Acrolentiginous melanoma/nail apparatus melanoma. The pigmented bands are not uniform in color and thickness (black arrows) with loss of parallelism (broken up line segments). Loss of parallelism is created by the atypical melanocytes that produce pigment irregularly. There is also Hutchinson sign (yellow arrows). (*Used with permission from Wilhelm Stolz.*)

  - High-risk dermoscopic criteria at this location in adults are usually not associated with high-risk pathology when seen in children
  - Disfiguring nail matrix biopsies can usually be avoided
  - Any rapidly changing scenario warrants a histopathologic diagnosis no matter how old or young the patient

Pearl

Digital monitoring is helpful to monitor pigmentation in the nail apparatus.

- ***Fungal melanonychia (Fig.31-26)***
  - Relatively rare
  - Twenty one plus species of dematiaceous fungi that produce melanin in their cell wall or secrete it extracellularly
  - Eight species of nondematiaceous fungi

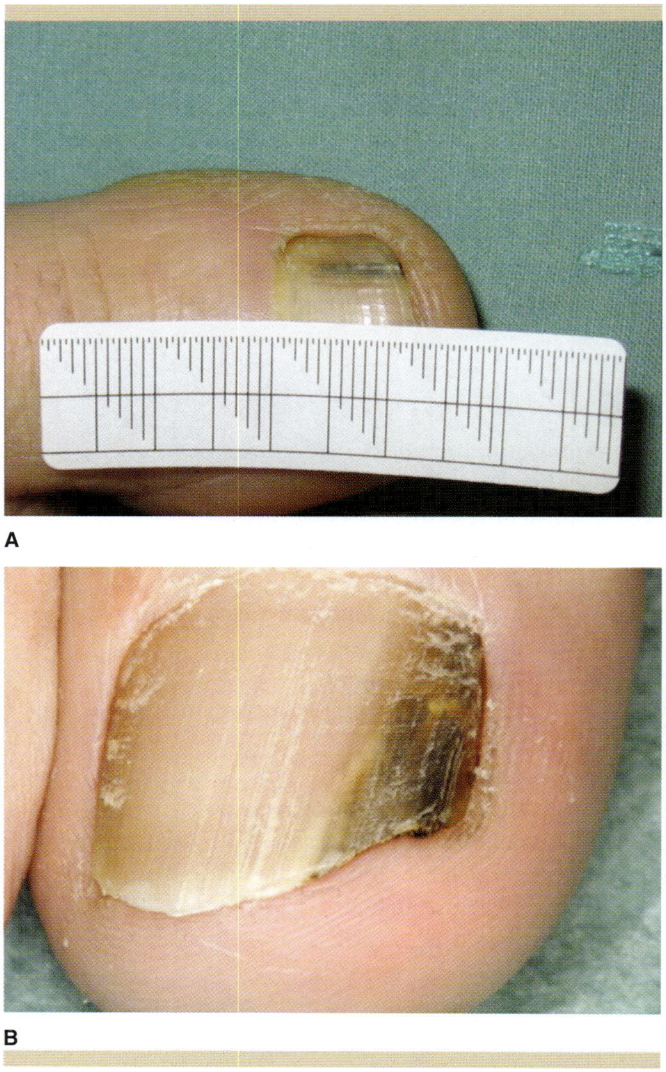

FIGURE 31-26 A and B Fungal Melanonychia created by demataceous fungi that produce melanin. (*Used with permission from Wilhelm Stolz.*)

    - Dematiaceous fungus *Scytalidium dimidiatum* and dermatophyte Trichophyton *rubrum* most frequently isolated agents of fungal melanonychia
    - There can be diffuse melanychia filling the entire nail or pigmented bands
    - The pigmented bands are wider distally and taper proximally, consistent with distal-to-proximal spread of infection
    - Components of the bands can be rounded proximally
- ***Micro-Hutchinson sign (Hutchinson sign)***
    - Pigmentation of the cuticle that can only be seen clearly with dermoscopy
    - A nonspecific dermoscopic finding that is often but not always associated with a nail apparatus melanoma
    - Pigmentation of the cuticle easily seen without dermoscopy
- ***Nonmelanocytic nail apparatus bands***
    - The history is important
    - Pregnancy
    - PUVA
    - Occupational exposure
    - Medications (chemotherapeutic agents, multiple nails)
    - Racial longitudinal melanonychia (multiple nails)
    - Nail trauma or inflammation (nail biting, friction, paranychia)
    - Exposure to exogenous pigments (chromonychia), tobacco, dirt, potassium permanganate, tar, iodine, silver nitrate (usually can be easily scratched off)
- **Uniform grayish lines/bands on a gray background can be seen in**
    - Lentigo
    - Ethnic pigmentation
    - Drug-induced pigmentation
    - Postinflammatory
    - Laugier-Hunziker syndrome
    - Represents epithelial hyperpigmentation without melanocytic hyperplasia
- ***Nail apparatus blood/subungual hematoma***
    - The color of blood seen in the nail apparatus depends how long the blood has been there
        - Fresh blood looks red or purple/violaceous
        - Older blood can look yellowish brown or black
    - A well-demarcated homogeneous area with parallel lines at the distal edge and globule-like blood spots/pebbles (Fig. 31-27)
    - Digital dermoscopy is helpful to follow nail apparatus blood that should slowly move distally over several months

Pearls

- Presence of blood does not rule out melanoma
- Search carefully for high-risk criteria that might also be present

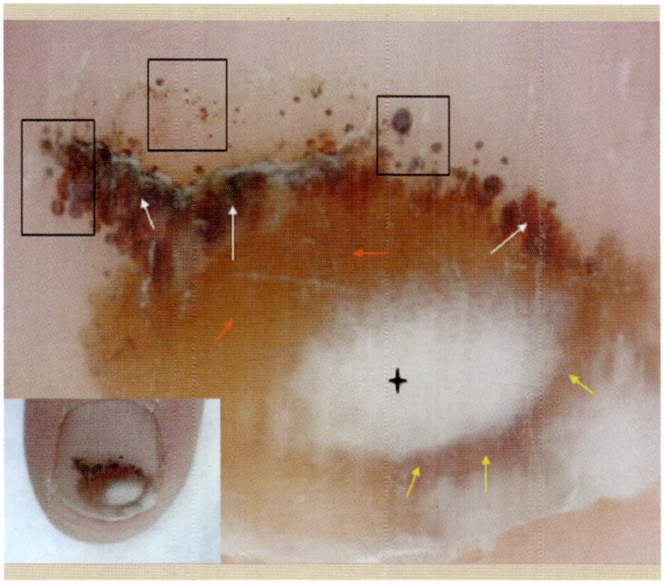

FIGURE 31-27 Subungual hematoma. Different colors plus purple blood pebbles (boxes) characterize this posttraumatic lesion. The white color (star) is secondary to trauma not regression. The brown (red arrows) and purple blotches (white arrows) result from the breakdown of blood. No melanoma-specific criteria are seen.

- Finding the Hutchinson sign and the parallel-ridge pattern on the surrounding skin adjacent to the nail can help make the diagnosis of nail apparatus melanoma
- An experienced surgeon and dermatopathologist plus a well-placed generous biopsy specimen are essential to make the correct diagnosis of nail apparatus pigmentation

Common Dermoscopic Patterns

- ***Congenital nevi***
    - Diffuse homogeneous brown color
    - Patchy or diffuse pigment network (target network may or may not be seen as network holes each with a small centrally located brown dot or pinpoint vessel)
    - Globular and/or cobblestone pattern (target globules may or may not be seen as globules with a smaller centrally located dot or vessel)
    - Islands of normal skin and islands of criteria such as network dots and globules
    - Multicomponent pattern with 3 or more distinct areas of criteria
    - Dark coarse terminal hairs (hypertrichosis) with or without surrounding hypopigmentation (perifollicular hypopigmentation) (Fig. 31-28)
    - Milia-like cysts and pseudofollicular openings most often found in seborrheic keratosis can be seen

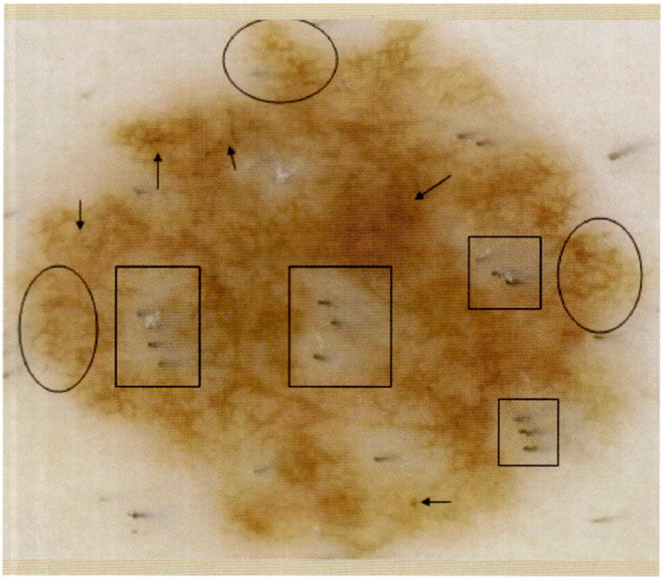

FIGURE 31-28 Congenital melanocytic nevus. Terminal hairs with perifollicular hypopigmentation (boxes), pigment network (circles), and brown dots (arrows) characterize this small congenital melanocytic nevus.

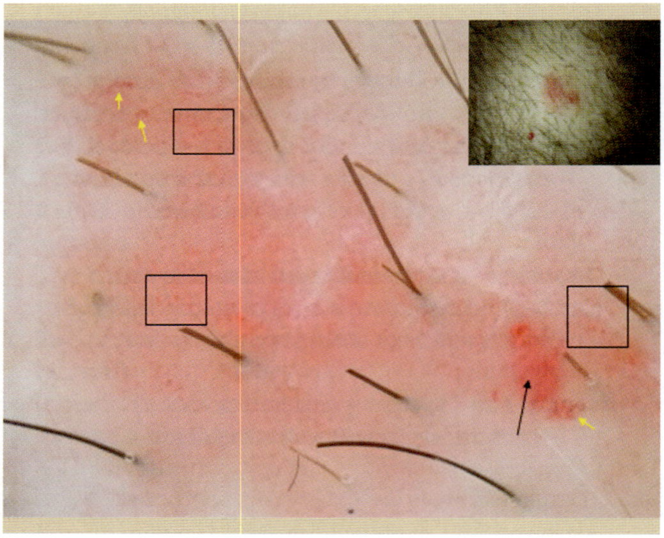

FIGURE 31-29 Acute pink lichen planus–like keratosis. This small papule was only found after a complete skin examination. There are different shades of pink color, pinpoint (boxes), and comma-shaped vessels (yellow arrows) plus a milky red area (black arrow). Amelanotic melanoma and Merkel cell carcinoma are in the clinical and dermoscopic differential diagnosis.

- ***Acquired nevi***
  - Light/dark brown or pink color
  - Regular pigment network filling the lesion
  - Sharp border demarcation
  - Globular or cobblestone global patterns (the most common patterns seen in children)
  - Symmetry of color and structure
  - Comma-shaped blood vessels
  - Hypopigmentation
  - Milia-like cysts, pseudofollicular openings, fissures, and ridges can be seen
  - Pink nevi can be featureless or feature poor and have a white/negative network
  - A solitary flat pink lesion is more worrisome than multiple soft and compressible pink lesions

Pearl

Dermoscopy might not be helpful to diagnose pink macules and papules which can be melanocytic, nonmelanocytic, benign, malignant, or inflammatory (Fig. 31-29)

- ***Blue nevi***
  - Blue, blue-gray, or blue-black homogeneous color (Fig. 31-3)
  - Variable number of subtle blue globular-like structures
  - Regression with white or gray areas commonly seen
  - Radiation tattoo, nodular, and cutaneous metastatic melanoma are in the dermoscopic differential diagnosis
  - The history is essential to help make the correct diagnosis
- ***Combined nevi***
  - Light/dark brown homogeneous color +/− other local criteria (regular nevus) and central blue blotch (blue nevus) with a "fried egg" clinical appearance
  - Diffuse brown homogeneous color with a blue border
  - Diffuse blue homogeneous color with a brown border
  - Variable combinations of blue and brown color
- ***Recurrent nevi/pseudomelanoma***
  - Sharp border
  - Irregular pigment network; irregular streaks
  - Irregular dots and globules
  - White scar-like areas with arborizing vessels
  - Any combination of criteria can be seen
  - Pigmentation centrally located in the scar; if the pigmentation goes out of the scar rule out melanoma
  - The history of previous surgery and histopathology is important (Fig. 31-30)
- ***Dysplastic nevi***
  - ABCD clinical lesions can look banal or high risk with dermoscopy
  - Being indistinguishable from melanoma

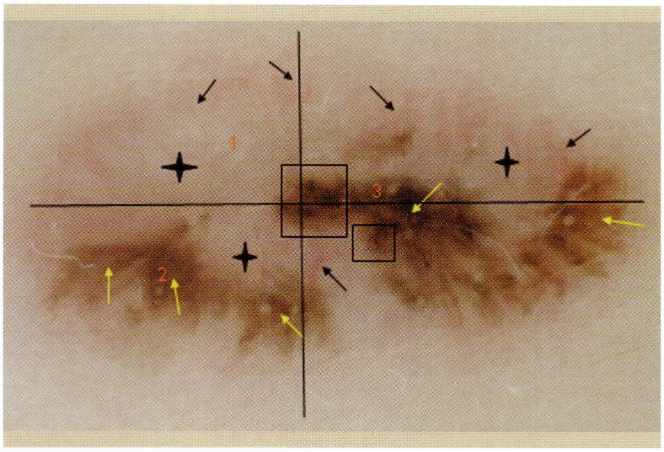

FIGURE 31-30 Recurrent nevus. Asymmetry of color and structure (+), the multicomponent global pattern (1, 2, 3) irregular brown globules (boxes), irregular dark blotches (yellow arrows), and scar tissue (stars) with arborizing vessels (black arrows) characterize this recurrent nevus. Regressive melanoma is in the dermoscopic differential diagnosis. Review the original pathology report to confirm the benign nature of this lesion.

- Evolving/changing might be the only clue that a lesion is high risk
- Asymmetry of color and structure
- Irregular pigment network
- Irregular blotches
- Irregular dots and globules
- Multifocal hypopigmentation (Fig. 31-31)

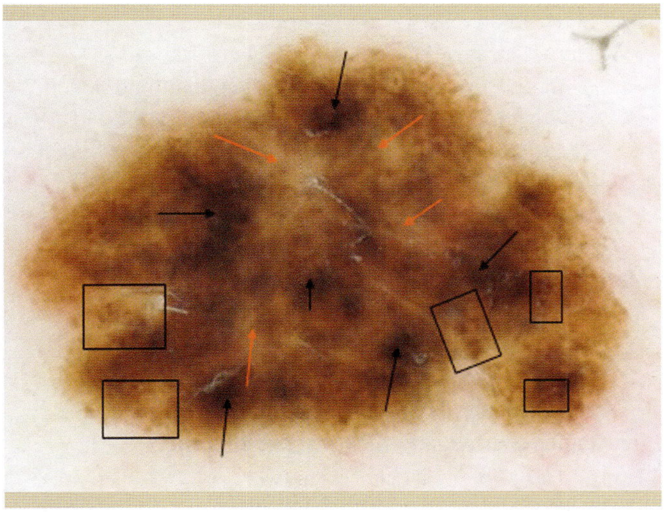

FIGURE 31-31 Dysplastic nevus. There are foci of irregular brown dots and globules (boxes), irregular dark blotches (black arrows), and multifocal hypopigmentation (red arrows). It might be hard to differentiate the hypopigmentation from regression.

- Regression, blue-white color/blue-white veil, polymorphous vessels, and streaks are not usually seen
- May look more malignant than benign but not definitely malignant
- Patients with multiple dysplastic nevi usually do not have many that look very atypical with dermoscopy
- Look for the clinical and/or dermoscopic "ugly duckling" to consider for biopsy or digital follow-up
- Pink dysplastic nevi can be feature poor or featureless with low- or high-grade histopathology

- ***Spitz nevi***
  - There are 6 patterns seen in Spitz nevi
    - Starburst
    - Globular
    - Homogeneous
    - Pink
    - Black pigment network
    - Atypical
  - Spitzoid is the term used when any of the different 6 patterns is seen
  - Starburst is the most common pattern (Fig. 31-32)
    - Streaks and/or dots and globules at the periphery
    - Light/dark brown, black, or blue color centrally
    - Regular or irregular pattern depends on the location of the streaks

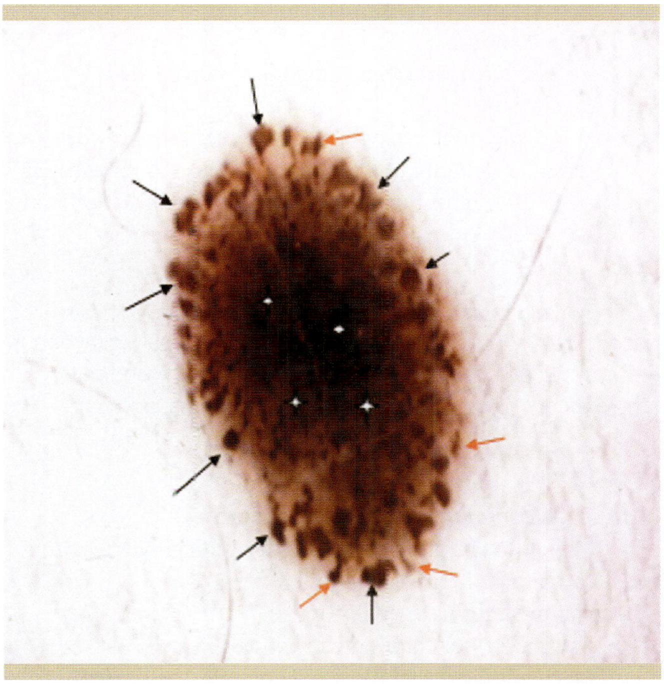

FIGURE 31-32 Spitz nevus. A central regular dark blotch (stars) plus brown globules (black arrows), and a few streaks (red arrows) at all points of the periphery characterize this classic symmetrical starburst/Spitzoid pattern. Beware, symmetrical starburst patterns can be seen in melanoma. Following this type of lesion with digital dermoscopy could be a very big mistake!

- Regular starburst pattern has symmetrical streaks around the lesion
- Irregular starburst pattern has foci of streaks at the periphery
- Symmetrical and asymmetrical starburst patterns can be seen in melanoma
- Globular is the second most common Spitzoid pattern
  - Filled with regular or irregular dots and/or globules
  - Blue color seen centrally is the clue that the lesion might be a Spitz nevus
- Homogeneous pattern
  - Featureless brown color
- Pink pattern
  - Featureless pink papule
    - ▲ Can have polymorphous vessels
    - ▲ Not to be mistaken for amelanotic melanoma
    - ▲ Not to be mistaken for a pyogenic granuloma
- Black network pattern
  - The lesion is composed totally of a prominent black pigment network
  - Ink spot lentigo and melanoma are in the differential diagnosis
- Atypical pattern
  - This can have any combination of melanoma-specific criteria similar to superficial spreading melanoma
  - The histopathologic diagnosis is usually a surprise
- White pigment network/negative pigment network/ reticular depigmentation can sometimes be identified
  - This is an important clue that the lesion is Spitzoid

> ***Pearl***
>
> Any Spitzoid pattern requires a histopathologic diagnosis especially in adults. Following these, lesions with digital dermoscopy have been reported but it is fool hardy and puts the patient's life at risk (i.e., missing spitzoid melanoma)!

- ***In situ melanoma*** **(trunk and extremities)**
  - May or may not demonstrate the clinical ABCD clinical criteria
  - Flat or slightly raised lesion
  - Asymmetry of color and structure
  - Black and/or dark brown irregular pigment network
  - Irregular dots and globules
  - Irregular dark blotches
  - Hypopigmentation
  - Lacks the criteria for deeper melanoma (pink, red, gray, or blue color, polymorphous vessels or regression)
  - May look more malignant than benign but not definitely malignant (Fig. 31-33)

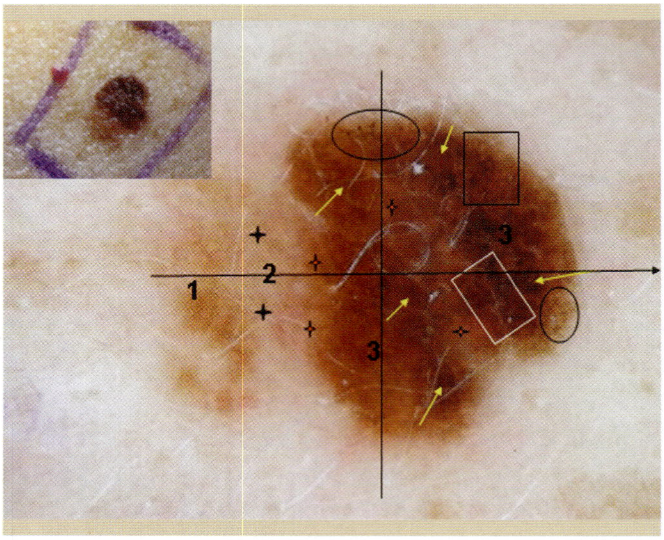

FIGURE 31-33 In situ melanoma. This is a melanocytic lesion because there is a pigment network (black box) and aggregated brown lobules (circles). There is asymmetry of color and structures (+), the multicomponent global pattern (1, 2, 3), irregular pigment network (black box), irregular brown dots and globules (circles), irregular dark blotches (yellow arrows), and reticular depigmentation (white box). The hypopigmentation (black stars) should not be confused with regression. There is diffuse erythema (red stars) and only 3 other colors.

- ***Superficial spreading melanoma***
  - Starts in an existing nevus or de novo
  - Demonstrates the clinical ABCD criteria
  - Contains a variable number of the melanoma-specific criteria found on the trunk and extremities (Figs. 31-19, 31-20, and 31-21)
- ***Nodular melanoma***
  - Starts in an existing nevus or de novo
  - May or may not be fast growing
  - Pigmented, hypomelanotic, or amelanotic
  - Can have symmetrical pigmentation and shape
  - Can be mistaken clinically for a banal nevus or squamous cell carcinoma
  - Usually lacks the clinical ABCD criteria
  - Due to the absence of the radial growth phase, there is a scarcity of local criteria (network, globules, streaks)
  - Remnants of local criteria may or may not be present at the periphery of the lesion
  - Large intense irregular dark black blotches
  - Multiple deeper skin colors seen such as blue, white, pink, milky red
  - Polymorphous vessels

Pearls

- The clinical appearance of a lesion (flat, palpable, or nodular, presence or absence of the ABCD criteria) plus the colors and structures seen with dermoscopy can help estimate if you are dealing with a thin, intermediate, or thick melanoma
- Flat melanomas are usually in situ or early invasive with black and/or brown color plus well-developed local criteria
- Thick melanomas tend to be elevated or nodular and can have a paucity or absence of local criteria such as pigment network, dots and globules plus blue-white color, regression, multiple other colors, and polymorphous vessels

- ***Amelanotic melanoma***
    - Flat, palpable, or nodular
    - Partially pigmented, hypopigmented, pink or red
    - May or may not have the melanoma-specific criteria typically seen in pigmented melanomas
    - Different shades of pink color and polymorphous vessels
    - Milky red areas are important clues to the correct diagnosis
    - Pediatric patients have a high proportion of amelanotic melanomas (Fig. 31-34)

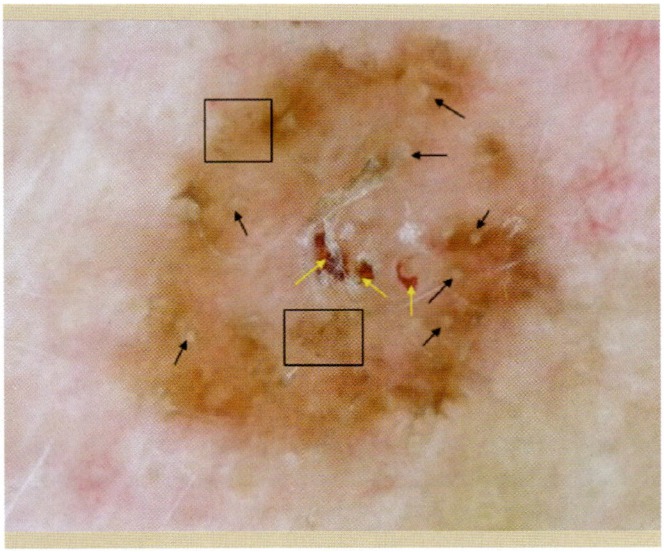

FIGURE 31-34 Amelanotic melanoma (feature poor melanoma). This is a melanocytic lesion because it has aggregated brown globules (boxes). There is an absence of melanoma-specific criteria found on the face with different shades of pink and brown color plus ulceration (yellow arrows). Follicular openings (black arrows) should not be confused with the milia-like cysts of a seborrheic keratosis.

- Amelanotic melanoma should always be in the differential diagnosis of a Merkel cell carcinoma, pyogenic granuloma or pink Spitz nevus
- Desmoplastic melanoma (DM)
    - Rare variant of cutaneous melanoma
    - Diagnosis often delayed
    - Most common clinical presentation palpable and/or indurated lesion on sun-exposed skin
    - Histopathology can be pure DM or mixed DM (associated with another subtype of melanoma, i.e., lentigo maligna)
    - Dermoscopically one can find one or more melanoma-specific criteria
    - Regression/white scar-like areas/peppering/gray color
    - Multiple colors
    - Polymorphous vessels
    - Milky red areas with or without milky red globules
    - Pink color/vascular flush
    - Crystalline structures

Pearl

A high index of suspicion and dermoscopic clues can increase the clinical diagnosis of dermoplastic melanoma

- **Pediatric melanoma**
    - Pediatric melanoma is rare yet the incidence is steadily increasing each year
    - Dermoscopic features of superficial spreading, pigmented nodular, or amelanotic melanoma
    - A significant number do not present with the ABCD clinical features
    - In many cases the conventional ABCD criteria are inadequate in children
    - Amelanosis, symmetry, regular borders, diameter less than 6 mm, bleeding, uniform color, variable diameter, de novo development are common

Pearls

- Additional ABCD detection criteria (amelanotic, bleeding bump, color uniformity, de novo, and diameter)
- At any age, E for evolution or any change is significant no matter what a lesion looks like

- ***Cutaneous metastatic melanoma***
    - Dermoscopy might not be as helpful to make the diagnosis as the history of a melanoma being previously excised
    - Single or multiple
    - Pigmented and/or nonpigmented macules, papules, and ulcerated or nonulcerated nodules can be seen in the same patient

- All different sizes, shapes, and colors can be seen in each patient with or without polymorphous vessels
- Any combination of criteria can be seen
- Benign patterns such as a hemangioma-like cutaneous metastatic melanoma (Fig. 31-17)

- ***Feature poor melanoma***
  - Melanoma without well developed melanoma specific criteria (Fig. 31-34)
  - Melanoma incognito/false negative melanoma
  - Clinically the lesion does not look like melanoma
  - With dermoscopy, there may be clues to help make the diagnosis
  - Clues to help make the diagnosis
    - History of dermoscopic change over time
    - A Spitzoid pattern in a lesion that does not look Spitzoid clinically
    - Areas of regression as the major high-risk criterion
    - Polymorphous vessels in a pink lesion
  - The *"Little Red Riding Hood Sign"* is when the lesion looks clinically benign from a distance but not close up with dermoscopy

Pearl

Dermoscopy should not only be used on clinically suspicious lesions if one wants to diagnose melanoma incognito

- ***Featureless melanoma***
  - Melanoma without dermoscopic criteria at all
  - Usually a pink or hypopigmented lesion
- **Nevi/Melanomas associated with decorative tattoos**
  - It is best not to cover melanocytic lesions with decorative tattoos
  - Malignant change could be camouflaged
  - The infiltration of tattoo pigment into melanocytic lesions can obscure dermoscopic features and makes an accurate dermoscopic diagnosis difficult
  - Laser removal of tattoos covering melanocytic lesions has been reported with invasive melanoma
  - It is not known if lasers have the potential to change benign nevi into melanoma
  - After Laser therapy, black pigment in tattoos can be found in regional lymph nodes and make the diagnosis of metastatic melanoma problematic

Pearls

- Avoid covering melanocytic lesions with decorative tattoos until there is more scientific evidence that is a safe procedure.
- One should excise a melanocytic lesion before covering the area with a tattoo.

- **Merkel cell carcinoma (MCC)**
  - Relatively rare tumor
  - Nonspecific clinical findings
  - Very few studied dermoscopically
  - High mortality rate
  - Often delay in diagnosis due to low index of suspicion
  - Amelanotic tumors are in the clinical and dermoscopic differential diagnosis (i.e., basal cell carcinoma, amelanotic melanoma, Bowen disease, acute lichen planus–like keratosis, and other benign lesions)
  - Variety of vascular patterns
  - Milky red areas with/without milky red globules
  - Polymorphous vessels (several different shapes)
  - Arborizing vessels (similar to basal cell carcinoma)
  - Pinpoint and glomerular vessels (similar to Bowen disease)

Pearl

An amelanotic tumor is nonspecific clinically and dermoscopically and can be melanocytic, nonmelanocytic, benign, malignant, or inflammatory. However, this set of clinical and dermoscopic features should raise a red flag for concern. Make a histopathologic diagnosis sooner than later. Add MCC to your differential diagnosis.

- ***Nail apparatus melanoma***
  - Amelanotic reddish diffuse color/amelanotic tumor
  - Diffuse melanonychia with different shades of black, brown, or gray color
  - Irregular pigmented bands (i.e., different colors, irregular spacing, thickness, loss of paralellism). See Fig. 31-25.
  - A single uniform band does not rule out melanoma
  - Irregular dots and globules
  - Blood can be found associated with other criteria
  - Nail plate destruction with advanced disease
  - +/− Hutchinson sign
  - The parallel-ridge pattern can be seen on the adjacent skin
- ***Ink spot lentigo***
  - Black macule or macules on sun-exposed areas
  - Prominent thickened black pigment network
  - Usually a very easy clinical and dermoscopic diagnosis
  - Melanoma could be in the clinical and dermoscopic differential diagnosis
  - Look for melanoma-specific criteria that should not be present in an ink spot lentigo
- **Solar lentigo**
  - Macules and/or patches
  - Different shades of homogeneous brown color
  - Moth-eaten concave borders
  - Fingerprint pattern with wavy parallel linear line segments can form arches, swirls, be hyphae-like

- ***Actinic keratosis***
  - Nonpigmented actinic keratosis
    - Scaly surface
    - Pinkish pseudonetwork and round white globules (follicular openings)
    - The pink pseudonetwork with roundish white structures has to be described as having a "strawberry-like" appearance
  - Pigmented actinic keratosis
    - Mimics lentigo maligna
  - Asymmetrical follicular pigmentation
  - Annular-granular structures
  - Rhomboid structures

Pearls

- Multiple scaly lesions (the neighbor sign) favor the diagnosis of actinic keratosis over lentigo maligna (single lesion). Both can have pigmented and nonpigmented variants
- Dermoscopic features of solar lentigo, actinic keratosis, and melanoma can be found in the same lesion
- Multiple biopsies might be needed to make the correct diagnosis
- Use the atypical features of melanoma when making an incisional biopsy

- *Bowen disease* (in situ squamous cell carcinoma)
  - Usually solitary pink or reddish scaly macule, papule, nodule, patch, plaque
  - On sun-exposed areas in elderly patients
  - Pinpoint and/or glomerular vessels
  - Clusters and/or diffuse distribution of vessels throughout the lesion
  - With or without homogeneous brown color and/or dark dots and globules (pigmented Bowen disease)

Pearls

- Clinically and dermoscopically a pink scaly lesion with pinpoint and/or glomerular vessels is not diagnostic of Bowen disease.
- The differential diagnosis includes amelanotic melanoma, acute lichen planus–like keratosis, psoriasis, and stasis changes
- Statistically, a pink lesion on sun-exposed skin with this vascular pattern usually turns out to be Bowen disease.

- ***Clear cell acanthoma (CCA)***
  - Rare tumor, very few have been studied
  - Pink macule or papule
  - 1 to 2 cm reddish-moist nodules with scale
  - Trunk and lower extremities
  - Diagnostic dermoscopic findings
    - Linear and/or curvilinear glomerular and/or pinpoint vessels
    - "String of Pearls" necklace-like circular arrangement of glomerular and/or pinpoint vessels
    - Other shaped telangiectatic vessels can be seen
- ***Keratoacanthoma/Invasive Squamous cell carcinoma***
  - Centrally located yellowish keratinous material/central keratin
  - White structureless zones
  - White circles
  - Hairpin/coiled and/or linear vessels at the periphery
- ***Sebaceous gland hyperplasia***
  - Delled yellow papules seen clinically
  - Multiple grouped white or yellow globules
  - Small caliber basal cell carcinoma–like vessels
  - The vessels have been termed crown or wreath-like vessels
  - Supposedly never to reach the center of the lesion
  - This is a misnomer because in reality the vessels rarely meet this criterion and can be found anywhere in the lesion

Pearl

The globules are the main dermoscopic feature used to differentiate sebaceous gland hyperplasia from basal cell carcinoma

- ***Collision tumor***
  - Lesion with the dermoscopic criteria for 2 different pathologies
  - Rarely one can find a triple collision lesion with 3 different pathologies
  - Collision tumors are commonly seen
  - Diagnostic criteria can be side by side or one can be seen within the other
  - Examples include
    - Seborrheic keratosis, basal cell carcinoma
    - Seborrheic keratosis, in situ or invasive squamous cell carcinoma
    - Seborrheic keratosis, amelanotic, or pigmented melanoma
    - Seborrheic keratosis, eccrine porocarcinoma
    - Basal cell carcinoma, seborrheic keratosis, clear cell acanthoma
  - Any combination is possible (Fig. 31-35)

OTHER DIAGNOSES MADE WITH DERMOSCOPY

Scabies

- Burrows appear as discrete linear whitish scaly areas
- Mites can be seen as a small *triangle/gray delta structure* that corresponds to the front section of the body with its mouth/biting apparatus and legs

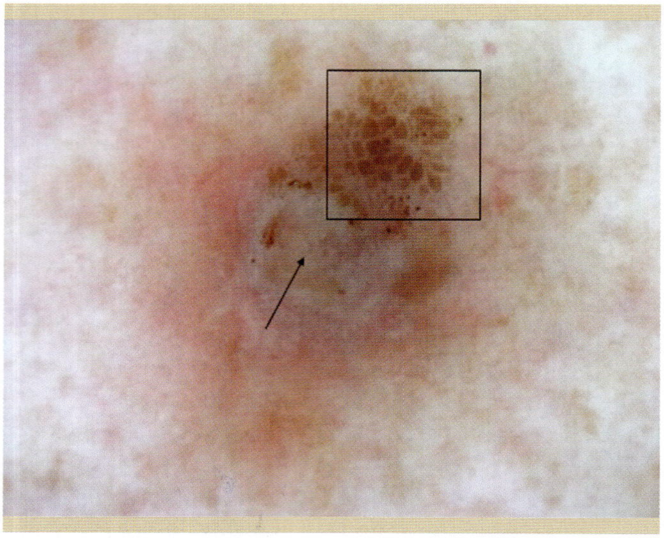

FIGURE 31-35 Collison tumor—squamous cell carcinoma and seborrheic keratosis. A rapidly growing nodule (arrow) representing a squamous cell carcinoma and the mountain and valley pattern of a seborrheic keratosis (box) characterize this lesion. The cobblestone pattern of a nevus is in the dermoscopic differential diagnosis.

- Higher magnification and oil increases the visibility of the mite, stool, and eggs

Lichen Planus

- Peppering
- Brown blotches
- White reticular areas (Wickham striae)
- Crystalline structures can be seen with polarized dermoscopy (Wickham striae)
- White network is in the dermoscopic differential diagnosis of Wickham striae

Warts

- Red and/or black dots (thrombosed capillaries)
- With or without a white halo

Psoriasis

- Red scaly plaque/plaques
- Diffuse distribution of glomerular and/or pinpoint vessels identical to Bowen disease
- Distribution of lesions will help differentiate Psoriasis from Bowen disease
- Both can have single or multiple lesions

Nail Folds

- Normal capillary loops are hairpin shaped and run parallel to the axis of the nail

Scleroderma Pattern

The triad of

- Rarefied capillaries (<6 loops per mm)
- Thin loops, megacapillaries
- Pearly shining sclerosis "cotton balls"

Dermatomyositis

Mega, twisted, branched loops, microhemorrhage

Lupus Erythematosus

Considerable variation of loops, branching, twisted microhemorrhage

INFESTATIONS

Pediculosis Capitis

- Direct visualization of the parasite and nits
- It is possible to see if the nits are full (vital nits) or empty which helps determine the success or failure of treatment

Pediculosis Pubis

It is possible to easily see the parasite attached to adjacent pubic hairs or hairs at other sites (i.e., eyelashes)

Trichoscopy

- The use of dermoscopy to evaluate scalp skin and hair follicles
- Any form of dermoscopy can be used (polarized, nonpolarized, contact, noncontact with or without fluid)
- Structures that can be visualized include
  - Hair shafts
  - Hair follicle openings
  - Perifollicular epidermis
  - cutaneous microvasculature

Criteria seen with trichoscopy

- Anisotrichosis: hair diameter variability greater than 20%
- Black dots (cadaverized hairs): black dots inside follicular openings and represent fragmented and destroyed hair shafts
- Brown halo(peripilar sign): brown macules surround emergence of the hair shafts from the scalp (follicular ostia) secondary to inflammation
- Circle hairs: thin short vellus hairs that form a circle
- Coiled hairs: telogen/catagen broken hairs that coil back
- Comma hairs: short c-shaped broken hair shafts with ectothrix parasitization
- Corkscrew hair: short spiral shape broken hair shafts
- Coudability hairs: hairs of normal length with a narrow proximal shaft
- Empty follicles: skin-colored small depressions without hairs
- Exclamation mark hairs: tapered telogen hairs with dark thick tip at the level of the skin

- Follicular keratotic plugging: keratotic masses plugging follicular ostia
- Follicular red dots: erythematous concentric structures in and around follicular ostia representing dilated vessels and extravasated blood
- Hair tufting: multiple hairs (6) emerging from the same ostium
- Honeycomb network–like structures: created by homogeneous brown rings, not a true pigment network created by elongated and hyperpigmented rete ridges
- Peripilar casts: concentrically arranged scales encircling emerging hair shafts
- Peripilar sign: brown halo surrounding follicular opening caused by inflammation
- Peripilar white halo: gray-white halo surrounding follicular ostia created by fibrosis
- Twisted red loops: multiple red dots at low magnification (x10, x20) and polymorphous beaded lines at higher magnification (x40) representing capillaries in the papillary dermis
- White dots: interfollicular acrosyringia and follicular openings
- White patches: well-demarcated irregular white patches seen in scarring alopecia devoid of follicular openings
- Yellow dots: round or polycyclic yellow to yellow-pink dots representing infundibula plugged with sebum and keratin. May be devoid of hairs or contain miniaturized, cadaverized, or dystrophic hairs

ACQUIRED HAIR/SCALP DISEASES

Seborrheic Dermatitis vs. Psoriasis

- Vascular patterns help make the diagnosis
- Psoriasis has pinpoint or glomerular vessels similar to skin plaques
- Seborrheic dermatitis lacks pinpoint or glomerular vessels but has arborizing and polymorphous vessels

Tinea Capitis

- Patchy alopecia, erythema, scale, cervical/posterior auricular/occipital adenopathy
- Comma hairs
- Corkscrew hairs: more commonly seen in African-American children
- Black dots
- Broken and dystrophic hairs

Trichosporosis (Piedra)

- Superficial mycosis of the hair shafts
    - White piedra (*Trichosporon beigelii*, *Trichosporon inkin*)
    - Hair shafts coated with yellow to beige sheaths
    - Distal fusiform nodules
    - Black piedra (*Piedraia hortae*)
    - Dark nodules along the hair shafts

Trichomycosis Capitis

- *Corynebacterium* species
- Scalp, axilla, pubic hairs
- Yellow sheaths attached to the hair shafts

Androgenic Alopecia

- Anisotrichosis
- Brown halo (peripilar sign)
- Yellow dots
- Honeycomb network
- White dots
- Circle vellus hairs
- Empty follicles

Alopecia Areata

- Yellow dots
- Black dots (cadaverized hairs)
- Circle hairs
- Exclamation mark hairs (mostly along the edges of the patches of alopecia)
- Coudability hairs
- Clustered vellus hairs
- Pseudomonilethrix hairs characterized by constrictions in the hair shaft
- Multiple depressed follicular osteo
- Fibrosis with white dots in long-standing cases
- Alopecia Areata Incognito
    - Subtype of alopecia areata with rapidly developing diffuse alopecia
    - Mimics telogen effluvium
    - Diffusely distributed yellow dots
    - Large number of short growing hairs (2–4 mm)

Trichotillomania

- Coiled hairs (not seen in alopecia areata)
- Broken hairs with different lengths
- Black dots
- Yellow dots
- Absence of exclamation mark hairs characteristic of alopecia areata

Traction Alopecia

- Marginal alopecia
- Traction due to hair styles
- Common African-Americans
- Hair casts around hair shafts at the periphery

Trichorrhexis Nodosa

- Mechanical, chemical, thermal damage
- White nodules along the hair shafts
- Fractured and frayed ends have a brush-like appearance

Bubble Hair

- High temperature from hair styling
- Gas formation creates bubbles that appear as white oval spaces with a Swiss-cheese appearance

Trichoptilosis (Split Ends)

- Longitudinal splitting at the distal ends of the hair shafts
- Two or multiple frayed ends at different lengths

Scarring Alopecia

- Primary and secondary types (i.e., lichen planopilaris, frontal fibrosing alopecia, discoid lupus, folliculitis decalvans)
- Decreased hair density
- Pinpoint white dots (follicular and acrosyringeal openings)
- Loss of follicular openings
- Cicatricial white patches

Congenital Hair Shaft Abnormalities

Monilethrix

- Hair shaft beading
- Elliptical nodes (normal shaft diameter)
- Narrow internodes (dystrophic hairs)
- Elliptical nodes regularly separated by narrow internodes
- "Regular bended ribbon sign"
- Hair shafts bend regularly at multiple locations in different directions
- **Trichorrhexis invaginata** ("bamboo hair")
  - Seen in Netherton syndrome (autosomal recessive, ichthyosiform erythroderma, atopic diathesis, trichorrhexis invaginata)
  - Invagination of the distal portion of the hair shaft into its proximal portion forming a ball in cup appearance
  - Bamboo/golf tee/matchstick hairs

Pili Annulati

- Alternating light and dark bands are seen clinically
- Light bands represent air-filled cavities

Pili Torti

- Flattened hair shafts
- Twisting at irregular intervals

Pili Trianguli and Canaliculi

- "Uncombable hair" dry unruly hair
- Triangular or reniform hair shafts
- Flattened hairs with longitudinal groves

Pili Bifurcati and Multigemini

- Hair shafts grow from the same papilla
- Split from a single tip
- Double tip (bifurcati)
- Several tips (multigemini)

QUIZ

Questions

1. Which criteria can be used to diagnose a melanocytic lesion?

   A. Milia-like cysts and pigmented pseudofollicular openings
   B. Arborizing vessels, ulceration, and pigmentation
   C. A central white patch plus fine peripheral pigment network
   D. Lacunae and black homogenous blotches
   E. Pigment network, brown globules, homogeneous blue color, or parallel patterns

2. Diagnosing a melanocytic lesion by default means that:

   A. There are high-risk criteria at the periphery of the lesion that are hard to identify.
   B. There are criteria for a seborrheic keratosis or basal cell carcinoma associated with pigment network and brown globules.
   C. There is an absence of criteria to diagnose a melanocytic lesion, seborrheic keratosis, dermatofibroma, pyogenic granuloma, or ink spot lentigo; therefore, the lesion should be considered melanocytic.
   D. There is an absence of criteria to diagnose a melanocytic lesion, seborrheic keratosis, basal cell carcinoma, dermatofibroma, or hemangioma; therefore, the lesion should be considered melanocytic.
   E. None of the above.

3. Which criteria can be used to diagnose a seborrheic keratosis?

   A. Milky red areas, irregular streaks, and pigmented follicular openings
   B. Streaks, irregular blotches, and regression
   C. Furrows, ridges, sharp border demarcation, milia-like cysts, pseudofollicular openings, fat fingers, and hairpin vessels
   D. Rhomboid structures and/or circle within a circle
   E. Diffuse brown color, glomerular vessels, and milia-like cysts

4. Which criteria can be used to diagnose a basal cell carcinoma?

   A. Pigment network and arborizing vessels
   B. Arborizing and pinpoint vessels plus multifocal hypopigmentation
   C. The absence of a pigment network, arborizing vessels, pigmentation, ulceration, spoke-wheel structures
   D. Glomerular vessels, ulceration, and blue ovoid nests of pigmentation
   E. Islands of black blotches, arborizing vessels, and moth-eaten borders

5. Vascular lesions can contain the following criteria:

   A. Out-of-focus lacunae-like globules
   B. A variable number of red, sharply demarcated vascular spaces called lacunae and fibrous septae
   C. Ten to twenty major and minor lacunae and thromboses
   D. A minimal of 2 well-developed glomerular vessels
   E. Fibrous septae, peppering, and blue dark lacunae

6. Dermatofibromas can be associated with the following criteria:
   A. Pigment network, arborizing vessels, and central white patch
   B. A central white patch that is never located at the periphery
   C. A central white patch and peripheral pigment network
   D. A complete absence of blood vessels and a few milia-like cysts
   E. Multifocal hypopigmentation, arborizing vessels, and a central bluish white veil

7. Melanoma-specific criteria on the trunk and extremities can contain this combination of criteria:
   A. Asymmetry of color and structure, a cobblestone global pattern, and regular globules or blotches
   B. A multicomponent global pattern, symmetry of color and structure, regular network, regular globules, and regression
   C. Polymorphous vessels, arborizing vessels, 2 colors, and regular streaks
   D. Irregular network, irregular globules, irregular blotches, and regression
   E. Rhomboid structures and the parallel-ridge pattern

8. Dysplastic nevi typically have the following combination of criteria:
   A. Symmetry of color and structure and no melanoma-specific criteria
   B. Asymmetry of color and structure, irregular network, regular blotches, and regular streaks
   C. Multifocal regression, peppering, regular pigment network, regular dots and globules
   D. Pinpoint, arborizing, and glomerular vessels plus several melanoma-specific criteria
   E. Asymmetry of color and structure plus several melanoma-specific criteria

9. Which statement is true about Spitz nevi?
   A. They can have 10 different patterns.
   B. A Spitzoid lesion only refers to the starburst or pink patterns.
   C. Melanoma is not in the differential diagnosis of regular starburst pattern.
   D. In an adult, most Spitzoid lesions do not need to be excised.
   E. Symmetrical and asymmetrical starburst patterns can be seen in melanoma.

10. Which of the following statement best describes the criteria seen in superficial spreading melanomas?
    A. Criteria associated with a benign nevus are never seen.
    B. They contain several well-developed melanoma-specific criteria such as symmetry of color and structure and one prominent color.
    C. Usually they have several well-developed melanoma-specific criteria such as asymmetry of color and structure, multicomponent global pattern, regular network, regular globules, and regular streaks.
    D. They contain a variable number of melanoma-specific criteria such as asymmetry of color and structure, multicomponent global pattern, irregular local criteria, 5 or 6 colors, and polymorphous vessels.
    E. They are usually feature poor or featureless.

Answers

1. E. Criteria to diagnose a melanocytic lesion include any variation of pigment network (regular and/or irregular), multiple brown dots and/or globules, homogeneous blue color of a blue nevus, and parallel patterns seen on acral skin. The default category is the last way to diagnose a melanocytic lesion. Milia-like cysts and follicular openings can be seen in melanocytic lesions but are not primary criteria to make the diagnosis. Answers A, B, and C diagnose a basal cell carcinoma, dermatofibroma, and hemangioma.
2. D. Diagnosing a melanocytic lesion by default means that one does not see criteria for a melanocytic lesion, seborrheic keratosis, basal cell carcinoma, dermatofibroma, or hemangioma. Default is an absence of criteria. One has to memorize all the criteria from each specific potential diagnosis to be able to diagnose a melanocytic lesion by default. Dermoscopy cannot be mastered by osmosis. It is essential to study and practice the technique routinely in ones daily practice. Ink spot lentigo and pyogenic granuloma are not in this algorithm.
3. C. All the criteria used to diagnose seborrheic keratosis are commonly seen in daily practice. Melanoma-specific criteria can also be seen in atypical seborrheic keratosis. Beware of seborrheic keratosis–like melanomas. Milky red areas, irregular streaks, regression, rhomboid structures, and circle within a circle are all melanoma-specific criteria that are more sensitive and specific for melanoma but could be found in seborrheic keratosis. Glomerular vessels are a primary criterion to diagnose Bowen disease and are not seen in seborrheic keratosis.
4. C. Basal cell carcinomas are usually a clinical diagnosis and dermoscopy is used to confirm ones clinical impression (on the spot dermoscopic second opinion). By definition, if one sees pigment network, the lesion could not be a basal cell carcinoma. A subset of melanomas can be undistinguished from basal cell carcinoma with pigmentation and arborizing vessels. Pinpoint and glomerular vessels could be seen but they would be out shadowed by arborizing vessels. If not, one could be dealing with a

basal cell–like melanoma. Moth-eaten borders are seen in lentigines and flat seborrheic keratosis, never in basal cell carcinomas.

5. B. The hallmark of vascular lesions are lacunae, vascular spaces with well-demarcated sharp borders. There is no set number of lacunae needed to make the diagnoses. At times one has to use their imagination to decide if the margins fit the criteria for vascular spaces. Different shades of red, blue, and even black are typically seen. Black homogeneous color usually represents thrombosis. Major and minor lacunae do not exist. Fibrous whitish septae and/or bluish white color are routinely seen in typical hemangiomas. At times it is not possible to differentiate lacunae and red color of a hemangioma from the milky red areas that can contain out-of-focus reddish globules seen in melanoma.
6. C. Dermatofibromas are ubiquitous benign tumors and in most cases dermoscopy is not needed to make the diagnosis. A central white patch and pigment network the primary criteria to make the diagnosis may or may not be present. It might not be possible to differentiate an atypical dermatofibroma from a melanoma if melanoma-specific criteria are identified. There are innumerable ways that the central white patch can appear, and in many cases it is not centrally located. Telectangietatic vessels with polymorphous shapes are commonly seen but basal cell–like arborizing vessels would make the diagnosis of a dermatofibroma unlikely.
7. D. Irregularity is the name of the game if criteria are to be considered melanoma specific. Melanoma-specific criteria can be seen in both benign and malignant pathology but are more sensitive and specific for melanoma. There is not a single melanoma-specific criterion that is pathognomonic for melanoma. One should learn their definitions and study as many classic textbook examples as possible. Rhomboid structures help diagnose melanoma on the face and the parallel-ridge pattern can be seen in acral melanomas.
8. E. Dysplastic nevi are ubiquitous in the light-skinned population and can be indistinguishable clinically and dermoscopically from melanoma. They usually look more benign than malignant with dermoscopy; however, there are melanomas that do not have well-developed melanoma- specific criteria. Vessels of any kind are not typically seen except in pink feature poor dysplastic nevi. They can have a variable number of melanoma- specific criteria (e.g., irregular pigment network, irregular dots and/or globules, irregular blotches) that are not as well developed as those seen in melanoma. Streaks, regression, and many colors are not usually seen and should raise a "red flag" of concern that the lesion might be a melanoma.
9. E. Spitzoid lesions are always a "red flag" for concern. Even symmetrical patterns can be seen in melanoma. There are only 6 patterns (starburst, globular, homogeneous, pink, black network, atypical). One often has to use their imagination to diagnose a Spitzoid lesion. Since symmetrical and asymmetrical Spitzoid patterns can be found in melanoma, they should all be excised in children as well as in adults. A dermatopathologist that specializes in melanocytic lesions is good, while one that has expertise in Spitzoid lesions is ideal. Even experienced dermatopathologists have trouble differentiating atypical Spitzoid lesions from melanoma, and atypical Spitzoid lesions have the potential to metastasize to regional lymph nodes and kill the patient.
10. D. Superficial spreading melanoma can have it all as far as the spectrum of melanoma-specific criteria goes. The criteria can be well developed or difficult to identify. Criteria associated with benign melanocytic lesions can also be seen. The more high-risk criteria identified in the lesion, the greater the chance that one is dealing with a melanoma. Nodular and amelanotic melanoma are more likely to be feature poor or featureless.

REFERENCES

Argenziano G et al. Dermoscopy features of melanoma incognito: indications for biopsy. *J Am Acad Dermatol* 2007;56(3):508–513.

Argenziano G et al. Dermoscopy of pigmented skin lesions. Results of a consensus meeting via the internet. *J Am Acad Dermatol* 2003;48:679–693.

Argenziano G et al. Vascular structures in skin tumors: a dermoscopy study. *Arch Dermatol.* 2004;140:1485–1489.

Blum A, Simionescu O, et al. Dermoscopy of pigmented lesions of the mucosa and mucocutaneous junction. *Arch Dermatol* Oct 2011;147(10):1181–1187.

Bowling J et al. Dermoscopy key points: recommendations from the international dermoscopy society. *Dermatology* 2007;214: 3–5.

Cari P et al. Improvement of the malignant/benign ratio in excised melanocytic lesions in the dermoscopy era: a retrospective study 1997–2001. *Br J Dermatol* 2004;150(4):687–692.

Haliasos EC, Kerner M, et al. Dermoscopy for the pediatric dermatologist part 1:dermoscopy of pediatric infectious and inflammatory skin lesions and hair disorders. *Pediatr Dermatol* Mar-Apr 2013;30(2):163–171.

Haliasos EC, Kerner M, et al. Dermoscopy for the pediatric dermatologist part 2: dermoscopy of genetic syndromes and cutaneous manifestations of pediatric vascular lesions. *Pediatr Dermatol* Mar-Apr 2013;30(2):172–181.

Haliasos EC, Kerner M, et al. Dermoscopy for the pediatric dermatologist part 3: dermoscopy of melanocytic lesions. *Pediatra dermatol* May-Jun 2013;30(3):281–293.

Jaimes N, Chen L, et al. Clinical and dermoscopic characteristics of desmoplastic melanoma. *JAMA Dermatol* Apr 2013; 149(4):413–421.

Johr, RH: Pink lesions. *Clin Dermatol* 2002;20:289–296.

Johr RH, Stolz W: *Dermoscopy: An Illustrated Self-Asessment Guide.* New York: McGraw Hill; 2010.

Kittler H et al. Diagnostic accuracy of dermoscopy. *Lancet Oncol* 2002;3:159–165.

Kittler H et al. Identification of clinically featureless incipient melanoma using sequential dermoscopy imaging. *Arch Dermatol* 2006;142(9):1113–1119.

Malvehy J, Puig S, Braun R, Marghoob A, Kopf AW: *Handbook of Dermoscopy*. London: Taylor and Francis; 2006.

Marghoob AA, Malvehy J, Braun PR, eds. *Atlas of Dermoscopy*, 2nd Ed. Informa Heathcare: London; 2012.

Menzies SW, Kreusch J, et al. Dermoscopic evaluation of amelanotic and hypomelanotic melanoma. *Arch Dermatol* Sep 2008; 144(9):1120–1127.

Menzies SW, Moloney FJ, et al. Dermoscopic evaluation of nodular melanoma. *JAMA Dermatol* Jun 2013;149(6):699–709.

Miteva M, Tosti A: Dermoscopy of hair shaft disorders. *J Am Acad Dermatol* Mar 2013;68(3):473–481.

Miteva M, Tosti A: Hair and scalp dermoscopy. *J Am Acad Dermatol* Nov 2012;67(5):1040–1048.

Stanganelli I, Argenziano G, et al. Dermoscopy of scalp tumors: a multi-center study conducted by the international dermoscopy society. *J Eur Acad Dermatol Venerol* Aug 2012;26(8):953–963.

Stolz W et al. *Color Atlas of Dermatoscopy*, 2nd Ed. Berlin: Blackwell Publishing; 2002.

Tosti A: *Dermoscopy of Hair and Scalp Disorders: With Clinical and Pathological Correlations*. Informa Healthcare; 2007.

CHAPTER 32

REFLECTANCE CONFOCAL MICROSCOPY: THE ERA OF NONINVASIVE IMAGING

MARIGDALIA K. RAMIREZ-FORT
DANIEL GAREAU
SAMER JALBOUT
GIOVANNI PELLACANI

BASIC PRINCIPLES OF REFLECTANCE CONFOCAL MICROSCOPY

History

- The confocal microscope was invented by Marvin Minsky in 1957
- The reflectance confocal microscope (RCM) was later modified and commercialized with the use of a laser light source and spinning polygon mirror

Utility

- In vivo RCM produces real-time optical sections, parallel to the skin surface, that are less than 5 μm in thickness, with a lateral resolution of 0.5 to 1.0 μm
- The cellular resolution allows for in vivo visualization of histological manifestations in the epidermis and superficial dermis such as architecture, cell size, shape, and occasionally organelles

Optical Principles

- The RCM consists of: a point source of light; condenser and objective lenses, scanning optomechanical components (polygon and galvanometric mirrors) and a point detector
- Creating an image
  - A 30x water immersion objective lens microscope is coupled with water to the skin such that the refractive index remains consistent (water, $n = 1.33$; epidermis, $n = 1.34$) and that aberrations are minimized
  - The device utilizes 830-nm coherent laser light (5–10 mW) to focus on diffraction-limited tissue of 0.5 μm in diameter
  - When an image is initiated, the laser is deflected off of a polygon scan mirror and the focused light is scanned in the tissue
  - The light then travels sequentially back through the optics to a conjugate focal plane within the microscope that contains a pinhole detector
  - The image by the objective lens is sequentially translated into 2-dimensional images of 500 μm, which are further composited into mosaics of 8 × 8 images, visualizing an entirety of a 4 × 4 mm area of tissue
  - Total imaging depth of RCM in normal skin is 200 to 300 μm, that is, the level of papillary dermis and upper reticular dermis
- Contrast and reflectance
  - Contrast is endogenous

- The mechanism of reflectance involves detection of backscattering of light
  - Structures that are bright (highly reflective) contain: (1) components with high refractive index (n) compared with surroundings, or (2) are similar in size to the wavelength of light
  - Highly reflective components of the skin include
    - ▲ Melanin (n = 1.72)
    - ▲ Hydrated collagen (n = 1.43)
    - ▲ Keratin (n = 1.51)
- Cells containing increased amounts of granules such as cells in a hypermetabolic state (i.e., neoplastic cells, inflammatory cells) will also present with high reflectivity when compared to surrounding nonpigmented cells and structures

Keratinocytic Tumors

- Seborrheic keratosis
  - Very common, benign epidermal tumors typically occurring after the third decade of life
  - These neoplasms are usually found on the trunk and extremities; anatomic regions subjected to greater amounts of friction over time tend to develop more seborrheic keratoses
  - Clinical features
    - Morphology ranges from skin-colored flat-topped papules to dark brown plaques
    - The neoplasms tend to have a "stuck-on" appearance and are characteristically verrucoid, with our without follicular plugs
  - Dermoscopic findings: vary vastly and correlate with degree of acanthosis
    - White dots/clods ("milia") are seen throughout all degrees of acanthosis but increase in size and frequency with degree of acanthosis
    - Mild acanthosis
      - ▲ Pattern: reticular lines, thin curved lines, circles, and dots
      - ▲ Colors: brown, yellow, and orange
    - Moderate acanthosis
      - ▲ Pattern: thick curved lines, structureless, and clods
      - ▲ Colors
        - △ Heavily pigmented lesions: black, brown (rarely, blue or gray), and orange
        - △ Less pigmented lesions: orange, yellow, or skin colored
  - Findings by RCM (Fig. 32-1)
    - Anastomosing acanthotic cords in the superficial epidermis will demonstrate highly refractive gyri contrasted to the faintly refractive sulci giving rise to a brain-like aspect
    - Stratum spinosum typically shows numerous brightly refractile keratinocytes; the keratinocytes

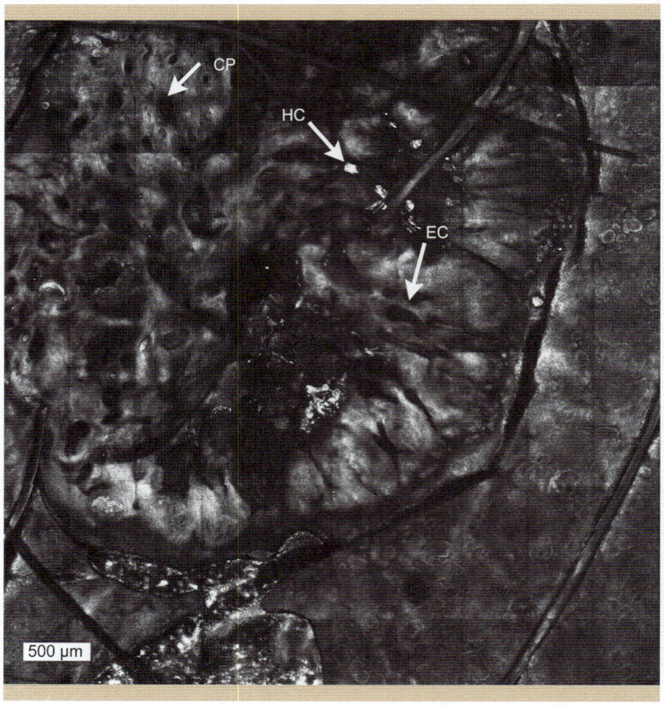

FIGURE 32-1 Seborrheic keratosis with corneal plugs (CP), horned cysts (HC), and elongated chords (EC). (*Used with permission from Giovanni Pellacani.*)

will demonstrate a regular cobblestone pattern (Note: Seborrheic keratoses tend to be more pigmented than surrounding normal skin, given the involved keratinocytes, greater refractive quality)
    - Dermal papillae at the dermal-epidermal junction (DEJ) may contain distorted papillary ring shape in the regular presentation—an enlargement of the papillary spaces is commonly present
    - Horn cysts appear as well defined, circular collections of brightly refractive material (keratin)
- Squamous neoplasia
  - Clinical features: rough, white hyperkeratosis on an erythematous base; lesions may erode and ulcerate
  - Dermoscopic findings: invasive squamous cell carcinoma is rarely pigmented, dermoscopically, the finding of numerous white circles is more suggestive of malignancy than the benign or precancerous counterparts (actinic keratosis and Bowen disease)
    - Patterns
      - ▲ Pigmented Bowen disease: structureless and dots arranged in lines,
      - ▲ Pigmented actinic keratosis: strucutureless, gray dots, white circles
    - Colors: brown, gray, pink (structureless)
    - Vessels: coiled vessels, clustered or arranged in lines
  - Findings by RCM (Fig. 32-2)
    - Superficial epidermis will demonstrate parakeratosis and detachment of keratinocytes

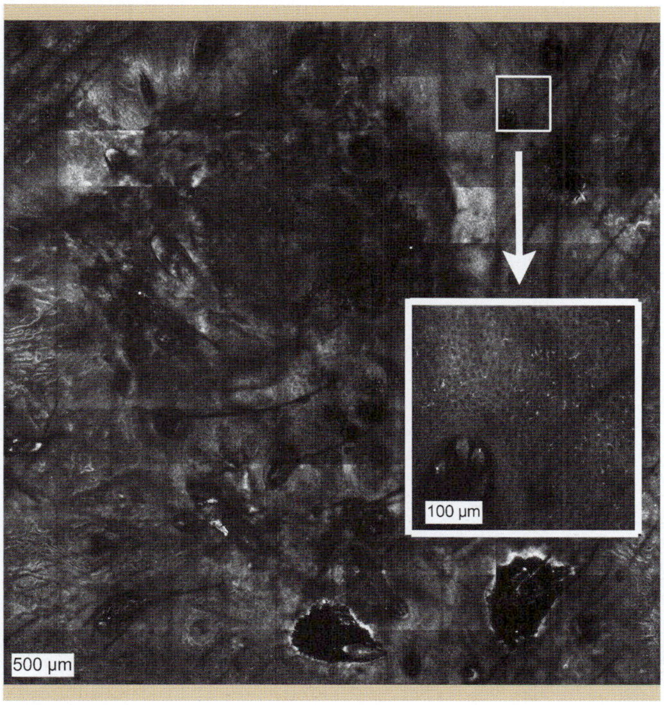

FIGURE 32-2 Squamous neoplasia: atypical honeycomb pattern outlined with broadened keratinocytes and cells of different size and shape (inset). Bright dots within keratinocytes correspond to inflammatory infiltrate (exocytosis). (*Used with permission from Giovanni Pellacani.*)

    - Frank disruption of cellular architecture and cellular pleomorphism are seen in the deeper epidermis (basal, spinous, and granular layers); degree of architectural disarray and cellular pleomorphism are the key features to determining a keratinocytic malignancy by RCM
    - The resolution of RCM is limited by depth; this limitation does not allow for direct evaluation of invasion across the DEJ
    - Inflammatory cells may be identified throughout the epidermis and dermis
- Basal cell carcinoma
  - Malignancy of the basal layer of keratinocytes
  - Occurs only on hair-bearing skin
  - Clinical features
    - More shiny (typically described as pearly) when compared to normal skin
    - Vascular neoplasms that bleed easily or may ulcerate
    - Malignant basal cells may be pigmented, presenting as a "pigmented basal cell carcinoma"
  - Dermoscopic findings
    - Pigmented basal cell carcinoma
      - ▲ Pigment patterns: blue or gray clods, radial lines that converge (reticular, branched, curved, and parallel lines are not seen in BCCs), blue or gray dots
      - ▲ Colors
        - △ Blue is the most common but brown, gray, and white may also be seen
        - △ Superficial malignant cells will appear brown; while deeper aggregates will appear blue
      - ▲ Blood vessels: these are highly angiogenic tumors; branching vessels or thin serpentine vessels are frequently encountered
  - RCM: findings are similar to the histopathology of these tumors (Fig. 32-3A-D)

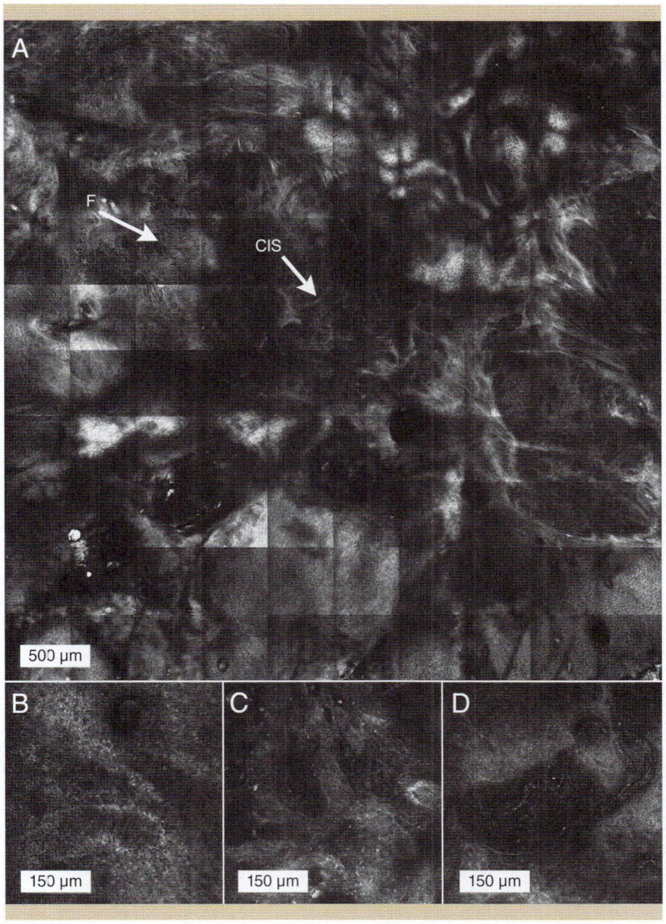

FIGURE 32-3 Basal cell carcinoma. (A) Discernable at the level of the superficial dermis, are bright tumor islands and dark silhouettes. (B) Here there is a lobulated bright basaloid island with a typical palisading structure as well as demarcated by surrounding cleft-like dark spaces; plump bright stellate structures (melanophages) are also visible. (C) Here we demonstrate elongated cord-like structures. (D) This figure demonstrates large vessels with blood cells and clearly visualizes the rolling of leukocytes. (*Used with permission from Giovanni Pellacani.*)

- Basal cells with large oval or elongated nuclei and scant cytoplasm arranged in nodules, islands, cords, or long strands
- Parakeratosis and mild disruption of keratinocytic architecture is noted throughout the epidermis
- An inflammatory infiltrate is typically identified in association to the aggregation of tumor cells
- Individual tumor cells frequently have peripheral palisading of nuclei
  - ▲ When the nuclei are organized along the same axis along the entire aggregate of tumor, they demonstrate streaming
  - ▲ When the nuclei are organized parallel to each other and perpendicular to the tumor aggregate, RCM visualizes peripheral palisading
- Increased angiogenesis and leukocyte trafficking is seen within the tumor; individual erythrocytes and leukocytes can be visualized in motion with the video capture feature

Melanocytic Tumors

- *Melanocytic nevi (Clark nevus and superficial congenital nevi): The common theme in evaluating benign nevi clinically, dermoscopically, or by RCM is that common nevi characteristically lack chaos and architectural disarray*
  - Clinical features
    - Clark nevi appear clinically as brown macules; there may be variation in shades of brown
    - Superficial congenital nevi appear clinically as lighter brown macules; may have hair
  - Dermoscopic findings
    - Patterns: reticular lines or small oval clods ("globules")
      - ▲ Clark nevi: often only reticular or with central structureless hyperpigmentation
      - ▲ Superficial congenital nevi: may also have reticular or branched lines; clods ("globules") are usually larger than in Clark nevi and may be light brown or skin colored
    - Colors: brown
      - ▲ Clark nevi: multiple shades of brown may be seen with central hyperpigmentation
      - ▲ Superficial congenital nevi: may be uniformly brown, have central hypopigmentation and white dots ("milia")
  - Findings by RCM (Figs. 32-4 and 32-5)
    - The resolution of RCM is limited by depth
      - ▲ The epidermis and superficial dermis are easily explored
      - ▲ Histopathological characterization of melanocytic tumors can be easily detected; however, evaluating certain benign entities such as Spitz nevi, deep penetrating nevi, and blue nevi, requires examination of the deeper dermis is necessary but is often not feasible

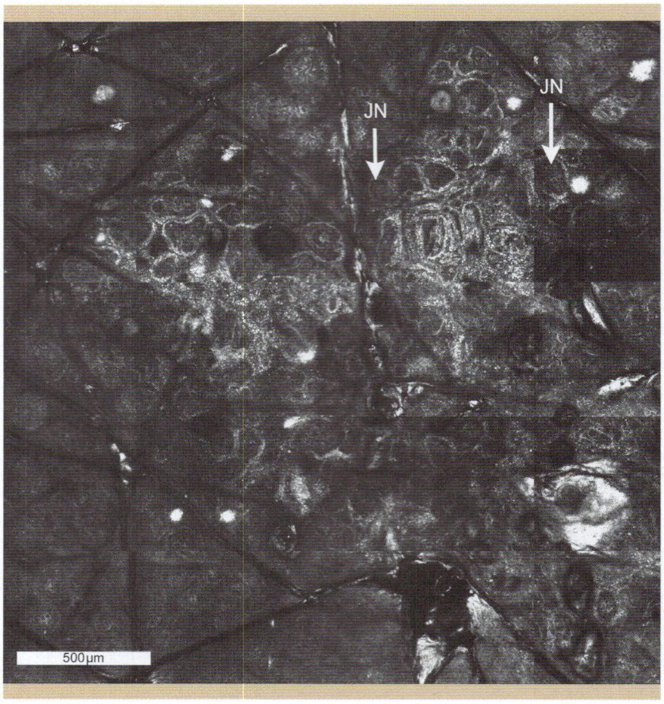

FIGURE 32-4 Junctional nevus at the dermal epidermal junction that appears symmetric and regular with ringed and edged papillae; junctional nests (JN) are found bulging into papillae openings. (*Used with permission from Giovanni Pellacani.*)

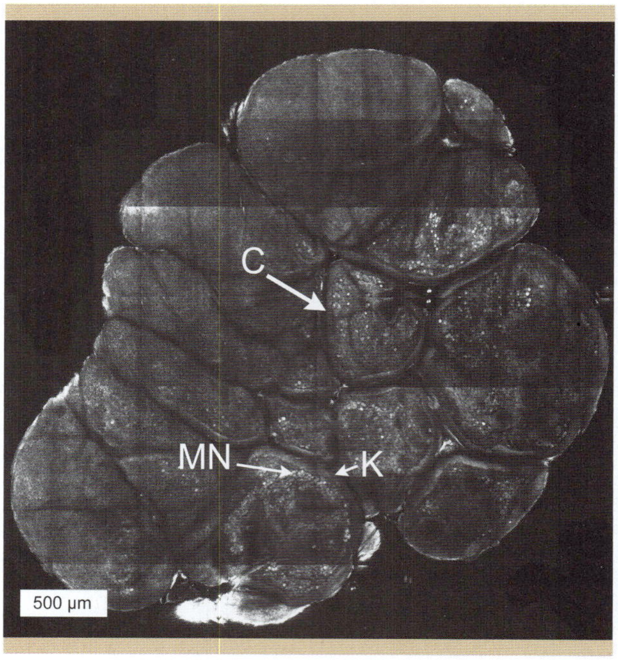

FIGURE 32-5 Intradermal nevus with grouped melanocytic nests (MN) or melanocytic clusters composing a general architecture of clods (C); each MN is separated by thin epidermal cristae. (*Used with permission from Giovanni Pellacani.*)

- Benign nevi display regular epidermal architecture
  - ▲ Individual keratinocytes in the superficial epidermis and deeper epidermis appear in 1 of 2 patterns: honeycomb (nonpigmented) or cobblestone (pigmented) patterns
  - ▲ Dermal papillary rings are all regular in size, shape, and distribution; in some nevi, these may be further characterized as "edged" papillae, caused by an accumulation of pigment in the keratinocytes and melanocytes lining the sides of the rete ridges
- Individual melanocytes are typically dispersed along the DEJ and appear as small polygonal cells, often not distinguishable from pigmented keratinocytes, with a highly refractile cytoplasm
- Nests of melanocytes appear as a refractile group or cluster of cells that are relatively uniform in size, shape, and distribution—these are typically encountered within or adjacent to the papillary rings, or forming ovoidal structures that enlarge the interpapillary spaces

- Malignant melanoma
  - Clinical features
    - Pigmented or nonpigmented (amelanotic) macules or papules with asymmetrical shape or color, with or without ulceration
  - Dermoscopic findings: any pattern or color may be found in a melanoma; typically all melanomas have more than 1 pattern or color arranged asymmetrically ("chaos")
    - Clues (adopted from Dr. Harald Kittler's revised pattern analysis)
      - ▲ Eccentric structureless zones of any color (except skin color)
      - ▲ Gray circles, lines, dots, or clods
      - ▲ Black dots or clods at the periphery
      - ▲ Segmental pseudopods or segmental radial lines at the periphery
      - ▲ White lines
      - ▲ Thick reticular lines
      - ▲ Polymorphous vessels
      - ▲ Parallel lines on the ridges
  - Findings by RCM (Fig. 32-6A-D)
    - Regular epidermal architecture of honeycomb or cobblestone patterns may be disrupted
    - Atypical melanocytes, including pagetoid melanocytes, may be encountered along the entire depth of the epidermis; these atypical melanocytes are characterized as large bright round cells with or without dendritic processes (note: irritated nevi, Spitz-Reed nevi, and dysplastic nevi may have benign pagetoid melanocytes as well—meaning that each of the individual features mentioned should be evaluated in the context of the entire lesion)

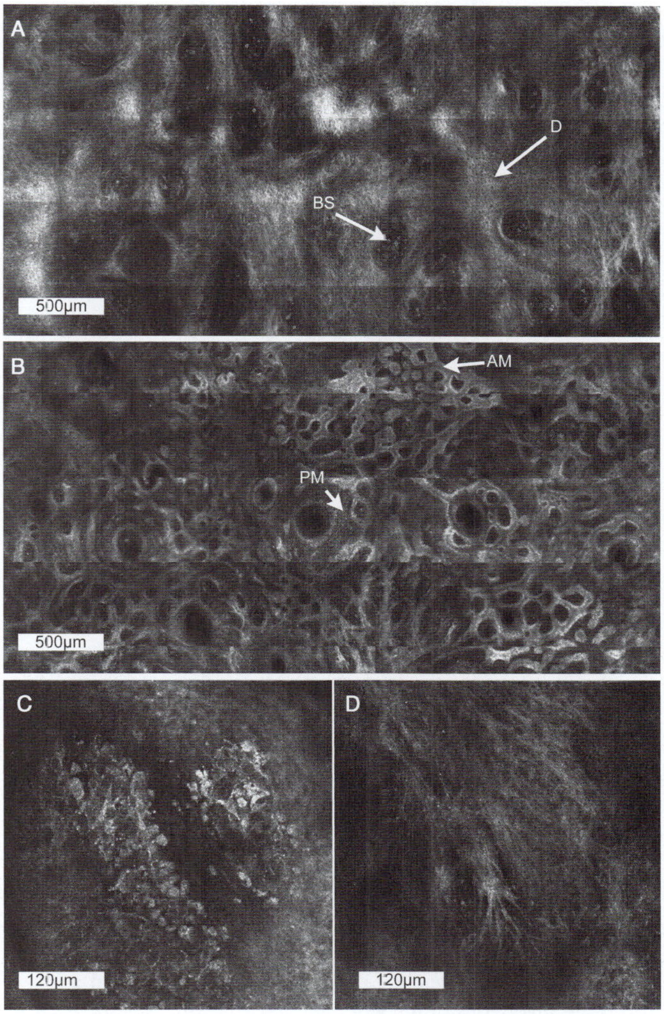

FIGURE 32-6 Malignant melanoma. (A) Superficial spreading melanoma with obvious disarray of the epidermal architecture; bright spots (BS) are noted within the papillae which signify hyper-reflective neoplastic melanocytes. (B) Malignant melanoma with an atypical meshwork (AM); pleomorphic dendritic (PM) and roundish cells are found throughout the tumor. (C) Here we see disarray of epidermal architecture with cellular aggregates that are irregular in size and distribution; note the dense aggregates of large atypical pagetoid cells. (D) The hyper-reflective tracts are found within the dermis; these correspond to atypical and thickened collagen fibers. (*Used with permission from Giovanni Pellacani.*)

- The dermal papillae may be disrupted and separated by large reflecting cells, termed nonedged papillae
- Melanocytic nests lose homogeneity and present as cell clusters with loose, chaotic morphology and

marked difference in size and shape of cells; the clusters are not equidistant from each other
- One may also encounter a sheet-like arrangement of melanocytes

Clinical Applications of Reflectance Confocal Microscopy

- The utility and clinical applications of RCM are continuously undergoing scrutiny for its use in
  - Aiding clinical and dermoscopic diagnosis
  - Guiding biopsies and margin mapping
  - Assessment of response to treatment

QUIZ

Questions

1. What is the approximate maximum depth of visualization of skin structures by confocal microscopy?
   A. 20-50 microns (epidermis)
   B. 200-250 microns (upper dermis)
   C. 500-1000 microns (deeper dermis)
   D. more than 2 mm (subcutis)

2. Which of the following descriptions corresponds to atypical keratinocytes in epithelial tumors visualized by confocal microscopy?
   A. Irregular honeycombed pattern, with poligonally shaped cells variable in size and shape and with pleomorphic nuclei
   B. Irregular cobblestone pattern, with bright large and nucleated cells
   C. Complete disarrangement of the epidermis with absence of any pattern
   D. Presence of amorphous material in the epidermal layers

3. Identify the following structures specific for the diagnosis of basal cell carcinoma:
   A. Dense and sparse nests
   B. Polycyclic papillary contours
   C. Islands and/or cords with palisading
   D. Meshwork pattern at the dermal epidermal junction

4. Confocal microscopy is most likely to detect the following features of a melanocytic nevi:
   A. Single melanocytes at the junction because of their dendritic appearance
   B. Melanocytic nests at the junction and in the upper dermis
   C. Nevocyte maturation
   D. Eumelanin and pheomelanin formation

5. The most characteristic confocal features of a melanoma are:
   A. Presence of large bright nucleated cells in the epidermis and atypical melanocytes in a disarranged junctional architecture
   B. Lack of maturation with depth
   C. Presence of mitoses
   D. Ulceration and neoangiogenesis

Answers

1. B. 200-250 microns (upper dermis)
2. A. Irregular honeycombed pattern, with poligonally shaped cells variable in size and shape and with pleomorphic nuclei
3. C. Islands and/or cords with palisading
4. B. Melanocytic nests at the junction and in the upper dermis
5. A. Presence of large bright nucleated cells in the epidermis and atypical melanocytes in a disarranged junctional architecture

REFERENCES

Ackerman AB, Kerl H, Sanchez J: A Clinical Atlas of 101 Common Skin Diseases. *Ardor Scribendi* 2000, www.derm101.com.

González S, Tannous Z: Real-time, in vivo confocal reflectance microscopy of basal cell carcinoma. *J Am Acad Dermatol* Dec 2002;47(6):869–874.

Guitera P, Menzies SW, Longo C, Cesinaro AM, Scolyer RA, Pellacani G: In vivo confocal microscopy for diagnosis of melanoma and basal cell carcinoma using a 2-step method: analysis of 710 consecutive clinically equivocal cases. *J Invest Dermatol* 2012;132(10):2386–2394. E-Pub 2012.

Kittler H, Rosendahl C, Cameron A, Tschandl P, eds. *Dermatoscopy.* Facultas Verlags- und Buchhandels AG: Australia; 2011.

Langley RG, Burton E, Walsh N, Propperova I, Murray SJ: In vivo confocal scanning laser microscopy of benign lentigines: comparison to conventional histology and in vivo characteristics of lentigo maligna. *J Am Acad Dermatol* Jul 2006;55(1):88–97.

Minsky M: Memoir on inventing the confocal scanning microscope. Scanning 1988;10:123–128.

Pellacani G, Cesinaro AM, Longo C, Grana C, Seidenari S: Microscopic in vivo description of cellular architecture of dermatoscopic pigment network in nevi and melanomas. *Arch Dermatol* 2005;141(2):147–154.

Pellacani G, Cesinaro AM, Seidenari S: In vivo assessment of melanocytic nests in nevi and melanomas by reflectance confocal microscopy. *Mod Pathol* 2005;18:469–474.

Pellacani G et al. The impact of in vivo reflectance confocal microscopy for the diagnostic accuracy of melanoma and equivocal melanocytic lesions. *J Invest Dermatol* 2007;127:2759–2765.

Pellacani G et al. In vivo confocal microscopy for detection and grading of dysplastic nevi: a pilot study. *J Am Acad Dermatol* 2011;66:e109–121.

Pellacani G et al. Spitz nevi: In vivo confocal microscopic features, histopathologic correlates and diagnostic significance. *J Am Acad Dermatol* 2009;60:236–247.

Rajadhyaksha M, Anderson RR, Webb RH: Video-rate confocal scanning laser microscope for imaging human tissues in vivo. *Appl Opt* 1999;38:2105–2115.

Rajadhyaksha M, Gonzalez S, Zavislan JM, Anderson RR, Webb RH: In vivo confocal scanning laser microscopy of human skin II: advances in instrumentation and comparison with histology. *J Invest Dermatol* 1999;113(3):293–303.

Rajadhyaksha M, Grossman M, Esterowitz D, Webb RH, Anderson RR: In vivo confocal scanning laser microscopy of human skin: melanin provides strong contrast. *J Invest Dermatol* 1995;104(6):946–52.

Rishpon A et al. Reflectance confocal microscopy criteria for squamous cell carcinomas and actinic keratoses. *Arch Dermatol* Jul 2009;145(7):766–72.

Scope A et al. In vivo reflectance confocal microscopy of shave biopsy wounds: feasibility for intraoperative mapping of cancer margins. *British J Dermatol* 2010;163:1218–1228.

CHAPTER 33

RADIOLOGIC FINDINGS

RIVA Z. ROBINSON,
SANA HASHMI,
MARIGDALIA K. RAMIREZ-FORT,
GUSTAVO PANTOL

Radiologic findings of various cutaneous disorders are organized and presented as follows (Table 33-1):

- Vesicular and bullous
- Connective tissue
- Cornification
- Hair and nails
- Hematologic
- Infectious
- Infectious, fungal
- Inflammatory
- Malignant potential
- Metabolic
- Pigmentation
- Vascular
- Other

TABLE 33-1 Radiological Findings in Skin Diseases and Related Conditions

Disease	Etiology	Clinical Features	Radiologic Findings
Vesicular and Bullous			
Junctional epidermolysis bullosa (Herlitz syndrome/epidermolysis bullosa letalis)	Autosomal recessive Defect in $\alpha6\beta4$-integrin	Generalized bullae, perioral granulation tissue, absent/shed nails, dysplastic teeth, respiratory edema	Pyloric atresia
Dermatitis herpetiformis	IgA against epidermal transglutaminase	Pruritic symmetric papules, vesicles, and occasionally bullae on extensor surfaces. Associated with Celiac disease	Atrophy of haustra in colon and ileum; atrophic spleen; Secondary hyperparathyroidism.
Pemphigus variants (vulgaris, paraneoplastic, erythematosus)	IgG against keratinocyte surface components: desmoglein 3 in vulgaris, multiple antigens in paraneoplastic, desmoglein 1 in erythematosus	Flaccid intraepidermal blisters	Pemphigus vulgaris: rarely intrathoracic solitary benign lymphoma (Castleman tumor) Paraneoplastic pemphigus: non-Hodgkin lymphoma Pemphigus erythematosus: sacroiliitis

TABLE 33-1 Radiological Findings in Skin Diseases and Related Conditions (Continued)

Disease	Etiology	Clinical Features	Radiologic Findings
Connective Tissue			
Buschke-Ollendorff syndrome (connective tissue nevus syndrome)	Autosomal dominant	Dermatofibrosis lenticularis disseminata, juvenile elastomas; involvement of phalanges, carpals, metacarpals most common	Osteopoikilosis
Ehlers-Danlos syndrome	Autosomal dominant Autosomal recessive (types VI and VIIC) Defective collagen (type V most commonly affected) and proteins involved in collagen production	Skin hyperextensibility, cigarette paper texture to scars, hypermobile joints; congenital dislocation of the hip (types I, IV, VIIA, and VIIB); kyphoscoliosis in type VI; dermatosparaxis in type VIIC	Mitral valve prolapse and aortic root dilation; wide joint spaces, arthrochalasis (abnormal joint laxity), calcified subcutaneous tissue
Goltz syndrome (focal dermal hypoplasia)	X-linked dominant Defect of PORCN gene	Fat herniation; cutaneous papillomas; punctate atrophy with telangiectasias in lines of Blaschko	Osteopathia striata (linear vertical opacities in metaphyses of the bones); lobster claw deformity of the hand
Lipoid proteinosis (hyalinosis cutis et mucosae, Urbach-Wiethe disease)	Autosomal recessive Defect of ECM gene	Hoarse cry at birth; early bullae with later pearly papules on face, eyelid, neck, mucosa, and extremities; alopecia, parotiditis, large wooden tongue, abnormal teeth, seizures	"Bean bag" hippocampal calcifications in the temporal lobe; deposits in vocal cords and other laryngeal structures; thickening of trachea and main stem bronchus
Marfan syndrome	Autosomal dominant Defect of fibrillin-1	Abnormalities of ocular, skeletal, and cardiovascular systems; abnormal dermal collagen architecture on electron microscopy	Kyphoscoliosis; pectus excavatum (depression of sternum), pectus carinatum (projection of sternum); mitral valve prolapse and aortic root dilation
Pseudoxanthoma elasticum	Autosomal dominant and recessive forms Defect in ABCC6 gene	Yellow pebbling of skin	Mitral valve insufficiency, and coronary artery disease, peripheral vascular disease; gastric or duodenal hemorrhage
Cornification			
Chondrodysplasia punctata (Conradi-Hünermann-Happle syndrome)	X-linked dominant Defect in emopamil-binding protein (EBP or 3β-hydroxysteroid-δ8-δ7-isomerase)	Ichthyosiform erythroderma in Blaschko lines, patchy alopecia, asymmetric focal cataracts	Stippled epiphyses (chondrodysplasia punctata), unilateral limb shortening, scoliosis
Congenital hemidysplasia with ichthyosiform and limb defects (CHILD)	X-linked dominant Defect in NSDHL gene encoding 3β-hydroxysteroid-dehydrogenase	Unilateral ichthyosiform erythroderma	Ipsilateral hypoplasia of limbs, bones and organs

(Continued)

TABLE 33-1 Radiological Findings in Skin Diseases and Related Conditions (Continued)

Disease	Etiology	Clinical Features	Radiologic Findings
Schimmelpenning syndrome	Unknown	Sebaceous nevi; seizures and mental deficiencies; colobomas and optic nerve defects	Frontal bossing, kyphoscoliosis, limb deformities; hemimegalencephaly, dysmyelination, cortical agyria
Palmoplantar keratoderma with periodontosis (Papillon-Lefévre syndrome)	Autosomal recessive Defect in cathepsin C	Palmoplantar keratoderma, psoriasiform hyperkeratotic plaques on elbows/knees, periodontitis, gingivitis	Calcification of dura mater; premature loss of deciduous teeth and sometimes permanent dentition
Hair and Nails			
Hypohidrotic ectodermal dysplasia (Christ-Siemens-Touraine syndrome)	X-linked recessive (ectodysplasin gene) Autosomal dominant (*EDAR* gene)	Smooth, dry skin; hypo/anhidrosis with concomitant pyrexia	Hypodontia or dental abnormalities (peg-shaped teeth)
Menkes syndrome (occipital horn syndrome)	X-linked recessive Defect of *ATP7A* gene	Pili torti, doughy skin; occipital horns develop from ectopic bone formation within the aponeuroses of the posterior neck muscles	Elongated and tortuous vessels, subdural hematomas, tumors and cysts of the epidermis and epidermal appendages, occipital bone calcium deposits; delayed myelination of white matter
Nail patella syndrome	Autosomal dominant Defect in LMX1B gene (chromosome 9q34)	Dysplastic nails (triangular lunula), nephropathy (may be subclinical), Lester iris (hyperpigmentation of pupillary margin), renal dysplasia	Hypoplastic or absent patellae; posterior iliac horns (Fong syndrome when isolated finding), renal calcifications, radial head dislocation
Cartilage-hair hypoplasia (McKusick syndrome)	Autosomal recessive, combined immunodeficiency	Cartilage hypoplasia (dwarfism), sparse fragile hair, small nails, hyperextensible digits, thin white skin	Widened sclerotic metaphysis of tubular bones; scoliosis, genu varum, joint laxity
Hematologic			
DiGeorge syndrome	Sporadic zinc finger anomaly TBX1 gene	Congenital absence of thymus and parathyroid; abnormal aorta, hypocalcemia, tetany; recurrent fungal and viral infections, cardiac problems most common cause of death	Absent thymic shadow
Fanconi syndrome (familial pancytopenia)	Autosomal recessive	Pigment abnormalities, severe anemia, thrombocytopenia, hyperreflexia, retinal hemorrhage, testicular hypoplasia	Radial aplasia or hypoplasia, absent thumbs

(Continued)

TABLE 33-1 Radiological Findings in Skin Diseases and Related Conditions (Continued)

Disease	Etiology	Clinical Features	Radiologic Findings
Infectious			
Congenital syphilis, early	*Treponema pallidum*	Clinical manifestations exhibited at birth or shortly thereafter	Epiphysitis of long bones (pain on motion, Parrot pseudoparalysis), osteochondritis, sawtooth lesion on x-ray in the metaphyses, onion skin periosteal reaction
Congenital syphilis, late	*Treponema pallidum*	Late skeletal findings usually manifest in the latter half of the first decade or in the second decade	Knee perisynovitis (Clutton joints), bulldog jaw (mandibular protuberance), gummas (skull, long bones), saber shins (anterior bowing of tibia), Higoumenaki sign (unilateral hyperostosis of the medial clavicle), scaphoid scapulae (concavity of vertebral border of scapulae)
Infectious, Fungal			
Aspergillosis	*Aspergillus* species	Disseminated disease seen in immunocompromised patients; saprophytic colonization in immunocompetent hosts	Aspergilloma: pulmonary nodule within a cavity. Semi-invasive aspergillosis: pulmonary nodules, consolidation. Invasive aspergillosis: pulmonary nodules, consolidation, fluid level within a cavity. Sinus disease, parenquimal lesions in the brain.
Blastomycosis	*Blastomyces dermatitis*	Atypical pulmonary disease with skin and bone involvement	Mass-like consolidation and lung nodules predominately in the upper lungs. Cavitations are common.
Coccidioidomycosis	*Coccidioides immitis*	Desert rheumatism, arthralgia; erythema multiforme or erythema nodosum may occur	HEAD: ring enhancing lesions, meningeal enhancement, vasculisits with infarcts. CHEST: Consolidations, nodules, cavitations, mediastinal or hilar adenopathy, pleural effusions
Cryptococcosis	*Cryptococcus neoformans*	Found in avian excreta and soil, may coexist with sarcoid	CHEST: Patchy air-space opacities, pulmonary nodules, cavitations, mediastinal lymphadenopathy, pleural effusions. HEAD: dilated perivascular spaces, parenchymal lesions, leptomeningeal enhancement.

(Continued)

TABLE 33-1 Radiological Findings in Skin Diseases and Related Conditions (Continued)

Disease	Etiology	Clinical Features	Radiologic Findings
Histoplasmosis	*Histoplasma capsulatum Histoplasma capsulatum var. duboisii*	Oral disease, Addision disease from adrenal infiltration	CHEST Histoplasmoma: large lung nodule. Acute: patchy airspace opacities. Disseminated: miliary pattern. Chronic: fibrosis, bullae and chronic opacities predominately in the upper lobes. HEAD: ring enhancing lesions, meningeal enhancement, vasculisits with infarcts.
Mucormycosis	*Rhizomucor Absidia Rhizomucor Rhizopus*	Often immunocompromised (organ transplantation, diabetic)	Invasive sinusitis.
Mycetoma (Madura foot)	Fungal or actinomycete infection of the subcutaneous tissue	Inoculation of foot with draining sinus formation and gross deformity	Soft tissue mass, bone erosion, osseous distortion. Extension to adjacent bones. Sinus disease.
Nocardiosis	*Nocardia asteroides*	Opportunistic infection	Consolidations, nodules, cavitations, reticulonodular opacities, pleural effusion. HEAD: parenchymal lesions.
Paracoccidioidomycosis	*Paracoccidioides brasiliensis*	Most common in Latin American countries, poor hygiene, malnutrition	Ground-glass opacities, centrilobular nodules, cavitations.
Inflammatory			
Dermatomyositis (Fig. 33-1)	Some association with various HLA subtypes	Proximal muscle weakness, Gottron papules, heliotrope rash, periungual telangiectasias	Osteoporosis, calcinosis, subcutaneous calcification; interstitial opacities.
Kawasaki syndrome (mucocutaneous lymph node syndrome)	Likely infectious cause	Most common in Japan; 5 of 6 criteria need to be met for diagnosis (fever unresponsive to antibiotics, conjunctivitis, erythema/edemas of palms, oral lesions, polymorphous eruption, cervical lymphadenopathy	Coronary artery aneurysm; coronary artery calcifications
Morphea	Likely autoimmune-induced inflammation	Localized scleroderma	Infiltration of skin, fascia, musculature, and bone with melorheostosis type bone lesions.
Reiter syndrome (reactive arthritis)	HLA-B27 increases susceptibility	Develops after enteric infections; seronegative spondyloarthritis, sacroiliitis	Enthesopathy, bone lucency, new bone formation; feet are involved with relative sparing of hands

(Continued)

TABLE 33-1 Radiological Findings in Skin Diseases and Related Conditions (Continued)

Disease	Etiology	Clinical Features	Radiologic Findings
SAPHO syndrome	Unknown	Eponym for the combination of synovitis, acne, pustulosis, hyperostosis, and osteitis	Sternoclavicular hyperostosis, osteolysis. Vertebral body sclerosis, endplate erosions, joint space narrowing. Long bones: aggressive type lesion with lucency and sclerosis.
Sarcoidosis	Unknown	Granulomatous multisystem disorder	Bilateral hilar adenopathy, interstitial pulmonary infiltrates, osteolytic lesions, dactylitis; splenomegaly, renal and bone involvement may be seen. Neurosarcoid: meningeal disease, parenchymal lesions, optic chiasm, infundibulum and cranial nerve lesions.
Psoriasis	Immune mediated inflammation, dysregulation of keratinocyte function and vascular structure. Th17 and Th1 cells are important	Erythematous papules and plaques with silver scale. Can have genital and nail involvement	Peripheral arthropathy with erosive changes predominately in the DIP joints, "pencil in cup" deformities of the fingers, acrosteolysis, sacroiliitis.
Gianotti- Crosti (papular acrodermatitis of childhood)	Association with viral infection (Epstein-Barr virus [EBV] and Hepatitis B virus [HBV] most commonly)	Self-limited nonpruritic, erythematous papules; may have lymphadenopathy or joint involvement (can progress to rheumatoid arthritis)	Generalized lymphadenopathy, persists for months after skin lesions have resolved; hepatosplenomegaly, polyarticular disease
Malignant Potential			
Cockayne syndrome (Fig. 33-2)	Autosomal recessive Defect in DNA helicase	Cachectic dwarfism, long limbs, contractures, photosensitivity, progressive neural degeneration, deafness, retinitis pigmentosum, cataracts, dental caries	Intracranial calcifications (Fig. 33-2) Thickened skull, microcephaly, normal pressure hydrocephalus, dysmyelination
Cowden disease	Autosomal dominant Defect in PTEN gene	Tricholemmomas, oral papillomas; Increased risk breast and thyroid cancer	Breast lesions; hamartomatous polyps; ovarian cysts; goiter
Dyskeratosis congenita	X-linked recessive Defect in dyskerin gene	Reticulated pigmentation of skin, dystrophic nails, premalignant oral leukoplakia	Pulmonary fibrosis
Gardner syndrome	Autosomal dominant Defect in AP C gene (β-catenin)	Epidermoid cysts, fibromas, desmoid tumors	Osteomas; odontomas/ supernumerary teeth, hyperostosis, thyroid tumors, intestinal adenomatous polyps

(*Continued*)

TABLE 33-1 Radiological Findings in Skin Diseases and Related Conditions (Continued)

Disease	Etiology	Clinical Features	Radiologic Findings
Gorlin-Goltz (basal cell nevus syndrome) (Fig. 33-3) (Fig. 33-4) (See also Chap. 23)	Autosomal dominant Defect in PATCHED1 gene	Basal cell carcinomas, palmoplantar pits, frontal bossing, medulloblastomas, ovarian fibromas, fibrosarcoma; Albright sign: short fourth metacarpal (Fig. 33-3)	Odontogenic jaw cysts, calcification of falx cerebri (Fig. 33-4), bifid ribs, kyphoscoliosis, long bone cysts
Peutz-Jeghers syndrome	Autosomal dominant Defect of STK11 gene	Periorificial mucocutaneous melanocytic macules (lentigenes)	Intestinal hamartomatous polyps most numerous in the jejunum and ileum
Metabolic			
Alkaptonuria (Fig. 33-5)	Autosomal recessive Deficiency of homogentisic acid oxidase	Blue-black discoloration of sclera and cartilage (ochronosis); dark sweat/urine/cerumen, arthropathy (large joints); deafness	Spine: osteoporosis, vertebral disc calcifications, calcification of anterior and posterior longitudinal ligaments. Joint space narrowing with fragmentation and osseous collapse of large joints.
Calcinosis cutis	Calcium deposition without bone formation	Three main types: dystrophic (damaged tissue with normal calcium/phosphorus levels); metastatic (normal tissue with abnormal calcium and phosphorous levels); idiopathic (no tissue damage or metabolic disorder)	Visceral and nonvisceral calcification; depends on type of cutaneous calcinosis
Gaucher disease	Autosomal recessive Deficiency of glucocerebrosidase	Type I (adults): hyperpigmentation, hepatosplenomegaly, lymphadenopathy, pancytopenia Type II (infancy): hepatosplenomegaly, rapid neurologic deterioration, chronic aspiration, pneumonia; bone marrow: Gaucher cells ("crumpled tissue paper")	Splenomegaly, osteoporosis bone infarcts, avascular necrosis of femoral head, Erlenmeyer flask deformity of long bones, periosteal new bone formation
Gout	Deposition of monosodium urate crystals	Tophi on helix of ears, elbows, fingers and toes	Soft-tissue tophi may calcify; juxta-articular punched out lytic lesions most frequent at the 1st metatarsophalangeal joint.
Graves disease (Fig. 33-6)	Hyperthyroidism due to TSH receptor stimulating autoantibodies	Diffuse goiter, exophthalmos, and dermopathy (pretibial myxedema)	Enarlgement of extraocular muscles, more common affecting the inferior medial and superior rectus muscles. (Fig. 33-6), increased orbital fat, optic nerve compression at the apex. Radioactive iodine uptake test: diffusely increased uptake

(*Continued*)

TABLE 33-1 Radiological Findings in Skin Diseases and Related Conditions (Continued)

Disease	Etiology	Clinical Features	Radiologic Findings
Hepatolenticular degeneration (Wilson disease)	Autosomal recessive Defect of ATB7B gene	Liver cirrhosis and failure; Kayser-Fleisher rings on cornea	Changes in the putamen and caudate nuclei may be found from copper deposition; osteoporosis and "fringed" appearance of articular surfaces; cirrhosis
Hypophosphatasia	Autosomal recessive, deficiency in alkaline phosphatase and defective osteogenesis	Symmetric skin dimples, early loss of teeth, arthritis	Metaphyseal dysplasia, osteopenia, bowing of long bones, "Erlenmeyer flask deformity"
Pigmentation			
Albright hereditary osteodystrophy (McCune-Albright syndrome)	Postzygotic mutation Defect in GNAS1 gene encoding alpha subunit of G stimulatory protein that regulates adenylate cyclase	"Coast of Maine" café-au-lait macules, precocious puberty, endocrine abnormalities (hyperthyroidism); dimpling over the metacarpophalangeal joints (Albright sign)	Polyostotic fibrous dysplasia, recurrent fractures, bowing of limbs, limb-length discrepancies, bone cysts, sclerosis at skull base; often with associated area of pigmentation
Hypomelanosis of Ito (incontinentia pigmenti achromians)	Unknown	Marbled cake hypopigmentation in Blaschko lines, seizures	Musculoskeletal abnormalities; asymmetry
Incontinentia pigmenti (Bloch-Sulzberger syndrome)	X-linked dominant Defect of NEMO gene	Arrangement of lesions in lines of Blaschko; appearance depends on stage of development (vesicular, verrucous, hyperpigmentation, hypopigmentation)	Peg- or conical-shaped teeth; brain atrophy
Neurofibromatosis I (Fig. 33-7)	Autosomal dominant Defect in neurofibromin	Café-au-lait spots often manifest first; intertriginous freckling; optic glioma most common intracranial tumor; Lisch nodules in iris	Optic glioma sphenoid wing dysplasia, cortical thinning of long bones, bowing of the tibia (Fig. 33-7), tibial pseudoarthrosis, scoliosis
Neurofibromatosis II (Fig. 33-8) (Fig. 33-9)	Autosomal dominant Defect in merlin	Cutaneous schwannoma; usually no more than 6 café-au-lait spots	Schwannomas, multiple meningiomas and ependymomas.
Tuberous sclerosis	Autosomal dominant Defect in hamartin (Chap. 9) or tuberin (Chap. 16)	Ash-leaf hypopigmented patches, connective tissue tumors	Hamartomas at multiple sites; phalangeal cysts, periosteal thickening, periventricular calcifications, cortical tubers, subependymal hamartomas; angiomyolipomas, pulmonary lymphangiomatosis, cardiac rhabdomyoma

(Continued)

TABLE 33-1 Radiological Findings in Skin Diseases and Related Conditions (Continued)

Disease	Etiology	Clinical Features	Radiologic Findings
Vascular			
Hereditary hemorrhagic telangiectasia (Osler-Weber-Rendu disease)	Autosomal dominant Defect in endoglin gene or AK1 gene	Telangiectasias, epistaxis	Pulmonary arteriovenous malformations; liver, kidney, splenic lesions, and intracranial vascular malformations.
Proteus syndrome	PTEN gene	Symmetrical overgrowth; capillary malformations and subcutaneous masses	Bony overgrowth of the cranium of facial structures, soft tissue and bony hypertrophy
Ataxia-telangiectasia (Louis-Bar syndrome)	ATM gene	Oculocutaneous telangiectasias, progressive cerebellar ataxia; noninfectious cutaneous granulomas; xerosis, gray hair	Sinopulmonary infections, thymus maldevelopment, subnormal bone age
Blue rubber bleb nevus syndrome (Bean syndrome)	Unknown	Multiple small, blue, rubbery lesions on palms/soles	GI venous malformation with endoscopy
Klippel-Trenaunay-Weber	Possibly due to persistent embryologic veins	Capillary-lymphaticovenous malformation, usually in lower extremity; Parkes-Weber variant: arteriovenous fistulas, high-output heart failure	Underlying bone and soft-tissue hypertrophy, varicosities, thromboses, destructive bone lesions, limb hypertrophy and abnormalities, compensatory scoliosis
Maffucci syndrome (enchondromatosis with hemangioma)	Unknown	Grapelike superficial and deep venous malformations (rarely malignant); between 15 and 30% of enchondromas transform to chondrosarcomas	Multiple enchondromas (phalanges, long bones), fractures, bowing, limb length discrepancies; phleboliths in hemangiomas; Ollier disease: multiple enchondromas without hemangiomas
Sturge-Weber (encephalotrigeminal angiomatosis)	Unknown	Facial capillary malformations (port-wine stain), seizures, hemiparesis, choroidal malformations, glaucoma	Tram track (double contour) calcifications of cerebral cortex, leptomeningeal angiomatosis; underlying soft-tissue and skeletal hypertrophy
Kaposi sarcoma	Angioproliferative disorder caused by HHV-8	Purple or dark macules, plaques, and nodules that may ulcerate; may also have associated lymphedema; can involve mucosa of mouth and GI tract	Bilateral pulmonary infiltrates in bronchovascular pattern; thickened septae between lobules; nodules within fissures; may have pleural or pericardial effusions or lymphadenopathy

(Continued)

TABLE 33-1 Radiological Findings in Skin Diseases and Related Conditions (Continued)

Disease	Etiology	Clinical Features	Radiologic Findings
Other			
Dermoid cyst	Sequestration of skin along embryonic closure lines	Present at birth on the head and neck most commonly	MRI to diagnose intracranial or intramedullary cysts
Langerhans cell histiocytosis (Figs. 33-10 to 33-12)	Unknown	Crusted purpuric papules and a scaly seborrheic-like eruption in the scalp and groin	Letterer-Siwe: honeycomb lung involvement with cystic cavities (Fig. 33-10); floating teeth, osteolytic bone lesions; Hand-Schüller-Christian: "punched out" osteolytic skull lesions (Fig. 33-11); eosinophilic granulomas in bones (Fig. 33-12)
Multicentric reticulohistiocytosis	Unknown	Destructive polyarthritis	Resorption of subchondral bone, arthritis mutilans, accordion hand (shortening of fingers and mutilation)
Rosai Dorfman disease (sinus histiocytosis with massive lymphadenopathy)	Non-Langerhans cell proliferative histiocyte disorder, possibly related to EBV	Yellow or purple macules, papules, nodules, or infiltrated plaques; associated with fever, cervical adenopathy, neutrophilia, polyclonal γ globulinemia	Massive lymphadenopathy; may involve CNS, bone, or salivary glands

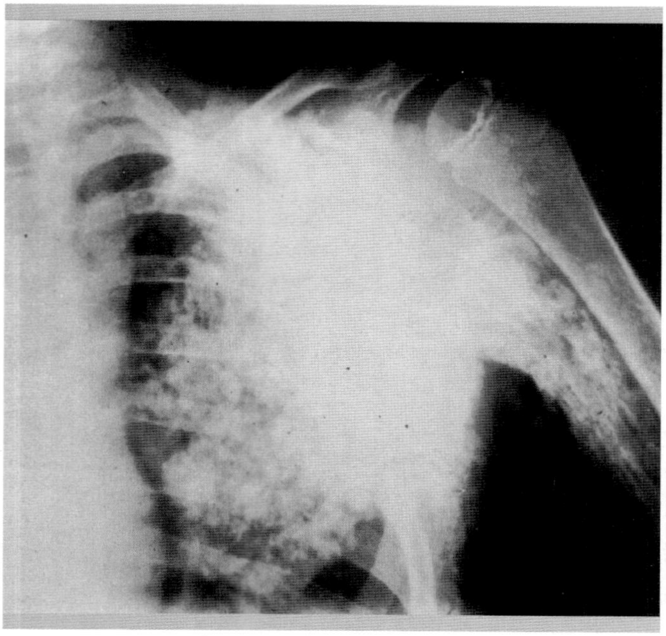

FIGURE 33-1 Dermatomyositis. (*Reprinted with permission from Freedberg IM et al. Fitzpatrick's Dermatology in General Medicine, 6th Ed. New York: McGraw-Hill; 2003.*)

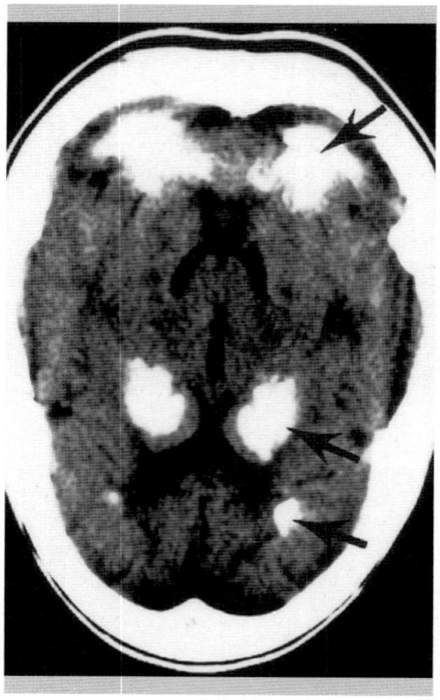

FIGURE 33-2 Intracranial calcifications of Cockayne syndrome. (*Reprinted with permission from Freedberg IM et al. Fitzpatrick's Dermatology in General Medicine, 6th Ed. New York: McGraw-Hill; 2003.*)

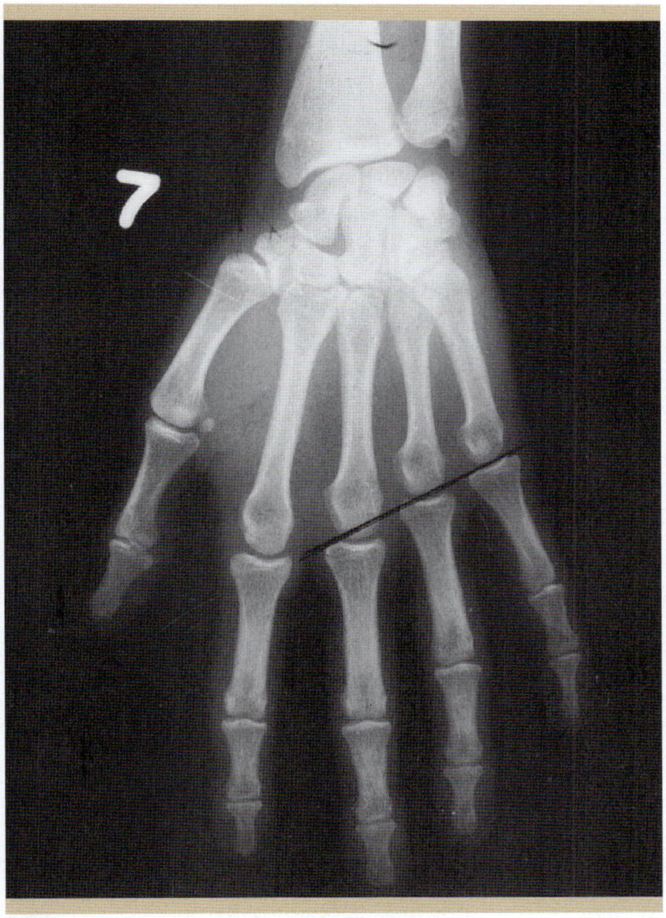

FIGURE 33-3 Albright sign of basal cell nevus sydrome. (*Reprinted with permission from Freedberg IM et al. Fitzpatrick's Dermatology in General Medicine, 6th Ed. New York: McGraw-Hill; 2003.*)

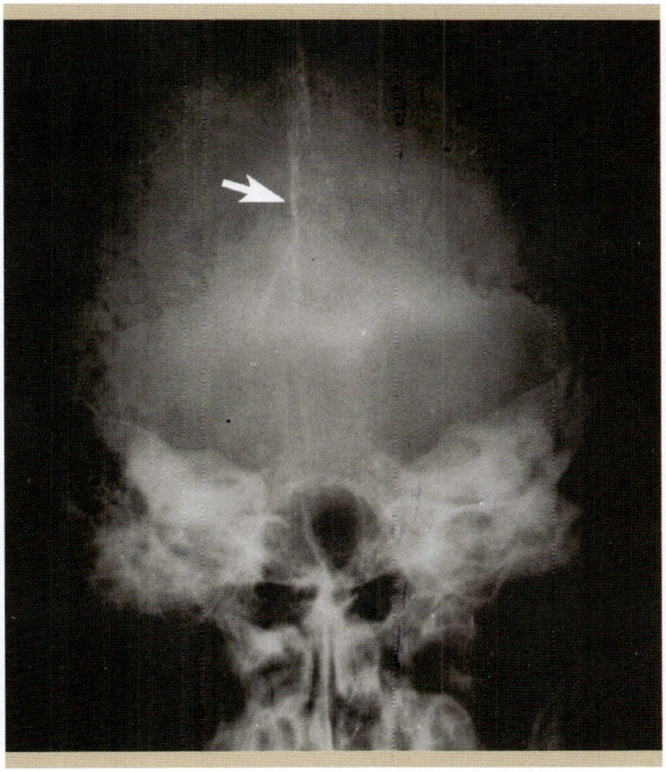

FIGURE 33-4 Calcification of falx cerebri in basal cell nevus syndrome. (*Reprinted with permission from Freedberg IM et al. Fitzpatrick's Dermatology in General Medicine, 6th Ed. New York: McGraw-Hill; 2003.*)

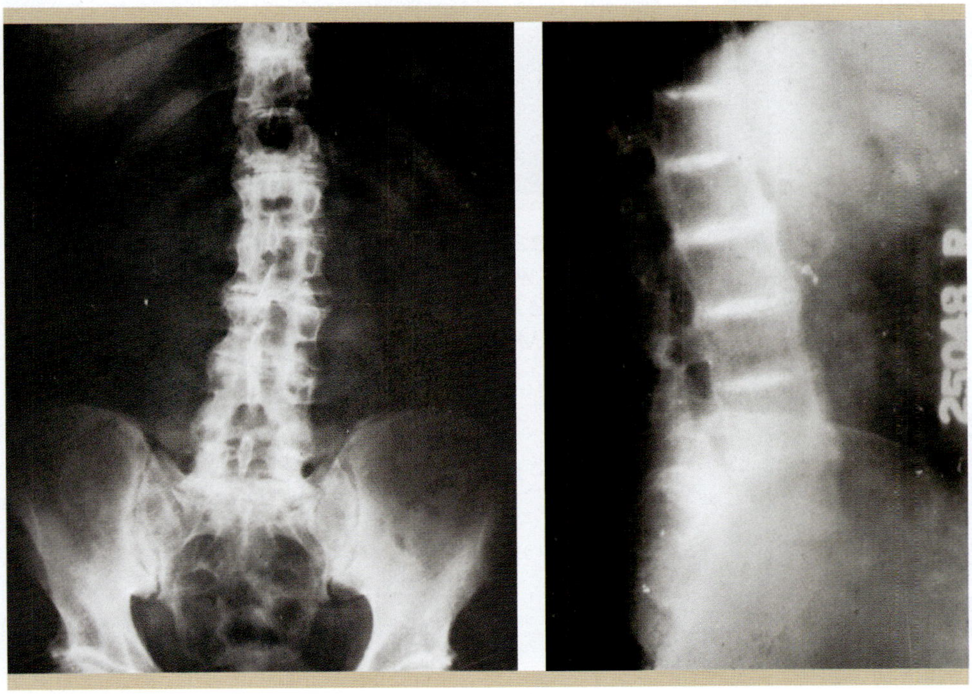

FIGURE 33-5 Radiologic findings in an alkaptonuric patient showing aortic and vertebral disk calcification. (*Reprinted with permission from Goldsmith LA et al. Fitzpatrick's Dermatology in Internal Medicine, 8th edition. New York: McGraw-Hill; 2012.*)

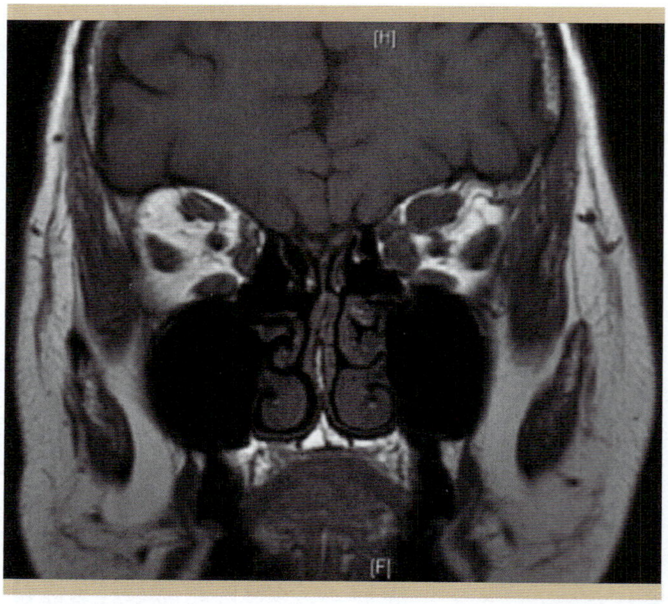

FIGURE 33-6 Head MRI shows thickening of the left superior and middle rectus muscle in a patient with thyroid ophthalmopathy.

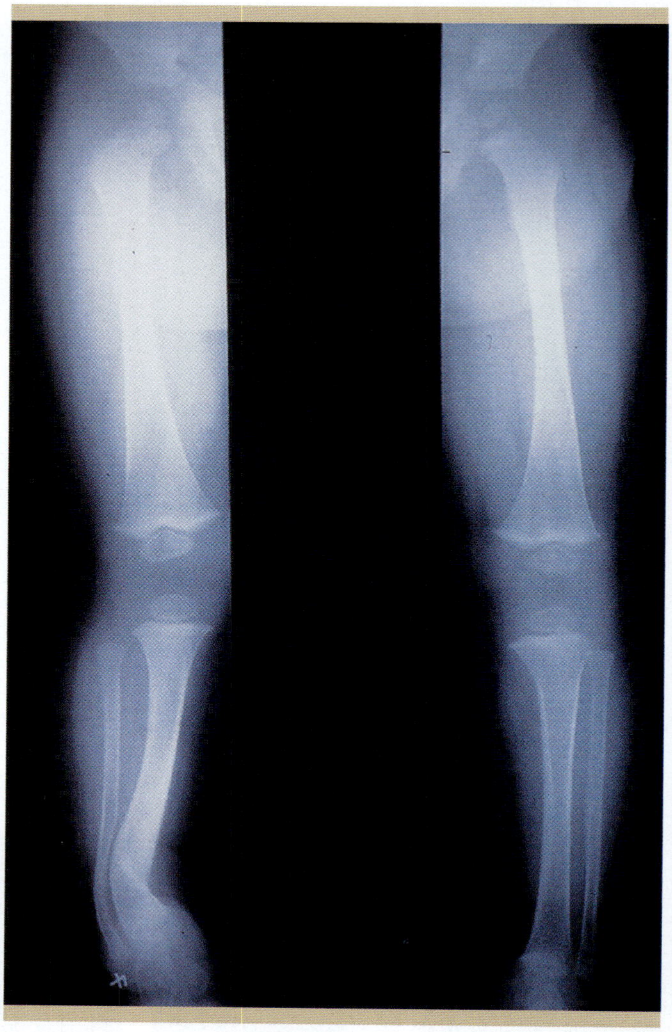

FIGURE 33-7 Tibial bowing seen in neurofibromatosis. (*Reprinted with permission from Freedberg IM et al. Fitzpatrick's Dermatology in General Medicine, 6th Ed. New York: McGraw-Hill; 2003.*)

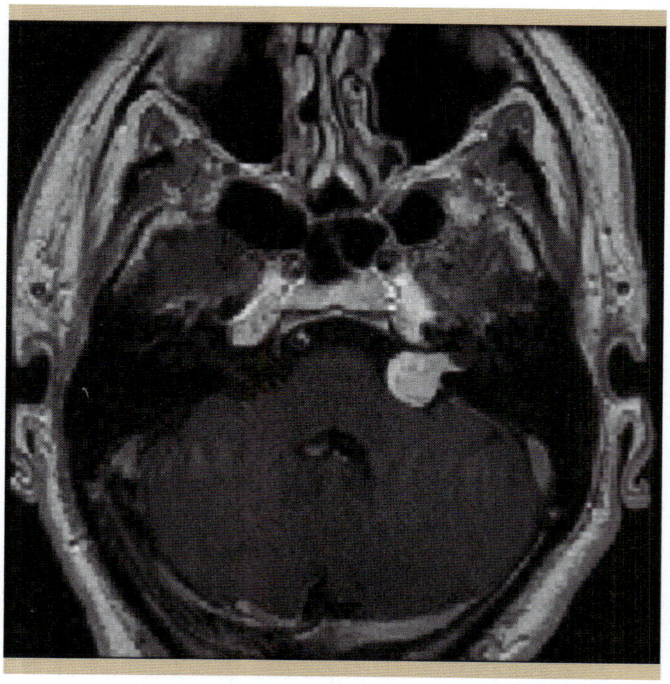

FIGURE 33-8 NF2, vestibular schwannoma.

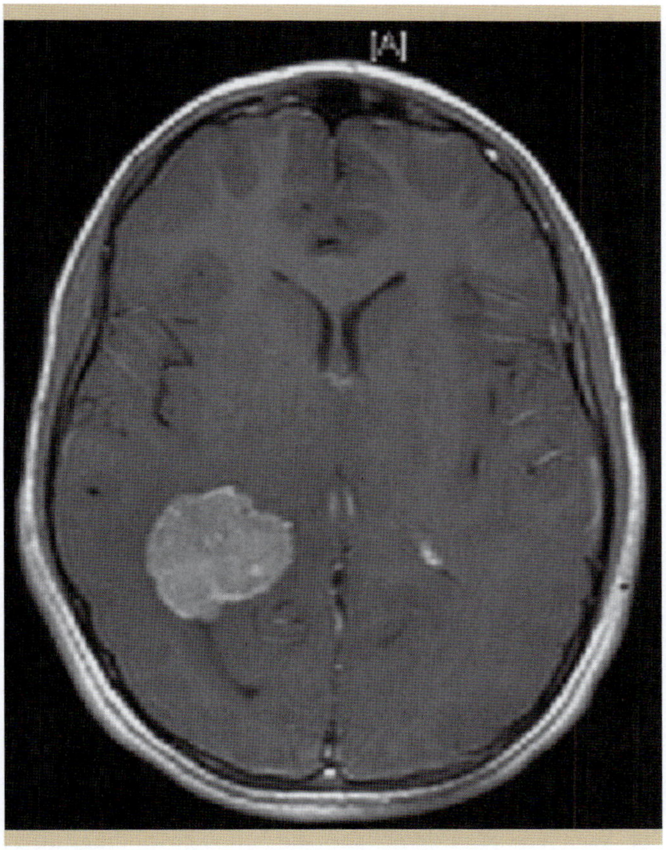

FIGURE 33-9 NF2, ventricular meningioma.

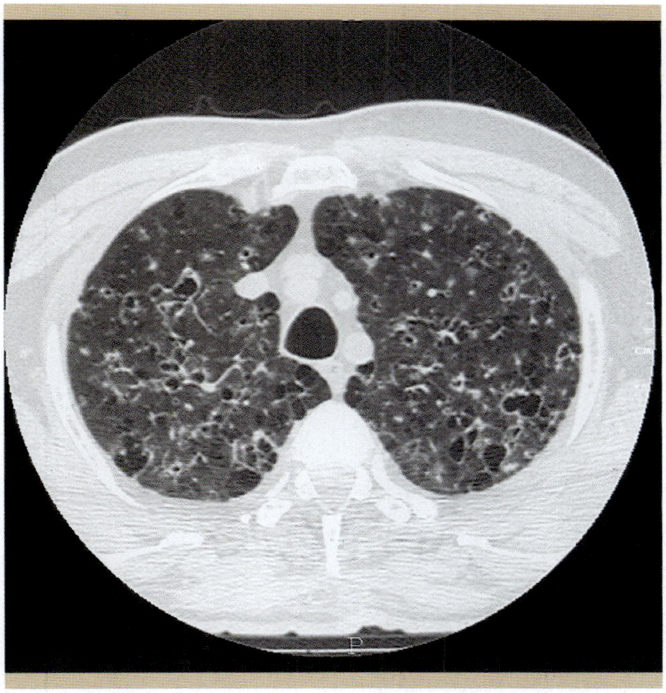

FIGURE 33-10 Letterer-Siwe disease, "honeycomb lung." (*Used with permission from E. De Juli, MD. Reprinted from Goldsmith LA et al. Fitzpatrick's Dermatology in Internal Medicine, 8th Ed. New York: McGraw-Hill; 2012.*)

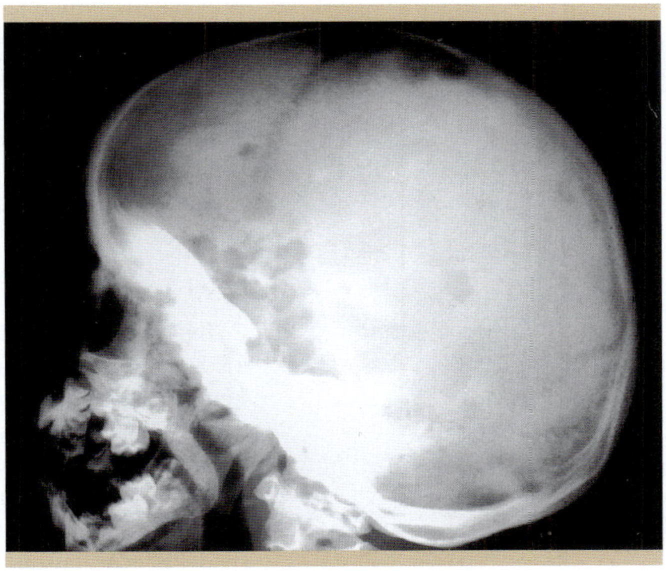

FIGURE 33-11 Hand-Schüller-Christian disease, osteolytic skull lesions. (*Reprinted with permission from Goldsmith LA et al. Fitzpatrick's Dermatology in Internal Medicine, 8th Ed. New York: McGraw-Hill; 2012.*)

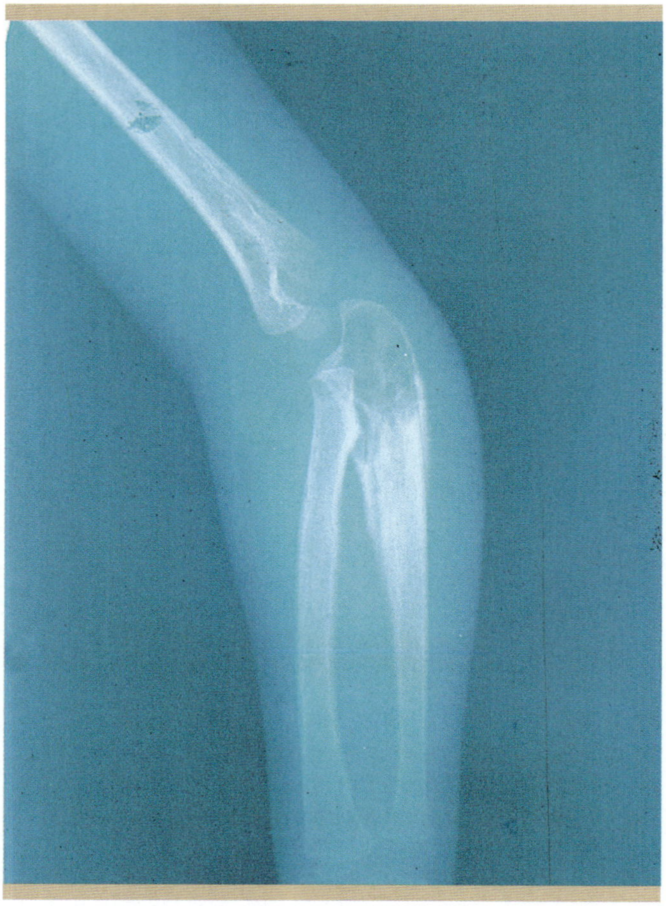

FIGURE 33-12 Eosinophilic granulomas. (*Reprinted with permission from Wolff et al. Fitzpatrick's Dermatology in Internal Medicine, 7th Ed. Mcgraw-Hill; 2008.*)

QUIZ

Questions

Use the following answer choices for the following set of questions:

A. Pyloric atresia
B. Osteopoikilosis
C. Honeycomb bone destruction
D. Stippled epiphyses
E. Absent patella and posterior iliac horns
F. Absent thymic shadow
G. Aplasia of radius
H. Coronary artery aneurysm and coronary artery calcifications
I. Odondogenic jaw cysts and calcification of falx cerebri
J. Intervertebral disk calcification
K. Erlenmeyer flask deformity of long bones
L. Polyostotic fibrous dysplasia
M. "Bullhead" sign in sternocostoclavicular region
N. Angiomyolipoma and rhabdomyoma
O. Enchondromas
P. Hamartomatous polyps of the jejunum and ileum
Q. Arthritis mutilans and accordion hand
R. Bean bag hippocampal calcification
S. "Whisker sign" on nuclear bone scan
T. Atrophy of colonic haustra

1. Which description matches the radiologic findings for a patient with draining sinus formation and gross deformity of the foot?
2. Which description matches the radiologic findings for a condition that may be indistinguishable from chronic osteomyelitis, hypervitaminosis A, and retinoid use?
3. Which description matches the radiologic findings for a patient with periorificial mucocutaneous melanocytic macules?
4. Which description matches the radiologic findings for a patient with lesions arranged in the lines of Blaschko that develop in stages from a vesicular, verrucous, hyperpigmented, then a final hypopigmented appearance?
5. Which description matches the radiologic findings caused by a defect in LMX1B gene (chromosome 9q34) and is associated with hyperpigmentation of the iris and renal dysplasia?
6. Which description matches the radiologic findings for a metabolic condition caused by a defect in homogentisic acid oxidase?
7. Which description matches the radiologic findings for a metabolic condition caused by the deficiency of alkaline phosphatase?
8. Which description matches the radiologic findings caused by a defect in emopamil binding protein?
9. Which description matches the radiologic findings for a patient with a connective tissue nevi with thickened elastin between normal collagen?
10. Which description matches the radiologic findings for a patient with a pruritic eruption of papules and vesicles on the extensor surfaces?

Answers

1. C. The condition is mycetoma (Madura foot), which follows traumatic inoculation of the foot with various fungal species or actinomycete bacteria. The organisms aggregate within abscesses and either drain onto the skin via sinus tracts or extend into the bones and joints causing osteomyelitis and arthritis.
2. M. The condition is SAPHO syndrome, which stands for synovitis, acne, pustulosis, hyperostosis, and osteitis. It is a rare condition of unknown etiology, mainly associated with hyperostosis of the anterior chest, palmoplantar pustulosis, hidradenitis suppurativa, and acne fulminans. As bone pain is a major symptom, prolonged retinoid use, hypervitaminosis A, and chronic osteomyelitis may also be suspected.

3. P. The condition is Peutz-Jeghers syndrome, an autosomal dominant condition caused by a defect of the STK11 gene. Patients have periorificial mucocutaneous melanocytic macules (lentigenes) and intestinal hamartomatous polyps that are most numerous in the jejunum and ileum. In contrast, Gardner syndrome patients have adenomatous polyps of the intestine, osteomas, supernumerary teeth, hyperostosis, and thyroid tumors.
4. O. The condition is incontinentia pigmenti, which is also known as Block-Sulzberger syndrome. It is an X-linked dominant disorder with a mutation in the NF κB essential modifier (NEMO) gene, and it may also be associated with brain atrophy. The lesions develop along the lines of Blaschko and progress in appearance from vesicular, to verrucous, hyperpigmented, and a final hypopigmented stage.
5. E. Caused by a defect in the LMX1B gene, this autosomal dominant disease is characterized by dystrophic nails without ridging, absent patellae, hyperpigmentation of the iris (Lester iris), renal dysplasia. Fong syndrome occurs with the iliac horns are present without any other abnormalities.
6. S. Metabolic condition caused by deficiency in homogentisic acid oxidase, causing oxidized homogentisic acid pigment to be deposited throughout body. Clinically, patients have cutaneous ochronosis, arthritis, and urine that darkens when exposed to light. Imaging shows osteoporosis. On the spine, articular cartilage is weakened, leading to prolapsed intervertebral disks. When imaged with nuclear bone scans, there is high uptake that extends from these disks laterally, giving the "whisker sign."
7. K. Autosomal recessive metabolic condition caused by alkaline phosphatase deficiency. It is characterized by skin dimpling, metaphyseal dysplasia, bowing of long bones, and early loss of teeth. Classic findings include the Erlenmeyer flask deformity on bones caused by defective mineralization and often multiple fractures or pseudofractures of long bones.
8. D. Chondrodysplasia punctata (Conradi-Hünermann-Happle syndrome) is an X-linked dominant disorder characterized by ichthyosiform erythroderma in Blaschko lines, patchy alopecia, and asymmetric focal cataracts.
9. B. Patients present with connective tissue nevus characterized by thickened elastic fibers in between normal collagen in the reticular dermis, as well as fibroblasts with large endoplasmic reticulum. Patients may also have osteopoikilosis caused by groups of tightly bound bony trabeculae and can be mistaken for bone metastases.
10. T. Often associated with Celiac disease (gluten sensitive enteropathy), the pruritic eruption is thought to be secondary to IgA deposits within the skin. Using contrast studies, atrophy of the colonic haustra or ileal villi may be present. Other radiologic findings include atrophic spleen and various hot spots on skeletal scintigraphy due to secondary hyperparathyroidism induced bone changes.

REFERENCES

Blauvelt A, Ehst B: *Pathophysiology of Psoriasis,* in UpToDate, Basow DS, ed. UpToDate, Waltham, 2012.

Brandt O, Abeck D, Gianotti R, Burgdorf W: Gianotti-Crosti syndrome. *J Am Acad Dermatol* 2006;54(1):136–145.

Diab M, Gallina K, Kurtz E, Bechtel M: Treatment of refractory pemphigus erythematosus with rituximab. *J Am Acad Dermatol* 2007;56(2):AB118.

Eisner JM, Russell M: Cartilage hair hypoplasia and multiple basal cell carcinomas. *J Am Acad Dermatol* 2006;54(2):S8–S10.

Goldsmith LA et al. *Fitzpatrick's Dermatology in General Medicine,* 8th Ed. New York: McGraw-Hill; 2012.

Happle R: The group of epidermal nevus syndromes: part I. Well defined phenotypes. *J Am Acad Dermatol* 2010;63(1):1–22.

Hiroko MH, Akaeda T, Maihara T, Ikenaga M, Horio T: Cockayne syndrome without typical clinical manifestations including neurologic abnormalities. *J Am Acad Dermatol* 1998;39(4): 565–570.

Hoger M, Fierlbeck G, Kuemmerle-Deschner J, et al. MRI findings in deep and generalized morphea (localized scleroderma). *AJR Am J Roentgenol* 2008;190(1):32–39.

Houser OW, Gomez MR: CT and MR imaging of intracranial tuberous sclerosis. *J Dermatol* 1992;19(11):904–908.

Jones J, Brenner C, Chinn R, Bunker CB: Radiological associations with dermatological disease. *Br J Radiol* 2005;78:662–671.

Kim GH, Dy LC, Caldemeyer KS, Mirowski GW: Buschke-Ollendorff syndrome. *J Am Acad Dermatol* 2003;48(4):600–601.

Kimonis VE, Mehta SG, Digiovanna JJ, Bale SJ, Pastakia B: Radiological features in 82 patients with nevoid basal cell carcinoma (NBCC or Gorlin) syndrome. *Genet Med* 2004;6(6):495–502.

Kirsch E, Hammer B, von Arx G: Graves' orbitopathy: current imaging. *Swiss Med Wkly* 2009;139(43–44):618–623.

Kormano M, Lindgren I: *Radiological Findings in Skin Diseases and Related Conditions.* New York: Thieme Medical; 1999.

Krown S, Chadha J.: *Classic Kaposi's Sarcoma: Clinical Features, Staging, Diagnosis, and Treatment,* in UpToDate, Basow DS, ed. UpToDate, Waltham, 2012.

Landim F, Rios H, Costa C, et al. Cutaneous Rosai-Dorfman disease. *Anais Brasileiros de Dermatologia* 2009;84(3):275–278.

McKee PH: *Pathology of the Skin: With Clinical Correlations* London: Mosby-Wolfe; 1996.

Robinson N, Hashimoto T, Amagai M, Chan L: The new pemphigus variants. *J Am Acad Dermatol* 1999;40(5):649–671.

Spitz JL: *Genodermatoses: A Full-Color Clinical Guide to Genetic Skin Disorders,* 2nd Ed. Philadelphia: Lippincott Williams & Wilkins; 2005.

Verhelst H, Van Coster R: Neuroradiologic findings in a young patient with characteristics of Sturge-Weber syndrome and Klippel-Trenaunay syndrome. *J Child Neurol* 2005;20(11):911–913.

Yanardag H, Pamuk ON: Bone cysts in sarcoidosis: what is their clinical significance? *Rheumatol Int* 2004;24(5):294–296. Epub 2003 Aug. 20.

CHAPTER 34

ELECTRON MICROSCOPY

ASRA ALI

INDICATIONS FOR ELECTRON MICROSCOPY

Ancillary to standard techniques (i.e., light microscopy) to resolve diagnostic difficulties in human histopathology through examination of ultrastructural findings at the cellular and organelle level

- Unclassifiable, undifferentiated neoplasms
- Supporting a diagnosis from a list of differential diagnosis
- Supporting a light microscopic diagnosis
- Determination of the primary site in metastatic neoplasms
- Medical disease of kidney
- Metabolic storage diseases
- Other congenital disorders
- Infectious agents
- Autoimmune diseases
- Certain cutaneous diseases
- Identification of foreign material in tissues

TECHNIQUE AND TISSUE PREPARATION

- Tissue preparation is similar to conventional wax embedding light microscopy: aldehyde fixation, dehydration, embedding, sectioning, and examination of sections exposed to some form of radiation
- Electron microscopy differences include
    - Image is formed by the scattering of electrons by heavy metal atoms (introduced as solutions of uranyl acetate and osmium tetroxide or lead citrate) selectively adherent to tissue sections
    - Tissue is embedded in epoxy, allowing for sectioning to a thickness of 100 nm
    - Tissue should be submitted in appropriate media (i.e., 2.5% glutaraldehyde; Karnovsky's [universal] solution)
- Fixation with glutaraldehyde provides the best structural preservation; unlike formaldehyde, glutaraldehyde is slowly penetrating. Therefore, only very small pieces of tissue are processed (i.e., 0.5–1 mm^3 or 2–3 mm^2 and thickness of about 0.5 mm)
- Although processing and staining are labor intensive, turn around time can be as short as 24 to 48 hours
- Electron microscopy may also be performed on formalin fixed material from deparaffinizing a wax block. Preservation may be sufficient for diagnostic purposes although results may be variable

DIAGNOSTIC CELLS AND ORGANELLES

Langerhans Cell (Fig. 34-1)

- Bone marrow–derived
- Antigen-processing and -presenting cells
- Indented nucleus with ropey nucleolus
- Rod- and racket-shaped (terminal expansion) cytoplasmic granules (Birbeck granules) with central dotted line
- Often seen at the cell surface when membrane-bound antigen is internalized by endocytosis
- Cytoplasm contains dispersed vimentin intermediate filaments

Merkel Cell (Fig. 34-2)

- Slowly adapting type I mechanoreceptors located in sites of high tactile sensitivity
- Present among basal keratinocytes
- Nucleus is lobulated
- Cytoplasm is electron lucent with prominent Golgi
- Margins of cells project cytoplasmic spines toward keratinocytes
- Typical granules (80–200 nm) have a dense core, halo, and a slightly ruffled membrane
- Granules contain neurotransmitter-like substances
- Intermediate filaments are numerous and assume a parallel or whorled arrangement near the nucleus (dot-like pattern)

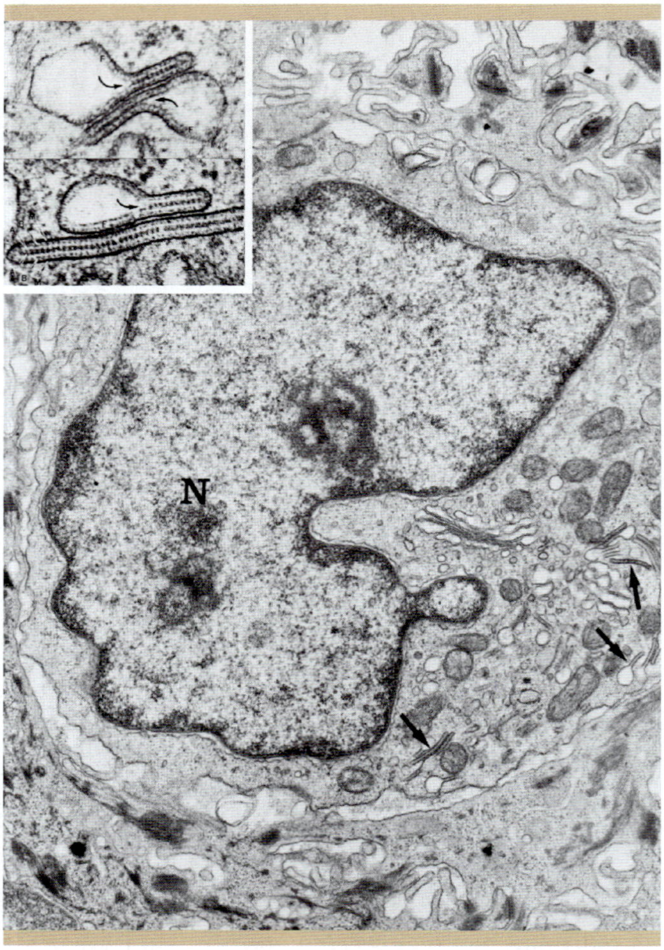

FIGURE 34-1 Langerhans cell. (*© 1967 Wolff. The Journal of Cell Biology, 1967, 35: 468–473. doi:10.1083/jcb.35.2.468.*)

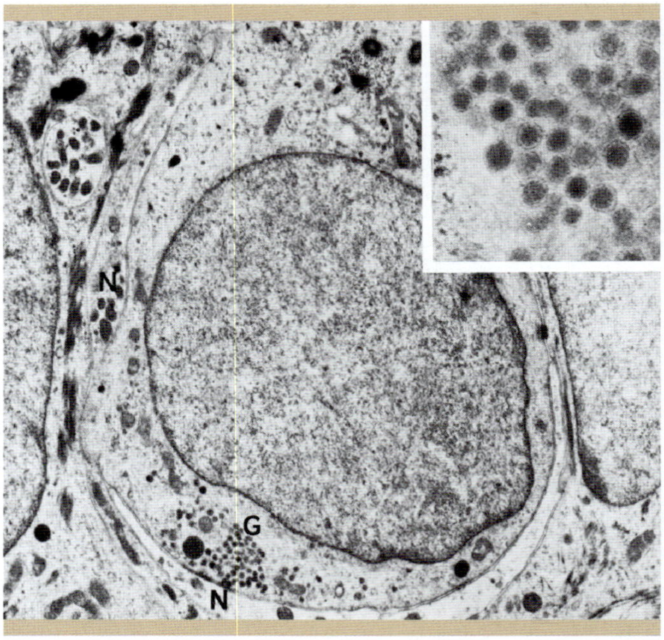

FIGURE 34-2 Merkel cell. (*Reprinted with permission from Goldsmith LA et al.* Fitzpatrick's Dermatology in General Medicine, *8th Ed. New York: McGraw-Hill; 2012.*)

Lamellar Granules (Fig. 34-3)

- In the intercellular space and cytoplasm of the granular cell
- 0.2 to 0.3 nm in diameter
- Membrane-bound secretory organelles containing a series of alternating thick and thin lamellae (folded sheets/disk-like/liposome-like structures)
- Contain glycoproteins, glycolipids, phospholipids, free sterols, acid hydrolases, and glucosylceramides

Dermal-Epidermal Junction (Fig. 34-4)

- Interface between epidermis and dermis
- LL = lamina lucida
- LD = lamina densa
- AFib = anchoring fibrils
- AFil = anchoring filaments
- HD = hemidesmosome
- KF = keratin filaments

Desmosome (Fig. 34-5)

- Calcium-dependent cell surface structures that function to promote adhesion of epidermal cells and aid in resistance to mechanical stresses
- Regularly organized submembrane plaque associated with intermediate filaments (see below)
- Intermediate line in the intercellular space
- Components of desmosome
- Desmosomal plaque
- Transmembrane glycoproteins (part of cadherin family)
- Desmosomal core

Intermediate Filaments (Fig. 34-4 [Upper Left Corner]: Dense Bundle of Tonofibrils)

- About 8 to 12 nm thick
- There are 5 main classes (cytokeratin, vimentin, desmin, neurofilament, and glial filament)
- Only cytokeratin filaments have a distinctive ultrastructure: bundle together to form tonofilaments or tonofibrils
- Other intermediate filaments are generally nonbundling
- Fibrin may closely resemble tonofibrils, appearing as masses of short fibers that on higher magnification demonstrate periodicity

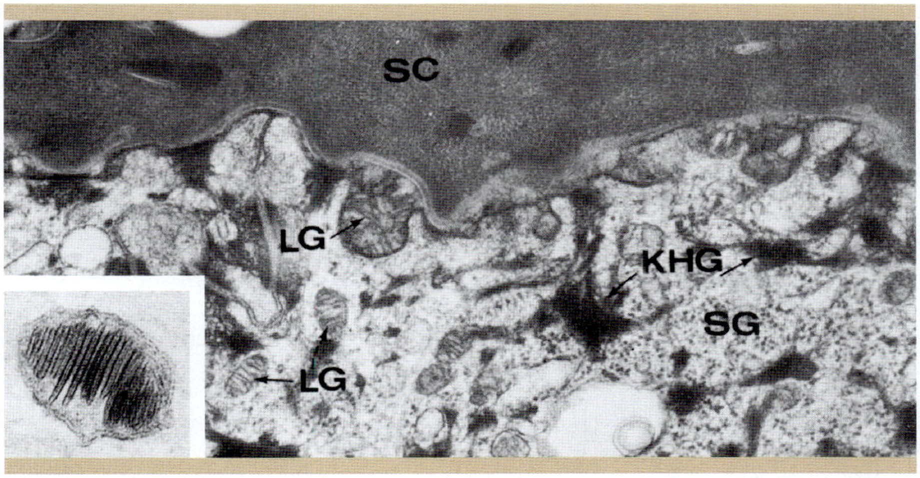

FIGURE 34-3 Lamellar granules. (*From Holbrook K: Structure and development of the skin, in* Pathophysiology of Dermatologic Disease, *2nd Ed., edited by Soter NA, Baden HP. New York: McGraw-Hill, 1991, p. 7, with permission. Inset used with permission from EC Wolff-Schreiner, MD. Reprinted from Goldsmith LA et al.* Fitzpatrick's Dermatology in General Medicine, *8th Ed. New York: McGraw-Hill; 2012.*)

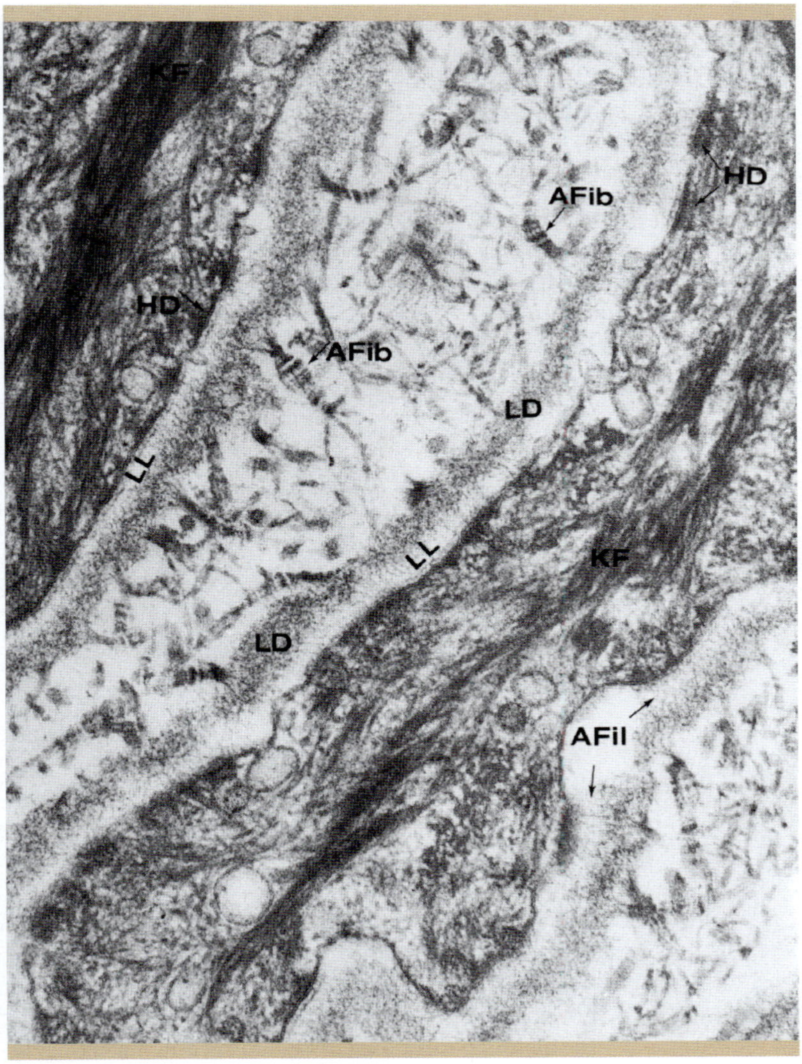

FIGURE 34-4 Dermal-epidermal junction. (*Reprinted with permission from Freedberg IM et al.* Fitzpatrick's Dermatology in General Medicine, *6th Ed. New York: McGraw-Hill; 2003.*)

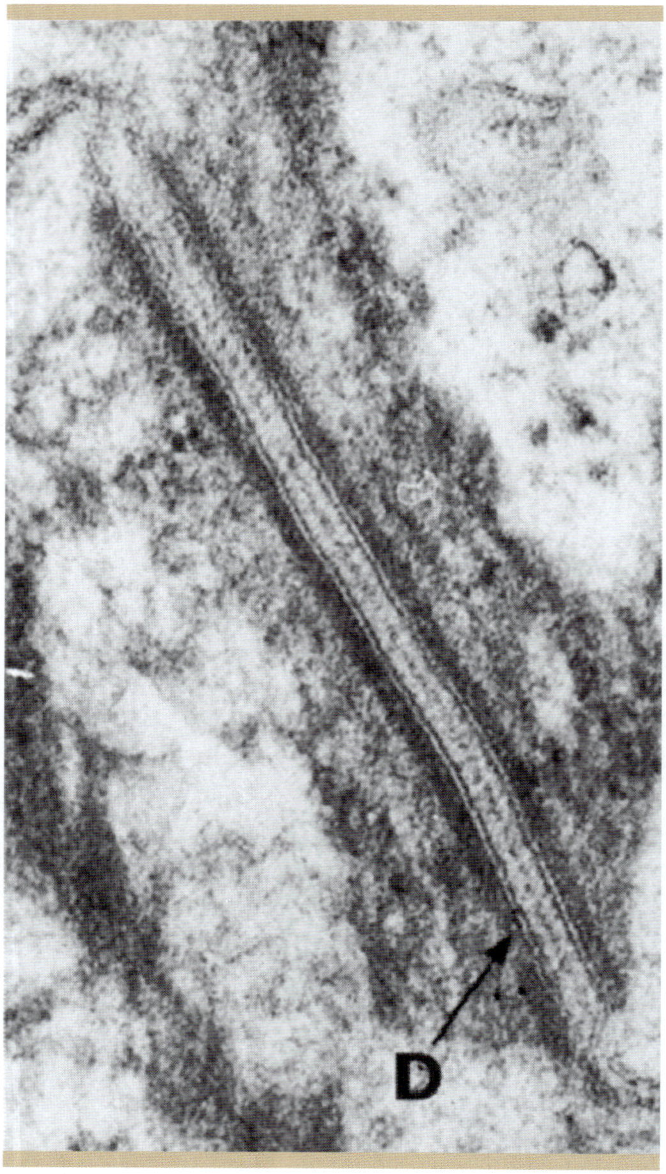

FIGURE 34-5 Desmosome. (*Reprinted with permission from Freedberg IM et al.* Fitzpatrick's Dermatology in General Medicine, *6th Ed. New York: McGraw-Hill; 2003.*)

Melanocyte (Fig. 34-6)

- Contains melanosomes in cytoplasm
- Single limiting membrane
- An aggregate of melanosomes confined within a single membrane is a compound melanosome
- Melanocytes project dendrites to adjacent keratinocytes which uptake melanosomes
- Melanocytes can be distinguished from keratinocytes by the absence of keratin filaments
- Melanosomes become elongated and form ordered cross-striated lattice in stage II of development
- Melanin does not appear until stage III
- Stage IV melanosomes are enriched with electron-dense melanin; the lattice is obscured

Macrophage (Fig. 34-7)

- Part of the mononuclear phagocytic system
- Derived from precursor cells of bone marrow that differentiates into monocytes in the blood
- Skin macrophages express CDIIc, CD6, and KiM8 antigens
- On electron microscopy: melanosomes within phagosomes

Mast cell (Fig. 34-8)

- Specialized secretory cells: originate in bone marrow from CD34 positive stem cells
- Proliferation depends on c-kit receptor and the stem cell factor (SCF) ligand
- Round/ovoid nucleus
- Granules can be secretory or lysosomal (0.2–0.5 nm)
- Mediators can be preformed and stored in granules (histamine, heparin, tryptase, chymase)
- Lattice-like structure of granules: found in mast cells of skin and intestinal submucosa
- Scroll-like structure of granules: found in mast cells of lung and intestinal mucosa

Collagen (Fig. 34-9)

- Fibers have regular banding pattern (periodicity) at approximately 70-nm intervals
- Regularly oriented fibers composed of fibrils and microfibrils
- Fibrils are aligned in a parallel manner, resulting in a pattern of cross-striations

Elastic Tissue (Figs. 34-10 and 34-11)

- Amorphous branching structures forming continuous sheets in some connective tissues
- Fibers composed of elastin with an electron-lucent core surrounded by thin, longitudinally oriented electron-dense microfibrils (Fig. 34-11)
- F = fibroblast; E = elastic tissue; C = collagen fibers (Fig. 34-10)

Eosinophil (Fig. 34-12)

- Nucleus has a deep groove and segment
- Granules contain electron-dense staining zone that is usually angulated or rectangular in shape surrounded by a lucent matrix
- Granules that contain the eosinophil basic proteins
  - Major basic protein (MBP)—only protein located in core
  - Eosinophilic cationic protein (ECP)—located in matrix
  - Eosinophil-derived neurotoxin (EDN)—located in matrix
  - Eosinophil peroxidase (EPO)—located in matrix

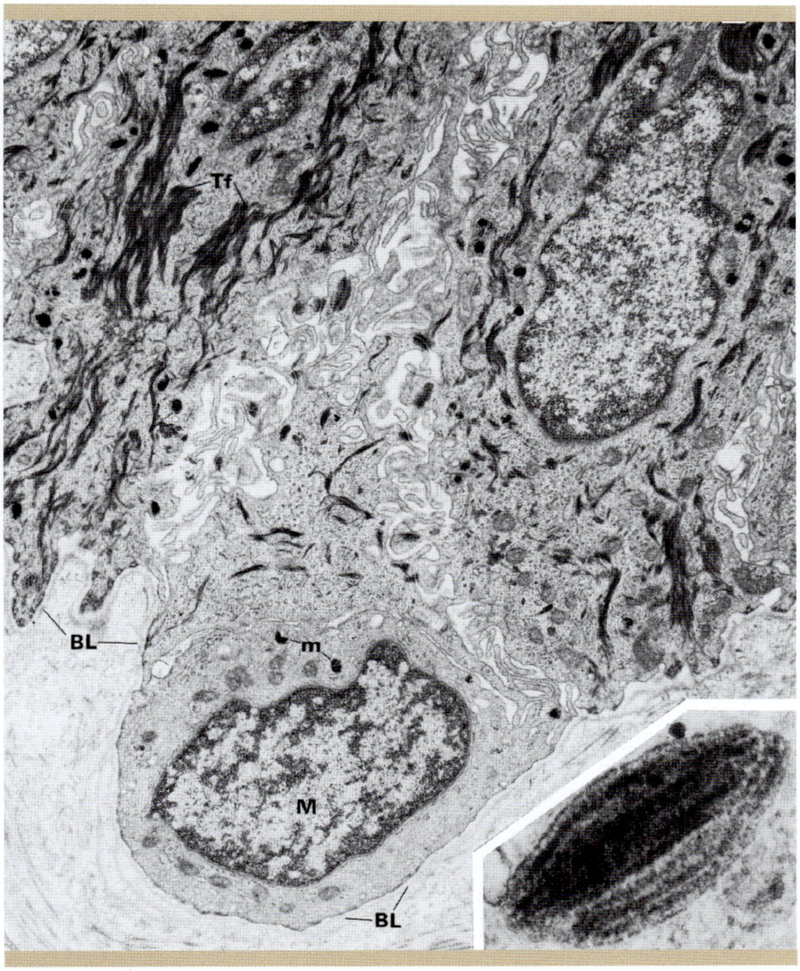

FIGURE 34-6 Melanocyte. (*Reprinted with permission from Freedberg IM et al.* Fitzpatrick's Dermatology in General Medicine, *6th Ed. New York: McGraw-Hill; 2003.*)

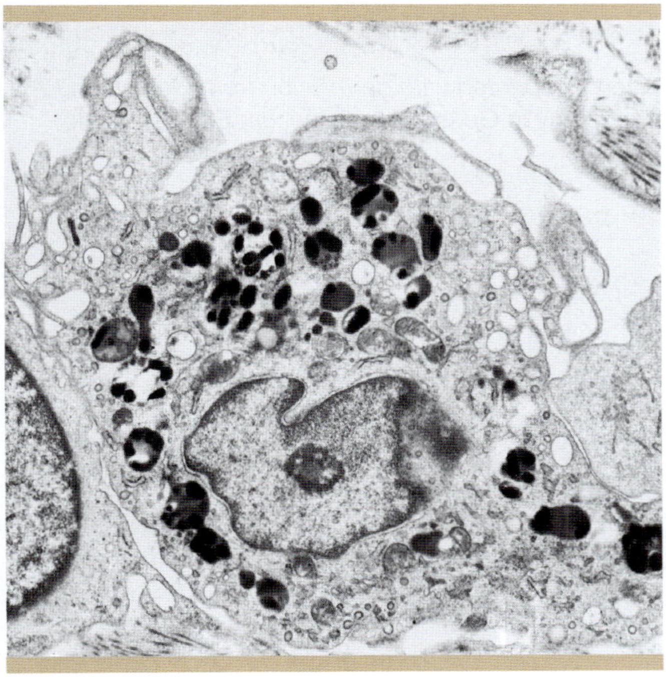

FIGURE 34-7 Macrophage. (*Reprinted with permission from Freedberg IM et al.* Fitzpatrick's Dermatology in General Medicine, *6th Ed. New York: McGraw-Hill; 2003.*)

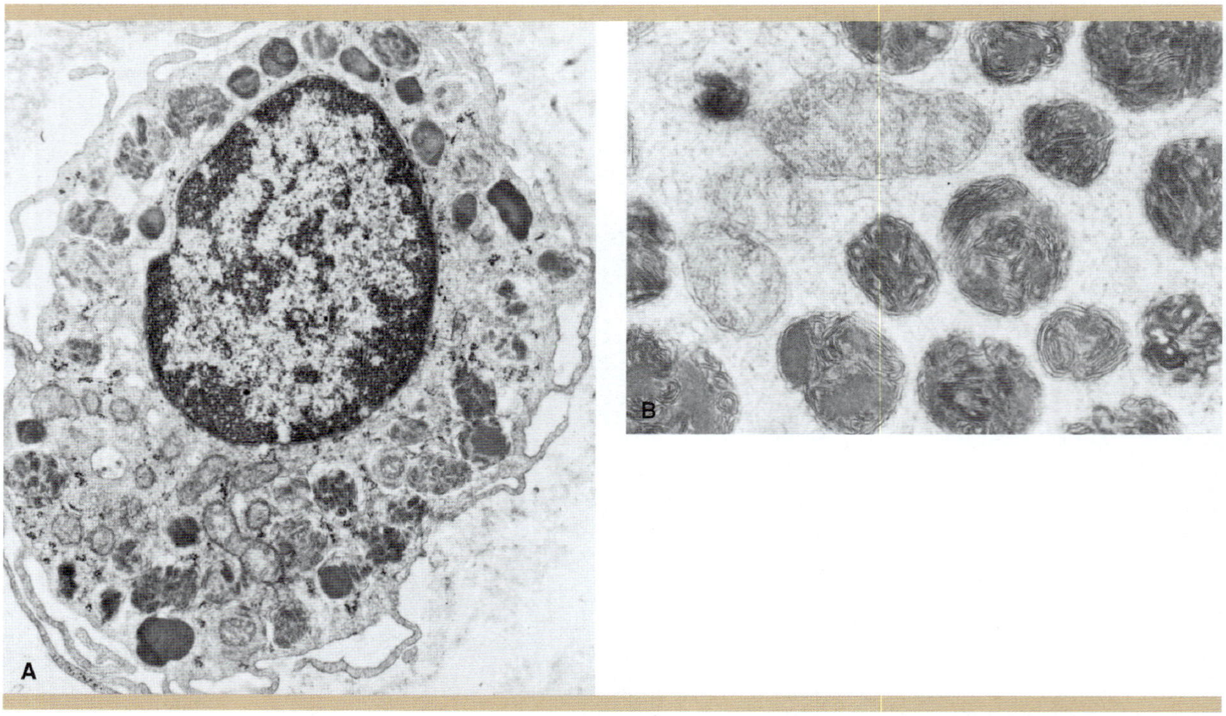

FIGURE 34-8 Mast cell. (*Reprinted with permission from Freedberg IM et al.* Fitzpatrick's Dermatology in General Medicine, *6th Ed. New York: McGraw-Hill; 2003.*)

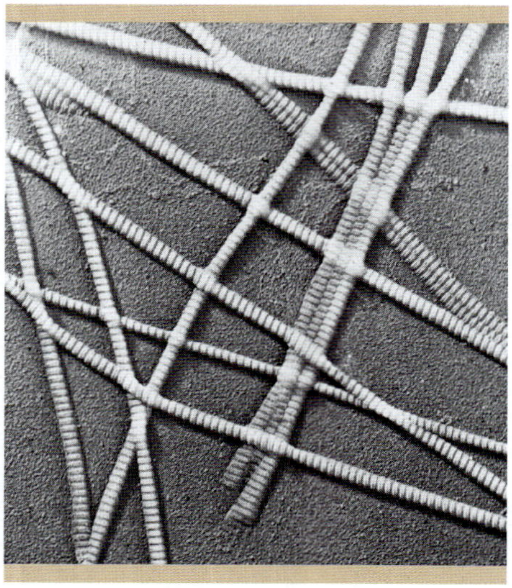

FIGURE 34-9 Collagen. (*Reprinted with permission from Goldsmith LA et al.* Fitzpatrick's Dermatology in General Medicine, *8th Ed. New York: McGraw-Hill; 2012.*)

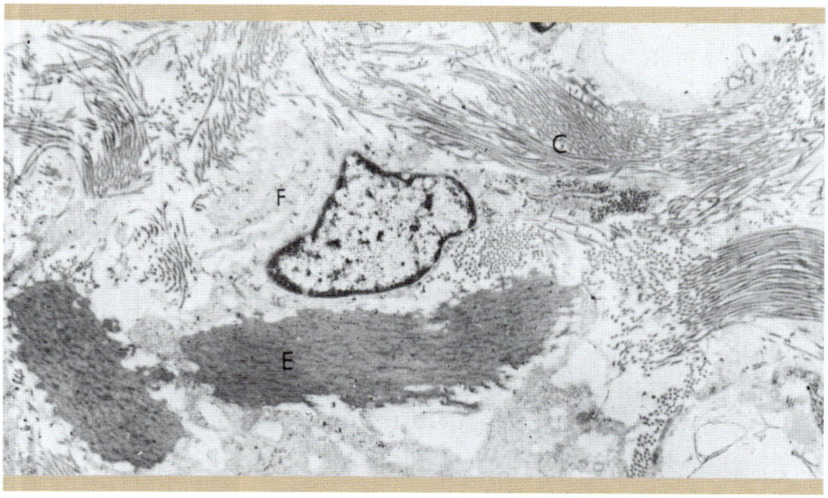

FIGURE 34-10 A fibroblast surrounded by elastic tissue. (*Reprinted with permission from Goldsmith LA et al.* Fitzpatrick's Dermatology in General Medicine, *8th Ed. New York: McGraw-Hill; 2012.*)

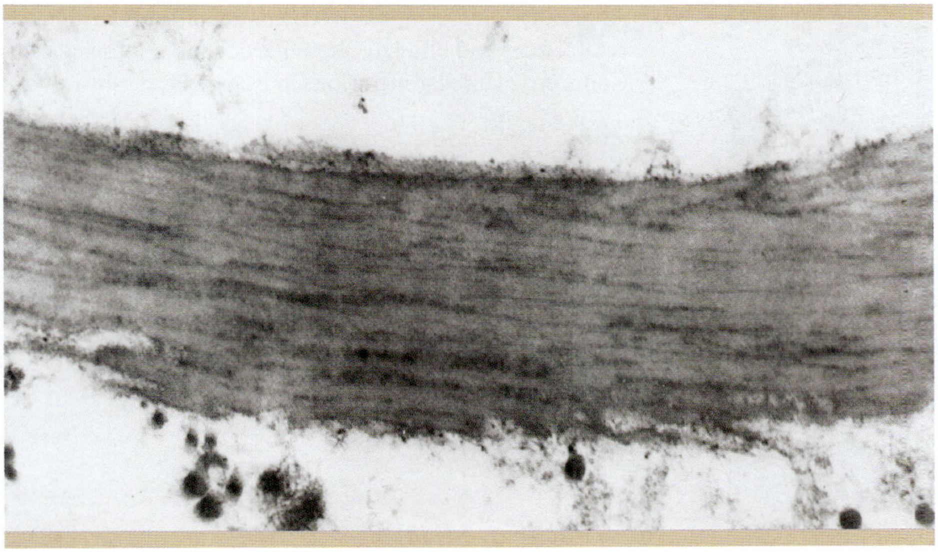

FIGURE 34-11 Elastic fibers in normal human skin. (*Reprinted with permission from Wolff et al.* Fitzpatrick's Dermatology in General Medicine, *7th Ed. New York: McGraw-Hill; 2008.*)

Amyloid

- Composed of nonfibrillary protein known as amyloid P component and a fibrillary component that is derived from various sources
- Has an antiparallel β-pleated sheet configuration
- Amorphous moderately dense material located in extracellular spaces
- At higher magnification, short and haphazardly arranged filaments (7–15 nm) can be observed, like straw strewn on the ground

ULTRASTRUCTURAL FINDINGS IN DERMATOLOGIC CONDITIONS

Fabry Disease (Fig. 34-13)

- Deficient activity of lysosomal enzyme α-galactosidase-A
- Inherited as X-linked recessive; heterogenous females are generally asymptomatic, but may have characteristic corneal opacities
- Manifestations include: angiokeratomas in bathing suit distribution, acroparesthesia, acute attacks of pain, cardiovascular and renal disease

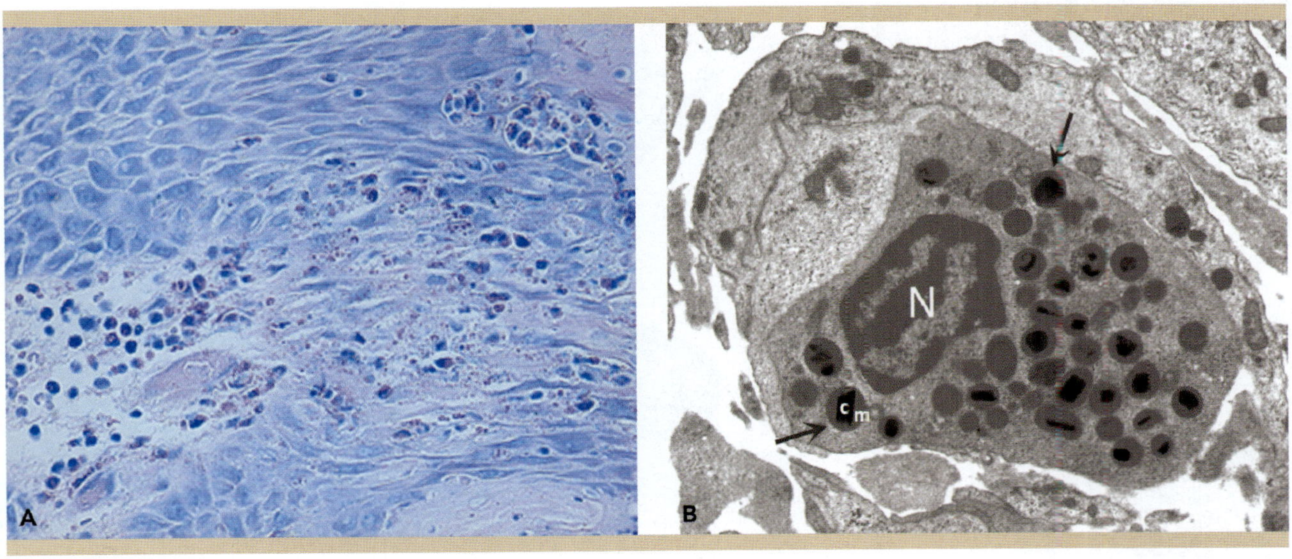

FIGURE 34-12 Eosinophil. (*From Freedberg IM et al.* Fitzpatrick's Dermatology in General Medicine, *6th Ed. New York: McGraw-Hill; 2003.*)

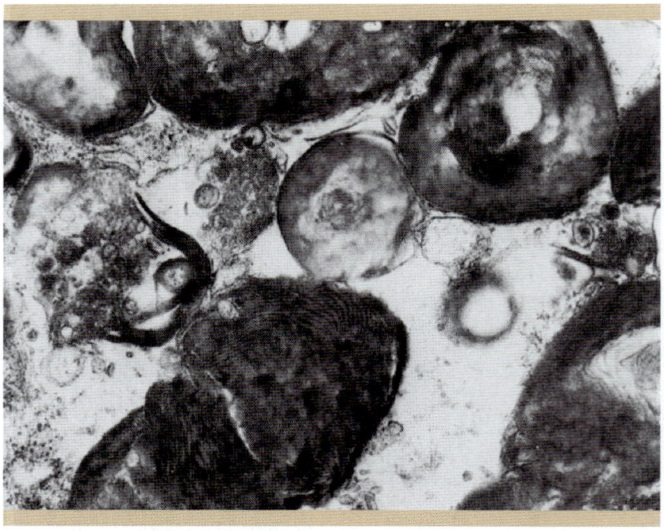

FIGURE 34-13 Mitral valve in Fabry disease. (*From Freedberg IM et al.* Fitzpatrick's Dermatology in General Medicine, *6th Ed. New York: McGraw-Hill; 2003.*)

- Accumulation of neutral glycosphingolipids in most visceral tissues and body fluids, in particular endothelial cells
- Concentric lamellar inclusions in lysosomes of fibrocytes

Mycosis Fungoides, Sézary Cell (Fig. 34-14)

- CD4+ T-helper lymphocytes
- Convoluted nucleus that is deeply indented (cerebriform)

Granular Cell Tumor

- Schwann cell origin
- Cytoplasmic granular appearance from numerous lysosomes, contain granular and membranous debris

INFECTIONS

Pox Virus (Fig. 34-15)

- Single molluscum contagiosum virus virion
- Size = 240 × 300 nm, no envelope

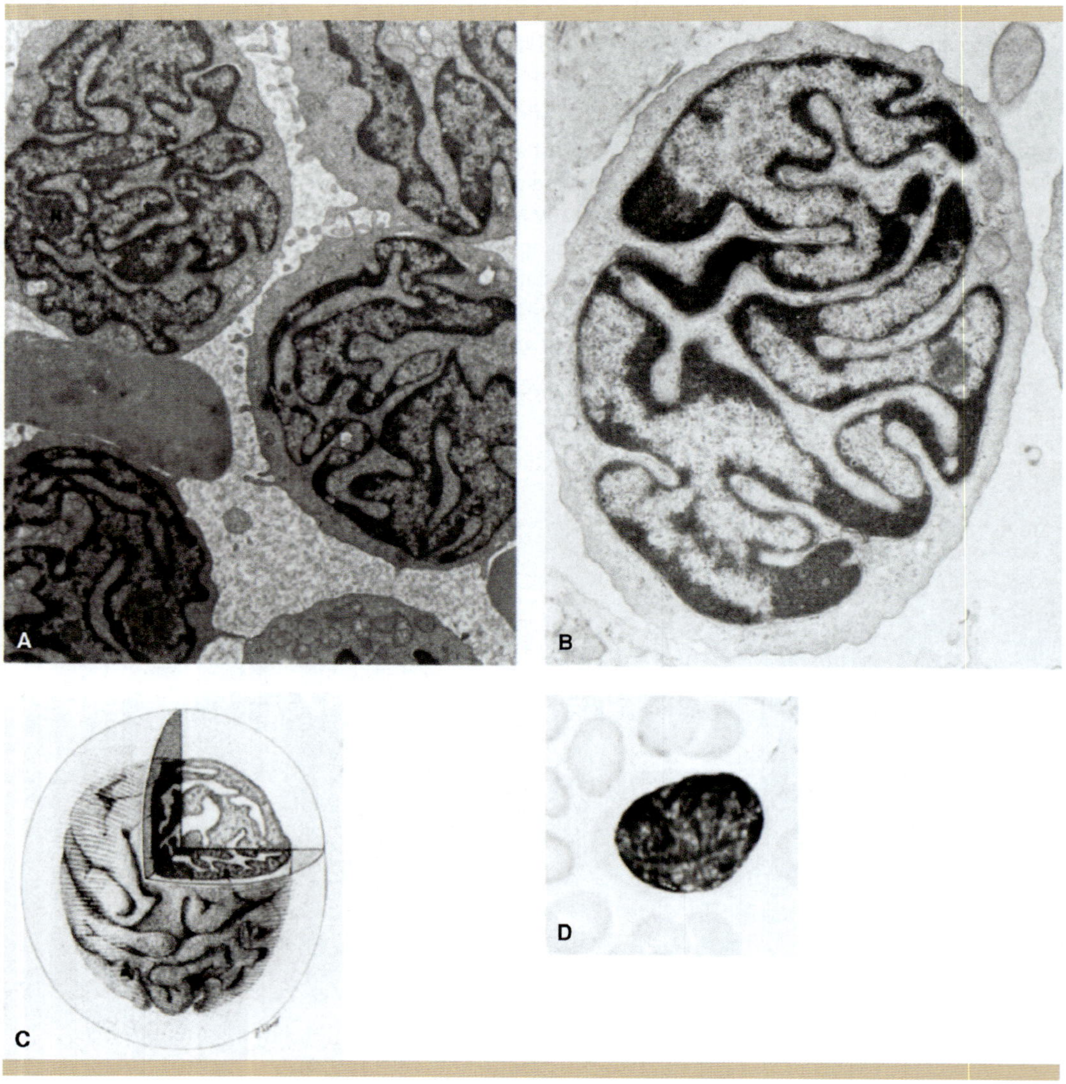

FIGURE 34-14 Sézary cell. (*From Freedberg IM et al.* Fitzpatrick's Dermatology in General Medicine, *6th Ed. New York: McGraw-Hill; 2003.*)

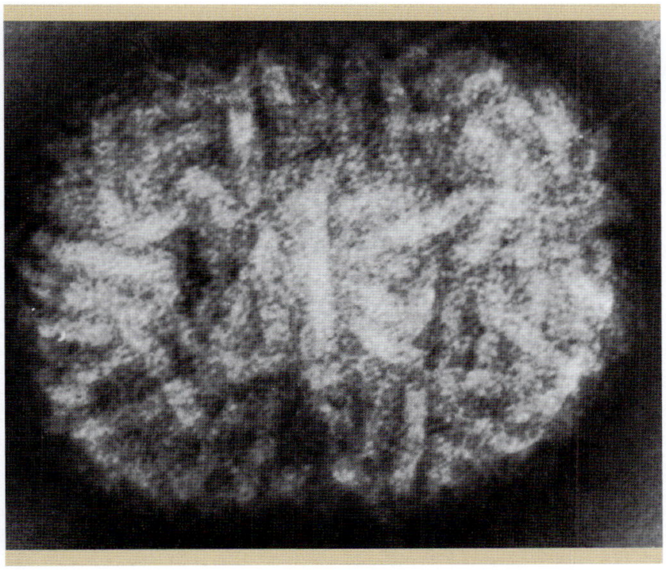

FIGURE 34-15 Pox virus. (*Reprinted from AF Howartson, JD Almeida, MG Williams: Morphology of varicella (chickenbox) virus.* Virology *1962;16:353. From Goldsmith LA et al.* Fitzpatrick's Dermatology in General Medicine, *8th Ed. New York: McGraw-Hill; 2012.*)

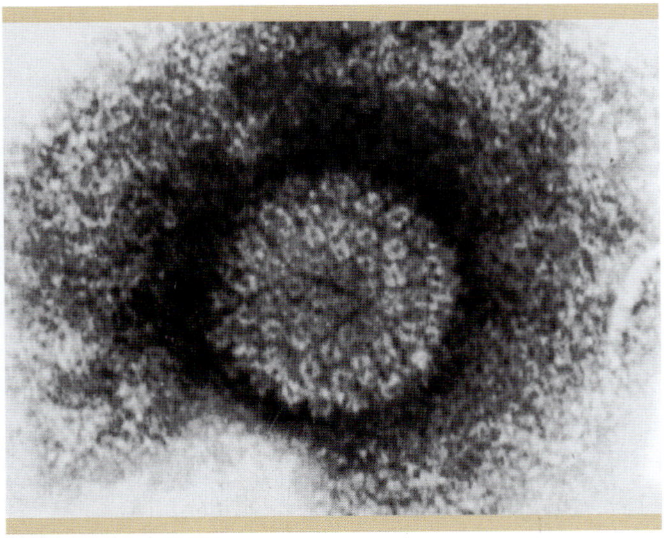

FIGURE 34-16 Herpes virus. (*Reprinted from AF Howartson, JD Almeida, MG Williams: Morphology of varicella (chickenbox) virus.* Virology *1962;16:353. From Goldsmith LA et al.* Fitzpatrick's Dermatology in General Medicine, *8th Ed. New York: McGraw-Hill; 2012.*)

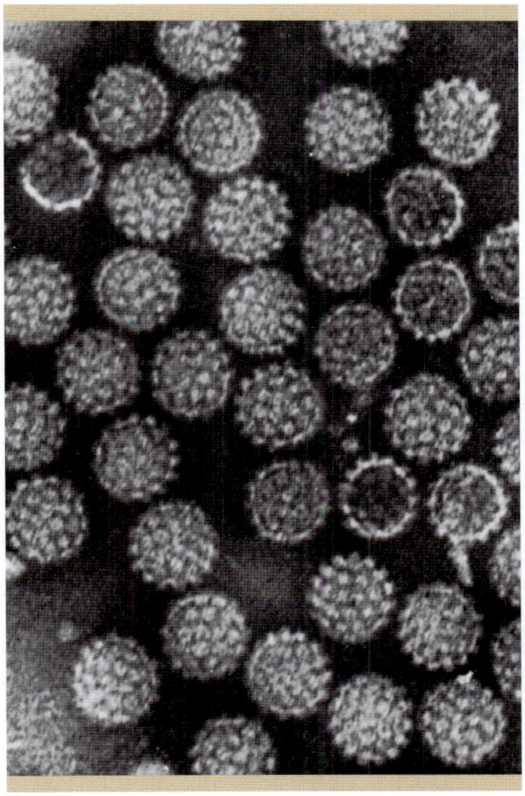

FIGURE 34-17 Papillomavirus. (*Reprinted from AF Howartson, JD Almeida, MG Williams: Morphology of varicella (chickenbox) virus.* Virology *1962;16:353. From Goldsmith LA et al.* Fitzpatrick's Dermatology in General Medicine, *8th Ed. New York: McGraw-Hill; 2012.*)

- Double stranded DNA (dsDNA) virus, capsid assembly in cytoplasm
- Also known to cause Orf, milkers' nodules, variola, and vaccinia

Herpes Family of Viruses (Fig. 34-16)

- Size = 120 to 200 nm
- Icosahedral, enveloped dsDNA
- Replicates in nucleus
- Herpes simplex (types 1 and 2) (human herpes virus [HHV] 1, HHV2), varicella-zoster (HHV3), Epstein-Barr virus (HHV4), cytomegalovirus (HHV5), HHV6 (roseola infantum), HHV8 (Kaposi sarcoma, body cavity lymphoma, Castleman disease)

Papillomavirus (Fig. 34-17)

- Multiple nonenveloped virions
- Size: 50 to 55 nm, icosahedral with capsid subunits (capsome)
- Nonenveloped dsDNA replicates in nucleus

QUIZ

Questions

1. Which study(s) should be performed to determine the precise location of separation in vesiculobullous conditions?
   A. Hematoxylin and eosin stained tissue sections
   B. Polarized light
   C. Heat-induced epitope retrieval
   D. Electron microscopy
   E. Laser microdissection

2. You have just seen a male patient that has numerous angiokeratomas and acroparesthesias. To confirm the diagnosis, a biopsy is performed. For optimal tissue preservation of celluar detail, how should the tissue to be submitted to pathology?
   A. In formalin
   B. In sterile saline
   C. In bacteriostatic saline
   D. In water
   E. In glutaraldehyde
   F. In Bouin solution

3. Which description matches the ultrastructural appearance of a patient with a brown macule that hives when stroked?
   A. Rod- and/or racquet-shaped cytoplasmic granule
   B. Homogenous dense core cytoplasmic granule
   C. Organized subepidermal plaque between 2 cells associated with keratin
   D. Organized subepidermal plaque between 1 cell and the dermis
   E. Scroll-like structure of granule
   F. Fibers with periodicity of approximately 70 nm and aligned in a parallel manner
   G. Granules with angulated or rectangular electron-dense area
   H. Convoluted nucleus with deep indentions (cerebriform)

4. Which description matches the ultrastructural appearance of a child with crusted purpuric papules and a scaly seborrheic-like eruption in the scalp and groin?
   A. Rod- and/or racquet-shaped cytoplasmic granule
   B. Homogenous dense core cytoplasmic granule
   C. Organized subepidermal plaque between 2 cells associated with keratin
   D. Organized subepidermal plaque between 1 cell and the dermis
   E. Scroll-like structure of granule
   F. Fibers with periodicity of approximately 70 nm and aligned in a parallel manner
   G. Granules with angulated or rectangular electron-dense area
   H. Convoluted nucleus with deep indentions (cerebriform)

5. Which description matches the ultrastructural appearance of an elderly person with tense bullae located on intertriginous areas and lower extremities that may be preceded by a hive without scarring?
   A. Rod- and/or racquet-shaped cytoplasmic granule
   B. Homogenous dense core cytoplasmic granule
   C. Organized subepidermal plaque between 2 cells associated with keratin
   D. Organized subepidermal plaque between 1 cell and the dermis
   E. Scroll-like structure of granule
   F. Fibers with periodicity of approximately 70 nm and aligned in a parallel manner
   G. Granules with angulated or rectangular electron-dense area
   H. Convoluted nucleus with deep indentions (cerebriform)

6. Which description matches the ultrastructural appearance of a fair-skinned, 70-year-old man with a solitary erythematous nodule on the face?
   A. Rod- and/or racquet-shaped cytoplasmic granule
   B. Homogenous dense core cytoplasmic granule
   C. Organized subepidermal plaque between 2 cells associated with keratin
   D. Organized subepidermal plaque between 1 cell and the dermis
   E. Scroll-like structure of granule
   F. Fibers with periodicity of approximately 70 nm and aligned in a parallel manner
   G. Granules with angulated or rectangular electron-dense area
   H. Convoluted nucleus with deep indentions (cerebriform)

7. Which description matches the ultrastructural appearance of a patient with persistent scaly patches in sun protected areas that respond poorly to topical steroids?
   A. Rod- and/or racquet-shaped cytoplasmic granule
   B. Homogenous dense core cytoplasmic granule
   C. Organized subepidermal plaque between 2 cells associated with keratin
   D. Organized subepidermal plaque between 1 cell and the dermis
   E. Scroll-like structure of granule
   F. Fibers with periodicity of approximately 70 nm and aligned in a parallel manner

G. Granules with angulated or rectangular electron-dense area
H. Convoluted nucleus with deep indentions (cerebriform)

8. Which description matches the ultrastructural appearance of a patient with hyperextensibilty of the skin, easy bruisability, poor healing with fish mouth scars?

A. Rod- and/or racquet-shaped cytoplasmic granule
B. Homogenous dense core cytoplasmic granule
C. Organized subepidermal plaque between 2 cells associated with keratin
D. Organized subepidermal plaque between 1 cell and the dermis
E. Scroll-like structure of granule
F. Fibers with periodicity of approximately 70 nm and aligned in a parallel manner
G. Granules with angulated or rectangular electron-dense area
H. Convoluted nucleus with deep indentions (cerebriform)

9. In which stage of development does the melanin appear in the melanosome?

A. Stage I
B. Stage II
C. Stage III
D. Stage IV
E. Stage V

10. Which protein is not an intermediate filament?

A. Desmin
B. Actin
C. Vimentin
D. Keratin
E. Neurofilament

Answers

1. D. Electron microscopy is an ancillary technique to resolve diagnostic difficulties in human histopathology through examination of ultrastructural findings at the cellular and organelle level, such as meticulous examination of the dermal-epidermal junction to determine the location of separation in vesiculobullous diseases. Immunofluorescence is also helpful. Hematoxylin and eosin stained tissue sections is the standard method of preparation of tissue for light microscopy. Polarized light is used to confirm the presence of polarizable material (i.e., amyloid). Heat-induced epitope retrieval may be necessary for immunohistochemistry of formalin fixed tissue.
2. E. Fixation with glutaraldehyde provides the best structural preservation; unlike formaldehyde, glutaraldehyde is slowly penetrating. Therefore, only very small pieces of tissue are processed (i.e., 0.5–1 mm^3 or 2–3 mm^2 and thickness of about 0.5 mm). Electron microscopy may also be performed on formalin fixed material from deparaffinizing a wax block. Preservation may be sufficient for diagnostic purposes although results may be variable. Formalin is used for routine tissue fixation. Sterile saline is often used to submit tissue for microbiology studies. Bouin solution may be used to help tissue dyes adhere.
3. E. The patient has a mastocytoma that demonstrates Darier sign (hives when stroked). The characteristic cell is mast cells that contain scoll like structure of granules on electron microscopy.
4. A. The patient has findings that suggest Langerhans cell histiocytosis. The characteristic cell is the Langerhans cell that contains rod- and/or racquet-shaped cytoplasmic granules on electron microscopy.
5. D. The patient has findings that suggest bullous pemphigoid, which affects proteins in the hemidesmosome.
6. B. The patient has findings that suggest Merkel cell carcinoma. The characteristic cell is the Merkel cell that contains homogenous dense core cytoplasmic granule on electron microscopy.
7. H. The patient has findings that suggest mycosis fungoides. The characteristic cell is the Sezary cell that contains a convoluted nucleus with deep indentions (cerebriform) on electron microscopy.
8. F. The patient has findings that suggest Ehlers-Danlos syndrome, which is a congenital abnormality of collagen. On electron microcopy, collagen appears as fibers with periodicity of approximately 70 nm and aligned in a parallel manner.
9. C. There are only 4 stages of melanosome development. Melanosomes become elongated and form ordered, cross-striated lattice in stage II of development. Melanin does not appear until stage III. In stage IV, melanosomes are enriched with electron-dense melanin; the lattice is obscured.
10. B. There are 5 main classes of intermediate filaments: cytokeratin, vimentin, desmin, neurofilament, and glial filament. Actin is a protein involved in the contractile apparatus of cells.

REFERENCES

Daróczy J, Rácz I: *Diagnostic Electron Microscopy in Practical Dermatology*. Budapest: Akadémiai Kiadó; 1987.
Elder DE, Elenitsas R, Johnson BL Jr, Murphy BG, ed. *Lever's Histopathology of the Skin*. Philadelphia: Lippincott Williams & Wilkins; 2005.
Fitzpatrick JE, Morellli JG: *Dermatology Secrets in Color*, 3rd Ed. Philadelphia: Mosby Elsevier; 2007.

Goldsmith LA et al. *Fitzpatrick's Dermatology in General Medicine*, 8th Ed. New York: McGraw-Hill; 2012.

Society for Ultrastructural Pathology: Handbook Committee: *Handbook of Diagnostic Electron Microscopy for Pathologists-In-Training*. New York: Igaku-Shoin Medical Publishers; 1996.

Wilborn WH, Hyde BM, Montes LF: *Scanning Electron Microscopy of Normal and Abnormal Human Skin*. Mahwah, New Jersey: Electron Optics Publishing Group; 1985.

Zelickson AS, Mottaz JH: *The Clinical Use of Electron Microscopy in Dermatology*, 4th Ed. Minneapolis: Bolger; 1985.

CHAPTER 35

HIGH-YIELD FACTS FOR THE DERMATOLOGY BOARDS

KIRAN MOTAPARTHI
KRISTY FLEMING

The purpose of this chapter is to present information that may be considered "high yield" for the dermatology board exam, mock boards, and recertification exam.

Table 35-1 identifies common factoids relating to genetic inheritance of diseases. Table 35-2 focuses on important disease-associated viruses. Table 35-3 focuses on histologic bodies. Table 35-4 discusses infectious diseases for which there are known vectors. Table 35-5 presents common contact allergens. Tables 35-6, 35-7, and 35-8 focus on common findings of the bones, eyes, and nails, respectively.

The information included herein should not be considered complete or exhaustive. Detailed descriptions of the topics are found in other chapters.

TABLE 35-1 Genes to Know

Disease	Gene/Protein		Gene Function
Incontinentia Pigmenti	XLD	(NEMO) NF-κB Essential modulator	Transcription factor
Autosomal Dominant Inheritance			
Angioedema, hereditary (Quincke's)	(C1INH) C1 esterase inhibitor		Inhibits first component of complement
Bannayan-Riley-Ruvalcaba	(PTEN) phosphatase and tensin homolog		Tumor suppressor
Bart syndrome	(COL7A1) type VII collagen		Anchoring fibril
Basal cell nevus syndrome (Gorlin)	(PTCH) patched homolog (Drosophila)		Inhibits "smoothened" signaling; this inhibition blocked by "hedgehog"
Bullous ichthyosiform erythroderma (epidermolytic hyperkeratosis)	Keratins 1 and 10		Intermediate filament
Bullous ichthyosis of Siemens	Keratin 2e		Intermediate filament

(*Continued*)

TABLE 35-1 Genes to Know (Continued)

Disease	Gene/Protein	Gene Function
Carney complex (LAMB [lentigenes, atrial myxomas, mucocutaneous myxomas, blue nevi], NAME [nevi, atrial myxomas, myxoid neurofibromas, ephilides])	(PRKAR1A)	R1 regulatory subunit of protein kinase A
Cowden syndrome (multiple hamartoma syndrome)	(PTEN)	Tumor suppressor
Darier disease (keratosis follicularis)	(SERCA2) calcium ATPase2A2	Calcium-dependent ATPase
Ectodermal dysplasia, hidrotic (Clouston's)	ED2 gene, HED gene/connexin-30	Gap junction protein
Ectodermal dysplasia with skin fragility	Plakophilin 1	Structural
Epidermolysis bullosa, dominant dystrophic (EB)	(Col7A1) Type VII collagen	Anchoring fibril
Epidermolysis bullosa simplex (EBS)	Keratins 5 and 14	Intermediate filament
Erythrokeratodermia variabilis (EKV)	Connexin-31	Gap junction protein
Gardner syndrome	(APC) adenomatosis polyposis coli	Tumor suppressor (cleaves β-catenin)
Hailey-Hailey disease	(ATPase2C1)	Calcium-dependent ATPase
Hereditary hemorrhagic telangiectasia (Osler-Weber-Rendu)	Endoglin, Alk-1 gene activin receptor-binding kinase	TGF-β signaling pathway
Lhermitte-Duclos syndrome	(PTEN)	Tumor suppressor
MEN I	(MEN1) menin gene	Tumor supressor
MEN IIa and IIb	(RET) receptor tyrosine kinase	Proto-oncogene
Milroy disease (Nonne-Milroy-Meige syndrome)	(FLT-4) a.k.a (VEGFr-3)	Growth factor receptor
Monilethrix	KRT hHb6 and hHb1, KRT86, KRT81, KRT83, DSG4 Type II human hair keratins, 6 & 1	Intermediate filament
Muir-Torre syndrome	MLH1, MSH2, MLH6	Mismatch repair gene
Nail-Patella syndrome	LMX1B gene	Homeobox domain transcription factor
Neurofibromatosis I	NF-1 (neurofibromin)	Increases GTPase activity of ras
Neurofibromatosis II	NF-2 (schwannomin or Merlin)	Tumor suppressor
NOMID syndrome (neonatal onset multisystem inflammatory disease); also called CINCA syndrome	CIAS1 gene	Cryopyrin gene, role in innate immune response
Pachyonychia congenita	K6, K16, or K17	Intermediate filament
Peutz-Jeghers syndrome	STK11	Tumor suppressor

(Continued)

TABLE 35-1 Genes to Know (Continued)

Disease	Gene/Protein	Gene Function
Piebaldism	(C-kit)	Proto-oncogene (tyrosine kinase)
Porphyria cutanea tarda	Uroporphyrinogen decarboxylase	
Porphyria, acute intermittent	Porphobilinogen deaminase	
Porphyria, erythropoietic protoporphyria (EPP)	Ferrochelatase	Mitochondrial gene
Porphyria, variegate	Protoporphyrinogen oxidase	Mitochondrial gene
Reed syndrome (cutaneous and uterine leiomyomatosis)	Fumarate hydratase	Tumor suppressor
Rubenstein-Taybi syndrome	(CBP) CREB-binding protein	Involved in cAMP-regulated gene expression
Striate PPK 1	Desmoglein 1	Structural protein
Striate PPK 2	Desmoplakin	Structural protein
Tuberous sclerosis	(TSC1) on Chrom. 9 hamartin gene (TSC2) on Chrom. 16 tuberin gene	GTPase-activating protein domain
Vohwinkel	Loricrin gene	Structural (cornified cell envelope)
Vohwinkel with deafness	Connexin-26	Gap junction protein
Vorner syndrome	Keratin 9	Intermediate filament
Waardenburg syndrome	(PAX3) (MITF) (EDN3/SOX10) – with Hirschsprung	Transcription factor Transcription factor endothelin
White sponge nevus	Keratins 4 and 13	Intermediate filament
Autosomal Recessive Inheritance		
Atrichia with papules ("alopecia universalis")	(HR) hairless gene	Zinc finger
Albinism I, oculocutaneous	TYR-tyrosinase	Melanin pathway
Albinism II, oculocutaneous	P gene–pink protein	Unknown
Albinism III, oculocutaneous (rufous)	(TYRP1) tyrosinase-related protein 1	Stabilizes tyrosinase
Alkaptonuria	(HGO) homogentisic acid oxidase	Phenylalanine and tyrosine breakdown pathway
Ataxia-telangiectasia (Louis-Bar)	(ATM/ATM protein) ataxia-telangiectasia mutated	Phosphatidylinos-itol-3-kinase-like domain
Bloom syndrome	(BLM)	DNA helicase
Chediak-Higashi syndrome	LYST/CHS1 gene/CHS protein	Lysosomal transport
Citrullinemia	(ASS) arginosuccinate synthetase gene	Enzyme in urea cycle
Cockayne syndrome	(CKN1) (ERCC6) XPB DNA helicase	DNA helicase—DNA repair

(*Continued*)

TABLE 35-1 Genes to Know (Continued)

Disease	Gene/Protein	Gene Function
Epidermolysis bullosa, generalized atrophic benign (GABEB)	(BPAg2) collagen XVII (LAMB3) laminin	Structural (hemidesmosome)
Epidermolysis bullosa, junctional (EB with pyloric atresia)	ITGB6 gene, ITBG4 gene/Integrin α6,b4	Structural (hemidesmosome)
Epidermolysis bullosa, junctional (EB letalis, Herlitz)	LAMA3, LAMB3, LAMC2 genes/ laminin 5	Structural (basement membrane)
EBS with muscular dystrophy	PLEC1 gene/plectin	Structural (hemidesmosome)
Familial Mediterranean fever	(MEFV)/pyrin	PMN inhibitor
Farber disease (lipogranulomatosis)	Acid ceramidase	Deficiency leads to ceramide accumulation
Gaucher disease	β-Glucocerebrosidase	Breakdown of glucosylsphingosine
Griscelli syndrome	(MTO5a) myosin Va	Melanosome transport to keratinocytes
Homocystinuria	Cystathionine synthetase	Condensation of homocysteine and serine
Hurler syndrome	α-L-iduronidase	Degradation of mucopolysaccharide in lysosomes
Hypotrichosis, localized autosomal recessive	(DSG4) desmoglein-4	Desmosomal cadherin
Ichthyosis, lamellar	Transglutaminase-1	Formation of cornified cell envelope
Naxos disease	Junctional plakoglobin	Structural protein
Niemann-Pick disease	Sphingomyelinase	Degradation of sphingomyelin
Netherton syndrome	SPINK5 gene	Serine protease inhibitor
Papillon-Lefevre syndrome	Cathepsin C	Lysosomal protease
Phenylketonuria	Phenylalanine hydroxylase	Hydroxylation of phenylalanine to tyrosine
PIBIDS syndrome, trichothiodystrophy	(XPD) (TFIIH) xeroderma pigmentosum D	DNA helicase
Porphyria, congenital erythropoietic (Gunther)	Uroporphyrinogen III cosynthase	
Porphyria, erythropoietic protoporphyria (EPP)	Ferrochelatase	Mitochondrial enzyme
Refsum syndrome	Phytanoyl-CoA hydroxylase	peroxisomal α-oxidative enzyme
Richner-Hanhart syndrome	Tyrosine aminotransferase	Degradation of tyrosine
Rothmund-Thomson (poikiloderma congenitale)	(RECQL4) DNA helicase	DNA helicase
Sjögren-Larsson syndrome	Fatty aldehyde dehydrogenase	oxidation of fatty acids to carboxylic acids

(Continued)

TABLE 35-1 Genes to Know (Continued)

Disease	Gene/Protein	Gene Function
Takahara disease	Catalase	Bacterial defense
Tangier disease (Familial α-lipoprotein deficiency)	(CERP)	Cholesterol efflux regulatory protein
Werner syndrome	(WRN) (ERCC) (XPB, D, and G)	DNA helicase
X-Linked Dominant Inheritance		
CHILD syndrome (congenital hemidysplasia with ichthyosiform erythroderma and limb defects)	(EBP gene) emopamil binding protein/(NSDHL gene) 3-β-hydroxy sterol dehydrogenase	Cholesterol biosynthetic pathway
Conradi-Hünermann syndrome	(EBP) (PEX7)	Sterol isomerase peroxisomal gene
Incontinentia pigmenti	(NEMO) NF-κB essential modulator	Transcription factor
X-Linked Recessive Inheritance		
Bruton agammaglobulinemia	(BTK gene)	Tyrosine kinase
Dyskeratosis congenita	(DKC1 gene) dyskerin (XLR) (TERC) telomerase, RNA component (AD)	rRNA processing Telomerase RNA component
Ectodermal dysplasia, hypohidrotic (Christ-Siemens-Touraine syndrome)	Ectodysplasin	Tumor necrosis factor
Fabry disease (angiokeratoma corporis diffusum)	α-galactosidase A	Hydrolyzes glycolipids and glycoproteins
Granulomatous disease of childhood, chronic	(CYBB gene) cytochrome B	NADPH-oxidase complex component (respiratory burst) needed to kill catalase-positive bacteria
Hunter syndrome	Iduronate sulfatase	Lysosomal degradation of heparan sulfate and dermatan sulfate
Ichthyosis, X-linked	Aryl sulfatase C (steroid sulfatase)	Conversion of sulfated steroid precursors to free steroid
Lesch-Nyhan syndrome	(HGPRT)	Purine salvage pathway enzyme
Menkes kinky-hair syndrome	MNK	Copper transporting ATPase
SCID (severe combined immunodeficiency disease)	(ADA) adenosine deaminase IL-2 receptor	common γ chain
Wiskott-Aldrich syndrome	(WASP) (sialoglycoprotein)	Binds GTPase and actin
Unknown or No Inheritance Pattern		
Atopic dermatitis	Filaggrin (FLG)	Filament aggregating protein
Beare-Stevenson syndrome	(FGFr2) FGF receptor 2	cell signaling
McCune-Albright syndrome	GNAS-1	Stimulates G protein increasing cAMP

TABLE 35-2 Viruses

Associated or Causative Virus	Disease	Description
Coxsackie virus A16	Hand-foot-mouth disease	Fever, ulcerovesicular stomatitis, acral erythematous vesicles, buttock lesions
Coxsackie viruses (A10)	Herpangina	Fever, painful ulcerations in mouth
EBV (Epstein-Barr virus)	Oral hairy leukoplakia	Corrugated white plaque on lateral tongue common in AIDS
EBV, HBV, echovirus 6	Unilateral laterothoracic exanthem	Asymptomatic to itchy unilateral morbilliform eruption
Echovirus 16	Boston exanthema	Mild exanthematous febrile illness with aseptic meningitis
Echovirus 25 and 32	Eruptive pseudoangiomatosis	Viral prodrome, then 2- to 4-mm blanchable red papules on the face and trunk
Enterovirus 71	Herpangina	Fever, painful ulcerations in mouth
Hepatitis B virus, and numerous other viral pathogens or vaccinations	Gianotti-Crosti syndrome	Children with sudden onset of lichenoid papules on face, extremities, and buttocks, sparing trunk
Hepatitis C virus	Lichen planus	Purple polygonal, plateau-shaped, pruritic, papules
HHV (human herpesvirus)-8	Castleman disease	Angiolymphoid hyperplasia usually plasmacytoid in lymph nodes
HHV-6	Rosai-Dorfman	Sinus histiocytosis with massive lymphadenopathy
HHV-6 and 7	Roseola infantum (exanthem subitum, sixth disease)	Infants with high fever followed by exanthema
HHV-7	Pityriasis rosea	salmon-colored patches on trunk
HHV-8	Kaposi sarcoma	Vascular tumor, various types
HPV (human papilloma virus)-16, 18, 31, 34	Bowen disease	Squamous cell carcinoma in situ
HPV (papovavirus-dsDNA) Low risk: Types 6 and 11 High risk: Types 16 and 18	Condyloma acuminata	Genital warts
HPV-1	Myrmecia Verruca plantaris	Large cup-shaped palmoplantar warts (Plantar warts)
HPV-13 and 32	Heck disease (focal epithelial hyperplasia)	Small white and pink papules in mouth
HPV-16	Bowenoid papulosis	Genital papules and plaques resembling Bowen disease
HPV-2	Verruca vulgaris	Common warts
HPV-23b	Stucco keratoses	White hyperkeratotic plaques on legs

(Continued)

TABLE 35-2 Viruses (Continued)

Associated or Causative Virus	Disease	Description
HPV-3, 10	Verruca plana	(Flat warts)
HPV-5, 8, 12, and others as well as common types	Epidermodysplasia verruciformis	Inherited disorder of HPV infection and SCCs
HPV-6 and 11	Buschke-Löwenstein	Giant condyloma
HPV-60	Ridged wart	Wart with preserved dermatoglyphics
HPV-7b	Butcher wart	Warty lesions seen in people who handle raw meat
HSV (herpes simplex virus)	Kaposi varicelliform eruption (eczema herpeticum)	Diffuse HSV ulcerations in eczematous dermatitis
MCV (molluscum contagiosum virus)-1 to MCV-4; MCV-2 in HIV	Molluscum contagiosum	Umbilicated lesions common in children and HIV
Nonspecific: hep. B, parvovirus B19, rubella	STAR complex	Sore throat, arthritis, rash
Paramyxovirus (RNA)	Measles (rubeola)	Viral prodrome, then enanthem (Koplik spots), then maculo-papular rash spreading craniocaudally
Parapoxvirus	Orf	Umbilicated nodule after farm animal exposure
Parvovirus B19	Erythema infectiosum (fifth disease)	Erythematous cheeks, reticular exanthem, anemia
Parvovirus B19	Papular purpuric stocking-glove syndrome	Pruritus, edema, and erythema of hands and feet
Togavirus (RNA)	Rubella	Viral prodrome, prominent lymphadenopathy, pain with superolateral eye movements, morbilliform rash, enanthem (Forschheimer spots)
Variola (poxvirus) (DNA)	Variola major (smallpox)	12-day incubation, fever and malaise, then centrifugal vesiculopustular rash

TABLE 35-3 Histologic Findings

Disease	Histologic Finding	Description
Type A-HSV, CMV, and VZV Type B-polio	Cowdry type A and B inclusion bodies	Type A: intranuclear eosinophilic, amorphous bodies surrounded by a clear halo Type B: in neuronal cells
Amiodarone hyperpigmentation	Lipofuscin granules	Yellow-brown granules in macrophages
Androgenic alopecia	Arao-Perkins bodies	Elastin bodies seen within "streamers" beneath vellus follicles
Benign cephalic histiocytosis	Comma-shaped bodies	Cytoplasmic bodies seen on EM
Café-au-lait macules, neurofibromatosis, Chediak-Higashi	Macromelanosomes	Large melanosomes
Chediak-Higashi	Giant liposomes in neutrophils	Large liposomal granules
Chromomycosis	Medlar/sclerotic bodies	Large (5–12 μm round, thick-walled brown cells seen in and out of giant cells)
Cutaneous meningioma	Psammoma bodies	Concentrically laminated calcified basophilic bodies
Cutaneous T-cell lymphoma	Pautrier microabscess	Clusters of lymphocytes within epidermis
Darier, Grover, warty dyskeratoma	Corps grains Corps ronds	Dyskeratotic keratinocytes with elongated nuclei seen in the granular zone Dyskeratotic keratinocytes with perinuclear halo and surrounding basophilic dyskeratotic material
Ehrlichiosis	Morulae	Leukocyte intracytoplasmic inclusions
Farber disease	Farber bodies	Curvilinear bodies seen in the cytoplasm of fibroblasts and endothelial cells on EM
Farber disease and other ganglioside storage diseases	Zebra bodies	Vacuoles with transverse membranes in endothelial cells on EM
Granular cell tumors	Pustulo-ovoid bodies	Round cytoplasmic eosinophilic inclusions
Granuloma inguinale	Donovan bodies	Intrahistiocyte inclusions comprise organisms that stain positively with Warthin-Starry stain or Giemsa
HTLV-1 (human T-cell lymphotrophic virus-1) and ATLL (adult T-cell lymphoma/leukemia)	Flower bodies/cells	Atypical CD4+ T cells
Interface dermatitis	Civatte/colloid bodies	Apoptotic keratinocytes that may be found in epidermis or extruded into papillary dermis
Interface dermatitis, especially LP	Max-Joseph space	Artifactual separation between dermis and epidermis
Langerhans cells	Birbeck granules	Racquet-shaped bodies seen on EM
Lepromatous leprosy	Globi	Collections of AFB (acid-fast bacilli) seen in foamy macrophages with Fite stain
Lipoid proteinosis	Onion skinning	Hyaline material surrounding blood vessels

(*Continued*)

TABLE 35-3 Histologic Findings (Continued)

Disease	Histologic Finding	Description
Malakoplakia	Michaelis-Gutmann bodies	Calcified lamellar eosinophilic bodies in foamy "von Hansemann" macrophages
Molluscum contagiosum	Henderson-Patterson bodies	Cytoplasmic eosinophilic inclusions in keratinocytes
Normal endothelial cells	Weibel-Palade bodies	Organelles seen on EM
Normal skin, absent in harlequin fetus	Lamellar/Odland bodies	Free fatty acid, ceramide, and cholesterol containing vacuoles released from the Golgi in the stratum granulosum seen on EM
Ochronosis	Banana bodies	Crescentic banana-shaped pigmented bodies in the upper dermis
Ovarian neoplasms	Psammoma bodies	Concentrically laminated calcified basophilic bodies
Plasmacytoid proliferations (e.g., multiple myeloma)	Dutcher bodies	Intranuclear inclusions of immunoglobulins
Pleomorphic lipoma	Floret cells	Multinucleated giant cells with radially arranged nuclei
Porphyria cutanea tarda, pseudoporphyria, and erythropoietic protoporphyria (EPP)	Caterpillar bodies	Eosinophilic wavy collection in basal layer of epidermis, found on roof of blister
Protothecosis	Mulberry bodies	Thick-walled spherical body containing organisms
Rabies	Negri bodies	Eosinophilic bodies within large neurons
Rhinoscleroma	Mikulicz cell	Foamy macrophage containing bacteria
Rhinoscleroma	Russell bodies	Immunoglobulin inclusions in plasma cells
Sarcoidosis, botryomycosis, sporotrichosis, actinomycosis, others	Asteroid bodies	Stellate collections of eosinophilic spicules in giant cells
Sarcoidosis and other granulomatous diseases	Conchoidal bodies (Schaumann bodies)	Shell-like calcium complexes within giant cells
Schwannoma	Antoni A tissue	Cellular areas with Verocay bodies
Schwannoma	Antoni B tissue	Loose stromal area with relative paucity of cells
Schwannoma	Verocay bodies	Palisading nuclei arranged in rows with peripheral eosinophilic cytoplasm
Sclerema neonatorum and subcutaneous fat necrosis of the newborn	Cholesterol clefts	Needle-like crystals in fat cells
Spitz nevus	Kamino bodies	Eosinophilic bodies composed of BMZ (basement membrane zone) material
Sporotrichosis	Cigar bodies	Budding cigar-shaped PAS+ yeast (rarely seen)
Thyroid neoplasms	Psammoma bodies	Concentrically laminated calcified basophilic bodies
Well syndrome, arthropod bites, other	Flame figures	Dermal eosinophils and eosinophilic granules surrounding central masses of brightly pink amorphous collagen

TABLE 35-4 Infectious Diseases and Their Vectors

Organism	Vector	Disease
Ancylostoma braziliense	Feces, animal	Cutaneous larva migrans
Arbovirus, RNA-virus	Mosquitoes (several species)	West Nile fever
Bartonella bacilliformis	*Lutzomyia verrucarum* (sandfly)	Carrion disease
Bartonella quintana	*Pediculosis humanus* (louse)	Trench fever
Borrelia afzelii	*Ixodes ricinus*	Acrodermatitis chronica atrophicans
Borrelia burgdorferi	*Ixodes scapularis (dammini)* (Northeast and Midwest United States) lxodes pacificus (Western United States)	Lyme disease
Borrelia duttonii, Borrelia recurrentis	*Ornithodoros tholozani* (tick) *Pediculus humanus* (louse)	Relapsing fever
Borrelia garinii and *B. afzelii*	*lxodes ricinus* (Europe)	Lyme disease
Burkholderia pseudomallei	Swamp water	Melioidosis (Whitmore disease)
Cercariae of Schistosomes (nonhuman)	Snails	Cercarial dermatitis
Dermatobia hominis (botfly) *and Cordylobia species*	Mosquito	Myiasis
Dracunculus medinensis	Cyclops water flea in drinking water	Dracunculiasis (guinea worm disease, medina worm)
Ehrlichia chaffeensis	Tick bites	Ehrlichiosis
Erysipelothrix rhusiopathiae	Found on pigs, shellfish, and turkeys	Erysipeloid of Rosenbach
Francisella tularensis	*Amblyomma americanum* (lone star tick) *Chrysops discalis* (deer fly) *Dermacentor andersoni* (tick) (from handling wild rabbits)	Tularemia (Ohara's disease, deer fly fever)
Leishmania mexicana; Leishmania braziliensis braziliensis; Leishmania braziliensis guyanensis; Leishmania braziliensis panamensis	*Lutzomyia* (sandfly)	Leishmaniasis, new world
Leishmania tropica; Leishmania major; Leishmania aethiopica; Leishmania infantum	*Phlebotomus perniciosus* (sandfly) Reservoir: Rodents (gerbils)	Leishmaniasis, old world
Leishmania mexicana	*Lutzomyia flaviscutellata*	Chiclero ulcer
Leptospira interrogans ictero haemorrhagiae	Rat urine	Weil disease
Loa loa	Chrysops species (mango fly or deer fly)	Loaiasis (Calabar, tropical and fugitive swelling)
Nocardia farcinica	Cattle	Bovine farcy
Onchocerca volvulus	*Simulium* species (black fly)	Onchocerciasis (river blindness)
Pseudomonas mallei	Horses, mules, and donkeys	Glanders (Farcy)

(*Continued*)

TABLE 35-4 Infectious Diseases and Their Vectors (Continued)

Organism	Vector	Disease
Rickettsia akari	*Allodermanyssus sanguineus* (house mouse mites) *Liponyssoides sanguineus* (house mouse mites) Reservoir: *Mus musculus* (house mouse)	ckettsialpox
Rickettsia conorii	*Rhipicephalus sanguineus* (dog tick)	Mediterranean fever (boutonneuse fever, South African tick bite fever)
Rickettsia prowazekii	*Pediculus humanus* (body louse) Reservoir: *Glaucomys volans* (flying squirrel)	Typhus, epidemic
Rickettsia rickettsii	*Amblyomma americanum* (lone star tick) *Dermacentor andersoni*, *Dermacentor variabilis Ixodid* ticks	Rocky Mountain spotted fever
Rickettsia tsutsugamushi	*Trombiculid* red mite (chigger)	Scrub typhus (tsutsugamushi fever)
Rickettsia typhi	*Xenopsylla cheopis* (rat flea)	Typhus, endemic
Schistosoma mansoni, Schistosoma haematobium, and Schistosoma japonicum	Snails	Schistosomiasis
Spirillum minor, Streptobacillus moniliformis	Rat bites	Rat-bite fever (Haverhill fever, Sodoku)
Spirometra (dog and cat tapeworm larvae)	Frogs and snakes (application or ingestion)	Sparganosis
Taenia solium	Contaminated food	Cysticercosis cutis
Toxoplasma gondii	Cat feces and undercooked meat	Toxoplasmosis
Trichinella spiralis	Pig, bear, and walrus meat	Trichinosis
Trypanosoma cruzi	Reduviid bug (assassin bug, kissing bug)	Chagas disease (American trypanosomiasis)
Trypanosoma gambiense, Trypanosoma rhodesiernse	Tsetse fly (*Glossina morsitans*)	African trypanosomiasis
Wuchereria bancrofti, Brugia malayi, Brugia timori	Culex, Aedes, and Anopheles mosquitos	Elephantiasis tropica
Yersinia pestis	Xenopsylla cheopis (rat fleas)	Plague

TABLE 35-5 Contact Allergens

Common Sources	Allergen	Other Information
Coral	*Tedania Ignis* (Bermuda fire sponge)	Contact erythema multiforme
Cement	Potassium dichromate	
Clothing	Formaldehyde	permanent-press textile products
Clothing snaps	Nickel sulfate	Eyelid dermatitis, dimethylglyoxime test (pink)
Coloring, blue	Cobalt dichloride	Nickel plating, hair dye, metal, vitamin B_{12}, cement, construction
Cosmetics	Ammonium persulfate	Hair bleach
	Benzalkonium chloride (Quaternium 15)	Shampoos
	Formaldehyde	
	Glyceryl thioglycolate	Permanent (hair) wave solutions
	Methyl methacrylate	Artificial nails, dental work
	Paraphenylenediamine	Dark hair dye, henna tattoo additive
	toluenesulfonamide/formaldehyde resin	Nail lacquer/hardener:eyelid dermatitis
	Imidazolidinyl urea (Germall 115)	Formaldehyde releaser found in cosmetics
Cyanoacrylate	Ethyl cyanoacrylate	
Flavoring; additives	Cinnamic aldehyde	Pastries, toothpaste, chewing gum, beverages, Bitters, lipstick
Food	Ammonium persulfate	Bleaching agent in flour
	Benzoyl peroxide	Bleaching agent in flour
	Diallyl disulfide	Garlic
	Eugenol	Cloves
	Sesamine	Sesame oil
Fragrance, adhesives, flavoring	Balsam of Peru	Cross-reacts with cinnamon, clove, orange peel, benzoin
Glues, plastics	Epoxy resin	
Jewelry	Na gold-thiosulfate	Best screen for allergy to gold; late and persistent positive reactions
Jewelry, clothing snaps	Nickel sulfate	Eyelid dermatitis, dimethylglyoxime test (pink)
Leather	Chromates potassium dichromate	
Medications	Benzocaine	Topical amide anesthetics
	Benzoyl peroxide	Acne medication
	Budesonide	Screening for Group B and D corticosteroids

(*Continued*)

TABLE 35-5 Contact Allergens (Continued)

Common Sources	Allergen	Other Information
	Ethylenediamine	Stabilizer in Mycolog; cross-reacts with aminophylline and hydroxyzine
	Glutaraldehyde	Cold sterilant
	Hydrocortisone-17-butyrate	Group B and D corticosteroids
	Neomycin sulfate	Topical antibiotic
	Tixocortol pivalate	Group A corticosteroids
Plants	Allyl isothiocyanate	Mustard, radish
	Calcium oxalate crystals	*Dieffenbachia* ("dumb cane")
	D-Usnic acid	Lichen
	Furocoumarin	Celery, dill, fig, lime, parsley, parsnip, meadow grass, St. John wort (Umbelliferae family)
	Limonene	Orange and lemon peel, tea tree oil
	Primin	Primrose (Primula obonica)
	ricin	Castor bean (Ricinus communis)
	Sesquiterpene lactone	Compositae family members (chrysanthemum, ragweed, artichoke)
	Tuliposide A	Peruvian lily, tulip
	Urushiol	Poison ivy, poison oak, poison sumac, Japanese lacquer tree, cashew nut, mango, ginkgo tree
Plaster	Potassium dichromate	
Preservatives	Kathon CG (methylchloroisothiazolinone)	Found in cosmetics, shampoo, moist wipes, formaldehyde-like
	Paraben mix	Low incidence of contact dermatitis
	Quaternium-15 (most common preservative cause of ACD)	Formaldehyde-releasing preservative, found in hair care products, moisturizers
	Thimerosal	Cosmetics, preservative in vaccines, contact lens solution, tuberculin skin test
Resin	p-tert-butylphenol	Formaldehyde resin adhesive in leather/rubber products
Rosin	Colophony (rosin) (abietic acid)	Solder, paper products, adhesives, paints, varnishes
Rubber products	2-Meroaptobenzothiazole (MBT)	Adhesive, pesticide, animal repellents, shoe allergy
	Black rubber mix (*N*-Phenyl-*N′* Isopropyl *p*-phenylenediamine, *N*-Phenyl-*N′* cyclohexylphenyle-nediamine, *N*,*N*-diphenyl-phenylenediamine)	

(*Continued*)

TABLE 35-5 Contact Allergens (Continued)

Common Sources	Allergen	Other Information
	Carbamates (zinc diethyldithiocarbamate, zinc dibutyldithiocarbamate)	
	Mercapto mix (4-morpholinyl-2-benzothiazyl disulfide, N-cyclohexyl-2-benzothiazolesulfenamide, 2,2-benzothiazyl disulfide)	
	Mixed dialkyl thioureas	Rubber accelerator, neoprene, tape, mouse pads, wet suits
	Tetramethylthiuram disulfide	Rubber accelerator, gloves, antimicrobial antioxidant in rubber products
Sunscreen	Oxybenzone	Photocontact
	Padimate O (PABA)	
Turpentine	Carene	

TABLE 35-6 Common Bone Findings in Disease

Disease	Finding
Acne fulminans	Osteolytic lesions
Albright osteodystrophy	Bradymetacarpalism
Apert syndrome	Synostosis
Buschke-Ollendorf syndrome	Osteopoikilosis
Cockayne syndrome	Dwarfism
Congenital syphilis	Osteochondritis, saber shins, saddle nose, mulberry molars, Hutchinson teeth
Conradi-Hünermann syndrome	Unilateral limb shortening, chondrodysplasia punctata
Ehlers-Danlos IX	Occipital horns
Fanconi syndrome	Absent radius or thumb
Franceschetti-Jadassohn syndrome	Malaligned great toes
Gardner syndrome	Craniofacial osteomatosis
Goltz syndrome	Osteopathia striata, lobster-claw deformity, scoliosis
Gorlin syndrome	Bifid rib, mandibular keratocysts, kyphoscoliosis, calcified falx cerebri, frontal bossing, etc.
Hallermann-Streiff syndrome	Bird-like facies, natal teeth
Homocystinuria	Marfanoid habitus, genu valgum
Linear morphea	Melorheostosis
Maffucci syndrome	Enchondromas, chondrosarcoma

(*Continued*)

TABLE 35-6 Common Bone Findings in Disease (Continued)

Disease	Finding
Marfan syndrome	Marfanoid habitus
McCune-Albright syndrome	Polyostotic fibrous dysplasia
MEN III	Marfanoid habitus
Multicentric reticulohistiocytosis	Mutilating arthritis
Nail-Patella syndrome	Posterior iliac horn, absent patella
Osteogenesis imperfecta	Fragile bones
Papillon-Lefèvre syndrome	Tentorial and chondroid plexus calcification
Rhizomelic dwarfism	Enchondromas
Von Recklinghausen (NF-1)	Sphenoid wing dysplasia

TABLE 35-7 Common Eye Findings in Disease

Condition	Eyes
Alkaptonuria	Pingueculae, Osler sign
Allezandrini syndrome	Unilateral retinitis pigmentosa
Argyria	Blue sclera
Ataxia-telangiectasia (Louis-Bar)	Bulbar telangiectasia
Behçet syndrome	Retinal vasculitis, uveitis, and hypopyon
CHIME syndrome (colobomas of eye; heart defects, ichthyosiform dermatosis, mental retardation, ear defects)	Colobomas of retina
Cicatricial pemphigoid	Symblepharon
Cockayne syndrome	Salt and pepper retinitis pigmentosa with optic atrophy
Congenital syphilis	Keratitis
Conradi-Hünermann syndrome	Asymmetric focal cataracts
Ehlers-Danlos VI	Keratoconus
Fabry disease	Whorl-like corneal opacities, spoke-like cataracts
Fanconi syndrome	Strabismus, retinal hemorrhages
Gardner syndrome	Congenital hypertrophy of retinal pigmented epithelium
Gaucher disease	Pingueculae
Goltz syndrome	Colobomas
Hallermann-Streiff syndrome	Microphthalmia, congenital cataracts, strabismus
Homocystinuria	Downward lens displacement
Incontinentia pigmenti (Bloch-Sulzberger)	Strabismus, atrophy, cataracts, optic coloboma

(*Continued*)

TABLE 35-7 Common Eye Findings in Disease (Continued)

Condition	Eyes
JXG	Hyphema, hypopyon
KID	Keratitis
Lamellar ichthyosis	Ectropion
LEOPARD	Hypertelorism
Lipoid Proteinosis (Urbach-Wiethe)	Eyelid "string of pearls"
Marfan syndrome	Upward lens displacement
Nail-patella syndrome	Lester iris
NF-2	Posterior subcapsular lenticular cataracts
Osteogenesis imperfecta	Blue sclera
PXE (Grönblad-Strandberg)	Angioid streak
Refsum syndrome	Salt and pepper retinitis pigmentosa
Richner-Hanhart	Pseudoherpetic keratitis
Sjögren-Larsson syndrome	Glistening dots, retinitis, pigmentosa
Tuberous sclerosis	Astrocytic hamartomas
Von Recklinghausen (NF-1)	Lisch nodules
Waardenburg syndrome	Dystopia canthorum, heterochromia, irides
Wilson disease	Kayser-Fleischer ring
X-linked ichthyosis	Posterior comma-shaped corneal opacities (Descemet membrane)

TABLE 35-8 Common Nail Findings in Disease

Condition	Nails
5-FU and AZT	Blue lunulae
Alopecia areata	Nail pits, red and spotted lunulae
Apert syndrome	1 large fingernail
Argyria	Slate blue lunulae
Arsenic	Mee lines
CHF, connective tissue disease	Red lunulae
Cirrhosis	Terry nails
Coffin-Siris syndrome	Fifth-nail dystrophy
Connective tissue disease and trauma	Pterygium inversum unguis
Darier-White disease	Red and white bands, V-nicking

(*Continued*)

TABLE 35-8 Common Nail Findings in Disease (Continued)

Condition	Nails
Fe^{2+} deficiency	Koilonychia
Hemochromatosis	Koilonychia
High fever, surgery, and meds (chemo)	Beau lines
Hyperthyroidism	Koilonychia
Hypoalbuminemia	Muehrcke nails
Lichen planus	Dorsal pterygium
Renal disease	Lindsay's nails
Retinoids, indinavir, and estrogen	Pyogenic granuloma
Trichinosis, endocarditis, and trauma	Splinter hemorrhages
Tuberous sclerosis	Koenen tumor
Wilson disease	Blue lunulae
Yellow nail syndrome	Yellow curved nails

QUIZ

Questions

1. What is the function of the affected gene in Cowden syndrome?

   A. Gap junction protein
   B. Tumor suppressor gene
   C. Transcription factor
   D. Growth factor receptor

2. Which of the following displays an autosomal recessive pattern of inheritance?

   A. Bullous ichthyosiform erythroderma
   B. Weber-Cockayne syndrome
   C. White sponge nevus
   D. Epidermolysis bullosa, junctional

3. Which of the following involves a defective enzyme located in mitochondria?

   A. Porphyria cutanea tarda (PCT)
   B. Porphyria, acute intermittent (AIP)
   C. Porphyria, erythropoietic protoporphyria (EPP)
   D. Hepatoerythropoietic porphyria (HEP)

4. Which of the following diseases is NOT due to a defective DNA helicase?

   A. Rothmund-Thomson (poikiloderma congenitale)
   B. Trichothiodystrophy
   C. Ataxia-telangiectasia (Louis-Bar syndrome)
   D. Bloom syndrome

5. What is the function of the defective gene product in Dyskeratosis congenita?

   A. Ribosomal RNA synthesis
   B. Telomerase
   C. Mismatch repair
   D. Both A and B

6. Which of the following storage diseases is inherited in an X-linked recessive manner?

   A. Farber disease (lipogranulomatosis)
   B. Gaucher disease
   C. Hurler disease
   D. Hunter disease

7. For a patient with Incontinentia pigmenti, what is the risk of having affected offspring?
   A. Fifty percent of females will be affected; no males will be affected
   B. Fifty percent of females will be affected; 50% of males will be affected
   C. Hundred percent of females will be affected; no males will be affected
   D. No females will be affected; 100% of males will be affected

8. What is the causative agent of hand-foot-mouth disease?
   A. Epstein-Barr virus (EBV)
   B. Coxsackie A16
   C. Human herpes virus-6 (HHV-6)
   D. Echovirus

9. Which of following types of human papilloma virus (HPV) are associated with focal epithelial hyperplasia?
   A. 3 and 10
   B. 5 and 8
   C. 6 and 11
   D. 13 and 32

10. Which of the following diseases is caused by a DNA virus?
    A. Measles (rubeola)
    B. Rubella
    C. Herpangina
    D. Erythema infectiosum (fifth disease)

11. Which of the following diseases is NOT transmitted by body lice?
    A. Trench fever
    B. Rickettsialpox
    C. Relapsing fever
    D. Epidemic typhus

12. Which of the following diseases is transmitted by the vector Lutzomyia (sandfly)?
    A. Leishmaniasis due to *Leishmania major*
    B. Leishmaniasis due to *Leishmania braziliensis*
    C. Carrion disease due to *Bartonella bacilliformis*
    D. Both B and C

13. Which of following allergens is associated with allergic contact dermatitis due to permanent (hair) wave solutions?
    A. Methyl methacrylate
    B. Glyceryl thioglycolate
    C. Ammonium persulfate
    D. Paraphenylenediamine

14. Which of the following allergens is associated with eyelid dermatitis?
    A. Toluene sulfonamide/formaldehyde resin
    B. Quaternium 15
    C. Cinnamic aldehyde
    D. Balsam of Peru

15. Which of the following plants is associated with phototoxicity due to forocoumarins?
    A. Peruvian lily
    B. Ragweed
    C. Primrose
    D. Celery

16. Which of the following is the most common cause of preservative-induced allergic contact dermatitis?
    A. Kathon CG
    B. Quaternium 15
    C. Thimerosal
    D. Parabens

17. Marfanoid habitus is a feature of all of the following diseases EXCEPT:
    A. Homocystinuria
    B. Multiple endocrine neoplasia type III
    C. Loeys-Dietz syndrome
    D. Cockayne syndrome

18. Which of the following diseases is associated with corneal opacities?
    A. X-linked ichthyosis
    B. Richner-Hanhart syndrome
    C. Fabry disease
    D. Both A and C

19. Which of the following diseases is associated with ventral pterygium?
    A. Scleroderma
    B. Lichen planus
    C. Darier disease
    D. Iron deficiency

20. Which of the following viral infections features intranuclear inclusion bodies?
    A. Molluscum contagiosum
    B. Varicella
    C. Rabies
    D. Small pox

21. Which of the following diseases is characterized by asteroid bodies?

    A. Sporotrichosis
    B. Rhinoscleroma
    C. Chromomycosis
    D. Granuloma inguinale

22. Flame figures may be seen in all of the following EXCEPT:

    A. Arthropod reaction
    B. Bullous pemphigoid
    C. Eosinophilic fasciitis
    D. Contact dermatitis

Answers

1. B. Cowden syndrome is associated with mutations in *PTEN*, a tumor suppressor gene. Mutations in gap junction proteins are associated with hidrotic ectodermal dysplasia, erythrokeratoderma variabilis, and Vohwinkel syndrome.
2. D. Junctional epidermolysis bullosa results from mutations in laminin 5 or $\alpha 6\beta 4$ integrin and displays and autosomal recessive pattern of inheritance. Bullous ichthyosiform erythroderma (epidermolytic hyperkeratosis), Weber-Cockayne syndrome (epidermolysis bullosa simplex), and white sponge nevus are due to mutations in keratins and are thus inherited in an autosomal dominant manner.
3. C. EPP is due to mutations in ferrochelatase, an enzyme present in mitochondria. Variegate porphyria is due to mutations in protoporphyrinogen oxidase, also present in mitochondria. The other porphyrias listed are due to mutations affecting cytoplasmic enzymes.
4. C. Ataxia-telangiectasia (Louis-Bar syndrome) is an autosomal recessive disease due to mutations in the *ATM* gene. Bloom syndrome, Cockayne syndrome, Rothmund-Thomson syndrome, Werner syndrome, and Trichothiodystrophy/PIBIDS are due to mutations in DNA helicases.
5. D. *DKC1* and *TERC* are genes involved in rRNA synthesis and telomerase function. Mismatch repair describes the function of MLH1, MSH2, and MLH6, genes mutated in Muir-Torre syndrome.
6. D. Hunter disease (due to a mutation in iduronate sulfatase) is inherited in an X-linked recessive manner. The other storage diseases display an autosomal recessive pattern of inheritance.
7. A. Incontinentia pigmenti is an X-linked dominant disease; females with this disease (heterozygotes) will pass on an affected X chromosome to 50% of female offspring. In contrast, since the disease is lethal in male hemizygotes, no male offspring will be affected.
8. B. Hand-foot-mouth disease is caused by Coxsackie A16. EBV is associated with oral hairy leukoplakia, unilateral thoracic exanthem, and Gianotti-Crosti syndrome. HHV-6 is associated with Rosai-Dorfman disease, roseola infantum, and pityriasis rosea. Echovirus is associated with unilateral thoracic exanthem, Boston exanthem, and eruptive pseudoangiomatosis.
9. D. HPV types 13 and 32 cause Heck disease (focal epithelial hyperplasia). HPV types 5 and 8 are associated with epidermodysplasia verruciformis. Types 6 and 11 cause condyloma accuminata.
10. D. Erythema infectiosum (fifth disease) is caused by parvovirus B19, a single-stranded DNA virus. Measles (paramyxovirus), rubella (togavirus), and herpangina (enterovirus 71, coxsackie A10) are caused by RNA viruses.
11. B. Rickettsialpox is caused by *Rickettsia akari*, transmitted by the bite of the house mouse mite (Allodermanyssus sanguineus). The human body louse transmits trench fever (Bartonella quintana), relapsing fever (Borrelia recurrentis), and epidemic typhus (Rickettsia prowazekii).
12. D. *Lutzomyia*, a sandfly, transmits Bartonella bacilliformis, the cause of Carrion disease (Oroya fever, acute phase) and Verruga peruana (chronic phase). *Lutzomyia* also transmits new world leishmaniasis. Old world leishmaniasis is transmitted by the sandfly *Phlebotomus*.
13. B. Glyceryl thioglycolate is found in permanent hair (wave) solutions. Ammonium persulfate is an allergen found in hair bleach. Paraphenylenediamine is associated with allergic contact dermatitis due to hair dye. Methyl methacrylate is found in artificial nails and dental materials.
14. A. Toluene sulfonamide/formaldehyde resin is found in nail lacquer/hardener and causes eyelid dermatitis.
15. D. Forocoumarins are associated with phototoxic reactions (phytophotodermatitis) and are present in celery, dill, fig, lime, parsley, parsnip, meadow grass, and St. John wort (members of the *Umbelliferae* or the *Apiaceae* family). Chrysanthemum, ragweed, and artichoke are members of the *Compositae* family and are associated with chronic photoallergic reactions. Primrose (primin) and peruvian lily (tuliposide A) are associated with allergic contact dermatitis.
16. B. All of the preservatives listed are potential causes of allergic contact dermatitis. Quaternium-15 is the most common cause of allergic contact dermatitis due to preservatives. Paraben mix is an uncommon cause of contact dermatitis.
17. D. Cockayne syndrome is a cause of dwarfism. Marfanoid habitus is a feature of Marfan syndrome, homocystinuria, MEN type III (IIb), and Loeys-Dietz syndrome. Loeys-Dietz syndrome shares features with Marfan syndrome and Ehlers-Danlos syndrome.
18. D. X-linked ichthyosis features posterior comma-shaped corneal opacities in Descemet membrane. Fabry disease

is associated with whorl-like corneal opacities. Richner-Hanhart syndrome (tyrosinemia type II) features pseudoherpetic keratitis and painful focal keratoderma.

19. A. Ventral pterygium (pterygium inversum unguis) is associated with trauma and connective tissue diseases, including scleroderma. Lichen planus is associated with dorsal pterygium. The nail findings in Darier disease are described as alternating red and white bands along with distal "v-nicking."
20. B. Intranuclear inclusion bodies are characteristic of herpes virus infections, including herpes simplex, varicella and herpes zoster, and cytomegalovirus. Rabies and poxvirus infections such as molluscum contagiosum (Henderson-Patterson bodies) and small pox (Guarnieri bodies) are characterized by intracytoplasmic inclusion bodies.
21. A. Asteroid bodies are stellate eosinophilic collections found in chronic granulomatous disorders including sporotrichosis, botryomycosis, actinomycosis, and sarcoidosis. Miculicz cells (parasitized histiocytes) and Russell bodies (immunoglobulin inclusions in plasma cells) are found in rhinoscleroma. Chromomycosis is characterized by medlar bodies (5–12 µm round, thick-walled brown cells). Granuloma inguinale features intracytoplasmic inclusions (Donovan bodies) that stain with Warthin-Starry stain or Giemsa.
22. C. Flame figures are collections of decomposed eosinophilic granules. This is a nonspecific histologic feature found in several disorders associated with abundant eosinophils, including arthropod reaction, bullous pemphigoid, and contact dermatitis. Eosinophilic fasciitis demonstrates a septal panniculitis and fasciitis on histology, with a polymorphous inflammatory infiltrate including eosinophils. Flame figures are not characteristic.

INDEX

Page numbers followed by "*f*" indicate figures and "*t*" indicate tables.

E

H